Cecil Essentials
of Medicine

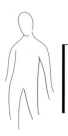

Cecil Essentials of Medicine
Fourth Edition

Thomas E. Andreoli, M.D., M.A.C.P.
The Nolan Chair in Internal Medicine
Professor and Chairman
Department of Internal Medicine
University of Arkansas College of Medicine
Chief of Medicine, University of Arkansas Hospital
Little Rock, Arkansas

Charles C. J. Carpenter, M.D., M.A.C.P.
Professor of Medicine
The International Health Institute
Brown University
Physician-in-Chief
The Miriam Hospital
Providence, Rhode Island

J. Claude Bennett, M.D., M.A.C.P.
Professor of Medicine and President
The University of Alabama at Birmingham
Formerly, Spenser Professor and Chair
Department of Medicine
University of Alabama School of Medicine
Birmingham, Alabama

Fred Plum, M.D.
University Professor
Department of Neurology and Neuroscience
Formerly, Anne Parrish Titzell Professor
  and Chairman of Neurology
Cornell University Medical College
Neurologist-in-Chief
The New York Hospital–Cornell Medical Center
New York, New York

W.B. Saunders Company
A Division of Harcourt Brace & Company
Philadelphia London Toronto Montreal Sydney Tokyo

W.B. SAUNDERS COMPANY
A Division of Harcourt Brace & Company

The Curtis Center
Independence Square West
Philadelphia, Pennsylvania 19106

Library of Congress Cataloging-in-Publication Data

Cecil essentials of medicine / Thomas E. Andreoli . . . [et al.].—4th ed.

p.   cm.

Includes bibliographical references and index.

ISBN 0–7216–6697–3

1. Internal medicine.   I. Cecil, Russell L. (Russell La Fayette).
   II. Andreoli, Thomas E. [DNLM: 1. Internal medicine.   WB 115 C388 1997]

RC46.C42   1997   616—dc20

DNLM/DLC   96–18701

Cecil Essentials of Medicine, fourth edition   ISBN 0–7216–6697–3

Printed in the United States of America.

Last digit is the print number: 9   8   7   6   5   4   3   2

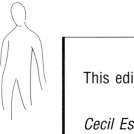

This edition of

Cecil Essentials

is dedicated to

Dr. Lloyd H. (Holly) Smith, Jr.

Holly originated the idea

for *Essentials* and nurtured it

through adolescence.

We thank you.

Contributors

Cardiovascular Disease

William M. Miles, M.D.
Associate Professor of Medicine, Indiana University School of Medicine; Krannert Institute of Cardiology, Indianapolis, Indiana

Eric S. Williams, M.D.
Professor of Medicine, Assistant Director, Division of Cardiology, Director, Cardiovascular Disease Fellowship Training Program, Indiana University School of Medicine; Krannert Institute of Cardiology, Indianapolis, Indiana

Douglas P. Zipes, M.D.
Distinguished Professor of Medicine, Pharmacology and Toxicology; Director, Division of Cardiology, Indiana University School of Medicine; Director, Krannert Institute of Cardiology, Indianapolis, Indiana

Respiratory Disease

Joseph H. Bates, M.D.
Professor and Vice Chairman, Department of Internal Medicine, University of Arkansas College of Medicine; Chief of the Medical Service, McClellan VA Hospital, Little Rock, Arkansas

Dennis W. McGraw, M.D.
Instructor, Department of Internal Medicine, University of Arkansas College of Medicine, Little Rock, Arkansas

Gary L. Templeton, M.D.
Instructor, Department of Internal Medicine, University of Arkansas College of Medicine, Little Rock, Arkansas

Pulmonary Critical Care

Joseph H. Bates, M.D.
Professor and Vice Chairman, Department of Internal Medicine, University of Arkansas College of Medicine; Chief of the Medical Service, McClellan VA Hospital, Little Rock, Arkansas

Dennis W. McGraw, M.D.
Instructor, Department of Internal Medicine, University of Arkansas College of Medicine, Little Rock, Arkansas

Gary L. Templeton, M.D.
Instructor, Department of Internal Medicine, University of Arkansas College of Medicine, Little Rock, Arkansas

Renal Disease

Sameh R. Abul-Ezz, M.D.
Assistant Professor of Internal Medicine, Division of Nephrology, University of Arkansas College of Medicine, Little Rock, Arkansas

C. Martin Bunke, M.D.
Associate Professor of Internal Medicine, Division of Nephrology, University of Arkansas College of Medicine, Little Rock, Arkansas

Harmeet Singh, M.D.
Assistant Professor of Internal Medicine, Division of Nephrology, University of Arkansas College of Medicine, Little Rock, Arkansas

Sudhir V. Shah, M.D.
Professor of Internal Medicine, Director, Division of Nephrology, University of Arkansas College of Medicine, Little Rock, Arkansas

Gastrointestinal Disease

Todd Baron, M.D.
Assistant Professor of Medicine, Division of Gastroenterology and Hepatology, University of Alabama at Birmingham, School of Medicine, Birmingham, Alabama

Stephen W. Lacey, M.D.
Assistant Professor of Internal Medicine, Division of Gastroenterology, University of Texas Southwestern Medical School, Dallas, Texas

Joel E. Richter, M.D.
Chairman, Department of Gastroenterology, Cleveland Clinic Foundation, Cleveland, Ohio

C. Mel Wilcox, M.D.
Associate Professor of Medicine, Division of Gastroenterology and Hepatology, University of Alabama at Birmingham, School of Medicine, Birmingham, Alabama

Diseases of the Liver and Biliary System

Gary A. Abrams, M.D.
Assistant Professor of Medicine, Division of Gastroenterology and Hepatology, Liver Center, University of Alabama at Birmingham, School of Medicine, Birmingham, Alabama

Michael B. Fallon, M.D.
Assistant Professor of Medicine, Division of Gastroenterology and Hepatology, Liver Center, University of Alabama at Birmingham, School of Medicine, Birmingham, Alabama

Hematologic Disease

Joseph O. Moore, M.D.
Professor of Medicine, Medical Director, Duke Oncology Consortium, Duke University School of Medicine, Durham, North Carolina

Thomas L. Ortel, M.D., Ph.D.
Assistant Professor of Medicine, Division of Hematology/Oncology, Duke University School of Medicine, Durham, North Carolina

Wendell F. Rosse, M.D.
Florence Reynaud McAlister Professor of Medicine and Medical Research, Division of Hematology/Oncology, Duke University School of Medicine, Durham, North Carolina

Oncologic Disease

Jerome B. Posner, M.D.
Professor of Neurology, Cornell University Medical College; George C. Cotzias Chair and Attending Neurologist, Memorial Sloan-Kettering Cancer Center, New York, New York

Metabolic Disease

Peter N. Herbert, M.D.
Professor of Medicine, Yale University School of Medicine; Chairman, Department of Medicine, Hospital of St. Raphael, New Haven, Connecticut

Endocrine Disease

Glenn D. Braunstein, M.D.
Professor of Medicine, University of California School of Medicine; Chairman, Department of Medicine, Cedars-Sinai Medical Center, Los Angeles, California

Theodore Friedman, M.D., Ph.D.
Assistant Professor of Medicine, University of California School of Medicine, Section of Endocrinology, Cedars-Sinai Medical Center, Los Angeles, California

Vivien Herman-Bonert, M.D.
Assistant Professor of Medicine, University of California at Los Angeles, School of Medicine; Section of Endocrinology, Cedars-Sinai Medical Center, Los Angeles, California

Anne L. Peters, M.D.
Clinical Assistant Professor of Medicine, University of California at Los Angeles School of Medicine; Section of Endocrinology, Cedars-Sinai Medical Center, Los Angeles, California

Diseases of Bone and Bone Mineral Metabolism

Joel S. Finkelstein, M.D.
Assistant Professor of Medicine, Harvard Medical School; Endocrine Unit, Massachusetts General Hospital, Boston, Massachusetts

Bruce H. Mitlak, M.D.
Clinical Research Physician, Eli Lilly and Company, Indianapolis, Indiana

David M. Slovick, M.D.
Assistant Professor of Medicine, Harvard Medical School; Endocrine Unit, Massachusetts General Hospital, Boston, Massachusetts

Musculoskeletal and Connective Tissue Disease

J. Claude Bennett, M.D.
Professor of Medicine and President, The University of Alabama at Birmingham, Birmingham, Alabama

Larry W. Moreland, M.D.
Associate Professor of Medicine, Division of Clinical Immunology and Rheumatology, University of Alabama at Birmingham, School of Medicine, Birmingham, Alabama

Infectious Disease

Charles C. J. Carpenter, M.D.
Professor of Medicine, Brown University; Physician-in-Chief, The Miriam Hospital, Providence, Rhode Island

Michael M. Lederman, M.D.
Professor of Medicine, Case Western Reserve University School of Medicine; Division of Infectious Diseases, University Hospitals of Cleveland, Cleveland, Ohio

Robert A. Salata, M.D.
Associate Professor of Medicine, Case Western Reserve University School of Medicine; Director, Division of Infectious Diseases, University Hospitals of Cleveland, Cleveland, Ohio

Neurologic Disease

Fred Plum, M.D.
University Professor, Department of Neurology and Neuroscience, Cornell University Medical College, New York, New York

Jerome B. Posner, M.D.
Professor of Neurology, Cornell University Medical College; George C. Cotzias Chair and Attending Neurologist, Memorial Sloan-Kettering Cancer Center, New York, New York

The Aging Patient

David A. Lipschitz, M.D., Ph.D.
Professor of Internal Medicine; Director, Division of Geriatrics, University of Arkansas College of Medicine; Director, GRECC, John L. McClellan Memorial VA Hospital, Little Rock, Arkansas

Dennis H. Sullivan, M.D.
Associate Professor of Internal Medicine, University of Arkansas College of Medicine; Staff Physician, GRECC, John L. McClellan Memorial VA Hospital, Little Rock, Arkansas

Substance Abuse

Timothy E. Holcomb, M.D.
Assistant Professor of Internal Medicine, University of Arkansas College of Medicine, Little Rock, Arkansas

Preface

This fourth edition of *Cecil Essentials of Medicine* recapitulates, in an entirely revised format, the characteristics of the first three editions of *Essentials.* Our intent, as in previous editions, is to provide a textbook that encompasses succinctly the core elements of internal medicine in a volume that can be readily understood by medical students, house officers, practitioners of general medicine, subspecialties of internal medicine and other medical disciplines, and other individuals involved either in preventive medicine or in delivering health care to ill individuals. This book considers, in a compact manner, the biologic basis for understanding disease processes, the clinical characteristics of diseases, and the compassionate and rational approaches to the diagnosis and treatment of diseases commonly encountered by practitioners of internal medicine and the medical subspecialties.

The fourth edition of *Essentials* remains about the same in size as preceding editions, but it has undergone substantial revision. All chapters have been revised thoroughly, and more than a third of the chapters have been rewritten entirely. Two new sections on key topics have been added, one on pulmonary critical care and one on alcohol and substance abuse. New section editors and authors have assumed the responsibilities for the sections Respiratory Disease, Pulmonary Critical Care, Gastrointestinal Disease, Diseases of the Liver and Biliary System, Hematologic Disease, Endocrine Disease, and Substance Abuse. Likewise, new contributors have also been added to the sections Cardiovascular Disease, Renal Disease, Metabolic Disease, Diseases of Bone and Bone Mineral Metabolism, and Infectious Disease.

There have also been significant changes in the format for illustrative material, both tabular and graphic. These include the use of four-color illustrations and a considerable expansion in the number of pathophysiologic, diagnostic, and therapeutic algorithms.

We are deeply indebted to a number of colleagues and collaborators. We are especially grateful to Dr. Lloyd H. (Holly) Smith, Jr., to whom this edition is dedicated. Holly not only helped formulate the idea for *Essentials* but also guided it gracefully through adolescence.

Dr. Susan S. Beland, Associate Professor of Internal Medicine at the University of Arkansas, reviewed all the graphic material for this edition, and Dr. Steven Frucht of the Neurology Department, Cornell Medical College, helped in the design and organization of the tabular and graphic material in Section XIV. Mr. Leslie E. Hoeltzel, Manager, Developmental Editors, and Ms. Lisette Bralow, Vice President and Editor-in-Chief, Medical Books, both of the W.B. Saunders Company, contributed their customary excellence in the design and preparation of the fourth edition of *Essentials.* Ms. Darlene D. Pedersen, former Senior Vice President and Editorial Director, Books Division, with W.B. Saunders, assisted with prior editions of *Essentials* and with the initial planning for this edition. Finally, we thank our very able secretarial staff members, Ms. Clementine M. Whitman (Little Rock), Ms. Dvora Aksler Konstant (Birmingham), Ms. Barbara S. Ryan (Providence), and Ms. Maureen P. O'Connor (New York).

THE EDITORS

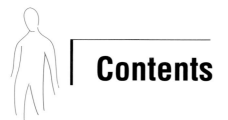

Contents

Cardiovascular Disease

Section I

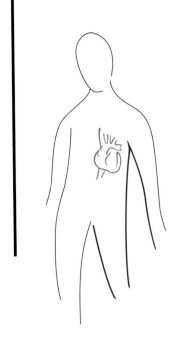

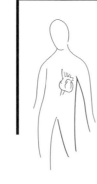

Structure and Function of the Normal Heart and Blood Vessels

GROSS ANATOMY

The heart includes two relatively thin-walled upper chambers, the right and left atria, and two thicker-walled lower chambers, the right and left ventricles (Fig. 1–1). The left ventricle must generate and pump against considerably higher pressure than must the right ventricle; therefore, it is thicker than the right ventricle. The interventricular septum separates the two ventricles. The lower and much larger part of the interventricular septum is termed the muscular interventricular septum and is composed of muscle of similar thickness to that of the left ventricular free wall. The uppermost portion of the septum, termed the membranous interventricular septum, also forms a portion of the right atrial wall.

Two atrioventricular (AV) valves separate the atria from the ventricles. The right-sided tricuspid valve is a three-leaflet structure. The left-sided mitral valve has only two leaflets. A fibrous ring called the annulus supports each valve and forms a portion of the fibrous structural skeleton of the heart. Chords of fibrous tissue, the chordae tendineae, extend from the ventricular surfaces of both AV valves and attach to the papillary muscles. Papillary muscles are bundles of cardiac muscle (myocardium) arising from the interior of the ventricular walls. As the ventricles contract, the papillary muscles also contract and contribute to effective valve closure.

The semilunar valves separate the ventricles from their respective outflow tracts. The pulmonic valve is composed of three fibrous leaflets or cusps that are forced open against the walls of the pulmonary artery during ventricular ejection of blood but fall back into the pulmonary outflow tract during diastole, their free edges coapting to prevent blood from returning into the right ventricle. The aortic valve is a thicker but similar three-cusp structure. The aortic wall behind each aortic valve cusp bulges outward, forming three structures known as sinuses of Valsalva. The two most anterior aortic cusps are known as the left and right coronary cusps because of the origins of the left and right coronary arteries from the respective sinuses of Valsalva, and the remaining posterior cusp is known as the noncoronary cusp.

The pericardium, a double-layered fibrous structure, encloses the heart. The visceral layer is immediately adjacent to the heart and forms part of the epicardium (outer layer) of the heart. The parietal layer is exterior to the heart and is separated from the visceral layer by a thin film of lubricating fluid (10 to 20 ml total) that allows the heart to move freely within the pericardial sac.

Venous blood returning from the body enters the right atrium through the inferior vena cava from below and the superior vena cava from above (Fig. 1–2). Most venous blood returning from the coronary circulation enters the right atrium via the coronary sinus. Blood from these three sources mixes and enters the right ventricle during diastole, when the tricuspid valve is open. The right ventricle subsequently contracts (systole), closing the tricuspid valve to prevent retrograde blood flow, and ejects blood through the pulmonic valve into the pulmonary artery. The pulmonary artery bifurcates into left and right branches that travel to the left and right lungs. The pulmonary artery has thinner walls than the aorta, and pulmonary arterial pressure is normally much lower than aortic pressure. The pulmonary artery progressively divides into smaller and smaller arteries, arterioles, and eventually capillaries, where carbon dioxide (CO_2) is exchanged for oxygen (O_2) via the pulmonary alveoli. The capillaries lead to pulmonary veins that coalesce to form the four larger pulmonary veins entering the left atrium posteriorly. Oxygenated blood from the pulmonary veins passes from the left atrium through the mitral valve to the left ventricle, which ejects blood during systole across the aortic valve into the aorta. The aorta divides into branches that deliver blood to the entire body. The division continues to form smaller arteries, arterioles, and eventually capillaries that deliver oxygen and metabolic substrates to the tissues in exchange for carbon dioxide and other waste products. Blood collected from the peripheral capillaries is returned to the right atrium via the venous system.

The right and left coronary arteries course over the epicardial surface of the heart to distribute blood to the myocardium (Fig. 1–3). The left main coronary artery bifurcates within a few centimeters of its origin into two major vessels. The left anterior descending coronary artery proceeds anteriorly in the anterior interventricular groove (between both ventricles) toward the apex of the heart, supplying the anterior free wall of the left ventricle and the anterior two thirds of the septum. The circumflex coronary artery travels posteriorly in the AV groove (between left atrium and ventricle) and usually supplies a portion of the posterolateral surface of the heart. The right coronary artery courses in the right AV groove (between right atrium and ventricle) and distributes several branches to the right ventricle before reaching the left ventricle, where the AV grooves meet the posterior interventricular groove (the "crux" of the heart). In 90% of patients the right coronary artery reaches the crux of the heart and supplies the branches to the AV node and the inferobasal third of the septum as the posterior descending artery. This pattern is termed "right dominant distribution" (even though the left coronary artery supplies the majority of the coronary circulation). In approximately 10% of patients, a relatively large circumflex coronary artery reaches the crux of the heart and gives rise to the posterior descending coronary artery and the branch to the AV node. This situation is termed "left dominant." Blood is supplied to the sinus node via a branch of the right coronary artery (55% of cases) or the circumflex coronary artery (45%). Most of the venous network of the heart coalesces to form the coronary sinus. A small amount of the right ventricular and atrial venous drainage occurs via much smaller anterior cardiac veins and tiny thebesian veins, most of which drain directly into the right atrium.

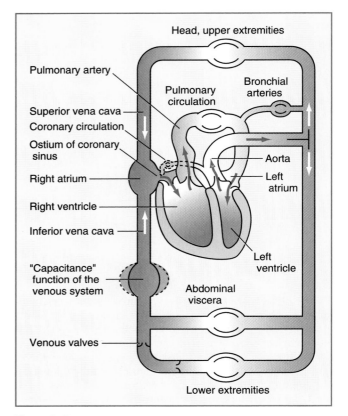

Figure 1-2

Schematic representation of the systemic and pulmonary circulatory systems. The venous system contains the greatest amount of blood at any one time and is highly distensible, accommodating a wide range of blood volumes (high capacitance).

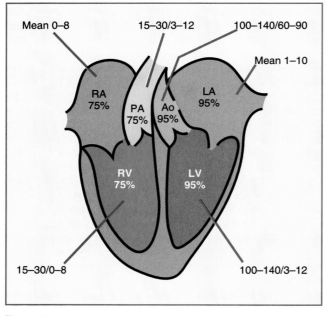

Figure 1-1

Orientation of cardiac chambers and great vessels with normal intracardiac pressures (mm Hg) and oxygen (O₂) saturations (%).

ELECTRICAL CONDUCTION SYSTEM (Fig. 1-4)

Cardiac electrical impulses originate in the sinus node, a spindle-shaped structure 10 to 20 mm long located near the junction of the superior vena cava and the right atrium. The role of specialized intra-atrial tracts in the conduction of the electrical impulse to the AV node is controversial. The AV node provides the only normal conduction pathway between the atria and the ventricles. It is situated just beneath the right atrial endocardium above the insertion of the septal leaflet of the tricuspid valve and anterior to the ostium of the coronary sinus. After conduction delay in the AV node, the electrical impulse travels to the His bundle, which descends posteriorly along the membranous interventricular septum to the top of the muscular septum. The His bundle gives rise to the right and left bundle branches. The right bundle branch is a single group of fibers that travels down the right ventricular side of the muscular interventricular septum. The left bundle branch is a larger, less discrete array of conducting fibers located on the left side of the interventricular septum. The left bundle branch may divide into two somewhat distinct pathways that travel toward the anterolateral (left anterior fascicle) and posteromedial (left posterior fascicle) papillary muscles. The left poste-

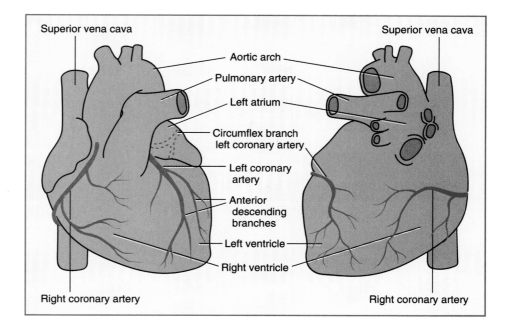

Figure 1-3

Major coronary arteries and their branches.

Superior vena cava

Superior vena cava

Aortic arch

Pulmonary artery

Left atrium

Circumflex branch left coronary artery

Left coronary artery

Anterior descending branches

Left ventricle

Right ventricle

Right coronary artery

Right coronary artery

rior fascicle is larger and most diffuse than the anterior fascicle and usually has a more reliable vascular supply than either the left anterior fascicle or the right bundle branch. The left and right bundle branches progressively divide into tiny Purkinje fibers that arborize and finally make intimate contact with ventricular muscle tissue.

MICROSCOPIC ANATOMY

In general, two functional cell types are present in cardiac tissue: those responsible for electrical impulse generation and transmission and those responsible for mechanical contraction. Nodal cells are thought to be the source of normal impulse formation in the sinus node and are richly innervated with adrenergic and cholinergic nerve fibers. Like the sinus node, the AV node and His bundle regions are innervated with a rich supply of cholinergic and adrenergic fibers. Purkinje cells are large clear cells found in the His bundle, bundle branches, and their arborizations. They have particularly well developed end-to-end connections that may facilitate rapid longitudinal conduction.

Atrial and ventricular myocardial cells, the contractile cells of the heart, consist of sarcomers containing thin actin filaments and thick myosin filaments (Fig. 1-5). Cyclic interaction between cross-bridges on the myosin filaments and specific sites on the actin filaments underlies muscle contraction. The thin filament contains the regulatory troponin-tropomyosin complex.

The surface membrane of the cell is termed the sarcolemma, and adjacent myocardial cells are connected end to end by a thickened portion of the sarcolemma termed the intercalated disc. The sarcolemma is a complex structure that contains ion pumps and channels, as well as hormone receptors and enzymes. It acts to maintain the resting transmembrane potential of cardiac cells and participates in the generation of the action potential

(see Chapter 8) and the triggering of contraction. Invaginations of the sarcolemma called T tubules come into close proximity to the sarcoplasmic reticulum. The sarcoplasmic reticulum is an internal membrane system that serves as a major intracellular storage site for calcium. When the cell is depolarized electrically, calcium is released from the sarcoplasmic reticulum. The amount of calcium entering the cell and that released from the sarcoplasmic reticulum determines the force of contraction. During muscle relaxation, calcium is taken up by the sarcoplasmic reticulum.

After fetal development, cardiac cells lose their ability to proliferate. Subsequent cardiac hypertrophy represents an increase in the size of myofibrillar units rather than an increase in cell number.

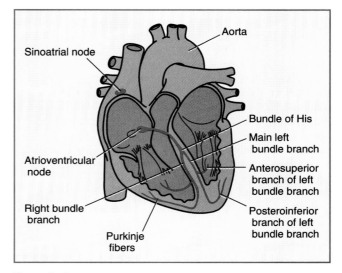

Aorta

Sinoatrial node

Bundle of His

Main left bundle branch

Atrioventricular node

Anterosuperior branch of left bundle branch

Right bundle branch

Posteroinferior branch of left bundle branch

Purkinje fibers

Figure 1-4

Schematic representation of the cardiac conduction system.

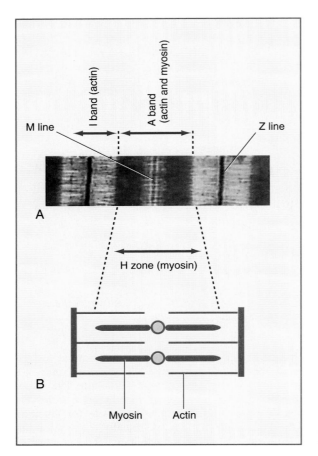

Figure 1-5

A, A sarcomere as it appears under the electron microscope. *B,* Schematic of the location and interaction of actin and myosin (see text).

FETAL CIRCULATION

The fetal circulation utilizes special vascular channels that normally disappear after birth. Oxygenated blood from the umbilical vein is shunted via the ductus venosus to the inferior vena cava. In the heart, it is shunted across the patent foramen ovale to the left atrium and systemic circulation. Blood returning from the upper portions of the fetus courses through the right atrium and ventricle, but most of it is shunted across the ductus arteriosus to the aorta. Thus, the right ventricular output is much greater than that of the left ventricle, but relatively little of the blood reaches the uninflated fetal lungs. Upon birth and lung inflation, the pulmonary vascular resistance is reduced, and pulmonary blood flow markedly increases. Pulmonary arterial pressures usually approach normal values after a few weeks. Systemic vascular resistance and pressure are increased, along with left atrial pressure. There is functional closure of the foramen ovale, which usually becomes permanently closed within a few months. In about 30% of normal individuals, a potential opening persists into adulthood.

MYOCARDIAL METABOLISM

The heart uses ATP, created primarily by metabolism of carbohydrates or fatty acids, to derive energy for contraction and electrical activity. ATP formation occurs via oxidative phosphorylation of adenosine diphosphate (ADP). Energy for electrical activity is minimal compared with that required for contraction. Stored energy reserves are scarce, and the heart must continually have a source of energy to function. The principal oxidative substrate for ATP production is fatty acid, but a variety of carbohydrates are also used, depending on the substrate concentration and other factors. Myocardial metabolism is aerobic, and a constant supply of O_2 must be available.

CIRCULATORY PHYSIOLOGY

Changes in cardiac output can be due to alterations of heart rate or stroke volume (cardiac output = heart rate × stroke volume). Factors that act to regulate ventricular function (and stroke volume) in the intact heart include contractility, preload, and afterload (Table 1–1). *Contractility* (or inotropic state) refers to the intrinsic strength of the muscle fibers. Preload is determined by the degree of ventricular filling during diastole. With increased filling, the ensuing contraction and stroke volume are augmented. Since ventricular filling volume is not readily measured clinically, ventricular filling pressure (or end-diastolic pressure) is used as an index of preload. Several factors can contribute to ventricular filling pressure (see Table 1–1).

The term *afterload* describes the "impedance" or resistance against which the heart must contract. Like pre-

TABLE 1-1	Factors Affecting Cardiac Performance
Preload (left ventricular diastolic volume)	Total blood volume Venous tone (sympathetic tone) Body position Intrathoracic and intrapericardial pressure Atrial contraction Pumping action of skeletal muscle
Afterload (impedance against which the left ventricle must eject blood)	Peripheral vascular resistance Left ventricular volume (preload, wall tension) Physical characteristics of the arterial tree (e.g., elasticity of vessels or presence of outflow obstruction)
Contractility (cardiac performance independent of preload or afterload)	Sympathetic nerve impulses ⎫ Circulating catecholamines ⎬ Increased contractility Digitalis, calcium, other inotropic agents Increased heart rate or postextrasystolic augmentation ⎭ Anoxia, acidosis ⎫ Pharmacologic depression ⎬ Decreased contractility Loss of myocardium Intrinsic depression ⎭
Heart Rate	Autonomic nervous system Temperature, metabolic rate

traction (Fig. 1–6): (1) During "isovolumic contraction," the intramyocardial pressure rises with no ejection of blood or change in ventricular volume; (2) when left ventricular pressure reaches that of the aorta, the aortic

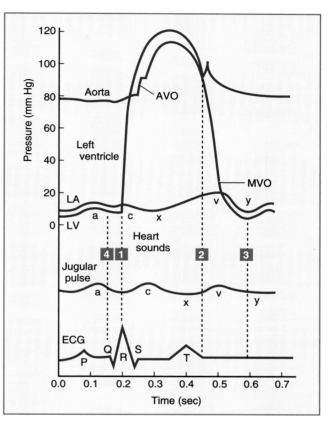

Figure 1–6

Simultaneous electrocardiogram (ECG) and pressures obtained from the left atrium, left ventricle, and aorta, and the jugular pulse during one cardiac cycle. For simplification, right-sided heart pressures have been omitted. Normal right atrial pressure closely parallels that of the left atrium, and right ventricular and pulmonary artery pressures time closely with their corresponding left-sided heart counterparts, being reduced only in magnitude. The normal mitral and aortic valve closure precedes tricuspid and pulmonic closure, respectively, whereas valve opening reverses this order. The jugular venous pulse lags behind the right atrial pressure.

During the course of one cardiac cycle, note that the electrical events (ECG) initiate and therefore precede the mechanical (pressure) events and that the latter precede the auscultatory events (heart sounds) they themselves produce. Shortly after the P wave, the atria contract to produce the a wave; a fourth heart sound may succeed the latter. The QRS complex initiates ventricular systole, followed shortly by left ventricular contraction and the rapid build-up of left ventricular (LV) pressure. Almost immediately LV pressure exceeds left atrial (LA) pressure to close the mitral valve and produces the first heart sounds. When LV pressure exceeds aortic pressure, the aortic valve opens (AVO), and when aortic pressure is once again greater than LV pressure, the aortic valve closes to produce the second heart sound and terminate ventricular ejection. The decreasing LV pressure drops below LA pressure to open the mitral valve (MVO), and a period of rapid ventricular filling commences. During this time a third heart sound may be heard. The jugular pulse is explained under the discussion of the venous pulse.

load, afterload can refer either to a single myofibril or to the heart as a whole. The afterload is approximated by the arterial pressure, the major determinant of the impedance to left ventricular contraction. In the intact heart, the afterload determines the amount of blood the heart can pump given a fixed preload and fixed state of contractility. The effects of afterload on cardiac performance are more prominent with failing ventricles. Examples of increased left ventricular afterload include systemic hypertension and aortic valve stenosis. Afterload is reduced in patients with mitral regurgitation.

The function of the ventricle during diastole has been increasingly recognized as an important determinant of cardiac function. Diastolic dysfunction generally refers to reduced ventricular compliance. This increased "stiffness" can limit ventricular filling and results in increased ventricular diastolic pressure at any given ventricular volume. Ventricular hypertrophy is a common cause of reduced ventricular compliance.

The autonomic nervous system plays an important role in the regulation of cardiac function, both directly and indirectly through effects on the peripheral circulation. A decrease in the cardiac output or blood pressure, for example, increases sympathetic and decreases parasympathetic discharge via baroreceptor mechanisms to increase heart rate. Likewise, an elevated blood pressure activates the carotid baroreceptors, augments vagal activity, and slows the heart rate.

Four phases of the cardiac cycle can be identified, beginning with initiation of ventricular myocardial con-

valve opens and blood is ejected from the contracting ventricle; (3) as the ventricle relaxes and left ventricular pressure decreases, the aortic valve closes and "isovolumic relaxation" occurs; (4) upon sufficient decrease in left ventricular pressure, the mitral valve opens and ventricular filling from the atrium occurs. The ventricle fills most rapidly in early diastole and again in late diastole when the atrium contracts. Loss of atrial contraction (e.g., atrial fibrillation or AV dissociation) can impair ventricular filling, especially into a noncompliant ("stiff") ventricle.

Normal intracardiac pressures are shown in Figure 1-1. Atrial pressure curves are composed of the a wave, which is generated by atrial contraction, and the v wave, which is an early diastolic peak caused by filling of the atrium from the peripheral veins. The x descent follows the a wave, and the y descent follows the v wave. A small deflection, the c wave, occurs after the a wave in early systole and probably represents bulging of the tricuspid valve apparatus into the left atrium during early systole. Ventricular pressures are described by a peak systolic pressure and an end-diastolic pressure, which is the ventricular pressure immediately before the onset of systole. Note that the minimum left ventricular pressure occurs in early diastole. Aortic and pulmonary artery pressures are represented by a peak systolic and a minimal diastolic value.

Cardiac output is a measure of the amount of blood flow in liters per minute. The cardiac index is the cardiac output divided by the body surface area and is normally 2.8 to 4.2 L/min/m². The pulmonary and systemic vascular resistances are also important parameters of circulatory function. Resistance is defined as the difference in pressure across a capillary bed divided by the flow across that capillary bed, usually the cardiac output: ($R = [P_1 - P_2]$/flow). For example, the pulmonary vascular resistance is the difference between the mean pulmonary arterial pressure and mean pulmonary venous pressure, divided by the pulmonary blood flow. Similarly, systemic vascular resistance is the difference between mean arterial pressure and mean right atrial pressure, divided by the systemic cardiac output. Note that an increase in arterial pressure may occur without necessarily causing an increase in vascular resistance. For example, if both pulmonary arterial and venous pressures are elevated to the same degree, pulmonary vascular resistance is unchanged; if pulmonary blood flow and pulmonary arterial pressure increase while pulmonary venous pressure remains the same, resistance is unchanged.

The most widely used parameter for quantitating overall ventricular function is the ejection fraction, defined as the diastolic volume minus the systolic volume (stroke volume), divided by the diastolic volume: ([DV − SV]/DV). These volumes may be estimated from either invasive (e.g., left ventriculography) or noninvasive (e.g., echocardiography or radionuclide ventriculography) tests. The ejection fraction may be a useful gross evaluation of ventricular function, but there are situations (e.g., when a large left ventricular aneurysm is present) in which the ejection fraction can give a misleading impression of overall ventricular function.

PHYSIOLOGY OF THE CORONARY CIRCULATION

Three major determinants of myocardial O_2 consumption are contractility, heart rate, and wall tension. Myocardial wall tension is directly proportional to the pressure within the ventricular chamber and the radius of the ventricular chamber (Laplace relationship). The myocardial mass is a determinant of wall tension and, therefore, myocardial O_2 consumption; the larger the muscle mass, the more O_2 is needed.

Oxygen (and nutrients) for the heart are delivered via the coronary circulation. Since O_2 extraction is nearly complete in the basal state, increased demand must be met by increased coronary blood flow. The coronary vascular bed is able to autoregulate, enabling myocardial O_2 and substrate delivery to equal the demand. Coronary vascular resistance is normally determined by the arterioles and is influenced by neural and metabolic factors. Both the sympathetic and parasympathetic nervous systems innervate the coronary arteries. Alpha receptor stimulation causes vasoconstriction, whereas stimulation of the beta₂ receptor as well as of the vagus (acetylcholine) causes vasodilation. Metabolic factors regulate regional perfusion. Several mediators, including O_2, CO_2, and metabolites such as adenosine, are important; adenosine is a potent coronary vasodilator formed by tissues in response to decreased coronary perfusion and is a critical mediator in coronary autoregulation. However, when coronary perfusion pressure falls to below 60 to 70 mm Hg, the vessels become maximally dilated and flow depends on perfusion pressure alone because capability for further autoregulation is lost. The normal coronary vascular bed has a capacity to increase its blood flow four- to fivefold during maximal exercise. Hemodynamic factors that affect coronary perfusion include arterial pressure (especially diastolic pressure because coronary flow occurs primarily in diastole), the time spent in diastole, and the intraventricular pressure (which exerts tension on the myocardial walls and diminishes coronary flow).

PHYSIOLOGY OF THE SYSTEMIC CIRCULATION

The aortic wall contains elastic fibers that allow it to expand with the expulsion of blood from the left ventricle, somewhat damping the pulse pressure generated and aiding diastolic flow to the coronary arteries with its recoil. The aorta successively branches into smaller and smaller vessels until arterioles, the major determinants of resistance in the systemic circulation, are reached. The arterioles contain a vascular sphincter that modulates blood flow dependent on regional metabolic needs; for example, acidosis and decreased O_2 tension increase regional perfusion, and vice versa. Autonomic and other neurohormonal influences affect arteriolar tone. The capillaries consist of a single endothelial cell layer and allow diffusion of O_2, nutrients, CO_2, and waste products. The capillaries lead into the venous system, where blood is eventually delivered back to the right atrium. The flow of blood returning to the heart is aided by the valves in the venous system, which prevent reverse flow, particularly in the larger veins of the legs. The "milking" action of the muscles of the arms and legs and the pressure changes in the thoracic cavity also help to return blood to the heart. The veins have considerably thinner walls than the arteries and can accommodate a larger blood volume under low pressures (capacitance vessels). Vasoconstriction or vasodilation of the venous system can control the amount of blood returning to the heart. More of the total blood volume is located in the venous than in the arterial portion of the circulation. The lymphatic vessels also contribute to the return of fluid from the periphery. The major terminal vessel of the lymphatic system is the thoracic duct, which usually empties into the left brachiocephalic vein.

PHYSIOLOGY OF THE PULMONARY CIRCULATION

The pulmonary circulation has a rich capillary network similar to that of the systemic circulation. The pulmonary alveoli are adjacent to the capillaries, permitting O_2 to diffuse into and CO_2 out of the capillary blood. O_2 is the major mediator of pulmonary autoregulation. In regions where the partial pressure of O_2 is high, pulmonary vasodilation occurs and blood flow is directed preferentially toward well-oxygenated areas of the lung. When the partial pressure of O_2 is low, pulmonary vasoconstriction occurs, preventing the perfusion of areas of the lung that have relatively poor O_2 availability. Acidemia potentiates the pulmonary vasoconstrictive effect of hypoxemia.

The lungs receive blood through the bronchial arteries as well as the pulmonary arteries (dual blood supply). The bronchial arteries supply arterial blood to the pulmonary tissue and drain into the bronchial veins, some of which drain into the systemic venous bed. Some bronchial veins drain into the pulmonary veins, creating a small physiologic right-to-left shunt.

Pulmonary vascular resistance is normally one-tenth that of systemic vascular resistance and accounts for the small pressure gradient required to propel blood across the pulmonary vascular bed. Because the pulmonary vasculature is very distensible (compliant), a relatively large left-to-right intracardiac shunt may exist with only a minimal rise in pulmonary arterial pressure (until or unless there are secondary structural and/or vasoconstrictive changes in the pulmonary vascular bed).

CARDIOVASCULAR RESPONSE TO EXERCISE

The heart responds to exercise principally by adrenergic stimulation and vagal withdrawal, which increase heart rate and contractility, and by peripheral circulatory alterations (Table 1–2). The increase in heart rate usually accounts for the majority of the increase in cardiac out-

TABLE 1–2	Physiologic Responses to Exercise
Response	**Mechanism**
↑Heart rate	↑Sympathetic stimulation
	↓Parasympathetic stimulation
↑Stroke volume	
↑Contractility	↑Sympathetic stimulation
↑Venous return	Sympathetic-mediated venoconstriction
	Pumping action of skeletal muscles
	↓Intrathoracic pressure with deep inspirations
	Arteriolar vasodilation in exercising muscle
↓Afterload	Arteriolar vasodilation in exercising muscle (mediated chiefly by local metabolites)
↑Blood pressure	↑Cardiac output
	Vasoconstriction (sympathetic stimulation) of nonexercising vascular beds
↑O_2 extraction	Shift in oxyhemoglobin dissociation curve due to local acidosis

put. Increased contractility contributes to the rise in cardiac output by increasing the stroke volume. Vessels supplying exercising muscles dilate, and there is some redistribution in cardiac output, whereas other vascular beds may vasoconstrict. Venous return is increased by several mechanisms. Isometric and isotonic exercises affect the cardiovascular system somewhat differently. The predominant response to isometric exercise (e.g., weight lifting) is an increase in peripheral vasoconstriction with a subsequent increase in arterial pressure. In contrast, isotonic exercise (e.g., jogging) reduces systemic vascular resistance primarily in exercising muscles, which improves cardiac output. Those who exercise regularly obtain a cardiac training effect, with a lower resting heart rate and a greater capacity to increase cardiac output during exercise.

CARDIOVASCULAR PHYSIOLOGY DURING PREGNANCY

See Chapter 12.

ELECTROPHYSIOLOGY

See Chapter 8.

REFERENCES

Berne RM, Levy MN: Cardiovascular Physiology. 6th ed. St. Louis, CV Mosby, 1991.

Hathaway DR, March KL, Lash JA, Adam LP, Wilensky RL: Vascular smooth muscle: A review of the molecular basis of contractility. Circulation 1991; 83:382.

Hurst JW, Anderson RH, Becker AE, Wilcox BR: Atlas of the Heart. New York, McGraw-Hill, 1988.

Katz AM: Physiology of the Heart. 2nd ed. New York, Raven Press, 1992.

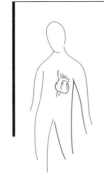

2

Evaluation of the Patient with Cardiovascular Disease

HISTORY

The history is a very important tool in the evaluation of patients with cardiovascular disease. In addition to aiding diagnosis, the history provides information about the patient's functional capacity. With many cardiac disorders, the functional capacity can be a determinant of prognosis and can play a role in determining the intensity of medical treatment or selection of surgical therapy. There are several classification schemes for functional capacity (Table 2–1). Despite the central role of the history, it must be recognized that the cardinal symptoms (Table 2–2) are not specific for cardiac disease. Alternative causes (e.g., gastrointestinal, pulmonary) often must be excluded. Also, some patients with cardiac disease may report atypical or no symptoms.

Chest pain is a common symptom. It may result from a variety of causes, both cardiac and noncardiac (Tables 2–3 and 2–4). It must be characterized carefully, including its quality, location, and duration, factors that precipitate and relieve it, and associated features. Ischemic cardiac pain is a visceral chest discomfort caused by insufficient oxygen delivery to an area of the heart. If the oxygen supply/demand mismatch is transient, angina pectoris may result. More profound and prolonged ischemia can lead to myocardial infarction. Angina pectoris (see Table 2–2) is usually the result of obstructive coronary disease. It is typically and predictably evoked by conditions or activities that increase myocardial oxygen demand (e.g., exertion, emotional stress). Activities in the morning, after meals, or in cold weather are especially likely to provoke discomfort (many patients insist angina is discomfort rather than pain). Angina pectoris usually lasts 2 to 10 minutes and is characteristically relieved by rest or sublingual nitroglycerin. Discomfort that has recently progressed in severity and/or intensity, particularly if accompanied by unprovoked rest pain, is considered unstable angina. Patients with Prinzmetal's angina due to coronary artery spasm characteristically experience unprovoked angina pain, with bouts often occurring in the early morning. The discomfort of acute myocardial infarction is characteristically more severe and prolonged (>30 minutes) than angina pectoris and is unrelieved by sublingual nitroglycerin. Nausea and diaphoresis often accompany the episode.

Pericarditis pain (see Table 2–3) is usually sharp and may radiate to the left trapezius area. It is often increased by inspiration and torso movement and improved by sitting upright and leaning forward. Acute aortic dissection causes sudden unrelenting and excruciating chest pain. Depending on the location of dissection, pain may radiate to the back, produce associated aortic insufficiency murmur, or lead to pulse or neurologic deficits.

Dyspnea is a subjective sensation of shortness of breath and often is a symptom of cardiac disease, especially in patients with congestive heart failure. Left ventricular failure typically results in increased left atrial and, thus, pulmonary venous pressures. Pulmonary compliance decreases, contributing to the sensation of dyspnea. As congestive heart failure worsens, transudative fluid accumulates in the alveoli. Because the supine position compared with the upright position augments venous return, patients with congestive heart failure demonstrate orthopnea, that is, shortness of breath in the supine position relieved by sitting up. They also may have paroxysmal nocturnal dyspnea, that is, awakening with shortness of breath 2 to 3 hours after falling asleep. It usually occurs only once nightly, is relieved by sitting or standing, and is probably related to central redistribution of fluid upon assuming the reclining position.

Occasionally, dyspnea can represent an anginal equivalent, a symptom of acute myocardial ischemia. Dyspnea is also a prominent feature of pulmonary disease, and at times the differentiation between pulmonary and cardiac causes of dyspnea is difficult. For example, patients with pulmonary dyspnea can exhibit orthopnea, whereas wheezes may be heard in patients with cardiac dyspnea (e.g., congestive heart failure). Sudden dyspnea is a common presentation of a pulmonary embolus.

Cyanosis is a bluish discoloration of the skin caused by an increased amount of nonoxygenated hemoglobin in the blood. Central cyanosis, often best seen on the oral mucous membranes, is due to right-to-left shunting of

TABLE 2–1	New York Heart Association Functional Classification	
Class I	No limitation	Ordinary physical activity does not cause symptoms
Class II	Slight limitation	Comfortable at rest Ordinary physical activity causes symptoms
Class III	Marked limitation	Comfortable at rest Less than ordinary activity causes symptoms
Class IV	Inability to carry on any physical activity	Symptoms present at rest

TABLE 2–2	Cardinal Symptoms of Cardiac Disease
	Chest pain or discomfort Symptoms of heart failure Palpitation Syncope, presyncope

blood or impaired pulmonary function. Peripheral cyanosis, best seen in the extremities, may be due to shunting or to local discoloration caused by vasoconstriction (e.g., low cardiac output, peripheral vascular disease, or exposure to cold).

Palpitation refers to an awareness of heart beat (see Chapter 8). Palpitations should be characterized by their onset and whether they are forceful, irregular, or rapid (it is often helpful to have patients "tap out" the palpitation). It is important to learn if the palpitations cause or are associated with other symptoms.

Syncope, or loss of consciousness, can result from a variety of causes, including cardiac and neurologic etiologies. Cardiac causes include aortic stenosis and hypertrophic cardiomyopathy, as well as cardiac arrhythmias and conduction disturbances. Cardiac syncope is often sudden. The absence of palpitations does not exclude arrhythmia as a cause. Orthostatic hypotension, at times aggravated by cardiac medications, is a cause of syncope. Vasovagal mechanisms can also underlie syncope (see Chapter 8).

Fatigue is a common cardiac symptom but is extremely nonspecific. Patients who have a reduced cardiac output often complain of fatigue.

Edema is common in patients with congestive heart failure. Edema of the lower extremities (or the sacral area in bedridden patients) often is a symptom of right ventricular failure. Other causes of peripheral edema include the

TABLE 2–3	Cardiovascular Causes of Chest Pain				
Condition	Location	Quality	Duration	Aggravating or Relieving Factors	Associated Symptoms or Signs
Angina	Retrosternal region; radiates to or occasionally isolated to neck, jaw, epigastrium, shoulder, or arms—left common	Pressure, burning, squeezing, heaviness, indigestion	<2–10 min	Precipitated by exercise, cold weather, or emotional stress; relieved by rest or nitroglycerin; atypical (Prinzmetal's) angina may be unrelated to activity, often early morning	S_4, or murmur of papillary muscle dysfunction during pain
Rest or unstable angina	Same as angina	Same as angina but may be more severe	Usually <20 min	Same as angina, with decreasing tolerance for exertion or at rest	Similar to stable angina, but may be pronounced. Transient cardiac failure can occur
Myocardial infarction	Substernal and may radiate like angina	Heaviness, pressure, burning, constriction	Sudden onset, 30 min or longer but variable	Unrelieved by rest or nitroglycerin	Shortness of breath, sweating, weakness, nausea, vomiting
Pericarditis	Usually begins over sternum or toward cardiac apex and may radiate to neck or left shoulder; often more localized than the pain of myocardial ischemia	Sharp, stabbing, knifelike	Lasts many hours to days; may wax and wane	Aggravated by deep breathing, rotating chest, or supine position; relieved by sitting up and leaning forward	Pericardial friction rub
Aortic dissection	Anterior chest; may radiate to back	Excruciating, tearing, knifelike	Sudden onset, unrelenting	Usually occurs in setting of hypertension or predisposition such as Marfan's syndrome	Murmur of aortic insufficiency, pulse or blood pressure asymmetry; neurologic deficit

TABLE 2-4	Noncardiac Causes of Chest Pain				
Condition	Location	Quality	Duration	Aggravating or Relieving Factors	Associated Symptoms or Signs
Pulmonary embolism (chest pain often not present)	Substernal or over region of pulmonary infarction	Pleuritic (with pulmonary infarction) or angina-like	Sudden onset; minutes to <1 hour	May be aggravated by breathing	Dyspnea, tachypnea, tachycardia; hypotension, signs of acute right heart failure, and pulmonary hypertension with large emboli; rales, pleural rub, hemoptysis with pulmonary infarction
Pulmonary hypertension	Substernal	Pressure; oppressive		Aggravated by effort	Pain usually associated with dyspnea; signs of pulmonary hypertension (see Table 5-3)
Pneumonia with pleurisy	Localized over involved area	Pleuritic localized		Painful breathing	Dyspnea, cough, fever, dull to percussion, bronchial breath sounds, rales, occasional pleural rub
Spontaneous pneumothorax	Unilateral	Sharp, well localized	Sudden onset, lasts many hours	Painful breathing	Dyspnea; hyperresonance and decreased breath and voice sounds over involved lung
Musculoskeletal disorders	Variable	Aching	Short or long duration	Aggravated by movement; history of muscle exertion or injury	Tender to pressure or movement
Herpes zoster	Dermatomal in distribution		Prolonged	None	Vesicular rash appears in area of discomfort
Esophageal reflux	Substernal, epigastric	Burning, visceral discomfort	10–60 min	Aggravated by large meal, postprandial recumbency; relief with antacid	Water brash
Peptic ulcer	Epigastric, substernal	Visceral burning, aching	Prolonged	Relief with food, antacid	
Gallbladder disease	Epigastric, right upper quadrant	Visceral	Prolonged	May be unprovoked or follows meal	Right upper quadrant tenderness may be present
Anxiety states	Often localized over precordium	Variable; often location moves from place to place	Varies; often fleeting	Situational	Sighing respirations, often chest wall tenderness

nephrotic syndrome, cirrhosis, and venous insufficiency. Peripheral edema may increase at the end of the day and decrease overnight as the dependent part is elevated and the fluid resorbed. Fluid within the peritoneal cavity is referred to as *ascites* and within the chest cavity as *pleural effusion.* Pleural effusion due to congestive heart failure is typically more prominent in the right side of the chest. Patients who have severe edema secondary to congestive heart failure may develop ascites, and ascites is especially frequent in patients who have constrictive pericarditis. Noncardiac causes of ascites such as cirrhosis, nephrosis, and peritoneal tumor must be excluded.

Cough and *hemoptysis* may be associated with cardiac disease, but it may be difficult to differentiate cardiac from pulmonary disease on the basis of these two symptoms alone. A cough, often orthostatic in nature, may be the primary complaint in some patients with pulmonary congestion. Hemoptysis can occur in congestive heart failure and is especially common in patients with mitral stenosis. Massive hemoptysis is generally not a cardiac symptom.

Nocturia, secondary to resorption of edema at night, is common in patients with congestive heart failure. Anorexia, abdominal fullness, right upper quadrant tenderness (secondary to hepatomegaly), and weight loss are also symptoms of advanced heart failure. Hoarseness may occasionally result from recurrent laryngeal nerve compression by an aortic aneurysm, dilated pulmonary artery, or large left atrium.

The history should include inquiry about prior illnesses (such as childhood rheumatic fever) or conditions that may predispose the patient to cardiac disorders. Women should be asked about problems during pregnancy, a state that stresses the cardiovascular system. The presence of risk factors for coronary artery disease (see Chapter 7) should be determined. The family history is important because some cardiac disorders are heritable. Medications can contribute to or simulate cardiac symptoms. Thus, medication history is important.

ARTERIAL PRESSURE AND PULSES

Arterial pressure is measured with a sphygmomanometer. Deflation of the arm cuff previously inflated above the systolic arterial pressure results in the sound of blood intermittently entering the artery (Korotkoff sounds) when cuff pressure falls to less than systolic pressure. As the cuff is progressively deflated to the diastolic pressure, the Korotkoff sounds disappear, signifying that blood is flowing within the artery in both systole and diastole. Spurious blood pressure measurements can be obtained if a cuff of incorrect diameter is used; a narrow blood pressure cuff used on an obese arm gives falsely elevated blood pressure readings, and a wide cuff on a thin arm gives falsely low readings. In such a patient, blood pressure can be obtained in the forearm with a regular-sized cuff, with the examiner listening over the radial artery. Blood pressure must be measured in the lower extremities to exclude coarctation of the aorta as a cause of upper extremity hypertension. The normal blood pressure in the leg is approximately 10 mm Hg higher than that in the arm.

Arterial pulses can be palpated over the carotid, axillary, brachial, radial, femoral, popliteal, dorsalis pedis, and posterior tibial arteries. The carotid pulses are most closely related to the aortic pressure in both timing and contour and provide the most information concerning cardiac function (unless local carotid disease is present). Representative carotid pulse contours are shown in Figure 2–1.

Arterial pulses are normally symmetric bilaterally. Inequalities may be explained by chronic atherosclerosis or more acute processes involving regional circulation, for example, dissection of the aorta, peripheral emboli, or vasculitis (e.g., Takayasu's disease). Strongly palpable pulses in the upper extremities with weakly palpable pulses in the lower extremities may suggest coarctation of the aorta. The amplitude of the carotid pulse increases with anemia, thyrotoxicosis, and aortic insufficiency because of the increased stroke volume and rate of left ventricular ejection. The carotid pulse amplitude is attenuated (pulsus parvus) in conditions associated with decreased left ventricular stroke volume (e.g., myocardial failure, tachycardia, hypovolemia, severe mitral stenosis, and constrictive pericarditis). Severe myocardial failure may result in pulsus alternans, an alternating intensity of

the arterial pulse. Pulsus parvus et tardus is a slowly rising, low-amplitude, late-peaking arterial pulse due to severe aortic outflow tract obstruction (see Fig. 2–1). In addition, severe aortic stenosis may be associated with a carotid shudder, coarse palpable carotid arterial vibrations associated with ejection. Pulsus parvus et tardus may not be present in older patients with aortic stenosis and a stiff, noncompliant arterial system or in patients with concomitant aortic insufficiency. Aortic insufficiency is associated with a high-amplitude pulse with a very rapid upstroke, referred to as a Corrigan or water hammer pulse. Severe aortic insufficiency with or without aortic stenosis may be associated with a bisferious pulse, a carotid arte-

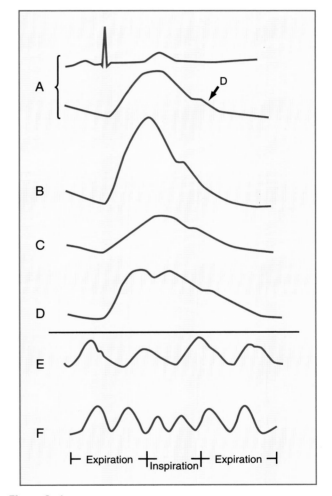

Figure 2–1

Normal and abnormal carotid arterial pulse contours. *A,* Normal arterial pulse with simultaneous ECG. The dicrotic wave (D) occurs just after aortic valve closure. *B,* Wide pulse pressure in aortic insufficiency. *C,* Pulsus parvus et tardus (small amplitude with a slow upstroke) associated with aortic stenosis. *D,* Bisferious pulse with two systolic peaks, typical of hypertrophic obstructive cardiomyopathy or aortic insufficiency, especially if concomitant aortic stenosis is present. *E,* Pulsus alternans characteristic of severe left ventricular failure. *F,* Paradoxical pulse (systolic pressure decrease of greater than 10 mm Hg with inspiration), most characteristic of cardiac tamponade.

rial pressure contour with two palpable systolic peaks. A bisferious pulse is also associated with hypertrophic obstructive cardiomyopathy (see Fig. 2–1). In this condition, a rapid initial upstroke of the carotid artery is attenuated in midsystole and followed by a second late systolic peak, indicative of a late systolic attempt by the ventricle to completely expel its blood. Pulsus paradoxus, a greater than normal decrease (>10 mm Hg) in systolic arterial pressure with inspiration, characteristically occurs in pericardial tamponade but may also be present in other conditions such as airway obstruction (acute exacerbation of chronic obstructive pulmonary disease or asthma). The mechanism of pulsus paradoxus is complex and multifactorial. A pulse of irregular intensity may occur in atrial fibrillation or other irregular arrhythmias.

EXAMINATION OF THE NECK VEINS

The purpose of neck vein examination is to estimate the right atrial pressure (central venous pressure) and to evaluate abnormalities in the venous pulse waveform. To estimate central venous pressure, the patient's torso should be at an angle so that the top of the internal jugular pulsation can be visualized. The vertical height of this column from the angle of Louis plus 5 cm (the distance from the angle of Louis to the right atrium at most angles is about 5 cm) approximates the actual venous pressure. Normal venous pressure is between 5 and 9 cm H_2O. Therefore, the normal vertical height of the jugular venous column is less than 3 to 5 cm above the sternal angle. Elevated jugular venous pressure occurs in patients who have right ventricular failure or an abnormality of right ventricular filling (e.g., tricuspid valve abnormality, constrictive pericarditis, or tamponade). The normal jugular venous pressure falls with inspiration and increases with expiration. If the opposite occurs (Kussmaul's sign), constrictive pericarditis or restrictive cardiomyopathy should be suspected.

The jugular venous pulse is composed of two large deflections (the a and v waves) and two negative deflections (the x and y descents) (Fig. 2–2). Although it is not usually appreciated on physical examination, a second positive deflection after the a wave, the c wave, is recordable. The a wave results from atrial contraction and is accentuated in patients with right ventricular hypertrophy, tricuspid or pulmonic stenosis, or contraction of the atrium against a closed tricuspid valve, as occurs in heart block (cannon a wave). Irregular cannon a waves occur with atrioventricular (AV) dissociation. Regular cannon a waves may occur in a junctional or ventricular rhythm that conducts retrogradely to the atrium or during some supraventricular tachycardias (see Chapter 8). The a wave is absent if atrial fibrillation is present. The c wave is due to transmitted pressure from the closed tricuspid valve thrust upward during right ventricular systole. The v wave is normally smaller than the a wave and is due to blood returning from the periphery to the right atrium during ventricular systole when the tricuspid valve is closed. The v wave may be the only visible positive deflection in patients with atrial fibrillation. Tricuspid regurgitation results in a large v wave with attenuation of

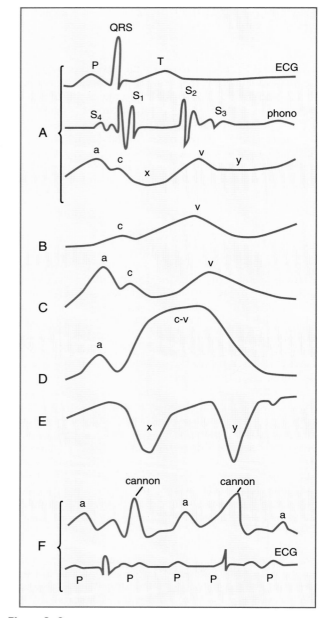

Figure 2–2

Normal and abnormal jugular venous pulse tracings. *A,* Normal jugular pulse tracing with simultaneous electrocardiogram (ECG) and phonocardiogram. *B,* Loss of a waves in atrial fibrillation. *C,* Large a waves in tricuspid stenosis. *D,* Large c-v waves in tricuspid regurgitation. *E,* Steep x and y descents in constrictive pericarditis. *F,* Jugular venous pulse tracing and simultaneous ECG during complete heart block demonstrating cannon a waves occurring when the atrium contracts against a closed tricuspid valve during ventricular systole.

the x descent. The y descent, representing atrial emptying, is decreased in the presence of tricuspid stenosis. Restricted filling of the right side of the heart (e.g., constrictive pericarditis or restrictive cardiomyopathy) produces a venous pulse with distinctive steep x and y descents. Right ventricular infarction can also cause prominent y descent.

PRECORDIAL EXAMINATION

Before auscultation, the precordium should be inspected and palpated. Inspection of the precordium should reveal any abnormalities of the bony structures (e.g., pectus excavatum) that may displace the heart and alter physical findings. The normal apical impulse occurs in early systole and is located within an area of approximately 1 cm^2 in the forth to fifth left intercostal space near the midclavicular line. Precordial palpation should begin with the point of maximal impulse and progress across the precordium, searching for abnormal impulses, palpable sounds, and thrills.

Left ventricular enlargement results in a laterally displaced and more diffuse apical impulse. If the ventricular enlargement is primarily dilation from volume overload (e.g., chronic aortic regurgitation), the impulse is characteristically increased in amplitude or hyperdynamic. If the enlargement results from pressure overload (e.g., aortic stenosis), the impulse is sustained. A palpable S_4 gallop is associated with pressure overload states, such as aortic stenosis or long-standing hypertension. A double systolic apical impulse is characteristic of obstructive hypertrophic cardiomyopathy. A systolic bulge medial to the point of maximal impulse is sometimes felt after a recent myocardial infarction and probably represents an area of left ventricular asynergy. A left parasternal lift generally indicates right ventricular dilation and/or hypertrophy. Vibrations (thrills) associated with the murmurs of valvular or congenital lesions may be palpable, as, for example, in aortic stenosis or ventricular septal defect. Occasionally, pulmonic closure (P_2) is markedly accentuated and palpable in patients with severe pulmonary hypertension. Systolic retraction of the apical impulse is a characteristic finding in constrictive pericarditis.

CARDIAC AUSCULTATION

Both patient and examiner should be physically comfortable to ensure adequate cardiac auscultation. The stethoscope diaphragm is used to analyze relatively high-frequency sounds, and the bell is used for low-frequency sounds. The diaphragm is applied with moderate pressure to the chest, whereas the bell should be applied very lightly. The examination may utilize several patient positions. The murmur of aortic insufficiency and the rub of pericarditis, for example, are best heard with the patient sitting upright and leaning forward at end expiration to bring the heart as close to the chest wall as possible. Apical gallop rhythms and the murmur of mitral stenosis may be best heard with the patient in the left lateral decubitus position. The click and late systolic murmur of mitral valve prolapse may be accentuated by standing. In some cases, the effects of respiration and certain maneuvers, such as the Valsalva maneuver, on heart sounds and murmurs can aid in proper identification of the underlying lesion.

There are four major auscultatory zones. The aortic listening area is the second intercostal space just to the right of the sternum, and the pulmonic area is opposite, at the second intercostal space just to the left of the sternum. The tricuspid area is the fourth intercostal space just to the left of the sternum, and the mitral area is at the point of maximal impulse. These areas provide general guidelines for auscultating pathology for each valve, but exceptions exist, and auscultation should not be limited to these sites.

The normal heart sounds consist of a first heart sound (S_1) and a second heart sound (S_2). S_1 occurs at the onset of systole and is generated by mitral and tricuspid valve closure. The closure of the aortic (A_2) and pulmonic (P_2) valves at end systole generates S_2. A_2 and P_2 occur almost simultaneously at end expiration. Upon inspiration, venous return increases to the right side of the heart because of decreased intrathoracic pressure and decreases to the left side of the heart because of increased pulmonary vascular capacitance. These changes delay P_2 and slightly advance A_2 so that A_2 and P_2 separate temporally during inspiration, becoming superimposed during expiration. P_2 is normally less intense than A_2 and is best heard at the second intercostal space to the left of the sternum.

An early diastolic gallop rhythm (S_3) is a low-pitched sound heard best with the bell of the stethoscope placed lightly over the point of maximal impulse, especially with the patient in the left lateral decubitus position. It is generated by rapid filling of the left ventricle in early diastole and is a physiologically normal sound in young people into the early 20s. Heard in older age groups, an S_3 signifies left or right ventricular failure or volume overload. An S_3 must be differentiated from other early diastolic sounds (e.g., a widely split S_2, the opening snap of mitral stenosis, a tumor plop from a left atrial myxoma, or the pericardial knock of constrictive pericarditis).

A soft, early-peaking systolic ejection murmur at the second left intercostal space can be a normal finding in some people, especially younger people and patients with high circulatory flow states, such as anemia, thyrotoxicosis, exercise, and pregnancy. It is probably generated by flow across the pulmonic outflow tract. Diastolic murmurs are never physiologic. Systolic and diastolic sounds can sometimes be heard over the cervical venous system (venous hums). These venous hums disappear with a change in position or light pressure over the vein. They are not pathologic but must be differentiated from cardiac murmurs or bruits.

ABNORMAL HEART SOUNDS (Fig. 2–3)

Variation in the intensity of S_1 may have diagnostic importance (Table 2–5). After a short PR interval, the mitral and tricuspid valves are wide open at the onset of systole (louder S_1), whereas after a long PR interval they are already almost closed at the onset of systole (softer S_1). S_1 may vary in intensity in patients with atrial fibrillation or some types of heart block, when the mitral and tricuspid valves are in various stages of closure at the onset of ventricular systole. S_1 is loud in patients who have mitral stenosis and a relatively pliable valve (the

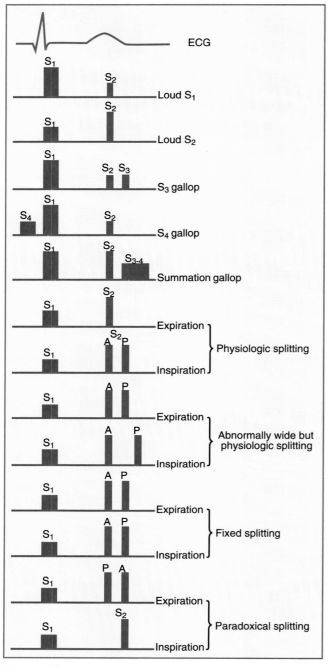

Figure 2–3

Abnormal heart sounds can be related to abnormal intensity, abnormal presence of a gallop rhythm, or abnormal splitting of S_2 with respiration.

mitral valve is wide open at the onset of left ventricular ejection). Splitting of S_1 is rarely of diagnostic significance.

Abnormalities in S_2 may be related to abnormal intensity or abnormal timing (Table 2–6; also see Table 2–5). A single S_2 is present in any condition in which the intensity of A_2 or P_2 is markedly attenuated. Persistent splitting of S_2 retaining normal respiratory variation oc-

curs when P_2 is delayed, or occasionally when A_2 is early, as in patients with mitral regurgitation or ventricular septal defect. Fixed splitting of S_2 is characteristic of atrial septal defect or lesions in which the right ventricle is unable to augment its stroke volume (e.g., severe pulmonic stenosis). Paradoxical splitting of S_2 (P_2 preceding A_2 during expiration and coincident with A_2 on inspiration) is usually caused by conditions that delay A_2. Examples include left bundle branch block and severe aortic stenosis.

The fourth heart sound (S_4 gallop) occurs during late diastolic ventricular filling due to atrial contraction. An S_4 is usually abnormal and is associated with reduced ventricular compliance (it is not indicative of systolic dysfunction). A left ventricular S_4 is characteristically found in patients with hypertension, aortic stenosis, hypertrophic cardiomyopathy, and myocardial infarction. A right ventricular S_4 is heard in pulmonary hypertension and pulmonic stenosis. An S_4 is not present in atrial fibrillation. A transient S_4 gallop coincident with chest pain may be suggestive of ischemia.

An early diastolic filling sound (S_3 gallop) may be physiologic in older children and young adults (see above), but in adults it occurs with impaired ventricular function and heart failure. It may be heard in volume overload states such as chronic aortic or mitral insufficiency, in which it probably also represents some degree of left ventricular dysfunction. Left ventricular gallop sounds are not heard in the presence of significant mitral stenosis. A right ventricular S_3 may be heard at the left lower sternal border or sometimes the epigastrium and is accentuated with inspiration.

When tachycardia is present and a diastolic gallop cannot be separated into a distinct S_3 and S_4, it is termed a summation gallop. It has a distinct cadence.

Normal valves make no sound as they open. However, an abnormal but pliable aortic or pulmonic valve may generate an opening sound called an ejection sound or click (Fig. 2–4). Ejection sounds are high pitched and occur early in systole, immediately upon completion of isovolumic contraction. More severe stenosis causes the ejection sound to occur earlier in systole, that is, closer to S_1. The cause of ejection sounds in pulmonary or sys-

TABLE 2–5	Abnormal Intensity of Heart Sounds		
	S_1	A_2	P_2
Loud	Short PR interval Mitral stenosis with pliable valve	Systemic hypertension Aortic dilation Coarctation of aorta	Pulmonary hypertension Thin chest wall
Soft	Long PR interval Mitral regurgitation Poor left ventricular function Mitral stenosis with rigid valve Thick chest wall	Calcific aortic stenosis Aortic regurgitation	Valvular or subvalvular pulmonic stenosis
Varying	Atrial fibrillation Heart block		

TABLE 2-6	**Abnormal Splitting of S$_2$**		
Single S$_2$	**Widely Split S$_2$ with Normal Respiratory Variation**	**Fixed Split S$_2$**	**Paradoxical Splitting of S$_2$**
Aortic stenosis Pulmonic stenosis Systemic hypertension Coronary artery disease Any condition that can lead to paradoxical splitting of S$_2$	Right bundle branch block Left ventricular pacing Pulmonic stenosis Pulmonary embolus Idiopathic dilation of the pulmonary artery Mitral regurgitation Ventricular septal defect	Atrial septal defect Severe right ventricular dysfunction	Left bundle branch block Right ventricular pacemaker Angina, myocardial infarction Aortic stenosis Hypertrophic obstructive cardiomyopathy Aortic regurgitation

temic hypertension is unclear but probably relates to the dilation of the aortic or pulmonary arterial root.

Mid- to late systolic clicks, often followed by a late systolic murmur, occur in patients with mitral valve prolapse. The clicks are thought to result from sudden tensing of the mitral valve apparatus as the valve prolapses. The clicks may be single or multiple and may occur at any time during systole, although they are generally later than ejection sounds. The behavior of these clicks and associated murmurs during physiologic maneuvers is summarized in Table 2–7.

The mitral and tricuspid valves also do not normally make an opening sound. However, with mitral or tricuspid stenosis, an early diastolic opening sound is heard if the valve is still pliable. The opening "snap" (OS) of mitral stenosis is earlier in diastole, is of higher pitch than an S$_3$ gallop, and is located somewhat medial to the point of maximal impulse. More severe stenosis causes the OS to occur earlier, that is, closer to S$_2$; the higher the left atrial pressure, the earlier the valve opens after the onset of isovolumic relaxation. OSs disappear as the stenotic AV valve calcifies and becomes immobile.

A pericardial knock is an early diastolic sound, sometimes difficult to distinguish from an S$_3$ gallop, heard in patients with constrictive pericarditis. Another abnormal early diastolic heart sound is the tumor "plop" of an atrial myxoma.

ABNORMAL MURMURS

Heart murmurs are vibrations of longer duration than the heart sounds and represent turbulent flow (see Fig. 2–4). Often, the turbulence results from flow across abnormal

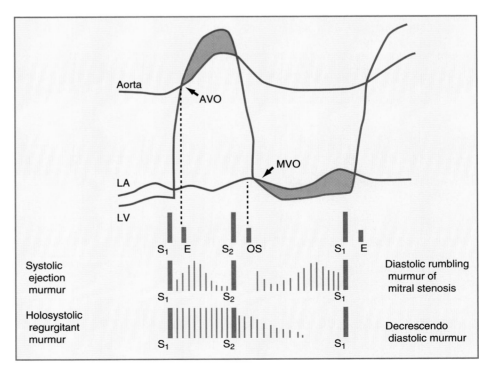

Figure 2-4

Abnormal sounds and murmurs associated with valvular dysfunction displayed simultaneously with left atrial (LA), left ventricular (LV), and aortic pressure tracings. AVO = Aortic valve opening; E = ejection click of the aortic valve; MVO = mitral valve opening; OS = opening snap of the mitral valve. The shaded areas represent pressure gradients across the aortic valve during systole or mitral valve during diastole, characteristic of aortic stenosis and mitral stenosis, respectively.

TABLE 2-7	Effects of Physiologic Maneuvers on Auscultatory Events

Maneuver	Major Physiologic Effects	Useful Auscultatory Changes
Respiration	↑ Venous return with inspiration	↑ Right heart murmurs and gallops with inspiration splitting of S_2 (Table 2-6)
Valsalva (initial ↑ BP, phase I; followed by ↓ BP, phase II)	↓ BP, ↓ venous return, ↓ LV size (phase II)	↑ HOCM ↓ AS, MR MVP click earlier in systole, murmur prolongs
Standing	↓ Venous return ↓ LV size	↑ HOCM ↓ AS, MR MVP click earlier in systole, murmur prolongs
Squatting	↑ Venous return ↑ Systemic vascular resistance ↑ LV size	↑ AS, MR, AI ↓ HOCM MVP click delayed, murmur shortens
Isometric exercise (e.g., handgrip)	↑ Arterial pressure ↑ Cardiac output	↑ Gallops ↑ MR, AI, MS ↓ AS, HOCM
Post PVC or prolonged RR interval	↑ Ventricular filling ↑ Contractility	↑ AS Little change in MR
Amyl nitrate	↓ Arterial pressure ↑ Cardiac output ↓ LV size	MVP click earlier in systole, murmur prolongs ↑ HOCM, AS, MS ↓ AI, MR, Austin Flint murmur
Phenylephrine	↑ Arterial pressure ↓ Cardiac output ↑ LV size	↑ MR, AI ↓ AS, HOCM MVP click delayed, murmur shortens

↑ = Increased intensity; ↓ = decreased intensity; AI = aortic insufficiency; AS = aortic stenosis; BP = blood pressure; HOCM = hypertrophic obstructive cardiomyopathy; LV = left ventricle; MR = mitral regurgitation; MS = mitral stenosis; MVP = mitral valve prolapse; PVC = premature ventricular contraction; RR = respiratory rate.

cardiac valves (see Fig. 2–4), but increased flow across a structurally normal valve can also give rise to certain murmurs. Murmurs are termed diastolic or systolic, and their intensity is graded (Table 2–8). The length of the murmur and its radiation (e.g., to the back, neck, axilla, or listening areas other than that of the valve primarily involved) should be described along with the quality of the murmur (e.g., blowing, harsh, rumbling, musical, or high or low pitched).

Systolic murmurs are usually divided into ejection and holosystolic types (Table 2–9). Systolic ejection murmurs are generated by either abnormalities within or increased flow across the aortic or pulmonary outflow tract. The systolic ejection murmur of coarctation of the aorta is late in systole compared with valvular ejection murmurs.

The murmur of significant mitral regurgitation is typically holosystolic and plateau in quality. Mitral regurgitation due to papillary muscle dysfunction may be confined to late systole. Mitral regurgitation due to the syndrome of mitral valve prolapse may be associated with a late systolic murmur that is often preceded by a systolic click. With Valsalva maneuver or prompt standing, the click moves toward S_1 and the murmur becomes longer. The murmur of tricuspid regurgitation, like most right-sided murmurs, increases in intensity with inspiration (unless there is associated right-ventricular failure). Ventricular septal defect can result in holosystolic murmur.

Early diastolic decrescendo murmurs are heard with aortic and pulmonic regurgitation. Aortic regurgitation can be due to valvular leaks or secondary to dilation of the valve ring (e.g., after aortic dissection). Pulmonic regurgitation also can be valvular or secondary to dilation

of the valve ring associated with pulmonary hypertension (Graham Steell murmur).

Although usually the result of mitral or tricuspid stenosis, low-pitched rumbles across AV valves can be heard in conditions of increased diastolic flow across a nonstenotic valve (e.g., tricuspid regurgitation or atrial septal defect) or nonvalvular obstruction to flow (e.g., atrial myxoma). A diastolic rumbling murmur may be heard in patients with severe chronic aortic insufficiency (Austin Flint murmur; see Chapter 6).

Continuous murmurs or "machinery murmurs" are caused by lesions that generate turbulent flow in both systole and diastole owing to a pressure gradient present throughout the cardiac cycle.

A pericardial friction rub accompanies pericarditis. It is a scratchy sound having one to three components. If all three components are present, one occurs during atrial systole, one during ventricular contraction, and one during rapid early diastolic ventricular filling. Pericardial friction rubs are usually best heard along the left sternal

TABLE 2-8	Grading System for Intensity of Murmurs
Grade 1	Barely audible murmur
Grade 2	Murmur of medium intensity
Grade 3	Loud murmur, no thrill
Grade 4	Loud murmur with thrill
Grade 5	Very loud murmur, stethoscope must be on the chest to hear
Grade 6	Murmur audible with stethoscope off the chest

TABLE 2–9	Classification of Heart Murmurs	
Class	**Description**	**Characteristic Lesions**
Ejection	Systolic Crescendo-decrescendo Often harsh in quality	Valvular, supravalvular, and subvalvular aortic stenosis Hypertrophic obstructive cardiomyopathy Pulmonic stenosis Aortic or pulmonary artery dilation Malformed but nonobstructive aortic valve ↑ Transvalvular flow (e.g., aortic regurgitation, hyperkinetic states, atrial septal defect, physiologic flow murmur)
Holosystolic	Extends throughout systole, relatively uniform intensity	Mitral regurgitation Tricuspid regurgitation Ventricular septal defect
Late systolic	Variable onset and duration, often preceded by a nonejection click	Mitral valve prolapse
Diastolic decrescendo	Begins with A_2 or P_2 Decrescendo with varying duration Often high pitched, "blowing"	Aortic regurgitation Pulmonic regurgitation

Mid-diastolic	Begins after S_2, often after an opening snap
	Low-pitched "rumble" heard best with bell of stethoscope
	With exercise or left lateral decubitus position
	Loudest in early diastole and upon atrial contraction (presystolic accentuation)
		Mitral stenosis
		Tricuspid stenosis
		↑ Flow across atrioventricular valves:
		  Tricuspid regurgitation
		  Mitral regurgitation
		  Atrial septal defect
		Atrial myxoma
		Austin Flint murmur

Continuous	Systolic and diastolic components "Machinery murmurs"	Patent ductus arteriosus Coronary AV fistula Ruptured sinus of Valsalva aneurysm into right atrium or ventricle

AV = Atrioventricular.

border while the patient is leaning forward in held expiration. Frequently only a single systolic component is audible and may be confused with a systolic murmur. A pleuropericardial friction rub involves not only the pericardial but also the pleural surfaces and varies with respiration.

PROSTHETIC VALVE SOUNDS

Metal valves of the ball and cage variety (e.g., Starr-Edwards valves) demonstrate loud, metallic opening and closing sounds that may be audible without a stethoscope. Tilting disc valves (e.g., the Bjork-Shiley valve) demonstrate a closing metallic sound but only a very soft opening sound. Porcine valves may generate no abnormal sounds, but a porcine valve in the mitral position sometimes has an OS as well as a soft diastolic rumble. Because there is a persistent gradient across any prosthetic valve, there is a systolic murmur across a prosthetic aortic valve and a soft diastolic rumble over a prosthetic mitral valve.

REFERENCES

Lembo NJ, Dell'Italia LJ, Crawford MH, O'Rourke RA: Bedside diagnosis of systolic murmurs. N Engl J Med 1988; 318:1572–1578.

Perloff JK: Physical Examination of the Heart and Circulation. 2nd ed. Philadelphia, WB Saunders, 1990.

Tavel ME: Clinical Phonocardiography and External Pulse Recording. 4th ed. Chicago, Mosby–Year Book, 1985.

3

Special Tests and Procedures in the Patient with Cardiovascular Disease

CARDIAC RADIOGRAPHY

The routine posteroanterior (PA) and lateral chest radiographs can provide information about cardiac size and contour (Fig. 3–1) and the status of the pulmonary vasculature. Cardiac enlargement is suggested when the maximum transverse diameter of the heart shadow is greater than one half of the maximum transverse thoracic diameter. The assessment can be misleading in some patients (e.g., due to body habitus or heart position). It is even less reliable with anteroposterior films (e.g., portable chest radiograph) because of magnification. Cardiac chamber sizes and detection of pericardial fluid are more accurately determined by other imaging techniques, such as echocardiography. The contour of the heart shadow on chest radiographs can suggest specific chamber dilation. Left atrial dilation, for example, can cause an upper posterior bulge on the lateral film and displace the left bronchus. Associated enlargement of the left atrial appendage, as with mitral stenosis, can produce a convex bulge below the pulmonary artery and the appearance of straightening of the left heart border on the PA film. A double-density appearance may also be present. Left ventricular dilation may displace the left heart apex downward and laterally and also posteriorly.

Increased pulmonary venous pressure, e.g., due to left heart failure, leads to enlargement of the pulmonary veins and redistribution of flow, such that the upper lobe vessels become more prominent. With progressive congestion, interstitial edema may cause blurring of hilar vessels along with increased horizontal linear markings of the lower lobes (Kerley B lines). Upon further increase in pulmonary venous pressure, transudation of fluid into alveolar spaces and pulmonary edema result. Cardiac pulmonary edema often preferentially involves the inner two thirds of the lung initially, giving rise to a "butterfly" or "bat wing" appearance.

Significant pulmonary arterial hypertension typically results in disproportionate dilation of the proximal pulmonary arteries. Increased pulmonary arterial blood in the setting of normal vascular resistance, e.g., due to uncomplicated atrial septal defect, causes dilation of both proximal and distal pulmonary arteries.

Fluoroscopy or plain films of the chest may reveal calcification in valves, coronary arteries, pericardium, or aorta. Other techniques (e.g., chest CT) can provide better assessment of coronary and pericardial calcification. Cardiac fluoroscopy can be used to determine if a tilting disk prosthetic heart valve opens and closes properly.

Specific radiographic signs of congenital and valvular lesions are discussed in their respective sections.

ELECTROCARDIOGRAPHY

It is beyond the scope of this text to provide a comprehensive discussion of electrocardiography; however, some basic principles are reviewed. The normal electrocardiogram (ECG) is produced by electrical activity of the heart recorded by skin electrodes. A diagrammatic representation of an ECG complex is depicted in Figure 3–2. The vertical axis represents amplitude in millivolts (10 mm = 1 millivolt). The horizontal scale represents time (5 mm = 0.20 second, 1 mm = 0.04 second). Routine ECG paper speed is 25 mm/sec, and thus one can determine the heart rate by measuring the interval separating two complexes (e.g., RR interval) in millimeters and dividing the number into 1500.

The first relatively low-amplitude and low-frequency deflection of the ECG, the P wave, represents atrial depolarization. The isoelectric portion of the ECG between the P wave and the next rapid deflection (QRS complex) is termed the PR segment. The PR interval is measured from the onset of the P wave to the onset of the QRS complex and is normally between 0.12 and 0.20 second in duration. The PR interval represents the time required for the electrical impulse to reach the ventricular myocardial cells and normally is largely due to conduction through the atrioventricular (AV) nodal area. A PR interval greater than 0.20 second is termed first-degree AV

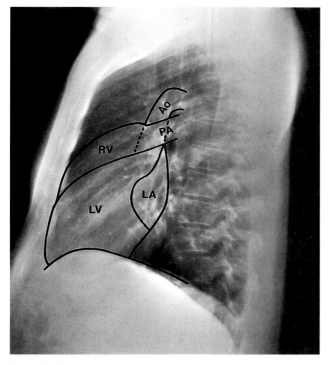

Figure 3–1
Schematic illustration of the parts of the heart, whose outlines can be identified on a routine chest radiograph. Ao = Aorta; LA = left atrium; LV = left ventricle; PA = pulmonary artery; RV = right ventricle.

block. The rapid, high-amplitude deflections following the PR segment are termed the QRS complex and represent ventricular depolarization. Atrial repolarization usually is not visible on the ECG because it is a low-amplitude, low-frequency event and occurs nearly simultaneously with ventricular depolarization. Ventricular depolarization begins in the septum, from left to right. Subsequently, the bulk of ventricular muscle is activated, followed lastly by depolarization of the base of the heart superiorly. An

initial negative deflection of the QRS is termed the Q wave; the initial positive deflection is termed the R wave; if a subsequent negative deflection is present, it is called the S wave. A positive deflection subsequent to the S wave is termed an R′ wave. The duration between the onset and the termination of the QRS complex is called the QRS interval and is normally less than 0.10 second. Upper and lower case letters are used to indicate the relative size of QRS deflections; for example, qRs refers to a small Q wave, large R wave, and small S wave. The isoelectric portion of the ECG following the QRS complex is the ST segment, followed by a low-frequency deflection, the T wave, which represents ventricular repolarization. The QT interval is measured from the beginning of the QRS complex to the end of the T wave. The QT interval is a measure of ventricular muscle refractoriness and varies with heart rate, decreasing as the heart rate increases. The QT interval is usually 0.35 to 0.44 second for heart rates between 60 and 100 beats/min, and one can estimate a corrected QT interval (normally less than 0.46 second in men and 0.47 second in women) by the Bazett formula, $QT_c = QT/\sqrt{RR}$ interval (all values must be expressed in seconds). In some patients, a broad, low-amplitude deflection follows the T wave and is called a U wave. The genesis of the U wave is not clear. The junction between the QRS and the ST segment is the J point.

Myocardial electrical activity can be represented with a vector, a value with both magnitude and direction, at any time during the cardiac cycle. A vector directed toward an exploring electrode of the ECG results in a positive deflection (above the baseline) in that lead. A vector directed away from a given exploring lead produces a negative deflection (below the baseline) in that lead. The mean QRS vector during depolarization is termed the electrical axis and can be identified using the surface ECG. Figure 3–3 illustrates the Einthoven triangle and the polarity of each of the six limb leads of the standard ECG. Electrodes are connected to the left arm, right arm, and left leg (the right leg lead is a ground). Lead I displays the potential difference between the left

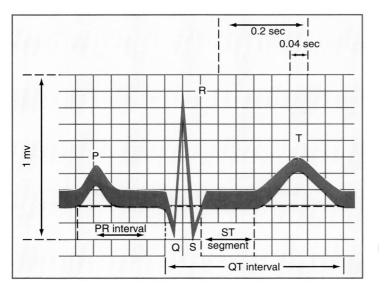

Figure 3–2
Normal electrocardiographic (ECG) complex with labeling of waves and intervals.

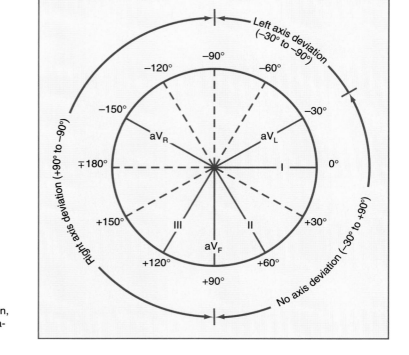

Figure 3–3

Hexaxial reference figure for frontal plane axis determination, indicating values for abnormal left and right QRS axis deviation.

and right arms (left arm positive); lead II, the potential difference between the right arm and left leg (left leg positive); and lead III, the potential difference between the left arm and left leg (left leg positive). Likewise, the augmented limb leads aV_L, aV_R, and aV_f are positive toward the left arm, right arm, and left leg, respectively. They are unipolar leads; that is, they measure the potential difference between the limb lead and a central point. When these six leads are taken together, they describe a full circle in the frontal plane at 30-degree intervals. Using this "hexaxial" frontal plane lead reference system, the frontal axis of any cardiac vector can be estimated. The mean QRS vector is normally between − 30 degrees and + 90 degrees. Mean QRS axes more superior than − 30 degrees are termed left axis deviation, and more rightward than + 90 degrees, right axis deviation. The T wave axis is normally within 30 to 45 degrees of the QRS axis. Leads displaying large positive or negative QRS deflections are generally parallel to the mean QRS axis; leads that are isoelectric, or have equal negative and positive deflections, are perpendicular to the QRS axis.

In addition to the six frontal plane leads, there are six standard precordial leads, V_1 through V_6, which are unipolar leads placed across the anterior chest. The precordial leads are considered positive, and a central reference point serves as the negative pole (unipolar lead). Leads V_1 and, to some extent, V_2 are close to the right ventricle and interventricular septum of the heart; leads V_4, V_5, and V_6 are close to the anterolateral wall of the left ventricle. Lead V_1 normally has a small R wave and large S wave, the midprecordial leads have equal R and S waves, and leads V_5 and V_6 have a large R wave and small S wave (often preceded by a small Q wave), reflecting the normal left ventricular predominance in the adult.

A vectorcardiogram is a two-dimensional recording of the vector loop generated by atrial and ventricular depolarization. Vectorcardiograms are infrequently used today.

ABNORMAL ECG PATTERNS

The normal P wave vector is positive in leads I, II, and aV_F and negative in aV_R. Criteria for left and right atrial enlargement are described in Table 3–1.

Left ventricular hypertrophy can result in increased QRS voltage, shift of the axis to the left, increased QRS duration, and shift of the ST segment and T wave in a direction opposite to that of the QRS complex (secondary ST-T wave changes). The ECG is relatively insensitive for the diagnosis of left ventricular hypertrophy. Several combinations of criteria have been utilized; one example is included in Table 3–1.

The ECG findings in right ventricular hypertrophy are summarized in Table 3–1. The degree of right axis deviation correlates somewhat with the degree of right ventricular hypertrophy, as do certain QRS configurations (e.g., a qR complex in V_1 is associated with right ventricular pressure exceeding left ventricular pressure).

Acute pulmonary embolus may be associated with transient and nonspecific ECG changes. These include right atrial abnormality, right axis deviation with clockwise rotation, incomplete or complete right bundle branch block, S waves in leads I, II, and III (S_1 S_2 S_3 pattern), and T wave inversion in the right precordial leads. Atrial arrhythmias are not uncommon.

ECG manifestations of chronic obstructive pulmonary disease are due to changes in lung volumes and to right ventricular hypertrophy. Right atrial abnormality,

TABLE 3-1	ECG Manifestations of Chamber Enlargement

Left atrial enlargement
P wave duration $\geq$ 0.12 sec
Notched, slurred P wave in leads I and II (P mitrale)
Biphasic P waves in V_1 with a wide, deep, negative terminal component
Mean P wave axis shifted to the left (between $+45$ and -30 degrees)

Right atrial enlargement
P wave duration $\leq$ 0.11 sec
Tall, peaked P waves of $\geq$ 2.5 mm in amplitude in leads II, III, or aV_F (P pulmonale)
Mean P wave axis shifted to the right ($\geq +70$ degrees)

Left ventricular enlargement
Voltage criteria:
  R or S wave in limb lead $\geq$ 20 mm
  S wave in V_1, V_2, or V_3 $\geq$ 30 mm
  R wave in V_4, V_5, or V_6 $\geq$ 30 mm
Depressed ST segments with inverted T waves in lateral leads ("strain" pattern); more reliable in the absence of digitalis therapy
Left axis of -30 degrees or more
QRS duration $\geq$ 0.09 sec
Left atrial enlargement
Time of onset of the intrinsicoid deflection (time from beginning of QRS to peak of R wave) $\geq$ 0.05 sec in lead V_5 or V_6

Right ventricular enlargement
Tall R waves over right precordium and deep S waves over left precordium (R : S ratio in lead V_1 > 1.0)
Normal QRS duration (if no right bundle branch block)
Right axis deviation
ST-T "strain" pattern over right precordium
Late intrinsicoid deflection in lead V_1 or V_2

right axis deviation, and clockwise rotation are often present. An S_1 S_2 S_3 pattern may be seen, and QRS voltage may be low. Right ventricular hypertrophy is sometimes present.

The common bundle of His divides into left and right bundle branches. Conduction delay or block in either of these bundle branches results in characteristic ECG patterns (Fig. 3–4, Table 3–2). In each of these, the QRS duration is 0.12 second or more. Left bundle branch block often is an indicator of organic heart disease. During left bundle branch block, initial septal activation is abnormal; therefore, the diagnosis of myocardial infarction, dependent upon Q waves in the first 0.04 second of the QRS, usually cannot be determined. Left ventricular hypertrophy cannot be diagnosed in the presence of left bundle branch block.

Right bundle branch block can be associated with organic heart disease but is sometimes seen in apparently normal hearts. The right ventricle is activated late, and therefore there is a terminal unopposed QRS vector directed rightward and anteriorly. Initial ventricular activation is normal (septal activation occurs normally from the left bundle branch), and thus myocardial infarction can be diagnosed in the presence of right bundle branch block.

The left bundle branch in many hearts appears to divide into two major divisions (fascicles), the left anterior (superior) fascicle and the left posterior (inferior) fascicle. A delay in conduction in either fascicle is termed a hemiblock or fascicular block and changes the sequence of left ventricular depolarization, reflected in a frontal axis shift. Because the left anterior fascicle is smaller and

more discrete than the left posterior fascicle, left anterior hemiblock is much more common than left posterior hemiblock; in fact, the presence of left posterior hemiblock is unusual without concomitant right bundle branch block. The ECG criteria for left fascicular blocks are listed in Table 3–3. The term *bifascicular block* refers to a right bundle branch block associated with a left anterior or left posterior fascicular block. If evidence of conduction delay or block exists in all three fascicles, trifascicular block is said to be present (e.g., alternating bundle branch block, left bundle branch block with infra-His first-degree AV block or complete infra-His heart block.)

Pre-excitation syndromes are discussed in Chapter 8.

The ECG is very useful in evaluating patients with ischemic heart disease (see Chapter 7). Ischemia may be manifested by downsloping or horizontally depressed (at least 1 mm) ST segments, which is the classic ischemic ST segment response seen with exercise testing. T wave inversion with or without ST depression may also indicate ischemia. ST depression and T wave changes, however, are nonspecific and must be correlated with the clinical setting. On the other hand, ST segment elevation is more specific and evokes a fairly narrow differential diagnosis. Localized ST elevation (current of injury) occurs with severe, usually transmural, ischemia (Fig. 3–5) and can accompany acute myocardial infarction (although the diagnosis of infarction requires the subsequent evolution of pathologic Q waves or enzyme evidence of infarction). Leads reflecting areas of the heart opposite the current of injury often demonstrate ST depression (reciprocal changes). Prinzmetal's angina, due to coronary artery spasm, can result in a reversible current of injury without infarction. Ventricular aneurysm can lead to a persistent ST segment elevation. Pericarditis is another cause of ST segment elevation. In this case, the elevation is typically diffuse and may be accompanied by depression of PR segment and sinus tachycardia.

Infarctions are localized by ECG to different areas of the heart (Table 3–4). Two types of infarction have been characterized electrocardiographically. Q wave infarctions (see Fig. 3–5) typically begin with a current of injury with the subsequent development of pathologic Q waves (generally $\geq$ 0.04 second in duration). As the current of injury resolves, T waves become inverted for a variable duration. Non–Q wave infarctions are characterized by ST segment depression and/or T wave inversion (Fig. 3–6). ST depression and T wave inversion are often nonspecific in themselves. Clinical correlation with cardiac isoenzyme determinations is necessary to verify the infarction.

Abnormal Q waves may be present in the absence of myocardial infarction. Examples include myocarditis, cardiac amyloidosis, neuromuscular disorders such as muscular dystrophy, myocardial replacement by tumor, sarcoidosis, chronic obstructive lung disease, hypertrophic cardiomyopathy, and certain varieties of Wolff-Parkinson-White syndrome.

Many patients have ECGs with nonspecific abnormal ST and T wave changes that preclude a definitive diagnosis. These are interpreted as "nonspecific ST and T wave changes" and must be correlated with the clinical status. A variety of metabolic and drug effects can cause ST

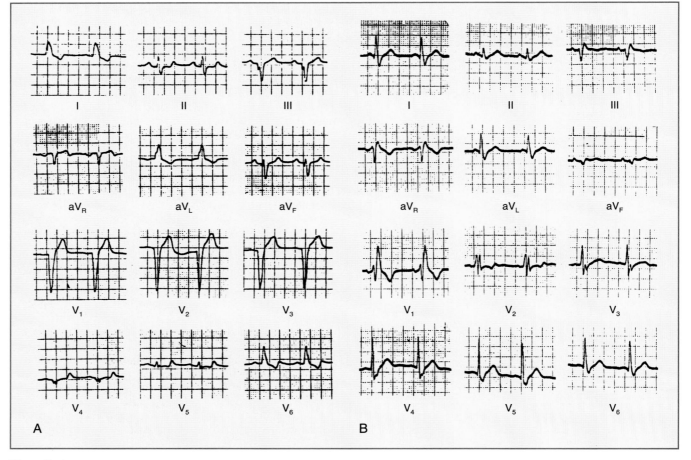

Figure 3–4
A, Left bundle branch block. B, Right bundle branch block. Criteria for bundle branch block are summarized in Table 3–3.

segment and T wave changes (Fig. 3–7). Hyperkalemia can be manifested as tall, peaked, narrow-based T waves.

Abnormalities of U waves include either increased amplitude of positive U waves or inverted (negative) U waves. Prominent positive U waves may be present normally in patients with bradycardia. They may also occur in hypokalemia and with some drugs, particularly digitalis

and antiarrhythmic agents such as amiodarone. Negative U waves can occur with left ventricular hypertrophy and with cardiac ischemia. A large U wave may sometimes be a manifestation of the delayed repolarization (prolonged QT) syndrome (see Chapter 8).

Electrical alternans refers to alternation of QRS voltage and sometimes even P wave and T wave voltage. The most common cause of electrical alternans is a large pericardial effusion.

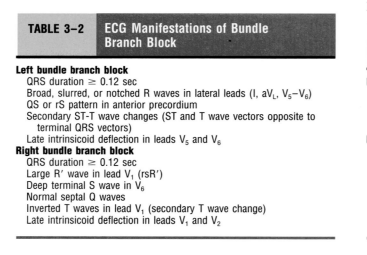

TABLE 3–2	ECG Manifestations of Bundle Branch Block

Left bundle branch block
  QRS duration ≥ 0.12 sec
  Broad, slurred, or notched R waves in lateral leads (I, aV$_L$, V$_5$–V$_6$)
  QS or rS pattern in anterior precordium
  Secondary ST-T wave changes (ST and T wave vectors opposite to terminal QRS vectors)
  Late intrinsicoid deflection in leads V$_5$ and V$_6$
Right bundle branch block
  QRS duration ≥ 0.12 sec
  Large R′ wave in lead V$_1$ (rsR′)
  Deep terminal S wave in V$_6$
  Normal septal Q waves
  Inverted T waves in lead V$_1$ (secondary T wave change)
  Late intrinsicoid deflection in leads V$_1$ and V$_2$

TABLE 3–3	ECG Manifestations of Fascicular Blocks

Left anterior fascicular block
  QRS duration ≤ 0.10 sec
  Left axis deviation (−45 degrees or greater)
  rS pattern in leads II, III, and aV$_F$
  qR pattern in leads I and aV$_L$
Left posterior fascicular block
  QRS duration ≤ 0.10 sec
  Right axis deviation (+90 degrees or greater)
  qR pattern in leads II, III, and aV$_F$
  rS pattern in leads I and aV$_L$
  Exclusion of other causes of right axis deviation (e.g., chronic obstructive pulmonary disease, right ventricular hypertrophy, lateral myocardial infarction)

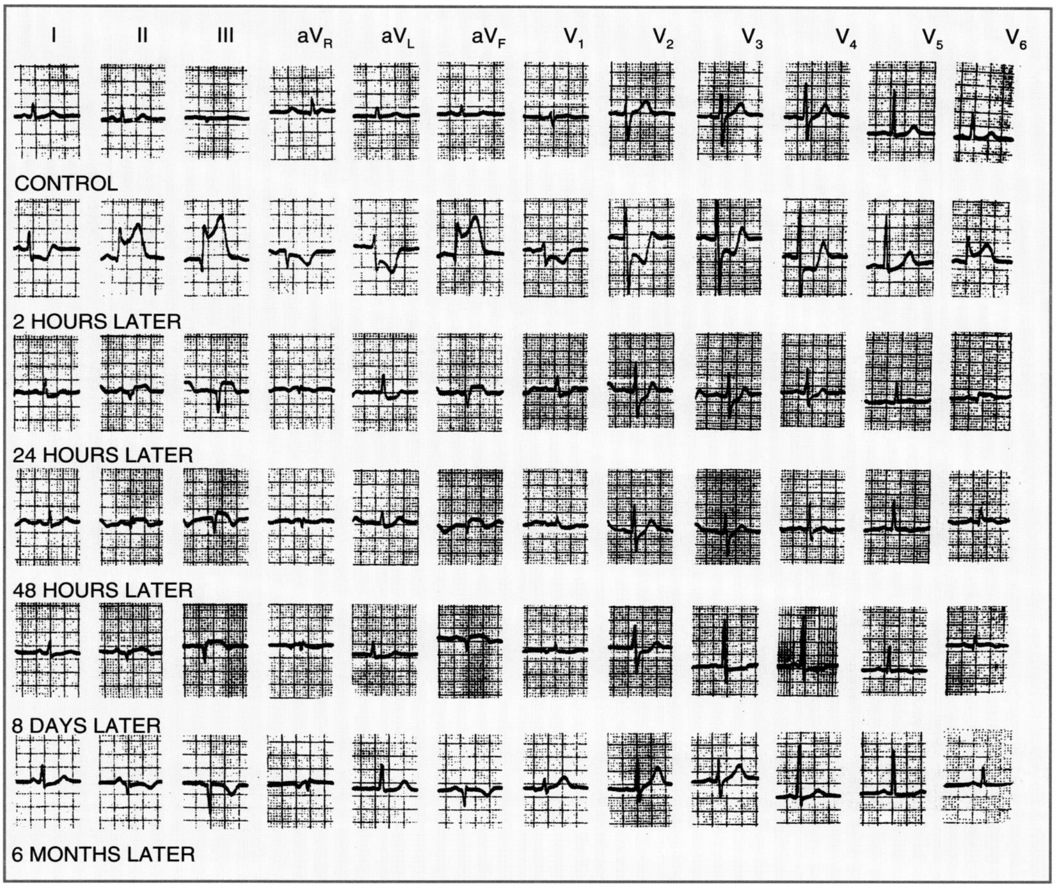

Figure 3-5
Evolutionary changes in a posteroinferior myocardial infarction. Control tracing is normal. The tracing recorded 2 hours after onset of chest pain demonstrated development of early Q waves, marked ST segment elevation, and hyperacute T waves in leads II, III, and aV$_F$. In addition, a larger R wave, ST segment depression, and negative T waves have developed in leads V$_1$ and V$_2$. These are early changes in indicating acute posteroinferior myocardial infarction. The 24-hour tracing demonstrates evolutionary changes. In leads II, III, and aV$_F$, the Q wave is larger, the ST segments have almost returned to baseline, and the T wave has begun to invert. In leads V$_1$ to V$_2$ the duration of the R wave now exceeds 0.04 second, the ST segment is depressed, and the T wave is upright. (In this example, electrocardiographic [ECG] changes of true posterior involvement extend past V$_2$; ordinarily only V$_1$ and V$_2$ may be involved.) Only minor further changes occur through the 8-day tracing. Finally, 6 months later the ECG illustrates large Q waves, isoelectric ST segments, and inverted T waves in leads II, III, and aV$_F$ and large R waves, isoelectric ST segment, and upright T waves in V$_1$ and V$_2$, indicative of an "old" posteroinferior myocardial infarction.

TABLE 3-4	ECG Localization of Myocardial Infarction	
Infarct Location	**Leads Depicting Primary ECG Changes**	**Likely Vessel* Involved**
Inferior	II, III, AVF	RCA
Septal	V$_1$–V$_2$	LAD
Anterior	V$_3$–V$_4$	LAD
Anteroseptal	V$_1$–V$_4$	LAD
Extensive anterior	I, AVL, V$_1$–V$_6$	LAD
Lateral	I, AVL, V$_5$–V$_6$	CIRC
High lateral	I, AVL	CIRC
Posterior†	Prominent R in V$_1$	RCA or CIRC
Right ventricular‡	ST elevation, V$_1$ and, more specifically, V$_4$R in setting of inferior infarction	RCA

*This is a generalization; variations occur.
†Usually in association with inferior or lateral infarction.
‡Usually in association with inferior infarction.
CIRC = circumflex artery; LAD = left anterior descending coronary artery; RCA = right coronary artery.

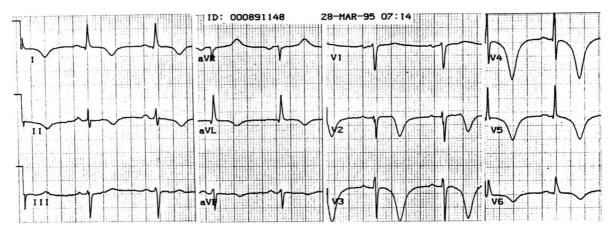

Figure 3-6
Non-Q wave myocardial infarction. There is deep broad-based T wave inversion.

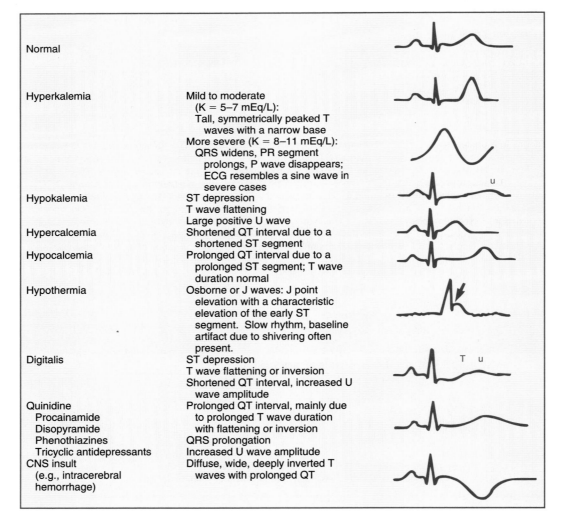

Normal		
Hyperkalemia	Mild to moderate (K = 5-7 mEq/L): Tall, symmetrically peaked T waves with a narrow base	
	More severe (K = 8-11 mEq/L): QRS widens, PR segment prolongs, P wave disappears; ECG resembles a sine wave in severe cases	
Hypokalemia	ST depression T wave flattening Large positive U wave	
Hypercalcemia	Shortened QT interval due to a shortened ST segment	
Hypocalcemia	Prolonged QT interval due to a prolonged ST segment; T wave duration normal	
Hypothermia	Osborne or J waves: J point elevation with a characteristic elevation of the early ST segment. Slow rhythm, baseline artifact due to shivering often present.	
Digitalis	ST depression T wave flattening or inversion Shortened QT interval, increased U wave amplitude	
Quinidine Procainamide Disopyramide Phenothiazines Tricyclic antidepressants	Prolonged QT interval, mainly due to prolonged T wave duration with flattening or inversion QRS prolongation Increased U wave amplitude	
CNS insult (e.g., intracerebral hemorrhage)	Diffuse, wide, deeply inverted T waves with prolonged QT	

Figure 3-7
Metabolic and drug influences on the electrocardiogram (ECG).

ECG manifestations of pericarditis are discussed in Chapter 8.

LONG-TERM AMBULATORY ECG RECORDING

Ambulatory continuous ECG recording (Holter monitor) or patient-activated ECG event recording is used to detect rhythm disturbances in patients with symptoms suggestive of arrhythmia or to document the efficacy of therapy for arrhythmias. Arrhythmia frequency and complexity can be quantitated and correlated with the patient's symptoms. Arrhythmias that occur infrequently or occur during a patient's normal daily activities can be documented. In addition, long-term ECG recording can document alterations in QRS morphology, ST segment, and T waves and thus may be useful for evaluation of ischemia that produces ECG changes; however, the efficacy of ambulatory ECG recordings for this purpose is controversial.

For continuous ambulatory ECG recording, two ECG leads are usually recorded simultaneously via electrodes attached to the patient's skin. A small box containing the tape recorder is carried for the period of recording, usually 24 hours, and the patient is encouraged to maintain his or her normal activities and to perform any activity that he or she feels may precipitate the arrhythmia. The tapes are scanned with a high-speed system with which a technician interacts, and examples are printed on ECG paper for the physician's interpretation.

In a patient whose arrhythmia is infrequent and difficult to document, recording for several days to weeks using a patient-activated recorder (event recorder) at the time of symptoms has replaced the Holter monitor in many situations in which correlation of infrequent symptoms with ECG findings is needed. The simplest type of event recorder can be carried with the patient; upon onset of symptoms it can be held to the chest and the ECG recorded and subsequently transmitted via telephone to a monitoring center. In patients with dizziness or syncope or in those whose symptoms are very fleeting, a continuous closed-loop event recorder is available, which is attached to the patient via skin electrodes; upon patient activation, the recorder saves several seconds of ECG monitoring prior to the event and several seconds after the event.

STRESS TESTING

Because symptoms of cardiovascular disease may not be evident in the resting state, exercise stress testing is sometimes necessary to demonstrate an abnormality and assess its severity. The most common type of exercise testing consists of continuous ECG monitoring while walking on a treadmill at increasing speeds and degrees of incline. Typically, the test is continued until the patient has reached 90% of the predicted maximal heart rate, has anginal chest pain that is progressive during exercise, has an excessive degree of ischemic ST segment depression or elevation during exercise, or has various arrhythmias (especially ventricular tachycardia or heart block) precipitated by exercise. The test is also stopped if there are any signs of circulatory failure (e.g., exhaustion, staggering gait, diminished pulse, or a decrease in systolic blood pressure). False-positive exercise ECG response can occur, and the predictability of the test is influenced by the pretest likelihood of coronary disease. Stress testing is most valuable diagnostically when typical ECG changes accompany reproduction of the patient's symptoms. In addition to treadmill testing, patients can be stressed with bicycle or arm exercise. Exercise testing results may be enhanced with nuclear (thallium scanning or radionuclide ventriculography) or echocardiographic techniques. Contraindications to stress testing include unstable symptoms, significant aortic stenosis, uncontrolled hypertension, congestive heart failure, or hemodynamic instability.

Exercise testing can aid in the differential diagnosis of chest pain. In addition, it can be used to evaluate prognosis and/or functional capacity in patients with known coronary heart disease or following myocardial infarction. In patients with coronary artery disease, an exercise test that results in significant ischemia at low workloads is indicative of increased risk, and further evaluation to include cardiac catheterization may be considered.

The normal response to exercise is an increase in heart rate and both systolic and diastolic blood pressure. The heart rate times maximal blood pressure may be calculated to estimate the workload obtained (double product). The respiratory oxygen uptake (metabolic equivalent or MET level) achieved can also be estimated.

The typical ECG response to exercise is a normal T wave polarity with either no change in the ST segment or mild depression of the J point with a rapidly upsloping ST segment. Abnormal ECG responses include at least a 1-mm depression of the J point and downsloping or horizontal depression of the ST segment similar to the ECG findings of ischemia (see Figs. 7–2 and 7–3). ST elevation is a markedly abnormal response to exercise unless it occurs in an area of old transmural infarction, in which case it may be related to regional wall dysfunction rather than ischemia. The precipitation of negative U waves with exercise is a positive ischemic response and usually indicates disease of the left anterior descending coronary artery. In addition to the reproduction of chest pain and ischemic ECG changes, non-ECG signs may be important; for example, the patient may develop an S_4 or S_3 gallop, a systolic murmur of papillary muscle dysfunction, or pulmonary congestion with exercise. A sustained decrease in blood pressure with exercise is a particularly grave finding indicative of extensive coronary artery disease.

The ECG cannot be considered diagnostically reliable in patients with pre-existing nonspecific ST-T wave abnormalities, left ventricular hypertrophy, left bundle branch block, digoxin treatment, electrolyte abnormalities (e.g., hypokalemia), and labile ST-T changes (abnormal ST-T changes occurring with hyperventilation or position changes). In these patients, one should consider nuclear or echocardiographic imaging techniques that can demonstrate regional perfusion or wall motion abnormalities with stress. Many physicians utilize stress-imaging techniques for women because of reduced ECG specificity. In patients who cannot exercise because of arthritic, neuromuscular, or peripheral vascular problems, imaging techniques may be used in conjunction with pharmacologic agents such as dipyridamole or dobutamine, which can mimic the effects of exercise and result in regional perfusion or wall motion defects.

ECHOCARDIOGRAPHY

Echocardiographic techniques utilize ultrasound to provide cardiovascular imaging and also hemodynamic assessment. The major techniques are two-dimension ultrasound imaging, doppler echocardiography, and color-flow doppler. Usually, the examination involves placing the ultrasound transducer on the chest (transthoracic echocardiography). In some situations, the transducer is inserted into the esophagus to obtain images from behind the heart (transesophageal echocardiography).

Ultrasound waves emitted from piezoelectric crystals in the transducer are reflected by structures with differing acoustic densities, particularly at the interface of structures, and return to the transducer where they are recorded. Ultrasound from a single transducer crystal yields an "ice-pick" view of the heart with high temporal resolution. If transducer crystals emit a moving beam, a larger portion of the heart is imaged in two dimensions. Two-dimensional echocardiography is the major technique for assessing cardiac chamber size, wall thickness, cardiac movement, and valve structure (Fig. 3–8).

Doppler echocardiography measures blood flow. Ultrasound frequency changes when reflected from a moving object (e.g., red blood cells), and the frequency change is directly proportional to the speed of the moving object. In turn, there is a mathematic relationship between blood velocity and pressure gradient. Doppler echocardiography can be used, for example, to estimate gradients across cardiac valves (Fig. 3–9). Valve area may also be calculated using the continuity equation. Color flow doppler provides a qualitative assessment of blood flow, superimposed on two-dimensional echocardiographic images. By convention, blood moving toward the transducer is given a red color, and blood moving away from the transducer is given a blue color. Turbulent blood flow results in a mosaic of colors. One use of color-flow doppler is to depict valve regurgitation and intracardiac shunts.

Transesophageal echocardiography provides high-resolution images and also permits examination of some areas not readily imaged by the transthoracic technique (e.g., left atrium, aorta). It is particularly valuable in the diagnosis of aortic dissection and the evaluation of some patients with suspected endocarditis. Other special echocardiographic procedures include contrast echocardiography (e.g., for detection of intracardiac shunts) and stress echocardiography (e.g., with exercise or pharmacologic stress).

NUCLEAR CARDIOLOGY

Through the use of various intravenously administered radiolabeled agents, either the myocardium or cardiac blood pools can be imaged. Studies can be performed at rest or following exercise or pharmacologic stress. With radionuclide angiography, the tracer (usually technetium 99m [^{99m}Tc] label) remains in the blood pool. Two basic

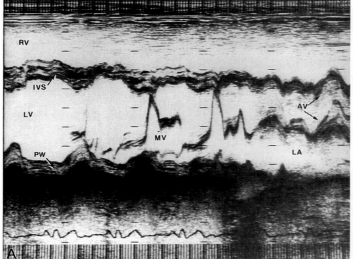
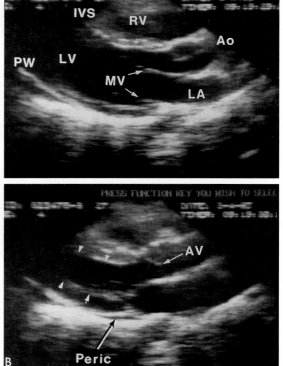

Figure 3–8

Portions of normal M-mode (A) and two-dimensional (B) echocardiograms. Ao = aorta; AV = aortic valve; IVS = interventricular septum; LA = left atrium; LV = left ventricle; MV = mitral valve; Peric = pericardium; PW = posterior LV wall; RV = right ventricle. The four white arrowheads indicate the left ventricular endocardium. (Courtesy of William F. Armstrong.)

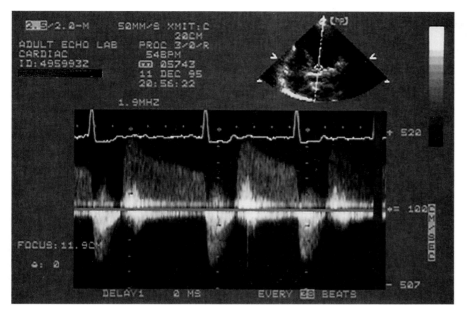

Figure 3-9
Doppler tracing in a patient with aortic stenosis and regurgitation. The velocity of systolic flow is related to the severity of obstruction.

techniques are available for radionuclide angiography: first-pass radionuclide method and equilibrium radionuclide method (MUGA). With the equilibrium radionuclide method, there is repetitive sampling of blood pool counts during portions of the cardiac cycle, as timed by the ECG. The averaged counts are displayed as one cardiac cycle, similar to contrast ventriculography. The major use is estimation of ventricular function, e.g., ejection fraction.

Myocardial perfusion imaging is usually performed in conjunction with stress testing. Thallium 201 (^{201}TL) is commonly employed, although other and newer agents (such as ^{99m}Tc sestimibi) are also available. Images may be planar or, more commonly, single-photon emission computed tomographic (SPECT). The ^{201}TL is injected intravenously just prior to termination of exercise testing, and images are obtained. An area of diminished ^{201}TL uptake indicates transient ischemia or myocardial scar. Images are repeated (e.g., 4 hours later). Reversibility of the defect, due to redistribution, denotes ischemia, whereas, persistence of the ^{201}TL defect suggests irreversible myocardial injury or scar. However, it is now clear that late reinjection with a second dose of ^{201}Tl or the additional acquisition of images 24 hours later can demonstrate reversibility (and hence viability) of some areas that appear irreversible using the standard protocol.

OTHER TECHNIQUES

Computed tomographic (CT) scanning is useful to detect aortic dissection or aneurysm and is probably the most sensitive method for detecting the pericardial thickening associated with constrictive pericarditis. Ultrafast CT scanning can detect calcification in the proximal coronary vessels, providing evidence of coronary artery disease.

Magnetic resonance imaging (MRI) can produce high-resolution tomographic images of the heart without employing ionizing radiation. MRI can provide informa-

tion about aortic aneurysm or dissection, pericardial constriction, and some vascular and congenital heart abnormalities. Positron emission tomographic (PET) scanning provides a noninvasive means of assessing regional myocardial metabolism. The detection of metabolic activity in areas with reduced perfusion and contractile function can indicate "hibernating" viable myocardium that may be salvageable with revascularization.

CARDIAC CATHETERIZATION

Cardiac catheterization involves introduction of hollow, fluid-filled catheters via the arterial and/or venous system into the heart to measure intracardiac pressures, blood flow, and oxygen saturation, and to inject contrast to perform cardiac angiography. The complexity of the procedure depends on the particular patient and lesion being investigated and ranges from extensive studies in patients with complex congenital and valvular heart disease to straightforward measurement of left heart pressures, ventriculography, and coronary arteriography in patients with coronary artery disease. The indications for cardiac catheterization depend on the type of cardiovascular disorder and associated clinical characteristics (as described in other chapters). Commonly, catheterization is employed when patients are being considered for therapeutic procedures, such as cardiac surgery or angioplasty. Cardiac catheterization is usually very safe, but procedure-related complications do occur. The overall mortality risk is in the range of 0.1% to 0.2%.

Fluid-filled catheters transmit pressure waves obtained in each vessel and cardiac chamber back to a transducer; pressure waveforms are displayed on an oscilloscope and recorded. Pressure differences across valves (gradient) are used to evaluate valvular stenosis (Fig. 3–10). The pulmonary capillary wedge pressure is measured after advancing a catheter as far into the pulmonary arterial tree as possible or inflating a balloon in a distal

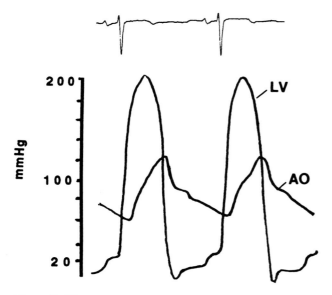

Figure 3–10

Electrocardiogram (ECG), left ventricular, and aortic pressure curves in a patient with aortic stenosis. There is a pressure gradient across the aortic valve during systole.

pulmonary artery, thus blocking pulmonary arterial pressure and allowing the distal catheter to record pulmonary capillary or venous pressure. This pressure, given a patent pulmonary venous system, reflects left atrial pressure, which in turn, given a normal mitral valve, reflects the left ventricular diastolic pressure. This measurement is useful not only in the catheterization laboratory but also during bedside right heart (Swan-Ganz) catheterization to estimate the left-sided filling pressures.

The cardiac output may be measured during catheterization by one of two basic techniques. Using the Fick method, the oxygen consumption of the patient is measured by collecting the expired air over a known period of time and simultaneously measuring arterial and mixed venous (pulmonary artery) oxygen content. The Fick equation states the following:

$$\text{Cardiac output} = \frac{O_2 \text{ consumption (ml/min)}}{\text{arterial } O_2 \text{ content} - \text{mixed venous } O_2 \text{ content (ml/L)}}$$

Cardiac output is expressed in liters per minute, and cardiac index, in liters per minute per square meter of body surface. In addition, cardiac output may be measured by an *indicator dilution technique,* using either a dye that is detected by colorimetric methods or temperature (thermodilution) as the indicator. When an indicator is injected into the circulatory system and detected downstream, a curve can be generated. The area under the curve is proportional to the cardiac output. Cardiac output and pressure data obtained during cardiac catheterization can be used to calculate systemic and pulmonary vascular resistance.

Intracardiac shunts can be detected by measuring oxygen saturations in various cardiac chambers. For example, an increase in oxygen saturation between the right atrium and right ventricle would occur in a ventricular septal defect in which oxygenated blood is shunted from the left to the right ventricle (oxygen "step-up"). If the cardiac output is known, the shunt can be quantitated. Secondly, indicator dilution methods similar to that used for cardiac output determination may be used to detect shunts. For example, if an indicator is introduced into the right atrium and detected sooner than expected in a systemic artery, a right-to-left shunt is present. In addition, indicator dilution methods can detect valvular regurgitation.

Cardiac catheterization can be used to detect and quantitate the severity of a stenotic valvular lesion. Valves that are regurgitant can be established (but are difficult to quantitate) by cardiac angiography, which involves injecting radiopaque contrast into various chambers of the heart. Upon coronary injection of contrast, atherosclerotic lesions appear as narrowings of the internal caliber of the vessels and are expressed in terms of percentage of diameter narrowing, for example, a 70% diminution in the luminal diameter. Lesions producing narrowings of 70% or greater are generally considered to be hemodynamically significant. However, coronary arteriography can underestimate the hemodynamic significance of some lesions, and the hemodynamic effect of a lesion can also be influenced by its length and geometry.

SPECIAL TECHNIQUES

Biopsies of ventricular endomyocardium can be obtained at the time of catheterization and are useful for diagnosing myocardial rejection in patients with cardiac transplants.

Bedside right heart catheterization with a balloon flow-directed (Swan-Ganz) catheter can be accomplished in an intensive care unit to assess intravascular volume status and to help guide drug therapy or fluid administration. Serial measurements of pulmonary arterial pressure, pulmonary capillary wedge pressure, right atrial pressure, and cardiac output using the thermodilution technique can be obtained (Fig. 3–11). Swan-Ganz catheterization is useful to help manage patients with cardiogenic, septic, and other forms of shock; during or after surgery in patients with significant cardiac disease; in patients with multiorgan failure in whom the fluid and hemodynamic management is complex; and during serial evaluation of pharmacologic or other interventions in patients with various cardiopulmonary abnormalities. It is useful in the differential diagnosis of cardiac versus noncardiac pulmonary edema and ventricular septal versus papillary muscle rupture in acute myocardial infarction and in patients with hypotension unresponsive to fluid administration. Swan-Ganz catheterization helps in the diagnosis of right heart abnormalities, such as pericardial tamponade or constriction and right ventricular infarction (Table 3–5).

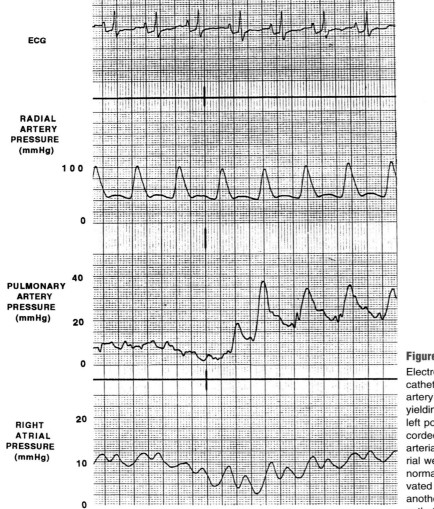

Figure 3–11

Electrocardiogram (ECG) and Swan-Ganz flotation catheter recordings. The left portion of the pulmonary artery tracing was obtained with the balloon inflated, yielding the pulmonary arterial wedge pressure. The left portion of the pulmonary arterial tracing was recorded with balloon deflated, depicting the pulmonary arterial pressure. In this patient, the pulmonary arterial wedge pressure (left ventricular filling pressure) is normal, and the pulmonary artery pressure is elevated because of lung disease. See Figure 7–10 for another example of Swan-Ganz balloon flotation catheter recording.

TABLE 3–5	Differential Diagnosis Using a Bedside Balloon Flow-Directed (Swan-Ganz) Catheter			
Disease State	**Thermodilution Cardiac Output**	**PCW Pressure**	**RA Pressure**	**Comments**
Cardiogenic shock	↓	↑	nl or ↑	
Septic shock (early)	↑	↓	↓	↓ Systemic vascular resistance; myocardial dysfunction can occur late
Volume overload	nl or ↑	↑	↑	
Volume depletion	↓	↓	↓	
Noncardiac pulmonary edema	nl	nl	nl	
Pulmonary heart disease	nl or ↓	nl	↑	↑ PA pressure
RV infarction	↓	↓ or nl	↑	
Pericardial tamponade	↓	nl or ↑	↑	Equalization of diastolic RA, RV, PA, and PCW pressure
Papillary muscle rupture	↓	↑	nl or ↑	Large v waves in PCW tracing
Ventricular septal rupture	↑ *	↑	nl or ↑	*Artifact due to RA → PA sampling of thermodilution technique; O₂ saturation higher in PA than RA; may have large v waves in PCW tracing

nl = Normal; PA = pulmonary artery; PCW = pulmonary capillary wedge; RA = right atrium; RV = right ventricle; ↑ = increased; ↓ = decreased.

REFERENCES

ACC/AHA Guidelines for Cardiac Catheterization and Cardiac Catheterization Laboratories. J Am Coll Cardiol 1991; 18:1149–1182.

Feigenbaum H: Echocardiography. 5th ed. Baltimore: Lea & Febiger, 1994.

Fisch C: Electrocardiography of Arrhythmias. Philadelphia: Lea & Febiger, 1990.

Marriott HJL: Practical Electrocardiography. 8th ed. Baltimore: Williams & Wilkins, 1988.

Pepine CJ, Hill JA, Lambert CR, (eds.): Diagnostic and Therapeutic Cardiac Catheterization. 2nd ed. Baltimore: Williams & Wilkins, 1994.

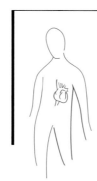

4 | Congestive Heart Failure

Heart failure refers to a state in which the heart cannot provide sufficient cardiac output to satisfy the body's metabolic needs or can do so only with elevated filling pressures. The latter commonly leads to pulmonary congestion and peripheral edema; hence, the term *congestive heart failure.*

Cardiac failure can result from a heterogeneous group of disorders (Table 4–1). Some (e.g., cardiomyopathy, myocardial infarction) directly impair myocardial contractility. Others impose an excess load on the ventricle, either volume overload (e.g., aortic regurgitation) or pressure overload (e.g., hypertension). Over time, excess load also results in secondary myocardial injury. Disorders that largely impair diastolic function (e.g., hypertrophic or restrictive cardiomyopathy) with or without associated contractile abnormalities can cause cardiac failure, as can restriction of ventricular filling due to mitral stenosis or constrictive pericarditis. Cardiac arrhythmias can be a primary cause of heart failure but more commonly contribute to cardiac dysfunction of patients with myocardial or valvular disorders. The manifestations and progression of cardiac failure are also influenced by the compensatory mechanisms that may be invoked when cardiac function is impaired. These include ventricular dilation, hypertrophy, and neurohormonal activation. Neurohormonal influences include the sympathetic nervous system and the renin-angiotensin system. The degree to which the individual compensatory mechanisms are evoked (and the associated clinical findings) depends in part on the underlying cardiac disorder and whether it is acute or chronic in onset.

Cardiac failure can also be classified as low or high output, primarily systolic or diastolic, and predominantly left or right ventricular. Most causes of heart failure (e.g., myocardial infarction, cardiomyopathy, valvular disease) are characterized by low-output failure, in which the cardiac output is insufficient at rest or with exertion. High-output failure refers to the inability of the heart to meet the abnormally elevated circulatory demands of conditions such as arteriovenous fistula, Paget's disease, anemia, hyperthyroidism, and beriberi. Systolic heart failure, the result of impaired contractile function, characterizes, for example, many congestive cardiomyopathies. Diastolic heart failure, reflecting reduced ventricular compliance, most typically occurs with hypertrophic cardiomyopathy and can also result from hypertension. But whereas systolic or diastolic dysfunction may predominate in individual patients, both are often present in patients with heart failure. Notable examples include heart failure due to myocardial infarction or long-standing hypertension. Some cardiac disorders primarily affect the left or right ventricle. Left heart failure from acute myocardial infarction, for example, typically results in pulmonary congestion and/or signs of reduced systemic cardiac output. By contrast, right heart failure secondary to severe lung disease leads to jugular venous distention and peripheral edema. Here too, however, the distinction is often relative. Most cardiac diseases impact both chambers, either directly or indirectly, since both ventricles share the intraventricular septum. Indeed, the most common cause of right heart failure is left heart failure.

By adjusting stroke volume and heart rate, the normal heart can increase cardiac output from approximately 5 L/min at rest to as much as 20 L/min during strenuous exercise. The stroke volume is dependent upon the contractile state of the ventricle, the preload (ventricular filling — estimated as end-diastolic pressure [EDP]), and the afterload (the resistance against which the ventricle empties). With systolic contractile dysfunction, the stroke volume for any given left ventricular filling pressure (LVEDP) is reduced and the ventricular filling curve is more flat (Fig. 4–1). Although the LVEDP is increased in heart failure (due to multifactorial mechanisms including renal salt/water retention and neurohormonal activation), the resultant increase in stroke volume is blunted. Moreover, the elevated LVEDP is also reflected in the left atrial and pulmonary venous pressures. Pulmonary congestion can ensue, including pulmonary edema as the pulmonary capillary pressure exceeds approximately 20 mm Hg. While the Frank-Starling curve depicted in Figure 4–1 primarily reflects systolic function, it is important to recognize the effects of diastolic dysfunction on it. As the ventricle becomes less compliant (or more "stiff"), the left ventricular diastolic pressure is higher at any given ventricular volume. This can limit ventricular filling (and, hence, stroke volume) and promote pulmonary vascular congestion.

As described previously, cardiac failure is accompanied by neurohormonal activation, one result of which is systemic vasoconstriction. This acts to increase venous return, and the enhanced arterial tone helps maintain blood pressure and perfusion of critical tissues. However, it also increases impedance to ventricular ejection. The abnormal ventricle may not be able to maintain output against this resistance (see Fig. 4–1). A vicious cycle can thus be established whereby declining stroke volume promotes more intense vasoconstriction, which, in turn, further impairs ventricular function. It is this relationship

TABLE 4–1	**Causes of Cardiac Failure**

A. Primary myocardial dysfunction (e.g., dilated cardiomyopathy, ischemic heart disease)
B. Excess ventricular load
   • Pressure overload (e.g., hypertension, aortic stenosis)
   • Volume overload (e.g., aortic or mitral regurgitation)
C. Restrictive disease
   • Myocardial (e.g., restrictive or infiltrative cardiomyopathy)
   • Pericardial (e.g., constriction, tamponade)
D. Electrical disorders (e.g., tachycardias, heart block)

that provides the rationale for vasodilator therapy for cardiac failure. Sympathetic nervous system activation also increases heart rate, a particularly important compensatory mechanism with acute heart failure. The cardiac effects of sympathetic nervous system stimulation can be blunted somewhat in advanced chronic heart failure. Circulating levels of catecholamines and peripheral arterial tone, however, remain elevated, and there is an inverse relationship between plasma catecholamine levels and prognosis. Excessive sympathetic tone can also heighten myocardial oxygen requirements and may contribute to myocardial injury. Activation of the renin-angiotensin system appears to be one of the major abnormalities of heart failure. Production of angiotensin II increases vasoconstriction and stimulates adrenal gland production of aldosterone. This, in turn, promotes renal sodium retention and potassium excretion. A number of other vasoactive substances can be activated in heart failure, including atrial natriuretic peptide (ANP) and arginine vasopressin. While vasopressin acts to reduce free water clearance,

ANP (produced in the atria in response to distention) promotes sodium and water excretion.

The salt and water retention characteristic of heart failure is the end result of several factors. Reduced renal blood flow due to pump failure along with renal vasoconstriction yields the physiologic perception of volume depletion. Neurohormonal substances further enhance sodium and water retention by the kidney. These actions overwhelm the counteractive effects of ANP.

Cardiac arrhythmias and conduction disturbances are common in patients with heart failure. Atrial fibrillation may be provoked by heart failure, and its development can precipitate or exacerbate heart failure (because of a rapid ventricular rate and loss of effective atrial contraction). Ventricular arrhythmias are also common, and sudden death is a major cause of mortality. The treatment of symptomatic or sustained arrhythmias is described in Chapter 8.

EVALUATION AND TREATMENT OF PATIENTS WITH HEART FAILURE

The patient's history is important in the diagnosis of heart failure and often aids in the identification of the underlying and/or precipitating cause. However, it is important to recognize that the individual symptoms are not specific for heart failure. Pulmonary congestion from left heart failure results in dyspnea. In chronic situations, it initially occurs with exertion but can progress to occur at rest. Cardiac dyspnea is also characteristically worsened by the recumbent position (orthopnea), as the added venous return from the no-longer-dependent lower extremities con-

Figure 4–1

Normal and abnormal ventricular function curves. When the left ventricular end-diastolic pressure is greater than 20 mm Hg (A), pulmonary edema often occurs. The effect of diuresis or venodilation is to move leftward along the same curve, with a resultant improvement in pulmonary congestion with minimal decrease in cardiac output. The stroke volume is poor at any point along this depressed contractility curve; thus, therapeutic maneuvers that would raise it more toward the normal curve would be necessary to improve cardiac output significantly. Unlike the effect of diuretics, that of digitalis or arterial vasodilator therapy in a patient with heart failure is to move the patient into

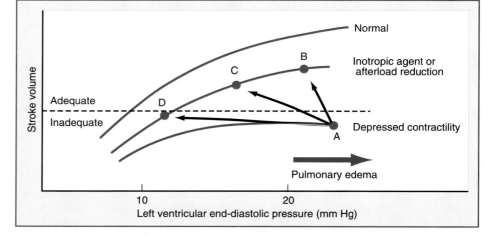

another ventricular function curve intermediate between the normal and depressed curves. When the patient's ventricular function moves from A to B by the administration of one of these agents, the left ventricular end-diastolic pressure may also decrease because of improved cardiac function; further administration of diuretics or venodilators may shift the patient further to the left along the same curve from B to C and eliminate the risk of pulmonary edema. A vasodilating agent that has both arteriolar and venous dilating properties (e.g., nitroprusside) would shift this patient directly from A to C. If this agent shifts the patient from A to D because of excessive venodilation or administration of diuretics, the cardiac output may fall too low, even though the left ventricular end-diastolic pressure would be normal (10 mm Hg) for a normal heart. Thus, left ventricular end-diastolic pressures between 15 and 18 mm Hg are usually optimal in the failing heart, to maximize cardiac output but avoid pulmonary edema.

tributes to an already engorged pulmonary vascular bed. A nonproductive cough may also occur. Left heart failure can also result in paroxysmal nocturnal dyspnea. When heart failure results in diminished cardiac output, fatigue results. If the heart disease develops slowly, patients may restrict their activities without awareness of specific symptoms. Thus, it is important to determine both the patient's symptoms and daily activity tolerance (functional capacity). Lower-extremity edema is a common complaint of patients with congestive heart failure. The pitting ankle and lower leg swelling typically involve both lower extremities, increasing in magnitude over the day and decreasing overnight. The history should also include inquiry about past cardiac and concomitant medical illnesses as well as risk factors and medications. Medication noncompliance is a potential cause of decompensation in a previously stable patient with chronic heart failure (Table 4–2).

The physical findings of heart failure are determined, in part, by the specific cause of the heart failure and are described in detail in other sections of the book. Increased heart rate may be present as a result of heightened sympathetic drive. The pulse pressure may also be narrowed. The detection of elevated jugular venous pressure can be an important finding in heart failure, at rest or in response to hepatojugular reflux testing. Careful analysis of the jugular pulse contour may also reveal a systolic regurgitant wave, indicative of tricuspid regurgitation. If overt pulmonary congestion is present, lung auscultation discloses rales, often bilateral or confined to the right lung base. It is unusual for cardiac failure to result in isolated left base rales. The finding of pleural effusion (usually right sided) may be present. Precordial palpitation may indicate left or right ventricular enlargement. An apical third heart sound gallop attests to left ventricular systolic dysfunction. A fourth heart sound is often heard too if sinus rhythm is present. However, a fourth heart sound, indicating reduced ventricular compliance, does not itself suggest cardiac failure. The murmur of mitral regurgitation is commonly present in patients with left heart failure. Signs of secondary pulmonary hypertension (e.g., increased P_2) may be found. If right ventricular dilation has developed, a right ventricular third sound may be heard at the left sternal border, as well as the murmur of tricuspid regurgitation. In ambulatory patients, pitting edema of the ankles can often be detected. In bedridden patients, edema may be more evident in the presacral area.

No electrocardiographic changes are specific for heart failure, but the electrocardiogram (ECG) may disclose signs of the underlying heart disease (e.g., myocardial infarction, ventricular hypertrophy, or rhythm disturbance). The chest radiogram can provide an estimate of ventricular chamber size, and the cardiac contour may be characteristic of some underlying cardiac causes. The chest film provides valuable information about the pulmonary vasculature (see Chapter 2). Pulmonary infiltrates and fibrosis can occasionally masquerade as heart failure. Clearing of the chest film in response to diuretic treatment supports the diagnosis of congestion. It is noteworthy that the radiographic manifestations of pulmonary

congestion may lag 12 to 24 hours following hemodynamic improvement. Noninvasive studies can be used to estimate cardiac chamber sizes and ventricular function. Echocardiography also demonstrates segmental and global wall motion abnormalities as well as chamber dimensions. Ventricular function can also be estimated by radionuclide ventriculography, including estimation of left and right ventricular ejection fractions.

Selected blood chemistry values can be altered by heart failure. A low serum sodium concentration suggests stimulation of the renin-angiotensin system as a compensatory mechanism. Elevated blood urea nitrogen and creatinine values can result either from intrinsic renal disease or functional impairment secondary to renal vasoconstriction and reduced cardiac output in heart failure. Hepatic congestion from heart failure can lead to abnormalities of blood liver function tests.

Since many of the clinical manifestations of cardiac failure involve the lungs, the differentiation between heart failure and pulmonary disease is sometimes difficult. In some cases, noncardiac pulmonary edema (adult respiratory distress syndrome [ARDS]) must be distinguished from cardiogenic pulmonary edema. A variety of processes can cause ARDS (e.g., infection, shock, neurologic injury, and drug toxicity). In part, ARDS results from leakage of plasma into the alveoli because of leaky capillaries; pulmonary venous (capillary wedge) pressures are normal (see Chapter 19).

Chronic congestive heart failure with peripheral edema must be differentiated from other edematous states, such as nephrotic syndrome, cirrhosis, and severe peripheral venous disease.

The ideal treatment of congestive heart failure is the removal or correction of the underlying cause, such as replacement of a severely stenotic aortic valve. Unfortunately, an underlying cause often cannot be removed, or secondary myocardial damage has also occurred. Factors precipitating or exacerbating heart failure should also be reversed to the degree possible. Patients should be instructed in dietary salt restriction and given guidelines about activity limitations and exercise. Adequate rest and avoidance of exertion that elicits symptoms is important. However, some regular dynamic exercise, for example, walking, may limit deconditioning and improve exercise capacity. Medical therapy for heart failure per se aims to control congestion, reduce the load on the heart, and improve the heart's pumping function (Table 4–3).

TABLE 4–2 Causes of Decompensation of Chronic Cardiac Failure

1. Lack of compliance with dietary or medication use
2. Development of cardiac arrhythmia (e.g., atrial fibrillation)
3. Uncontrolled hypertension
4. Superimposed medical illness (e.g., pneumonia, pulmonary embolus)
5. Medication side effect or drug interaction
6. Worsening renal function
7. New cardiac abnormality (e.g., myocardial infarction, mitral regurgitation)

TABLE 4-3	Principles of Management of Congestive Heart Failure*

Objective	Potential Means
Reduce cardiac workload	Adequate physical and emotional rest Vasodilator therapy Assisted circulation (e.g., intra-aortic balloon pump)
Improve cardiac pumping performance	Digitalis Other positive inotropic agents (e.g., dobutamine, dopamine) Correct cardiac rhythm abnormality
Control excess salt and retention	Dietary sodium restriction Diuretic therapy Mechanical fluid removal (e.g., thoracentesis, dialysis/ultrafiltration)

* The use of specific components is determined by the type and severity of the heart failure (see text). The management also includes, to the degree possible, the removal of the underlying cause of the heart failure.

TREATMENT

Diuretics (see Chapter 26)

Although not present in every patient, congestion (pulmonary or peripheral) is a major manifestation of heart failure. When congestion is present, diuretic therapy is indicated. If heart failure is mild and renal function preserved, a mild thiazide-type diuretic may be effective. More pronounced heart failure or associated renal dysfunction usually requires a loop diuretic, for example, furosemide. Congestion that is refractory to generous doses of furosemide (e.g., > 160 mg/day) may require the addition of a second diuretic with a different site of action, such as metolazone or hydrochlorothiazide. Diuretics can induce hypokalemia, metabolic alkalosis, and azotemia. Monitoring and replacement of potassium is especially important, along with periodic monitoring of other electrolytes and indices of renal function. Fluid restriction (e.g., 1000 to 2000 ml/day) can be of value in patients with dilutional hyponatremia. Potassium and volume loss can be especially pronounced with combination diuretic treatment; careful clinical and laboratory monitoring is required. A diuretic-induced potassium loss may be mitigated if an angiotensin-converting enzyme (ACE) inhibitor is also being administered for heart failure. Potassium-sparing diuretics, such as triamterene, are also available. Use of these agents with an ACE inhibitor can induce dangerous levels of hyperkalemia. If these agents are used together, close monitoring of potassium levels is mandatory. Torsemide is a recently available loop diuretic with oral and intravenous bioequivalence (compared with the approximate 2:1 dose equivalence of oral and intravenous furosemide). Its oral form may offer an advantage in the edematous patient who does not exhibit satisfactory absorption and effects of furosemide. Regardless of the diuretic selected, it is important to avoid overdiuresis, which can further limit stroke volume, lead to orthostatic symptoms, and worsen renal function. Daily home weight recording can be useful for some patients.

Vasodilators

Venous and arteriolar vasodilators reduce cardiac filling pressure and increase stroke volume in patients with left ventricular systolic dysfunction (see Fig. 4–1). They have become an integral part of the treatment of heart failure (Table 4–4). In addition to symptom improvement, they also provide improved survival in selected groups of patients. One of the ACE inhibitors, for example, captopril or enalapril, is commonly selected for chronic treatment. The major side effects are hypotension and azotemia. Hyperkalemia can also result, and ACE inhibitors can cause allergic reactions, including angioedema. The most troublesome side effect is cough. Treatment is usually initiated with a small "test" dose, with monitoring of blood pressure response. Blood pressure is proportional to stroke volume and peripheral vascular resistance; a desired ACE inhibitor effect is that a fall in resistance will be accompanied by an increase in stroke volume such that blood pressure remains stable. However, therapy is ultimately limited by the blood pressure in many patients. The lower acceptable limits vary somewhat among heart failure patients. Often, systolic pressures of approximately 90 mm Hg are tolerated without orthostatic lightheadedness or worsening of fatigue. Vasodilator therapy offers added advantage for patients with associated aortic or mitral regurgitation. Reduction of left ventricular outflow

TABLE 4-4	Vasodilating Drugs for Congestive Heart Failure			
Agent	Predominant Site of Action	Administration Route		Usual Dose
Nitroglycerin	V ≫ A	IV		Initially 5–10 μg/min titrate upward to desired effect as tolerated by BP and HR
Nitroprusside	A, V	IV		Initially 10 μg/min titrate upward to desired effect as tolerated by BP
Isosorbide dinitrate	V ≫ A	Oral		Initially 5–10 mg tid (up to 40 mg tid)
Hydralazine	A	Oral		Initially 10 mg qid (up to 75 mg qid)
Captopril	A, V	Oral		Target: 25–50 mg tid (often begin with 6.25 mg test dose)
Enalapril	A, V	Oral		Target: 10 mg bid (often initial dose 2.5–5.0 mg)
Ramipril	A, V	Oral		5 mg bid
Lisinopril	A, V	Oral		5–20 mg/day

A = Arterial dilator; bid = twice a day; BP = blood pressure; HR = heart rate; IV = intravenous; qid = four times a day; tid = three times a day; V = venous dilator.

resistance favors forward over regurgitant flow. By contrast, arteriolar vasodilation can be dangerous in the setting of aortic or mitral stenosis, in which the output is not limited by myocardial dysfunction but rather is fixed by the stenotic valve orifice. The combination of isosorbide dinitrate and hydralazine provides veno- and arteriolar vasodilation, respectively. It offers an alternative to ACE inhibitor therapy. Nitrate/hydralazine therapy may be less likely than an ACE inhibitor to induce hypotension and usually does not adversely affect renal function. The dosages, side effects, and contraindications of these and other vasodilators are described in other sections of the text. Other oral vasodilating drugs are currently being evaluated in clinical trials of heart failure patients.

Acutely ill patients with severe heart failure may require intravenous infusions of vasodilating drugs. In such patients, hemodynamic monitoring with bedside catheterization of the right side of the heart may be useful, particularly if concomitant inotropic therapy is necessary. If blood pressure is satisfactory, the potent short-acting veno- and arteriolar vasodilator sodium nitroprusside can be begun at 5 to 10 μg/min. The dosage is then increased every 10 to 15 minutes until there is hemodynamic improvement or an unacceptable decline in closely monitored blood pressure. If the latter occurs or inadequate perfusion persists, then inotropic therapy with dobutamine or dopamine infusion can be added (see Sympathomimetic Amines). Intravenous nitroglycerin can be used in heart failure patients and may be particularly useful with underlying ischemic heart disease. Nitroglycerin's predominant vasodilating effect is on the venous circulation, with lesser arteriolar vasodilation. Thus, pulmonary congestion may be improved with only a modest increase in cardiac output.

Digitalis

Digitalis augments cardiac output in the setting of myocardial failure, primarily by increasing the inotropic state of the heart (see Fig. 4-1). No drug has been used longer for the treatment of patients with heart failure. Nonetheless, its role in patients with sinus rhythm has been somewhat controversial, in part because of its modest inotropic action and the risk of drug toxicity. Recent trials have confirmed a clear symptomatic benefit of digitalis in heart failure with systolic dysfunction (e.g., S$_3$, dilated left ventricle). Digitalis is especially beneficial when heart failure is accompanied by atrial fibrillation, as digitalis' electrophysiologic effects include slowing of atrioventricular conduction and resultant ventricular rate. The effect of chronic digitalis treatment on mortality in heart failure patients is being tested in ongoing trials. Digitalis is not beneficial in the setting of ventricular hypertrophy and preserved systolic function (e.g., hypertrophic cardiomyopathy) and may be detrimental.

Digoxin is most frequently prescribed; a daily maintenance dose of 0.25 mg is adequate for most patients. Its bioavailability appears to differ significantly among several preparations. Digoxin undergoes renal excretion in proportion to the creatinine clearance. The dosage must be reduced with renal insufficiency and is also usually reduced in the elderly and individuals of small stature. Digoxin is highly protein bound and is not removed by hemodialysis. Digoxin blood levels are increased by concomitant quinidine or amiodarone; the dose should be reduced (often by one half) in this setting. Digitalis blood levels can be helpful, particularly in the setting of altered excretion or absorption or suspected overdose. However, blood levels have limitations, and digitalis toxicity remains primarily a clinical diagnosis. Digoxin blood levels should be determined at least 6 hours after the last dose.

The most important manifestations of digitalis toxicity are ventricular arrhythmias and atrioventricular conduction abnormalities. Paroxysmal atrial tachycardia with block and accelerated junctional rhythm can also indicate serious toxicity. Other manifestations may include anorexia, nausea, vomiting, confusion, and visual changes.

Sympathomimetic Amines

In patients with advanced or refractory cardiac failure, intravenous inotropic therapy (e.g., with dobutamine or dopamine infused over 24 to 96 hours) may promote diuresis and stabilization. These agents enhance contractility through stimulation of cardiac beta receptors. At low doses, dopamine also stimulates the renal dopaminergic receptor, which may facilitate diuresis. Dobutamine is less likely than dopamine to increase heart rate. It also exerts less alpha-adrenergic effect. These characteristics may be of particular benefit when the cardiac failure is the result of ischemic (coronary) heart disease. Dobutamine does not directly stimulate the dopaminergic renal receptor. In patients with satisfactory blood pressure, the usual dobutamine dose range is 2.5 to 10 μg/kg/min.

In patients with satisfactory blood pressure, dopamine may be administered at 2 to 5 μg/kg/min, beginning with a low dose that is increased as necessary and as tolerated. Dopamine can increase heart rate and can precipitate arrhythmias in some patients. At high doses (e.g., $\geq$ 5 to 10 μg/kg/min), it stimulates alpha receptors, which increases peripheral vascular resistance, and, hence, afterload. If cardiac failure is accompanied by hypotension, dopamine is usually given at moderate doses (e.g., 4 to 5 μg/kg/min) and increased as necessary. If hypotension persists despite dopamine doses greater than 15 μg/kg/min, then other measures, such as balloon counterpulsation, can be considered. In some cases, norepinephrine may be required to maintain acceptable blood pressure. This agent has potent alpha-adrenergic stimulating effects, and the blood pressure increase is largely due to vasoconstriction. The evaluation and management of shock is described in Chapter 19.

Cardiovascular Assist Devices

Support of the failing heart can be provided by mechanical assist devices, the most common of which is intra-

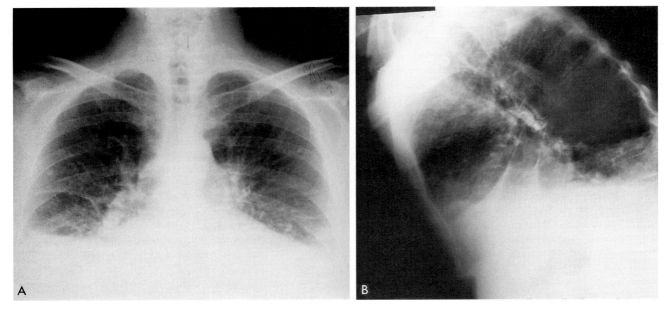

Figure 4–2
Posteroanterior chest radiographs showing cardiomegaly *(A)* and pulmonary vascular congestion typical of pulmonary edema *(B)*.

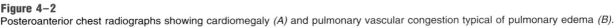

aortic balloon counterpulsation. The intra-aortic balloon is usually inserted percutaneously via the femoral artery and advanced into the descending thoracic aorta. Timed from the ECG, the balloon is inflated during diastole. This maintains proximal aorta (and, hence, coronary artery) perfusion pressure, and enhances distal blood flow. The balloon is deflated just prior to ventricular ejection, substantially reducing aortic impedance. Maintaining coronary perfusion pressure along with marked ventricular unloading can also improve cardiac ischemia. Balloon counterpulsation can be useful in stabilizing patients prior to coronary angioplasty or surgical revascularization or surgical correction of severe mitral regurgitation or acquired ventricular septal defect. It is used in some patients in the early postoperative period following cardiac surgery. Balloon counterpulsation is sometimes used in severely ill patients as a bridge until cardiac transplantation can be accomplished. New cardiovascular assist devices are currently being developed and/or tested in clinical trials. The role of cardiac transplantation is described in Chapter 12.

Other complications of chronic heart failure can include thromboembolism. Many physicians recommend warfarin anticoagulation for heart failure patients with a very dilated left ventricle and severely reduced ejection fraction, especially if there is ECG evidence of intraventricular thrombus. Patients with concomitant atrial fibrillation should receive anticoagulation.

ACUTE PULMONARY EDEMA

Initial measures for acute cardiogenic pulmonary edema (Fig. 4–2) usually include oxygen supplementation and sublingual nitroglycerin (which can be of value even with nonischemic etiologies because of its unloading action).

Furosemide (20 to 80 mg intravenously, based on the patient's clinical characteristics) is standard therapy. Morphine (3 to 5 mg intravenously) can be effective in helping control acute symptoms; care must be taken to avoid respiratory depression in patients with chronic pulmonary insufficiency.

If systemic blood pressure is satisfactory (generally, systolic pressure ≥ 90 to 100 mm Hg), nitroglycerin can be given as intravenous infusion (see Table 4–4). If there is adequate response and/or the underlying etiology is severe mitral or aortic regurgitation or marked systemic hypertension, then sodium nitroprusside may be chosen for unloading therapy. Careful monitoring of blood pressure, along with clinical assessment of peripheral perfusion, is mandatory.

Evaluation of the patient's status and treatment response includes digital pulse oximetry and arterial blood gas analysis. If severe hypoxia does not respond rapidly to treatment or the patient has respiratory acidosis, then

TABLE 4–5	Left Ventricular Diastolic Dysfunction

Examples of Causes

Coronary artery disease
Systemic hypertension
Aortic stenosis
Hypertrophic cardiomyopathy
Infiltrative cardiomyopathy

Pathophysiology

Impaired ventricular filling due to diminished diastolic relaxation and/or compliance; leads to elevated left ventricular filling, left atrial, and pulmonary venous pressures

Manifestations

Dyspnea, pulmonary edema in the setting of normal or near-normal ventricular systolic function

intubation and mechanical ventilation are required. Pulmonary artery balloon catheter monitoring is often used in patients who do not respond to treatment or require vasoactive drugs to maintain blood pressure. This technique is also indicated if there is uncertainty about the cardiogenic cause of severe pulmonary edema. For some patients with refractory pulmonary edema, intra-aortic balloon counterpulsation can be of value.

The management of the patient with pulmonary edema includes assessment of the cause and its removal to the degree possible. In addition to the physical examination, ECG, chest radiography, and cardiac enzymes, the evaluation includes echocardiography. Blood studies include complete blood count, electrolytes (with particular care to maintain normal potassium levels), and blood urea nitrogen and creatinine values.

DIASTOLIC HEART FAILURE

Most patients with left heart failure have reduced left ventricular systolic function along with variable degrees of diastolic dysfunction. However, some patients have predominant diastolic dysfunction in the setting of normal or near-normal systolic function (Table 4–5). The noncompliant ventricle leads to elevated ventricular, atrial, and pulmonary venous pressures. Dyspnea is the major symptom, and pulmonary edema can occur. Causes of diastolic dysfunction can include coronary heart disease, systemic hypertension, aortic stenosis, hypertrophic cardiomyopathy, and infiltrative cardiomyopathies. Diastolic dysfunction should be suspected in patients with heart failure but normal or near-normal systolic function. Echocardiography plays an important role in the assessment. Doppler echocardiography and radionuclide imaging can also aid in the detection of diastolic dysfunction.

Treatment of diastolic heart failure includes efforts toward identification and correction of its cause, for example, cardiac ischemia or hypertension. Diuretics and nitrates can be cautiously employed to reduce the elevated left ventricular filling pressure (and dyspnea). However, patients with diastolic dysfunction require higher-than-normal pressure to adequately fill the noncompliant ventricle. Excessive diuretic action can lower cardiac output and blood pressure. Calcium channel–blocking drugs and beta-adrenergic–blocking drugs may improve diastolic function. Their role in patients with hypertrophic cardiomyopathy is described in Chapter 9. Inotropic agents are not beneficial in patients with isolated diastolic function and in some clinical situations may be detrimental.

REFERENCES

ACC/AHA Task Force: Guidelines for the evaluation and management of heart failure. Circulation 1995; 92:2764–2784.

Bonow RO, Udelson JC: Left ventricular diastolic dysfunction as a cause of congestive heart failure. Mechanisms and management. Ann Intern Med 1992; 117:502–510.

Cody RJ, Kubo SH, Pickworth KK: Diuretic treatment for the sodium retention of congestive heart failure. Arch Intern Med 1994; 154: 1905–1914.

Cohn JN, Johnson G, Ziesche S, et al.: A comparison of enalapril with hydralazine-isosorbide dinitrate in the treatment of chronic congestive heart failure. N Engl J Med 1991; 325:303–310.

5

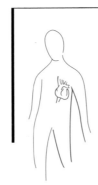

Congenital Heart Disease

Congenital heart disease refers to cardiac abnormalities present at birth. It occurs in approximately 6 to 8 of every 1000 live births. The abnormalities vary greatly in type as well as in the magnitude and timing of their effects on cardiac function. The lesions and their circulatory effects may be modified by the profound circulatory adjustments at birth (see Chapter 1), and further structural changes may occur over subsequent weeks, months, or years. Some lesions, for example, ventricular septal defect, may disappear spontaneously. Conversely, a bicuspid aortic valve may function normally at birth and not become clinically manifest until secondary thickening and calcification over decades leads to aortic stenosis.

In most cases of congenital heart disease, a specific cause for the defect cannot be determined. Some congenital cardiac lesions are heritable, but a recognized chromosomal abnormality and distinct pattern of inheritance occur in only a minority of patients. Examples include the autosomal dominant Holt-Oram syndrome, which commonly consists of a hypoplastic thumb (or other upper limb anomaly) and ostium secundum atrial septal defect, and the trisomy 21 Down syndrome, which can include endocardial cushion defect. Exposure to teratogens, environmental factors, and maternal infections (e.g., rubella) during pregnancy can lead to development of congenital heart lesions.

Congenital heart disease can be classified in several different ways. This chapter focuses on congenital heart disease encountered in adults (Table 5–1). It includes those lesions whose natural history may permit survival, as well as lesions for which surgical therapy in infancy or childhood enables survival into adulthood. The latter group has grown remarkably and presents special problems that are best addressed with input from physicians and ancillary personnel with particular interest and training in this area. In some adult patients with cyanotic congenital heart disease, the management must also address secondary hematologic disorders (e.g., polycythemia). Patients may also be at risk for endocarditis, and prophylactic antibiotic treatment is required for dental work and other procedures associated with bacteremia. Echocardiography (including Doppler and color-flow techniques) plays a prominent role in the evaluation of patients with congenital cardiac disease.

BICUSPID AORTIC VALVE

A congenitally bicuspid aortic valve may be present in nearly 2% of the population and is more common in men than in women. It may function normally throughout life. Alternatively, it may undergo progressive fibrosis and calcification, leading to aortic stenosis and requiring surgical replacement, typically in the fourth or fifth decade. In other cases, progressive aortic regurgitation results. Aortic regurgitation can also complicate infective endocarditis of a bicuspid valve. The evaluation and treatment of aortic stenosis and of aortic regurgitation is described in Chapter 6. A satisfactorily functioning bicuspid valve can be associated with a short grade 1 or 2 mid-systolic ejection murmur at the right base. The diagnosis is strengthened by the presence of a systolic ejection sound and by a concomitant soft diastolic murmur of aortic regurgitation. The diagnosis can often be confirmed by echocardiography. Even if the function is essentially normal, recognition of bicuspid valve is important so that endocarditis prophylaxis can be employed and appropriate follow-up assured.

It should be noted that there are other uncommon types of congenital left ventricular outflow obstruction, including supravalvular and subvalvular aortic stenosis. The latter includes a discrete membranous obstruction. Whereas an ejection sound may herald the onset of the murmur of valvular aortic stenosis, an ejection sound is not typically present with nonvalvular obstruction.

COARCTATION OF THE AORTA

Coarctation denotes a localized narrowing of the aorta from eccentric infolding of the media. It is usually located just beyond the origin of the left subclavian artery or just after insertion of the ligamentum arteriosum. About a quarter of the patients have an associated bicuspid aortic valve. Aneurysm of the circle of Willis can also be present; rupture of the aneurysm is a catastrophic complication. Most patients are asymptomatic when coarctation is diagnosed and can survive into adulthood even if surgery is withheld. However, longevity is re-

TABLE 5–1	Findings in Selected Uncomplicated Congenital Cardiac Defects*

Type	Physical Findings	ECG	Chest Radiograph
Atrial septal defect	Ejection murmur across pulmonic valve Widely and fixed split S_2 Diastolic flow murmur across tricuspid valve Parasternal (RV) impulse	rSr' or rSr's'; left axis with ostium primum defect	Large pulmonary artery and increased pulmonary vascular markings (pulmonary plethora)
Ventricular septal defect	Holosystolic left parasternal murmur ± thrill Normal or moderately split S_2 Diastolic flow murmur and S_3 Apical impulse prominent and displaced laterally; also parasternal impulse	Biventricular or left ventricular hypertrophy	Cardiomegaly Prominent pulmonary artery and pulmonary plethora
Patent ductus arteriosus	Widened arterial pulse pressure Hyperdynamic apical impulse Continuous "machinery" murmur	LV hypertrophy	Prominent pulmonary artery and pulmonary plethora; enlarged LA, LV; occasionally calcified ductus
Congenital valvular aortic stenosis	Decreased pulse pressure and carotid upstroke Sustained apical impulse S_4; systolic ejection murmur ± thrill Single or paradoxical splitting of S_2 Concomitant aortic regurgitation common	LV hypertrophy	Poststenotic aorta dilation Prominent LV
Valvular pulmonic stenosis	Large jugular a wave RV parasternal impulse Pulmonic ejection sound Systolic ejection murmur ± thrill at second left intercostal space Widely split S_2 with soft (or inaudible P_2) Right ventricular S_4	RV hypertrophy RA abnormality	Pulmonary blood flow normal or reduced Poststenotic dilation of main or left pulmonary artery RA and RV enlargement
Coarctation of aorta	Reduced lower extremity blood pressure; delayed, diminished femoral pulses Mid-systolic coarctation murmur at left sternal border or posterior left intrascapular area Continuous murmur from collaterals Sustained apical impulse; S_4 Evidence of associated bicuspid aortic valve common	LV hypertrophy	Prominent ascending aorta; LV enlargement Poststenotic aortic dilation Notching of inferior rib Surfaces from collateral flow in intercostal arteries
Ebstein's anomaly	Acyanotic or cyanotic (right-to-left shunt due to increased RA pressure) Increased jugular pressure and regurgitant wave Systolic murmur of tricuspid regurgitation increased with inspiration Wide splitting of S_2; S_4 and S_3	RA abnormality Right bundle branch block PR prolongation Ventricular pre-excitation	Enlarged RA Pulmonary vascularity normal or decreased
Tetralogy of Fallot	Usually cyanotic Clubbing may be present Prominent ejection murmur at left sternal border Soft or absent P_2	RV hypertrophy RA abnormality	"Boot"-shaped heart due to RV hypertrophy, small pulmonary artery, and small LV Pulmonary vascularity normal or reduced

*Findings vary depending on severity of lesions and associated abnormalities (see text).
ECG = Electrocardiogram; LA = left atrium; LV = left ventricle; RA = right atrium; RV = right ventricle.

duced, and without surgery, only a minority reach 40 years of age. Major complications include congestive heart failure, aortic dissection or rupture, infective endocarditis or endarteritis, and cerebral hemorrhage. Elective surgical repair is recommended for children (often at age 5 or 6 years) or young adults with significant coarctation. The decision to employ surgical therapy can be more difficult for uncomplicated coarctation in patients older than 50 years. Hypertension may persist or recur following coarctation surgery.

Coarctation is typically suspected when a patient with systemic hypertension is found to have delayed femoral pulse (radial-femoral pulse lag) and 30 mm Hg or greater systolic pressure difference between the right arm and the legs. Signs of left ventricular hypertrophy are present.

PULMONIC VALVE STENOSIS

Congenital obstruction to right ventricular ejection usually occurs at the level of the pulmonic valve (supravalvular and subvalvular stenosis are much less common). Valvular pulmonic stenosis can also lead to hypertrophy of the right ventricular infundibulum, producing secondary subvalvular infundibular stenosis. The stenotic pulmonic valve is typically dome shaped. The murmur is present from birth. Symptoms and physical findings are determined by the severity of stenosis and the right ventricular response to the pressure overload. Symptomatic patients may report dyspnea or fatigue. With moderate or severe stenosis, the jugular a wave is prominent and there is a right ventricular lift along the left sternal border. The second heart sound is widely split (reflecting prolonged ejection from the right ventricle). The mid-systolic ejection murmur is best heard at the left sternal border. Valvular pulmonic stenosis may be accompanied by an ejection sound. As stenosis worsens, the ejection sound moves toward the first heart sound and the murmur becomes longer.

The treatment of patients with mild pulmonic stenosis may be limited to endocarditis prophylaxis. For those with significant obstruction (e.g., greater than 50 mm Hg pressure gradient), percutaneous balloon valvuloplasty has largely replaced surgical valvuloplasty.

ATRIAL SEPTAL DEFECT

Atrial septal defects are classified by their location. Ostium secundum defects occur in the region of the fossa ovalis. Ostium primum defects involve the inferior portion of the septum and may be associated with other endocardial cushion abnormalities, such as ventricular septal defect. Sinus venosus atrial septal defects are located in the superior portion of the septum. These very infrequent lesions may be accompanied by partial anomalous pulmonary venous return to the superior vena cava or right atrium. Uncomplicated atrial septal defect subjects the right ventricle to a volume overload. The magnitude of the left-to-right shunt is determined by the size of the defect and the relative compliance of the right and left ventricles.

Atrial septal defect is one of the more common congenital cardiac lesions in adolescents and adults. Ostium secundum is the most common type. Patients are often asymptomatic during childhood and early adulthood. Significant pulmonary hypertension and the development of pulmonary vascular disease are uncommon but do occur in a small percentage of patients with a large shunt. Although patients with atrial septal defect may live into advanced years, the life expectancy with significant defects is reduced. Older patients may deteriorate as concomitant disorders (such as coronary disease or hypertension) reduce the left ventricular compliance and thereby increase the shunting to the already overloaded right ventricle. Congestive heart failure may develop. Atrial fibrillation and other supraventricular arrhythmias also complicate the course.

The murmur associated with uncomplicated atrial septal defect is an ejection murmur, resulting from the increased flow from the right ventricle. The left and right atrial pressures are similar, and the flow across the septal defect does not directly contribute to the murmur. The right ventricular volume overload also leads to prolonged right ventricular ejection. Hence, the second heart sound is widely and persistently split. Transthoracic and, especially, transesophageal echocardiography can demonstrate atrial septal defect, and intravenous injection of saline (contrast echocardiography) may visualize shunting at the atrial level. Echocardiography also demonstrates right ventricular size and can reveal motion consistent with right ventricular volume overload. Most patients with atrial septal defect and pulmonary-to-systemic shunt ratios greater than 1.5 are referred for surgical repair, preferably during childhood.

VENTRICULAR SEPTAL DEFECT

There is a tendency for smaller ventricular septal defects to close spontaneously during childhood and for large defects to result in childhood symptoms and complications requiring surgical repair. Hence, it is uncommon to encounter adult patients with ventricular septal defect. With some large defects, the large pulmonary blood flow from the left-to-right shunt along with secondary pulmonary vascular disease produces significant increases in pulmonary artery pressure and vascular resistance. In this setting, the left-to-right shunt is replaced by right-to-left shunting with resultant arterial oxygen desaturation and cyanosis (Eisenmenger's complex). Although Eisenmenger's complex was initially described as a complication of ventricular septal defect, Eisenmenger's physiology can complicate other congenital disorders in which an initial

TABLE 5-2	Findings of Eisenmenger's Physiology*

Signs of pulmonary arterial hypertension
  Prominent jugular a wave (decreased ventricular compliance due to RV hypertrophy)
  Jugular regurgitant wave (if functional tricuspid regurgitation present)
  Left parasternal (right ventricular) lift
  Palpable pulmonary artery pulsation (second left intercostal space)
  Pulmonic ejection murmur
  Loud P_2
  Diastolic decrescendo murmur of pulmonic insufficiency (Graham Steell murmur)
  Holosystolic murmur of tricuspid regurgitation
Cyanosis
Clubbing of fingers
Erythrocytosis

*Not all findings are present in each case.
RV = Right ventricle.

left-to-right shunt is replaced by a right-to-left shunt because of the development of significantly elevated pulmonary vascular resistance and pulmonary hypertension. Patients with Eisenmenger's physiology may experience syncope, hemoptysis, and chest pain and develop polycythemia (Table 5–2). With the development of Eisenmenger's physiology, surgical repair of the defect is usually of limited benefit, the pulmonary vascular resistance is largely irreversible, and the operative mortality is high.

The murmur associated with a small or moderate ventricular septal defect is holosystolic—often with a thrill—and is most prominent at the left sternal border. Doppler echocardiography, including intravenous injection of contrast, aids in evaluation of ventricular septal defect. Patients with a small defect and shunt may require only endocarditis prophylaxis. Adults with larger defects and pulmonary-to-systemic shunt ratios greater than 1.5 may be considered for surgical repair in the absence of prohibitively elevated pulmonary vascular resistance.

PATENT DUCTUS ARTERIOSUS

Normally, the ductus arteriosus functionally closes several hours after birth, and it anatomically closes within 4 to 8 weeks. Failure of the ductus to close results in a persistent communication between the aorta and pulmonary artery. Patent ductus arteriosus (PDA) is more common in premature infants and those born at high altitudes. PDA can be accompanied by other congenital cardiac lesions, such as coarctation and ventricular septal defect.

The amount of shunting across a PDA and the resultant hemodynamic effects are largely determined by the size of the ductus and the level of pulmonary vascular resistance. The normal fall in pulmonary vascular resistance following birth is accompanied by increased left-to-right shunting. If the ductus is small, the prognosis from a cardiac standpoint is very good and the major risk is infective endarteritis. If the ductus is large, this can result in volume overload of the left ventricle and pulmonary congestion. Persistence of a large PDA can be subsequently complicated by the development of pulmonary vascular changes with Eisenmenger's physiology and elevated pulmonary vascular resistance. If pulmonary vascular resistance equals or exceeds systemic vascular resistance, the left-to-right shunt is replaced by right-to-left shunting. This can lead to "differential" cyanosis, confined to the lower extremities (since the nonoxygenated blood enters the aorta distal to the left subclavian artery). The elevated right-sided cardiac pressure can result in right ventricular failure.

The characteristic murmur of uncomplicated PDA is continuous and "machinery" in quality, most prominent in the first to third parasternal spaces. If the shunt is large, left ventricular enlargement may be present. If Eisenmenger's physiology complicates the course, signs of pulmonary arterial hypertension are evident and the ductus murmur may be no longer audible. PDA can be assessed by Doppler echocardiographic techniques.

Patients with PDA should receive antibiotic endarteritis prophylaxis for dental work and other procedures associated with bacteremia. Essentially all PDA patients (unless elderly or with serious concomitant illness) with persistent left-to-right shunt should undergo surgical interruption of the PDA (which also reduces the endarteritis risk). The operation carries low risk and does not require cardiopulmonary bypass. Surgery is contraindicated in patients with severe pulmonary arterial hypertension and Eisenmenger's physiology.

TETRALOGY OF FALLOT

Tetralogy of Fallot is the most common cyanotic congenital cardiac anomaly in adults. Its components include ventricular septal defect, pulmonic stenosis, rightward displacement of the aorta (overriding the ventricular septal defect), and right ventricular hypertrophy. The ventricular septal defect is nonrestrictive, and the right ventricular pressures are at systemic levels. Occasionally, the pulmonic stenosis is mild and the patient acyanotic. More commonly, the pulmonic stenosis is greater and there is right-to-left shunting across the ventricular septal defect. Exercise and other situations associated with decreased systemic vascular resistance can worsen the right-to-left shunting and cyanosis. Complications can include infective endocarditis and brain abscess. Polycythemia can be marked in some patients.

Patients with tetralogy of Fallot usually undergo palliative or corrective surgery during childhood. Survival beyond age 20 to 30 years without surgery is uncommon but does occur. Selected adults may also benefit from surgical repair.

Uncommon congenital cardiac defects compatible with survival into adulthood include situs inversus, Ebstein's anomaly, congenitally corrected transposition of the great arteries, and ectopic origin of the coronary arteries. Congenital complete atrioventricular heart block and right ventricular dysplasia (which can be associated with ventricular tachycardia) are described in Chapter 8.

In Ebstein's anomaly, the tricuspid leaflets do not attach normally to the valve annulus and are displaced downward into the right ventricle. A portion of the right ventricle is thus functionally right atrium (atrialized right ventricle). Consequences include tricuspid regurgitation and impaired right ventricular function. The right atrial pressure is elevated, and if there is associated atrial septal defect or patent foramen ovale, right-to-left shunting can result. Patients with Ebstein's anomaly can experience supraventricular arrhythmias (including atrial fibrillation or flutter). Ebstein's anomaly can also be associated with ventricular pre-excitation (Wolff-Parkinson-White syndrome), as described in Chapter 8.

Congenitally corrected transposition of the great arteries is characterized by transposition of the aorta and pulmonary artery and by inversion of the ventricles. Thus, systemic venous blood passes from the right atrium through the mitral valve to the morphologic left but functionally right ventricle and then into the pulmonary artery. Conversely, the morphologic right but functional left ventricle receives blood from the left atrium and ejects it into the aorta. Survival and function into adulthood occurs, but failure of the systemic ventricle can also develop.

Other complications include the development of atrioventricular heart block. Congenitally corrected transposition can also be accompanied by other lesions, including ventricular septal defect and Ebstein's anomaly of the tricuspid valve.

Congenital coronary artery anomalies include origin of the circumflex vessel from the right sinus of Valsalva. If an aberrant coronary artery courses between the aorta and pulmonary trunk (e.g., left coronary artery arising from the right coronary sinus), angina pectoris, myocardial infarction, or sudden death can result, particularly with physical exertion. Coronary arteriovenous fistulae can drain into a cardiac chamber (e.g., right ventricle), the vena cava, or a pulmonary vein and can give rise to a continuous murmur. Depending on the amount of fistula flow and the site to which it flows, cardiac ischemia can result. Echocardiographic techniques can detect the dilated fistulous vessel in some cases.

GENERAL CONSIDERATIONS IN THE EVALUATION AND MANAGEMENT OF ADULTS WITH CONGENITAL HEART DISEASE

The care of patients with complex congenital heart disease increasingly includes that of individuals who have undergone surgical procedures during infancy or childhood. They, as well as patients who have not undergone surgery, can present a number of additional problems and issues, including activity and exercise guidelines, genetic and pregnancy considerations, and insurability/employment issues. Some patients are also at risk for the development of secondary abnormalities and cardiac arrhythmias or conduction disturbances. Patients with cyanotic congenital heart disease may have secondary erythrocytosis; when decompensated and symptomatic (e.g., hyperviscosity symptoms), cautious phlebotomy may be indicated (after exclusion of dehydration and iron deficiency). Hyperuricemia and mild bleeding diathesis can also occur. Because of the complexity of these issues, they are best addressed by individuals and facilities with particular experience and expertise in adult congenital heart disease.

REFERENCES

American College of Cardiology Bethesda Conference Report: Recommendations for determining eligibility for competition in athletes with cardiovascular abnormalities, B26, 1994.

O'Fallon WM, Weidman WH (Eds.): Report from the Second Joint Study on the Natural History of Congenital Heart Defects (NHS-2). Circulation 1993; 87(Suppl I):1–126.

Perloff JK, Child JS: Congenital Heart Disease in Adults. Philadelphia: WB Saunders, 1991.

6 Acquired Valvular Heart Disease

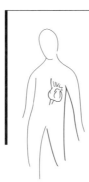

GENERAL CONSIDERATIONS

Many heart valve disorders place an excess load on the heart. With aortic or pulmonic stenosis, for example, it is a pressure overload, and ventricular hypertrophy is a major compensatory mechanism. Other disorders, such as aortic regurgitation, subject the ventricle to a volume overload, and ventricular dilation is the major compensatory change. When the valve dysfunction develops slowly, the compensatory mechanisms may help maintain overall cardiac function for some time. Ultimately, the excess load can lead to secondary and largely irreversible myocardial dysfunction. In many patients with heart failure due to chronic valve disease, the heart failure is the result of both the mechanical effect of the valve lesion and secondary myocardial dysfunction. When the valve dysfunction is acute and severe, for example, aortic regurgitation due to endocarditis, heart failure can result despite normal myocardial (contractile) function.

Echocardiographic and Doppler techniques are important tools in the diagnosis of valvular heart disease and estimation of its severity. In some cases, they may obviate the need for cardiac catheterization. However, cardiac catheterization remains the standard means of evaluating most patients when surgical therapy is being considered. This is particularly the case when multivalve disease is present and when concomitant coronary disease must be assessed because of the patient's symptoms or age.

The decision about whether and when to employ surgical therapy to repair or replace an abnormal valve rests on several considerations and can be difficult. Often, it is based on the patient's symptoms and clinical findings, along with a knowledge of the natural history of the specific valve lesion. The functional status of the left ventricle is an important determinant also. Ideally, corrective therapy should be employed before significant secondary myocardial injury has occurred. With some lesions, the myocardial damage may occur before limiting symptoms develop. Surgical therapy may involve repair of the native valve in some cases, but in most adults who require surgery the valve is replaced with a prosthesis. Beyond the operative risk, prosthetic heart valves can be associated with complications and dysfunction (discussed later). Thus, it is important that surgical therapy be recommended at a time when its benefits outweigh the risks and when it can be expected to result in significant symptomatic improvement and/or improved prognosis.

Patients with valvular heart disease (including those with prostheses) are at risk for the development of infective endocarditis. Oral hygiene is important along with antibiotic prophylaxis for dental work or other procedures associated with bacteremia.

AORTIC STENOSIS

Aortic stenosis can result from congenital (e.g., bicuspid valve) and rheumatic disease and from degeneration and calcification of a tricuspid valve (Table 6–1). When aortic valve disease is rheumatic, associated mitral valve disease is expected. In young and middle-aged adults, a bicuspid aortic valve with progressive scarring and calcification is most common. Patients presenting after age 65 years usually have calcification of a tricuspid valve. Aortic stenosis is more common in men. The outflow obstruction leads to left ventricular hypertrophy. Symptoms are not usually present until the obstruction is advanced. The cardinal symptoms are angina pectoris, syncope, and dyspnea. Angina can occur in the absence of obstructive coronary disease because of the heightened oxygen demand associated with hypertrophy and high wall tension, coupled with decreased diastolic coronary flow. Dyspnea can result from diastolic dysfunction associated with the increased afterload and noncompliant hypertrophied ventricle. Late in the course, systolic dysfunction can also develop. The development of any of the cardinal symptoms in the setting of severe aortic stenosis indicates substantial mortality risk (Fig. 6–1) and is an indication for surgical therapy. The average life expectancy after symptom onset is 2 to 3 years (less if the symptoms are due to heart failure). Although symptoms play an important role in the timing of surgical repair, sudden death may be the only symptom in a small percentage of patients. Because symptoms (and perhaps sudden death) often accompany physical exertion, vigorous activities and competitive sports should be avoided by patients with aortic stenosis, even if it is only mild to moderate in severity.

The ejection murmur of aortic stenosis is typically harsh, heard well at the aortic area, and radiates to the base of the neck (Table 6–2). Although often loud, the murmur's intensity may decrease in advanced cases as the cardiac output is reduced. The duration of the murmur is related to the obstruction severity. A fourth heart sound is

TABLE 6–1	Causes of Cardiac Valvular Disease in Adults

Aortic stenosis
    Bicuspid aortic valve
    Calcified tricuspid valve
Aortic regurgitation
    Bicuspid aortic valve
    Aortic root dilation
    Rheumatic (if associated mitral stenosis present)
    Endocarditis
Mitral stenosis
    Rheumatic
Mitral regurgitation
    Mitral valve prolapse
    Ischemic heart disease (e.g., papillary muscle dysfunction)
    Left ventricular dilation
    Mitral annulus calcification
    Rheumatic
Tricuspid regurgitation
    Functional, e.g., due to right ventricular dilation/failure
    Tricuspid valve prolapse
    Endocarditis

expected if sinus rhythm is present. Chest palpation may reveal the sustained impulse of left ventricular hypertrophy. The carotid pulse (Fig. 6–2) is characteristically reduced in amplitude and prolonged in duration (pulsus parvus et tardus). A carotid "shudder" may also be palpated in some cases. However, these findings may be influenced by intrinsic changes in the carotid vessels in the elderly. The electrocardiogram (ECG) often demonstrates changes consistent with left ventricular hypertrophy.

Echocardiography and Doppler techniques can confirm the presence of aortic valve disease and the status of the left ventricle. The severity of the obstruction can also be estimated using Doppler flow velocity to determine valve gradient and by calculation of valve area by the continuity equation. It is important to recognize that the

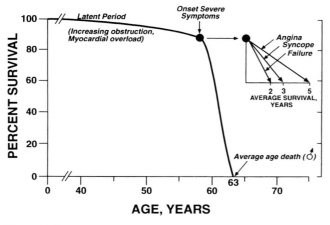

Figure 6–1
Natural history of aortic stenosis without surgical therapy. (Reproduced with permission from Ross J Jr, Braunwald E: Aortic stenosis. Circulation 1968; 38[Suppl V]:61. Copyright 1968 American Heart Association.)

gradient across a stenotic valve is dependent on the cardiac output as well as on the severity of obstruction. If cardiac output is reduced from associated left ventricular dysfunction, a lesser gradient may still represent significant valve obstruction. Most symptomatic patients with suspected severe aortic stenosis undergo cardiac catheterization to confirm the severity of valve disease and determine if concomitant coronary disease is present. A calculated valve area ≤ 0.7 cm^2 defines critical aortic stenosis and is usually associated with a transvalvular gradient of ≥ 50 mm Hg (if left ventricular function is preserved). Surgical therapy is indicated for symptomatic patients with severe aortic stenosis. In most adult patients, this entails replacement with a prosthetic valve. Although the operative risk and prognosis are best in patients with normal left ventricular function, the presence of left ventricular dysfunction does not contraindicate aortic valve replacement. Unlike some other valvular lesions, aortic stenosis relief usually results in improved left ventricular function.

AORTIC REGURGITATION (see Tables 6–1 and 6–2)

Chronic aortic regurgitation can result from dilation of the aortic root as well as from disorders of the aortic valve. Disorders of the aortic valve include bicuspid aortic valves, rheumatic disease, and prior endocarditis. Depending on the etiology, aortic regurgitation and stenosis may both be present. Some connective tissue disorders that affect the ascending aorta, such as Marfan's syndrome, are associated with aortic regurgitation.

Aortic regurgitation results in a volume overload of the left ventricle with ventricular dilation. The stroke volume is increased, as the left ventricle ejects both the forward output and the blood that regurgitates into the ventricle during diastole. As regurgitant volume increases, the left ventricular diastolic pressure rises. Although chronic aortic regurgitation may be tolerated for a long time, significant regurgitation ultimately results in secondary myocardial dysfunction that may persist after surgical repair of the valve.

Patients with mild to moderate aortic regurgitation usually do not have associated symptoms. Even patients with severe regurgitation may be asymptomatic. Some patients report palpitations or pounding in the head or chest from the hyperdynamic circulation. Dyspnea results from elevated pulmonary venous pressure. When congestive failure occurs, patients may also complain of fatigue and weakness. Patients with aortic regurgitation can also experience angina pectoris—even with normal coronary arteries—because of reduced diastolic coronary perfusion pressure gradient.

The large stroke volume and diastolic runoff produce the wide pulse pressure characteristic of chronic aortic regurgitation. The cardiac impulse is hyperdynamic and laterally displaced (see Fig. 6–2). The diastolic decrescendo murmur is high pitched and heard best with the patient sitting upright and leaning forward. A systolic ejection murmur, reflecting the increased stroke volume across the abnormal valve, is often present, as is a third

TABLE 6–2	Characteristic Physical, ECG, and Chest Radiographic Findings in Chronic Acquired Valvular Heart Disease		
	Physical Findings	**ECG**	**Radiograph**
Aortic stenosis	Pulsus parvus et tardus (may be absent in older patients or with associated aortic regurgitation); carotid "shudder" (coarse thrill) Ejection murmur radiates to base of neck; peak late in systole if stenosis severe Sustained but not markedly displaced LV impulse A_2 decreased, S_2 single or paradoxically split S_4 gallop, often palpable	LV hypertrophy; left bundle branch block also common Rare heart block from calcific involvement of conduction system	LV prominence without dilation Poststenotic aortic root dilation Aortic valve calcification
Aortic regurgitation	Increased pulse pressure Bifed carotid pulses Rapid pulse upstroke and collapse LV impulse hyperdynamic and displaced laterally Diastolic decrescendo murmur; duration related to severity Systolic flow murmur S_3G common	LV hypertrophy, often with narrow deep Q waves	LV and aortic dilation
Mitral stenosis	Loud S_1 Opening snap (OS) (S_2-OS interval inversely related to stenosis severity) S_1 not loud, and OS absent if valve heavily calcified Signs of pulmonary arterial hypertension	Left atrial abnormality Atrial fibrillation common RV hypertrophy pattern may develop if associated pulmonary arterial hypertension	Large LA: double-density, posterior displacement of esophagus, elevation of left mainstem bronchus Straightening of left heart border due to enlarged left appendage Small or normal size LV Large pulmonary artery Pulmonary venous congestion
Mitral regurgitation	Hyperdynamic LV impulse S_3 Widely split S_2 may occur Holosystolic apical murmur radiating to axilla (murmur may be atypical with acute mitral regurgitation, papillary muscle dysfunction, or mitral valve prolapse—see text)	Left atrial abnormality LV hypertrophy Atrial fibrillation	Enlarged LA and LV Pulmonary venous congestion
Mitral valve prolapse	One or more systolic clicks—often mid-systolic—followed by late systolic murmur Auscultatory findings dynamic—see text Patients may exhibit tall thin habitus, pectus excavatum, straight back syndrome	Often normal Occasionally ST-depression and/or T wave changes in inferior leads	Depends on degree of valve regurgitation and presence or absence of those abnormalities
Tricuspid stenosis	Jugular venous distention with prominent a wave if sinus rhythm Tricuspid OS and diastolic rumble at left sternal border—may be overshadowed by concomitant mitral stenosis Tricuspid OS and rumble increased during inspiration	Right atrial abnormality Atrial fibrillation common	Large RA
Tricuspid regurgitation	Jugular venous distention with large regurgitant (systolic) wave Systolic murmur at left sternal border, increased with inspiration Diastolic flow rumble RV S_3 increased with inspiration Hepatomegaly with systolic pulsation	RA abnormality Findings often related to cause of the tricuspid regurgitation	RA and RV enlarged Findings often related to cause of the tricuspid regurgitation

*Findings are influenced by the severity and chronicity of the valve disorder.
ECG = Electrocardiogram; LA = left atrium; LV = left ventricle; RA = right atrium; RV = right ventricle.

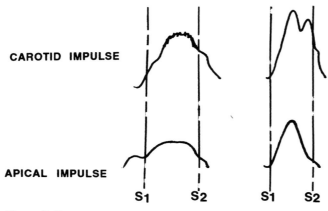

CAROTID IMPULSE

APICAL IMPULSE

S₁ S₂ S₁ S₂

Figure 6-2

Diagrammatic depiction of carotid and apical impulses with aortic stenosis *(left panel)* and aortic regurgitation *(right panel)*. (See text for more information.)

heart sound. With severe aortic regurgitation, a diastolic low-pitched murmur (Austin-Flint murmur) that can be confused with mitral stenosis may be heard at the apex. This murmur presumably reflects the effects of the aortic regurgitant jet and increased ventricular diastolic pressure on the mitral valve. In some cases of severe aortic regurgitation, the mitral valve leaflets may be prematurely closed. The peripheral signs of severe aortic regurgitation include rapid rise and quick collapse of the arterial pulse and a double impulse during systole (bisferious pulse) of the carotid artery.

The natural history of chronic aortic regurgitation is variable. Mild regurgitation may not progress in severity. Progression is more likely when moderate regurgitation is present. Even patients with severe chronic aortic regurgitation may remain asymptomatic for a long time, but once symptoms develop, deterioration can be rapid. Important predictors of the development of symptoms and worse prognosis are the degree of left ventricular dilation and the presence of left ventricular systolic dysfunction. Accordingly, asymptomatic patients with chronic aortic regurgitation should have periodic noninvasive studies of left ventricular function to detect early signs of systolic dysfunction. Echocardiographic techniques can also provide information about the cause of aortic regurgitation in many cases, and the regurgitation can be demonstrated by Doppler and color flow studies.

The major indications for surgical aortic valve replacement are evidence of left ventricular systolic dysfunction and onset of symptoms. It is important that patients be followed closely and surgery employed before systolic dysfunction is significant, since dysfunction due to myocardial damage may not improve postoperatively. For asymptomatic patients with significant aortic regurgitation and normal systolic function, oral vasodilator therapy can be of benefit. By reducing systemic resistance, forward flow is enhanced and the regurgitant volume reduced. Vasodilator therapy is also used for symptomatic patients who refuse surgical therapy or are not candidates for surgery because of concomitant medical problems.

Acute aortic regurgitation differs from chronic aortic regurgitation in several ways. Causes of acute aortic regurgitation include infective endocarditis, prosthetic aortic valve dysfunction, and proximal dissection of the aorta. Severe acute aortic regurgitation places a volume overload on a left ventricle that has not had time to dilate in a compensatory manner. The increased ventricular diastolic pressure leads to increased left atrial pressure and pulmonary congestion. Because of ventricular size, the stroke volume cannot increase to the degree necessary, and forward stroke volume is reduced. The patients usually have sinus tachycardia. Although the arterial pulse may have a rapid rise, the systolic pressure is normal. The diastolic pressure is not reduced to the extent seen with chronic aortic regurgitation. Therefore, the pulse pressure may be normal or only mildly increased, and the associated peripheral arterial signs of chronic aortic regurgitation are usually absent. The diastolic murmur may be less prominent and shorter. A third heart sound gallop can be heard. Echocardiographic and Doppler studies can be especially valuable in assessing the aortic regurgitation, its cause, and the underlying left ventricular function. With severe regurgitation, there may be premature diastolic closure of the mitral valve because of the elevated left ventricular pressure.

The medical treatment of heart failure due to acute aortic regurgitation includes vasodilator therapy. If the heart failure is severe, this may involve intravenous nitroprusside. Surgical therapy, often urgent, is the definitive treatment for significant heart failure due to acute aortic regurgitation.

MITRAL STENOSIS

Although mitral stenosis can be congenital in origin, virtually all cases are the result of rheumatic valve disease. Two thirds of mitral stenosis patients are women. There is progressive thickening of the valve leaflets and fusion of the commissures. Calcification contributes to the valve immobility and stenosis. The chordae tendineae also may thicken and fuse and shorten. The valve scarring progresses slowly and takes at least several years before the valve dysfunction becomes hemodynamically significant. Deformation of the valve and its supporting structures can also cause associated mitral regurgitation. Mitral stenosis leads to elevated left atrial pressure, which rises further during exertion. The left atrium is enlarged. In the absence of a coexistent regurgitant lesion, the left ventricle is normal in size. The elevated left atrial pressure leads to pulmonary venous congestion that causes the major symptoms in mitral stenosis: exertional dyspnea, orthopnea, and paroxysmal nocturnal dyspnea. Later in the course, cardiac output is reduced, leading to fatigue and weakness. Elevated left atrial and pulmonary venous pressures can contribute to variable degrees of pulmonary arterial hypertension. A reactive increase in pulmonary vascular resistance can also contribute to pulmonary arterial hypertension, and in some patients with severe longstanding mitral stenosis, obliterative changes in the pulmonary vascular bed can occur. Pulmonary congestion and pulmonary arterial hypertension can provoke right ventricular failure and functional tricuspid regurgitation.

Diastolic filling of the ventricle is determined not only by the pressure gradient across the stenotic valve, but also by the duration of diastole. As heart rate increases, diastole shortens more than systole. Thus, situations that increase heart rate, for example, exertional or emotional stress, may not be tolerated by mitral stenosis patients. This is most dramatic with the onset of atrial fibrillation, a common complication of mitral stenosis. (With atrial fibrillation there is also loss of effective atrial contraction.) A patient's first episode of pulmonary edema often occurs with uncommon physical exertion or with the onset of atrial fibrillation.

Symptoms from mitral stenosis usually do not develop for a decade or more after acute rheumatic fever. In the United States, symptom onset is most common in the third or fourth decade of life. In addition to the cardinal symptoms of dyspnea and orthopnea, some patients experience hemoptysis. Mitral stenosis can also be complicated by embolism of thrombus from the enlarged left atrium and cause stroke, particularly when atrial fibrillation is also present.

Characteristic findings of mitral stenosis (see Table 6–2) include a loud first heart sound because the valve is at its maximal (albeit reduced) opening until rapidly closed by the onset of ventricular systole. The high-pitched opening snap of the mitral valve follows the second heart sound. As the severity of mitral stenosis increases, the interval between the second sound and opening snap decreases (the higher the left atrial pressure, the earlier it will meet the falling left ventricular pressure curve). If the valve is heavily calcified and immobile, the first sound may not be loud and the opening snap may not be audible. The low-pitched rumbling murmur of mitral stenosis is heard best at the cardiac apex with the patient in the left lateral decubitus position. The murmur is loudest in early diastole (during the rapid ventricular filling phase). If sinus rhythm is present, the murmur intensity increases again with atrial contraction (presystolic accentuation). The murmur can be difficult to hear in some cases; it may be accentuated by exercise. If pulmonary artery pressures are elevated, a palpable impulse may be detected at the left sternal border and the second heart sound is prominent upon auscultation.

Echocardiography can detect mitral valve thickening and stenosis and provides information about valve mobility and degree of calcification. Doppler echocardiography permits indirect estimation of mitral valve area using the rate of pressure fall (pressure half-time). The severity of mitral stenosis and associated hemodynamic changes can be determined at cardiac catheterization, along with calculation of valve area using the Gorlin formula. The normal valve area is 4 to 6 cm². Severe mitral stenosis represents a valve area of less than 1 cm².

Patients with class I to II symptoms and mild-to-moderate mitral stenosis can usually be managed medically. This includes control of heart rate; some patients benefit from beta-adrenergic blocking drugs. Control of ventricular rate is especially important with atrial fibrillation, and more than one drug may be required (digitalis, beta blocker, or calcium channel blocker). Anticoagulation is also indicated in cases such as this to reduce the risk of thromboembolism. Patients with limiting symptoms and severe mitral stenosis should be referred for consideration of percutaneous mitral valve balloon valvuloplasty, surgical commissurotomy, or mitral valve replacement. Balloon valvuloplasty is usually limited to patients with pliable noncalcified valves and no evidence of left atrial thrombus or significant mitral regurgitation. In appropriate patients, mitral valve commissurotomy is associated with low operative mortality risk and good hemodynamic result and may spare the patient a prosthetic value for many years. If commissurotomy is not feasible (e.g., due to heavy valve calcification or significant mitral regurgitation), the valve can be replaced with a prosthesis.

MITRAL REGURGITATION

Mitral regurgitation can result from a number of causes (see Table 6–1), including myxomatous degeneration of the mitral valve, mitral valve prolapse (see below), and rheumatic heart disease. It can occur in patients with left ventricular dilation because of annular stretching or papillary muscle dysfunction and in patients with hypertrophic cardiomyopathy. Patients with coronary heart disease can develop mitral regurgitation due to papillary muscle ischemia or infarction. Calcification of the mitral annulus can cause mitral regurgitation. Congenital forms also occur, such as in association with ostium primum atrial septal defect. Acute mitral regurgitation can result from rupture of chordae tendineae or papillary muscle and from infective endocarditis.

Chronic mitral regurgitation produces a volume overload. Unlike aortic regurgitation, however, the left ventricular afterload is reduced as blood flows during systole into the low-pressure left atrium, which dilates to variable degrees to accommodate the volume. Left ventricular pressure and volume do not increase to the degree seen with chronic aortic regurgitation. In some patients with chronic mitral regurgitation, the left atrium is markedly enlarged, and pressures in the atrium and pulmonary vascular bed are near normal. Commonly, however, the left atrium is moderately enlarged and there is elevation of left atrial pressure, which can lead to pulmonary congestion and dyspnea. Chronic mitral regurgitation can also provoke variable degrees of pulmonary arterial hypertension. Ultimately, chronic mitral regurgitation of sufficient severity results in myocardial contractile dysfunction.

The characteristic murmur of chronic mitral regurgitation is holosystolic, beginning immediately after a soft first heart sound (see Table 6–2). It is high pitched and heard best at the apex with radiation to the axilla. Mitral regurgitation can also result in a murmur confined to late systole, for example, from papillary muscle dysfunction. Mitral regurgitation associated with late-systolic murmurs is usually only mild to moderate in severity. Echocardiography can assess mitral valve structure, cardiac chamber sizes, and left ventricular function. Doppler echocardiography and color flow studies provide some information about the severity of mitral regurgitation. At cardiac catheterization, mitral regurgitation severity is estimated by the amount of contrast regurgitated into the left atrium after injection of the contrast into the left ventricle. This qualitative assessment can be difficult at times. It is important to recognize that echocardiographic or ejection fraction determinations can overestimate the systolic function of the left ventricle because the ventricle is unloaded by the mitral regurgitation.

The medical treatment of significant chronic mitral regurgitation includes afterload reduction with vasodilating drugs, such as angiotensin-converting enzyme inhibitors. Patients with limiting symptoms despite medical therapy are referred for consideration of surgery. However, the development of symptoms in patients with chronic mitral regurgitation is often associated with left ventricular dysfunction. Surgical results are much less satisfactory when left ventricular systolic function is impaired. Thus, left ventricular function should be monitored periodically (by ejection fraction or echocardiographic techniques) so that surgical therapy can also be considered in patients with early evidence of left ventricular function change even if they are only mildly symptomatic. In some cases, the mitral valve can be repaired at surgery. If the valve disease is severe or the annulus very dilated or if there is extensive calcification, then mitral valve replacement is required. Acute severe mitral regurgitation results in marked increase in left atrial pressure and pulmonary vascular congestion and usually is not well tolerated. Emergency surgery is often required. Echocardiography may reveal the underlying cause (e.g., flail mitral leaflet from chordal rupture or signs of endocarditis). Afterload reduction with intravenous nitroprusside may aid in stabilization until surgery can be performed.

MITRAL VALVE PROLAPSE

Mitral valve prolapse (MVP) is common and can cause mitral regurgitation ranging from trivial to severe. It can be an isolated finding or occur in association with other disorders, including heritable connective tissue disorders such as Marfan's syndrome. It is more common in women. Many patients with MVP exhibit some features, such as sternal abnormalities or tall thin stature, that are similar to features of patients with the heritable connective tissue states. MVP may be inherited as an autosomal dominant phenotype. For most patients, MVP is benign, but significant valve regurgitation and a variety of complications occur in a minority of patients. In some cases, there can be associated prolapse of the tricuspid valve.

In patients with significant mitral regurgitation, the mitral valve usually is large, "floppy," and redundant and the chordae are elongated. Histologic changes include loose myxomatous connective tissue, along with collagen dissolution.

Most patients with MVP are asymptomatic, but a variety of symptoms have been associated with MVP in some patients, including atypical chest pain, palpitations, fatigue, anxiety, postural phenomena, and neuropsychiatric symptoms. It has been proposed that an associated neuroendocrine or autonomic dysfunction state occurs in some patients (MVP syndrome) and may contribute to the symptoms. If the mitral regurgitation is significant, car-

diac symptoms as described previously with mitral regurgitation can be present.

The characteristic cardiac findings of MVP include a mid-systolic click and late systolic regurgitant murmur (see Table 6–2). An important feature of MVP is the dynamic nature of its symptoms. At times, repeated examinations are required to detect the physical findings. Maneuvers that reduce ventricular size, such as prompt standing or Valsalva maneuver, cause the floppy valve to prolapse into the left atrium earlier and to a greater extent during ventricular systole. Thus, the click moves toward the first heart sound and the murmur is longer. Echocardiography is used to confirm the diagnosis of MVP.

In most patients with MVP, the mitral valve structural changes are not advanced, the associated mitral regurgitation is mild, and there are no complications. Reassuring the patient is an important part of treatment. However, mitral regurgitation is progressive in some patients and can become severe. Middle-aged or older men may be more likely to develop severe regurgitation or complications. Rupture of chordae tendineae can lead to acute worsening. Other complications of MVP include infective endocarditis, cardiac arrhythmias, and thromboembolism. Sudden death in the absence of hemodynamically significant mitral regurgitation does occur but is rare. Antibiotic endocarditis prophylaxis is indicated in all MVP patients with structural valve changes and/or murmur of regurgitation. Beta-adrenergic blocking drugs can be effective for some symptomatic patients. The treatment of symptomatic or sustained arrhythmias is described in Chapter 8. If significant valve regurgitation is present, the treatment approach is as described in the previous section.

TRICUSPID STENOSIS (see Table 6–2)

Tricuspid stenosis is usually rheumatic in etiology and does not occur as an isolated lesion. Like mitral stenosis, it is gradually progressive, is more common in women, and usually becomes symptomatic in mid-adulthood. Tricuspid stenosis can occasionally be caused or simulated by carcinoid syndrome, endomyocardial fibroelastosis, congenital valvular malformations, or right atrial myxoma.

Because it is such a low-pressure system, relatively small gradients across the tricuspid valve (5 mm) may indicate significant tricuspid stenosis. Echocardiographic diagnosis is probably more accurate than catheterization because of the small gradient involved.

TRICUSPID REGURGITATION
(see Tables 6–1 and 6–2)

Tricuspid regurgitation is most commonly functional, due to dilation of the tricuspid annulus related to right ventricular dilation. Other causes include rheumatic disease, tricuspid valve prolapse, Ebstein's anomaly, carcinoid syndrome, intracardiac tumors, penetrating or nonpenetrating cardiac trauma, and infective endocarditis. Normal tricuspid valves may be affected by endocarditis, particularly in drug addicts.

Functional tricuspid regurgitation may regress after associated lesions are corrected and pulmonary hypertension resolves. At times, plication of the tricuspid annulus is required to improve functional tricuspid regurgitation. If annuloplasty is unsuccessful or if significant tricuspid stenosis is present, tricuspid valve replacement can be performed.

PULMONIC STENOSIS AND REGURGITATION

Pulmonic stenosis is usually congenital and is discussed in Chapter 5. It can occasionally occur in an acquired form with hypertrophic cardiomyopathy (caused by bulging of the septum into the right ventricular outflow tract) or secondary to pericardial tumor involvement in the area.

Acquired pulmonary regurgitation is usually associated with pulmonary hypertension caused by left heart valvular disease (Graham Steell murmur) or pulmonary disease. The murmur sounds similar to that of aortic insufficiency and is heard best at the second left intercostal space. This murmur is high pitched, early diastolic, and decrescendo in character. In distinction, isolated congenital pulmonic regurgitation results in a lower-pitched murmur that occurs later in diastole, is heard best at the third to fourth left intercostal space, and resembles more the murmur of tricuspid stenosis.

MULTIVALVULAR DISEASE

Combined valvular lesions are common, especially in rheumatic heart disease. In addition to organic lesions, development of mitral and tricuspid regurgitation or pulmonic regurgitation may occur secondary to the hemodynamic disturbance of other valvular lesions. In general, the manifestations of the more proximal valve lesions are the more prominent. For example, in patients with mitral and aortic valvular lesions of similar severity, mitral valve manifestations may predominate and the degree of aortic stenosis may be underestimated. Failure to correct all significant valvular lesions at the time of surgery may lead to an inadequate clinical result and illustrates the importance of excluding concomitant lesions at the time of catheterization. The surgical risk for double valve replacement is greater than that for single valve replacement.

RHEUMATIC FEVER

Rheumatic fever usually occurs in children 5 to 15 years of age. It is caused by group A beta-hemolytic streptococcal pharyngitis that occurs 1 to 3 weeks prior to the clinical manifestations of rheumatic fever. It is believed that an immune response to the *Streptococcus* is responsible for the disease. Males and females are equally affected. It is more common in patients of lower socioeco-

nomic level. The incidence of rheumatic fever in the United States has declined in recent years.

Aschoff's nodules in the myocardium are the characteristic pathologic feature of rheumatic fever. The most serious manifestation of rheumatic fever is a pancarditis that may involve the endocardium, myocardium, and pericardium. Usually the mitral valve is involved; less frequently, the aortic, and even less frequently, the tricuspid valves are involved. Pulmonic valve involvement is extremely rare. Valvulitis is recognized by a new insufficiency murmur. Aortic and mitral stenosis murmurs are not heard acutely. Myocarditis may manifest with heart failure. Pericarditis may produce a friction rub, and the PR interval on the ECG may be prolonged. Because of the difficulty in diagnosing rheumatic fever, guidelines (modified Jones criteria) for establishing the diagnosis were developed. Major manifestations include carditis, polyarthritis, chorea, erythema marginatum, and subcutaneous nodules. Minor manifestations include fever, arthralgia, previous rheumatic fever or rheumatic heart disease, elevated acute phase reactants, and a prolonged PR interval. There should also be laboratory evidence of a preceding streptococcal infection (positive throat culture or increased antistreptolysin-O [ASO] titer).

Penicillin should be administered to eradicate streptococcal infection. Salicylates are effective for treating fever and arthritis but probably have no effect on carditis. The usefulness of steroids is unproven. Congestive heart failure is treated traditionally.

The relatively high recurrence rate of rheumatic fever after streptococcal infection continues for at least 5 to 10 years after the initial infection; therefore, rheumatic fever prophylaxis should be discontinued only in adults 5 to 10 years after the acute episode and then only if the risk of the streptococcal infection is low. Adults working with school-age children, those in the military service, those exposed to large numbers of people, and those in the medical or allied health professions should receive prophylaxis indefinitely. Patients with a significant degree of rheumatic heart disease or a history of repeated occurrences should have prophylaxis indefinitely. The recommended regimen for prophylaxis is 1.2 million units of benzathine penicillin monthly. Oral penicillin, erythromycin, or sulfadiazine can be used, but because of noncompliance, these agents are somewhat less effective than the parenteral regimen.

PROSTHETIC VALVES (Fig. 6–3)

The two basic types of available prosthetic valves are mechanical (e.g., tilting disk or bileaflet) and bioprosthetic (also called tissue valves). The mechanical valves are more likely to result in long-lasting function but require careful anticoagulation because of thromboembolic risk. Bioprostheses are less likely to be complicated by thromboembolic disease, but the functional lifetime of the valve can be much less, particularly when placed in young individuals. The selection of a specific prosthesis is beyond the scope of this text, but considerations may include the patient's age, expected lifetime, the risk of

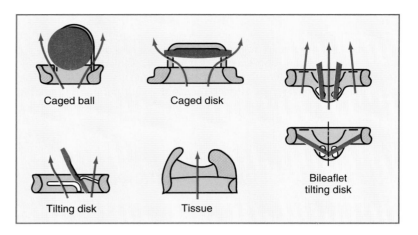

Figure 6-3

Designs and flow patterns of major categories of prosthetic heart valves: caged-ball, caged-disk, tilting-disk, bi-leaflet tilting-disk, and bioprosthetic (tissue) valves. While flow in mechanical valves must course along both sides of the occluder, bioprostheses have a central flow pattern. (Reprinted with permission from Annals of Biomedical Engineering, Vol 10, FJ Schoen et al, Bioengineering aspects of heart valve replacement, copyright 1982, Pergamon Press, Ltd.; and from Schoen FJ: Pathology of cardiac valve replacement. *In* Morse D, Steiner RM, Fernandez J [eds.]: Guide to Prosthetic Cardiac Valves, p 209. New York, Springer-Verlag, 1985. Copyright Springer-Verlag, Inc., 1985.)

chronic anticoagulation therapy, and the presence of other factors mandating chronic anticoagulation independent of the prosthetic valve type.

All prosthetic heart valves are somewhat stenotic. Prosthetic dysfunction (secondary to thrombosis or calcification) can lead to increased obstruction or the development of regurgitation. Regurgitation can also result from a perivalvular leak, that is, in the area of the sewing ring of the valve. Turbulence associated with valve dysfunction can cause hemolysis. Even normally functioning prosthetic valves can cause hemolysis in some patients. Endocarditis is another potential complication in patients with prosthetic heart valves. Antibiotic prophylaxis should be administered prior to dental, gastrointestinal, and genitourinary surgery and other procedures associated with bacteremia.

Echocardiographic and Doppler studies can aid in the evaluation of prosthetic valve function. Additional information can be obtained from transesophageal echocardiography, particularly if prosthetic valve endocarditis is suspected. The excursion of mechanical valve disks can be examined by fluoroscopy.

REFERENCES

Bonow RO, Lakatos E, Maron BJ, Epstein SE: Serial long-term assessment of the natural history of asymptomatic patients with chronic aortic regurgitation and normal left ventricular systolic function. Circulation 1991; 84:1625–1635.

Boudoulas H, Kolibash AJ, Baker PB, et al.: Mitral valve prolapse and the mitral valve prolapse syndrome. Am Heart J 1989; 118:796–818.

Boudoulas H, Vavuranakis M, Wooley CF: Valvular heart disease: The influence of changing etiology on nosology. J Heart Valve Dis 1994; 3:516–526.

Reyes VP, Raju BS, Wynne J, et al.: Percutaneous balloon valvuloplasty compared with open surgical commissurotomy for mitral stenosis. N Engl J Med 1994; 331:961–967.

7

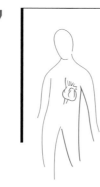

Coronary Heart Disease

Coronary heart disease is a major cause of morbidity and the leading cause of death in the United States and in most industrialized countries. The clinical manifestations of coronary heart disease can include sudden cardiac death, stable and unstable angina pectoris, acute myocardial infarction, and congestive heart failure. It is noteworthy that there has been a progressive decline in morbidity and mortality from coronary heart disease since the late 1960s. A number of factors probably contribute to this change, including population efforts related to risk factor reduction, such as detection and treatment of hypertension, as well as medical and surgical treatments of the clinical manifestations of coronary heart disease.

ATHEROSCLEROSIS

Coronary heart disease is most often the result of atherosclerosis in the epicardial coronary vessels. Atherosclerosis is a complex disorder, and many factors play roles in its pathogenesis. Preventable risk factors (Table 7–1), genetic susceptibility, local arterial and hemodynamic factors, and sex influence the development of atherosclerosis. Initially, there is an influx of low-density lipoproteins (LDL) and blood monocytes into the subintimal area of the vessel wall, presumably at a site of injury to the vascular endothelium. Some of the LDL is oxidized and ingested by macrophages, contributing to the formation of foam cells. Subsequently, a central core of necrotic extracellular lipid develops, covered by a fibrous cap. The process involves smooth muscle migration and proliferation and collagen synthesis. A variety of endothelial-, blood cell–, and platelet-related factors contribute to the inflammatory and healing processes. Calcification occurs as the lesion progresses. The resultant atherosclerotic plaque narrows the arterial lumen. Although the effect of a plaque on blood flow is also influenced by length and geometry of the lesion, a reduction of lumen diameter by 70% is generally required to significantly limit blood flow (Fig. 7–1).

Atherosclerotic plaques are also subject to disruption (or fissuring) of the fibrous cap, exposing circulating blood to thrombogenic plaque lipid and vessel wall collagen. Hemorrhage may occur into the plaque and/or vessel wall. The resultant platelet activation and thrombus formation further compromise blood flow. Plaque disruption with platelet and fibrin and subsequent thrombus formation is the major mechanism underlying the acute coronary syndromes, that is, unstable angina pectoris and acute myocardial infarction.

RISK FACTORS

Epidemiologic studies have demonstrated that many factors contribute to the development and progression of atherosclerosis. Advancing age, sex, and genetic predisposition are unalterable. Although male sex is an important risk factor, coronary heart disease is also a major problem for women and is the leading cause of death in women older than 50 years. On average, women manifest symptoms about 10 years later than men. Coronary heart disease risk increases with the use of oral contraceptives and with menopause but is decreased with postmenopausal hormone replacement.

Systemic arterial hypertension (e.g., persistent diastolic blood pressure ≥ 90 mm Hg and systolic blood pressure ≥ 140 mm Hg) is a major risk factor for cardiovascular disease. The higher the diastolic or systolic pressure, the greater the risk. Effective treatment of even mild hypertension (diastolic pressure 90 to 104 mm Hg) reduces risk. The treatment of patients with hypertension includes nonpharmacologic or lifestyle modification measures, such as weight control, sodium restriction, and exercise.

Serum cholesterol levels are related to the risk of developing coronary heart disease, and the relationship is continuous over a wide range of cholesterol values. The relationship between elevated serum total cholesterol and coronary heart disease is primarily due to high levels of LDL cholesterol. By contrast, there is an inverse correlation of high-density lipoprotein (HDL) cholesterol with coronary heart disease. Guidelines have been developed for the population at large and for higher-risk patients with established coronary heart disease or multiple risk factors (see Chapter 61). Recent large intervention trials have established the effectiveness of cholesterol reduction by dietary and drug management. Elevated triglyceride levels are often associated with excessive caloric intake, obesity, and diabetes. An independent association between serum triglyceride levels and coronary heart disease has been more controversial, but high levels probably do confer some risk, especially in women.

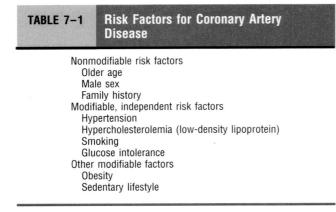

TABLE 7-1	Risk Factors for Coronary Artery Disease

Nonmodifiable risk factors
 Older age
 Male sex
 Family history
Modifiable, independent risk factors
 Hypertension
 Hypercholesterolemia (low-density lipoprotein)
 Smoking
 Glucose intolerance
Other modifiable factors
 Obesity
 Sedentary lifestyle

NONATHEROSCLEROTIC CAUSES OF CORONARY ARTERY OBSTRUCTION

Although uncommon, several nonatherosclerotic causes of coronary artery obstruction exist. Emboli to coronary arteries can occur in endocarditis, from mural thrombi in the left atrium or ventricle, from prosthetic valves, or from cardiac myxomas or can be associated with cardiopulmonary bypass or coronary arteriography. Trauma to coronary arteries can result from penetrating and non-penetrating injuries and can also complicate cardiac catheterization. Various forms of arteritis (syphilis, polyarteritis nodosa, Takayasu's disease, disseminated lupus erythematosus, and rheumatoid arthritis) can affect the coronary arteries. The mucocutaneous lymph node syndrome (Kawasaki's disease) can be accompanied by vasculitis in several organ systems; the most significant feature is a vasculitis involving intima, media, and adventitia of the coronary arteries that results in aneurysm and, sometimes, thrombus formation. Radiation therapy can result in coronary disease.

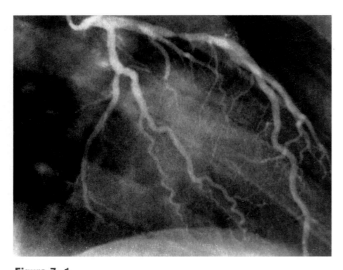

Figure 7-1
Angiogram of the left coronary system. There is an obstructive lesion in the left anterior descending artery.

Dissection of the proximal aorta can interrupt coronary flow. Rarely, *in situ* coronary thrombosis may occur in hematologic disorders such as polycythemia vera, thrombocytosis, and disseminated intravascular coagulation. Cocaine use can lead to coronary artery spasm and/or thrombosis and may accelerate atherosclerosis. Spasm of a coronary artery (Prinzmetal's angina, discussed further on) is another cause of coronary obstruction. The spasm may occur in association with atherosclerosis, or, rarely, in the absence of demonstrable underlying coronary disease.

NONOBSTRUCTIVE CAUSES OF ISCHEMIC HEART DISEASE

Conditions associated with increased left ventricular pressure and wall tension, a decrease in diastolic perfusion pressure, and/or an increase in left ventricular mass (e.g., aortic stenosis) may cause myocardial ischemia by altering the balance of oxygen supply and demand. In addition, conditions in which substrate delivery is decreased (e.g., hypotension, anemia, and carbon monoxide poisoning) may cause myocardial ischemia, especially if pre-existing coronary lesions are present.

A syndrome of myocardial infarction with angiographically normal coronary arteries exists. Approximately 2% of patients with myocardial infarction demonstrate no obstructive lesions on coronary arteriography. These patients tend to be young, have a low incidence of coronary risk factors, and often have no history of angina pectoris prior to infarction. The prognosis for survival after the acute event is usually good. The cause is unknown, but possible etiologies include coronary emboli, coronary artery spasm, coronary artery disease in smaller vessels beyond the resolution of coronary arteriography, and coronary arterial thrombosis with recanalization.

PATHOPHYSIOLOGY OF ISCHEMIC HEART DISEASE

The manifestations of coronary heart disease occur when myocardial oxygen demand exceeds oxygen supply. Under normal conditions, increased demand is met by increased coronary blood flow. The regulation occurs at the arteriole level (resistance vessels). The arterioles dilate in response to increased demand. In the presence of a significant obstruction in a more proximal epicardial coronary vessel, the distal arterioles in its distribution may be maximally or near-maximally dilated to meet basal demand. The coronary reserve is reduced, and flow may not increase sufficiently under conditions of increased demand. Myocardial ischemia results. In addition to fixed obstruction, transient localized increases in epicardial coronary tone can contribute to limitation of blood flow. In its most dramatic form, spasm can result and be the dominant cause of reduced blood flow (Prinzmetal's angina). Coronary tone is mediated, in part, by vasoactive substances synthesized by vascular endothelium. The synthe-

TABLE 7-2	Angina Pectoris			
Type	**Pattern**	**ECG**	**Usual Coronary Abnormality**	**Medical Therapy**
Stable	Chronic unchanged pattern of precipitation and relief Induced by physical activity or emotional stress; lasts 5–10 min, relieved by rest or sublingual nitroglycerin	Baseline often normal or nonspecific ST-T changes, or signs of prior myocardial infarction ST depression or T wave inversion during angina	≥70% stenosis due to atherosclerotic plaque in one or more coronary arteries	Aspirin Sublingual nitroglycerin Anti-ischemic medications*
Unstable	Recent increase in angina frequency or severity, especially with rest pain; new-onset angina if at low activity level May last longer and be less responsive to sublingual nitroglycerin	As with stable angina, though changes during discomfort may be more pronounced Occasionally, ST elevation during discomfort	Fissured plaque with platelet and fibrin-thrombus contribute to stenosis	Aspirin, heparin (e.g., PTT 1.5–2 × normal) Anti-ischemic medications
Prinzmetal's or variant angina	Typically unpredictable rest pain, often in early morning hours	Transient ST segment elevation during pain (ST depression and/or T wave inversion can also occur)	Coronary artery spasm at a region of fixed but often nonstenotic lesion; can also occur in angiographically normal vessel	Calcium channel blockers Nitrates Aspirin

*Long-acting nitrates, beta-adrenergic blocking drugs, calcium channel–blocking drugs—see text.
PTT = Activated partial thromboplastin time.

sis of these substances and the vessels' response to them may be altered by atherosclerosis. Vasoactive substances (e.g., thromboxane) released from platelets at the site of an atherosclerotic lesion can also contribute to a localized increase in coronary tone.

As noted previously, myocardial oxygen demand can occasionally exceed oxygen supply in the absence of coronary artery obstruction. An example is severe aortic stenosis, in which the hypertrophied muscle and increased wall tension increase oxygen demand, while the increased intramural pressure may limit distal blood flow.

Cardiac ischemia can alter myocardial contraction and relaxation, leading to systolic and diastolic dysfunction. The dysfunction can be transient, as in stress-induced angina, or permanent, as in myocardial infarction. Severe but reversible ischemia may lead to myocardial stunning, in which systolic and diastolic dysfunction persist for hours to days following the episode. Chronic ischemia can also be associated with hibernating myocardium, in which reduced flow is sufficient to maintain cell viability but not adequate for normal contractile function.

Severe prolonged ischemia can result in myocardial injury, with release of enzymes and other markers of acute myocardial infarction. Following interruption of coronary flow, irreversible myocardial injury in its distribution generally begins within 20 to 30 minutes. The amount of injury is related to the degree of obstruction, its duration, and also to the presence or absence of collateral blood vessels. The latter small vessels coursing from a nonobstructed coronary artery to the distal portion of an obstructed coronary artery provide some perfusion and hence protection to the ischemic area. In some acute myocardial infarction patients, changes in ventricular size

and geometry continue to develop after the acute event. Both infarct expansion and ventricular dilation may occur. This ventricular remodeling can be associated with increased complication and mortality risk.

Cardiac ischemia can also alter electrical function of the heart because of changes in ion transport, neural influences, and myocardial scarring. A variety of arrhythmias and conduction disturbances can result.

ANGINA PECTORIS (Table 7–2)

Angina pectoris is the visceral chest discomfort that results from transient myocardial ischemia. It is often described as a substernal discomfort (many patients insist it is not a pain) perceived as a pressure or tightness or a fullness sensation. It may radiate to the neck, jaw, shoulder, or arm—often the left arm. Some patients report dyspnea rather than discomfort, a situation termed angina-equivalent dyspnea. Because angina is usually the result of atherosclerotic coronary artery obstruction, it is typically elicited by physical exertion or emotional stress that transiently increases myocardial oxygen demand beyond that which can be delivered. Most patients can describe situations likely to evoke discomfort. Common precipitating factors include hurrying and climbing stairs. Many patients find activities in the morning or cold air or after meals more likely to elicit angina. Typical angina comes on over a few seconds or minutes, lasts 5 to 15 minutes, and resolves with rest or sublingual nitroglycerin.

Angina is termed stable in the setting of a chronic course of predictable transient stress-induced discomfort. Angina that has significantly progressed in frequency, severity, or duration, particularly if accompanied by un-provoked rest pain, is deemed unstable angina. New-onset angina, if occurring with low levels of exertion, is also considered unstable angina. Unstable angina with rest pain warrants hospitalization and intensive medical therapy.

In the appropriate clinical setting, the history permits the presumptive diagnosis of angina pectoris. Unfortunately, angina is atypical in one or more of its features in some patients, rendering the diagnosis more difficult. In addition, other disorders (see Table 2–2) at times lead to symptoms that can be confused with angina pectoris. Pain that is focal, inframammary, stabbing, and fleeting is not likely to be angina. Although assessment of cardiac risk factors is important in the evaluation, their presence alone does not prove that a patient's discomfort is angina, nor does their absence exclude it.

Physical examination between episodes of discomfort may reveal normal findings. During angina, the heart rate and blood pressure are often somewhat increased. An S_4 is often present, attesting to reduced ventricular compliance with ischemia. If a substantial amount of myocardium is ischemic during the episode, signs of transient left ventricular dysfunction (S_3, pulmonary congestion) may develop, as well as the murmur of mitral regurgitation from papillary muscle ischemia. Between episodes of discomfort, the electrocardiogram (ECG) may be normal, demonstrate nonspecific ST-T wave changes, or show signs of prior infarction. The characteristic (though not invariably present) ECG changes during angina include ST segment depression and/or T wave inversion (Fig. 7–2). With more profound ischemia, transient ST segment elevation may occur.

For patients with suspected stable angina pectoris, stress testing can provide objective signs of ischemia (stress testing should not be performed in the patient with unstable angina until symptoms have been stabilized). For many patients with stable angina, the major benefit of stress testing is assessment of functional capacity and the detection of signs indicating more extensive coronary disease or high-risk state (Fig. 7–3). For many patients with angina with normal resting ECG, treadmill exercise ECG is employed (see Chapter 3). The addition of an imaging technique (thallium perfusion scintigraphy or echocardiography) increases the sensitivity and specificity of stress testing but also the cost. These studies are most valuable in patients whose ECG may not provide reliable signs of ischemia, such as those with resting or hyperventilation-induced ECG abnormalities. Many physicians also choose imaging studies for patients with atypical symptoms and for women (in whom false-positive ECG changes may be more common). If stress testing is necessary for a patient who cannot exercise, pharmacologic stress tests, such as dipyridamole thallium or dobutamine echocardiography, are available.

The prognosis of patients with chronic stable angina is influenced by a number of factors, including the patient's functional capacity, the level of exertion necessary to elicit ischemia, and the extent of ischemia as reflected by the magnitude of associated ECG, thallium, or echo-

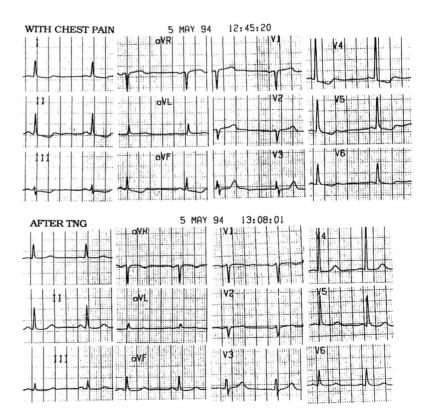

Figure 7–2
Electrocardiogram (ECG) obtained during angina pectoris *(top tracing)* and following administration of sublingual nitroglycerin and relief of discomfort *(bottom tracing)*. During angina in this patient, there is transient ST segment depression and T wave changes.

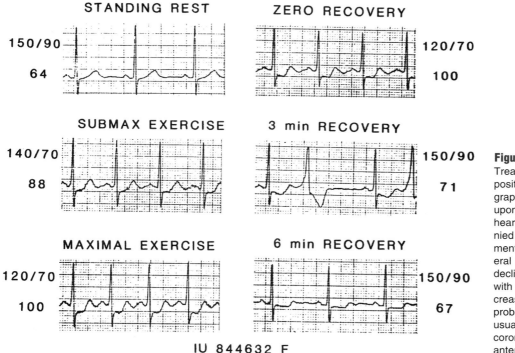

STANDING REST

150/90
64

ZERO RECOVERY

120/70
100

SUBMAX EXERCISE

140/70
88

3 min RECOVERY

150/90
71

MAXIMAL EXERCISE

120/70
100

6 min RECOVERY

150/90
67

IU 844632 F

Figure 7–3
Treadmill exercise test. Strongly positive exercise electrocardiographic test. The test was stopped upon reproduction of angina at low heart rate and workload, accompanied by marked (>2 mm) ST segment depression that persisted several minutes into recovery. The decline in systolic blood pressure with exercise also denotes increased risk. Negative u waves are probably present also with exercise, usually indicating that the obstructive coronary disease involves the left anterior descending artery.

cardiographic changes. One of the most important determinants is functional status of the left ventricle. Left ventricular function can be assessed noninvasively by echocardiography or radionuclide estimation of ejection fraction. The concomitant presence of peripheral vascular disease also is associated with more pronounced coronary heart disease. For patients who undergo coronary cineangiography, the extent and severity of obstructive coronary disease is related to prognosis.

Coronary angiography (see Chapter 3) provides the most definitive assessment of the extent and severity of coronary artery disease. But even this test has some limitations, and interpretation of results is usually best when correlated with functional studies (e.g., stress testing). Coronary angiography also carries risk (albeit small) and is expensive. It is indicated for patients with unacceptable symptoms despite medical therapy to assess the potential for revascularization (Table 7–3). Patients whose stress tests indicate high risk or extensive coronary disease also

generally undergo coronary angiography. Angina patients with reduced functional capacity or left ventricular dysfunction undergo the procedure as well. Many physicians recommend coronary angiography for patients with unstable angina, whereas others reserve the test for patients whose symptoms do not stabilize or who have inducible ischemia on stress testing performed after stabilization. Occasionally, coronary angiography is performed for diagnosis if the clinical picture and/or stress test results are inconclusive.

MEDICAL MANAGEMENT OF ANGINA

Management of the patient with angina includes instruction about activity guidelines, proper use of medications, and warning signs that should prompt medical attention. The latter includes discomfort not responsive to two or three sublingual nitroglycerin pills, each given 5 minutes apart. Situations likely to evoke angina should be avoided, along with exertion after meals and in cold weather. Regular activity that is tolerated, such as a walking program, is encouraged to maintain conditioning. Control of risk factors, including high blood pressure and smoking, are important, as is relief of aggravating factors such as anemia and congestive heart failure. Aspirin (160 to 325 mg/day) is recommended for its antiplatelet effects. Sublingual nitroglycerin should be used when angina occurs; it also is effective prophylactically when an activity likely to evoke angina must be undertaken.

The available anti-ischemic medications to prevent episodes of angina include long-acting nitrates, beta-adre-

TABLE 7–3	Indications for Coronary Angiography in Patients with Stable Angina Pectoris

1. Unacceptable angina despite medical therapy (for consideration of revascularization)
2. Stress testing results suggesting high-risk or extensive coronary disease
3. Angina in setting of left ventricular dysfunction or reduced functional capacity
4. Certain patients for diagnosis (e.g., equivocal stress testing results)

TABLE 7-4	Nitrate Preparations for Angina			
Preparation	**Indication**	**Onset (min)**	**Duration**	**Usual Dose**
Sublingual nitroglycerin	Acute anginal episode; prophylaxis before necessary activity likely to evoke angina	2–5	10–30 min	0.4 mg (can be repeated at 5-min intervals if BP acceptable)
Isosorbide dinitrate	Angina prophylaxis	15–30	3–6 hr	Initial dose often 10 mg tid, increased as necessary to 40 mg tid
Isosorbide mononitrate	Angina prophylaxis	30–60	6–8 hr	Two 20-mg doses given 7 hr apart
Nitroglycerin 2% ointment	Angina prophylaxis	20–60	4–6 hr	0.5–2 in applied q6h
Transdermal nitroglycerin	Angina prophylaxis	30–60	>12 hr	5- to 15-mg patch; removed overnight to retard tolerance
Intravenous nitroglycerin infusion	Unstable angina			Initial dose 5–15 μg/min titrated upward as necessary and as tolerated by BP

BP = blood pressure.

nergic blocking drugs, and calcium channel–blocking drugs. There is no single optimal regimen for every patient. Rather, the regimen is determined by the frequency of angina, patient characteristics such as heart rate, blood pressure, and ventricular function, and concomitant disorders that may increase the likelihood of intolerance or side effect of a given drug.

The smooth muscle relaxant effect of nitrates (Table 7–4) promotes dilation of systemic veins and, to a lesser extent, the arterial system. A decrease in venous return to the heart reduces preload and subsequently decreases ventricular wall tension and afterload (and blood pressure). These are important determinants of myocardial oxygen demand. Nitrates can also dilate the larger conductance coronary arteries and may thus increase myocardial blood supply. The most common side effect is headache. The use of long-acting nitrates can lead to the development of tolerance. This can be minimized by prescribing the medicine such that there is a nitrate-free interval (oral isosor-

bide dinitrate given three times a day or a transdermal patch removed overnight).

Beta-adrenergic blocking drugs slow heart rate, blunt the exercise-induced increase in heart rate, decrease myocardial contractility, and can reduce elevated blood pressure, all actions that reduce oxygen consumption. Beta-adrenergic blocking drugs (Table 7–5) available for use vary in several characteristics, including lipid solubility, duration of action, and the degree to which they affect beta-receptor subtypes. The beta$_1$ receptor mediates the major cardiac actions of the sympathetic nervous system, whereas beta$_2$ receptors promote vasodilation and dilation of pulmonary bronchi. Beta$_2$-receptor blockade can exacerbate asthma as well as the manifestations of peripheral vascular disease in some patients. Thus, beta blockers that predominantly act on beta$_1$ receptors may be more useful in patients with chronic obstructive lung disease or peripheral vascular disease. However, the beta$_1$ selectivity is relative; at the higher doses often necessary for effective

TABLE 7-5	Selected Beta-Adrenergic Blocking Drugs			
Drug	**Cardioselectivity**	**Lipid Solubility**	**Intrinsic Agonist Activity**	**Usual Dosage**
Propranolol	−	+	−	Oral: 80–320 mg/day (given in 2–4 divided doses)*
Metoprolol	+	+	−	Oral: 50–100 mg bid IV: 5 mg × 3 at 2–5 min intervals
Atenolol	+	−	−	Oral: 50–100 mg/day IV: 5 mg given over 5 min, may be repeated 10 min later
Nadolol	−	−	−	Oral: 40–160 mg/day
Timolol	−	+	−	Oral: 10–20 mg bid
Acebutolol	+	−	+	Oral: 200–600 mg bid
Labetalol (combined alpha and beta blocking)	−	+	−	Oral: 100–300 mg bid
Pindolol	−	+	+	Oral: 5–30 mg bid
Esmolol	+	−	−	IV: 50–200 μg/kg/min after a loading dose

*Long-acting preparations are also available.
+ = Present; − = absent; IV = intravenous.

cardiac result, the selectivity may be lost. Even these beta blockers cannot be used in patients with overt bronchospasm. Beta blockers can affect atrioventricular conduction as well as heart rate. Thus, they are contraindicated in the presence of significant resting bradycardia or atrioventricular conduction disturbance. Other potential side effects may include fatigue, sleep disturbance, and exacerbation of depression. Some of these side effects may be less prominent with hydrophilic beta blockers that are less likely to penetrate the central nervous system. Beta blockers can lead to a small reduction of HDL cholesterol and some increase in serum triglycerides.

Calcium ions play important roles in vascular smooth muscle constriction, myocardial contraction, and the genesis of the cardiac action potential. Calcium channel–blocking drugs can affect each of these actions. The calcium channel–blocking drugs, however, are structurally distinct and vary in the degree to which they directly or reflexly alter heart rate, vascular tone, contractility, and atrioventricular conduction. Verapamil and, to a somewhat lesser degree, diltiazem, slow heart rate. Verapamil may thus offer an advantage for the angina patient who cannot take a beta blocker because of bronchospasm. Verapamil and diltiazem also reduce atrioventricular conduction and myocardial contractility. They should not be used in the setting of bradycardia, conduction disturbance, or left ventricular dysfunction. The dihydropyridine nifedipine is a more potent vasodilator (and antihypertensive) and does not significantly impair cardiac contractility or atrioventricular conduction. The lack of much direct electrophysiologic effect plus potent vasodilation can lead to a reflex increase in heart rate. In some clinical syndromes, nifedipine as monotherapy has been associated with worsening of coronary heart disease symptoms. The reflex actions of nifedipine may be blunted by concomitant beta-blocking therapy. The reflex actions may be less likely with long-acting nifedipine preparations and with newer (second-generation) dihydropyridines.

Combination drug therapy with a nitrate and beta blocker is commonly used for patients with angina. Some patients with more severe angina may benefit from the addition of a drug from each of the three classes (with appropriate avoidance of electrophysiologic or negative inotropic side effects). It is also important that combination therapy not result in excessive lowering of blood pressure, leading to orthostatic symptoms.

Patients with unstable angina and pain at rest should be hospitalized for intensive medical therapy. Aspirin and heparin for anticoagulation should be given in the absence of contraindication and have been demonstrated to reduce progression to myocardial infarction and mortality. Anti-ischemic medications, commonly nitrates and beta blockers, are also administered. In the presence of pain during rest or severe pain, the nitrate is often given initially as intravenous nitroglycerin. A calcium channel blocker can be added if necessary or if there is intolerance or contraindication to a beta blocker. However, as suggested previously, nifedipine as monotherapy has been associated with an adverse outcome in patients with unstable angina, and diltiazem or verapamil should not be given if there is associated left ventricular dysfunction.

Patients with unstable angina whose symptoms do not promptly stabilize with medical therapy in the hospital or who experience recurrent ischemia represent high-risk patients. Coronary angiography is recommended for consideration of revascularization. Increased risk is also indicated by transient ECG changes and ischemic episodes accompanied by pulmonary congestion, S_3, or a transient mitral regurgitation murmur. For patients with severe refractory symptoms, intra-aortic balloon counterpulsation (IABP) may be helpful until revascularization is undertaken. The IABP reduces impedance to left ventricular ejection and also maintains diastolic coronary perfusion pressure.

Most patients with unstable angina stabilize with medical therapy and can then undergo stress testing for further risk stratification. Those with positive tests are referred for coronary angiography. Many physicians routinely recommend coronary angiography, even if symptoms have stabilized, if the patient's age is not advanced and there are no serious concomitant illnesses.

CORONARY BYPASS SURGERY AND CORONARY ANGIOPLASTY FOR ANGINA PECTORIS

Coronary artery bypass surgery (CABPS) is very effective in reducing or eliminating symptoms in patients with angina pectoris. In certain subgroups, CABPS improves prognosis. For stable patients with preserved left ventricular function, the operative mortality risk is ≤ 1%; the risk of clinically apparent perioperative myocardial infarction is about 2.5%. Left ventricular dysfunction increases the operative risk. However, patients with left ventricular dysfunction also have increased risk with medical therapy and are most likely to derive mortality benefit from surgery if the dysfunction is not so severe that the operative risk is prohibitive. Other factors that can influence the decision about CABPS include the size of the coronary vessels and whether there is diffuse or distal coronary disease that would reduce the effectiveness of the bypasses. Conduits used for bypass include saphenous veins from the lower extremities and the internal mammary artery.

Coronary bypass surgery is often considered for patients with unacceptable angina despite medical therapy. It should also be considered for patients with stenosis of the left main coronary artery and those with triple vessel disease accompanied by left ventricular dysfunction, inducible ischemia, or poor functional capacity. In these patients, CABPS has been associated with improved prognosis, compared with medical therapy.

Unfortunately, CABPS does not halt coronary disease. Obstructive lesions can subsequently develop in native vessels not subjected to bypass and in the bypasses themselves. By 7 to 10 years after bypass surgery, angina recurs in 40% to 50% of patients. Internal mammary arteries are more likely than saphenous veins to maintain long-term patency. Aspirin therapy is given to bypass surgery patients to increase graft patency. Careful attention to risk factor reduction, including lipid levels is important. If refractory angina or unstable symptoms develop in patients who previously underwent a bypass, percutaneous coronary angioplasty or repeat CABPS can be considered. The risk of repeat revascularization is higher than that of the first operation.

Percutaneous transluminal coronary angioplasty (PTCA) involves passing a balloon catheter into a coronary artery, positioning the balloon portion across a stenotic lesion, and inflating the balloon with several atmospheres of pressure to dilate the stenosis. The procedure disrupts the intima, splits the atherosclerotic plaque, and often results in a small local dissection. PTCA is successful in ≥90% of cases. Acute coronary occlusion can complicate PTCA and can lead to acute myocardial infarction (~4%) and/or to the need for emergent coronary bypass surgery (~3%). The mortality rate associated with PTCA is about 1%. PTCA can also be complicated by restenosis at the site of dilation, usually in the weeks to months following the procedure. In published series of elective PTCAs, the restenosis rate at 6 months ranges from 30% to 40%. The mechanism of restenosis is complex and involves vascular smooth muscle hyperplasia as a response to the dilation injury. A second PTCA procedure is successful in many of these patients. PTCA is most effective for patients with unacceptable angina despite medical therapy and a discrete proximal stenosis in a major coronary artery. PTCA is not used for patients with left main coronary disease. Selected patients with multivessel obstructive coronary disease (generally involving two vessels) can benefit from PTCA. Results of PTCA in patients with unstable angina are similar to those in stable patients, but the risk of acute coronary occlusion is higher, presumably because of the disrupted plaque and associated thrombus. It is desirable to treat unstable angina patients initially with heparin and aspirin before moving to PTCA unless recurrent or refractory ischemia requires earlier PTCA.

A number of newer catheter-based techniques have been developed for use with PTCA in selected patients. These include catheter-delivered coronary artery stents, which may be particularly beneficial in patients with abrupt closure after PTCA and for obstructive lesions in saphenous vein grafts.

VARIANT ANGINA

In 1959, Prinzmetal described a syndrome of chest pain unrelated to exertion with associated transient ST segment elevation on the ECG. The episodes are more common in the early morning hours and may be accompanied by cardiac arrhythmias, including ventricular tachycardia or heart block. Sudden death can occur. There can be spontaneous variability in the frequency of variant angina episodes. Variant angina is the result of localized intense spasm, usually in the proximal portion of a major coronary artery (hence, the profound ischemia and ST segment elevation). Some patients exhibit a more generalized arterial hypersensitivity and may experience migraine headache or Raynaud's phenomenon. There is an association between cigarette smoking and variant angina. Although the classic ECG finding is ST segment elevation, ST depression or T wave inversion can also occur. Usually the spasm occurs at the site of an atherosclerotic plaque, although the plaque itself may not be obstructive. In some cases, the coronary artery is angiographically normal between episodes. Detection of objective evidence of ischemia can be difficult because of the unpredictable nature of the episodes. In some cases, demonstration of transient ST segment elevation during symptoms on ambulatory ECG monitoring (Fig. 7–4) can aid in the diagnosis. Coronary spasm with reproduction of symptoms and ECG changes may follow cautious provocative testing with ergonovine during coronary angiography. Ergo-

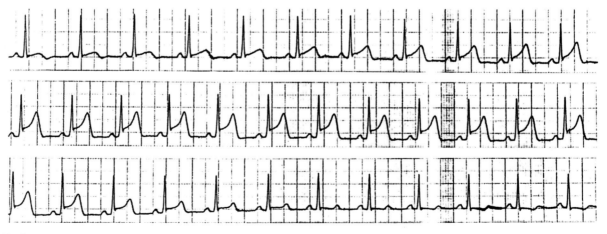

Figure 7–4
Continuous electrocardiographic recording in a patient with Prinzmetal's (variant) angina. Spontaneous onset of chest discomfort began during the *top strip* accompanied by transient ST segment elevation. By the *bottom strip* (several minutes later), both discomfort and ST elevation have resolved.

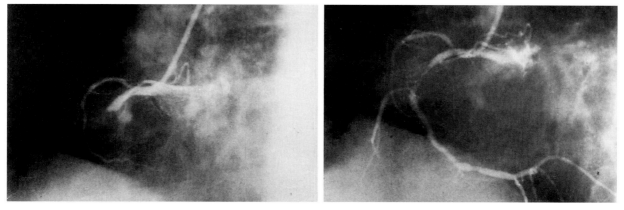

Figure 7–5

Right coronary artery angiogram in a patient with acute inferior myocardial infarction. The *left panel* demonstrates total obstruction of the right coronary artery. The *right panel* depicts restoration of flow 90 minutes after the intravenous administration of tissue-type plasminogen activator.

novine is an ergot alkaloid with alpha-adrenergic and serotoninergic effects. Vessels prone to spasm are supersensitive to its vasoconstrictive properties. The resultant spasm can be both intense and prolonged, leading to significant cardiac ischemia and arrhythmias. Intracoronary administration of vasodilating drugs (nitroglycerin) may be required for relief. Provocative testing is not employed if there are obstructive coronary artery lesions. The therapy of variant angina centers on the use of vasodilating drugs (calcium channel blockers and nitrates). Beta-adrenergic blocking drugs may have the potential to be detrimental by promoting unopposed alpha-adrenergic vasoconstriction.

ACUTE MYOCARDIAL INFARCTION

Acute myocardial infarction (AMI) often develops at rest or with normal activity. In many cases, it is the patient's first clinical manifestation of coronary heart disease. These observations are consistent with the prominent role of acute thrombotic occlusion of a coronary artery at the site of a disrupted atherosclerotic plaque (Fig. 7–5). Large databases have demonstrated a diurnal pattern of onset, with a peak occurrence about 6 a.m. Clinical experience holds and evidence supports that vigorous physical exertion, especially in an otherwise sedentary individual, can contribute to triggering of AMI, as can emotional stresses such as anger. The stresses associated with surgical procedures or cardiac arrhythmias (atrial fibrillation with rapid ventricular response) can provoke AMI in some patients with underlying coronary heart disease.

Typically, AMI results in severe chest pain lasting >30 minutes and unrelieved by sublingual nitroglycerin. Nausea, diaphoresis, and dyspnea are common. However, patients vary considerably in the intensity or even presence of symptoms. About 20% of AMIs are unrecognized, because symptoms are atypical, mild, or even ab-

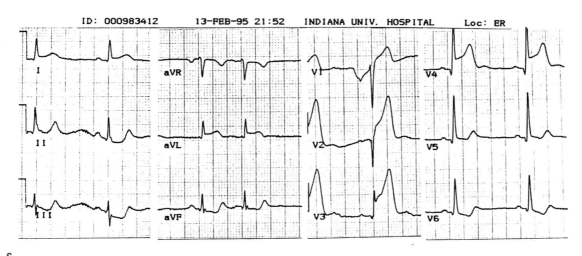

Figure 7–6

Acute anteroseptal myocardial infarction. There is a current of injury in leads V_1–V_4, I, AVL. Q waves have developed in the anterior leads.

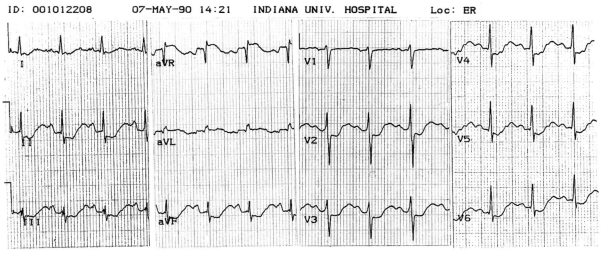

ID: 001012208   07-MAY-90 14:21   INDIANA UNIV. HOSPITAL   Loc: ER

Figure 7-7

Marked ST segment depression in a patient with prolonged chest pain due to acute non-Q wave myocardial infarction. ST segment depression is not specific for infarction (e.g., it can result from transient myocardial ischemia and other causes). Confirmation of non-Q wave infarction rests on serial cardiac enzyme determination. See Figure 3-6 for the deep T wave inversion that also can accompany non-Q wave infarction.

sent. Patients with diabetes mellitus may be more likely to experience silent myocardial infarction. Some patients present not with pain but with symptoms due to an AMI complication, such as pulmonary edema. In the uncomplicated AMI, the heart rate and blood pressure are often somewhat increased, although bradycardia frequently accompanies acute inferior myocardial infarction. A fourth heart sound, attesting to the reduced ventricular compliance, is expected if sinus rhythm is present. An apical systolic murmur due to mitral regurgitation from papillary muscle ischemia may be detected. With a large infarction, systolic dysfunction with an S_3 may be heard.

An ECG should be obtained immediately in any patient with suspected AMI, both to aid in diagnosis and to help identify patients who may be candidates for thrombolytic therapy or emergent angioplasty. AMI can be designated electrocardiographically as Q wave or non-Q wave. (The past designations of *transmural* and *subendocardial,* respectively, are no longer used, since pathologic studies failed to show a consistent relation of the ECG pattern with the intramural location of infarction.) Q wave infarction typically begins with a localized current of injury (ST segment elevation), with the subsequent development of a pathologic Q wave, generally $\geq .04$ seconds in duration (Fig. 7-6; also see Fig. 3-5 and Table 3-4). The typical ECG findings of non-Q wave infarction include ST segment depression and/or T wave inversion (Fig. 7-7). About 90% of patients with evolving Q wave infarction have total occlusion of the infarct artery. By contrast, the obstruction is high grade but with some residual flow in most patients with the non-Q wave pattern. Despite the central role of the ECG, it must be recognized that the first ECG is diagnostic in only about one half of AMI patients. The initial tracing may show nonspecific findings, and in about 10% of patients, the first tracing is normal. By performing serial tracings, the

ECG contribution to diagnosis rises substantially. Myocardial injury leads to the release of enzymes into the blood. Creatine kinase MB (CK-MB) isozyme is the most sensitive and specific conventional marker of myocardial injury. With AMI, CK-MB blood levels usually exceed normal limits by 6 to 8 hours, peak at 12 to 48 hours, and return to normal 24 to 48 hours later (Fig. 7-8). Thus, the level upon presentation may still be normal.

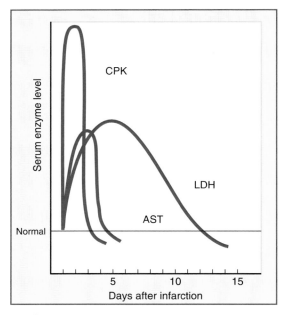

Figure 7-8

Typical time course for detection of enzymes released from the myocardium upon necrosis. AST = Serum aspartate aminotransferase; CPK = creatine kinase; LDH = lactic dehydrogenase.

Serum lactate dehydrogenase (LDH) levels rise later with AMI and may remain elevated for several days. Thus, LDH isozyme analysis can be useful for the patient who presents a couple of days after suspected AMI, when CK-MB levels may have returned to normal. LDH can be fractionated into five isozymes. Cardiac LDH is principally LDH_1. With myocardial infarction, LDH_1 exceeds levels of LDH_2.

Although CK-MB is disproportionately present in cardiac muscle, blood levels can be elevated in some patients with other disorders, including substantial skeletal muscle injury. In light of this and the delay between AMI onset and diagnostic CK-MB values, there is interest in other markers, including blood levels of cardiac troponins.

The evaluation of AMI patients includes chest radiograph. Although there are no characteristic findings of infarction, the study aids in the assessment of pulmonary vascularity and may demonstrate signs of disorders that can complicate or simulate AMI. Echocardiography may demonstrate a segmental wall motion abnormality (although this is not diagnostic of infarction) and also provides assessment of overall ventricular function. Many of the complications of AMI can also be detected or confirmed by echocardiography.

TREATMENT OF ACUTE MYOCARDIAL INFARCTION

Most deaths associated with AMI occur during the first hours following the onset of symptoms, the result of ventricular fibrillation. Because of this and the benefit of early AMI treatment, it is important that patients know the warning signs and seek medical care promptly when they develop. Many cities employ emergency medical technicians who can recognize the symptoms of AMI, initiate ECG monitoring, and treat ventricular tachyarrhythmias, terminating them with electrical defibrillation if necessary. Airway management, intravenous drug delivery, and cardiopulmonary resuscitation can be administered if needed. Prehospital emergency cardiac care, especially the rapid treatment of life-threatening ventricular arrhythmias, improves survival after AMI.

The early hospital treatment includes supplemental oxygen administration, continuous ECG rhythm monitoring, and insertion of an intravenous line so that necessary medications can be given. A 12-lead ECG should be obtained without delay. If blood pressure is acceptable, a sublingual nitroglycerin is administered. The early treatment should include aspirin, 160 to 325 mg, which has been shown to reduce mortality. Morphine, 2 to 4 mg intravenously and repeated every 5 to 15 minutes if necessary, is given to aid in the control of pain, again if blood pressure is satisfactory. Morphine exerts vagotonic effects and can decrease blood pressure and also depress respiratory drive. An intravenous infusion of nitroglycerin is often administered for its anti-ischemic and unloading effects, particularly if blood pressure is elevated or if there is associated pulmonary congestion.

Sinus bradycardia occurs in some AMI patients, particularly with inferior myocardial infarctions (Fig. 7–9), where it may be accompanied by hypotension (because of enhanced vagal tone and right coronary artery supply of the sinus node). If the bradycardia is asymptomatic and hemodynamically tolerated, no specific treatment is required. If symptoms or hemodynamic changes mandate treatment, atropine, 0.5 mg IV, can be administered. For AMI patients with elevated heart rate and blood pressure, the cautious use of intravenous beta blocker therapy, such as metoprolol, may be beneficial if there are no contraindications, including significant heart failure, hypotension, bradycardia, and significant atrioventricular conduction disturbance. If there is particular concern about these complications, the short-acting agent esmolol may offer advantage.

THROMBOLYTIC THERAPY AND PRIMARY CORONARY ANGIOPLASTY FOR ACUTE MYOCARDIAL INFARCTION

Myocardial necrosis occurs progressively following acute coronary occlusion. Timely restoration of coronary blood flow by thrombolytic therapy or direct PTCA salvages myocardial tissue and reduces mortality risk in appropriately selected patients.

Inclusion criteria (Table 7–6) for intravenous thrombolytic therapy include chest pain characteristic of AMI with associated ECG current of injury (ST segment elevation). Clinical trials indicate benefit also for AMI patients with new or presumably new left bundle branch block ECG pattern. Thrombolytic therapy is not routinely indicated for AMI patients with ST segment depression or T wave inversion. Time is of central importance—the earlier the treatment, the greater the benefit. The early trials clearly established the value of treatment in patients presenting within 6 hours following symptom onset. Patients who present between 6 and 12 hours also derive some benefit if there is ongoing ischemia and ST segment elevation. The risk of stroke in thrombolytic-treated patients is increased in the elderly. However, the mortality risk of AMI is also higher in these patients. Many elderly patients (65 to 70 years of age) can benefit from thrombolytic therapy. It may be best to focus on "physiologic" rather than chronologic age.

The contraindications for thrombolytic therapy are listed in Table 7–7. They center on characteristics that may increase the risk of bleeding complications. The most important complication is stroke due to intracranial hemorrhage. (Ischemic stroke can also complicate AMI, even in the absence of thrombolytic therapy.) Stroke risk is increased in patients with hypertension (particularly in the elderly) and in patients with cerebrovascular disease. The risk varies somewhat with the specific thrombolytic regimen used (e.g., it is greater with tissue-type plasminogen activator than streptokinase) and is increased by the concomitant use of heparin. Overall stroke risk with commonly used regimens is in the range of 1.0% to 1.7%.

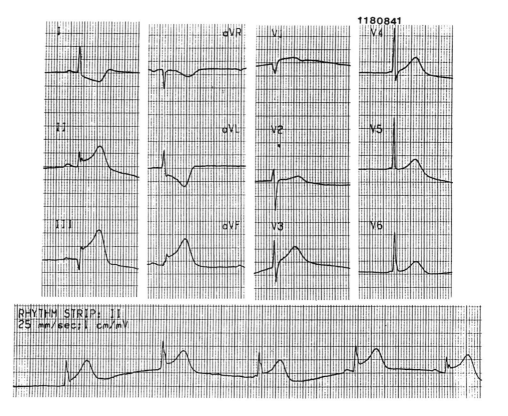

1180841

Figure 7–9

Acute inferior myocardial infarction. There also is some ST segment elevation in lead V_1, which can be indicative of associated right ventricular involvement. The rhythm strip demonstrates marked sinus bradycardia with junctional escape rhythm (the last complex is a conducted sinus beat).

Thrombolytic agents currently approved for intravenous use in AMI include streptokinase (SK), tissue-type plasminogen activator (tPA), and anistreplase. Streptokinase produces a more profound systemic lytic state. Because it is more antigenic, SK can result in allergic symptoms, and its use is occasionally accompanied by hypotension. The latter usually responds to interruption or slowing of the infusion. Because of the induction of antibodies, it should not be chosen for patients who have previously received SK. Streptokinase is administered as 1.5 million units over 1 hour. tPA is more fibrin specific. Allergic reactions are rare. It is considerably more expensive than SK. As indicated previously, the risk of stroke is slightly higher with tPA than with SK. The conventional tPA regimen was 100 mg, administered as 60 mg IV infusion over the first hour, the first 6 to 10 mg of which was given as intravenous bolus over the first 2 to 3 minutes, followed by 20 mg intravenous infusion per hour over the second and third hours. More recently, tPA has been administered via a "front-loaded" approach, as tested in the large GUSTO clinical trial (Table 7–8). This regimen includes an initial 15-mg bolus, followed by 0.75 mg/kg (maximum 50 mg) over 30 minutes, followed by 0.5 mg/kg (maximum 35 mg) over 60 minutes.

There has been considerable controversy about the best thrombolytic regimen. Angiographic studies indicate that early restoration of coronary patency is greater with

TABLE 7–6	Selection Criteria for Thrombolytic Therapy in Acute Myocardial Infarction

1. Chest pain consistent with acute myocardial infarction
2. ECG changes:
   ST segment elevation >1 mm in two or more limb or contiguous precordial leads
   New or presumed new left bundle branch block
   ST segment depression with prominent R wave in leads V_2–V_3 *if* felt to represent posterior infarction
3. Time from onset of symptoms:
   <6 hours: most beneficial
   6–12 hours: less benefit but worthwhile if continued ischemic pain
   >12 hours: little apparent benefit unless "stuttering" course with ongoing chest pain
4. Age—"physiologic" age more important than chronologic age:
   <75 years: definite benefit
   >75 years: benefit less clear cut

TABLE 7–7	Contraindications for Thrombolytic Therapy in Acute Myocardial Infarction

Absolute
  Active bleeding
  Major surgery, organ biopsy, or major trauma within 6 weeks
  Stroke or symptomatic cerebrovascular disease; intracranial tumor; recent head trauma
  Suspected aortic dissection
  Suspected pericarditis
  Bleeding diathesis
  Severe hypertension
Relative
  Puncture of a noncompressible vessel
  Prolonged (e.g., >10 min) cardiopulmonary resuscitation
  History of gastrointestinal bleeding

TABLE 7-8	Accelerated (Front-Loaded) Tissue-Type Plasminogen Activator and Streptokinase Regimens Utilizing Intravenous Heparin as Tested in the GUSTO Trial

Streptokinase (SK)	Tissue-Type Plasminogen Activator (tPA)
Aspirin ≥160 mg	Aspirin ≥160 mg
SK: 1.5 million units IV over 60 min	tPA: 15-mg bolus IV, followed by 0.75 mg/kg body weight (not to exceed 50 mg) over 30 min, followed by 0.5 mg/kg (not to exceed 35 mg) over 60 min
Heparin 5000-unit bolus IV, then 1000 units/hr*	Heparin 5000-unit bolus IV, then 1000 units/hr*

*Adjusted by PTT determinations.
IV = Intravenous.

tPA than SK, but some clinical trials have demonstrated comparable clinical results when comparing the two. In the GUSTO trial, which also used adjunctive heparin, as is commonly employed in the United States, there was a 1% absolute mortality reduction in front-loaded tPA-treated patients compared with those receiving SK. The relative benefit appeared to be most prominent in younger patients (<65 years) and in those with anterior or large infarctions. The adjunctive use of heparin to enhance thrombolysis and reduce early reocclusion increases the bleeding risk. Heparin appears to be important with tPA, which is shorter acting and induces a more modest systemic lytic state. Although heparin has also commonly been used with SK, it is not established that its benefits outweigh the associated risk. The optimal duration of heparin therapy following thrombolytic treatment is also not clear. It is often given for 24 to 48 hours in the uncomplicated patient.

Coronary flow can also be re-established with emergent (direct) PTCA. The residual stenosis is less than with thrombolytic treatment, and there appears to be lower incidence of recurrent ischemia. The stroke risk is also less. Studies from highly experienced angioplasty centers indicate a mortality and ventricular function benefit of PTCA over thrombolysis in patients treated within 6 hours of symptom onset. PTCA offers particular value for patients with a contraindication to thrombolytic treatment. PTCA may also be particularly beneficial for AMI patients with evolving cardiogenic shock. Because most hospitals do not provide emergent PTCA, thrombolytic therapy remains the primary means of restoring coronary flow in most AMI patients. Patients who experience recurrent ischemia following thrombolytic therapy generally undergo prompt cardiac angiography for consideration of PTCA or surgical revascularization.

OTHER MEASURES

Traditionally, the patient with uncomplicated AMI is confined to bed for the first 24 to 36 hours, except for the use of bedside commode. Activity is then cautiously and progressively increased, often with guidance and supervision from a rehabilitation program. Patients are usually transferred out of the cardiac care unit after 3 days. Many patients require stool softeners or laxatives to avoid constipation and straining. Uncomplicated patients are usually discharged about 1 week following infarction. Predischarge exercise testing for uncomplicated patients aids in assessing activity tolerance and guidelines. It is also used to identify patients at higher risk for recurrent events and more extensive coronary disease. Patients with inducible ischemia and those whose clinical characteristics indicate high risk are referred for coronary angiography. This decision must also take into account the patient's general medical condition and age.

Large trials have demonstrated that routine treatment with beta-adrenergic blocking drugs (metoprolol, timolol, propranolol) reduces overall mortality, sudden death, and/or reinfarction following AMI. Absent of contraindications such as significant heart failure, bradycardia, or conduction disturbance, they are begun in the hospital and continued in the long term. Some authorities have questioned the value of long-term beta blocker treatment in low-risk AMI patients, that is, those without large infarction, recurrent ischemia, or complication. Aspirin is also continued long term. Anticoagulation with coumadin is reserved for patients with a specific indication (echocardiographic evidence of intraventricular thrombus, a condition more likely to accompany anteroapical infarction). Recent trials have demonstrated long-term benefit of angiotensin-converting enzyme inhibitor treatment in AMI patients with left ventricular dysfunction or large infarction.

NON-Q WAVE MYOCARDIAL INFARCTION

The natural history of non-Q wave infarction appears to be somewhat different than that of Q wave infarction. For most non-Q wave patients, the acute thrombus is not totally obstructive or undergoes early spontaneous thrombolysis or there is generous collateral flow. Studies in the prethrombolytic era demonstrated that the resultant acute myocardial injury was less and the in-hospital prognosis better than for patients with Q wave infarction. However, the non-Q wave patients were at greater risk for recurrent ischemic events, and the long-term prognosis was comparable to that of the Q wave patients. As indicated previously, thrombolytic therapy does not routinely benefit and is not recommended for non-Q wave patients. Their early treatment commonly involves aspirin, heparin, and anti-ischemic medications. Because of the risk of recurrent ischemic events, many physicians are more likely to employ coronary angiography as part of the postinfarction evaluation. Non-Q wave myocardial infarction patients with recurrent ischemia, either spontaneous or exercise test induced, are at particular risk and should undergo angiographic study for consideration of revascularization. Non-Q wave myocardial infarction patients with persistent ST segment depression also appear to be at increased risk. Some trial data suggest that the routine use of diltiazem in survivors of non-Q wave infarction with preserved left ventricular function may reduce the incidence of reinfarction. Diltiazem can have deleterious effects and should not be used in patients with left ventricular dysfunction.

COMPLICATIONS OF MYOCARDIAL INFARCTION AND THEIR MANAGEMENT

Cardiac arrhythmias and conduction disturbances can complicate AMI. They generally require treatment when they cause hemodynamic compromise, worsen myocardial ischemia, or predispose to more malignant arrhythmias, such as sustained ventricular tachycardia or fibrillation. The approach should also include reversal of conditions that can exacerbate arrhythmias, such as hypokalemia, hypomagnesemia, hypoxia, or medication side effect.

The risk of ventricular fibrillation is greatest during the first few hours of AMI. Prompt electrical defibrillation with 200 to 400 joules should be performed. Ventricular fibrillation or ventricular tachycardia during the early hours of myocardial infarction does not carry the same adverse prognostic implication as when they occur later in the recovery period. Sustained ventricular tachycardia often requires electrical cardioversion. If the ventricular tachycardia is tolerated, an initial attempt with intravenous lidocaine may be tried. If ventricular tachycardia is not suppressed by lidocaine, intravenous procainamide can be substituted or added to lidocaine. Intravenous bretylium may also be useful to prevent recurrence of sustained ventricular tachyarrhythmias. The treatment of ventricular arrhythmias is described in detail in Chapter 8. Accelerated idioventricular rhythm (60 to 100 bpm) is a relatively common occurrence in AMI patients and can also accompany reperfusion in some of them. It is often well tolerated and usually does not require specific antiarrhythmic therapy.

The use of lidocaine infusion as prophylactic treatment in AMI patients is not recommended. Premature ventricular complexes do not reliably predict progression to ventricular tachycardia or fibrillation; they usually do not require specific antiarrhythmic therapy. Some physicians feel that very frequent premature ventricular beats or nonsustained ventricular tachycardia in the early hours of AMI warrant institution of lidocaine therapy. Lidocaine toxicity is more likely in patients with impaired hepatic function and in the elderly. Lidocaine blood levels can be helpful in monitoring therapy.

Supraventricular arrhythmias also occur in many AMI patients. An associated rapid ventricular response with atrial fibrillation can worsen myocardial ischemia and hemodynamic status. If not contraindicated, beta-adrenergic blocking drugs may be effective for rate control in patients with atrial fibrillation. However, if there is associated ischemic pain or hemodynamic compromise, prompt electrical cardioversion is indicated in patients with sustained supraventricular tachyarrhythmia (other than sinus tachycardia). The treatment of atrial tachyarrhythmias is discussed in Chapter 8.

Second-degree atrioventricular (AV) block of the

Mobitz I (Wenckebach) type is common in patients with inferior myocardial infarction because of increased vagal tone and/or ischemia of the AV node. It is usually temporary and, if asymptomatic, requires no therapy. If it impairs hemodynamic status, atropine is usually effective. If Wenckebach block progresses to complete heart block, the escape rhythm usually is junctional at reasonable rates (40 to 60 per minute). By contrast, Mobitz type II second-degree AV block is an uncommon complication, usually of a large anterior infarction. The risk of progression to complete heart block is greater with Mobitz II block, and the escape is less reliable and slower, arising from a ventricular focus. A temporary pacemaker is indicated in patients in the Mobitz type II second-degree AV block.

Temporary pacemaker placement is usually recommended also for AMI patients with third-degree (or complete) heart block, especially if the infarction is anterior and the site of block is in the ventricular His-Purkinje system. Complete AV block should be differentiated from other types of AV dissociation, such as that seen in inferior infarction due to sinus bradycardia with independent junctional escape or accelerated rhythm. Other conditions for which a temporary pacemaker has been inserted because of the risk of progression to high-degree AV heart block include new bifascicular block (right bundle branch block with left anterior or posterior fascicular block, or alternating right and left bundle branch block). Some physicians rely on standby external pacemakers for some asymptomatic patients with new bifascicular block. For some AMI patients (those with complete heart block or Mobitz type II block), permanent pacemaker insertion may be indicated. However, it is noteworthy that the mortality risk of such patients is primarily related to the extent of myocardial injury rather than to the conduction disturbance. Conduction abnormalities and pacemaker use is described in Chapter 8.

Several types of hemodynamic disturbances can complicate AMI. Early hypotension with bradycardia in patients with inferior infarction has been described previously. In other patients, isolated signs of peripheral hypoperfusion (reduced blood pressure, cool skin, reduced urine output) result from hypovolemia. The hypovolemia can be relative, from diminished ventricular compliance, or absolute, from diaphoresis, vomiting, or diuretics. Cautious fluid administration can be beneficial. The development of congestive heart failure is an adverse prognostic sign. Isolated pulmonary congestion is treated with diuretics (furosemide) and vasodilator therapy (nitroglycerin). The role of angiotensin-converting enzyme inhibitors is discussed elsewhere. For patients with both pulmonary congestion and peripheral hypoperfusion, therapy often includes an inotropic drug (dobutamine or dopamine) and a vasodilator (nitroglycerin) (see Chapter 4). If this is not successful or tolerated, an intra-aortic counterpulsation device may enhance stabilization. Cardiogenic shock, in the absence of a mechanical complication, usually indicates that 40% or more of myocardium has been injured; mortality risk is high. For selected AMI patients with cardiogenic shock, emergent PTCA may improve prognosis.

In patients with severe heart failure or shock, hemodynamic monitoring with a bedside right heart balloon

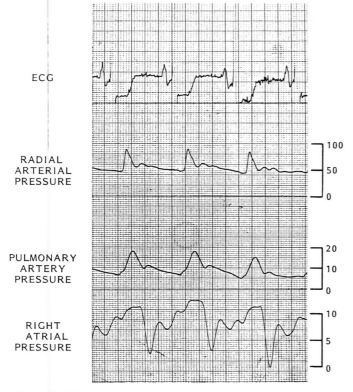

Figure 7–10

Electrocardiogram (ECG), arterial and Swan-Ganz bedside catheter recordings in a patient with right ventricular infarction. Hypotension is present, and cardiac output estimated by thermodilution (not shown) is reduced. The pulmonary artery pressures are normal. There is elevation of the right atrial pressure with a prominent y descent.

(Swan-Ganz) catheter is usually employed to aid in assessment of the patient's volume status and response to treatment. The left ventricular filling pressure (pulmonary capillary wedge pressure), thermodilution-estimated cardiac output, and systemic vascular resistance can be calculated. The normal pulmonary capillary wedge pressure is 10 to 12 mm Hg, but the optimal wedge pressure in AMI patients with noncompliant left ventricle is usually in the 16 to 18 mm Hg range. As pressures rise about 20 mm Hg or so, pulmonary congestion may result. Swan-Ganz monitoring also can be helpful in the patient with suspected ventricular septal rupture (see later).

Acute inferior myocardial infarction can be accompanied by right ventricular infarction. The ECG findings include ST segment elevation in right precordial leads, especially V_4R. The characteristic clinical findings include jugular distention (at times with waveform that can simulate pericardial constriction [Fig. 7–10] with prominent y descent), low blood pressure, and clear lung fields, unless there is associated left ventricular failure. Fluid administration, despite jugular distention, is usually required to adequately fill the left ventricle and restore blood pressure to acceptable levels. With these measures and time, right ventricular function subsequently improves in many patients.

Mechanical complications of AMI include left ventricular free wall rupture, ventricular septal rupture, and papillary muscle rupture. Free wall rupture usually develops 3 to 5 days following AMI, produces sudden hemodynamic collapse (at times with electromechanical dissociation), and is usually fatal. Rare patients have survived after pericardiocentesis and emergent surgical repair. Also rare is when the course is less acute and blood is walled off within the pericardial space, producing a pseudoaneurysm. The diagnosis is usually made by the echocardiographic demonstration of a narrow-based communication between the pseudoaneurysm and ventricular cavity. In contrast to true ventricular aneurysm, a pseudoaneurysm may rupture. Prompt surgical therapy should be considered. Rupture of the intraventricular septum is an uncommon complication that can occur with anterior or inferior infarction. It also typically occurs 3 to 5 days following AMI. It usually results in severe heart failure and a new holosystolic murmur, often with an associated thrill. At times, the murmur can be difficult to distinguish from mitral regurgitation. The diagnosis can usually be confirmed by color-flow Doppler echocardiography. Septal rupture results in an oxygen "step-up" that can be detected using samples from right atrial and pulmonary artery ports of the Swan-Ganz catheter. Intensive medical therapy and insertion of an intra-aortic counterpulsation device are used in an attempt to stabilize the patient, but emergent surgical repair is usually required. Rupture of a papillary muscle usually results in severe sudden heart failure. An apical holosystolic murmur also results, but it may be relatively soft because of reduced cardiac output. Color-flow Doppler echocardiography can confirm the diagnosis. Large V waves may be evident in the pulmonary capillary wedge pressure recordings. In addition to intensive medical therapy, including vasodilators if blood pressure is adequate, intra-aortic balloon counterpulsation may be employed in preparation for surgical therapy. In contrast to papillary muscle rupture, papillary muscle dysfunction due to ischemia is relatively common in AMI. The resultant mitral regurgitation and its effect on cardiac function may range from mild to severe.

A left ventricular aneurysm is a discrete, thin, bulging segment of noncontracting ventricular myocardium. It is most common with anteroapical myocardial infarctions, and can be detected by echocardiography. Aneurysm formation is partly a consequence of ventricular remodeling, as described previously. Limitation of infarct size by early reperfusion and the use of angiotensin-converting enzyme inhibitors in patients at risk for the development of aneurysm appear to reduce the frequency of this complication. Complications of left ventricular aneurysm can include congestive heart failure and ventricular arrhythmias. In selected patients with refractory congestive heart failure or ventricular arrhythmias, aneurysmectomy is indicated as part of the surgical treatment of the patient.

Mural thrombi can form in left ventricular aneurysms and also in larger anteroapical Q wave infarctions, even in the absence of discrete aneurysm. Such patients are at increased risk for systemic embolic events. In light of this, it is generally recommended that patients with large anterior myocardial infarction receive therapeutic anticoagulation with heparin during hospitalization. Longer-term anticoagulation with coumadin is then employed in patients with echocardiographic evidence of mural thrombus. Anticoagulation is also often continued for patients with very dilated and hypokinetic left ventricle.

A pericardial friction rub indicating pericarditis can accompany or follow AMI. It is more common with Q wave infarctions of substantial size. Associated pain may be confused with postinfarction unstable angina. The classic ECG signs of pericarditis may not be evident. The rub may be transient or wax and wane in intensity. Symptoms and signs of infarct-related pericarditis may respond to aspirin. Nonsteroidal anti-inflammatory agents and corticosteroids are generally not used during the acute stage of myocardial infarction because they may impair infarct healing and perhaps increase the risk of cardiac rupture.

The development of recurrent ischemia (postinfarction unstable angina) identifies a high-risk patient. Coronary angiography is recommended for consideration of PTCA or surgical revascularization. Other clinical factors indicating increased risk, including congestive heart failure, reduced left ventricular function, and complex ventricular arrhythmias after the very early stage, have been described earlier. For the uncomplicated patient, risk stratification usually includes predischarge stress testing. Patients with symptoms or signs of ischemia at low or moderate workload and those with reduced functional capacity usually undergo full evaluation to include coronary cineangiography. It is important to emphasize again efforts to control risk factors, including lipid levels, in survivors of AMI.

REFERENCES

ACC/AHA Task Force: Guidelines and indications for coronary bypass surgery. J Am Coll Cardiol 1991; 17:543–589.

ACC/AHA Task Force: Guidelines for the early management of patients with acute myocardial infarction. J Am Coll Cardiol 1990; 16:249–292.

AHCPR Clinical Practice Guidelines: Unstable angina: diagnosis and treatment, 1994.

Brown BG, Zhao XQ, Sacco DE, Albers JJ: Lipid lowering and plaque disruption. New insights into prevention of plaque disruption and clinical events in coronary disease. Circulation 1993; 87:1781–1791.

Fibrinolytic Therapy Trialists Collaborative Group: Indications for fibrinolytic therapy in suspected acute myocardial infarction. Lancet 1994; 343:311–321.

GUSTO Investigators: An international randomized trial comparing four thrombolytic strategies for acute myocardial infarction. N Engl J Med 1993; 329:673–682.

Pryor DB, Bruce RA, Chaitman BR, et al.: Determination of prognosis in patients with ischemic heart disease. J Am Coll Cardiol 1989; 14:1016–1042.

8

Arrhythmias

MECHANISMS OF ARRHYTHMOGENESIS

If a microelectrode is introduced into a single myocardial cell, an action potential (Fig. 8–1) can be recorded by measuring the potential difference between the inside and the outside of the cell (inside negative). The resting membrane potential of a normal Purkinje cell is approximately − 90 millivolts (mv) with respect to the outside of the cell. When the membrane potential is depolarized to a certain threshold level, an action potential occurs with a rapid upstroke (phase 0); a return toward zero from the initial overshoot or early rapid repolarization (phase 1); a plateau (phase 2); final rapid repolarization (phase 3); and resting membrane potential and diastolic depolarization (phase 4). The normal resting potential is maintained by the active (i.e., energy-requiring) exclusion of sodium and the accumulation of potassium inside the cell. Phase 0 or rapid depolarization is due chiefly to the opening of the sarcolemmal channels to sodium entrance in atrial and ventricular muscle and cells in the His-Purkinje system. Calcium is important in the maintenance of the action potential plateau of fast sodium channel–dependent cells and in the generation of the action potential upstroke in slow calcium channel–dependent cells such as those of the sinus and atrioventricular (AV) nodes. Phase 3 is mediated chiefly by an outward potassium current, and the membrane returns to its negative resting potential during electrical diastole.

Automaticity is a property of some cardiac tissues that allows them to undergo gradual phase 4 depolarization spontaneously until threshold potential is reached and the cell initiates an action potential that is propagated from one cell to another. Normal automaticity is present in sinus nodal tissue, some atrial and junctional tissues, the bundle branches, and Purkinje fibers. The sinus node discharges more rapidly than the other cells and is the normal pacemaker of the heart. *Conduction* is the propagation of a cardiac impulse and is most closely influenced by the amplitude and upstroke velocity of phase 0 of the action potential. *Refractoriness* is a property of cardiac tissue during which a stimulus occurring soon after a previous action potential fails to elicit another normal action potential; it is most closely related to the duration of phase 3 of the cardiac action potential in most cardiac tissues.

Although the autonomic nervous system may affect atrial and ventricular tissue to a small extent, the most prominent autonomic effects are observed on the sinus and the AV nodes. Sympathetic stimulation increases the rate of automaticity and increases conduction velocity, whereas parasympathetic (vagal) activation does the opposite. Baroreceptors in the carotid sinus, located at the bifurcation of the internal and external carotid arteries, activate the vagus nerve when blood pressure increases and reflexively decrease heart rate and AV nodal conduction velocity.

The genesis of cardiac arrhythmias is divided into disorders of impulse formation, disorders of impulse conduction, and combinations of the two (Table 8–1). One cannot unequivocally determine the mechanism for most clinical arrhythmias, but each arrhythmia may be most consistent with or best explained by a particular electrophysiologic mechanism. Disorders of impulse formation are defined as an inappropriate discharge rate of the normal pacemaker (the sinus node) or abnormal discharge from an ectopic pacemaker that usurps control of the atrial or ventricular rhythm. An appropriate discharge rate of a subsidiary pacemaker that takes control of the cardiac rhythm upon sinus slowing is termed an escape beat or rhythm, whereas an inappropriately rapid discharge rate of an ectopic pacemaker (abnormally increased automaticity) that usurps control of the cardiac rhythm from the normal sinus mechanism is termed a premature complex or, when they occur in a series, an ectopic tachycardia.

Parasystole may be due to abnormal automaticity and refers to an ectopic atrial or ventricular pacemaker that discharges regularly and appears to be protected from the dominant cardiac rhythm by entrance block into the area of abnormal automaticity. Therefore, it may depolarize the myocardium intermittently whenever the myocardium is excitable, but it is not discharged by the dominant rhythm. In addition, the abnormal focus may demonstrate variable degrees of exit block, and thus it may intermittently fail to depolarize the myocardium at a time when it would be expected. Characteristic features of ventricular parasystole are (1) parasystolic premature ventricular complexes (PVCs) that are a multiple of a common integer; (2) coupling of PVCs to preceding normally conducted complexes that is not fixed, as it often is in

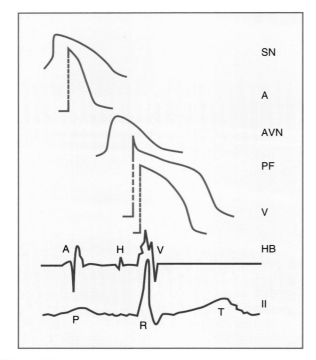

Figure 8–1
Action potentials recorded from different tissues in the heart remounted with a His bundle recording and scalar electrocardiogram (ECG) from a patient to illustrate the timing during a single cardiac cycle. A = Atrial muscle potential; AVN = atrioventricular nodal potential; HB = His bundle recording; II = lead II; PF = Purkinje fiber potential; SN = sinus nodal potential. The AH interval measured in the His bundle recording approximates AV nodal conduction time, and the HV interval approximates His-Purkinje system conduction time.

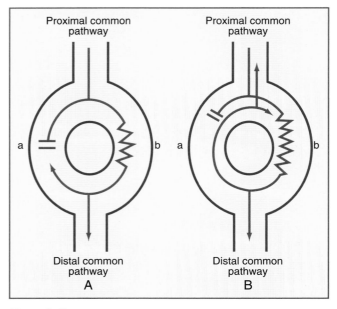

Figure 8–2
Mechanism of re-entry. Re-entry requires the presence of two separate pathways that join proximally and distally. *Panel A* illustrates a premature impulse that blocks antegradely in pathway a *(double bars)* but conducts down pathway b, albeit with a moderate conduction delay *(serpentine arrow)*. The impulse attempts to return up pathway a but meet refractory tissue. In *Panel B,* a more premature impulse blocks earlier in pathway a and experiences more conduction delay in pathway b. This impulse finds pathway a recovered from its previous activation and returns retrogradely to the proximal common pathway. If able to again travel antegradely over pathway b, it would activate the distal common pathway prematurely. If this cycle were to continue, a circus movement or re-entrant tachycardia would result.

TABLE 8–1	Genesis of Arrhythmias
Disorders of Impulse Formation	**Disorders of Impulse Conduction**
Atrial tachycardia with or without block	Heart block
Accelerated junctional rhythm	Re-entry:
Nonparoxysmal AV junctional tachycardia	AV nodal re-entrant tachycardia
Accelerated idioventricular rhythm	Reciprocating tachycardia using an accessory pathway (Wolff-Parkinson-White syndrome)
Parasystole	Atrial flutter
	Atrial fibrillation
	Ventricular tachycardia
	Ventricular flutter
	Ventricular fibrillation

Either or Both

Atrial, junctional, or ventricular extrasystoles
Flutter and fibrillation
Ventricular tachycardia

AV = Atrioventricular.

patients with nonparasystolic PVCs; and (3) periodic fusion complexes between the parasystolic and the normally conducted beat.

Disorders of impulse conduction include conduction delay and block that can result in bradyarrhythmias and provide the basis for re-entry, the most common mechanism responsible for arrhythmia development. Re-entry can occur at any level of the cardiac electrical system, including the sinus node, the atria, the AV node, the His-Purkinje system, and the ventricular myocardium. Normal cardiac tissue has relative homogeneity of conduction and refractoriness so that an impulse starts at the sinus node, travels through the atrium, the AV node, and the His-Purkinje system, and terminates with organized depolarization of ventricular muscle. Once all tissues are depolarized, the impulse is extinguished because there is no further tissue to activate. However, a re-entrant or reciprocating rhythm can occur within various tissues if certain criteria are met, giving rise to a continuous reactivation of tissue and generating a tachycardia. For re-entry to occur (Fig. 8–2) there must be two functionally dissociated pathways, permitting the impulse to travel in one direction down one pathway but blocking it in the other pathway. Thus, the pathway with longer refractoriness may block a premature impulse traveling antegradely. The first pathway, having shorter refractoriness but slower conduction, conducts the impulse to the distal common pathway with a delay that permits it to travel retrogradely up the second pathway and find the proximal tissue re-excitable. If this circus movement continues, a tachycardia occurs.

APPROACH TO THE PATIENT WITH SUSPECTED OR CONFIRMED ARRHYTHMIAS

History-taking in patients with suspected or confirmed rhythm abnormalities should be aimed at detecting the presence of cardiac or noncardiac disease that may be linked causally to the genesis of a rhythm abnormality. Common symptoms that prompt patients with rhythm disturbances to consult a physician are palpitations, syncope, presyncope, and congestive heart failure. The ability of a patient to sense an irregular, slow, or rapid heart rhythm varies greatly; some patients are completely unaware of a marked arrhythmia, whereas others feel every premature impulse. In addition, some patients may complain of palpitations when they have no detectable rhythm disturbance or merely sinus tachycardia. Dizziness is a common complaint in people with tachy- or bradyarrhythmias but also may be due to nonarrhythmic causes. Syncope refers to complete but transient loss of consciousness and also has a variety of causes (see Table 8–8). Exacerbation of congestive heart failure may occur with arrhythmias. If a patient senses palpitations, the physician should determine whether the patient senses a slow heart beat, a rapid heart beat, a regular or irregular heart beat, its rate, and whether the onset and termination of the palpitations are sudden or gradual.

The physical examination is useful in detecting evidence of underlying cardiac disease. In addition, abnormalities of the pulse may be noted, and clues regarding AV dissociation during an arrhythmia may be detected (e.g., intermittent cannon a waves in the jugular venous pulse or varying intensity of S_1 during a regular tachyarrhythmia).

The resting electrocardiogram (ECG) may reveal the specific arrhythmia responsible for symptoms or give clues regarding a tachyarrhythmia; for example, short episodes of nonsustained ventricular tachycardia may be recorded in a patient who has presented with syncope or cardiac arrest due to a sustained ventricular tachycardia. In addition, indirect evidence may be obtained from the ECG that may suggest the cause of the arrhythmia; for example, the presence of a delta wave should alert the physician to the possibility that a tachycardia due to Wolff-Parkinson-White syndrome may be present. The ECG may also provide evidence of the cause of the arrhythmia, such as the presence of ischemic heart disease documented by ECG evidence of myocardial infarction.

Twenty-four–hour ambulatory ECG (Holter monitoring) and patient-activated event recorders (given to the patient for weeks at a time) are important tools for evaluating patients with suspected arrhythmias. They permit quantitation of arrhythmia frequency and complexity, cor-

relation with the patient's symptoms, potential diagnosis of an unknown arrhythmia, and evaluation of the effect of antiarrhythmic therapy. They can record arrhythmias while patients are engaged in their normal daily activities; can document alterations in the QRS, ST, and T waves; and may be useful in documenting pacemaker function or malfunction. Certain arrhythmias are common during prolonged ECG monitoring in normal patients and may be of no clinical significance. In many patients, symptoms are very infrequent and difficult to detect even with prolonged ECG monitoring. Exercise testing can be used to precipitate arrhythmias in some patients.

Invasive electrophysiologic procedures are useful and involve introducing catheter electrodes into the heart to record electrical activity from the atria, ventricles, and His bundle, and to stimulate the atria or ventricles electrically. Supraventricular or ventricular tachycardias may be induced by programmed electrical stimulation. The test may be used diagnostically to determine whether a particular rhythm disorder exists or to determine the mechanism of a known arrhythmia. The test may also be used therapeutically to terminate a tachycardia, to determine the efficacy of drug or other therapy, or to deliver electrical energy via the catheter to ablate a pathway or focus responsible for a recurrent arrhythmia. Electrophysiologic testing is important in patients with resistant tachyarrhythmias undergoing either surgical resection or ablation of a tachycardia focus or pathway. Patients considered candidates for antitachycardia pacemaker devices or implantable cardioverter-defibrillator devices require electrophysiologic study to confirm the mechanism and origin of the arrhythmia and the efficacy and safety of this mode of therapy. Electrophysiologic study may be helpful in discovering patients with sinus nodal dysfunction or AV block.

Esophageal electrocardiography is sometimes a useful noninvasive technique to diagnose arrhythmias. An electrode introduced approximately 40 cm from the patient's nares into the esophagus can record an atrial electrogram and often can be used to pace the atrium.

Autonomic and pharmacologic manipulations sometimes aid in diagnosing arrhythmias. Most commonly, vagal maneuvers (e.g., carotid sinus massage), adenosine, or administration of verapamil to slow AV nodal conduction is used. Carotid sinus massage is performed with the patient in the supine position. With the neck hyperextended and the head turned away from the side being tested, light pressure is applied to the carotid impulse at the angle of the jaw. If no change occurs, pressure is more firmly applied with a gentle rotating motion for approximately 5 seconds on one side and then on the other; both sides are not stimulated simultaneously. Prior to carotid sinus massage, the carotid artery should be auscultated; massage should not be performed in patients who have carotid bruits.

Head-up tilt table testing is useful in evaluating patients with suspected neurally mediated syncope. This entity is believed to be due to exaggerated vagal activation and sympathetic withdrawal in response to a sympathetic stimulus, resulting in vasodilation, hypotension, and relative bradycardia. Head-up passive tilt of 60 to 80 degrees for 15 to 60 minutes can reproduce these signs and symptoms in susceptible individuals, especially if provoked by the administration of intravenous isoproterenol during tilting.

MANAGEMENT OF CARDIAC ARRHYTHMIAS

Before initiating antiarrhythmic therapy, one must determine whether the arrhythmia should be treated. Any arrhythmia that causes symptomatic hypotension or sudden death should be suppressed. However, the situation in which the arrhythmia occurs dictates whether chronic, long-term therapy is necessary. For example, an episode of ventricular fibrillation in a patient at the onset of an acute myocardial infarction does not necessarily require long-term drug therapy because of the low likelihood of recurrence. However, ventricular fibrillation in a patient without an acute myocardial infarction carries a high risk of recurrence. Some patients may have arrhythmias that, while not life threatening, produce disabling symptoms of dizziness or palpitations and require therapy. Rhythms that are tolerated well in patients with structurally normal hearts (e.g., paroxysms of supraventricular tachycardia) may not be tolerated in patients with diseased hearts (e.g., ischemic heart disease or mitral stenosis) and may require therapy. The decision to treat a patient with an asymptomatic tachyarrhythmia is more difficult. Certain arrhythmias, such as short episodes of asymptomatic nonsustained ventricular tachycardia, are in themselves harmless but may be forerunners of more serious sustained ventricular tachyarrhythmias. The decision to treat is complicated by the side effects, occasionally life threatening, of antiarrhythmic drugs, such as exacerbation of ventricular arrhythmias in 5 to 15% of cases. Although patients with premature ventricular complexes and complex nonsustained ventricular ectopy after myocardial infarction are at increased risk of subsequent sudden death, no antiarrhythmic drugs other than beta blockers have been shown to improve survival, and some drugs may make it worse.

Before beginning chronic antiarrhythmic therapy, factors contributing to the occurrence of the arrhythmia should be considered. These include digitalis excess, hypokalemia, hypomagnesemia, hypoxia, thyrotoxicosis, and other severe metabolic derangements. Congestive heart failure, anemia, or infection should be corrected. Smoking, excessive alcohol intake, caffeine- or theophylline-containing beverages or foods, fatigue, emotional upset, and some over-the-counter drugs (e.g., nasal decongestants) may exacerbate arrhythmias.

Drugs

"Therapeutic" serum concentrations of antiarrhythmic drugs are those that usually exert therapeutic effects without adverse effects in most patients. However, dosage and blood concentrations must be adjusted for any particular patient, and the measured serum concentration is of secondary importance if the response to the drug is appropriate and side effects are absent. The therapeutic-to-toxic ratio of most antiarrhythmic drugs is relatively narrow, and knowledge of drug pharmacokinetics is important to avoid toxic peak and subtherapeutic trough concentrations. Most antiarrhythmic drugs can be administered at intervals equal to the elimination half-life of the drug after an initial loading dose. At a constant dosing interval without a loading dose, the time required to reach steady state is a function of the elimination half-life of the drug. Ninety-four percent of steady-state level is achieved after four half-lives and 99% after seven half-lives. The same principle applies to the decrease in drug levels after discontinuation of the drug. Therefore, a drug with a longer half-life takes longer to reach steady state and longer to be eliminated than does one with a shorter half-life. Drugs with shorter half-lives are inconvenient to administer orally because of more frequent dosing requirements. Some medications with relatively short half-lives can be given in long-acting forms that release the drug gradually and result in adequate blood concentrations for a longer period without a high peak level immediately upon administration of the drug. The pharmacokinetics of drug distribution and elimination are often important; for example, lidocaine blood concentrations may be high after an intravenous bolus but drop very quickly as the drug is redistributed throughout the body. Once this early redistribution phase occurs, blood concentrations fall much less precipitously during the elimination phase, at which time the lidocaine is metabolized by the liver. Therefore, to avoid very high serum concentrations within the first 10 minutes and a subtherapeutic nadir after redistribution has occurred, lidocaine therapy may be initiated in two or more boluses, 5 to 10 minutes apart, instead of as one larger bolus. The organ responsible for elimination of a particular drug, usually the kidneys or liver, must be known, and dosage adjustments must be made in patients with organ dysfunction. The percent of gastrointestinal absorption of some drugs is important to estimate intravenous versus oral dosages; for example, digoxin is only about 80% absorbed orally, compared with 100% availability of an intravenous dose. Some drugs are metabolized to compounds that also demonstrate antiarrhythmic activity, such as *N*-acetyl procainamide, which is the active metabolite of procainamide. Drug interactions may necessitate dosage adjustments. For example, quinidine increases digoxin serum concentrations. Changes in pharmacokinetics may occur in some groups of patients, such as decreased lidocaine requirements in elderly patients or those with congestive heart failure. Disparity in drug absorption and metabolism may occur in different patients owing to genetically controlled enzyme systems that allow some patients to metabolize drugs such as procainamide quickly (rapid acetylators). The amount of drug bound to serum proteins affects the activity and metabolism of a drug and also may affect the interpretation of serum drug concentrations, because many assays measure both free and protein-bound drug.

Although *in vitro* electrophysiologic properties are known for each drug, and certain drugs are known to be more useful for one type of arrhythmia than another, much of antiarrhythmic drug therapy is trial and error. Even drugs grouped within the same class (Table 8–2)

TABLE 8–2	Vaughn Williams (Modified) Classification of Antiarrhythmic Drugs

Class I   Predominantly reduce the maximum velocity of the upstroke of the action potential (phase 0):
    IA: Quinidine
        Procainamide
        Disopyramide
    IB: Lidocaine
        Phenytoin
        Tocainide
        Mexiletine
    IC: Flecainide
        Propafenone
        Moricizine (?)

Class II   Inhibit sympathetic activity: propranolol and other beta blockers

Class III   Predominantly prolong action potential duration:
    Amiodarone
    Sotalol
    Bretylium

Class IV   Block the slow inward current: verapamil and other calcium antagonists

may vary in their clinical electrophysiologic effects, and when one is unsuccessful in a particular patient, another drug from the same class may be effective. It is important to remember that this classification serves a useful communication purpose but cannot be applied rigidly for several reasons. Not all drugs assigned to a single group exhibit entirely similar actions, and some drugs have properties of more than one class. The classification is based on *in vitro* electrophysiologic effects on normal Purkinje fibers; drug effects on diseased *in vivo* tissues may be different, or the mechanism of action may even have nothing to do with its direct electrophysiologic actions. Tables 8–3, 8–4, and 8–5 summarize the currently available antiarrhythmic agents. It is important to remember that a potential adverse effect of any antiarrhythmic agent is arrhythmia exacerbation.

Lidocaine

Lidocaine has minimal effects on automaticity or conduction *in vitro* unless marked abnormalities are pre-existent. Lidocaine affects fast channel–dependent tissues (atrial and ventricular muscle and His-Purkinje tissue) but usually not slow calcium channel–dependent tissues (sinus

TABLE 8–3	Antiarrhythmic Drugs: Dosage and Pharmacokinetics*

	Usual Dose Ranges (mg)				Effective Serum or Plasma Concentration (μg/ml)	Elimination Half-Life After Oral Dose (hr)	Major Route of Elimination
	Intravenous		Oral				
Drug	Loading	Maintenance	Loading	Maintenance			
Lidocaine	1–3 mg/kg at 20–50 mg/min	1–4 mg/min	—	—	1–5	1–2	Liver
Quinidine	6–10 mg/kg at 0.3–0.5 mg/kg/min	—	600–1000	300–600 q6h	3–6	5–9	Liver
Procainamide	6–13 mg/kg at 0.2–0.5 mg/kg/min	2–6 mg/min	500–1000	2000–6000 qd (q3–4h doses for procainamide, q6h doses for sustained release form)	4–10	3–5	Kidneys
Disopyramide	—	—	300–400	100–400 q6–8h	2–5	8–9	Kidneys
Phenytoin	100 mg q5min for ≤1000 mg	—	1000	100–400 q12–24h	10–20	18–36	Liver
Propranolol	0.25–0.5 mg q5min for ≤0.15–0.20 mg/kg	—	—	10–200 q6–8h	—	3–6	Liver
Bretylium	5–10 mg/kg at 1–2 mg/kg/min	0.5–2.0 mg/min	—	—	0.5–1.5	8–14	Kidneys
Verapamil	10 mg over 1–2 min	0.005 mg/kg/min	—	80–120 q6–8h	0.10–0.15	3–8	Liver
Amiodarone	150 mg over 10 min (can be repeated); then 1 mg/min × 6h, then 0.5 mg/min	—	800–1600 qd for 1–3 wk	100–400 qd	1.0–2.5	30–50 days	Liver
Tocainide	—	—	400–600	400–600 q8–12h	4–10	11	Liver
Mexiletine	—	—	400–600	150–300 q6–8h	0.75–2.0	10–17	Liver
Flecainide	—	—	—	100–200 q12h	0.2–1.0	20	Liver
Propafenone	—	—	600–900	150–300 q8–12h	0.2–3.0	5–8	Liver
Moricizine	—	—	300	200–300 q8h	—	—	—
Adenosine	6–12 mg (rapidly)	—	—	—	—	—	—
Sotalol	—	—	—	80–160 q12h	—	10–15	Kidneys

* Results presented may vary according to doses, disease state, and intravenous or oral administration.

TABLE 8–4	Antiarrhythmic Drugs: Electrocardiographic Effects			
Drug	**Sinus Rate**	**PR**	**QRS**	**QT**
Lidocaine	0	0	0	0
Quinidine	0 ↑	↓ 0 ↑	↑	↑
Procainamide	0	0 ↑	↑	↑
Disopyramide	0 ↑	0	↑	↑
Phenytoin	0	0	0	0 ↓
Propranolol	↓	0 ↑	0	0 ↓
Bretylium	0 ↓	0 ↑	0	0 ↑
Verapamil	0 ↓	↑	0	0
Amiodarone	↓	0 ↑	0	↑
Tocainide	0 ↓	0	0	0 ↓
Mexiletine	0	0	0	0 ↓
Flecainide	0 ↓	↑	↑	↑
Propafenone	0 ↓	↑	↑	0 ↑
Moricizine	0 ↓	0 ↑	0 ↑	0
Adenosine	↓ then ↑	↑	0	0
Sotalol	↓	0 ↑	0	↑

duction time in the AV node, its vagolytic actions may shorten conduction time, and the overall result is a balance between the two effects. Quinidine has alpha-adrenergic blocking effects that may cause significant hypotension, especially if vasodilators are administered concomitantly. If given slowly, quinidine may be administered intravenously. Intramuscular quinidine is incompletely absorbed and may cause tissue necrosis.

Quinidine prolongs the effective refractory period of atrial and ventricular muscle and accessory pathways. It may be effective in treating patients with AV nodal reentry and tachycardias in Wolff-Parkinson-White syndrome. Quinidine may prevent supraventricular tachycardias not only by its effects on tissue refractoriness but also by preventing the atrial or ventricular premature

and AV nodes). It appears to be particularly potent at altering electrophysiologic parameters in ischemic tissue. Lidocaine rarely causes clinically significant hemodynamic effects. It is used only parenterally because of extensive first-pass hepatic metabolism upon oral administration. Its metabolism is decreased in elderly patients and those with hepatic disease, heart failure, and shock. Maintenance doses should be reduced by one third to one half in patients with low cardiac output. Prolonged infusion of lidocaine can reduce its clearance, and dosage may have to be decreased after a day or so. Intramuscular administration has been advocated for use by emergency medical technicians when caring for a patient with an acute myocardial infarction before reaching the hospital, but lidocaine is usually administered intravenously. The ability to achieve rapid effective plasma concentrations and a fairly wide toxic-to-therapeutic ratio with a low incidence of hemodynamic complications make lidocaine a very useful antiarrhythmic drug. It is effective against a variety of ventricular arrhythmias but is generally ineffective against supraventricular arrhythmias. The use of lidocaine prophylactically in patients with acute myocardial infarction is controversial (see Chapter 7). Lidocaine is usually the parenteral drug of first choice in patients with ventricular arrhythmias. Although lidocaine may decrease ventricular response in some patients with Wolff-Parkinson-White syndrome and atrial fibrillation, it usually has no effect on or can even accelerate the ventricular response in patients with rapid ventricular responses.

Quinidine

Quinidine is useful for long-term oral treatment of both atrial and ventricular arrhythmias. Quinidine has little effect on normal automaticity but depresses automaticity from abnormal cells. It prolongs conduction time and refractoriness in most cardiac tissues, and it increases the threshold of excitability in atrial and ventricular tissue. Although the direct effect of quinidine is to prolong con-

TABLE 8–5	Antiarrhythmic Drugs: Side Effects
Drug	**Major Side Effects**
Lidocaine	CNS: dizziness, paresthesias, confusion, delirium, stupor, coma, seizures
Quinidine	Hypotension
	GI: nausea, vomiting, diarrhea, anorexia, abdominal pain
	"Cinchonism": tinnitus, hearing loss, visual disturbances, confusion, psychosis
	Rash, fever, anemia, thrombocytopenia
	"Quinidine syncope"
Procainamide	Drug-induced lupus erythematosus
	Nausea, vomiting
	Hypotension
	Giddiness, psychosis
Disopyramide	Anticholinergic; urinary retention, constipation, blurred vision, closed-angle glaucoma
	Congestive heart failure
Phenytoin	CNS: nystagmus, ataxia, drowsiness, stupor
	Nausea, anorexia
	Rash, gingival hypertrophy, megaloblastic anemia, lymph node hyperplasia, peripheral neuropathy, hyperglycemia, hypocalcemia
Propranolol	Bronchoconstriction, exacerbation of congestive heart failure, bradycardia, ischemia upon withdrawal, fatigue, depression, impotence
Bretylium	Orthostatic hypotension
	Transient hypertension, tachycardia, and worsening of arrhythmias (initial catecholamine release)
	Nausea, vomiting
Verapamil	Left ventricular failure, bradycardia, AV block
Tocainide	CNS: dizziness, tremor, paresthesias, ataxia, confusion
	GI: nausea, vomiting
Amiodarone	Agranulocytosis, pulmonary fibrosis, elevation of hepatic enzymes, corneal microdeposits, bluish-gray skin discoloration, hyper- or hypothyroidism, nausea, constipation, anorexia, bradycardia, exacerbation of heart failure; elevates plasma levels of digoxin, quinidine, procainamide; potentiates effects of warfarin (side-effects minimized by maintenance doses ≤ 300 mg/d); hypotension with IV administration.
Mexiletine	CNS: dizziness, tremor, paresthesias, ataxia, confusion
	GI: nausea, vomiting
Flecainide	Congestive heart failure, sinus node dysfunction, dizziness, blurred vision, incessant ventricular tachycardia
Propafenone	Dizziness, blurred vision, disturbances in taste
Moricizine	Nausea, dizziness, headache
Adenosine	Transient flushing, chest discomfort, dyspnea
Solatol	Same as propranolol, prolonged QT

AV = Atrioventricular; CNS = central nervous system; GI = gastrointestinal; IV = intravenous

complexes that may trigger the arrhythmia. Quinidine can terminate existing atrial flutter or fibrillation in about 10 to 20% of patients, especially if the arrhythmia is recent in onset and the atria are of normal size. Because quinidine slows the rate of atrial flutter and also exerts a vagolytic effect on AV nodal conduction, it may increase the ventricular response in patients with atrial flutter. Therefore, the patient should be treated with digitalis, a beta-blocker, verapamil, or diltiazem to control the ventricular rate before quinidine is administered. Prior to electrical cardioversion, quinidine may be administered to attempt chemical conversion of atrial fibrillation or atrial flutter, and it may also help maintain sinus rhythm once it is achieved, either chemically or electrically.

Quinidine may produce syncope in 0.5 to 2% of patients, thought most often to result from a polymorphic ventricular tachyarrhythmia termed *torsades de pointes* when associated with a long QT interval. Many patients with quinidine syncope have significantly prolonged QT intervals and are also receiving digitalis. Treatment for quinidine syncope entails discontinuation of the drug and avoidance of similar antiarrhythmic agents. Drugs that do not prolong the QT interval, such as lidocaine, tocainide, or phenytoin, may be tried. Phenobarbital or phenytoin and related drugs that induce hepatic enzyme production shorten the duration of quinidine's action by increasing its elimination. Quinidine elevates serum digoxin and digitoxin concentrations.

Procainamide

Electrophysiologic effects of procainamide resemble those of quinidine. Procainamide exerts less intense anticholinergic effects than disopyramide and quinidine. It has a major metabolite, *N*-acetyl procainamide (NAPA), that exhibits much weaker electrophysiologic effects than does procainamide. In patients with renal failure, NAPA levels increase more than procainamide levels and must be monitored to prevent toxicity. A sustained-release form is available that can be administered every 6 hours instead of every 3 to 4 hours; the total daily dose of both procainamide and the sustained-release form of procainamide should be the same. Procainamide depresses myocardial contractility only in high doses. It may produce peripheral vasodilation, probably via a mild ganglionic blocking action. The clinical indications for procainamide are very similar to those for quinidine. Although the effects of both drugs are similar, an arrhythmia not suppressed by one drug may be suppressed by the other. Conduction disturbances and ventricular tachyarrhythmias similar to those caused by quinidine can occur.

Procainamide does not increase serum digoxin levels. A systemic lupus erythematosus–like syndrome including arthralgia, fever, pleuropericarditis, hepatomegaly, and hemorrhagic pericardial effusion with tamponade has been described. The brain and kidneys are usually spared, and hematologic complications are unusual. Sixty to 70% of patients who receive procainamide develop antinuclear antibodies (ANA), but clinical symptoms occur in only 20 to 30% and are reversible when the drug is stopped. A positive ANA titer is not necessarily a reason to stop procainamide therapy.

Disopyramide

Disopyramide has electrophysiologic actions similar to those of quinidine and procainamide but exerts greater anticholinergic effects than either, without antiadrenergic effects. Disopyramide has prominent negative inotropic effects, and patients who have evidence of abnormal ventricular function should receive the drug either not at all or only with extreme caution.

The role of disopyramide in the treatment of atrial and ventricular arrhythmias is similar to that of quinidine. Like quinidine, it can cause a 1:1 conduction during atrial flutter if the patient is not adequately digitalized. Disopyramide does not alter digitalis metabolism.

Phenytoin

Phenytoin is a potent medication to treat central nervous system seizures, but its antiarrhythmic actions are limited. It effectively abolishes abnormal automaticity caused by digitalis toxicity. Sinus nodal automaticity and AV conduction are only minimally affected by phenytoin. Phenytoin's electrophysiologic effects *in vitro* appear similar to those of lidocaine. It exerts minimal hemodynamic effects. Phenytoin may be successful in treating atrial and ventricular arrhythmias due to digitalis toxicity but is much less effective in treating arrhythmias of other etiologies.

Tocainide

Tocainide is an analogue of lidocaine that undergoes negligible hepatic first-pass metabolism and therefore approaches 100% oral bioavailability. It is effective for ventricular tachyarrhythmias, but its efficacy appears to be less than that of lidocaine. Currently, its use has been curtailed owing to the occasional occurrence of granulocytosis.

Mexiletine

Mexiletine is similar to lidocaine in many of its electrophysiologic actions. It is effective for ventricular but not supraventricular tachyarrhythmias and may be useful when combined with type IA antiarrhythmic agents such as quinidine. Adverse effects and efficacy are similar to those of tocainide. Like tocainide, the toxic effects occur at plasma concentrations only slightly higher than therapeutic levels; therefore, effective use of this drug requires careful titration of dosage. A patient's response to intravenous lidocaine may help predict his or her response to oral mexiletine.

Beta Blockers

Propranolol is discussed here as a prototype beta-adrenergic receptor blocker. Differences in the pharmacokinetics, beta-adrenergic receptor selectivity, and antagonist/agonist actions have been discussed in Chapter 7.

Propranolol slows the sinus nodal discharge rate and lengthens AV nodal conduction time (PR interval increases) and refractoriness. These effects may be marked if the heart rate or AV conduction is particularly dependent on sympathetic tone or if sinus or AV nodal dysfunction is present. There is no effect on refractoriness or conduction in the His-Purkinje system at usual doses, and the QRS complex and QT interval do not change. It appears that the beta-blocking activity of propranolol is responsible for its antiarrhythmic effects because a local anesthetic (or quinidine-like) effect of propranolol is present only at doses 10 times those causing the beta-blocking effect. Serum concentrations vary from patient to patient, and the appropriate dose is determined by the patient's physiologic response, such as changes in resting heart rate or prevention of an increase in heart rate with exercise. If one beta blocker is ineffective against arrhythmias, the other beta blockers are usually also ineffective.

Propranolol is used most commonly to treat supraventricular tachyarrhythmias. Sinus tachycardia due to thyrotoxicosis, anxiety, and exercise may be slowed by propranolol. Propranolol does not usually terminate atrial flutter or fibrillation but may, by itself or combined with digitalis, control the ventricular response by prolonging AV nodal conduction time or refractoriness. Re-entrant supraventricular tachycardias using the AV node as one limb of the pathway (e.g., AV nodal re-entrant tachycardia and reciprocating tachycardias associated with the Wolff-Parkinson-White syndrome) may be prevented by propranolol alone or combined with other drugs. Propranolol is useful in treating ventricular arrhythmias associated with the prolonged QT syndrome and mitral valve prolapse. It usually does not prevent chronic recurrent ventricular tachycardia in patients with ischemic heart disease if the tachyarrhythmia occurs without acute ischemia. A new short-acting beta blocker, esmolol, has a half-life of only 9 minutes after intravenous infusion and may be useful for the acute termination of supraventricular tachycardias such as AV nodal re-entry.

Bretylium Tosylate

Bretylium tosylate initially releases norepinephrine stores from adrenergic nerve terminals but subsequently prevents further norepinephrine release. This initial catecholamine release may aggravate some arrhythmias and produce transient hypertension. Although the chemical sympathectomy-like state may be antiarrhythmic, other electrophysiologic properties may also contribute to the antiarrhythmic properties of bretylium. Bretylium does not depress myocardial contractility or affect vagal reflexes. After the initial increase in blood pressure, the drug may subsequently cause hypotension, usually orthostatic and controlled if the patient is supine. Bretylium is poorly absorbed orally and is commonly administered intravenously. Bretylium has been reported to induce spontaneous termination of ventricular fibrillation. Bretylium is indicated in patients with life-threatening ventricular arrhythmias that have not responded to lidocaine and possibly to other drugs.

Calcium Antagonists

The calcium antagonists have been discussed in Chapter 7. Verapamil and diltiazem do not affect cells with normal fast response characteristics (atrial and ventricular muscle, His-Purkinje system), but in fast channel–dependent cells rendered abnormal by disease, they may suppress electrical activity. Slow channel–dependent tissue (sinus and AV nodes) exhibits an increase in conduction time and refractoriness after verapamil or diltiazem administration. Therefore, they prolong the AH interval without affecting His-Purkinje conduction or the QRS interval. Sinus rate may decrease, but in intact animals it often does not change significantly because of counteraction by sympathetic reflexes activated by peripheral vasodilation. Verapamil and diltiazem do not affect directly refractoriness of atrial or ventricular muscle or the accessory pathway. Combined therapy with a beta blocker and verapamil can be attempted in patients with normal cardiac contractility, but the patient should be observed for the development of heart failure and/or symptomatic bradycardias because the compensatory sympathetic response to slow channel blockade is blocked. Calcium infusion or isoproterenol may counteract some of the adverse effects of verapamil until temporary pacing can be initiated.

Intravenous verapamil or diltiazem is effective for terminating sustained paroxysmal supraventricular tachycardias that are not terminated by vagal maneuvers, such as those reciprocating tachycardias employing the AV node or sinoatrial (SA) node in the tachycardia circuit. These drugs can decrease the ventricular response in patients with atrial fibrillation or flutter but convert only a small number of these rhythms to sinus rhythm. Verapamil or diltiazem may be used in patients with congestive heart failure and supraventricular tachycardia if it is thought that termination of the arrhythmia will relieve the heart failure. Verapamil may increase the ventricular response in patients with atrial fibrillation associated with the Wolff-Parkinson-White syndrome, and the drug is relatively contraindicated in that situation. Verapamil is usually not effective in patients with recurrent ventricular tachyarrhythmias and can result in hemodynamic collapse when given intravenously to patients with sustained ventricular tachycardia. A rare patient may have a verapamil-sensitive ventricular tachycardia believed due to triggered activity.

Amiodarone

Amiodarone is an antiarrhythmic agent initially introduced as an antianginal coronary vasodilator. It has a broad spectrum of antiarrhythmic efficacy against supraventricular and ventricular arrhythmias. Even though it prolongs the QT interval, it may suppress arrhythmias in patients with the long QT syndrome. It is effective in AV nodal re-entry, reciprocating tachycardias associated with the Wolff-Parkinson-White syndrome, atrial flutter, and atrial fibrillation, as well as ventricular tachyarrhythmias. Antiarrhythmic efficacy develops after several days of oral administration but may occur earlier with intravenous administration. Intravenous amiodarone may be life saving in cases of drug-refractory ventricular fibrillation or ventricular tachycardia. Amiodarone prolongs action potential duration and refractoriness in all cardiac tissues, slows sinus discharge, and prolongs AV nodal conduction time. Because of a variety of adverse effects, amiodarone should be administered only to patients with highly symptomatic or life-threatening arrhythmias and only if conventional drug therapy has failed.

Sotalol

Sotalol has both nonspecific beta-adrenoreceptor–blocking properties and class III effects, prolonging atrial and ventricular refractoriness by interfering with potassium currents. It is a racemic mixture of *d*- and *l*-isomers; the *l*-isomer has almost all of the beta-blocking action, while both isomers have the class III effects. Sotalol is effective for both atrial and ventricular tachyarrhythmias. It must be used with caution or avoided in patients with congestive heart failure, bradycardia, hypotension, or other contraindication to beta blockade. Excessive QT prolongation may occur (especially in the setting of renal insufficiency) and is dose dependent. *Torsades de pointes* occurs in about 2% of patients, usually those with severe underlying heart disease and prolonged QT interval initially.

Flecainide

Flecainide profoundly slows conduction in all cardiac fibers but only minimally increases refractoriness. It modestly depresses the cardiac inotropic state and should be used with caution in patients with heart failure. It is useful for ventricular tachyarrhythmias and is especially effective at suppressing PVCs or runs of nonsustained ventricular tachycardia. Therapy should begin in the hospital while the ECG is monitored because of the high incidence of aggravation of existing ventricular arrhythmias or onset of new ventricular arrhythmias (5 to 25% of patients). This proarrhythmic effect is especially prominent in patients who have sustained ventricular tachycardia and poor left ventricular function and receive higher doses of the drug. Dose increases should not be made more frequently than every 4 days. Flecainide has resulted in increased mortality in patients with asymptomatic ventricular arrhythmia following myocardial infarction, apparently a late proarrhythmic effect. Its use for ventricular arrhythmias should therefore be reserved for patients with refractory, sustained, life-threatening ventricular tachyarrhythmias with electrophysiologic study guidance. Flecainide may be very useful in patients with structurally normal hearts and AV nodal re-entry, tachycardias involving accessory pathways, or atrial fibrillation.

Moricizine

Moricizine is a type 1 antiarrhythmic agent that reduces the maximum velocity of the action potential upstroke with potency comparable to that of quinidine, but unlike quinidine, it does not prolong repolarization of atrial or ventricular muscle. It is therefore difficult to subclassify moricizine within class 1. It prolongs both AV nodal and His-Purkinje conduction and has no effect on left ventricular function. It is effective for both ventricular and supraventricular tachyarrhythmias.

Propafenone

Propafenone has electrophysiologic effects similar to those of flecainide but also has mild beta-blocking properties. It must therefore be used with caution in patients with poor left ventricular function, sinus nodal or AV conduction defects, or bronchospastic asthma. Propafenone is effective for ventricular and supraventricular arrhythmias. Its long-term proarrhythmic potential has never been established in a study similar to that described for flecainide.

Adenosine

Adenosine is an endogenous nucleoside available for intravenous administration for termination of paroxysmal supraventricular tachycardias due to AV nodal re-entry or AV re-entry associated with an accessory pathway. It causes marked but transient slowing of AV nodal conduction and sinus nodal discharge. Its half-life is less than 10 seconds, metabolized by erythrocytes and vascular endothelial cells. Therefore, adenosine must be given as a very rapid injection followed by a saline flush. The initial dose is 6 mg, followed, if necessary, in 2 minutes by 12 mg. It is antagonized competitively by methylxanthines such as caffeine and theophylline and potentiated by blockers of nucleoside transport such as dipyridamole. Adenosine terminates more than 95% of AV nodal re-entrant or AV re-entrant tachycardias within 30 seconds of administration. During atrial tachycardias or atrial flutter it often results in transient higher-degree AV block, aiding the differential diagnosis of the tachycardia mechanism. Symptoms of flushing, chest discomfort, and shortness of breath are common but transient.

Direct-Current Cardioversion and Defibrillation

Direct-current (DC) electrical cardioversion or defibrillation is the method of choice for terminating tachyarrhythmias that result in hemodynamic deterioration and those unresponsive to pharmacologic termination. Cardioversion refers to the delivery of a DC shock, usually of relatively low energy, synchronized with the QRS complex of an organized tachyarrhythmia. QRS synchronization is important to avoid delivering a shock during ventricular repolarization (T wave) that may precipitate ventricular fibrillation. Defibrillation refers to an asynchronously delivered, relatively high-energy shock to terminate ventricular fibrillation. Most supraventricular and ventricular tachyarrhythmias terminate with DC shock, although rhythms due to abnormally increased automaticity, especially if associated with digitalis intoxication, may not.

Prior to elective cardioversion the procedure should be explained to the patient and a physical examination, including palpation of all pulses, performed. Metabolic parameters (i.e., blood gases, electrolytes) should be normal, and ideally the patient should have fasted for 6 to 8 hours prior to the procedure. Digitalis should be withheld on the morning of cardioversion. Patients receiving digitalis without clinical evidence of toxicity are at very low risk for digitalis-induced complications. A short-acting barbiturate or benzodiazepine can be used for anesthesia. Intravenous access should be available, and resuscitation equipment should be at hand. Paddles should be lubricated with an electrolyte jelly and placed firmly to contact with the chest wall, either one paddle in the left infrascapular region and the other over the upper sternum at the third interspace, or one paddle to the right of the sternum at the first or second interspace and the other in the left midclavicular line at the fourth or fifth interspace. Shocks of 25 to 50 joules terminate most tachyarrhythmias except for atrial fibrillation, which may require 100 to 200 joules, and ventricular fibrillation, which may require 100 to 400 joules. If the first low-energy shock fails to terminate the arrhythmia, the energy should be titrated upward.

Tachycardia that produces complications of hypotension, congestive heart failure, or angina and does not response promptly to medical management should be terminated electrically. DC shock should be avoided if possible in patients with tachyarrhythmias caused by digitalis toxicity because of the risk of precipitating life-threatening refractory ventricular tachyarrhythmias. The administration of an antiarrhythmic drug prior to electrical termination of the arrhythmia may help maintain sinus rhythm after cardioversion. Many arrhythmias, especially chronic atrial fibrillation, commonly recur, and maintenance of sinus rhythm is sometimes a difficult problem.

Ventricular fibrillation due to an improperly synchronized or at times a properly synchronized shock is a complication of DC cardioversion. Immediate electrical defibrillation is mandatory. Systemic emboli occur, and patients with atrial fibrillation, especially those with a high risk for emboli (e.g., mitral stenosis, atrial fibrillation of recent onset, a history of emboli, a prosthetic mitral valve, enlarged left ventricle or left atrium, or congestive heart failure), may require anticoagulation for 3 weeks before cardioversion to lower the risk of emboli. Anticoagulation should be continued for several weeks after cardioversion. Elevation of myocardial enzyme fractions after cardioversion is not common.

Cardiac Pacemakers

Cardiac pacemakers are devices either implanted permanently or inserted temporarily, consisting of a pulse generator and an electrode that is either placed transvenously into the right ventricle and/or atrium or sutured directly into the epicardium at the time of surgery. Small electrical impulses, generated by the pulse generator and delivered via the electrode catheter, depolarize local cells to threshold potential and cause the entire chamber to depolarize. Pacemakers are widely used for treating bradyarrhythmias but can also be useful for treatment of some tachyarrhythmias. Indicators for temporary and permanent pacing are summarized in Table 8–6.

A pacemaker code has been developed to describe the pacing modalities available in any particular pacemaker. The first letter is the chamber paced (V = ventricle, A = atrium, and D = atrium and ventricle). The second letter is the chamber in which sensing occurs (V = ventricle, A = atrium, D = atrium and ventricle, and O = none). The third letter indicates the mode of response: sensed spontaneous activity inhibiting pacemaker output (I), trigger discharge into the refractory period (T), or trigger ventricular pacing in response to a sensed atrial event as well as inhibition of ventricular pacing during a sensed ventricular event (D). Some examples are illustrated in Table 8–7. An R added as a fourth letter indicates that the pacemaker is rate responsive; that is, it increases the pacing rate in response to physiologic need. Sensors used to measure physiologic need include activity (vibration), blood temperature, and respiratory rate (thoracic impedance).

The main advantages of dual-chamber pacing modes are the preservation of AV synchrony and the ability to increase ventricular paced rate with an increase in atrial rate. Safeguards are built into the VDD and DDD modes so that the ventricular response cannot exceed a predetermined upper rate, should an atrial tachyarrhythmia occur. Newer models can detect the onset of an atrial tachyarrhythmia and automatically switch from the DDD to the VVIR mode (mode-switching). A problem unique to dual-chamber pacing modes (DDD or VDD) that trigger ventricular depolarization from sensed atrial activity is pacemaker-mediated tachycardia. During pacemaker-mediated tachycardia, the pacemaker senses a retrograde P wave conducted after a paced ventricular beat or a PVC and triggers a subsequent ventricular depolarization after the programmed AV delay. This paced ventricular complex can again conduct retrogradely to the atrium, creating a sensed P wave that generates another paced ventricular complex. If this continues, a sustained "reciprocating" tachycardia that utilizes the pacemaker as the antegrade limb may occur. Extensive programmability of the newer pacemaker models, particularly that of atrial refractoriness, avoids pacemaker-mediated tachycardia in most cases.

For patients in whom a pacemaker is implanted only for an occasional symptomatic bradycardia or in whom optimal hemodynamic function is of no consequence, a simple VVI pacemaker may be sufficient. However, there are many patients in whom maintenance of physiologic AV synchrony may be advantageous. The normal increase in heart rate with exercise may be preserved either by dual-chamber, atrial-synchronous pacing (e.g., DDD mode), or, if the sinus node is incompetent, by a VVIR or DDDR pacemaker that is able to sense a physiologic event such as activity and increase its discharge rate appropriately. Pacemaker malfunction may be manifested by

TABLE 8–6	Indications for Temporary and Permanent Pacing

	Definitely Indicated	Probably Indicated	Probably Not Indicated	Definitely Not Indicated
Complete AV block				
Congenital (AV nodal)				
Asymptomatic				X
Symptomatic	T,P			
Acquired (His-Purkinje)				
Asymptomatic		T,P		
Symptomatic	T,P			
Surgical (persistent)				
Asymptomatic	T	P		
Symptomatic	T,P			
Second-degree AV block				
Type I (AV nodal)				
Asymptomatic				X
Symptomatic	T,P			
Type II (His-Purkinje)				
Asymptomatic		T,P		
Symptomatic	T,P			
First-degree AV block				
AV nodal				
Asymptomatic				X
Symptomatic			X	
His-Purkinje				
Asymptomatic				X
Symptomatic			X	
Bundle branch block (BBB)				
Asymptomatic				X
Symptomatic		P*		
Left BBB during right heart catheterization	T			
Acute myocardial infarction				
Newly acquired bifascicular BBB	T			
Pre-existing BBB				X
Newly acquired BBB plus transient complete AV block	T	P		
Second-degree AV block				
Type I (asymptomatic)				X
Type II	T	P		
Complete AV block	T	P		
Atrial fibrillation with slow ventricular response				
Asymptomatic				X
Symptomatic	T,P			
Sick sinus syndrome (bradytachy syndrome)				
Asymptomatic			X	
Symptomatic	T,P			
Hypersensitive carotid sinus syndrome				
Asymptomatic			X	
Symptomatic	T,P			

*No other cause found for symptoms.
AV = Atrioventricular; P = permanent; T = temporary; X = not indicated.

(1) failure to capture (activate myocardium), (2) abnormal sensing (oversensing or undersensing), or (3) abnormal discharge rate. Malfunction may be intermittent. Many pacemakers alter their discharge rate when the battery approaches depletion.

Nonpharmacologic Therapy of Tachyarrhythmias

Nonpharmacologic therapy of both supraventricular and ventricular tachyarrhythmias has become commonplace, especially in light of the incomplete efficacy and proarrhythmic potential of drug therapy, as well as the advances in nonpharmacologic techniques. Antitachycardia pacing techniques to terminate supraventricular tachycardias have become less important as catheter ablation techniques for AV nodal re-entrant tachycardia and AV re-entrant tachycardia associated with accessory pathways have improved. Antitachycardia pacing for ventricular tachyarrhythmias has become more important as the technique has been incorporated into implantable cardioverter-defibrillators (ICDs). Antitachycardia pacing can terminate many slower monomorphic ventricular tachycardias; the major hazard is acceleration of the ventricular tachycardia to a rapid, hemodynamically unstable rhythm, and therefore immediate defibrillation capability must also be available in the implanted device. If successful, antitachy-

TABLE 8-7	Common Pacemakers

Pacemaker Type	Code	Chamber Paced	Chamber Sensed	Mode
Ventricular asynchronous	VOO	V	None	Continuous pacing
Ventricular demand	VVI	V	V	Ventricular pacing inhibited by spontaneous QRS
Atrial demand	AAI	A	A	Atrial pacing inhibited by spontaneous P wave
Atrial synchronous, ventricular inhibited	VDD	V	A,V	Ventricular pacing follows a sensed P wave after a preset AV delay; ventricular pacing inhibited by spontaneous QRS; no atrial pacing
AV sequential	DVI	A,V	V	Ventricular pacing follows atrial pacing after a preset AV delay; ventricular and atrial pacing inhibited by spontaneous QRS; no P wave sensing
Optimal sequential	DDD	A,V	A,V	Ventricular pacing follows sensed P waves or atrial pacing after a preset AV delay; ventricular pacing inhibited by spontaneous QRS; atrial pacing inhibited by spontaneous P wave
Rate responsive	VVIR	V	V	Same as VVI or DDD, but pacing rate increases with physiologic demand
	DDDR	A, V	A, V	

A = Atrial; AV = atrioventricular; V = ventricular.

cardia pacing to terminate ventricular tachycardia is more desirable than delivery of a shock.

ICDs may improve survival in patients resuscitated from sudden cardiac death not associated with a myocardial infarction and in patients with hemodynamically unstable drug-resistant ventricular tachycardias. These devices automatically sense a rapid heart rhythm and deliver a 30- to 40-joule discharge to restore sinus rhythm. They can recycle and deliver subsequent shocks if the first shock is unsuccessful. Current devices also deliver stimuli to treat bradycardias and terminate tachycardias. They are implanted using a transvenous technique where the generator is placed under the skin in the upper abdominal or pectoral region, and electrodes for defibrillation, pacing, and sensing are passed through the subclavian veins to the right side of the heart. Drug therapy may be required after implantation of an ICD to limit the number of arrhythmia episodes or modify the arrhythmia so that syncope does not result prior to device activation, or to control supraventricular arrhythmias such as atrial fibrillation.

Catheter ablation of arrhythmias has assumed major importance. Radiofrequency energy delivered via a catheter provides a safe and effective means of creating small, discrete lesions to ablate either an arrhythmia focus or a pathway associated with an arrhythmia. Catheter ablation should be offered as an early therapy for patients with arrhythmias associated with Wolff-Parkinson-White syndrome and successfully eliminates the tachycardia in more than 95% of patients. In addition, selective ablation of the slow or fast AV nodal pathway responsible for AV nodal re-entrant tachycardia, while preserving anterograde AV nodal conduction, is also possible in more than 95% of patients. Inadvertent complete AV block occurs in <1%. The AV node can be modified or completely ablated in patients who have refractory atrial fibrillation or other atrial tachyarrhythmias with a rapid ventricular response. Complete AV junctional ablation leaves the patient pacemaker dependent but eliminates the rapid ventricular response. Catheter ablation for ventricular tachycardia is more difficult, but selected patients with monomorphic ventricular tachycardias associated with minimal or no structural heart disease may be good candidates for cathe-

ter ablation of ventricular tachycardia. Ablation of the circuit responsible for typical atrial flutter is successful in 80 to 90% of patients. Direct ablation of atrial tachycardia foci or the circuit responsible for atrial flutter may be possible in selected patients.

With the advent of catheter ablation techniques, surgery for patients with Wolff-Parkinson-White syndrome and AV nodal re-entrant tachycardia is performed less often, although it is occasionally used after a failed catheter ablation or in a patient with a concomitant indication for cardiac surgery. Surgical ablation of ventricular tachycardia can be performed in selected patients with sustained ventricular tachycardia unresponsive to medical therapy who have aneurysm formation with otherwise preserved left ventricular function. The operation consists of aneurysmectomy and endocardial resection and/or cryoablation of the tachycardia focus. Surgery eliminates ventricular tachycardia in about 70% of such patients. An additional 20% have ventricular tachycardia suppressed with previously ineffective drug therapy. Surgery for other varieties of ventricular tachycardia can occasionally be performed using direct excision of the focus, for example, the infundibulectomy scar after repairs of tetralogy of Fallot. A surgical procedure for atrial fibrillation (the maze procedure) may be useful in selected drug-refractory patients, and catheter ablation techniques for elimination of atrial fibrillation are under development.

SPECIFIC ARRHYTHMIAS

Sinus Nodal Rhythm Disturbances (Fig. 8-3)

Normal sinus rhythm refers to impulse formation beginning in the sinus node and, in adults, having a rate of between 60 and 100 beats/min. The P wave is upright in leads 1, 2, and aV_F and negative in lead aV_R. The rate of sinus nodal discharge is under autonomic control and increases with sympathetic and decreases with parasympathetic stimulation. *Sinus tachycardia* refers to a tachycardia of sinus origin with a rate exceeding 100 beats/min. Sinus tachycardia occurs with stresses such as fever, hypotension, thyrotoxicosis, anemia, anxiety, exertion, hy-

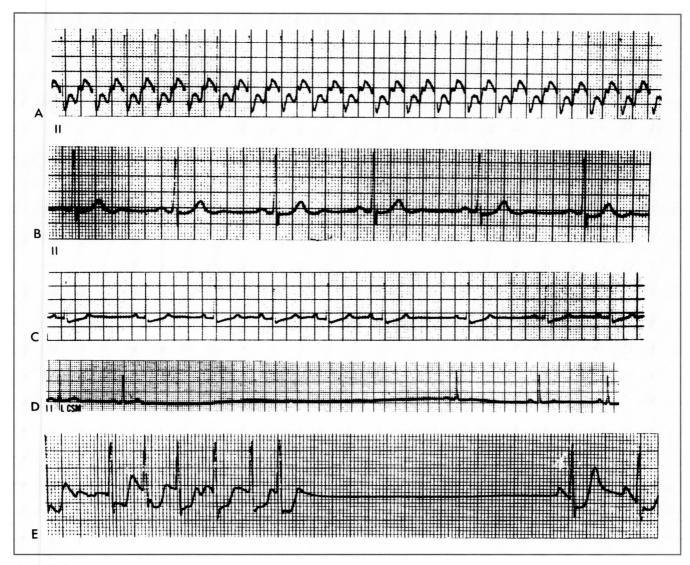

Figure 8–3

A, Sinus tachycardia (rate, 150 beats/min) in a patient during acute myocardial ischemia; note ST segment depression. *B,* Sinus bradycardia (rate, 46 beats/min) in a patient receiving propranolol. *C,* Respiratory sinus arrhythmia. The phasic variation in heart rate corresponds to a respiratory rate of approximately 12/min. *D,* Hypersensitive carotid sinus syndrome. Gentle left carotid sinus massage produced a prolonged period of asystole. *E,* Bradycardia-tachycardia syndrome. A fairly long period of asystole results before restoration of sinus rhythm upon termination of an episode of atrial fibrillation.

povolemia, pulmonary emboli, myocardial ischemia, congestive heart failure, shock, drugs (e.g., atropine, catecholamines, thyroid, alcohol, caffeine), or inflammation. Therapy should be focused on the cause of the tachycardia. If the sinus tachycardia must be treated directly, beta blockers may be used. Rarely, severely symptomatic drug-refractory inappropriate sinus tachycardia may be treated by ablation of the sinus node. *Sinus bradycardia* refers to sinus node discharge at a rate <60 beats/min. The P wave contour is normal, but sinus arrhythmia is often present. Sinus bradycardia frequently occurs in young adults, especially well-trained athletes, and is common at night. Sinus bradycardia can be produced by a variety of conditions, including eye manipulation, increased intracranial pressure, myxedema, hypothermia,

sepsis, fibrodegenerative changes, vagal stimulation, and vomiting, and the administration of parasympathomimetic drugs, beta-adrenergic–blocking drugs, or amiodarone. It occurs commonly in the acute phase of myocardial infarction, especially inferior myocardial infarction. Treatment of asymptomatic sinus bradycardia is usually not necessary. If cardiac output is low or tachyarrhythmias occur owing to the slow heart rate, atropine or, if necessary, isoproterenol may be effective. There is no drug that effectively and safely increases the heart rate over a long period, and therefore electrical pacing is the treatment of choice chronically if symptomatic sinus bradycardia is present.

Sinus arrhythmia refers to phasic variation in the sinus cycle length by greater than 10%. P wave morphology is normal. Respiratory sinus arrhythmia occurs when the PP interval shortens during inspiration as a result of reflex inhibition of vagal tone and lengthens during expiration. Nonrespiratory sinus arrhythmia refers to sinus arrhythmia not associated with the respiratory cycle. Symptoms are unusual and treatment not necessary.

In *sinus pause (sinus arrest)* and *sinoatrial exit block,* a sudden unexpected failure of a P wave occurs. In sinoatrial exit block, the PP interval surrounding the absent P wave is a multiple of the P to P intervals, implying that the sinus impulse was generated but did not propagate through the perinodal tissue to the atrium. If no such cycle relationship can be found, the term *sinus pause* or *sinus arrest* is employed. Acute myocardial infarction, degenerative fibrotic changes, digitalis toxicity, or excessive vagal tone can produce sinus arrest or exit block. Therapy involves searching for the underlying cause. Patients are not treated if they are asymptomatic. If they are symptomatic and the arrhythmia is not reversed by correcting the underlying causes, pacing is employed.

Wandering atrial pacemaker involves a transfer of the dominant pacemaker from the sinus node to latent pacemakers in other atrial sites or in the AV junction. The change from one pacemaker focus to another occurs gradually, associated with a change in the RR interval, PR interval, and P wave morphology. Treatment is usually not necessary except if symptoms occur from bradyarrhythmias.

The *hypersensitive carotid sinus syndrome* is characterized by cessation of atrial activity due to sinus arrest or SA exit block with light pressure over the carotid baroreceptors. In addition, AV block may be observed. Adequate junctional or ventricular escape complexes may not occur. Cardioinhibitory carotid sinus hypersensitivity is arbitrarily defined as ventricular asystole exceeding 3 seconds during carotid sinus stimulation. Vasodepressor carotid sinus hypersensitivity is defined as a fall in systolic blood pressure of 30 to 50 mm Hg without cardiac slowing, usually with reproduction of a patient's symptoms. The treatment in symptomatic patients is pacemaker implantation (to include at least a ventricular lead, because the sinus node slowing is usually also associated with AV block). Neither atropine nor pacing prevents the vasodepressor manifestations of carotid sinus hypersensitivity. Severe vasodepressor carotid sinus hypersensitivity occasionally requires denervation of the carotid sinus.

The term *sick sinus syndrome* is applied to a variety of sinus nodal and AV nodal abnormalities that occur alone or in combination. They include (1) persistent spontaneous sinus bradycardia not caused by drugs and inappropriate to the physiologic circumstances, (2) sinus arrest or exit block, (3) combinations of sinus and AV conduction disturbances, and (4) alternation of paroxysms of atrial tachyarrhythmias with periods of slow atrial and ventricular rates (bradycardia/tachycardia syndrome). The sick sinus syndrome may be associated with AV nodal or His-Purkinje conduction disturbances. If symptoms are present from bradyarrhythmias, pacemaker implantation is appropriate. Pacing for the symptomatic bradyarrhythmia combined with drug therapy for the tachyarrhythmia is often needed.

Sinus nodal re-entrant tachycardia accounts for 5 to 10% of paroxysmal supraventricular tachycardias. Its mechanism is presumed to be re-entry within the sinus node and the perinodal tissues, giving rise to a tachycardia, usually with a rate of 130 to 140 beats/min and containing P waves very similar to sinus P waves. AV block may occur without affecting the tachycardia. Vagal activation may slow and then abruptly terminate the tachycardia by its action on sinus nodal tissue. Tachycardia may be induced and terminated at electrophysiologic study with premature atrial stimulation. Treatment with a beta blocker, verapamil, or digitalis is effective therapy in most patients; otherwise, ablation can be employed.

Atrial Rhythm Disturbances (Fig. 8-4)

Premature atrial complexes (PACs) are characterized by a premature P wave, usually of differing morphology from the sinus P wave. PACs occurring very early in diastole may be followed by either aberrantly conducted QRS complexes or no QRS complexes (nonconducted PAC). In general, the shorter the interval from the last QRS to the P wave, the longer the PR interval after the PAC. PACs are less likely to be followed by a fully compensatory pause than are PVCs (see discussion further on). PACs are common in normal people but may occur in a variety of situations, such as infection, inflammation, myocardial ischemia, psychological stress, tobacco or alcohol use, or caffeine ingestion. PACs can be the forerunner of a sustained supraventricular tachyarrhythmia. They do not require therapy unless they produce symptoms or precipitate tachyarrhythmias.

In *atrial flutter,* the atrial rate is usually 250 to 350 beats/min. Ordinarily, the ventricular rate is half of the atrial rate. If AV block is greater than 2 : 1 in the absence of drugs, abnormal AV conduction is suggested. In children with pre-excitation syndrome or in patients with hyperthyroidism, 1 : 1 AV conduction can occasionally occur. Drugs such as quinidine, procainamide, or disopyramide may reduce the atrial rate to the range of 200 beats/min, raising the danger of 1 : 1 AV conduction. The atrial activity appears as regular sawtooth waves without an isoelectric interval between flutter waves. Flutter waves are commonly inverted in leads 2, 3, and aV_F. Ventricular response to atrial flutter may be irregular, generally of a Wenckebach nature, or regular. Chronic atrial flutter is usually associated with underlying heart disease, but paroxysmal atrial flutter may occur in patients without organic heart disease. Toxic and metabolic conditions such as thyrotoxicosis, alcoholism, and pericarditis may be associated with atrial flutter. There are fewer systemic emboli in patients with atrial flutter than in patients with atrial fibrillation, presumably because of the atrial contraction. Carotid sinus massage may decrease the ventricular response but does not terminate the arrhythmia. Cardioversion (< 50 joules) usually restores sinus rhythm. If atrial fibrillation ensues, a second shock of higher energy may be necessary. Rapid atrial pacing also terminates atrial flutter, although some patients develop atrial fibrillation instead of sinus rhythm; however, atrial fibrillation is usually an easier arrhythmia in which to control the ventricular response.

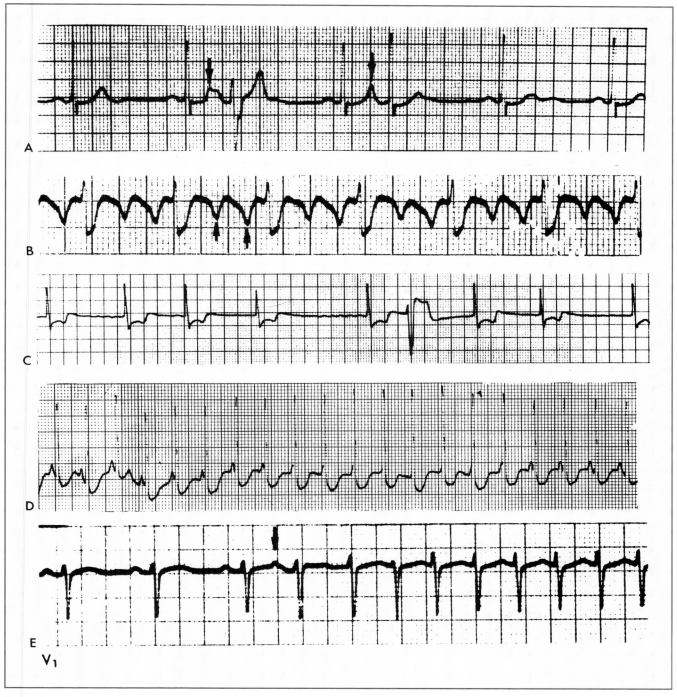

Figure 8-4

A, Premature atrial systoles with and without aberrancy. The first premature atrial systole *(arrow)* occurs at a shorter PR interval than does the second premature atrial systole *(arrow)* and conducts with a bundle branch block contour. The first premature atrial systole conducts with aberrancy, but the second does not because the first reaches the bundle branch system before complete recovery of repolarization. *B,* Atrial flutter. Flutter waves are indicated by *arrows*. The conduction rate is 3:1; i.e., three flutter waves to one QRS complex, and is a less common conduction ratio. *C,* Atrial fibrillation. Atrial activity is present as the undulating wavy baseline seen in the midportion of the electrocardiogram (ECG) strip. The premature ventricular complex (PVC) must be differentiated from aberrant supraventricular conduction. *D,* Nonparoxysmal junctional tachycardia with atrioventricular (AV) dissociation. *E,* Paroxysmal supraventricular tachycardia. Three sinus beats are interrupted by a premature atrial systole *(arrow),* which conducts with PR prolongation and initiates the supraventricular tachycardia. The most common mechanisms of this arrhythmia are AV nodal re-entry and AV re-entry using an accessory pathway as the retrograde limb.

Intravenous verapamil, beta blockers, or digitalis may slow the ventricular response to atrial flutter, and in a few patients may restore sinus rhythm. Type I antiarrhythmic drugs (such as quinidine, procainamide, or disopyramide) or type III drugs (sotalol or low-dose amiodarone) may terminate atrial flutter in some patients and are often useful in preventing recurrences. These drugs should not be administered unless AV nodal block has been previously achieved, because slowing the atrial flutter rate combined with the vagolytic effects of disopyramide or quinidine may lead to 1 : 1 AV conduction. Ablation of the atrial flutter circuit is very effective for typical atrial flutter if there is little or no associated atrial fibrillation.

Atrial fibrillation is characterized by totally disorganized atrial activation without effective atrial contraction. The ECG shows small, irregular baseline undulations of variable amplitude. The ventricular response is irregularly irregular, usually between 100 and 160 beats/min in the untreated patient with normal AV conduction. It is easier to slow the ventricular response with drugs in patients with atrial fibrillation than in patients with atrial flutter because of the greater number of atrial impulses reaching the AV node and decreasing the overall number of impulses that conduct to the ventricles. Chronic atrial fibrillation is usually associated with underlying heart disease, whereas paroxysmal atrial fibrillation may occur in apparently normal hearts. Atrial fibrillation commonly results from rheumatic heart disease (especially with mitral valve involvement), cardiomyopathy, hypertensive heart disease, pulmonary emboli, pericarditis, coronary heart disease, thyrotoxicosis, or heart failure from any cause. Episodes of atrial fibrillation may cause decompensation of patients with borderline cardiac function, especially those with mitral or aortic stenosis. Patients with chronic atrial fibrillation are at a greatly increased risk of developing systemic emboli, particularly if mitral valve disease is also present. Left atrial diameter tends to be smaller in patients with paroxysmal atrial fibrillation or in patients whose atrial fibrillation is easily terminated with cardioversion. Physical findings in patients with atrial fibrillation include a variation in the intensity of the first heart sound, absence of a waves in the jugular venous pulse, and an irregular ventricular rhythm. A pulse deficit may appear with faster ventricular rates; that is, the auscultated apical rate exceeds the palpable radial rate owing to failure of many of the ventricular contractions to generate a palpable peripheral pulse. Although atrial fibrillation with a very rapid ventricular response can sometimes seem regular, it is always irregular upon careful measurement, and true regularization of the ventricular rhythm in patients with atrial fibrillation should suggest development of sinus rhythm, atrial flutter, junctional rhythm, or ventricular tachycardia (the latter two may be manifestations of digitalis intoxication).

It is important to correct any precipitating causes of atrial fibrillation such as thyrotoxicosis, mitral stenosis, pulmonary emboli, or pericarditis. If the onset of atrial fibrillation is associated with acute hemodynamic decompensation, DC cardioversion should be employed (usually requires 100 to 200 joules). In the absence of decompensation, the patient should be treated with digitalis, a beta blocker, verapamil, or diltiazem to maintain a resting apical rate of 60 to 80 beats/min that does not exceed 100 beats/min after mild exercise. Quinidine or other type I antiarrhythmic drugs, or one of the type III drugs (sotalol or amiodarone) may be useful either to convert atrial fibrillation to sinus rhythm or to maintain sinus rhythm once it is restored with electrical cardioversion. The risks of chronic antiarrhythmic drug therapy must be balanced against the potential benefits of maintaining sinus rhythm. Patients with atrial fibrillation of less than 12 months' duration or without markedly enlarged left atria are more likely to remain in sinus rhythm after cardioversion. Anticoagulation prior to drug or electrical cardioversion is definitely indicated in patients at high risk of emboli (i.e., those with mitral stenosis, previous emboli, a prosthetic mitral valve, or cardiomegaly) and is probably indicated in any patient with atrial fibrillation of >1 week's duration. Anticoagulation therapy should be administered 2 to 3 weeks prior to cardioversion and continued for 2 to 4 weeks afterward. If termination of atrial fibrillation is urgent, a transesophageal ECG may be obtained prior to cardioversion to exclude a thrombus in the left atrial appendage. Patients with chronic atrial fibrillation or those with paroxysmal episodes of atrial fibrillation despite drug therapy are at increased risk of embolic stroke, especially if there is underlying heart disease. These patients should receive warfarin (international normalized ratio [INR] 2.0 to 3.0) if no contraindications exist, or possibly aspirin therapy. Rapid atrial pacing does not terminate atrial fibrillation.

In *atrial tachycardia with AV block,* the atrial rate is usually 150 to 200 beats/min, and variable degrees of AV conduction are present. This rhythm is often associated with digitalis excess and occurs most commonly in patients with significant organic heart disease, such as coronary heart disease, cor pulmonale, and digitalis intoxication. Isoelectric intervals are present between P waves in contrast to atrial flutter. Carotid sinus massage should be performed with caution in patients suspected of having digitalis toxicity. If the patient is not receiving digitalis, the rhythm may be treated with digitalis to slow the ventricular response, and subsequently type I or III agents may be added. If atrial tachycardia occurs in a patient receiving digitalis, digitalis toxicity should be suspected. Usually the ventricular response is not rapid, and withholding digitalis is sufficient therapy.

Chaotic or *multifocal atrial tachycardia* is characterized by atrial rates between 100 and 130 beats/min with marked variation in P wave morphology and irregular PP intervals. It occurs commonly in patients with pulmonary disease and in diabetics or older patients who eventually may develop atrial fibrillation. Digitalis is usually not helpful in this arrhythmia, but verapamil may be effective. Therapy is directed toward the underlying disease.

Atrioventricular Junctional Rhythm Disturbances

If suprajunctional pacemakers fail, a *junctional escape rhythm* may emerge at a rate of 35 to 60 beats/min. The junctional escape rhythm is usually fairly regular, but the rate may increase gradually when the escape rhythm first begins (warm-up phenomenon). A junctional rhythm may be associated with retrograde P waves for each QRS complex, or AV dissociation may be present.

Premature junctional complexes arise from the AV junction. A retrograde P wave is usually present but may be prevented by a sinus P wave. They usually do not require therapy.

A regular junctional rhythm with a rate exceeding 60 beats/min (usually between 70 and 130 beats/min) is considered an accelerated junctional rhythm or *nonparoxysmal AV junctional tachycardia*. The gradual onset and termination account for the term *nonparoxysmal* and may imply that the mechanism of the tachycardia is increased automaticity. Retrograde activation of the atria or AV dissociation may be present. Nonparoxysmal AV junctional tachycardia occurs most commonly in patients with underlying heart disease, such as inferior myocardial infarction, myocarditis, and acute rheumatic fever, or after open heart surgery. The most common cause is digitalis excess. Therapy is directed toward the underlying etiologic factor.

The *paroxysmal supraventricular tachycardias* (PSVTs) are regular tachycardias that occur and terminate suddenly. They are due to a variety of mechanisms, the most common of which are AV nodal re-entry (approximately 60% of cases) and AV re-entry using a concealed accessory bypass tract (approximately 30% of cases). Sinus nodal re-entry, intra-atrial re-entry, and automatic atrial tachycardias account for the remaining PSVTs.

AV nodal re-entry is characterized by narrow QRS complexes (unless functional aberration has occurred), sudden onset and termination, and regular rates, usually between 150 and 250 beats/min. Carotid sinus massage may slow the tachycardia slightly, and if termination occurs, it is abrupt. AV nodal re-entry commonly occurs in patients with no organic heart disease. Symptoms vary according to the rate of the tachycardia and the presence of organic heart disease. In some patients, rest, reassurance, and sedation may abort an attack. Vagal maneuvers including Valsalva, carotid sinus massage, and gagging may terminate the tachycardias and should be repeated after each pharmacologic intervention. Intravenous adenosine, 6 to 12 mg, or verapamil, 5 to 10 mg, terminates AV nodal re-entry in over 95% of cases and is the treatment of choice, should vagal maneuvers fail. If the patient is experiencing hemodynamic compromise, DC cardioversion with low energies is effective. Digoxin, beta blockers, verapamil, and diltiazem are the initial drug choices for chronic therapy, and the type IA, IC, or III agents are also effective in resistant cases. In patients with drug inefficacy or intolerance, or who prefer to avoid long-term drug therapy, selective catheter ablation of the slow or fast AV nodal pathway should be considered.

Paroxysmal supraventricular tachycardia may be caused by re-entry utilizing a retrograde concealed accessory pathway. The presence of the accessory pathway is not evident during sinus rhythm because antegrade accessory pathway conduction is not present, and therefore the

ECG manifestations of the Wolff-Parkinson-White syndrome are not evident. However, the mechanism of tachycardia is the same as that in most patients with the Wolff-Parkinson-White syndrome, that is, antegrade conduction over the AV node and retrograde conduction over the accessory pathway. Because it takes a relatively long time for the impulse to travel through the ventricular tissue to the accessory pathway and back to the atrium, the retrograde P wave during this form of tachycardia occurs after completion of the QRS complex, usually in the ST segment or early T wave. In distinction, patients with AV nodal re-entrant tachycardias usually have their retrograde P wave inscribed during or just after the QRS complex, although longer retrograde conduction intervals can occur in AV nodal re-entry. Tachycardia rates tend to be somewhat faster than those in AV nodal re-entry (≥ 200 per minute), but a great deal of overlap exists. Vagal maneuvers, adenosine, verapamil, and diltiazem are excellent choices for prompt termination. Chronic therapy often involves combinations of drugs that prolong accessory pathway conduction time and refractoriness (e.g., quinidine or flecainide) and drugs slowing AV nodal conduction. Catheter ablation of the accessory pathway is an excellent option.

Pre-Excitation Syndromes (Fig. 8–5)

Pre-excitation syndromes occur when ventricular activation occurs earlier than would be expected using the normal AV conduction system. There are several varieties of anomalous AV connections; the most common is the Wolff-Parkinson-White syndrome, in which an accessory AV pathway connects atrium with ventricle, short-circuiting the normal AV conduction system. A portion of the ventricle is activated via conduction over the accessory pathway before the remainder of the ventricle is activated via the normal AV conduction system, and the resultant QRS is a fusion of activation initiated by each of the two (normal and abnormal) AV pathways. Therefore, the PR interval is usually shortened (<0.12 second), and the duration of the QRS is increased (>0.12 second). The initial slurring of the QRS secondary to ventricular pre-excitation is referred to as the delta wave. Although the Wolff-Parkinson-White syndrome has been divided into type A (positive delta wave in V_1 and V_6) and type B (negative delta wave in V_1 and positive delta wave in V_6), this classification system is a gross oversimplification of the many ECG varieties produced by AV connections at different sites and is not very useful clinically. Accessory AV pathways may be located anywhere along the AV ring on either the left or right side or along the septum and are occasionally multiple.

The most common arrhythmia caused by an abnormal AV connection is termed *orthodromic* reciprocating tachycardia: the antegrade limb of the re-entrant circuit is the AV node, and the retrograde limb is the accessory pathway. The more unusual *antidromic* tachycardia utilizes the accessory pathway for the antegrade limb and the AV node as the retrograde limb. In the orthodromic variety, the QRS complexes either are normal or exhibit

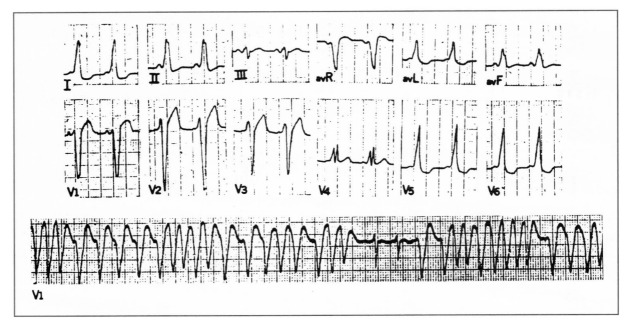

Figure 8-5
Pre-excitation syndrome is apparent in the 12-lead electrocardiogram (ECG) (short PR interval, wide QRS, delta wave). During atrial fibrillation the ventricular rate is extremely rapid, at times approaching 350 beats/min. The gross irregularity of the cycle lengths, wide QRS complexes interspersed with normal QRS complexes, and very rapid rate should suggest the diagnosis of atrial fibrillation and an atrioventricular (AV) bypass tract.

functional left or right bundle branch block. In the antidromic variety, the QRS complexes are totally pre-excited and consist of a wide, bizarre QRS. Similar pre-excited QRS complexes can occur when an atrial tachyarrhythmia (e.g., atrial fibrillation) results in an extremely rapid ventricular response via the accessory AV connection. Most adults with pre-excitation have normal hearts, although Ebstein's anomaly has an increased incidence of pre-excitation. Sudden death occurs rarely but may be a threat in patients with atrial fibrillation and rapid ventricular responses or in patients with associated congenital anomalies.

Patients who have frequent episodes of tachyarrhythmias and/or in whom the arrhythmias cause significant symptoms should receive therapy. Drugs that prolong refractoriness of the accessory pathway (e.g., quinidine, procainamide, disopyramide, and flecainide) or the AV node (e.g., digitalis, verapamil, and propranolol) may be effective in treating the reciprocating tachycardia; long-term therapy may require one drug from each group or drugs with both properties (propafenone, sotalol, or amiodarone). Drugs that prolong accessory pathway refractoriness are effective in slowing the ventricular rate during atrial flutter or atrial fibrillation. Because digitalis has been reported to shorten refractoriness in the accessory pathway and accelerate the ventricular response in some patients with atrial fibrillation, it is advisable not to use digitalis as a single drug in patients with the Wolff-Parkinson-White syndrome. Lidocaine and intravenous verapamil have also been reported to increase the ventricular response during atrial fibrillation in some patients with the Wolff-Parkinson-White syndrome. Termination of an acute episode of orthodromic reciprocating tachycardia may be approached as for AV nodal re-entry, but intravenous verapamil should not be given in patients with atrial fibrillation or flutter. Catheter ablation of accessory pathways is highly effective and safe; it should be considered in any patient with Wolff-Parkinson-White syndrome and symptomatic arrhythmias. Patients with delta waves on their ECG but with no history of tachycardia should generally not be treated.

Ventricular Rhythm Disturbances (Fig. 8-6)

Premature ventricular complexes are premature, bizarrely shaped QRS complexes of prolonged duration differing in contour from the dominant QRS complex. The T wave is large and oriented in the opposite direction from the major QRS deflection. The sinus node and atria are usually not activated prematurely by retrograde conduction from the PVC, and therefore a "compensatory pause" results; that is, the pause after the PVC is sufficiently long that the interval between the two normally conducted QRS complexes flanking the PVC equals two sinus cycle lengths. A PVC that does not produce a pause is termed interpolated. Two successive PVCs are termed a pair or couplet, and three or more successive PVCs are arbitrarily termed ventricular tachycardia. If PVCs have different contours, they are called multifocal, multiform, polymorphic, or pleomorphic. If PVCs are not coupled to the previous QRS, parasystole should be considered; however, many nonparasystolic PVCs do not exhibit fixed coupling. The prevalence of PVCs increases with age. They are often asymptomatic but can give rise to palpitations, or if present in long runs of bigeminy, may pro-

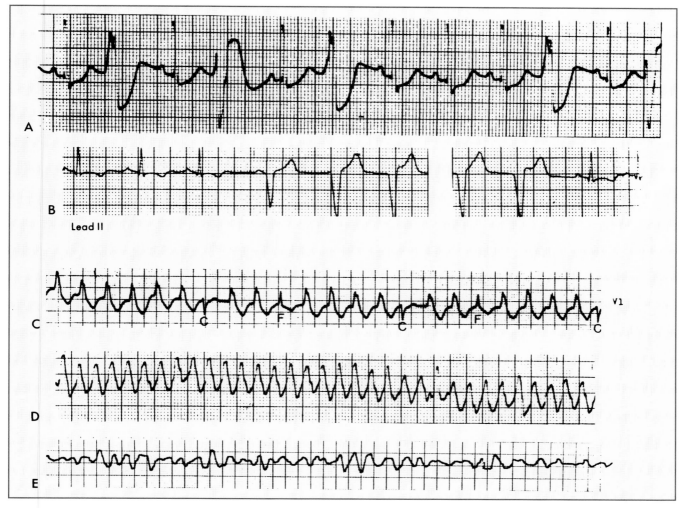

Figure 8–6

A, Multiform premature ventricular systoles. Each sinus beat is followed by premature ventricular complexes (PVCs) that have two contours, one predominantly upright and the other predominantly negative. *B,* Accelerated idioventricular rhythm. The sinus rate slows slightly and allows the escape of an idioventricular rhythm. A fusion beat with a short PR interval results. Subsequently the sinus node once again regains control of the ventricular rhythm. *C,* Ventricular tachycardia. A regular wide complex tachycardia is present. Atrial activity is not readily apparent. The complexes marked C and F most likely represent capture and fusion complexes that confirm the ventricular origin of the arrhythmia. *D,* Ventricular flutter. Ventricular depolarization and repolarization appear as a sine wave with regular oscillations. The QRS complex cannot be distinguished from the ST segment or T wave. *E,* Ventricular fibrillation. The baseline is irregular and undulating without any electrical evidence of organized ventricular activity.

duce hypotension, because they are premature and relatively ineffective at ejecting blood. The number of PVCs may increase during infection, ischemia, anesthesia, psychological stress, and excessive use of tobacco, caffeine, or alcohol. In the absence of underlying heart disease, the presence of PVCs probably has no significance regarding longevity or limitation of activity, and antiarrhythmic therapy is not indicated. The presence of PVCs identifies patients at an increased risk of cardiac death if they have coronary artery disease, hypertrophic cardiomyopathy, or mitral valve prolapse; however, treatment of PVCs has not been demonstrated to decrease sudden death. If drug therapy is indicated (usually only in patients with symptoms), lidocaine can be used acutely, and any type I or III agent may be considered for chronic therapy.

Ventricular tachycardia occurs when three or more consecutive PVCs occur with a rate exceeding 100/min. The QRS complexes usually have a prolonged duration and bizarre shape, with ST and T vectors opposite to the major QRS deflection. Atrial activity may be independent of ventricular activity (AV dissociation), or the atrium may be depolarized by the ventricles retrogradely (ventriculoatrial association). QRS contours may be unchanging (uniform) or may vary. The differentiation between sustained and nonsustained ventricular tachycardia is somewhat arbitrary but clinically useful; one guideline is that sustained ventricular tachycardia lasts at least 30 seconds or requires termination prior to 30 seconds because of hemodynamic decompensation.

The ECG distinction between supraventricular tachycardia with abnormal intraventricular conduction and ventricular tachycardia can be difficult. Supraventricular tachycardia may be associated with prolonged QRS complexes when pre-existing bundle branch block is present, functional aberration exists, or conduction over an accessory pathway is present. When fusion or capture QRS complexes occur during a wide-complex tachycardia (that is, early, narrow complexes that are either partially [fusion] or completely [capture] caused by activation from a supraventricular source), the ventricular origin of the tachycardia can be assumed. The identification of AV dissociation, sometimes requiring esophageal or intracardiac recordings to determine atrial activity, is much more characteristic of ventricular than supraventricular tachycardia. However, only about 50% of ventricular tachycardias demonstrate complete AV dissociation. In addition, the following characteristics favor a supraventricular origin: slowing or termination of the tachycardia by increased vagal tone, onset after a premature P wave; RP interval ≤ 100 msec, more atrial impulses than ventricular impulses (e.g., $2:1$ AV conduction), initiation of wide complexes after a long/short cycle sequence; and rsR′ in V_1. With preceding normal QRS conduction, if left axis deviation or QRS duration of ≥ 140 msec is present during tachycardia, ventricular tachycardia is likely.

Ventricular tachycardia occurs in patients with ischemic heart disease, congestive and hypertrophic cardiomyopathy, mitral valve prolapse, valvular heart disease, and primary electrical disease (no identifiable structural heart disease). Even short runs of ventricular tachycardia may be important when detected in the late hospital phase of acute myocardial infarction, because the 1-year mortality rate of this group appears to be much greater than for patients without tachycardia.

Deciding when to treat patients with ventricular tachycardia is sometimes difficult. Patients with chronic recurrent sustained ventricular tachycardia and those with symptomatic nonsustained ventricular tachycardia are treated. Treatment of patients with asymptomatic nonsustained ventricular tachycardia is controversial. Acute therapy of ventricular tachycardia is achieved with intravenous lidocaine; if unsuccessful, intravenous procainamide, bretylium, or amiodarone may be used. If hypotension, shock, angina, congestive heart failure, or symptoms of cerebral hypoperfusion are present, the rhythm should be terminated promptly with DC cardioversion, beginning with very low energies (10 to 50 joules) synchronized with the QRS. DC cardioversion of digitalis-induced ventricular tachycardia may be hazardous but is sometimes necessary. If ventricular tachycardia is recurrent despite drug therapy, pacing may occasionally be useful for termination. Before chronic drug therapy is instituted, a search for reversible conditions contributing to the arrhythmia should be done; for example, metabolic abnormalities, hypoxia, digitalis excess, and congestive heart failure should be corrected. Effective drugs for chronic therapy include quinidine, procainamide, disopyramide, mexiletine, sotalol and amiodarone. Phenytoin is usually not successful unless digitalis toxicity is present, and propranolol is usually unsuccessful unless the ventricular tachycardia is related to ischemia or catecholamine stimulation. Amiodarone is commonly utilized in patients with left ventricular dysfunction because of its high efficacy and the proarrhythmic potential of many of the other drugs. Combinations of drugs are sometimes necessary. Implantable cardioverter-defibrillators, catheter ablation, or surgery may be considered in patients with ventricular tachycardia refractory to drug therapy.

Accelerated idioventricular rhythm refers to impulse formation originating in the ventricle with a rate of approximately 60 to 110 beats/min. It often competes with the sinus node for control of the heart, and fusion and capture complexes occur commonly. The onset of the arrhythmia is often gradual (nonparoxysmal), and enhanced automaticity is presumed to be the mechanism. Precipitation of more rapid ventricular arrhythmias is not common. The arrhythmia usually occurs in patients with acute myocardial infarction or digitalis toxicity, and suppressive therapy is usually not necessary. If symptoms occur or if more malignant tachyarrhythmias result, therapy as noted above is indicated. Often simply increasing the sinus rate with atropine or atrial pacing suppresses the accelerated idioventricular rhythm.

Ventricular fibrillation generates little or no blood flow and is usually fatal within 3 to 5 minutes unless terminated. Ventricular fibrillation is recognized by the presence of irregular undulations of varying contour and amplitude without distinct QRS complexes, ST segments, or T waves. *Ventricular flutter* appears as a sine wave with regular, large oscillations occurring at a rate of 150 to 300 per minute. Ventricular fibrillation occurs in a variety of situations, including coronary artery disease, antiarrhythmic drug administration, hypoxia, ischemia, atrial fibrillation with rapid ventricular rates in the pre-excitation syndromes, accidental electrical shock, and poorly timed cardioversion. Most patients resuscitated from out-of-hospital cardiac arrest have ventricular fibrillation as their arrhythmia, often without acute myocardial infarction. Treatment is an immediate nonsynchronized DC shock using 200 to 400 joules. If ventricular fibrillation has been present for more than a few minutes, correction of metabolic abnormalities may aid in electrically converting the rhythm, although DC shock should not be delayed to await correction of hypoxia or acidosis. Once ventricular fibrillation has been terminated, medications to prevent recurrence of ventricular fibrillation should be initiated (e.g., lidocaine). Ventricular fibrillation rarely, if ever, terminates on its own and is lethal unless DC shock is applied.

Long QT Syndrome

The term *torsades de pointes* refers to a ventricular tachyarrhythmia characterized by QRS complexes of changing amplitude that appear to twist around the isoelectric line, occurring in the setting of a prolonged QT interval. Episodes of torsades de pointes often terminate spontaneously, but ventricular fibrillation may supervene. The syndrome may be either congenital or acquired. Acquired forms may be caused by any antiarrhythmic drug that prolongs the QT interval (e.g., quinidine, procainamide, disopyramide, or sotalol) or by psychoactive drugs such as phenothiazines and tricyclic antidepressants. In addition, potassium or magnesium depletion, liquid protein

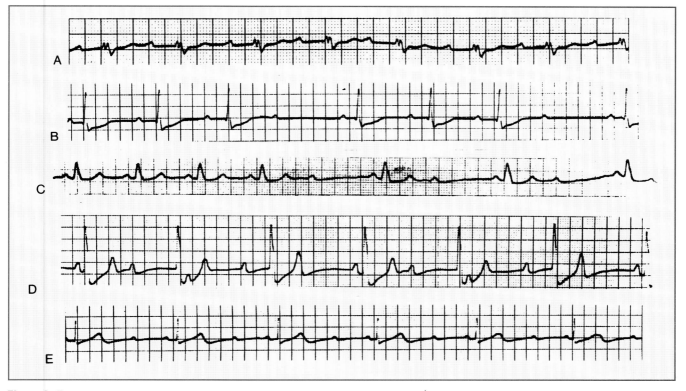

Figure 8–7
A, First-degree atrioventricular (AV) block. The PR interval is prolonged. *B,* Second-degree AV block (type I, Wenckebach), characterized by progressive PR prolongation preceding the nonconducted P wave. In the setting of a normal QRS complex, Wenckebach almost always occurs at the level of the AV node. *C,* Second-degree AV block, type II. Left bundle branch block is present in this recording of lead I. Sudden failure of AV conduction results, without antecedent PR prolongation. *D,* Acquired third-degree (complete) AV block. Complete AV dissociation is present owing to complete AV heart block. Atria and ventricles are under control of separate pacemakers, the sinus node and an idioventricular escape rhythm, respectively. *E,* Congenital third-degree (complete) AV block in a young adult at the level of the AV node. The QRS complex is normal.

diet, and other metabolic abnormalities may be associated with the long QT syndrome. Acute therapy involves withdrawing the offending drug and correcting metabolic abnormalities. Antiarrhythmic agents that prolong the QT interval may worsen the arrhythmia. Intravenous magnesium, 1 to 2 gm over 5 to 10 minutes, often eliminates the tachycardia. Temporary ventricular or atrial pacing is also effective therapy for suppressing the bursts of polymorphic tachycardia. Isoproterenol has been reported to be effective until pacing is instituted. If a polymorphic ventricular tachycardia resembling torsades de pointes is present but the QT interval is normal, standard antiarrhythmic drugs may be given.

Patients with congenital prolonged QT syndrome who are at increased risk for sudden death include those who have family members who died suddenly at an early age and those who have experienced syncope or torsades de pointes. ECGs should be obtained from all family members when a patient presents with suspected congenital long QT syndrome. Auditory stimuli, psychological stress, and exercise may provoke an arrhythmia in susceptible patients. For patients who have idiopathic long QT syndrome but no syncope, complex ventricular arrhythmias, or family history of sudden cardiac death, no therapy is recommended. In asymptomatic patients with long QT syndrome who have complex ventricular arrhythmias or a family history of premature sudden cardiac death, beta blockers at maximally tolerated doses are recommended. In patients with syncope, beta blockers at maximally tolerated doses, combined with phenytoin or phenobarbital if necessary, are suggested. For patients who continue to have syncope despite drug therapy, left-sided cerviocothoracic sympathetic ganglionectomy has been effective, because sympathetic imbalance appears to be important in the pathogenesis of this syndrome. An ICD is indicated in patients who continue to have ventricular tachyarrhythmias despite these therapies.

Heart Block (Fig. 8–7)

Heart block refers to a disturbance of impulse conduction and should be distinguished from interference, a normal phenomenon in which impulse conduction is blocked owing to physiologic refractoriness in the wake of a preceding impulse. Heart block may occur anywhere in the heart but is commonly recognized by ECG in the AV node, His bundle, or bundle branches. In *first-degree AV heart block,* AV conduction time is prolonged (PR interval ≥ 0.20 second), but all impulses are conducted. *Second-degree heart block* occurs in two forms: *type I second-degree heart block* (Wenckebach) is characterized by a progressive lengthening of the PR interval until a P wave is not conducted. *Type II second-degree AV heart block* denotes occasional or repetitive sudden block of a P wave without prior measurable lengthening of the PR interval. Type II AV block often antedates the development of Stokes-Adams syncope and complete AV block, whereas type I AV block with a normal QRS complex is usually more benign and does not progress to advanced forms of AV conduction disturbances. In the patient with acute myocardial infarction, type I AV block usually accompanies inferior infarction, is transient, and does not require temporary pacing, whereas type II AV block usually accompanies anterior myocardial infarction, may require temporary or permanent pacing, and is associated with a high mortality, mostly due to pump failure. First-degree or type I second-degree AV block can occur in healthy young people, especially well-trained athletes. Any medication that affects AV nodal conduction (e.g., digitalis, beta blockers, or verapamil) may cause first- or second-degree AV block.

Type I AV block with a normal QRS complex is usually at the level of the AV node proximal to the His bundle. Type II AV block usually occurs in association with a bundle branch block and is localized to the His-Purkinje system. Type I AV block in a patient with a bundle branch block may represent block in either the AV node or the His-Purkinje system. Type II AV block in a patient with a normal QRS complex may be due to intra-His block but is more likely to be type I AV nodal block that exhibits small increments in AV conduction time. Note that 2:1 AV block may represent either AV nodal or His-Purkinje block.

Complete AV block occurs when no atrial activity conducts to the ventricles. The atria and ventricles are controlled by independent pacemakers, and thus complete AV block is one cause of AV dissociation. The ventricular rhythm is usually regular. If the AV block is at the level of the AV node (e.g., congenital AV block), the QRS complexes are normal in morphology and duration, with rates of 40 to 60 per minute, and respond to autonomic influences. If the AV block is in the His-Purkinje system (usually acquired), the escape rhythm originates within the ventricle, has a wide QRS and a slower rate, and is less reliable and under less autonomic influence. Causes of AV block include surgery, electrolyte disturbances, endocarditis, tumor, Chagas' disease, rheumatoid nodules, calcific aortic stenosis, myxedema, polymyositis, infiltrative processes such as amyloid, sarcoid, or scleroderma, drug toxicity, coronary disease, and degenerative processes. In children the most common type of AV block is congenital and is usually asymptomatic; in some, however, symptoms eventually develop, requiring pacemaker implantation. The indications for pacemaker therapy in heart block are summarized in Table 8–6. Atropine (for AV nodal block) and isoproterenol (for heart block at any site) may be used transiently while preparations are made for ventricular pacing. Drugs cannot be relied on to increase the heart rate for more than several

hours to a few days without producing significant side effects.

The term *AV dissociation* describes independent depolarization of the atria and ventricles. AV dissociation is not a primary disturbance of rhythm but is a "symptom" of an underlying rhythm disturbance produced by one or a combination of three causes that prevent the normal transmission of impulses from atrium to ventricle:

1. Slowing of the dominant pacemaker of the heart (usually the sinus node), allowing escape of a subsidiary or latent pacemaker. This is AV dissociation by default of the primary pacemaker and is often a normal phenomenon, for example, sinus bradycardia and a junctional escape rhythm.
2. Acceleration of a latent pacemaker that usurps control of the ventricles. This abnormally enhanced discharge rate of a usually slower subsidiary pacemaker is pathologic, for example, junctional or ventricular tachycardia.
3. Block at the AV junction that prevents impulses formed at a normal rate in a dominant pacemaker from reaching the ventricles so that the ventricles beat under the control of a subsidiary pacemaker, for example, complete AV block with a ventricular escape rhythm. It is important to remember that complete AV dissociation is not synonymous with complete AV block.

Syncope (See also Chapter 114)

Syncope refers to sudden transient loss of consciousness, usually due to transient cerebral hypoperfusion. Presyncope is described as a light-headed spell that, if more prolonged, would cause loss of consciousness. Both may occur in the same patient and have similar etiologies. The causes of syncope are summarized in Table 8–8.

Cardiac syncope is due either to lesions that obstruct outflow of blood from the heart or to arrhythmias. In patients with severe aortic stenosis or other causes of obstructive syncope, when the systemic vascular resistance decreases upon exercise, the heart is unable to augment cardiac output sufficiently to maintain perfusion and syncope results. Both tachyarrhythmias and bradyarrhythmias that result in cerebral hypoperfusion can cause cardiac syncope. The hypersensitive carotid sinus syndrome, described earlier, is a well-recognized cause of syncope.

The history and physical examination are valuable in excluding many causes of syncope (see Table 8–8). Even though the ECG may not reveal the actual arrhythmia causing syncope, ECG clues (e.g., the presence of simple or complex ventricular ectopy, evidence of a previous myocardial infarction, or the delta wave of the Wolff-Parkinson-White syndrome) may suggest potential arrhythmic causes. Prolonged ECG recording may be the cornerstone of diagnosis in arrhythmic syncope. On most occasions, more than 24 hours of recording are required to detect the responsible arrhythmia and a patient-activated event recorder is necessary. Exercise testing is also valuable in some patients whose arrhythmias are exercise induced. Patients with obstructive syncope such as aortic stenosis should not undergo exercise testing. Reproduc-

TABLE 8–8	Causes of Syncope

Cause	Features
Peripheral Vascular or Circulatory	
Vasovagal syncope (neurally mediated)	Prodrome of pallor, yawning, nausea, diaphoresis; precipitated by stress or pain; occurs when patient is upright, aborted by recumbency; fall in blood pressure without appropriate rise in heart rate
Micturition syncope	Syncope with urination (probably vagal)
Post-tussive syncope	Syncope after paroxysm of coughing
Hypersensitive carotid sinus syndrome	Vasodepressor and/or cardioinhibitory responses with light carotid sinus massage (see text)
Drugs	Orthostasis
	Occurs with antihypertensive drugs, tricyclic antidepressants, phenothiazines
Volume depletion	Orthostasis
	Occurs with hemorrhage, excessive vomiting or diarrhea, Addison's disease
Autonomic dysfunction	Orthostasis
	Occurs in diabetes, alcoholism, Parkinson's disease, deconditioning after a prolonged illness
Central Nervous System	
Cerebrovascular	Transient ischemic attacks and strokes are unusual causes of syncope; associated neurologic abnormalities are usually present
Seizures	Warning aura sometimes present, jerking of extremities, tongue biting, urinary incontinence, postictal confusion
Metabolic	
Hypoglycemia	Confusion, tachycardia, jitteriness prior to syncope; patient may be taking insulin
Cardiac	
Obstructive	Syncope is often exertional; physical findings consistent with aortic stenosis, hypertrophic obstructive cardiomyopathy, cardiac tamponade, atrial myxoma, prosthetic valve malfunction, Eisenmenger's syndrome, tetralogy of Fallot, primary pulmonary hypertension, pulmonic stenosis, massive pulmonary embolism
Arrhythmias	Syncope may be sudden and occurs in any position; episodes of dizziness or palpitations; may be a history of heart disease; brady- or tachyarrhythmias may be responsible—check for hypersensitive carotid sinus

tion of symptoms with upright tilt testing (see Approach to the Patient with Suspected or Confirmed Arrhythmias, last paragraph) is valuable in patients with vasovagal syncope. In selected patients, especially those with structural heart disease, invasive electrophysiologic studies may be useful to delineate the etiology of the syncope.

TABLE 8–9	Selected Causes of Sudden Death

Noncardiac
Central nervous system hemorrhage
Massive pulmonary embolus
Drug overdose
Hypoxia secondary to lung disease
Aortic dissection or rupture

Cardiac
Ventricular tachycardia
Bradyarrhythmias, sick sinus syndrome
Aortic stenosis
Tetralogy of Fallot
Pericardial tamponade
Cardiac tumors
Complications of infective endocarditis
Hypertrophic cardiomyopathy (arrhythmia or obstruction)
Myocardial ischemia
    Atherosclerosis
    Prinzmetal's angina
    Kawasaki's arteritis

Sudden Cardiac Death

The most commonly used definition of sudden death is unexpected, nontraumatic death occurring within an hour after the onset of symptoms. Sudden cardiac death claims approximately 1200 lives daily in the United States and is the leading cause of death among men between the ages of 20 and 60. By far the most common cause of sudden death is cardiac, and within that group, the most common cause is ventricular tachyarrhythmias.

Nonarrhythmic causes of sudden death are listed in Table 8–9.

Ventricular tachyarrhythmias, generally related to ischemic heart disease, are the most common cause of sudden cardiac death. Although 75% of patients resuscitated from ventricular fibrillation have extensive coronary artery disease, only 20% have evidence of acute transmural myocardial infarction at the time of sudden death. Approximately 75% of patients who experience sudden death have a previous history of cardiac disease; sudden death is the first manifestation of cardiac disease in the remainder. The difference in recurrence of sudden death in patients whose initial episode occurred with (2% at 1 year) and without (22% at 1 year) acute myocardial infarction may be due to different arrhythmia mechanisms. Patients with ventricular fibrillation at the time of an acute myocardial infarction probably do not need long-term antiarrhythmic therapy unless chronic late ventricular tachycardia is documented. The risk of recurrent ventricu-

TABLE 8–10	Risk Factors for Sudden Cardiac Death After Myocardial Infarction

1. Decreased left ventricular function (ejection fraction <40%)
2. Residual ischemia
3. Complex ventricular ectopy
4. Late potentials on signal-averaged ECG
5. Evidence of decreased vagal effect (blunted sinus cycle length variability or carotid baroreceptor sensitivity)
6. Induction of sustained monomorphic ventricular tachycardia with programmed ventricular stimulation

ECG = Electrocardiogram.

lar fibrillation is higher if there is evidence of left ventricular dysfunction or evidence of previous myocardial infarction. Nonatherosclerotic etiologies of ventricular tachyarrhythmias associated with sudden death are mitral valve prolapse, hypertrophic or other cardiomyopathies, antiarrhythmic drugs, myocarditis, prolonged QT syndrome, and Wolff-Parkinson-White syndrome with rapid antegrade conduction over an accessory pathway.

The identification of patients at high risk for sudden cardiac death can be difficult (Table 8–10). The occurrence of complex ventricular ectopy, including multiform PVCs, pairs, and ventricular tachycardia in survivors of myocardial infarction, is associated with a two- to threefold increase in subsequent sudden death; however, suppression of ventricular ectopy with antiarrhythmic agents has not been proven to decrease and possibly could increase the incidence of sudden death. The risk of sudden cardiac death and the incidence of complex ectopy are greater in patients with poor left ventricular function.

The signal-averaged ECG is a computerized technique that averages multiple QRS complexes to reduce noise and allow detection of low-amplitude, high-frequency potentials occurring just after the inscription of the QRS complex; these "late potentials" correspond to delayed and fragmented conduction in areas of the ventricle that are responsible for ventricular tachycardia. They are present in 73 to 92% of patients with sustained and inducible ventricular tachycardia after myocardial infarction, 0 to 6% of normal volunteers, and 7 to 15% of patients after myocardial infarction who do not have ventricular tachycardia. Late potentials after myocardial infarction constitute an independent risk factor that detects patients prone to develop ventricular tachycardia and can be combined with other data such as ejection fraction, spontaneous ventricular ectopy, or responses to stress testing to recognize with high sensitivity and specificity patients at risk for ventricular tachycardia or sudden cardiac death. It can also be used to detect patients with nonsustained ventricular tachycardia or syncope who may develop sustained ventricular tachycardia at electrophysiologic study.

The patient who has suffered sudden cardiac arrest in the absence of acute myocardial infarction and the patient with recurrent symptomatic ventricular tachyarrhythmias must be treated with antiarrhythmic therapy. The end point of antiarrhythmic therapy to be used to judge efficacy is often unclear. The mere attainment of

"therapeutic" serum levels of an antiarrhythmic agent is not sufficient to guard against recurrent ventricular tachyarrhythmias. Prolonged ECG monitoring is noninvasive, simple, and widely available. However, many patients with sudden death demonstrate very little spontaneous ectopy between episodes; therefore, suppression of spontaneous ectopy cannot be used as an end point in these patients. In addition, even in patients with spontaneous ectopy, it is not clear whether an appropriate end point would be elimination of all ventricular tachycardia, all complex ectopy, or all PVCs. Drug evaluation using exercise testing and prolonged ambulatory recording to judge efficacy has been reported to decrease the incidence of recurrent malignant tachyarrhythmias but can be used only in patients with spontaneous high-grade ventricular ectopy between episodes of sustained tachyarrhythmia. Likewise, serial electrophysiologic testing to guide antiarrhythmic therapy can be used in a subset of patients in whom ventricular tachycardia is inducible by programmed electrical stimulation. The suppression with a drug of ventricular tachycardia inducible by electrical stimulation provides an indicator of drug success that is better than suppression of spontaneous ectopy and can be used in patients with little or no spontaneous ectopy. If arrhythmias cannot be suppressed or slowed with drug therapy, or if there is no reliable indicator of drug efficacy, then either an ICD or empiric amiodarone therapy can be employed. Coronary artery revascularization alone is usually not sufficient to prevent recurrent ventricular tachyarrhythmias unless the episode was closely related to acute ischemia and left ventricular function is good.

Antiarrhythmic therapy in patients after myocardial infarction as prophylaxis for malignant cardiac arrhythmias has not been proven effective. Several large multicenter studies have demonstrated a decrease in the incidence of sudden death in patients treated with beta-adrenergic receptor blocking agents after myocardial infarction, and these drugs probably should be considered if no contraindication to their administration exists.

PRINCIPLES OF CARDIOPULMONARY RESUSCITATION

Cardiopulmonary resuscitation consists of basic and advanced life support. Upon evaluating a patient with suspected cardiac arrest, one should first quickly establish that the patient is truly unresponsive and not breathing. If a pulse is not present, a precordial thump to the midsternum may be tried. Subsequently, the "ABCs" of basic life support should be observed: Airway, Breathing, and Circulation. The mouth and pharynx should be examined to ensure that no obstruction is present. The tongue should be removed from the posterior pharynx by tilting the head backward and hyperextending the neck. This maneuver can sometimes cause resumption of spontaneous respiration. If no breathing is noted, mouth-to-mouth or mouth-to-nose breathing should be initiated in four quick breaths. Time is often wasted trying to intubate a patient when adequate ventilation could be accomplished immediately via mouth or mask ventilation. One should check to see that the chest rises with each ventilation. If a carotid pulse is not present after the initial ventilations, external cardiac compression over the lower half of the sternum (not over the xiphoid process) should be initiated. The sternum should be depressed 3 to 5 cm, with the patient lying on a hard surface. Compressions should be approximately 80 to 100 per minute, with a ratio of five compressions to one ventilation if two rescuers are present. A single rescuer must give 15 chest compressions alternating with two ventilations.

Advanced life support should be initiated while basic life support continues. Defibrillation should be applied if indicated as soon as possible and *is the single most definitive treatment available for most cardiac arrests.* Oxygen should be administered, and an adequate intravenous access should be established. If circulation has not been restored quickly, sodium bicarbonate (1 mEq/kg intravenously) is given to treat metabolic acidosis and is repeated after 10 minutes; further administration of sodium bicarbonate should be guided by blood gas and pH measurements once effective circulation is restored. Epinephrine (5 to 10 ml of a 1 : 10,000 solution administered via an intravenous, intracardiac, or endotracheal route every 5 minutes as needed) is useful in treating asystole and also in aiding defibrillation of fine (low-amplitude) ventricular fibrillation. Atropine (boluses of 0.5 mg IV at 5-minute intervals to a total dose of approximately 2 to 4 mg) can be administered for profound bradycardia. Isoproterenol given as a constant infusion (2 to 20 μg/min) and titrated according to response may be used to treat bradyarrhythmias if atropine is ineffective. Emergency cardiac pacing may be attempted for bradyarrhythmias if atropine and isoproterenol are unsuccessful.

Lidocaine, procainamide, bretylium tosylate, or intravenous amiodarone can be administered to help terminate ventricular tachyarrhythmias and prevent their recurrence. Intravenous furosemide and/or morphine may be used to relieve pulmonary edema. Calcium chloride (2.5 to 5 ml of a 10% solution repeated, if necessary, in 10 minutes) is given to increase myocardial contractility, especially if electromechanical dissociation is present. Calcium should be used with caution in a patient with known digitalis excess. Calcium chloride precipitates if given in the same intravenous line with sodium bicarbonate.

Electromechanical dissociation refers to the presence of cardiac electrical activity without appropriate mechanical activity. It may be caused by decreased filling of the heart (e.g., hypovolemia, cardiac tamponade, pulmonary embolus) or severe myocardial pump depression that may respond to calcium. Emergency pericardiocentesis may be attempted if cardiac tamponade is suspected.

The widespread application of cardiopulmonary resuscitation via education of the public and extensive emergency care systems in many cities has increased both the number of cardiac arrest victims who reach the hospital and the number who survive to be discharged. Survival critically depends on the time from arrest to the initiation of resuscitation and is best if basic life support can be initiated within 3 to 4 minutes and more definitive therapy (i.e., defibrillation) shortly thereafter.

REFERENCES

Driefus LS (Chairman): ACC/AHA Task Force. Guidelines for implantation of cardiac pacemakers and antiarrhythmia devices. J Am Coll Cardiol 1991; 18:1.

Emergency Cardiac Care Committee and Subcommittees, American Heart Association Guidelines for cardiopulmonary resuscitation and emergency cardiac care. JAMA 1992; 268(16):2171.

Fisch C: Electrocardiology of Arrhythmias. Philadelphia: Lea & Febiger, 1990.

Laupacis A, Albers G, Dunn M, Feinberg W: Antithrombotic therapy in atrial fibrillation. Chest 1992; 102(suppl):426S–433S.

Miles WM, Zipes DP: Pre-excitation syndromes. *In* Hurst JW (ed.): Current Therapy in Cardiovascular Disease. 4th ed. St. Louis: Mosby–Year Book, 1994, pp 77–83.

Naccarelli GV (ed.): Electrophysiology Self Assessment Program. Bethesda, MD: American College of Cardiology, 1996.

Zipes DP (Chairman): ACC/AHA Task Force. Guidelines for intracardiac electrophysiological and catheter ablation procedures. J Am Coll Cardiol 1995; 26:555.

Zipes DP: Cardiac arrhythmias. *In* Braunwald E (ed.): Heart Disease. A Textbook for Cardiovascular Medicine. 4th ed. Phildelphia: WB Saunders, 1992.

Zipes DP, Jalife J (eds.): Cardiac Electrophysiology. From Cell to Bedside. 2nd ed. Philadelphia: WB Saunders, 1995.

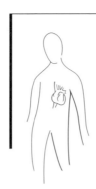

9 | Myocardial and Pericardial Disease

MYOCARDIAL DISEASE

Myocarditis

Myocarditis indicates involvement of the heart in an inflammatory process. Often the inflammation is caused by an infectious agent. In North America, it is typically viral (e.g., Coxsackie virus), whereas in South America, Chagas' disease due to the parasite *Trypanosoma cruzi* is more common. Infectious agents can cause myocardial damage by direct invasion of the myocardium, by production of a toxin (e.g., diphtheria), or by immunologic mechanisms. The latter is felt to be most important in viral myocarditis, with immunologic reaction to changes in cell surface or a new viral-related antigen. The inflammatory process may also involve the pericardium.

Myocarditis exhibits a broad range of manifestations, from an inapparent asymptomatic and self-limited process to uncommon fulminant inflammation and severe heart failure. Cardiac dysfunction may resolve or be persistent. Previous viral myocarditis is often suspected in patients with idiopathic dilated cardiomyopathy. However, this relationship is difficult to establish with certainty.

Myocarditis may be suspected when cardiac symptoms and signs develop in the setting of recent flulike syndrome. The symptoms are nonspecific and may include fatigue, dyspnea, and palpitations. Chest pain usually is from associated pericardial involvement but can simulate acute myocardial infarction. Tachycardia is common. If ventricular dysfunction is present, a third heart sound and mitral regurgitation murmur may be detected. Signs of overt congestive heart failure develop in severe cases. The most common electrocardiogram (ECG) changes are ST segment and T wave alterations. Echocardiography may demonstrate ventricular dysfunction, which in some cases appears regional rather than global. Myocardial injury can lead to elevated MB-creatine kinase blood levels. Evidence of myocarditis may be found on endomyocardial biopsy, although a negative biopsy does not exclude the diagnosis. At present, biopsy is not routinely employed for suspected myocarditis since it generally does not alter treatment decisions. Routine immunosuppressive therapy has not been proven to be effective, although future studies may identify patients who will benefit from this form of treatment. Therapy is usually supportive and includes adequate rest. Congestive heart failure is treated in the routine manner. Arrhythmias can complicate myocarditis. Their evaluation and treatment guidelines are described in Chapter 8.

Cardiomyopathy

Cardiomyopathy refers to a group of diseases involving the heart muscle itself. A number of classification schemes have been proposed. The cardiomyopathies are often divided into dilated, hypertrophic, and restrictive categories (Table 9–1). However, these distinctions are not rigid, and some cardiomyopathies exhibit characteristics of more than one group.

Dilated Cardiomyopathy

Dilated cardiomyopathy is characterized by impaired systolic function and dilation of one or both ventricles. Dilated cardiomyopathy often occurs without an identifiable cause and is termed idiopathic (Table 9–2). Dilated cardiomyopathy can also be secondary in response to a large number of causes, including ethanol and anticancer drugs such as anthrocyclines. Cardiac toxicity of the anthrocyclines appears related to the cumulative dose. Peripartum cardiomyopathy is a dilated cardiomyopathy occurring during the last month of pregnancy or within 6 months of delivery. It is more common in older multiparous patients.

The clinical manifestations of dilated cardiomyopathy are related to congestive heart failure. The ECG findings are often nonspecific. Left bundle branch block is also common. Echocardiography confirms ventricular dilation and reduced systolic function. Although cardiomyopathy is typically a diffuse process, some degree of regional wall motion abnormality can occur. If coronary artery disease is a potential cause of or contributor to an apparent cardiomyopathic process, coronary angiography is usually performed. Treatment of overt heart failure is described in Chapter 4. Vasodilator therapy with an angiotensin converting enzyme inhibitor plays a prominent role. It can help relieve symptoms and improve prognosis in many patients. The course of dilated cardiomyopathy is usually, but not invariably, progressive deterioration. Supraventricular (e.g., atrial fibrillation) and ventricular ar-

TABLE 9-1	Classification of Cardiomyopathy		
	Dilated (Congestive)	**Hypertrophic**	**Restrictive**
Symptoms	Dyspnea, orthopnea fatigue, leg edema	Dyspnea, angina, syncope after exertion, palpitations	Dyspnea, fatigue, leg edema
Characteristic cardiac physical findings	Cardiomegaly; S_3 and S_4 common; murmur of mitral and tricuspid regurgitation	Bifed apical impulse with palpable S_4; ejection murmur at LSB (increased with Valsalva); often associated mitral regurgitation murmur	Normal size or slightly enlarged heart; S_3 common; S_4; murmur of tricuspid or mitral regurgitation; elevated jugular venous pressure, inspiratory increase in venous pressure
Electrocardiogram	Sinus tachycardia; left bundle branch block common	Left ventricular hypertrophy; abnormal Q waves	Low voltage; abnormal Q waves; conduction abnormalities
Echocardiogram	Dilated cardiac chambers; generalized reduced ventricular wall motion and systolic function	Normal or small left ventricular cavity; left ventricular hypertrophy; asymmetric septal thickening; systolic anterior motion of anterior mitral valve leaflet	Thick walls, reduced systolic function; glistening appearance of left ventricular in amyloid
Treatment	Diuretics; unloading agents; digoxin	Beta-adrenergic–blocking drugs or selected calcium channel–blocking drugs; sequential atrioventricular (DDD) pacing for selected patients with refractory symptoms; surgical septal myectomy for refractory obstructive symptoms	Treatment of underlying cause; diuretics

DDD = Atrial synchronous ventricular pacemaker; LSB = left sternal border.

rhythmias are relatively common in dilated cardiomyopathy. Many of the deaths are sudden, presumably the result of ventricular tachycardia or fibrillation.

Hypertrophic Cardiomyopathy

Hypertrophic cardiomyopathy is characterized by inappropriate myocardial hypertrophy. Typically, the hypertrophy is asymmetric, predominantly involving the intraventricular septum. In a minority of patients, the hypertrophy is more concentric. The hypertrophied muscle bundles usually appear disorganized histologically, with a bizarre whorled appearance. Both familial (antosomal dominant) and sporadic forms of the disorder exist. Elderly patients with hypertension may present with a clinical picture consistent with hypertrophic cardiomyopathy. With hypertrophic cardiomyopathy, the left ventricular end-systolic volume is reduced and the ventricle often appears hypercontractile. In some patients, the hypertrophied septum, along with systolic anterior movement of the anterior mitral leaflet, results in a subvalvular left ventricular outflow tract gradient (hypertrophic cardiomyopathy with obstruction). In these cases, the gradient is characteristically dynamic and varies with physiologic or pharmacologic maneuvers. In some patients, a measurable gradient is present only with these maneuvers. In susceptible patients, the gradient (and associated murmur) may be increased by provocations that reduce ventricular volume (hypovolemia, Valsalva, or prompt standing) or that further increase contractility (e.g., digitalis). Although marked outflow obstruction can occur, it is the reduced ventricular compliance (diastolic dysfunction) and volume that play major pathophysiologic roles in most patients. The abnormal stiffness of the ventricle limits filling and increases pulmonary venous pressure. The clinical manifestations of hypertrophic cardiomyopathy are quite variable, ranging from asymptomatic status to sudden death.

In symptomatic patients, dyspnea is most common. Anginal chest pain can occur, as can syncope. Syncope and sudden death have been associated with competitive sports and other vigorous exertion; vigorous exertion should be avoided in patients with hypertrophic cardiomyopathy. Risk factors for sudden death include prior syncope, onset at young age, family history of sudden death, and complex ventricular arrhythmias. Atrial fibrillation is an important and common complication. It can lead to marked clinical deterioration as ventricular filling is further reduced by the loss of atrial contraction and the shortening of diastole due to tachycardia.

The symptoms and cardiac findings of hypertrophic cardiomyopathy are summarized in Table 9–1. In some patients, the carotid arterial upstroke is initially brisk but may then be followed by a midsystolic dip (as the dynamic gradient develops) and a second late systolic rise. The mid-systolic ejection murmur is typically harsh and

TABLE 9-2	Causes of Dilated Cardiomyopathy

Idiopathic
Toxin-induced
  Alcohol
  Anthracycline
  Cobalt
  Catecholamine
Radiation
Infectious
  Viral
  Parasitic (e.g., Chagas' disease)
Metabolic
  Starvation
  Thiamine deficiency (beriberi)
  Thyrotoxicosis
Sarcoidosis
Hemochromatosis
Peripartum or postpartum cardiomyopathy
Genetic

prominent between the left sternal border and apex. Augmentation of the murmur upon prompt standing or during Valsalva maneuver straining is characteristic (Table 9–3). An associated mitral regurgitant murmur is often present. A prominent fourth heart sound, attesting to reduced ventricular compliance, is typically audible and palpable. The ECG may demonstrate signs of ventricular hypertrophy and Q waves simulating myocardial infarction. The Q waves are often deep and relatively narrow. In an uncommon form of hypertrophic cardiomyopathy in which the hypertrophy is confined to the cardiac apex (apical hypertrophic cardiomyopathy), giant negative T waves may be recorded in leads $V_4 - V_6$.

Echocardiographic/Doppler examination is the most important laboratory study, permitting detection of the extent and location of hypertrophy, as well as chamber sizes, valve function, and estimation of outflow gradient. It also is useful for screening family members of patients with hypertrophic cardiomyopathy.

Beta-adrenergic–blocking drugs and the calcium channel–blocking drugs verapamil or diltiazem can improve symptoms in many patients. A survival benefit, however, has not been demonstrated. In selected patients, the use of dual-chamber cardiac pacing has been reported to improve outflow gradient and clinical status. For patients with refractory symptoms from outflow obstruction despite medical therapy, surgical myectomy to thin the ventricular septum and widen the outflow tract can be considered. For patients with atrial fibrillation or with sustained or symptomatic ventricular arrhythmias, antiarrhythmic therapy (e.g., with amiodarone) is employed, as outlined in Chapter 8. Patients with serious arrhythmias and survivors of cardiac arrest should undergo evaluation by electrophysiology specialists. In selected high-risk patients, an implantable cardiac defibrillator is used. Hypertrophic cardiomyopathy patients should receive endocarditis prophylaxis.

Restrictive Cardiomyopathies

This is the least common type of cardiomyopathy (see Table 9–1). It is characterized by abnormal diastolic function with impaired ventricular filling and elevated filling pressure. It can be caused by infiltrative processes such as amyloidosis, esosinophilic endomyocardial disease, hemochromatosis, and sarcoidosis. Radiation-induced heart muscle disease can also underlie restrictive cardiomyopathy. Although diastolic dysfunction is a hallmark of restrictive cardiomyopathy, some underlying causes can also impair systolic function. Often, signs of right-heart failure (jugular venous distention, edema, ascites) are prominent, and the differential diagnosis may include constrictive pericarditis. In both disorders, early ventricular filling is rapid, but late filling is limited or absent, yielding a "square-root" sign in ventricular pressure recordings. The atrial pressure is elevated and typically demonstrates prominent y and x descents, yielding an M-shaped waveform. Both right and left ventricular filling pressures are elevated, but the left is often greater than the right in restrictive cardiomyopathy patients. This is in contrast to constrictive pericarditis with characteristic

TABLE 9–3	Effect of Selected Maneuvers on Dynamic Outflow Gradient and Murmur in Hypertrophic Cardiomyopathy	
Maneuver	**Mechanism**	**Effect on Gradient and Murmur**
Valsalva (during strain)	↓ LV cavity size (↓ preload and ↓ afterload)	↑
Standing	↓ LV cavity size (↓ preload)	↑
Postextrasystolic beat	↑ Contracticity, (also ↑ preload)	↑
Squatting	↑ LV cavity size (↑ preload and ↑ afterload)	↓
Isometric hand-grip exercise	↑ Afterload	↓

LV = Left ventricle.

equalization of pressures. For most causes of restrictive cardiomyopathy, there is no specific treatment beyond symptomatic measures for heart failure.

Amyloid heart disease results in a thickened, firm, rubbery ventricular muscle. Although diastolic dysfunction is prominent, systolic dysfunction can also occur. The ECG typically demonstrates low voltage. Abnormal Q waves can simulate myocardial infarction. Conduction disturbances and arrhythmias are not uncommon. Echocardiography typically demonstrates small left ventricular cavity along with thickening of the walls (often including the atrial septum). Bright sparkling appearance of the myocardium may be present, although this finding is not specific for amyloid heart disease. With generalized disease, amyloid deposits may be detected on rectal or gingival biopsies, and if the associated clinical and echocardiographic findings are sufficient, a diagnosis of amyloid heart disease can be made. If the findings are less conclusive, myocardial biopsy may be required.

PERICARDIAL DISEASE

Acute Pericarditis

Inflammation of the heart's pericardial lining can result from a variety of causes (Table 9–4). The most common causes are viral and idiopathic (many of which are also presumed to be postviral). Typical manifestations include sudden anterior chest pain, pericardial friction rub, and ECG changes. The pain is usually substernal, at times with radiation to the left shoulder or trapezius ridge. It characteristically has a pleuritic component and is worsened by coughing, deep inspiration, and recumbent position. It may be relieved by sitting up and leaning forward. The friction rub is diagnostic. Classically, the scratchy high-pitched rub has three components, corresponding to movement of the heart with atrial systole, ventricular systole, and early diastolic filling. However, in some patients only one or two components can be heard (the ventricular systole component is most common), and the rub may be intermittent and variable in intensity. Its absence does not exclude the diagnosis.

The ECG signs (Fig. 9–1) include a current of injury (ST segment elevation). With pericarditis, the current of injury is characteristically diffuse, concave upward, and is not accompanied by reciprocal ST segment depression. Associated inflammation of the atrial pericardium can result in PR segment depression. Sinus tachycardia is common. With time, the ST segment elevation resolves, and there may be T wave inversion of variable duration. Supraventricular arrhythmias, including atrial fibrillation, are recognition complications.

The chest radiogram does not provide direct evidence of pericarditis, but cardiomegaly may result from an associated pericardial effusion. Echocardiography is much more sensitive and is the laboratory test of choice for the detection of pericardial fluid, which is expected with pericardial inflammation. At times, signs indicating hemodynamic effects of the pericardial fluid can be identified by echocardiography (see later).

Nonspecific laboratory indicators of inflammation, such as an elevated erythrocyte sedimentation rate and leukocytosis, are usually present. The selection of other laboratory studies depends in part on the clinical setting.

TABLE 9–4	Causes of Pericarditis

Idiopathic
Viral (e.g., Coxsackie B, echovirus, adenovirus, infectious mononucleosis, hepatitis B, acquired immunodeficiency syndrome)
Fungal (e.g., histoplasmosis)
Tuberculosis
Acute bacterial (purulent)
Acute myocardial infarction
Postpericardiotomy syndrome
Radiation
Neoplasm (e.g., metastatic lung or breast carcinoma; leukemia, lymphoma, melanoma)
Uremia
Autoimmune disorders (e.g., systemic lupus erythematosus, rheumatoid arthritis, scleroderma)
Drug reaction/hypersensitivity syndromes (e.g., procainamide, hydralazine)
Myxedema

Tests that may aid in the exclusion of specific diagnoses include fungal serology (e.g., histoplasmosis), purified protein derivative skin testing, thyroid and renal function studies, and connective tissue screens such as antinuclear antibody, rheumatoid factor, and complement levels. Acute and convalescent viral serologic studies can support a diagnosis of viral pericarditis, but they do so retrospec-

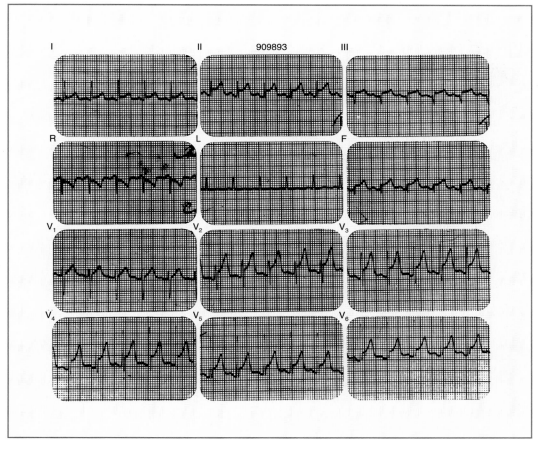

Figure 9–1
Typical electrocardiogram in pericarditis, showing diffuse ST elevation.

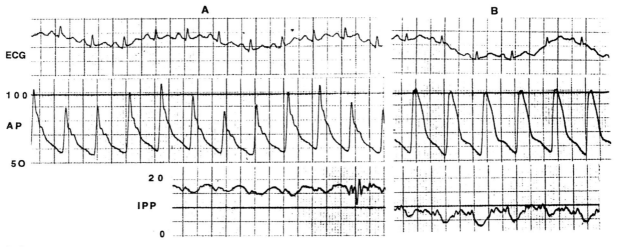

Figure 9–2

Electrocardiogram (ECG), systemic arterial and intrapericardial pressures (recorded in the catheterization laboratory) in a patient with cardiac tamponade. The left tracings *(A)* demonstrate sinus tachycardia and pulsus paradoxus. The intrapericardial pressure is elevated at about 15 mm Hg. After pericardiocentesis *(B; right panels)*, the heart rate has slowed, the pulsus paradoxus is no longer present, and the elevated intrapericardial pressure has resolved.

tively and are not commonly used in the elevation of individual patients. If purulent pericarditis is suspected, blood cultures are obtained.

The treatment of patients with acute pericarditis ideally focuses on its cause. For viral or idiopathic pericarditis, the treatment often includes salicylates or other nonsteroidal anti-inflammatory agents. Colchicine also may be beneficial. When standard treatment fails, a short course of tapered corticosteroid therapy may be required for symptomatic relief. However, this can be associated with a steroid dependency syndrome in some patients. Anticoagulants should generally not be administered during acute pericarditis because of the risk of developing hemopericardium. Most causes of pericarditis are self-limited, and the inflammation resolves within a several-week interval. A recurrent episode of pericarditis occurs in some patients, and a small percentage experience more chronic relapsing pericarditis. This can be very difficult to effectively treat and can be complicated by steroid dependency, necessitating very gradual withdrawal of the medication. Constrictive pericarditis rarely develops after an episode of idiopathic or viral pericarditis.

Pericardial Effusion

Pericardial effusion can result from any cause of pericarditis. Some causes, such as breast or lung carcinoma or lymphoma, can lead to chronic pericardial effusion without any clinical signs of pericardial inflammation. In these cases, the effusion may be detected incidentally or when a complication such as tamponade develops. Effusions are characterized by the amount of fluid—small, moderate, or large. Most surround the heart but can be localized. In the setting of large effusion, the apical impulse may not be palpable, and the heart sounds may be diminished in intensity. ECG may demonstrate diminished voltage. As indicated previously, pericardial effusion can lead to cardiomegaly on chest radiogram, and a large effusion may produce a water bottle– or flash-shaped heart contour. But echocardiography is the test of choice to detect pericardial effusion and permits a more accurate estimation of the amount and location of the fluid. With some large effusions, particularly those associated with neoplasm, the heart may demonstrate a pendulum or swinging motion within the pericardial space. This can be accompanied by electrical alternans on the ECG, in which there is alternating amplitude or morphology of the complexes of every other beat.

The hemodynamic consequences of pericardial effusion depend on the volume of fluid and the rate of its development. If fluid accumulates slowly, as is often the case with neoplastic causes, the pericardium may expand and accommodate a large amount of fluid before intrapericardial pressure rises significantly. In acute settings, such as secondary to trauma, lesser amounts of fluid may be tolerated. In either case, once intrapericardial pressure begins to rise, a small amount of additional fluid can lead to marked hemodynamic effects and rapid clinical deterioration. Tamponade develops when pericardial fluid under pressure compresses the heart. The venous pressure rises, and stroke volume falls. With hemodynamic compromise, the jugular pressure is elevated, and tachycardia is present. Tamponade is characterized by pulsus paradoxus, a fall in systolic blood pressure during inspiration > 10 mm Hg (Fig. 9–2). The pulse may also diminish or be undetectable during inspiration. It should be noted, however, that pulsus paradoxus is not specific for tamponade. It can occur, for example, with respiratory distress associated with chronic pulmonary disease or acute asthma. The echocardiographic detection of right atrial or right ventricular systolic collapse strongly supports the hemodynamic effects of a pericardial effusion (i.e., manifest or impending tamponade) but is not entirely specific.

Cardiac tamponade is a medical emergency, and fluid drainage is usually indicated when pericardial effusion has resulted in a significant rise in central venous pressure. The fluid can be removed by pericardiocentesis or pericardiostomy. The latter is usually performed surgically, but balloon catheter techniques have been developed. Patients with tamponade and hypotension should receive intravenous fluids until pericardial drainage is accomplished. The removed pericardial fluid should be carefully examined for bacteria, abnormal cells, and glucose and protein content. Suspicion of purulent pericarditis is also an indication for pericardial drainage. By contrast, pericardial fluid removal for diagnosis of pericardial effusion cause in the absence of elevated venous pressure or suspected purulent pericarditis (i.e., "diagnostic tap") is unlikely to yield diagnostic information.

Constrictive Pericarditis

Constrictive pericarditis results from insidious and progressive scarring of the pericardium in response to a prior insult. Calcification of the pericardium is often present. Almost all of the causes of pericarditis can lead to constriction, as can radiation therapy for cancer and cardiac surgery. However, in most cases, the underlying cause of this uncommon disorder cannot be identified and it is termed idiopathic. Venous pressures are elevated as the stiff noncompliant pericardium limits ventricular filling. In contrast to tamponade, in which ventricular filling is impeded throughout diastole, constriction limits filling primarily in mid- and late diastole. This underlies the prominent y descent in the jugular venous waveform and the right ventricular square root sign seen during cardiac catheterization.

The clinical manifestations are similar to those of right heart failure. Peripheral edema and abdominal distention with ascites can be marked. Hepatic congestion can lead to palpably enlarged liver and abnormal liver chemistries. The key that primary hepatic disease with cirrhosis is not the etiology lies in the identification of substantially elevated jugular venous pressure with a prominent y descent. An inspiratory increase in jugular venous pressure, Kussmaul's sign, may also be present. Pulsus paradoxus is typically absent in chronic constriction. An early diastolic sound termed a pericardial knock may be heard at the cardiac apex. In long-standing cases,

a rim of pericardial calcium may be evident on the chest radiogram, especially the lateral view. Thickening of the pericardium and associated calcification is best detected by computed tomography or magnetic resonance imaging. Such a study is indicated if constriction is suspected. Although echocardiography is the test of choice for identification of pericardial effusion, standard echo techniques are of limited value for the evaluation of pericardial thickening and constriction.

The differential diagnosis often includes restrictive cardiomyopathy, and its exclusion is sometimes difficult. In selected cases, endomyocardial biopsy is required to exclude a restrictive process such as amyloid heart disease.

Although typically chronic, constrictive pericarditis can at times present with a subacute course over months rather than years. Also, in some cases, patients present both with effusion and signs of pericardial constriction. With such effusive-constrictive pericarditis, evidence of impaired ventricular filling persists after removal of pericardial fluid.

The most definitive treatment of patients with symptomatic constrictive pericarditis is surgical pericardiectomy. However, the operation can be especially difficult and carry significant risk if delayed until marked calcification has occurred. Also, cardiac function may not normalize postoperatively because of inability to completely remove the pericardium or because of fibrosis and atrophy of the underlying myocardium.

REFERENCES

Bonow RO, Udelson JE: Left ventricular diastolic dysfunction as a cause of congestive heart failure. Mechanisms and management. Ann Intern Med 1992; 117:502–510.

Cannan CR, Reeder GS, et al: Natural history of hypertrophic cardiomyopathy: A population-based study, 1976 through 1990. Circulation 1995; 92:2488–2495.

Dec GW, Fuster V: Idiopathic dilated cardiomyopathy. N Engl J Med 1994; 331:1564–1575.

Fowler NO: Cardiac tamponade. A clinical or an echocardiographic diagnosis? Circulation 1993; 87:1738–1741.

Sugrue DO, Rodeheffer RJ, Codd MD, et al: The clinical course of idiopathic dilated cardiomyopathy. A population-based study. Ann Intern Med 1992; 117:117–123.

Vaitkus PT, Kussmaul WG: Constrictive pericarditis versus restrictive cardiomyopathy: A reappraisal and update of diagnostic criteria. Am Heart J 1991; 122:1431–1441.

10

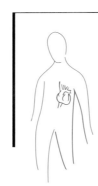

Cardiac Tumors and Trauma

CARDIAC TUMORS

Tumors involving the heart may be primary or metastatic; both types are rare (Table 10–1). Myxoma is the most common primary tumor of the heart and is usually benign. Early detection of resectable cardiac tumors is particularly important because of the heart's limited capacity to tolerate space-occupying lesions. Cardiac tumors may also carry the risk of embolization. Most malignant cardiac tumors are sarcomas, with angiosarcoma and rhabdomyosarcoma being the most frequent. Prior to histologic examination, it is not possible to distinguish benign from malignant tumors, but malignant tumors are more likely to present with evidence of metastases, invasion, or rapid growth. Tumor type may be identified occasionally from tissue at the time of peripheral embolectomy. Malignant primary tumors of the heart are associated with a very poor prognosis. Ventricular tachyarrhythmias may be the presenting symptom in some patients with ventricular tumors. Cardiac metastases usually involve pericardial effusions. Masses within the heart chambers occur much less often. The most common cardiac metastatic lesions are bronchogenic carcinoma, breast cancer, lymphoma, and leukemia. Malignant melanoma is particularly likely to result in cardiac metastases.

Echocardiography plays a central role in the evaluation of patients with cardiac tumors. Transesophageal echocardiography can be especially helpful in examination of the left atrium. Magnetic resonance imaging can contribute to the diagnostic evaluation in some patients.

Myxomas can arise from the endocardial surface of any cardiac chamber, but the majority arise from the left atrium, most commonly in the region of the fossa ovalis. They are usually pedunculated. As a general rule, 10% of cardiac myxomas manifest malignant characteristics, and 10% arise in locations other than the left atrium. Occasionally, they can be bilateral. Myxomas usually present in one of three general ways: (1) progressive interference with mitral valve function that causes decreased exercise tolerance, dyspnea on exertion, and pulmonary edema, with syncope or presyncope possibly occurring; (2) stroke or occlusion of a major systemic artery due to an embolus; or (3) systemic manifestations that include fever, wasting, arthralgias, malaise, anemia, or Raynaud's phenomenon.

If the left myxoma interferes with mitral valve func-

tion, a regurgitant valvular murmur may occur. A murmur resembling that of mitral stenosis may be present owing to obstruction of the valve orifice during diastole. The intensity of the murmur may change with changes in body position. An early diastolic sound termed a "tumor plop" may occur secondary to movement of the tumor toward the left ventricle in early diastole. The erythrocyte sedimentation rate, gamma globulins, and white blood cell count may be elevated. The cause of the systemic manifestations is not clear, but they may result from products secreted by the tumor, necrotic tumor debris, or an immunologic reaction.

Cardiac myxoma is usually diagnosed by echocardiography. Two-dimensional echocardiography shows the tumor location and movement with the cardiac cycle. Cardiac catheterization with angiocardiography usually is not necessary when the diagnosis has been established noninvasively and may be associated with risk of tumor embolus.

Cardiac myxomas should be excised surgically once identified. A recurrent myxoma follows resection in a small number of patients. Thus, follow-up evaluation is important, including echocardiographic study.

NONPENETRATING TRAUMA

Blunt chest trauma is especially common after steering wheel impact from an automobile accident. It may produce myocardial contusion, resulting in myocardial hemorrhage and, at times, some degree of necrosis. Often, there is little or no residual myocardial scar once healing is complete. Large contusions may lead to myocardial scars, cardiac or septal rupture, congestive heart failure, or formation of true or false aneurysms. Necrosis or hemorrhage involving the cardiac conduction system can produce intraventricular or atrioventricular block. Coronary artery laceration, valvular damage, or pericardial tears may occasionally occur after blunt trauma. The chest pain of myocardial contusion is similar to that of myocardial infarction and is often confused with musculoskeletal pain from the chest trauma. The echocardiogram (ECG) at the time of injury may show a diffuse injury pattern similar to that of pericarditis. Later, the ECG may reveal serial development of Q waves similar to that of acute myocardial infarction if significant necrosis has occurred. Brady-

TABLE 10–1	Examples of Tumors of the Heart and Pericardium

Primary	Metastatic
Benign	Melanoma
Myxoma*	Leukemia
Lipoma	Lung
Papillary fibroelastoma	Breast
Rhabdomyoma	Lymphoma
Fibroma	Renal
Malignant	
Angiosarcoma	
Rhabdomyosarcoma	
Mesothelioma	
Fibrosarcoma	

*In some series, these make up a quarter or more of the cases.

arrhythmias and tachyarrhythmias are common. Contractile abnormalities are usually not severe unless concomitant injury to a valve or the septum has occurred. The mesiobuccal fraction of creatine kinase is elevated, but its specificity may be reduced if there is marked total creatine kinase elevation from associated skeletal muscle injury. Newer markers of myocardial injury, such as cardiac troponins, may be more specific in this situation. Echocardiography may reveal a wall motion abnormality and aid in the evaluation of associated pericardial effusion. Myocardial contusion is usually treated similarly to myocardial infarction, with initial monitoring and subsequent progressive ambulation. Anticoagulants should not be administered to patients with myocardial contusion. If the patient survives the acute episode, the long-term prognosis is usually good, although late complications such as ventricular arrhythmias occasionally occur.

Rupture of the aorta is a common consequence of blunt trauma, such as seen in vehicular accidents. It is often fatal. It most commonly occurs just distal to the take-off of the left subclavian artery. The patient may complain of pain in the back or chest similar to that of aortic dissection. The chest radiograph usually reveals widening of the mediastinum. Patients may demonstrate increased arterial pressure in the upper extremities and decreased arterial pressure and pulse pressure in the lower extremities. Signs of decreased renal or spinal cord perfusion may become evident. The diagnosis is usually confirmed by aortography, and the treatment is surgical.

PENETRATING TRAUMA

Penetrating cardiac injuries may be due to external objects such as bullets or knives and also bony fragments resulting from chest injury. Because of its anterior location, the right ventricle is most commonly involved. Iatrogenic causes of cardiac penetrating injury include perforation of the heart during catheterization and cardiac trauma from cardiopulmonary resuscitation.

Penetrating injury to the heart may present as exsanguinating hemorrhage with hemothorax or cardiac tamponade if hemorrhage has been limited to within the pericardial sac. Immediate pericardiocentesis and administration of large volumes of fluids may be performed as preparations are being made for emergency surgery. A "postpericardiotomy" type of pericarditis, infection, arrhythmias, aneurysm formation, and ventricular septal defects are late complications of penetrating cardiac injury. The risk of bacterial endocarditis, infection from a retained foreign body, and foreign body embolus are complications peculiar to penetrating injuries.

REFERENCES

Cheitlin MD: Cardiovascular trauma. Circulation 1982; 65:1529; 1982; 66:244.

Reeder GS, Khandheria BK, Seward JB, Tajik AJ: Transesophageal echocardiography and cardiac masses. Mayo Clinic Proc 1991; 66: 1107–1109.

Salcedo EE, Cohen GI, White RD, Davison MD: Cardiac tumors: Diagnosis and management. Curr Probl Cardiol 1992; 17:73–137.

11

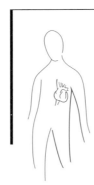

Aortic and Peripheral Vascular Disease

AORTIC ANEURYSMS (Table 11–1)

Aortic aneurysms, localized areas of increased aortic diameter, may occur in the ascending aorta, aortic arch, descending thoracic aorta, or abdominal aorta, depending on the etiology. The most common cause of aortic aneurysm is atherosclerosis, and the majority involve the abdominal aorta. They typically begin just below the renal arteries and extend to or involve the aortic bifurcation. Abdominal aneurysms are usually asymptomatic when detected. Some patients experience a sensation of abdominal fullness or pulsation or back pain. Pain may develop with enlargement or impending rupture of the aneurysm. Aortic rupture is associated with acute abdominal and back pain with tenderness. Abdominal aneurysm may be suspected by palpation of a pulsatile abdominal mass. However, aortic pulsation can be detected in some normal thin individuals, and aortic aneurysm may not be palpable in patients who are obese or have muscular abdominal walls. Abdominal aortic aneurysms can be detected and followed by ultrasound or computed tomography with contrast. Aortography is usually needed when surgery is being planned.

Aneurysm complications include rupture and distal embolism (thrombus or atheroembolism). Aneurysms usually enlarge progressively, and there is a strong relationship between aneurysm size and risk of rupture. Many authorities recommend elective surgery for good-risk patients if an abdominal aneurysm is larger than 4 cm. Serial observation, e.g., with ultrasound, can be used in asymptomatic patients with aneurysms smaller than 4 cm. The development of symptoms or aneurysm enlargement under observation is also an indication for surgery.

Thoracic aortic aneurysms can result from atherosclerosis. Other causes include Marfan's syndrome or cystic medial necrosis. Surgical therapy is usually recommended for symptomatic or enlarging thoracic aneurysms and for those 6 cm or larger in diameter.

AORTIC DISSECTION

Aortic dissection (see Table 11–1) is caused by a tear of the aortic intima with formation of a false channel within the aortic media. Blood in the false channel may re-enter the true aortic channel via a second intimal tear or rupture through the adventitia into the periaortic tissues. Most dissections arise either in the ascending aorta within several centimeters of the aortic valve or in the descending thoracic aorta just beyond the origin of the left subclavian artery in the region of the ligamentum arteriosum. Hypertension plays an important role in most cases of aortic dissection. Marfan's syndrome also predisposes patients to aortic dissection. Aortic dissection typically results in sudden severe chest pain. Depending on the location of the dissection, pain may radiate to the back. Dissection can lead to pulse deficits and neurologic signs, and proximal dissection may lead to aortic regurgitation. Aortic dissection can result in widening of the mediastinum on chest radiograph, but a normal chest radiograph does not exclude the diagnosis. The most important initial study is transesophageal echocardiography or computed tomography, which should be obtained immediately if the diagnosis is suspected. Emergent treatment includes beta-adrenergic–blocking drugs and agents to control blood pressure while the diagnosis is being confirmed. Prompt surgery generally is indicated in proximal (type I and type II) dissections, whereas medical therapy may be the initial treatment of choice for uncomplicated distal dissection (type III). Medical therapy must be administered to surgical patients both during the preoperative period and chronically postoperatively to prevent progression or repeat dissection. Aortic size should also be reassessed (e.g., by computed tomography) at periodic follow-up.

AORTIC ARTERITIS

Aortic arteritis, or aortitis, is an inflammatory process of the aortic wall that may be caused by several disease processes. When it involves the origin of various aortic branches (e.g., the innominate artery, the left common carotid artery, and the left subclavian artery), it is termed the "aortic arch syndrome" and is characteristically produced by Takayasu's syndrome. Takayasu's arteritis, or pulseless disease, appears to be most common in Japanese females and is an aortic panarteritis that leads to eventual luminal obliteration from the thickened walls and superimposed thrombus. Localized aneurysm formation may occur. The process may involve the coronary ostia or any of the branches of the aortic arch. Although rare today, tertiary syphilis can cause an aortic arteritis that may lead

TABLE 11–1	Aortic Aneurysms*					
Aneurysm Type	Etiology	Location	Clinical Features	Potential Physical Findings	Laboratory Findings	Treatment
Atherosclerotic	Atherosclerosis	Usually abdominal (between renal arteries and aortic bifurcation)	Often older males Often asymptomatic until rupture Abdominal fullness or pulsations; back or epigastric pain, worse prior to rupture.	Palpable, pulsatile abdominal mass; abdominal bruit Peripheral emboli Associated peripheral vascular disease	Size estimated by abdominal ultrasound or CT	Symptomatic, enlarging or > 6 cm: surgery Less than 4 cm and asymptomatic observe Control of blood pressure and other risk factors
Aortic dissection	Hypertension Marfan's syndrome Cystic medial necrosis Aortic coarctation Trauma	Type I: Proximal ascending thoracic aorta to descending aorta. Type II: Confined to ascending thoracic aorta. Type III: Begins in descending aorta and extends distally	Severe, sudden unrelenting tearing chest pain; depending on dissection location, may radiate to back or abdomen Rarely severe pain absent Aortic branch occlusions, e.g., causing stroke or spinal cord ischemia, limb or bowel ischemia, or renal impairment Aortic root involvement, e.g., causing aortic valve regurgitation, or rupture into pericardium with tamponade	Hypertension Asymptomatic pulses Pulse or neurologic deficit Aortic regurgitation	Wide mediastinum on chest x-ray (not always present or reliable); TEE, CT, or MRI usually diagnostic Angiography may be necessary to define surgical anatomy	Beta-blocker and antihypertensive (e.g., intravenous nitroprusside) Urgent surgery for proximal dissection Surgery consideration for complicated distal dissection

* See text.
CT = Computed tomography; MRI = magnetic resonance imaging; TEE = transesophageal echocardiography.

to an ascending aortic aneurysm, aortic valvulitis with insufficiency, and/or coronary ostial stenosis. It is a late manifestation of syphilis, usually occurring 10 to 30 years after the primary infection. Involvement is much more prominent in the aortic root than in the distal aorta, in contrast to atherosclerotic aortic aneurysms. This whole process is often asymptomatic and detected by eggshell calcification of the ascending aorta on chest radiograph.

MISCELLANEOUS AORTIC DISEASE

Large peripheral arterial emboli may obstruct the abdominal aortic bifurcation, resulting in so-called saddle emboli. These usually originate from the left side of the heart but, rarely, may originate from the aorta itself in the area of an atherosclerotic lesion. Other, rarer causes are "paradoxical emboli" (from the right side of the heart or venous system in patients with right-to-left shunts), atrial myxomas, or infective endocarditis (very large emboli can occur in acute endocarditis and fungal endocarditis). Obstruction at the aortic bifurcation is characterized by the sudden onset of severe pain in both legs, peripheral neurologic abnormalities, and evidence of decreased perfusion occurring bilaterally. It must be differentiated from acute atherosclerotic aortic thrombosis and aortic dissection. The diagnosis is confirmed by angiography. Surgical removal of the clot with subsequent anticoagulation and/or treatment of the underlying cause is necessary.

Infected aortic aneurysms are rare. The most common congenital aortic anomaly is coarctation of the aorta

(see Chapter 5). Congenital aortic aneurysms of the sinus of Valsalva may rupture into the right atrium or ventricle, producing a continuous murmur. Sinus of Valsalva aneurysms can occasionally produce coronary occlusion, conduction disturbances, or valvular malfunction. Infective endocarditis can be complicated by sinus of Valsalva aneurysm.

PERIPHERAL VASCULAR DISEASE (Table 11–2)

Chronic occlusive peripheral arterial disease is usually the result of atherosclerosis. Involvement of the lower extremities is most common. The characteristic presenting symptom is claudication, provoked by walking and relieved by standing still. It can be confused with pseudoclaudication (due to lumbar spinal stenosis), but pseudoclaudication is positional, requiring sitting or lying down for relief. Progression of peripheral arterial occlusive disease can lead to ischemic rest pain, typically involving the foot or toes and being worse at night. Advanced disease can also result in painful ischemic foot ulcers. Evaluation of the patient includes careful palpation of the pulses and auscultation for bruits. Measurement of the ankle and brachial systolic blood pressures (ankle/brachial index) can provide objective evidence. Arteriography is employed when surgical therapy or balloon angioplasty is contemplated. Patients with claudication may benefit from a regular walking program, stopping as needed at onset of symptoms. Pentoxifylline may improve the microcirculation and exercise tolerance in some pa-

Table 11–2	Peripheral Vascular Diseases

Disease	Pathology	Clinical Features	Physical Findings	Laboratory Findings	Treatment
Atherosclerotic occlusive peripheral vascular disease	Atherosclerotic narrowing of large and medium-sized arteries of lower extremities; segmental with skip areas; occasionally involves upper extremities	Male > female Common in diabetics Exertional leg pain relieved with rest (claudication); rest pain implies severe compromise Buttock claudication and impotence with aortoiliac obstruction (Leriche's syndrome)	Decreased or absent lower extremity pulses Aortic, iliac, or femoral bruit Limb ischemia: cool, pale, cyanotic; shiny dry skin without hair; nail changes, ulcerations, gangrene	Ankle, brachial blood pressure Doppler and arteriography locate obstructions	Intermittent claudication: • Exercise (stop when claudication occurs) • Stop smoking • Avoid peripheral vasoconstricting drugs, e.g., propranolol • Meticulous skin and nail care • Pentoxyifylline Severe claudication or rest ischemia: • Percutaneous transluminal angioplasty or surgical bypass; amputation if gangrenous
Thromboangiitis obliterans	Intimal proliferation and thrombi in small to medium-sized vessels with inflammatory infiltrates Segmental involvement of arteries and veins Upper and lower extremity involvement	Male > female Usually occurs before age 30 Etiology not understood but related to smoking Cool extremities Raynaud's phenomenon Distal limb claudication (e.g., instep or hand)	Cool extremities Digital ulcers Migrating thrombophlebitis		Stop smoking Sympathectomy to prevent vasospasm Amputation of distal extremities for gangrene
Arterial embolism	Can arise from the heart or aorta	Sudden onset of painful extremity (occasionally more gradual)	Cold, pale extremity with absent pulses distal to embolus	Pathologic examination of embolus may reveal etiology Doppler examination helps localize embolus	Heparin Surgical embolectomy for larger vessels Chronic anticoagulation if embolic source cannot be eliminated
Atheromatous embolism	Atheromatous ± thrombus debris usually from aorta, producing arteriolar occlusion		Blue digits and livedo reticularis; renal insufficiency		Removal of source of debris, if possible
Raynaud's phenomenon	Vasospasm of digital vessels precipitated by cold and relieved by heat	Underlying causes: Arterial occlusive diseases Connective tissue diseases Neurologic diseases Ingestion of vasoconstricting drugs Nerve compression syndromes Cryoglobulinemia or cold agglutinins Post frostbite or trench foot Raynaud's disease (female > male)	White, cyanotic digit upon exposure to cold or emotional upset; hyperemic upon resumption of circulation Normal pulses Chronic nail and skin changes (sclerodactyly) in severe cases: small areas of distal gangrene but digital amputation rare		Limitation of cold exposure Stop smoking Vasodilators Regional sympathectomy

tients. In all patients with peripheral arterial disease, avoidance of trauma, careful foot and toe hygiene, and attention to injuries are important. Management should also include efforts toward control of atherosclerosis risk factors, including cessation of smoking.

Thromboangitis obliterans, or Buerger's disease, is a less common type of occlusive peripheral vascular disease that can involve small and medium-sized arteries and veins. Most patients are men, and symptoms may begin before age 30 years. Smoking is a prominent characteristic of patients with this disorder; cessation of smoking is a central goal of its treatment.

Acute peripheral arterial occlusion can result from thrombosis or embolism. Sudden pain may occur, accompanied by pallor, paresthesia, paralysis, and pulselessness of the involved extremity. Peripheral arterial emboli usually originate from thrombi either in the left atrium or the left ventricle or from atheromatous emboli located in atherosclerotic plaques in the aorta. A "paradoxical embolus" refers to an embolus originating from the venous system, passing through a right-to-left intracardiac shunt, and lodging in the systemic arterial tree. Septic emboli may occur with endocarditis and tumor emboli, with cardiac myxoma. Acute thrombosis of a vessel is sometimes difficult to distinguish from embolism but should be suspected if no source for emboli is present and if the patient has concomitant severe atherosclerotic disease.

Raynaud's phenomenon is associated with vasospasm of the small arteries and arterioles of the skin and digits. Intermittent pallor and cyanosis, typically of the fingers and often precipitated or worsened by cold temperature, result. Raynaud's phenomenon can accompany a variety of disorders, including occlusive arterial disease. Raynaud's changes can occur in the absence of other disease (primary or Raynaud's disease). Primary Raynaud's is more likely to involve both fingers and toes and occur bilaterally.

PERIPHERAL ANEURYSMS AND FISTULAS

Peripheral aneurysms are usually secondary to atherosclerosis. Less common causes include heritable connective tissue disorders, infection, arteritis, congenital defects, and trauma. Aneurysm symptoms may result from rupture, distal embolization, or local pressure on adjacent structures such as nerves or veins. Infection is an uncommon complication. Surgical treatment is usually indicated for symptomatic aneurysms. Peripheral aneurysms are located most commonly in the popliteal artery but can occur elsewhere, including the iliac and femoral arteries. Aneurysm formation in the upper extremities is usually the result of trauma. Aneurysms of the popliteal and femoral arteries are often palpable. Diagnosis can be confirmed with ultrasound study. Elective surgery is usually indicated because of the risk of complication, including thromboembolism. False (or pseudo-) aneurysm refers to a persistent tear in the arterial wall allowing a contained accumulation of blood in the perivascular space. False aneurysms generally have a greater risk of rupture. They usually result from trauma, such as catheterization of the

femoral artery. In this case, ultrasound confirms the diagnosis, and ultrasound-directed local pressure can often be effective treatment. If not effective, surgical therapy may be employed.

Arteriovenous (AV) fistulas are acquired or congenital abnormal communications between arteries and veins without an intervening capillary network. Acquired fistulas may be created to facilitate hemodialysis or may occur after trauma such as a gunshot or stab wound. Increased blood flow leads to venous dilation and makes the region of the fistula abnormally warm; the area distal to the fistula may be cool. If the fistula is large, a high cardiac output state may occur and may contribute to heart failure. Because of the low-resistance pathway, diastolic blood pressure tends to decrease, and systolic blood pressure and pulse pressure increase. A bruit and thrill may be present over the fistula. If the artery serving the fistula is compressed, shunting via the low-resistance circuit is prevented, and a prompt decrease in the pulse rate may occur (Branham's sign). Acquired fistulas are best treated surgically. Congenital AV fistulas are often multiple and small and may be accompanied by cutaneous birthmarks. Enlargement of the entire limb may occur, since the fistulas are present during the period of rapid bone growth. Bruits and pulsatile masses are uncommon, since the fistulas are small and multiple. Treatment is less satisfactory than that of large acquired AV fistulas.

ARTERIAL TRAUMA

Arterial trauma occurs with penetrating or blunt injuries, including fractures and dislocations. Swelling within a compartment of an extremity after blunt trauma can cause both arterial and neurologic damage and responds to decompression of the compartment. Arterial trauma is usually a surgical emergency. Arterial injury may be iatrogenic from catheterization of brachial or femoral arteries. Loss of local pulse after a catheterization procedure should be approached surgically with early thrombectomy and/or repair, since waiting may necessitate more complicated procedures.

PERIPHERAL VENOUS DISEASE

Varicose veins of the lower extremities is a common disorder that can be primary or secondary to deep venous obstruction. Nonspecific treatment includes support stockings. Sclerotherapy or vein stripping can be used for patients for whom conservative measures fail or who develop complications such as recurrent superficial thrombophlebitis. Other causes of superficial thrombophlebitis include indwelling venous catheters in the arm. Superficial thrombophlebitis typically results in a firm, tender, red cord. Cellulitis often must be excluded. Treatment includes warm moist packs and aspirin to reduce inflammation. If related to indwelling catheter, the catheter should be removed.

DEEP VEIN THROMBOSIS (see Chapter 53)

Swelling of an extremity can also occur from obstruction of the lymphatic outflow (lymphedema). Lymphedema may be idiopathic (primary) or, more commonly, secondary (e.g., due to lymphangitis, neoplasms, adenopathy, or surgical removal of lymph nodes). Lymphedema is typically more firm than venous-related edema and pits poorly. Lymphedema of the lower extremity usually involves the foot and toes, whereas venous edema spares the toes. The treatment of lymphedema is properly fitted elastic support.

REFERENCES

Spittell JA Jr: Diagnosis and management of occlusive arterial disease. Curr Probl Cardiol 1990; 15:1–35.

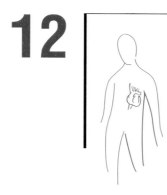

12

Other Cardiac Topics

A. Transplantation

Cardiac transplantation was first performed in humans in 1967 but was accompanied by a high graft rejection rate. The subsequent availability of cyclosporine immunosuppression beginning in the mid-1980s sharply reduced the number of patients with graft rejection and led to increased and more successful transplantations in patients with end-stage heart disease. Current 1- and 5-year survival rates approach 90% and 80%, respectively. The major limitation to cardiac transplantation is donor availability.

The inclusion and exclusion criteria for cardiac transplantation continue to evolve and vary somewhat in different centers. Currently, the upper age limit for candidates at most centers is 60 to 65 years. Exclusion criteria include factors or coexistent illnesses that would increase morbidity or mortality of the transplant procedure or independently lead to poor prognosis (e.g., pulmonary hypertension with irreversible high pulmonary vascular resistance, insulin-dependent diabetes mellitus with end-stage organ disease, and irreversible renal or hepatic dysfunction.

For orthotopic transplantation, the patient's heart is removed, leaving the posterior walls of the atria with their venous connections to suture to the donor atria. The great vessels are then anastomosed. Immunosuppression regimens vary but often include combinations of cyclosporine, azathioprine, and prednisone. Newer agents and combinations are also being evaluated. Post-transplant complications include rejection, which is monitored by right ventricular endomyocardial biopsies, and infection. After the first year, the leading cause of death is the development of coronary artery disease in the transplanted heart. This progressive disease includes diffuse myointimal proliferation and is not typical of atherosclerotic coronary disease. Its mechanism is not clearly established but may be an immune-mediated process in the graft vasculature. Angina is not provoked by the denervated heart, and standard stress testing techniques may not identify the disease process. Periodic angiographic study can be used but can be difficult to interpret in some cases. Hypertension is very common in transplant patients. Cyclosporine can be associated with hypertension and can also cause nephrotoxicity.

Left ventricular assist devices are means of circulatory support for patients whose hemodynamics cannot be sustained by either pharmacologic therapy or intra-aortic balloon counterpulsation. Left ventricular assist devices consist of a pump with an intake from the left ventricle and output into the ascending thoracic aorta. They are used in patients for temporary support after cardiac surgery if pump-oxygenator dependence develops in spite of conventional measures or if refractory cardiogenic shock occurs early after operation, situations in which recovery of left ventricular function is anticipated. In addition, they may be used as "bridges" in patients awaiting availability of a suitable donor heart for cardiac transplantation.

B. Surgery

Major noncardiac surgery in some patients with pre-existing heart disease can be associated with an increased risk of death or complications. The burdens of anesthesia, surgical trauma, wound healing, infection, hemorrhage, and pulmonary insufficiency may overwhelm the diseased heart. The internist is often asked to assess cardiovascular risk in patients undergoing noncardiac surgery and to aid in their preoperative and postoperative management. The preoperative evaluation includes clinical assessment of the patient's history, current symptoms, functional capacity, ventricular function, electrocardiogram, and chest radiograph. For patients with certain cardiac disorders and/or clinical characteristics, the preoperative evaluation may include additional studies, such as stress imaging tests.

General anesthetics reduce myocardial contractility and also have autonomic nervous system effects that may cause either hypotension or hypertension. Regional, spinal, or epidural anesthesia minimizes myocardial depression, but sympathetic blockade and hypotension still may result. In general, there appears to be no difference in risk between general anesthesia and spinal anesthesia in cardiac patients. The anesthesiologist must maintain adequate ventilation, oxygenation, and blood pH throughout the procedure. The electrocardiogram is routinely monitored throughout surgery. If cardiac disease is significant, arterial blood pressure, central venous pressure, and/or pulmonary arterial wedge pressure may need to be monitored throughout the procedure. Cardiac arrhythmias are particularly likely in patients with heart disease and occur most commonly during induction of anesthesia and intubation. Excessive vagal tone can cause bradyarrhythmias and usually responds to adjusting the depth of anesthesia or administering atropine. Antiarrhythmic agents may be administered if needed (see Chapter 8).

Some patients have life-threatening indications for surgery, and cardiac risk does not affect whether the surgery should be performed. Emergency surgery is associated with greater risk than nonemergency surgery because there is no time to optimize the patient's cardiac status. In elective surgery, however, the timing of the operation or even whether the operation should be done may depend upon a preoperative estimation of surgical risk. Cardiac risk is strongly associated with the type of surgical procedure. Herniorrhaphy and transurethral resection of the prostate carry relatively low risk, whereas chest, abdominal, and retroperitoneal surgery have a relatively high risk.

Ischemic heart disease is one of the major determinants of cardiac risk. The risk is particularly high if surgery is performed after recent myocardial infarction (e.g., within 6 months) or if the patient has unstable symptoms. Elective surgery should be deferred. In stable patients with known coronary disease and significant symptoms or reduced functional capacity, the preoperative evaluation commonly includes stress testing. If the patient is unable to exercise, this may involve a pharmacologic test such as dipyridamole-thallium scintigraphy or dobutamine echocardiography. If these tests are positive, preoperative angiography may be indicated for further risk assessment and/or consideration of revascularization.

Decompensated congestive heart failure is another major operative risk factor and should be treated vigorously prior to noncardiac surgery.

Patients with symptomatic heart block may need prophylactic pacing prior to surgery. Those with chronic bifascicular block or asymptomatic type I second-degree atrioventricular block probably do not require prophylactic pacemaker placement prior to anesthesia.

Patients with valvular heart disease tend to tolerate the operation according to their pre-existing functional status. Patients with critical aortic or mitral stenosis are at particularly high risk. Treatment of heart failure should be optimized preoperatively, and those with severe valvular lesions should be considered for corrective surgery prior to elective noncardiac operation. In patients with valvular disease or prosthetic heart valves, endocarditis prophylaxis should be administered if appropriate.

Mild to moderate hypertension does not alter surgical risk. Severe hypertension should be controlled prior to surgery, as should heart failure or angina associated with it.

Patients with congenital heart disease are at increased risk according to their functional disability. Patients with cyanotic congenital heart disease and polycythemia have an increased risk of hemorrhage due to coagulation defects and thrombocytopenia, and they may tolerate hypotension and hypoxia poorly. Appropriate endocarditis prophylaxis should be administered. Patients with right-to-left shunts are at risk for paradoxical emboli.

C. Pregnancy

Marked changes in normal circulatory physiology occur during pregnancy. The cardiac output rises by the end of the first trimester, peaking at a level in the 20th to 24th week that is maintained until after delivery. Increases in stroke volume, heart rate, and blood volume accompany this, along with decreases in systolic blood pressure and the systemic and pulmonary vascular resistances. Oxygen consumption and minute ventilation increase. Easy fatigability, decreased exercise tolerance, dyspnea, peripheral edema, a third heart sound, and a mid-systolic murmur may be normal in pregnancy. The mechanical pressure of a gravid uterus on the inferior vena cava may decrease venous return and reduce cardiac output. The hemodynamic stresses of pregnancy can exacerbate a pre-existing cardiac abnormality with adverse effects on the mother and in some cases the fetus. The clinical differentiation of worsening heart disease from the normal symptoms and findings of pregnancy can be difficult. Echocardiography can often aid in the assessment.

Careful management of many pregnant patients with pre-existing heart disease can permit completion of pregnancy and delivery without serious harm to mother or fetus. However, some pre-existing heart diseases carry such high risk that consideration should be given to therapeutic abortion in the first trimester. This can include patients with pulmonary hypertension (either primary or secondary to Eisenmenger's syndrome), cardiomyopathy with pre-existing overt heart failure, and Marfan's syndrome with dilated aortic root.

Rheumatic valvular disease in young women usually involves mitral stenosis. Mitral stenosis is aggravated by the increased cardiac output and heart rate of pregnancy. The incidence of heart failure increases as pregnancy progresses. These patients have an increased risk of complications from atrial fibrillation, emboli, or endocarditis during pregnancy. Nevertheless, most of these patients can be managed carefully through pregnancy. Right ventricular failure may increase the peripheral edema, venous stasis, and risk of pulmonary embolism. For pregnant patients with mitral stenosis and refractory heart failure, balloon mitral valvuloplasty may offer an alternative to surgical commissurotomy.

Women with significant mitral or aortic valvular disease who desire children may require surgical correction of the lesion before conception. Cardiac surgical intervention during pregnancy carries increased risks for both mother and fetus (especially during the first 4 months, before organogenesis is complete). Patients with prosthetic heart valves, especially those requiring anticoagulation, face additional problems. There is some gradient across normal prosthetic valves, and the increased circulatory demands of pregnancy can result in relative stenosis. The mother's anticoagulation must be switched from warfarin to heparin, which does not cross the placenta. Warfarin is teratogenic. Heparin is discontinued, and, if necessary, protamine is administered upon the onset of labor. Patients given warfarin should not breast-feed, since it is excreted in breast milk. Patients with valvular heart disease should receive peripartum endocarditis prophylaxis.

Survival to reproductive age in patients with congenital heart disease has become more common since the advent of surgical intervention. The risk of pregnancy in patients after surgical correction of congenital heart lesions depends on the completeness of their repair and residual defects such as left ventricular dysfunction or pulmonary hypertension. Patients with uncomplicated cardiac lesions such as ostium secundum atrial septal defects usually tolerate pregnancy without problem. Patients with uncorrected cyanotic heart disease are at high risk with pregnancy. They often are marginally compensated and may not tolerate the hemodynamic stresses of pregnancy. Adverse hemodynamics may result in increased right-to-left shunt and increasing maternal cyanosis, magnifying the risk to both mother and child. Women with coarctation of the aorta have an increased risk of aortic dissection during pregnancy. Women with persistent cardiomegaly following peripartum cardiomyopathy are at high risk during subsequent pregnancies.

Maternal and fetal complications and mortality are directly related to functional class, and therapy should be optimized throughout pregnancy. Medication selection must include consideration of potential effects on the fetus. Digitalis, diuretics, and direct-acting vasodilators such as hydralazine for heart failure are usually well tolerated. The safety of angiotensin-converting enzyme inhibitors has not been established. Heart failure treatment should include decreased activity and salt intake along with removal—to the degree possible—of factors that may exacerbate heart failure. Patients with heart failure may need to be hospitalized during the final weeks of pregnancy. If needed because of serious cardiac arrhythmia, beta-adrenergic blocking drugs, calcium antagonists, and type I antiarrhythmic drugs such as quinidine and procainamide are generally well tolerated. Amiodarone has been associated with neonatal abnormalities and should be avoided if at all possible. Chest radiographs and cardiac catheterization should be avoided if possible because of the radiation risks to the fetus. Most women with heart disease should undergo a spontaneous term vaginal delivery, although cesarean section may be necessary in selected seriously ill patients.

REFERENCES

Cardiac Transplantation 24th Bethesda Conference. J Am Coll Cardiol 1993; 22:1–64.

Mangana DT, Goldman L: Pre-operative assessment of patients with known or suspected coronary disease. N Engl J Med 1995; 333: 1750–1756.

McAnulty JH, Morton MJ, Ueland K: The heart and pregnancy. Curr Probl Cardiol 1988; 13:589–665.

Perloff JK: Pregnancy and congenital heart disease. J Am Coll Cardiol 1991; 18:340–342.

Respiratory Disease

Section II

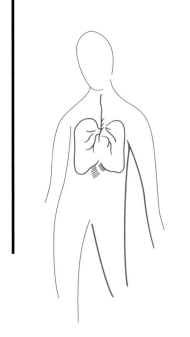

13

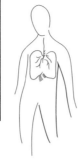

Approach to the Patient with Respiratory Disease

Although the most important function of the lungs is to provide gas exchange, the lungs also serve as an important phagocytic organ, an endocrine organ, and a filter to collect emboli. The epithelial lining of the lungs, like the skin, is exposed to the environment; thus, environmental injuries are commonly expressed as respiratory disorders. The lungs serve a paramount role in regulating blood pH, and the lungs and upper airways serve to warm and humidify inhaled air. Heat and water loss, therefore, are constants of lung function, and disease and injury to the lung usually affect several of these functions since they are interrelated. To arrive at the correct diagnosis of a pulmonary disorder, these intertwining roles must be considered. Of all the information the clinician may collect in coming to a decision regarding diagnosis and treatment, a careful history provides the most important data.

COMMON PRESENTING COMPLAINTS

Shortness of breath, dyspnea, is perhaps the most common pulmonary complaint. It is important to discover how the dyspnea was first noted and how it may have changed over time. In chronic disorders, the onset is insidious, and the patient may attribute the dyspnea to aging or deconditioning. In acute disorders, such as pneumothorax or pulmonary embolism, the onset may be very sudden. The dyspnea should be quantitated, and this is done by asking the patient to estimate how far he or she can walk at an average pace. The dyspnea may be episodic, occurring only at night, at work, or when lying down. Details regarding these episodes should be carefully explored. Many patients with markedly compromised lung function have more dyspnea when lying than sitting because the vital capacity falls in the supine position. Patients with congestive heart failure may note dyspnea when lying, but most times this does not occur immediately. Instead the patient may awake with dyspnea and cough several hours after retiring. In this instance, the dyspnea results from a progressive redistribution of intravascular and extravascular fluid secondary to the change in body position. Asthma may cause episodic dyspnea and is frequently worse in the evening hours. Occupational asthma may manifest as dyspnea on return-

ing to work after a relatively comfortable weekend or long holiday away from work.

Cough is perhaps the most understated pulmonary symptom. In general, it should be considered abnormal to cough. Healthy persons living under normal conditions go for days or weeks without a cough. A nonproductive cough is the most common early suggestion of chronic bronchitis secondary to tobacco abuse. These patients may deny cough at all, even though they may cough several times during an interview. When this fact is pointed out, the patient excuses this cough as "sinus drainage" or may consider that all people have a cough. Cough may be the only symptom of early-onset asthma; such patients frequently cough with exercise or at night. The cough may not produce sputum, either because there are no excess secretions in the airways (dry cough) or because the cough is ineffective in producing the high-velocity airflow in the trachea necessary to propel secretions through the larynx and into the oral pharynx. This ineffective cough is seen in patients with advanced obstructive lung disease, severe asthma, and in diseases associated with profound weakness of the muscles of respiration as in quadriplegia and in neurologic disorders such as advanced myasthenia gravis.

Sputum production should be carefully characterized—when it was first noted and how it progressed. Many patients deny raising sputum even though they may later acknowledge sputum production. A common pattern is that seen in chronic bronchitis, when the patient raises sputum with vigorous coughing only upon arising—the cough throughout the remainder of the day may fail to produce sputum. The volume of sputum produced should be estimated—the patient can help with this by judging the amount. Ask him or her "How much do you produce in 24 hours—a teaspoon full, a tablespoon full, a half cup, or more?" The character of the sputum should be noted, and its character may change as the illness progresses. Most common pulmonary disorders produce clear sputum of a mucoid nature. At times it may appear green or yellow, and blood may be present. When there is an associated hemoptysis, the character of the blood and the volume should be described. The most common cause of hemoptysis varies by geographic region. In the United States it is due to chronic bronchitis; in developing countries it is most often due to tuberculosis. Hemoptysis is most often noted as a small fleck of blood mixed with the mucoid or yellow sputum. In pulmonary edema, the sputum may be frothy and pink or red in color, with the blood more evenly mixed with the sputum. Uncommonly, the hemoptysis may be mostly blood, and the patient may cough bright red or dark red blood in large amounts. When the blood volume is large, with or without clots, malignancy, tuberculosis, or pulmonary cavity disease due to infection is most likely. Massive hemoptysis is defined as ≥ 600 ml in 24 hours. Such an episode is an emergency and may be fatal. In some instances, hemoptysis is a result of bleeding from the upper airways, even though the blood is produced after coughing. Some patients confuse hematemesis with hemoptysis.

Chest pain is among the most common complaints seen by general physicians. In many instances the cause is never found, even after a careful search; in these instances the patient can usually be reassured that the pain is not indicative of a serious illness. Chest pain may be produced by disease of the musculoskeletal system, the heart and aorta, the esophagus, the nerves innervating the chest wall and its contents, the mediastinal structures, the pleura, and the pericardium.

The lungs are not sensitive to pain. Pleuritic pain is very characteristic—the patient notes a sharp, severe pain over the rib cage or upper abdomen associated with deep breathing or coughing. The patient may "splint" the chest by selectively restricting chest expansion on the affected side. Pleuritic pain may be seen with rib fractures; diseases of the pleura or lung such as pneumonia, pleural effusion, empyema, or pneumothorax. Pain associated with esophageal disease or spasm of the esophagus may closely mimic angina pectoris. Anterior chest wall pain that can be reproduced with firm pressure over the costochondral junctions is generally attributed to inflammation at these sites (Tietze's syndrome). When the pleural surfaces over the diaphragm are a source of pain, the pain may be noted in the shoulder since these surfaces are innervated by the phrenic nerve. When the intercostal nerves are involved with herpes zoster infection, the first symptom may be severe, constant, unilateral chest pain, and when there is no associated skin eruption, the cause may escape detection until the characteristic rash appears.

A careful history regarding tobacco smoking is essential. The details must include the age when the patient began to smoke and an estimation of the number of cigarettes smoked per day over the years. This is important even if the patient quit smoking years before. A careful occupational history is important when chronic disease of the airways and the lung interstitium is found. This is best done by asking the patient to begin by describing the first job he or she ever had and then sequentially each job after that until the present or last work has been described. Careful attention to possible exposures to toxic fumes and inhaled particulate such as asbestos fibers and other silicates is required. Place of residence and recent travel to distant geographic regions must be noted. Hobbies may be associated with exposure to potentially toxic dusts and solvents. Congenital diseases may cause chronic disorders with early onset of symptoms, such as may be seen with the immotile cilia syndrome, which produces repeated episodes of pneumonia and bronchitis,

or the α_1-antitrypsin deficiency syndrome, which produces dyspnea in mid- to early adulthood.

PHYSICAL EXAMINATION

Physical examination of the chest can provide a wealth of useful information to assist in diagnosis and management in the clinic, emergency department, and hospital. Full development of skills in chest examination requires that the examiner be a good observer and careful about noting small details (Table 13–1). The first step is to observe the patient breathe and, if possible, listen for a cough. The sound of a cough can tell many things. A vigorous cough indicates that the individual can keep the upper airways clear of secretions, and if secretions are present in the upper airways the cough will produce sputum. The sound of a cough can provide the trained ear with an estimate of the vital capacity and the rate of expiratory air flow. Many times the cough reveals audible wheezing, not heard on quiet breathing. A weak cough may reveal the rattling sound of secretions in the upper airways and trachea even though no sputum is produced because the force of the cough is so reduced. Finally, it is notable that repeated deep breaths frequently induce coughing in patients who have inflamed airways as in asthma and bronchitis. Thus, coughs may be as individualized and as characteristic as cardiac murmurs.

As one observes the patient breathe, the respiration rate is noted. Most normal adults breathe at rates < 18 per minute and do so by symmetric expansion of the rib cage and abdomen (due to a downward motion of the diaphragm). As the respiratory effort increases, the patient

TABLE 13–1	Systematic Approach to Physical Examination of the Chest

I. Inspection
  Initial impression—distress, wheeze, malnourishment, etc.
  Respiratory rate, depth, and pattern
  Asynchronous motion of the rib cage and abdomen
  Recession of the intercostal, supraclavicular, or suprasternal
    spaces
  Tracheal tug
  Cyanosis
  Finger clubbing or nicotine stains
  Accessory muscle employment
  Pursed-lip breathing
  Chest wall shape and deformity
II. Palpation
  Tracheal deviation
  Chest expansion (globally/locally)
  Vocal fremitus
  Pleural rub
  Lymphadenopathy
  Subcutaneous emphysema
III. Percussion
  Normal, dull, or increased
IV. Auscultation
  Breath sounds (over small airways)—vesicular sounds are heard
  Bronchial breath sounds over small airways associated with whispered pectoriloquy and egophony indicate lung consolidation
  Added sounds—can be only absent, wheezes, crackles, or pleural
    rub

may use the intercostal muscles and diaphragm more extensively, and if greater effort is required, the scalene muscle group will be recruited for use. The examiner cannot see the scalene muscles contract. To detect this, the examiner should place the tips of the second, third, and fourth digits in the supraclavicular space and press firmly downward. Holding the hand in this position for a few respiratory cycles allows one to feel these muscles contract and become firm with each inspiration. These muscles are used almost continuously by patients with advanced chronic obstructive lung disease and are used in almost all patients during episodes of moderate to marked dyspnea. The last muscle to be recruited for bellows activity is the sternocleidomastoid. When this muscle is contracting with each inspiration (best detected by palpation rather than observation), the patient is making a near-maximal effort to breathe. Such patients cannot continue such maximal efforts to breathe for prolonged periods; they tire quickly, and this may lead to respiratory failure. Patients with obstructive lung disease due to emphysema may use pursed-lip breathing to provide symptomatic relief of dyspnea.

Abnormal movements of the chest wall can give important clues about diagnosis. When the rib cage and abdomen do not expand synchronously, diaphragmatic and/or intercostal paralysis may be present. Patients with advanced obstructive lung disease or severe asthma may have flattened diaphragms. As the diaphragm becomes flat, it pulls the lower rib cage inward on inspiration—a sign that can be visually noted when extreme. More often, it is detected by the observer placing his or her hands over the lower anterior rib cage and observing whether the hands move apart or together on inspiration. When the hands move together, the diaphragm is flat, which

indicates that the chest is markedly overexpanded. The trachea may deviate from the midline when there is a mediastinal shift, as seen with a large pneumothorax or a massive pleural effusion. Vocal fremitus is the palpable vibration associated with the spoken word, detected by placing the hands against the chest wall as the patient repeats a word or number. Fluid in the pleural space or lung collapse with a pneumothorax markedly reduces the transmission of these vibrations. Chest wall percussion is most helpful in detecting when the air-filled lung is replaced by fluid or a solid structure. Increased fremitus, as is seen in pulmonary consolidation, is most difficult to detect and is seldom helpful.

During auscultation, the examiner should compare the two sides of the chest at equidistant points from the midline. The breath sounds should be evaluated first. All normal persons have three types of breath sounds: listening over the trachea reveals a bronchial breath sound, listening just lateral to the midline near the tracheal bifurcation reveals bronchovesicular breath sounds, and listening over the peripheral lung areas where only small airways and alveoli are present reveals vesicular breath sounds. In lung diseases, the normal vesicular sound is usually replaced by a bronchovesicular sound and, uncommonly, by a bronchial breath sound. The type of breath sound heard is determined while the examiner listens when the patient is sitting, breathing with the mouth open, taking relatively deep breaths. A bronchial sound is characterized by the sound of expiration being longer than that of inspiration, in sharp contrast to the vesicular breath sound, where the duration of inspiration is three to five times longer than the sound of expiration. A bronchovesicular breath sound is one for which the duration of inspiration and expiration is approximately equal. A

TABLE 13–2	Physical Findings in Common Pulmonary Disorders						
Disorder	Mediastinal Displacement	Chest Wall Movement	Vocal Fremitus	Percussion Note	Breath Sounds	Added Sounds	Voice Sounds
Pleural effusion	Heart displaced to opposite side	Reduced over affected area	Absent or markedly decreased	Dull	Absent over fluid; bronchial at upper border	Absent; pleural rub may be found above effusion	Absent over effusion; increased with egophony at upper border
Consolidation	None	Reduced over affected area	Increased or normal	Dull	Bronchial	Crackles	Increased with egophony and whispered pectoriloquy
Pneumothorax	Tracheal deviation to opposite side if under tension	Decreased over affected area	Absent	Resonant	Absent or decreased	Absent	Absent
Atelectasis	Ipsilateral shift	Decreased over affected area	Variable	Dull	Absent or diminished	Crackles may be heard	Absent
Bronchospasm	None	Decreased symmetrically	Normal or decreased	Normal or decreased	Bronchovesicular	Wheeze	Normal or decreased
Interstitial fibrosis	None	Decreased symmetrically	Normal or increased	Normal	Bronchovesicular	End-inspiratory crackles unaffected by cough or posture	Normal

vesicular breath sound of normal intensity heard throughout the lung fields is a highly reliable sign of normal lung tissue. Bronchovesicular breath sounds heard over the peripheral airways are abnormal but nonspecific; almost all abnormalities of the lung produce this effect. When bronchial breath sounds replace vesicular sounds, the lung may be consolidated (no air in the alveolar spaces). Bronchial sounds are also heard at the upper margin of a pleural effusion. When consolidation is present, the examiner may also detect that vocal sounds are well transmitted to the chest wall. Normally when the patient is asked to count off numbers in a whispered voice, the words cannot be understood as one listens through a stethoscope with the diaphragm placed firmly on the chest wall. Over consolidated areas, these whispered words or numbers are clearly heard (whispered pectoriloquy). Small areas of consolidation are best found by asking the patient to repeat the letter "e." Over consolidated areas, the sound of a spoken long "e" is heard as long "a" with a marked nasal quality (egophony).

After the breath sounds are evaluated, the next step is to listen for any extra sounds not present normally. There may be crackles (rales), wheezes, or pleural sounds. Wheezes may be high or low pitched and may occur during inspiration, expiration, or both. The high-pitched wheeze is a musical sound, and when it is localized it suggests partial bronchial obstruction, as seen with a mass, stricture, or foreign body. Diffuse wheezing is noted in asthma, chronic obstructive lung disease, chronic bronchitis, and, at times, in pulmonary edema. Wheezing not heard on normal breathing may be brought out when the subject is asked to expire forcefully, as when making a vital capacity effort, or when asked to breathe in and out rapidly, taking short breaths each time (panting).

Crackles are short sequences of discontinuous sounds that are almost always heard on inspiration and rarely on expiration. When secretions pool in the trachea, a rattling sound is produced that can be heard at the bedside without the use of the stethoscope. Crackles heard only with a stethoscope are generally produced as small airways pop open during inspiration. Although terms such as "coarse" and "fine" are used to describe these crackles, these adjectives are nonspecific and do not provide reliable, useful information. The recommended approach is to describe the moment during inspiration when the crackle is heard. Crackles heard only at end inspiration are heard at the lung bases in most normal individuals when they reach their 50s and 60s. Obesity produces end-inspiratory crackles, as do pulmonary edema, pneumonia, and atelectasis. Lung disease states that decrease lung compliance most often produce end-inspiratory crackles. Crackles heard in mid-inspiration that terminate prior to end inspiration are heard in bronchitis and chronic obstructive lung disease.

Pleural sounds are produced when the visceral and parietal pleura are inflamed. As these surfaces move against each other during the respiratory cycle, a typical crunching sound is heard. The sound is likened to that created by walking in fresh-fallen snow. At times the sound is heard only in inspiration or expiration. When the mediastinal pleura is involved, the cardiac motion may produce the same sound, as is found with pneumomediastinum.

The typical findings of some common pulmonary disorders are listed in Table 13–2.

REFERENCES

Braman SS (ed.): Pulmonary signs and symptoms. Clin Chest Med 1987; 8:177–334.

Nath AR, Chapel LH: Inspiratory crackles early and late. Thorax 1974; 29:223–227.

Sapria JD: About egophony. Chest 1995; 108:867.

14

Anatomic and Physiologic Considerations

The most important function of the lung is to accept blood exiting from the right ventricle, decrease its carbon dioxide content, and then return blood to the left atrium. This demand varies dramatically, from basal levels of 3 to 4 ml of O_2 or CO_2 kg$^{-1} \cdot$ min^{-1} to as much as 60 ml of O_2 or CO_2 kg$^{-1} \cdot$ min^{-1} at maximum exercise capacity. To accomplish this, sufficient blood and gas must be brought together at a sufficiently large surface area to allow for rapid and adequate gas exchange.

THE AIRWAY

Structure

The inspired air travels through a complex pathway on its way to the alveoli. The nose and pharynx heat, humidify, and filter the air of particulates and water-soluble gases. Air then passes through the larynx, a complex group of muscles and cartilages, which remains patent during inspiration and closes during swallowing and maneuvers that require an increase in intrathoracic pressure, such as defecation and vomiting. As the inspired air exits the larynx and enters the trachea, it has been warmed to 37°C, humidified to 100%, and filtered free of almost all particulate matter > 10 μm in diameter.

The trachea is a 10- to 12-cm tube supported by U-shaped cartilages and a fibrous posterior membrane. The trachea divides into two mainstem bronchi at the carina. The right mainstem bronchus is a more direct continuation of the trachea; thus, aspirated foreign bodies tend to lodge on the right side. The airways continue to branch, and in the smaller airways the cartilage becomes incomplete and disappears when the airways are 1 to 2 mm in diameter. The first 19 branches, ending at the terminal bronchioles, provide a rapid and enormous expansion of the total airway cross-sectional area, increasing from 2.5 cm^2 in the trachea to approximately 900 cm^2 (Fig. 14–1). Beyond this are three generations of respiratory bronchioles whose walls are made up of increasing proportions of alveoli. This anatomic arrangement progresses into the alveolar ducts and culminates in the alveolar sacs. At this point, the cross-sectional area of the alveolar capillary membrane has increased to 70 to 80 m^2.

The epithelial surface of the alveolar capillary membrane, the site of gas exchange, is lined primarily by flat, type I pneumocytes, which rest on a thin basement membrane. Interspersed between the type I cells are the columnar type II cells, which produce surfactant, the surface tension–lowering substance lining the alveoli and alveolar ducts. After a significant injury to the alveolar-capillary membrane, this cell proliferates and is probably responsible for the repair.

VENTILATION

During inspiration, respiratory muscle contraction increases intrathoracic volume, which in turn decreases airway pressure below atmospheric and causes air to enter the lungs. Expiration is passive, as the intrinsic elasticity of the lungs and chest wall returns the volume of the system to its resting position. With increased ventilatory requirements, the expiratory muscles may be enlisted to assist in lung emptying.

The respiratory muscles include the diaphragm, the intercostal and accessory muscles, and the abdominal muscles. The diaphragm is the major muscle of inspiration, and when it contracts, it pushes down against the abdominal contents, causing the ribs to move upward and outward. The increase in abdominal pressure causes an outward motion of the abdominal wall, the clinical hallmark of diaphragmatic contraction. The intercostal and accessory muscles not used in normal quiet breathing, primarily the sternocleidomastoid and the scalene muscles, facilitate inspiration by directly elevating the chest wall. In advanced emphysema, the diaphragm assumes a flat position rather than being dome shaped. This markedly alters the chest wall movement; rather than moving the lower rib cage upward and outward on inspiration, the flat diaphragm pulls the rib cage inward during inspiration. The abdominal muscles increase abdominal pressure and drive the relaxed diaphragm upward during expiration and other situations requiring increases in intrathoracic pressure, such as coughing. As expiration is normally passive, expiratory muscle activity is not necessary unless ventilatory requirements are high or significant airway obstruction is present.

The respiratory muscles, like other skeletal muscles, will, if stressed sufficiently, fatigue. Proper training can induce a small but significant increase in their strength and endurance. The typical relations between resting

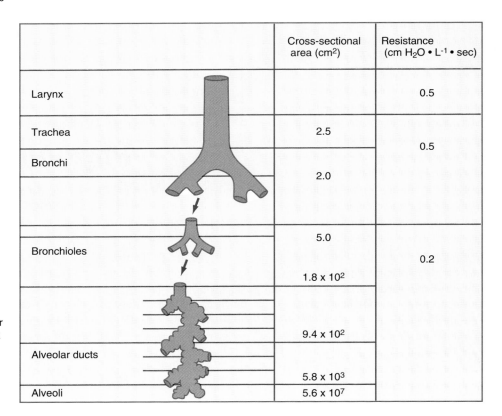

	Cross-sectional area (cm²)	Resistance (cm $H_2O \cdot L^{-1} \cdot$ sec)
Larynx		0.5
Trachea	2.5	0.5
Bronchi	2.0	
Bronchioles	5.0	0.2
	1.8×10^2	
	9.4×10^2	
Alveolar ducts		
	5.8×10^3	
Alveoli	5.6×10^7	

Figure 14–1

The subdivision of the airways and their nomenclature. The cross-sectional area increases dramatically as we reach the peripheral, small airways. (Adapted from Weibel ER: Morphometry of the Human Lung. Berlin, Springer, 1963; with permission.)

length and the amount of tension developed also exist. For the respiratory muscles, length can be translated into lung volume, and when length is increased, as in emphysema, inspiratory muscle efficiency is decreased (Fig. 14–2).

To increase intrathoracic volume, the respiratory muscles must overcome elastic and resistive forces. If the lungs of a normal individual were removed from the chest, they would collapse, while the volume of the chest wall would expand to about 80% of the total capacity of the thoracic space. Thus, when combined, the lungs and chest wall pull in opposite directions, with the resting volume of the system, the functional residual capacity (FRC), occurring at the volume at which the outward pull of the chest wall equals the inward pull of the lungs, which is normally less than 50% of total lung capacity (TLC).

Changes in elasticity are commonly considered in terms of inverse function: Compliance equals the change in volume or change in pressure. In normal lungs, near FRC, it takes an average of 1 cm H_2O to inflate the lungs by 200 ml (Fig. 14–3); that is, compliance at this volume is 200 ml/cm H_2O. However, near TLC, the lung and chest wall get stiffer, requiring greater inflationary pressure. Compliance decreases with pulmonary fibrosis or pulmonary edema and increases with emphysema. The normal compliance of the chest wall is also 200 ml/cm H_2O, and this may be decreased by skeletal abnormalities such as scoliosis or increased by the loss of respiratory muscle tone in neuromuscular disease.

The second force that must be overcome by the respiratory muscles is airway resistance, defined as the

driving pressure divided by air flow, normally 1 to 2 cm H_2O $L^{-1} \cdot sec^{-1}$. It is greatly dependent on the total cross-sectional areas of the airways, and thus, even though the individual peripheral airways are narrow, their contribution to overall airway resistance is small because of the increase in total cross-sectional area (see Fig. 14–1). Many factors influence airway resistance. An increase in lung volume decreases resistance because of the tethering effect of the alveoli on the airways. Other factors that influence airway resistance include bronchial smooth muscle contraction (bronchospasm), intrinsic or extrinsic airway compression, and the dynamic compression of a forced expiration.

The work of breathing is the product of the pressure generated and the change in volume. In normal subjects, this represents a tiny fraction of the overall energy utilized by the body (4 to 5%), even with high ventilatory requirements such as exercise. However, in the presence of lung disease, as the work of breathing increases, the O_2 requirements of the respiratory muscles can become inordinately high, as much as 30% of total-body O_2 consumption. Under these circumstances, the benefit of any increase in gas exchange achieved by increasing ventilation may be offset, or even exceeded, by the increased O_2 consumption and CO_2 production of the respiratory muscles.

Gas entering the lungs is divided into that entering the gas-exchanging regions of the lung, the alveolar volume (VA), and that remaining in the conducting airways, the dead space (VD). At end expiration, VD is filled with gas that has already equilibrated with pulmonary capillary blood; thus, on the subsequent inspiration, the amount of

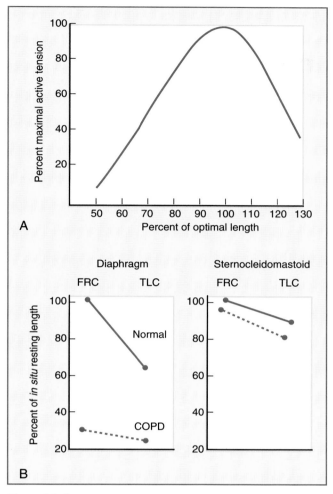

Figure 14-2

A, The length-tension curve for the diaphragm. At lengths above or below the optimal *in situ* resting length, the amount of tension generated decreases. *B,* The change in the length of the diaphragm and sternocleidomastoid muscles at functional residual capacity (FRC) and total lung capacity (TLC) in a normal subject and a patient with chronic obstructive lung disease (COPD) and hyperinflation. Increased FRC shortens the resting length of the diaphragm so that contraction during inspiration becomes inefficient. Consequently, rib cage expansion becomes more dependent on accessory muscle contraction. (From Druz WS, Danon J, Fishman HC, et al: Approaches to assessing respiratory muscle function in respiratory disease. Am Rev Respir Dis 1979; 119:145; with permission.)

fresh gas reaching the alveoli is equal to the tidal volume (VT) minus VD. VD makes up 20 to 40% of a normal VT.

Distribution of VA within the lung depends on the regional pleural pressure. Normally, pleural pressure is most negative at the apex of the lung and becomes less negative as we move toward the lung base. This gradient is caused by a combination of gravity due to the weight of the lung and the different stresses imposed by the shape of the lung and chest wall. As a result of this gradient, the lung bases are better ventilated than the apices.

Control of Ventilation

The precise adjustment in ventilation necessary to meet changing metabolic demands is made by balancing tidal volume and respiratory frequency through the integrative function of the three components of the respiratory control system: respiratory control centers, respiratory sensors, and respiratory effectors (Fig. 14–4).

Respiratory Control Centers

The neurons controlling respiration are located at several levels in the brain stem. The most important network resides in the medulla oblongata, where respiratory rhythm originates. These medullary neurons receive input from the pons, which, while not necessary for rhythmic breathing, appears to fine tune the respiratory pattern. The brain stem centers are responsible for the automatic control of ventilation, but the cerebral cortex can override them during wakefulness to permit speech and other actions requiring voluntary control of ventilation.

Respiratory Sensors

The respiratory sensors consist of the central and peripheral chemoreceptors and the chest wall and intrapulmonary sensory receptors. The central chemoreceptors, lo-

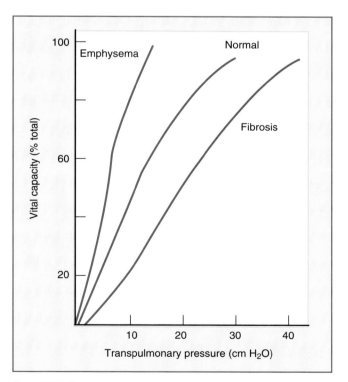

Figure 14-3

The compliance curves for normal subjects and patients with emphysema and pulmonary fibrosis. An elevation in the transpulmonary pressure required to achieve a given lung volume increases the work of breathing.

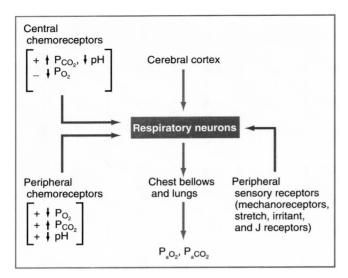

Figure 14-4
Schematic representation of the respiratory control system. The respiratory neurons in the brain stem receive information from the chemoreceptors, peripheral sensory receptors, and cerebral cortex. This information is integrated, and the resulting neural output is transmitted to the chest bellows and lungs.

cated on the ventral surface of the medulla oblongata, rapidly respond to any increase in CO_2 or hydrogen ion concentration by increasing ventilation (Fig. 14-5*A*). Under normal circumstances, these receptors are very sensitive, keeping the Pa_{CO_2} constant despite marked variability in CO_2 production. In contrast, hypoxia does not act as a central respiratory stimulant but instead depresses the central chemoreceptors. Conversely, the peripheral chemoreceptors, located in the carotid bodies, are activated mainly by hypoxia and less so by CO_2 and hydrogen ions. They are also sensitive to a fall in blood pressure, which may partly account for hyperventilation seen in shock. Unlike linear response to P_{CO_2}, the ventilatory response to hypoxemia is hyperbolic, and a fall in PO_2 causes little increase in ventilation until there is significant hypoxemia (PO_2 less than 60 mm Hg) (Fig. 14-5*B*).

Mechanoreceptors in the chest wall respond to stretch of the intercostal muscles and reflexively modulate the rate and depth of breathing. Tidal volume and respiratory frequency may also be reflexively affected by stimuli arising in (1) airway irritant receptors, which respond to physical or chemical stimulation; (2) pulmonary stretch receptors, which respond to marked increases in lung volume (Hering-Breuer reflex); or (3) J receptors found in the juxtacapillary junctions, which respond to vascular engorgement and congestion.

Effectors of the Respiratory System

Signals are transmitted from the respiratory center to the respiratory muscles by (1) the phrenic nerves, which supply the diaphragm; (2) the intercostal nerves, which innervate the intercostal and abdominal muscles; (3) the acces-

sory cranial nerves, which supply the sternomastoid muscles; and (4) the lower cervical nerves, which supply the scalene muscles. In addition, a variety of muscles acting on the soft palate, tongue, and hyoid bone maintain upper airway patency and offset the collapsing effect of the negative pressures generated by the respiratory muscles. During wakefulness, both the upper airway and the chest wall muscles display rhythmic inspiratory activity. During sleep, upper airway muscle activity wanes, whereas diaphragmatic activation changes little.

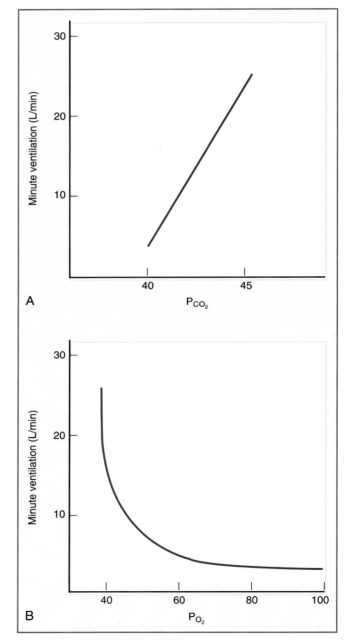

Figure 14-5
A rising P_{CO_2} leads to a linear increase in minute ventilation *(A)*. The ventilatory response to hypoxemia *(B)* is less sensitive and is clinically relevant only when the PO_2 has dropped significantly.

THE BLOOD VESSELS

Structure

The lungs receive blood from two vascular systems—the bronchial and pulmonary circulations. The nutritive blood flow to all but the alveolar structures comes from the bronchial circulation, which originates from the aorta. About one third of the venous effluent of the bronchial circulation drains into the systemic veins and back to the right ventricle. The remainder drains into the pulmonary veins and, along with the contribution from the thebesian veins in the heart, represents a component of the 1 to 2% right-to-left shunt found in normal subjects.

The pulmonary arterial system runs alongside the airways from the hila to the periphery. The arteries down to the level of the subsegmental airways (2 mm in diameter) are thin-walled, predominantly elastic vessels. Beyond this, the arteries become muscularized until they reach diameters of 30 μm, at which point the muscular coat disappears. Most of the arterial pressure drop takes place in these small muscular arteries, which are responsible for the active control of blood flow distribution in the lung. The pulmonary arterioles empty into an extensive capillary network and drain into thin-walled pulmonary veins, which eventually join with the arteries and bronchi at the hilum and exit the lung to enter the left atrium.

Perfusion

The pulmonary vascular bed serves as a source of nutritive blood to the alveolar membrane, but its most important role is in pulmonary gas exchange. It delivers the entire systemic venous return to the pulmonary capillary bed, where exchange of O_2 and CO_2 occurs. Although it receives the same blood flow per minute as the systemic circulation, there are differences between the vascular beds. First, since the pulmonary vascular resistance, calculated as (pulmonary arterial pressure/left atrial pressure) cardiac output, is only about one tenth of systemic vascular resistance, the pressure in the pulmonary vascular bed is only one tenth of that in the systemic circulation. Second, all structures within the thorax, including the pulmonary vascular bed, the heart, and the great vessels, are exposed to the surrounding pressures, both pleural and alveolar, which vary during respiration. Mean intraluminal esophageal pressure closely reflects mean pleural pressure.

The distribution of blood flow within the lung is greatly dependent on the interaction between vascular and alveolar pressure. Alveolar pressure is relatively constant throughout the lung. However, like any column of fluid, pulmonary vascular pressure is lower at the top and greater at the bottom of the lung (Fig. 14–6). At the apex, pulmonary arterial pressure is usually just able to overcome alveolar pressure. However, a fall in arterial pressure or any rise in alveolar pressure (positive pressure breathing) may cause alveolar pressure to exceed arterial pressure, with cessation of flow. This is known as zone 1

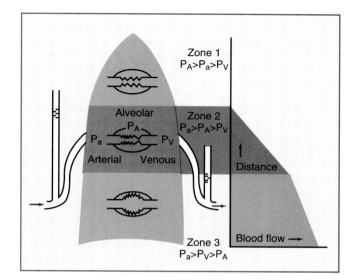

Figure 14–6
The zonal model of blood flow in the lung. Because of the interrelationship of vascular and alveolar pressures, the lung base receives the most flow (see text for explanation). (From West JB, Dollery CT, Naimark A: Distribution of blood flow in isolated lung; relation to vascular and alveolar pressures. J Appl Physiol 1964; 19:713, with permission.)

conditions. Below this lies zone 2, where the alveolar pressure is less than arterial pressure but greater than venous pressure. Blood flow in zone 2 depends on the difference between arterial pressure and alveolar pressure. Blood flow continues to increase down zone 2 because of rising arterial pressure and eventually reaches a point, zone 3, at which venous pressure finally exceeds alveolar pressure and flow becomes dependent on arterial-venous pressure difference. Blood flow increases progressively down zone 3 because of increasing distention and recruitment of the pulmonary vessels.

Many factors affect the overall pressure-flow relations in the pulmonary circulation. When cardiac output increases in normal upright humans, as during exercise, pulmonary vascular resistance actually falls because of the ability to recruit new vessels and distend the ones already open. This allows large increases in blood flow with lesser increases in pressure, thus preventing the transudation of fluid into the lungs, owing to a higher microvascular pressure. Pulmonary vascular resistance is also affected by lung volume. It is lowest at FRC and increases at lower lung volumes because there is less distention of the pulmonary arteries, which, like the airways, are tethered by the lung parenchyma. At higher lung volumes, pulmonary vascular resistance also falls, owing to compression of capillaries by the distending alveoli.

In addition to these passive influences, a number of factors actively affect pulmonary vascular tone. The most important is alveolar hypoxia, which results in constriction of the perfusing artery by mechanisms as yet unknown. This factor may be useful when alveolar hypoxia is localized, since reduction in perfusion to poorly ventilated alveoli reduces the abnormality of gas exchange,

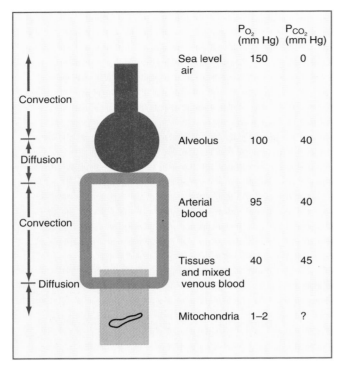

Figure 14–7
The transfer of O_2 and CO_2 from the atmosphere to the mitochondria.

which is otherwise inevitable. During generalized hypoxia, its beneficial nature is not always apparent, as in sojourners at high altitude, in whom it may be a major cause of pulmonary edema. Acidosis causes a vasoconstrictor response of lesser magnitude. Other vasoactive compounds produced in the body, such as prostaglandins and adrenergic substances, may also alter pulmonary vascular tone.

Gas Transfer

Carbon dioxide and O_2 are transported between the environment and the tissues by convection and diffusion (Fig. 14–7). In the blood, O_2 combines with hemoglobin, and the resulting O_2 saturation is determined by the oxyhemoglobin dissociation curve (Fig. 14–8A). More than 98% of O_2 in the blood is combined with hemoglobin; the remainder is dissolved in the plasma. Above a Pa_{O_2} of 150 mm Hg, hemoglobin is totally saturated and carries 1.34 ml O_2/gm hemoglobin; further rises in Pa_{O_2} increase only the amount of O_2 dissolved in the plasma at the rate of 0.003 ml O_2/100 ml blood/mm Hg P_{O_2}. CO_2 is carried in the blood in three forms: bicarbonate (90%), dissolved in plasma, or combined with protein, predominantly hemoglobin. The relation between the P_{CO_2} and the CO_2 content is described by the CO_2 dissociation curve (Fig. 14–8B), which is steeper and more linear than the oxyhemoglobin dissociation curve.

A number of factors influence the relations between P_{O_2} and P_{CO_2} and their contents, which can be described

as changes in the position of the respective dissociation curves. Increased P_{CO_2} and temperature and decreased pH shift the oxyhemoglobin dissociation curve to the right, decreasing affinity of hemoglobin for O_2 and expediting its release to the tissues. Converse changes in these factors have the opposite effect. Increased levels of 2,3-diphosphoglycerate (2,3-DPG), produced during chronic hypoxemia or anemia, also shift the curve to the right,

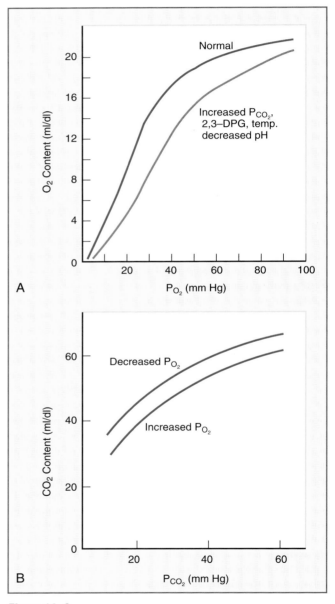

Figure 14–8
A, The oxyhemoglobin dissociation curve. The bulk of the O_2 is carried combined with hemoglobin. The various factors that decrease the hemoglobin O_2 affinity are shown. Opposite changes increase hemoglobin O_2 affinity, shifting the curve to the left. B, The CO_2 dissociation curve. It is more linear than the oxyhemoglobin curve throughout the physiologic range. Increased P_{O_2} shifts the curve to the right, which decreases CO_2 content for any given P_{CO_2} and thus facilitates CO_2 off-loading in the lungs. The shift to the left at a lower P_{O_2} facilitates CO_2 on-loading at the tissues.

whereas carbon monoxide shifts it to the left and also reduces the O_2 content by competitively binding to hemoglobin. The most important influence on the CO_2 dissociation curve is PO_2; increased PO_2 shifts the curve to the right, thus reducing the affinity of hemoglobin for CO_2 and assisting in the unloading of CO_2 in the lungs.

PULMONARY GAS EXCHANGE

The arterial blood gas values are determined by the composition of alveolar gas and its successful equilibration with the blood in the pulmonary capillaries. In turn, the PO_2 and PCO_2 in the alveoli are determined by the inspired gas tensions, the mixed venous PO_2 and PCO_2, the total ventilation, the blood flow, and, most important, the success with which the lung is able to match ventilation and blood flow. Abnormality of any of these factors leads to hypoxemia and/or hypercapnia.

HYPOVENTILATION. Minute ventilation and the arterial PCO_2 are inversely related. Hypoventilation is defined as a minute ventilation that, for a given metabolic demand, is inadequate to keep the arterial PCO_2 in the normal range. Since ventilation is normally closely coupled to metabolic CO_2 production, hypoventilation usually represents a failure of respiratory control or of the ventilatory pump to respond. Hypoventilation is commonly due to pharmacologic depression of or structural damage to the respiratory center, a neuromuscular disease, or a chest wall abnormality.

The increase in PCO_2 leads to a concomitant fall in the PO_2, as described in the alveolar gas equation

$$PA_{O_2} = (PB - PH_2O)\, FI_{O_2} - \frac{Pa_{CO_2}}{R}$$

where PA_{O_2} is alveolar PO_2, PB is atmospheric pressure (usually 760 mm Hg), PH_2O is the partial pressure of water vapor (47 mm Hg), FI_{O_2} is the fractional concentration of inspired O_2, and R is the respiratory exchange ratio (which can be estimated at 0.8). We see that any rise in Pa_{CO_2} leads to a concomitant fall in PA_{O_2} and thus in Pa_{O_2}.

ABNORMAL DIFFUSION. Under normal conditions, blood spends about 0.75 second in the pulmonary capillaries. Since it ordinarily takes only about one third of this time for the blood to equilibrate with alveolar gas, there is a wide safety margin before abnormal pathology results in nonequilibration, that is, a diffusion impairment. It has been estimated that the diffusing capacity of the lung must fall to less than 10% of normal before it affects Pa_{O_2} at rest. Three factors may stress the system sufficiently to interfere with complete equilibration: increased diffusion distance due to a thickening of the alveolar capillary membrane; increased rate of blood flow or a reduction in the number of open capillaries, decreasing the time the blood spends in the process of equilibration; and reduced driving pressure from alveolus to blood, as

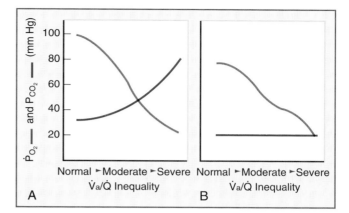

Figure 14–9

A, The effect of increasing ventilation-perfusion ($\dot{V}a/\dot{Q}$) inequality on arterial PO_2 and PCO_2 when cardiac output and minute ventilation are held constant. The change in gas tensions when ventilation is allowed to increase is shown in *B.* Increased ventilation can maintain a normal PCO_2 but can only partially correct the hypoxemia. (Adapted from Dantzker DR: Gas exchange abnormalities. *In* Montenegro H [ed.]: Chronic Obstructive Pulmonary Disease. New York, Churchill Livingstone, 1984, pp 141–160; with permission.)

seen at extreme altitudes. Diffusion impairment almost never plays a role in the hypoxemia of disease.

VENTILATION-PERFUSION INEQUALITY. The proper matching of ventilation and blood flow within the lung is necessary for the adequate uptake of O_2 and elimination of CO_2. While the lung is sometimes regarded as a single gas-exchanging unit, it really contains units that differ in their relative amounts of blood flow and ventilation. In normal persons, the span of ventilation-perfusion ($\dot{V}a/\dot{Q}$) ratios is very small, varying from about 0.5 to 3.0, with an average of 0.8. As lung disease develops, the range increasingly widens, with some units receiving very little ventilation relative to perfusion, while others are excessively ventilated. If $\dot{V}a/\dot{Q}$ inequality develops, the arterial PO_2 will fall and the PCO_2 will rise (Fig. 14–9*A*). In patients with normal respiratory drive and without severe limitation in ventilatory capacity, the increasing PCO_2 leads to a progressive increase in ventilation. This increase in ventilation is capable of keeping the PCO_2 normal but only minimally attenuates the fall in the PO_2 (Fig. 14–9*B*) because of the different shapes of the oxyhemoglobin and carboxyhemoglobin dissociation curves (see Fig. 14–8). The oxyhemoglobin dissociation curve plateaus at a high PO_2; thus, the increased PO_2 in alveoli receiving increased ventilation fails to increase the O_2 content of blood leaving that unit. Since no additional O_2 has been added, it cannot compensate for the poorly ventilated lung units. The carboxyhemoglobin dissociation curve, on the other hand, is linear throughout the physiologic range. Any decrease in PCO_2 is accompanied by a fall in CO_2 content, allowing the overventilated alveoli to offset the failure of poorly ventilated lung units to eliminate CO_2. As $\dot{V}a/\dot{Q}$ inequality worsens with progression of the underlying disease, further increases in ventilation eventually become impossible, and both hypoxemia and hyper-

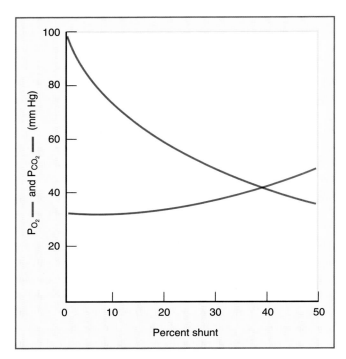

Figure 14-10
The effect of increasing shunt on the arterial Po_2 and Pco_2. The minute ventilation has been held constant in this example. Under normal circumstances, the hypoxemia would lead to an increased minute ventilation and a fall in the Pco_2 as the shunt increases. (From Dantzker DR: Gas exchange abnormalities. *In* Montenegro H [ed.]: Chronic Obstructive Pulmonary Disease. New York, Churchill Livingstone, 1984, pp 141–160; with permission.)

capnia result. $\dot{V}a/\dot{Q}$ inequality is the characteristic abnormality of gas exchange in chronic obstructive and restrictive lung diseases.

SHUNT. Intrapulmonary or intracardiac shunt, where blood bypasses ventilated lung units, is a most potent source of hypoxemia, but hypercapnia is not seen (Fig. 14–10). In fact, as the hypoxemia progresses, hypocapnia is usually found, owing to the stimulatory effects of the low Pa_{O_2} on ventilatory drive. Shunting is the major mechanism of hypoxemia in pulmonary edema, pneumonia, and atelectasis.

NONPULMONARY FACTORS

Abnormalities other than alterations in lung function may influence the Pa_{O_2} through their effect on the mixed venous PO_2 (Pv_{O_2}). The Pv_{O_2} is decreased when cardiac output is inappropriately low, when O_2 consumption ($\dot{V}O_2$) is increased (as with exercise or fever), or when the hemoglobin concentration or O_2 saturation is low. For any lung unit, the resultant end-capillary PO_2 is influenced by the Pv_{O_2}, although the magnitude of this effect on the arterial O_2 content will be greatest in lungs with $\dot{V}a/\dot{Q}$ inequality or shunt (Fig. 14–11). The importance of this phenomenon is the recognition that a fall in Pa_{O_2} in a patient with lung disease may be due to one of these

nonpulmonary factors rather than to deterioration in lung function, thus requiring a very different intervention.

GROWTH AND AGING OF THE NORMAL LUNG

The lung grows by alveolar multiplication up to about 8 years, and thereafter no additional alveoli are formed; the number of conducting airways is complete at birth. The conducting airways grow in length and diameter according to body size. There are approximately 24×10^6 alveoli at birth and 300×10^6 in the adult. At an early age, the maximum number of alveoli is reached, and after this the alveoli increase in diameter. This gives a marked increase in the alveolar surface area, which reaches its maximum of 70 to 80 m^2 at about age 20.

The lung volumes all increase in proportion to body growth. The maximums for volume are reached for both sexes at about age 20. Thereafter with aging, the normal lung shows a progressive loss of alveolar surface area, together with a concurrent decrease in elastic recoil. Aging is associated with alveolar septal membranes that weaken and stretch and with loss of alveolar septal membranes, so that by 80 years the surface area of the lung is reduced by about 30%. Loss of surface areas brings a decrease in the elastic recoil at all lung volumes. Flow resistance during forced expiration increases with age, resulting in reduced maximal flow rates and reduced timed forced expiratory volumes. The decrease in elastic

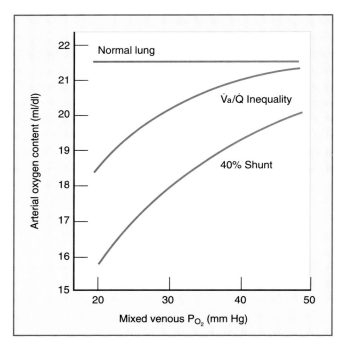

Figure 14-11
The effect of altering mixed venous PO_2 (Pv_{O_2}) on the arterial oxygen content under three assumed conditions: a normal lung, severe ventilation-perfusion ($\dot{V}a/\dot{Q}$) inequality, and the presence of a 40% shunt. For each situation the patient is breathing 50% O_2 and the PV_{O_2} is altered, keeping all other variables constant. (From Dantzker DR: Gas exchange in the adult respiratory distress syndrome. Clin Chest Med 1982; 3:57; with permission.)

recoil results in a decrease in the negative pressure measured in the pleural space. In the normal young adult studied in the upright position at functional residual capacity, the pleural pressure is about -10 cm of H_2O near the lung apex and about -6 cm of H_2O at the lung base. In the normal 70-year-old person, these measurements under the same conditions show pressures of -6 cm of H_2O at the apex, and at the lung base the value may be 0 or slightly positive. These pressure changes are of great importance and explain why in older persons small airways in the lower lung zone collapse during expiration. Thus, lower zone airway closure occurs during tidal volume breathing in seated subjects over age 65. This leads to uneven gas distribution in the basal lung units and contributes to the progressive increase in the alveolar-arterial oxygen gradient observed with aging. It also explains the frequent observation that normal elderly individuals have persistent early inspiratory crackles at the lung bases; on deep inspiration these closed airways open, producing the crackling sounds.

The muscle strength of the respiratory apparatus declines with age, resulting in significant decreases in both maximal inspiratory and maximal expiratory pressures, as compared with young adults. In addition, aging produces a stiffening of the chest wall; elderly persons have weaker muscles to act on a chest wall that has grown stiffer. Aging produces a decreased sensitivity of the carotid body chemoreceptors; the hypoxic ventilatory drive is reduced by about 50% and the hypercapnic drive to a comparable extent as persons reach their 60s. The population most often exposed to the threats of hypoxemia and hypercarbia is least able to detect these changes and is poorly prepared to respond.

NONRESPIRATORY FUNCTIONS OF THE LUNG

In addition to its central role in gas exchange, the lung is active in both the metabolism and the degradation of many substances. Surfactant production by the alveolar type II cell is an important metabolic function of the lungs. The lung is also involved in the biosynthesis of arachidonic acid into products of both the lipoxygenase and cyclooxygenase pathways. Although a myriad of physiologic functions have been ascribed to these agents, a clear relation to pulmonary function is still lacking. In addition, the lung is capable of removing or inactivating a large number of biologically active substances, including serotonin, bradykinin, and prostaglandins. It is also the principal site of the conversion of angiotensin I to angiotensin II.

REFERENCES

MacNee W: Pathophysiology of cor pulmonale in chronic obstructive lung disease. Am J Respir Crit Care Med 1994; 150:1158–1168.
Rubin LJ: Primary pulmonary hypertension. Chest 1993; 104:236–250.
West JB: Respiratory Physiology—The Essentials. 3rd ed. Baltimore, Williams & Wilkins, 1985.

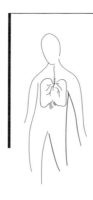

15

Diagnostic Techniques and Their Indications

IMAGING PROCEDURES

The standard chest roentgenogram complements the history and physical examination as the starting point for the diagnosis of pulmonary disorders. The chest radiograph may demonstrate a density that only physical examination can distinguish as being either consolidation or loculated fluid. Conversely, the chest radiograph may show dramatic involvement of the upper lung zone by tuberculosis, while the physical examination may yield unremarkable findings. Standard views include the posteroanterior (PA) and the left lateral projections; they reduce disproportionate magnification of the heart and anterior mediastinal structures. These films allow visualization of the air-containing lung, vascular markings, heart and mediastinal structures, pleura, lymph nodes, ribs, spine, and soft tissues of the thorax. Correct interpretation requires that the film be taken as close to total lung capacity as possible. A correctly exposed film allows the vertebral bodies to be barely visible behind the heart. A number of specialized views and procedures can be added to the standard PA and lateral films (Table 15–1).

Significant improvement in visualization of chest structures has occurred with the use of computed tomography (CT), which provides excellent visibility of areas previously difficult to see and has 10 times the contrast resolution of conventional radiography. Excellent evaluation of the mediastinum makes it valuable in the work-up of bronchogenic neoplasms. Differentiating pleural from parenchymal densities, a common problem on the routine film, has been improved. CT has virtually replaced the standard tomograms for evaluating the presence of early metastatic spread to the lung parenchyma. Unfortunately, specificity is low, and 20 to 60% of nodules visualized on the CT scan but not on the radiograph are benign. In addition, CT is useful for detecting calcification in pulmonary nodules. High-resolution CT scanning of the lung parenchyma, possible with newer-generation CT scanners, is more sensitive in detecting interstitial disease than are plain chest radiographs or standard CT scans. While high-resolution CT scanning can yield findings specific for certain interstitial lung diseases, confirmatory clinical and biopsy data remain essential for diagnosis in most cases. Currently, the greatest utility of this technique may be in the evaluation of clinically suspected diffuse interstitial lung disease when specific findings are absent on standard imaging tests.

Ultrasonography is useful in helping to differentiate between solids and fluids in pleural opacities and to localize loculated pleural effusions. The utility of magnetic resonance imaging for most pulmonary diseases remains to be determined.

PULMONARY FUNCTION EVALUATION

Routine studies performed in the pulmonary function laboratory can be grouped into four categories: lung volumes, air flow, diffusing capacity, and maximal pressures.

One problem in interpreting pulmonary function tests is establishment of normative values. Reference studies demonstrate that test results are "normally" distributed. Normal individuals may vary from day to day and from hour to hour in their ability to exert a maximum effort when performing these tests. These variations become even greater when testing an ill patient, especially when there is weakness and/or confusion. Values ranging within 1.64 standard deviations of the mean encompass 90% of individuals and are considered normal. However, an arbitrary percentage of the mean cannot be used to define normal for all studies, since the width of the normal distribution varies from test to test. In addition, because of the broad range of normal values, patients with results "within normal limits" may still have pulmonary disease if a change is noted upon serial testing.

The lung is conveniently divided into four volumes and three capacities, each capacity consisting of a number of volumes (Fig. 15–1). The components of the vital capacity can be obtained with routine spirometry. The residual volume (RV), however, must be measured indirectly, since it represents air left in the lungs at completion of a full expiration. In fact, we actually measure functional residual capacity (FRC) rather than RV, since the former, that is, the volume at the end of a normal expiration, is a more reproducible point. The expiratory reserve volume (ERV) is then subtracted from FRC to obtain the RV.

Two techniques are commonly used to measure FRC: helium dilution and body plethysmography. Helium dilution is limited by the ability of the test gas to equili-

TABLE 15-1	Specialized Radiographic Techniques	
Study or View	**Indication**	**Comment**
Oblique	Visualization of hilum and pleural plaques; contralateral oblique is best view for apical disease	Better done with CT
Lordotic	Right middle lobe and lingular disease	
Lateral decubitus	Identification of pleural effusions, air-fluid levels, and fungus balls	Both left and right should always be done
Upright-supine	Differentiation of pleural from parenchymal disease in critically ill patients requiring portable radiography	
Inspiratory-expiratory	Obstruction of bronchus or air trapping in enclosed pleural or lung spaces	
Bronchograms	Diagnosis of bronchiectasis	Indicated only in the rare situation when surgery is contemplated; can now be diagnosed by CT
Pulmonary angiogram	Detection of congenital anomalies of the pulmonary vasculature; diagnosis of pulmonary emboli	
Fluoroscopy	Diaphragmatic movement; differentiation between chest wall lesions and lung parenchymal lesions	

CT = Computed tomography.

brate completely with all portions of the lung. In the presence of significant airway obstruction, this will not occur and the FRC will be significantly underestimated. Body plethysmography eliminates this problem and measures the total thoracic gas volume, whether it is located in a bulla or is in direct communication with the airway, and thus provides a truer reflection of the FRC.

The dynamics of air flow can be evaluated during a forced expiratory maneuver by recording the change in volume against time to calculate flow rate or by directly measuring volume and flow (Figs. 15-2 and 15-3). The flow-volume loop is particularly useful in demonstrating the presence of central airway obstruction, which, by affecting primarily the peak inspiratory and expiratory flows, gives a characteristic loop (see Fig. 15-3). An estimate of total airway resistance can be determined by body plethysmography.

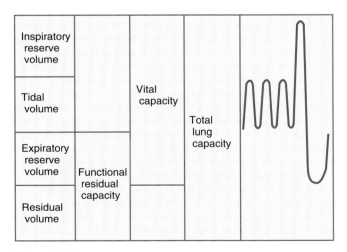

Figure 15-1
Lung volumes and capacities. While vital capacity and its subdivision can be measured by spirometry, calculation of residual volume requires measurement of functional residual capacity by body plethysmography, helium dilution technique, or nitrogen washout.

The measurement of the diffusing capacity for carbon monoxide (DL_{CO}) is an indicator of the adequacy of the alveolar-capillary membrane and so is reduced when the latter is decreased, as in pulmonary fibrosis, emphysema, and pulmonary vascular disease. In patients with a restrictive physiologic defect, diffusing capacity helps to differentiate chest bellows (DL_{CO} normal) from parenchymal disease (DL_{CO} decreased). It should be recognized that decreased hemoglobin concentration can reduce measured DL_{CO} in the absence of pulmonary parenchymal abnormalities and that correction of the measured DL_{CO} is required when anemia is present.

Measurements of maximal static respiratory pressure are important methods of detecting respiratory muscle dysfunction in patients with neuromuscular disease. Maximal inspiratory pressure is obtained by recording mouth pressure during a maximal inspiratory effort from residual volume, and maximal expiratory pressure is recorded during a maximal expiratory effort at total lung capacity.

Measurement of lung volumes and flow rates after certain challenges such as methacholine, exercise, cold air, or exposure to organic or inorganic substances helps in the diagnosis of bronchospasm. Acute reversibility is determined by the repetition of these challenges after bronchodilator administration. However, failure of flow to improve following a single dose of a bronchodilator does not necessarily indicate irreversible disease and does not exclude the possibility of a clinical response to bronchodilator treatment.

More complex testing is occasionally required to answer specific questions. Exercise studies are valuable in judging the degree of disability as well as in elucidating the cause of dyspnea on exertion. Expired gas, minute ventilation, heart rate, and arterial oxygenation are measured during increased workloads. The degree of limitation and the relative contribution of ventilatory and cardiovascular factors can be assessed. Polysomnography is an essential tool in the diagnosis of sleep apnea (see Chapter 21), and measurement of CO_2 sensitivity is used to assess the regulation of breathing.

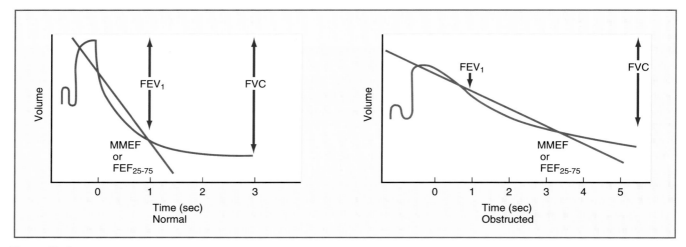

Figure 15–2

Spirometry in a normal subject and a patient with obstructive lung disease. FEV_1 represents the forced expired volume in 1 second, and FVC represents the forced vital capacity. The slope of the line connecting the points at 25% and 75% of the FVC represents the forced expired flow, FEF_{25-75}, or maximum midexpiratory flow (MMEF). The FEF_{25-75} is less reproducible and less specific than the FEV_1.

Clinical Assessment of the Regulation of Ventilation

The respiratory control system activates the ventilatory pump, as well as upper airway pharyngeal dilator muscles, and is a crucial determinant of the arterial blood gases. Primary dysfunction of the ventilatory control system should be suspected when hypercapnia is present in the absence of significant lung or chest bellows disease (Table 15–2). However, control system dysfunction may also result in an inadequate compensatory response for coexisting lung or chest wall disease and may contribute to the development of hypercapnia or the exaggeration of hypoxemia in these diseases.

Clinical assessment of ventilatory control focuses on the response to hypercapnia and hypoxia. The rebreathing test is the most common clinical method of assessing CO_2 sensitivity. Normally, minute ventilation increases by an average of 2 L/min/mm Hg CO_2 (range, 1 to 8 $L^{-1} \cdot min^{-1} \cdot mm^{-1}$ Hg CO_2) (see Fig. 14–5A). Blunting of the CO_2 response occurs in idiopathic hypoventilation, obesity-hypoventilation syndrome, narcotic or sedative ingestion, hypothyroidism, metabolic alkalosis, and primary neurologic disorders. The reduced response in patients with chronic obstructive pulmonary disease (COPD), and CO_2 retention is discussed later. Chemosensitivity to hypoxia is technically more difficult to measure, and generally there is a good relationship between reduced chemosensitivity to O_2 and that to CO_2. Individuals in their 60s

Figure 15–3

A, The maximum expired flow-volume curve in a normal subject. The peak expiratory flow (PEF) and forced expiratory flows at 50% and 75% of the exhaled vital capacity (FEF_{50} and FEF_{75}) are indicated. PIF = Peak inspiratory flow. *B,* In obstructive lung disease (OLD), hyperinflation pushes the position of the curve to the left, and there is characteristic scalloping on expiration. In restrictive lung disease (RLD), lung volumes are reduced, but flow for any one point in volume is normal. The flow-volume curve displays different patterns with various forms of upper airway obstruction (UAO), with reduction in respiratory flow if the obstruction is outside the thoracic cavity and, additionally, in expiratory flow if the obstruction is due to a fixed deformity.

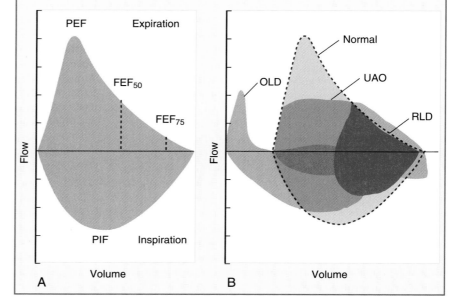

TABLE 15–2	Detection of Primary Ventilatory Control System Dysfunction

Suspect impaired chemosensitivity in the presence of hypercapnia and the following:
1. Disproportionately small reduction in FEV_1
2. Normal alveolar-arterial PO_2 gradient
3. Ability to achieve normocapnia with voluntary hyperventilation
4. Ability to generate a negative inspiratory pressure of at least − 30 mm Hg, which eliminates muscle weakness as a cause of hypercapnia

or older who are in good health show decreased sensitivity to hypoxemia, as compared with healthy young adults.

Assessing the Efficiency of Pulmonary Gas Exchange

The arterial blood gases are the most valuable indices of pulmonary gas exchange because they are simple to obtain and provide important information to guide patient management. The pH defines the presence and magnitude of acid-base disorders, and the PCO_2 helps to differentiate a metabolic from a respiratory etiology. In addition, the PCO_2 assesses the adequacy of ventilation. The PO_2, measured while the patient is breathing room air, is a sensitive index of lung disease, although it may be influenced by overall ventilation and nonpulmonary factors that alter the mixed venous PO_2 (see Chapter 14). In addition, the arterial PO_2 decreases with age, probably owing to a gradually increasing ventilation-perfusion inequality. Normal values are listed in Table 15–3.

A number of simple relationships can help one use the arterial blood gases to correctly interpret acid-base disorder:

For metabolic acidosis, the expected PCO_2
$$= 1.5 \, (HCO_3) + 8$$

For metabolic alkalosis, the expected PCO_2
$$= 0.7 \, (HCO_3) + 20$$

If the PCO_2 is higher or lower than expected, an additional respiratory acidosis or alkalosis is present.

For primary respiratory abnormalities, the expected change in pH depends on whether renal compensation has occurred:

For acute increases or decreases in the arterial PCO_2, there should be a change of 0.008
$$\text{pH units/mm Hg } PCO_2$$

TABLE 15–3	Normal Values for Arterial Blood Gases

$$PO_2 = 104 - 0.27 \times age$$
$$PCO_2: 36-44$$
$$pH: 7.35-7.45$$
$$\text{Alveolar-arterial } O_2 \text{ difference} = 2.5 + 0.21 \times age$$

For chronic increases or decreases in the arterial PCO_2, the expected change is 0.003
$$\text{pH units/mm Hg } PCO_2$$

When patients breathe an increased fractional concentration of O_2 (FI_{O_2}), the arterial PO_2 may be a less sensitive guide to the degree of underlying lung disease, since the relationship between FI_{O_2} and Pa_{O_2} differs depending on the type of abnormal gas exchange that is present (Fig. 15–4). Measuring arterial blood gases while the patient is breathing room air and while he or she is breathing an FI_{O_2} of 1.0 can help to differentiate between $\dot{V}A/\dot{Q}$ inequality, with which the Pa_{O_2} will reach above 500 mm Hg, and shunt, with which a much lower Pa_{O_2} will be achieved (see also Fig. 23–3). This test is subject to major technical error unless great care is used to ensure that the patient is breathing 100% oxygen. Small undetected leaks allowing room air to enter the respiratory circuit will markedly lower the alveolar oxygen tension and give a lower Pa_{O_2} value, suggesting falsely that a shunt is present.

A number of indices are derived from the arterial blood gases. The most useful is the alveolar-arterial O_2 difference (A-aD_{O_2}). The ideal Pa_{O_2} is calculated from the alveolar gas equation (see Chapter 14). If gas exchange is optimal, then calculated Pa_{O_2} should be close to measured Pa_{O_2}. Any factor making gas exchange less efficient will widen the A-aD_{O_2}. In normal persons, this is usually less than 10 mm Hg, increasing to as much as 20 mm Hg in older normal subjects. When hypoxemia is due to hypoventilation, the A-aD_{O_2} remains normal, since the fall in PO_2 is due to the rise in PCO_2, and the calculated Pa_{O_2} should fall to the same degree as the Pa_{O_2}. Thus, the A-aD_{O_2} is of practical value in differentiating hypoventilation from the other causes of hypoxemia.

Additional indices provide essentially the same information as the alveolar-arterial O_2 gradient: the arterial-alveolar tension ratio and the arterial PO_2/FI_{O_2} ratio. The most complex index is the venous admixture ($\dot{Q}s/\dot{Q}t$),

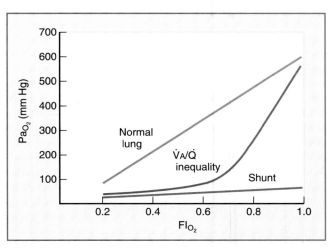

Figure 15–4

The relationship between Pa_{O_2} and fractional concentration of O_2 (FI_{O_2}) in individuals with normal lungs, ventilation-perfusion ($\dot{V}A/\dot{Q}$) inequality, and shunt.

which requires the measurement of mixed venous P_{O_2} in addition to arterial P_{O_2}. This provides an estimate of the true shunt when measured on an $F_{I_{O_2}}$ of 1.0 and the true shunt plus the functional shunt from low $\dot{V}_A/\dot{Q}$ units when measured on room air. A number of nomograms and abbreviated equations do not require the mixed venous P_{O_2}. However, the assumptions inherent in these "shortcuts" make them no more useful than the alveolar-arterial gradient.

A commonly calculated index is the dead space–tidal volume ratio (V_D/V_T). It is measured using the Bohr equation

$$V_D/V_T = \frac{Pa_{CO_2} - PE_{CO_2}}{Pa_{CO_2}}$$

where Pa_{CO_2} and PE_{CO_2} are the arterial and mixed expired P_{CO_2}, respectively. In normal individuals, V_D is 20 to 40% of V_T and consists almost entirely of anatomic dead space (i.e., the conducting airways). Increase of V_D/V_T indicates an additional component of alveolar dead space due to the presence of ventilation-perfusion inequality.

Noninvasive Oximetry

Oximeters measure O_2 saturation (Sa_{O_2}) on the basis of the different absorption spectra of oxyhemoglobin and deoxyhemoglobin. User calibration is not required, since the instruments automatically compensate for variations in skin thickness and slight differences in pigmentation and vascular perfusion. Accuracy of the various commercial oximeters differs but is generally about ± 4% for Sa_{O_2} levels above 80%; falsely high readings are common below this level. Other factors that may alter accuracy of oximetry readings include elevated carboxyhemoglobin levels, jaundice, deep skin pigmentation, and decreased local perfusion to the ear or fingertip. In addition, oximetry is not a sensitive guide to gas exchange in patients with high baseline Pa_{O_2} values because of the peculiar shape of the O_2 dissociation curve (see Fig. 14–8), whereby large changes in Pa_{O_2} may result in little change in Sa_{O_2}.

Invasive Diagnostic Techniques

Bronchoscopy. This is used to visualize the airways, to sample secretions, and to perform forceps biopsy. The rigid scope remains the instrument of choice when a wide channel is required, such as in massive hemoptysis or removal of large foreign bodies. Otherwise, the flexible scope is preferable because it is easy to maneuver and it provides much-improved visualization of the airways beyond the first bronchial division. The latter is invaluable in the evaluation and biopsy of endobronchial lesions or in localizing the site of hemoptysis. In conjunction with fluoroscopy, bronchoscopy can be used in the biopsy of peripheral lung lesions.

Transthoracic Needle Aspiration. Aspiration of lung tissue through a thin needle inserted percutaneously with CT guidance is most useful with peripheral lesions, with which the bronchoscope has its least success. It provides material for cytologic examination or microbial studies rather than histologic examinations. A larger cutting needle, capable of providing a histologic specimen, may be useful in pleurally based lesions when the cytologic specimen is not helpful. The major complication is pneumothorax, which occurs in 20 to 30% of cases; chest tube drainage is required in only 1 to 15% of cases. Hemoptysis may occur but is rarely of clinical significance.

Thoracentesis and Pleural Biopsy. Pleural fluid examination and interpretation are covered in Chapter 19. Parietal pleural biopsy can be accomplished if sufficient fluid separates the lung from the chest wall. Histologic examination reveals granulomas in more than 60% of cases of suspected tuberculosis effusion, and when histology is combined with culture of the tissue sample, the yield may be 90%. Biopsy is positive in 39 to 75% of cases of suspected malignancy, which is a lower rate than for cytologic examination of the fluid. Thoracoscopy with biopsy of pleural lesions under direct vision can be performed when the pleural effusion remains undiagnosed after thoracentesis and biopsy.

Transbronchial Needle Aspiration and Mediastinoscopy. During mediastinoscopy, a small tube is passed into the mediastinum through an incision in the sternal notch. Biopsies can be done on lymph nodes in the anterior mediastinum and the right peritracheal region.

Transbronchial needle biopsy may be a useful technique for sampling mediastinal lymph nodes, especially in the subcarinal and pretracheal regions, and may avoid the need for more invasive procedures, such as mediastinoscopy and mediastinotomy.

Lung Biopsy. When the procedures just described yield negative findings, an open lung biopsy may be indicated. In the immunocompromised host, as well as in other patients with diffuse interstitial lung disease, open lung biopsy has a greater diagnostic yield than does transbronchial biopsy using a fiberoptic bronchoscope, but still a proportion of patients have nonspecific findings. Despite the critical nature of the patients' illness, the mortality rate in large series of open lung biopsy is less than 0.5%. Thoracoscopy with lung biopsy is very useful for the diagnosis of diffuse lung diseases or localized small lesions that cannot be diagnosed by bronchoscopy, and for larger mass lesions when an open thoracotomy is refused or not medically indicated.

REFERENCES

American Thoracic Society: Single-breath carbon monoxide diffusing capacity (transfer factor). Am J Respir Crit Care Med 1995; 152: 2185–2198.

Crapo RO: Pulmonary function testing. N Engl J Med 1994; 331:25–30.

Miniati M, Filippi E, Falaschi F: Radiologic evaluation of emphysema in patients with chronic obstructive pulmonary disease. Am J Resp Crit Care Med 1995; 151:1359–1367.

16

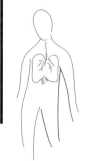

Obstructive Lung Disease

The obstructive lung diseases are characterized by reduction of expiratory flow rates and include common disorders such as asthma and chronic obstructive pulmonary disease (COPD) and less common ones such as bronchiectasis and cystic fibrosis. Multiple factors contribute to the development of the airway obstruction in these disorders, and some of them may be common to more than one disease. However, recent studies have provided enough insight into the pathophysiology of obstructive airway disease to allow a sufficiently clear definition of the various entities to accommodate clinical needs (Table 16–1).

PATHOPHYSIOLOGY OF AIRWAY OBSTRUCTION

Air flow in the lungs is directly proportional to the driving pressure and inversely related to the airway resistance. The effective driving pressure during forced expiration is derived primarily from the elastic recoil of the lung. The reduction in elasticity, which is characteristic of emphysema, therefore leads to a decrease in the maximum expiratory flow. In other diseases, the decrease in air flow is due to an increase in resistance caused by factors that reduce the cross-sectional area of the airway.

Bronchial inflammation is a common cause of increased airway resistance. Irritants such as cigarette smoke, external pollutants, recurrent infection, or chronic immunologic stimulation may induce inflammatory goblet cell metaplasia of the bronchiolar epithelium, mucosal edema, and the production of excessive, thick secretions in susceptible patients. If untreated, this inflammatory process may result in the loss of ciliated epithelium, squamous metaplasia, and eventual peribronchial fibrosis.

Another cause of increased airway resistance is bronchoconstriction. The airway is enclosed by smooth muscle that is innervated by both adrenergic (bronchodilating) and cholinergic (bronchoconstricting) pathways. Cholinergic control is mediated by a vagal reflex, via irritant receptors lying just beneath the mucosa of the large airways, trachea, and upper respiratory tract. Stimulation of these receptors by inhaled irritants or inflammation produces bronchoconstriction. Adrenergic-mediated bronchodilation, however, is primarily due to stimulation of $\beta2$-adrenergic receptors by circulating catecholamines rather than direct innervation. Nonadrenergic, noncholinergic endogenous mediators such as histamine and prostaglandins may also dilate or constrict bronchial smooth muscle directly or reflexively by exciting the irritant receptors. These pathways, which function to protect the lungs of normal subjects from noxious agents, may contribute to airway hyperreactivity in patients with obstructive lung disease.

Airway obstruction leads to characteristic changes in lung volumes (Table 16–2), with an increase in residual volume (RV) and functional residual capacity (FRC) and a normal or increased total lung capacity (TLC). The vital capacity (VC) is decreased as the RV takes up more and more of the thoracic gas volume. A number of factors may contribute to the increase in RV and FRC. Decrease in the elastic recoil of the lungs in patients with emphysema moves the FRC closer to the relaxed volume of the chest wall (about two thirds of TLC). The greater tendency of abnormal airways, particularly at the lung base, to collapse during expiration traps air behind the closed airways. The marked resistance to expiratory flow may not permit complete exhalation during the time available for expiration. Finally, certain patients with asthma have persistent activity of the inspiratory muscles during expiration, which actively maintains a high FRC.

There are three major consequences of these changes in lung volume. Because of the nonlinear nature of the pressure-volume relationship of the lung, breathing at high lung volumes along the flat portion of the curve requires a greater pressure for the same change in volume (see Fig. 14–3), further increasing the work of breathing. In addition, the higher the resting lung volume, the shorter the inspiratory muscles are at the beginning of the breath (see Fig. 14–2). This places them at a disadvantaged position on their length-tension curve, diminishing their ability to alter transpulmonary pressure and predisposing them to fatigue. Hyperinflation, however, has one beneficial effect. Because of the tethering effect of the lung parenchyma on the airways, there is an inverse relationship between lung volume and airway resistance. Thus, hyperinflation is the one strategy immediately available in asthmatics to minimize sudden changes in airway caliber.

Abnormal pulmonary gas exchange is an inevitable consequence of obstructive lung disease. Airway obstruction and the breakdown of alveolar walls produce ventilation-perfusion mismatch that interferes with the efficient

TABLE 16–1	Obstructive Lung Diseases	
Disorder	**Major Clinical Criteria**	**Distinctive Laboratory Findings**
Chronic obstructive lung disease	Chronic progressive dyspnea	Decreased expiratory flow rates, hypoxemia ± hypercapnia
Emphysema	Little or no sputum, cachexia	Hyperinflation, increased lung compliance, and low carbon monoxide diffusing capacity
Chronic bronchitis	Cough and sputum production, history of chronic irritant exposure (mostly smoking, occasionally industrial exposure)	By itself, no significant physiologic impairment
Asthma	Episodic dyspnea; may be associated with allergy to environmental agents	Marked airway hyperreactivity
Bronchiectasis	Large volume of sputum production, clubbing	Chest x-ray findings of dilated bronchi with thickened walls, decreased lung volumes, and decreased expiratory flow
Immotile cilia syndrome	Associated with situs inversus or dextrocardia, sinusitis, and infertility	Abnormal sperm anatomy
Hypogammaglobulinemia		Abnormal decrease in one or more immunoglobulins
Cystic fibrosis	Bronchiectasis associated with gastrointestinal disease, sinusitis, and infertility	Increased sweat Cl and Na, abnormal pancreatic function

transfer of both oxygen (O_2) and carbon dioxide (CO_2). Up to a certain point, patients with obstructive lung disease can increase their minute ventilation sufficiently to prevent the development of hypercapnia, despite worsening hypoxemia (see Chapter 14). However, with continued progression of the disease, a point is reached beyond which further increase in ventilation is impractical because of the high energy requirements or the development of muscle fatigue. It then becomes more efficient, physiologically, to allow the Pa_{CO_2} to rise, eliminating it at a higher concentration but lower minute ventilation and metabolic cost. The onset of hypercapnia is not always clearly related to the degree of mechanical impairment, and it appears that some patients prefer to work harder to maintain normocapnia, whereas others with the same degree of impairment are satisfied to breathe less and allow worse gas exchange (see Chapter 21).

Acute exacerbations of the chronic process brought on by increased bronchospasm, infection, or congestive heart failure may lead to worsening ventilation-perfusion inequality or the development of intrapulmonary shunt and further worsen gas exchange. Gas exchange may also worsen during sleep, owing to a characteristic reduction in minute ventilation. A patient with adequate arterial blood gases during the day may develop significant hypercapnia and arterial desaturation at night.

ASTHMA

Asthma is a common disease of the airway that affects 3 to 5% of the United States population. The underlying etiology remains unclear, but three basic characteristics have been identified: airway inflammation, airway hyperresponsiveness to a variety of stimuli, and airway obstruction that is at least partially reversible spontaneously or with treatment. The inflammatory response, characterized pathologically by cellular infiltration, epithelial disruption, mucosal edema, and mucous plugging, is thought to underlie airway hyperreactivity and bronchospasm. Infiltration of the bronchial mucosa and submucosa by eosinophils, activated T lymphocytes, mast cells, and other inflammatory cells is a feature commonly seen in asthma of all severities. These cells are a source of cytokines, arachidonic acid metabolites, bradykinins, and other factors believed to contribute to the pathophysiology of asthma. The stimulus initiating the inflammatory response may be immunologic in origin, as in classic extrinsic asthma, in which mast cells, sensitized by IgE antibodies, degranulate and release bronchoactive mediators following exposure to a specific antigen. In other patients, there is no identifiable cause, as in adult-onset asthma, in which patients frequently show no evidence of allergy. Recognized categories of asthma are listed in Table 16–3. Clinical differentiation among these types is important only in situations in which there are clear-cut, easily identifiable, and avoidable extrinsic factors, such as drugs or industrial substances.

The diagnosis of asthma is typically based on the presence of episodic dyspnea associated with wheezing. Intermittent cough is also common and may be the sole presenting symptom in some patients. Symptoms are frequently worse at night or in the early morning, paralleling

TABLE 16–2	Abnormalities of Lung Volume		
	Pulmonary Disorder		
Lung Volume	**Obstructive Disease**	**Restrictive Disease**	**Neuromuscular Disease**
Vital capacity	D	D	D
Functional residual capacity	I	D	N
Residual volume	I	D	I
Total lung capacity	N or I	D	D

D = Decreased; I = increased; N = normal.

TABLE 16–3	Types of Asthma
Classification	**Initiating Factors**
Extrinsic	IgE-mediated external allergens
Intrinsic	?
Adult onset	?
Exercise induced	Alteration in airway temperature and humidity; mediator release
Aspirin-sensitive (associated with nasal polyps)	Aspirin and other nonsteroidal anti-inflammatory drugs
Allergic bronchopulmonary aspergillosis	Hypersensitivity to *Aspergillus* species (not infection)
Occupational	Metal salts (platinum, chrome, and nickel)
	Antibiotic powder (penicillin, sulfathiazole, tetracycline)
	Toluene di-isocyanate (TDI)
	Flour
	Wood dusts
	Cotton dust (byssinosis)
	Animal proteins

the diurnal cycle of forced expiratory flow rates. Other precipitating factors include exercise, cold air, irritating gases, and viral infections. Bacterial infection is a less common cause of an asthma exacerbation.

Laboratory studies are usually nonspecific but may occasionally help detect specific types of asthma (Table 16–4). The chest radiograph may be normal during asymptomatic periods or demonstrate hyperinflation in the

TABLE 16–4	Diagnostic Studies in Asthma
1. Routine pulmonary function test	Decreased FEV_1; hyperinflation; improvement with bronchodilator
2. Special pulmonary function test	
a. Methacholine, histamine, or cold-air challenge	Indicates the presence of nonspecific bronchial hyperreactivity; bronchoconstriction occurs at lower dose in asthma
b. Challenge with specific agents: occupational, drugs, etc.	Occasionally performed
c. Portable peak flow measurements	Helpful in diagnosis of occupational asthma and outpatient management of brittle asthmatic
3. Chest x-ray	Fleeting infiltrates and central bronchiectasis in ABPA
4. Skin tests	Demonstrate atopy; little value except prick test to *Aspergillus fumigatus* positive in ABPA
5. Blood tests	Eosinophils and IgE usually increased in atopy; levels may be very high in ABPA; *Aspergillus* precipitins increased in many but not all patients with ABPA

ABPA = Allergic bronchopulmonary aspergillosis; FEV_1 = forced expiratory volume in 1 second.

symptomatic patient. In patients with allergic bronchopulmonary aspergillosis, serial films may show infiltrates that change location or features suggestive of central bronchiectasis. Pulmonary function studies may also be normal or show the findings of obstruction, which usually improves significantly following the acute administration of bronchodilators. In cases where the diagnosis is not clear, bronchoprovocation testing with histamine or methacholine can be used to detect the presence of airway hyperreactivity.

Acute severe asthma (status asthmaticus) refers to an attack of increased severity that is unresponsive to routine therapy. Although the attack is sometimes prolonged, fatal episodes may occur unexpectedly with overwhelming suddenness. A history of increasing bronchodilator use is commonly obtained. Clinical signs of severe exacerbation include pulsus paradoxus, use of accessory respiratory muscles, diaphoresis, orthopnea, and decreased mental status. The degree of physiologic disturbance is best appreciated by a measure of expiratory flow rates, using either spirometry or a peak expiratory flowmeter. Such indices are also helpful in assessing the response to acute and chronic therapy, because they provide immediate quantitative information and can be obtained at frequent intervals without discomfort. Complementary information can be obtained by measurement of arterial blood gases. Hypoxemia is usually, but not invariably, present and does not correlate closely with airway obstruction. Pa_{CO_2} is typically reduced early in an attack. With increasing severity, Pa_{O_2} falls and Pa_{CO_2} returns to normal and then rises, accompanied by a mixed respiratory and metabolic acidosis. In these circumstances, intubation and mechanical ventilation may become necessary. Hypercapnia at presentation is not an absolute indication for intubation because most patients improve with vigorous treatment, but careful monitoring is essential. In general, arterial blood gas measurements are less sensitive and specific than assessment of airway obstruction in judging the response to therapy.

CHRONIC OBSTRUCTIVE PULMONARY DISEASE (COPD)

Patients with COPD have slowly progressive airway obstruction. The course of the disease is punctuated by periodic exacerbations resulting in an increase in dyspnea and sputum production or, occasionally, the precipitation of acute respiratory failure. These exacerbations are often due to pulmonary infection, the development of heart failure, or poor patient compliance with prescribed therapy. Until recently, an episode of acute respiratory failure was associated with a poor long-term prognosis, but with modern management such an episode does not appear to alter overall prognosis.

Chronic obstructive pulmonary disease generally affects middle-aged and older individuals. Patients usually present with dyspnea and exercise intolerance. Cough and sputum production are other common complaints but may be absent in many patients. Physical examination reveals signs of lung overinflation, prominent use of accessory respiratory muscles, diminished breath sounds, and diffuse wheezing, especially during a forced expiration. Patients may vary in their appearance from thin and even cachectic looking ("pink puffer") to being overweight, edematous, and cyanotic ("blue bloater"). In the past these two extremes of clinical presentation have been associated with specific pathologic entities, emphysema and bronchitis, respectively. However, recent clinicopathologic correlations have not supported this impression.

In COPD's early stages, the physical examination may be normal, and the diagnosis will depend on laboratory studies documenting reduced expiratory flow rates. A decreased VC and expiratory flow rates with increased RV, FRC, and TLC are characteristic of COPD. Marked temporal variability in the degree of airway obstruction associated with asthma is not present in COPD. However, as is the case with asthma, bronchospasm is usually present, and expiratory flow can often be increased acutely by bronchodilators. The usual improvement in patients with COPD, on the order of 15 to 20% of the prebronchodilator value, is less than that observed in asthma. Arterial blood gases generally evidence hypoxemia of varying severity. Hypercapnia is typically not seen until advanced stages of the disease. The degree of hypoxemia may not correlate very well with either the severity of the air flow obstruction or the degree of dyspnea, and some severely limited patients have relatively well preserved blood gases. Hypoxia may worsen during sleep and with exercise. When the degree of hypoxemia becomes severe (Pa_{O_2} less than 60 mm Hg), hypoxic vasoconstriction with subsequent anatomic remodeling of the pulmonary arteries leads to the development of pulmonary hypertension and subsequent right heart failure (cor pulmonale). It may also result in significant polycythemia.

Three pathophysiologic disorders are recognized as a part of the syndrome of COPD: emphysema, small airway disease, and chronic bronchitis. In any given patient, one or more of these manifestations may predominate.

EMPHYSEMA

Emphysema is characterized anatomically by an abnormal enlargement of the air spaces distal to the terminal bronchioles, as a result of destructive changes in the alveolar walls. The degree of airway obstruction in patients with COPD correlates most closely with the severity of emphysema, and patients who have significant functional impairment usually have at least a moderate degree of emphysema.

The pathogenesis of emphysema has yet to be determined with certainty, although most theories favor an imbalance of proteases and antiproteases in the lung, with resultant lung destruction. These theories are based on the discovery of a small number of patients with an inherited deficiency of alpha$_1$-antiprotease, the major antiprotease, who develop emphysema even without other risk factors. Cigarette smoke, the major etiologic factor in the development of emphysema, has been shown to increase the numbers of alveolar macrophages and neutrophils in the

lung, enhance protease release, and impair the activity of antiproteases. However, other factors must determine susceptibility to emphysema because fewer than 10 to 15% of smokers develop clinical evidence of airway obstruction.

The diagnosis of emphysema is usually inferred from the clinical and laboratory findings. Chest roentgenograms demonstrate hyperinflation with depressed diaphragms, increased anteroposterior diameter, and widened retrosternal air space. These findings, however, are seen whenever hyperinflation is present, and more specific features in emphysema include attenuation of the pulmonary vasculature and the presence of hyperlucent areas. The one finding that correlates well with the anatomic presence of emphysema is a reduction in diffusing capacity because of the loss of alveolar capillaries. High-resolution computed tomography (CT) scanning can also detect the presence of emphysema but is not routinely indicated because of its expense.

SMALL AIRWAY DISEASE

The earliest manifestation of COPD appears to be in the peripheral airway. Abnormalities that have been identified include inflammation of the terminal and respiratory bronchioles, fibrosis of the airway walls leading to narrowing, and goblet cell metaplasia. These lesions undoubtedly contribute to airway obstruction, although the correlation is not as close as with the degree of emphysema. Furthermore, only a small proportion of cigarette smokers with these pathologic abnormalities go on to develop symptomatic COPD.

CHRONIC BRONCHITIS

Chronic bronchitis is defined as a persistent cough resulting in sputum production for more than 3 months in each year over the previous 3 years. Diagnosis requires exclusion of other conditions associated with cough and sputum production, such as bronchiectasis. As with emphysema, cigarette smoke is the major etiologic factor, although exposure to other pollutants such as dusts may play a role by causing chronic irritation. Cough and sputum production do not appear to have an independent effect on the development of airway obstruction. The airway obstruction seen in the setting of chronic bronchitis is due to associated emphysema, bronchospasm, and obstruction of the peripheral airway. The findings on physical examination, pulmonary function assessment, and radiography depend on the degree of associated airway obstruction.

BRONCHIECTASIS

Bronchiectasis is an abnormal and persistent dilation of the bronchi due to destructive changes in the elastic and muscular layers of the walls. It may be widespread or localized to a single lung segment. Before the introduction of antibiotics and immunoprophylaxis of common childhood viral illnesses, bronchiectasis was usually a consequence of severe necrotizing lung infection. In developing countries, it is still most commonly a sequela of gram-negative pneumonia, but in developed nations it is more likely to be associated with other systemic diseases. Inadequately treated patients with allergic bronchopulmonary aspergillosis may develop bronchiectasis due to persistent inflammation. Immunodeficiency states such as hypogammaglobulinemia predispose to frequent respiratory tract infections and the development of bronchiectasis. Interference with the normal clearance mechanisms may also cause chronic inflammation and bronchiectasis. Cystic fibrosis (discussed later) is the most common example of this. An unusual congenital cause of decreased lung clearance and bronchiectasis is the immotile cilia syndrome, which is due to structural abnormalities in the microtubular system. This is often associated with sinusitis, situs inversus or dextrocardia, and infertility.

The diagnosis of bronchiectasis is made by a history of long-standing chronic cough and the production of large quantities of foul sputum, occasionally blood tinged, and physical findings of persistent crackles over the affected lung regions. With severe, long-standing disease, there may be digital clubbing, cor pulmonale, and massive hemoptysis. The chest radiograph may be normal or may display minor nonspecific features, such as increased markings or linear atelectasis. On occasion, the radiograph demonstrates bronchiectasis, showing thickening of the bronchial walls well out to the lung periphery and even cystic lesions. A definitive diagnosis in less-advanced cases can be made by high-resolution CT. Pulmonary function studies invariably show obstruction and occasionally significant hyperinflation, although restricted lung volumes may be present with severe disease.

CYSTIC FIBROSIS

Cystic fibrosis is a common generalized disorder of exocrine gland function, which impairs clearance of secretions in a variety of organs (Table 16–5). It is associated with abnormal chloride transport in the apical membrane of epithelial cells. This autosomal recessive disorder occurs in about 1 in every 200 white births. The defective gene responsible for cystic fibrosis, located on the long arm of chromosome 7, encodes a protein called the cystic fibrosis transmembrane conductance regulator (CFTR), believed to be a chloride channel. A deletion in the CFTR gene that results in the loss of a phenylalanine residue at position 508, termed the ΔF508 mutation, is found in approximately 70% of patients with cystic fibrosis. More than 170 other mutations in this gene account for the remaining 30%. As more mutations are described, milder and less debilitating forms of cystic fibrosis are being recognized.

The pathophysiology of cystic fibrosis is a result of the mutated CFTR gene product creating a lesion in epithelial cells that impairs the secretion of chloride into the airway lumen. In addition, there is increased sodium reabsorption from the airway lumen. Water follows the movement of NaCl into the cells, and this concentrates airway secretions, which become more viscous. Mucociliary

TABLE 16–5	Cystic Fibrosis—Organ Involvement

I. Pulmonary

Cough and sputum production
Recurrent pneumonias
Bronchial hyperreactivity
Hemoptysis
Pneumothorax
Marked digital clubbing
Cor pulmonale

II. Upper Respiratory Tract

Nasal polyps
Chronic sinusitis

III. Gastrointestinal

Meconium ileus in the neonate
Meconium ileus equivalent (childhood, adult)
Rectal prolapse
Hernias
Chronic pancreatic dysfunction causing steatorrhea, malnutrition, and vitamin deficiency
Acute pancreatitis (rare)
Diabetes mellitus
Cirrhosis and portal hypertension
Salivary gland inflammation

IV. Genitourinary

Sterility in men
Low fertility rate in women

clearance becomes impaired, and this leads to recurrent infections, chronic inflammation, and bronchial wall destruction.

The disease is usually discovered in childhood and diagnosed by an elevated sweat chloride level (greater than 60 mEq/L). Some patients escape diagnosis until their late teens, and with genetic analysis, increasingly older patients are being recognized. They usually have minimal extrapulmonary symptoms and only mild respiratory complaints, often labeled asthma or recurrent bronchitis. When it is found in infants, cystic fibrosis usually presents with gastrointestinal symptoms, particularly steatorrhea and bowel obstruction (see Table 16–5). However, the pulmonary features eventually pose the biggest problem. Classically, *Staphylococcus aureus* in childhood and the mucoid strain of *Pseudomonas aeruginosa* in later years cause recurrent respiratory infections that are particularly difficult to treat because of chronic colonization of the airways. The course is usually one of gradual but progressive respiratory failure. Recent improvements in antibiotics, nutritional therapy, and supportive care, however, have improved the prognosis such that the median survival has increased from less than 2 years in the 1940s up to more than 20 years in the 1990s.

Treatment of cystic fibrosis includes vigorous bronchopulmonary toilet, antibiotics, bronchodilators, and nutritional support, including pancreatic enzyme replacement. Recombinant human DNase given by aerosol decreases sputum viscosity and improves forced expiratory flow by 10 to 20%. Inhaled amiloride and other therapies to improve hydration of airway secretions have also shown promise. Double lung transplantation may be an alternative for patients with advanced disease who are nearing a terminal state.

Identification and cloning of the CFTR gene have offered the potential for gene therapy. Delivery and expression of the normal gene product in the airway epithelium have been successful in animals, demonstrating the feasibility for this mode of therapy, and human trials are now underway. Genetic screening can detect approximately 85% of carriers and is available to those with a family history of cystic fibrosis.

TREATMENT

For the most part, specific therapy aimed at basic pathophysiologic mechanisms of each of the obstructive lung diseases is not yet available. Specific replacement therapy with alpha$_1$-antiprotease is available for patients with emphysema and a homozygous absence of the required gene, but the efficacy of such treatment is not established. The treatment of all forms of obstructive lung disease is otherwise symptomatic and directed toward the reduction of abnormal airway tone, the treatment of inflammation, and specific complications such as infection, excessive bronchial secretions, hypoxemia, and cor pulmonale.

PHARMACOLOGIC THERAPY

Drugs used in the treatment of obstructive lung disease can be categorized into two major groups: bronchodilators and anti-inflammatory agents (Table 16–6). Of the bronchodilators, the sympathomimetics are the most potent. The development of selective β_2-adrenergic receptor agonists has improved the specificity of the sympathomimetic agents for the adrenergic receptor found in airway smooth muscle. Although these agents can be given orally or parenterally, inhalation is the preferred route of administration because the side effects are lower for any degree of bronchodilation. Most of these agents have a duration of action of 3 to 6 hours. However, newer agents effective up to 12 hours have become available. These long-acting agents are currently indicated only for maintenance therapy in the treatment of asthma. Their role in COPD has not been determined. Inadequate clinical response to β_2-adrenergic agonists may be indicative of an insufficient dose or ineffective use of the metered-dose device or nebulizer. Decreased effectiveness in the face of increasing use is a signal of worsening airway inflammation.

Anticholinergic agents were the first clinically available bronchodilators, but their use declined because of unwanted side effects. As the importance of vagally mediated bronchospasm has been elucidated, these agents have received renewed interest. A new anticholinergic agent, ipratropium bromide, has been developed; unlike atropine, its systemic absorption is poor, and therefore it has fewer extrapulmonary effects. Ipratropium is particularly effective in patients with COPD and in selected patients with exacerbations of asthma.

Methylxanthines such as theophylline are about 50% as potent as the sympathomimetics. Effectiveness is related to the blood level and is optimal between 8 and 15 μg/ml. Above these concentrations, the incidence of

TABLE 16–6	Pharmacologic Therapy for Airway Obstruction

Sympathomimetics
 Beta$_2$-specific agents: metaproterenol, terbutaline, albuterol
 Epinephrine
Methylxanthines
 Theophylline
 Aminophylline
Anticholinergics
 Atropine
 Ipratropium bromide
Anti-inflammatory drugs
 Corticosteroids
 Cromolyn sodium

gastrointestinal, cardiac, and neurologic toxicity is unacceptable. The usual adult dose is 10 to 12 mg/kg/day but may vary widely, depending on the presence of factors that alter the metabolism of theophylline (Table 16–7). In patients with COPD it is difficult to demonstrate that the addition of theophylline provides additional bronchodilation to that achieved by optimal doses of beta$_2$-specific sympathomimetics. However, some patients obtain symptomatic improvement that may relate, in part, to the additional small beneficial effects theophylline has on cardiac and respiratory muscle function. In asthma, theophylline is indicated mainly to reduce the wide swings in airway smooth muscle tone seen especially in the early morning hours when blood levels of other bronchodilators are low and normal circadian variation causes increased airway tone. In addition, when sympathomimetics are not sufficient, theophylline may decrease symptomatic complaints.

Corticosteroids are invaluable to reduce airway inflammation, although they do not work acutely to relieve airway obstruction. Their usage early and in sufficient doses in the treatment of acute asthma or the acute exacerbation of COPD has been shown to lessen the degree of airway obstruction (over 12 to 24 hours), to decrease the total time of hospitalization, and to reduce recurrence. The complications of chronic administration limit their

TABLE 16–7	Factors Affecting Theophylline Clearance

Clearance increased by	Cigarette smoking
	Marijuana smoking
	Charcoal-broiled meat
	Phenobarbital
Clearance decreased	
by 25%	Erythromycin
	Propranolol
	Allopurinol
	Oral contraceptives
by 50%	Cimetidine
	Phenytoin
	Influenza vaccine
	Infection
by 100% or more	Heart failure
	Heptatic cirrhosis

usefulness, although the introduction of potent, inhaled corticosteroids (beclomethasone and triamcinolone) has significantly reduced this problem. Inhaled corticosteroids have become first-line therapy for patients with asthma who require more than occasional use of β-agonists for symptom control. Suppression of airway hyperresponsiveness often requires larger doses than currently recommended in the United States (e.g., 1600 to 2600 μg instead of 400 to 800 μg of beclomethasone per day). Local oropharyngeal side effects (hoarseness and candidiasis) can be reduced or eliminated by the use of a large-volume "spacer."

Inhaled sodium cromolyn and nedocromil prevent bronchospasm in some asthmatics but are not helpful in the management of an acute asthmatic attack. Although stabilization of the mast cell membrane and the prevention of mediator release are the major proposed mechanisms of action, these agents are also effective in forms of asthma without an atopic association, probably because of an anti-inflammatory effect. In people whose asthma is difficult to control, it is a useful drug to try before turning to chronic oral steroid therapy. The drug should be used for 3 to 4 weeks before deciding on its efficacy. It may also be used intranasally to relieve the symptoms of allergic rhinitis.

A suggested scheme for the administration of the bronchodilators is shown in Figure 16–1.

OXYGEN

The hypoxemia complicating obstructive lung disease has two major deleterious consequences: decreased O_2 delivery to the tissues and hypoxic pulmonary vasoconstriction with resultant cor pulmonale. O_2 therapy is thus an integral part of the treatment of patients with obstructive lung disease and should be used whenever the arterial saturation falls below 90%. In some patients, O_2 may be required only with acute exacerbations, but in those with chronic disease it may be needed during sleep, with exercise, or continuously, depending on when desaturation occurs. Because of the mechanism of the hypoxemia, namely, ventilation-perfusion inequality, the desaturation can be corrected by small increases in the inspired fractional O_2 concentrations, achieved with less than 4 L/min of nasal flow. It has been clearly demonstrated that COPD patients having a resting Pa_{O_2} below 55 mm Hg (≤ 60 mm Hg if cor pulmonale or polycythemia is present) benefit from long-term O_2 therapy. Such patients have improved survival when O_2 is delivered throughout the 24 hours of the day. Patients should be re-evaluated after 2 months, as up to 40% may have improvement sufficient to make continued supplementation unnecessary (Fig. 16–2).

ANTIBIOTICS AND VACCINES

Some exacerbations of airway obstruction are secondary to acute infections. In patients with obstructive airway diseases, airway colonization with putative bacterial pathogens is common. However, in the absence of systemic

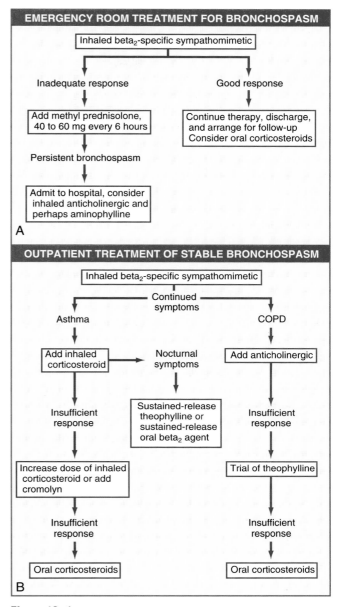

Figure 16–1
Scheme for treatment of bronchospasm in the emergency department *(A)* and in patients with stable disease *(B)*.

signs of infection or a clear-cut change in the quality and quantity of sputum, there is no indication for antibiotics. In patients with bronchiectasis or cystic fibrosis, the specific organism responsible, usually *S. aureus* or *Pseudomonas,* is easily identifiable. However, in patients with COPD or asthma, a specific bacterial pathogen is usually not found, although *Hemophilus influenzae* and *Streptococcus pneumoniae* are sometimes present in great number. In the first case, the appropriate antibiotic can be chosen, whereas in the latter case it is often more cost efficient to administer a broad-spectrum antibiotic such as ampicillin, trimethoprim-sulfamethoxazole, or tetracycline. The route of administration, oral or intravenous, depends on the specific agent and the acuteness of the process.

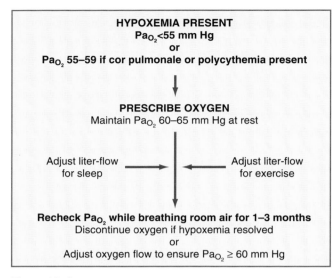

Figure 16-2
Decision tree for administration of long-term oxygen therapy.

Immunization with influenza vaccines directed at specific epidemic strains is the single most effective intervention available for reducing morbidity and mortality. The value of the pneumococcal vaccine for older patients with COPD has not been as firmly established. However, its use for these patients is generally recommended.

SMOKING CESSATION

It is of utmost importance that patients with COPD stop smoking. Susceptible smokers who develop COPD have an increased rate of decline in lung function measured as forced expiratory volume in 1 second (FEV_1) (80 ml/yr)

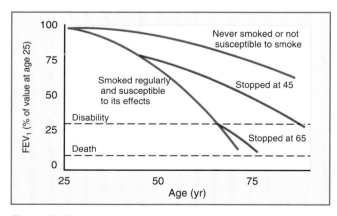

Figure 16-3
Pattern of decline in forced expiratory volume in 1 second (FEV_1), with risk of morbidity and mortality from respiratory disease in a susceptible smoker compared with a normal subject or nonsusceptible smoker. Although cessation of smoking does not replenish the lung function already lost in a susceptible smoker, it decreases the rate of further decline. (Adapted from Fletcher C, Peto R: The natural history of chronic airflow obstruction. Br Med J 1977; 1: 1645; with permission.)

compared with nonsusceptible smokers and nonsmokers (FEV_1, 30 ml/yr) (Fig. 16-3). Following cessation of smoking, the rate of decline in the susceptible smoker is reduced to that in the nonsmoker (30 ml/yr). Drugs that decrease the physical craving for cigarettes, such as nicotine gum and transdermal nicotine patches, along with behavioral modification and long-term physician support, increase the success of cessation attempts.

PHYSICAL THERAPY AND REHABILITATION

Chest physiotherapy (percussion and postural drainage) is employed on the assumption that sputum retention has undesirable consequences. Although this is a reasonable but unproven assumption, and although physiotherapy increases the immediate volume of sputum cleared, there is no evidence that it affects the natural history of any disease or is better than coughing at clearing secretions. Patients with pulmonary disease of sufficient severity to prevent normal daily living commonly demonstrate an improved quality of life when enrolled in a properly run rehabilitation program. However, pulmonary rehabilitation has not been shown to alter the rate of decline in pulmonary function or improve survival. Finally, nutritional needs in these patients must be addressed. This is important in cystic fibrosis, as supplemental pancreatic enzymes and vitamins are necessary. The debilitated patient with emphysema must also be considered for nutritional support because poor nutrition may render him or her susceptible to respiratory failure through decreased muscle strength.

VOLUME REDUCTION SURGERY AND LUNG TRANSPLANTATION

Lung volume reduction surgery has recently received interest as a surgical option for the treatment of selected patients with COPD. The size of the overexpanded lung is reduced by removing 20 to 30% of the most diseased portions of the lung. This allows the diaphragm, rib cage, and chest wall to return to a more normal shape and thereby work more efficiently. Patients considered for this procedure should have quit smoking at least 6 months prior to surgery, have no other major disease, and be willing to participate in both a pre- and postoperative lung rehabilitation program. A marked improvement in symptoms and pulmonary function has been observed in some patients following volume reduction surgery. However, not all patients benefit from the procedure, and significant complications such as a bronchopulmonary fistula can occur. Lung volume reduction surgery has not been proven to prolong survival, and prospective clinical trials, now underway, are needed.

In selected patients with end-stage chronic respiratory failure, lung transplantation may also be a viable therapeutic option. Single lung transplantation has been successfully performed in patients with end-stage emphysema, with reversal of physiologic abnormalities. Patients with cystic fibrosis have undergone successful transplantation, although they generally require bilateral transplantation because of the risk of infecting a single lung transplant from the remaining native lung.

REFERENCES

Cystic fibrosis—from the gene to the cure. Am J Resp Crit Care Med 1995; 151:S45–S82.

Lemanske RF Jr: Mechanisms of airway inflammation. Chest 1992; 101(Suppl):372S–377S.

National Asthma Education Program: Guidelines for the Diagnosis and Management of Asthma. Bethesda, MD, National Institutes of Health. DHMS publication No. (NIH) 92-3042, 1991.

Standards for the diagnosis and care of patients with chronic obstructive pulmonary disease. Am J Resp Crit Care Med 1995; 152:S77–S120.

Stephen PT, Celli BR: Long-term oxygen therapy. N Engl J Med 1995; 333:710–714.

17

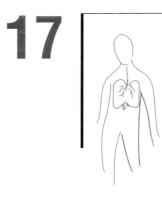

Diffuse Infiltrative Diseases of the Lung

A large number of lung diseases are characterized by the replacement or infiltration of normal lung by abnormal tissue (Fig. 17–1). On rare occasions, the insulting agent may be well recognized, as in silicosis. More often, the causative process is unknown and only the response is obvious. The insult may cause injury by direct toxicity, as a result of an inflammatory response, or through an immunologically mediated reaction. Regardless of the mechanism of injury, the influx of inflammatory cells into the lung interstitium, perivascular space, and alveolar space results in the development of an alveolitis or vasculitis and, if carried to completion, lung fibrosis.

CLINICAL MANIFESTATIONS

The majority of patients present with an insidious onset of dyspnea, exercise limitation, and dry nonproductive cough. A very thorough history of exposures and symptoms is the essential part of the evaluation of patients with diffuse lung disease. Examination of the chest characteristically reveals mid to late inspiratory crackles and tachypnea. Physical findings of pulmonary hypertension, cor pulmonale, and cyanosis are usually late manifestations. Evidence of extrathoracic disease is valuable in suggesting a specific diagnosis, such as the skin lesions of sarcoidosis or the arthritis of a collagen vascular disease. The chest radiograph may confirm the presence of diffuse infiltrative disease but is rarely diagnostic on its own.

As fibrosis replaces normal lung structures, there is a decrease in all lung volumes (see Table 16–2), a fall in lung compliance, and a decline in the diffusing capacity. The loss of alveolar space and airway abnormalities produce ventilation-perfusion inequality, but hypoxemia is usually mild until the disease progresses to a significant degree, and hypercapnia is uncommon. However, patients with interstitial fibrosis often demonstrate oxygen desaturation on exercise despite only mild hypoxemia at rest.

A specific diagnosis, when not clear from the presentation, depends on lung biopsy findings. In certain diseases, such as sarcoidosis, sufficient tissue can be obtained using a fiberoptic bronchoscope and a transbronchial biopsy, but this may be insufficient in others, such

as idiopathic pulmonary fibrosis, and an open lung biopsy may be indicated.

SPECIFIC ENTITIES

Diseases with Known Etiologies

Pneumoconioses

Pneumoconioses are lung diseases produced by the inhalation of inorganic dust. These dusts may be fibrous minerals, such as asbestos, or nonfibrous minerals, such as silica or metals. The clinical spectrum varies widely according to the nature of the inhaled substance and the type of response it evokes in the lung. Some substances such as asbestos lead to progressive fibrosis, whereas others such as iron dust produce little or no reaction even when deposited in large amounts. The common inorganic dusts are listed in Table 17–1 and are divided according to their structure and fibrogenic potential.

Among the fibrous minerals, asbestos is the most important health hazard (Table 17–2). The pulmonary fibrosis (asbestosis) is dose dependent, whereas diseases in the pleural space do not seem to be related to the intensity of exposure. In addition to pulmonary fibrosis and benign pleural disease, there is a fivefold increase in the rate of bronchogenic carcinoma among nonsmoking asbestos workers compared with a nonsmoking control population. Among smoking asbestos workers, the risk is 60- to 90-fold. Malignant mesotheliomas of the pleura and peritoneum are also associated with asbestos exposure but bear no apparent relationship to smoking. There is a prolonged latency period between the exposure and the tumors, usually at least 20 years and sometimes as long as 30 to 40 years. Several studies have indicated that the shape, length, and diameter of asbestos fibers are important characteristics in determining carcinogenic potential.

Deposition of coal dust around the first- and second-order respiratory bronchioles causes coal workers' pneumoconiosis, or "black lung." This may be accompanied by minimal inflammation but is insufficiently severe to cause symptoms or measurable physiologic derangement in most workers. Simple pneumoconiosis consisting of a fine, diffuse, reticulonodular pattern seen on chest roent-

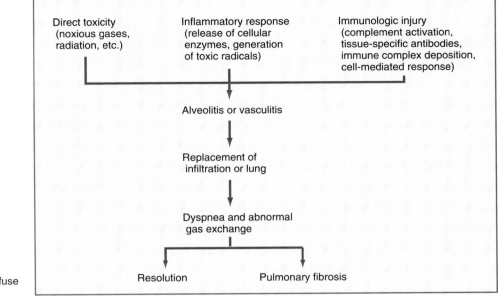

Figure 17–1
Pathophysiology and outcome of diffuse infiltrative lung disease.

genogram and the development of a productive cough occur in 5% of coal workers. Physiologic impairment, when present, is slight. In a smaller number of miners, perhaps 0.4%, nodular densities of 1 cm or greater may be visible on chest radiograph, representing dense collagenous nodules (complicated coal workers' pneumoconiosis). Unlike the simple form, this can eventually result in progressive massive fibrosis and restrictive lung disease.

The pulmonary response to a more fibrogenic dust, such as silica, is dramatically magnified. Silica exposure occurs in most mining operations, sandblasting, pottery working, brick making, and foundry work. In most cases, silicosis develops after at least 20 years of exposure, although it can develop in 5 years or less with intense exposure to a high concentration of dust. Roentgenographic gradation of disease ranges from small diffuse nodules with minimal hilar node enlargement to large nodules, predominantly in the upper lobes, which vary from about 1 cm to conglomerate masses occupying most of a lobe (progressive massive fibrosis). Eggshell calcification of the hilar nodes is characteristic. The chest radio-

graphic findings do not correlate well with the symptoms and physiologic impairment in silicosis. The course of the disease may be modified by other factors such as coexisting smoking or superinfection with mycobacterial disease, either *Mycobacterium tuberculosis, M. intracellulare,* or *M. kansasii.*

No specific treatment exists for any pneumoconiosis, and only removal from the offending environment may modify the eventual progression to respiratory failure. A careful and repeated search for mycobacterial disease is mandatory in silicosis, especially with sudden worsening of the condition. Cessation of smoking, aggressive treatment of routine bacterial infections, and the use of oxygen to treat complicating cor pulmonale may improve function and prolong life.

Hypersensitivity Pneumonitis

Hypersensitivity pneumonitis, or extrinsic allergic alveolitis, occurs in individuals who have developed an abnormal sensitivity to some organic agent. Four to 6 hours following exposure in a sensitized subject, there is the onset of cough, dyspnea, fever, and malaise; wheezing is usually absent. Diffuse crackles are heard on auscultation, and the chest radiograph reveals nodular or reticulonodular infiltrates with relative sparing of the apices. In most cases, these symptoms gradually resolve but recur on subsequent exposure. The duration of symptoms may gradually increase with repeated exposure and eventually result in the development of pulmonary fibrosis and restrictive lung disease.

A vast array of substances can cause this disorder (Table 17–3), the prototype being farmer's lung, a hypersensitivity to thermophilic *Actinomyces,* an organism found in moldy hay. Patients with these disorders have serum precipitins to specific proteins, although the pres-

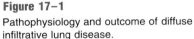

Substance	Fibrogenicity	Occupation
I. Fibrous minerals		
Asbestos	High	Asbestos mining, shipyard and boiler work, insulation installation
Talc	High	Talc mining and milling
Fiberglass	Low	Insulation
II. Nonfibrous minerals		
Silica	High	Mining, sandblasting, etc.
Coal	Low	Mining
III. Metals		
Iron	Low	Mining, refining, and fabricating
Aluminum	Uncertain	Mining, refining, and fabricating
Beryllium	High	Mining and fabricating

TABLE 17–2	Asbestos-Related Respiratory Disease

Form	Comment
Asbestosis	Interstitial fibrosis; long latent period; clubbing; crackles
Pleural thickening	Calcified plaques; intensity proportional to exposure; only significant in that it indicates prior exposure
Benign effusions	Hemorrhagic; asymptomatic; spontaneous remission and recurrence
Pleural mesothelioma	Latent interval 20 to 40 years; not dose related; probably unrelated to smoking; median survival 12 months
Bronchogenic carcinoma	Fivefold increased risk in exposed non-smoker and 60- to 90-fold risk in exposed smoker

TABLE 17–4	Common Drug-Induced Lung Disease

Drug	Dose Relation	Pathologic and Clinical Appearance
I. Cancer chemother-apeutic agents		
Bleomycin	Both acute and dose dependent	Pulmonary fibrosis
Busulfan	> 600 mg	Pulmonary fibrosis
Chlorambucil	> 2 g	Pulmonary fibrosis
Methotrexate	None	Pneumonitis
II. Analgesics and hypnotics		
Aspirin	Serum level > 45 mg/dl	Pulmonary edema
Ethchlorvynol, propoxyphene hydrochloride, heroin	Overdose	Pulmonary edema
Opiates and other psychotropic drugs	Chronic intravenous abuse	Pulmonary fibrosis and vasculitis
III. Antibiotics		
Nitrofurantoin	Acute	Hypersensitivity pneumonitis
Sulfonamides	Chronic	Pulmonary fibrosis, Löffler's syndrome

ence of precipitins does not, by itself, define the disease, because 50% of similarly exposed subjects develop precipitins but remain asymptomatic. The disorder is believed to result from both immune complex and cell-mediated immune mechanisms.

The treatment is to remove or avoid the offending agent. Occasionally, in the acute situation corticosteroids are required. The efficacy of corticosteroids in the chronic phase, once fibrosis has set in, however, is less clear, although a trial in symptomatic patients is indicated.

Other Clearly Extrinsic Causes of Diffuse Infiltrative Lung Disease

External radiation in doses in excess of 5000 rads over a 4- to 6-week period frequently produces radiation pneumonitis within the first 6 months following exposure, and almost always by a year after exposure. Many drugs cause diffuse lung disease (Table 17–4). Some cancer chemotherapeutic agents, such as chlorambucil, produce dose-related toxicity, whereas others, like methotrexate, produce hypersensitivity reactions. Both phenomena occur with bleomycin in an acute syndrome; chronic illness is

almost inevitable when more than 400 to 500 units are used. Synergism between bleomycin and other causes of lung injury, such as radiation and high concentrations of oxygen, has been suspected. Antimicrobials, especially nitrofurantoin and sulfonamides, may cause hypersensitivity lung disease, and a number of sedatives and hypnotics have been implicated in noncardiogenic pulmonary edema, especially with intravenous abuse. Exposure to noxious gases such as chlorine, ammonia, phosgene, ozone, hydrogen sulfide, and nitrogen dioxide can cause severe lung injury. The nature of the injury depends upon the reactivity of the gas, its concentration, and the length of exposure and ranges from tracheobronchitis to adult respiratory distress syndrome.

Diffuse Lung Disease of Unknown Etiology

Collagen Vascular Diseases

Rheumatoid arthritis is associated with five different pulmonary manifestations present in a high percentage of seropositive cases: exudative pleural effusion characterized by a very low glucose concentration; pulmonary nodules varying from a few millimeters to more than 5 cm in diameter; rheumatoid nodules in association with coal workers' pneumoconiosis (Caplan's syndrome); diffuse interstitial fibrosis; and pulmonary vasculitis. With the exception of the nodules and the low glucose in the pleural fluid, patients with systemic lupus erythematosus (SLE) may have many of the same manifestations. Pleuri-

TABLE 17–3	Hypersensitivity Pneumonitis

Antigen	Source	Disease Examples
Thermophilic bacteria	Moldy hay and other organic material, heated humidifiers	Farmer's lung, bagassosis, humidifier lung
Other bacteria, particularly *Bacillus subtilis*	Water	Detergent worker's and humidifier lung
Fungi	Moldy organic material, water	Maple bark-stripper's lung, suberosis, sequoiosis
Animal protein	Bird droppings, animal dander	Pigeon breeder's lung, rodent handler's disease
Amoeba	Water	Humidifier lung

tis and pneumonitis have also been described in Sjögren's syndrome, polymyositis, and dermatomyositis. The lung is commonly involved in scleroderma presenting as pulmonary fibrosis and/or pulmonary hypertension. Last, granulomatous inflammation of the pulmonary parenchyma has been demonstrated in temporal arteritis and polymyalgia rheumatica.

Pulmonary Vasculitis

Pulmonary vasculitis may occur as a part of one of the aforementioned connective tissue disorders or in the course of a systemic granulomatous or hypersensitivity vasculitis.

The granulomatous vasculitides include classic Wegener's granulomatosis, limited Wegener's granulomatosis, and lymphomatoid granulomatosis. Wegener's granulomatosis is a necrotizing vasculitis initially described as involving three organ systems: the lung, the upper respiratory tract, and the kidneys. However, many other organs in the body may be affected. Lung involvement usually takes the form of single or multiple nodular lesions that have a propensity to cavitate. In the limited form of Wegener's granulomatosis, patients have a similar pathology but are free of renal disease. The serum from 90% of patients with classic Wegener's contains antineutrophil cytoplasmic antibody (c-ANCA). However, false-positive c-ANCA results have been reported in a number of disorders, and a positive c-ANCA does not obviate the need for a tissue diagnosis. Both Wegener's variants respond well to cyclophosphamide in combination with prednisone. Rapid and accurate diagnosis of Wegener's granulomatosis is essential because the disease is often fatal without cyclophosphamide treatment. Lymphomatoid granulomatosis resembles Wegener's but differs in the frequent central nervous system involvement. It is now clear that this disease is really an angiocentric lymphoma and not a true vasculitis. Combination chemotherapy regimens are used, but the prognosis is poor.

In hypersensitivity vasculitis, pulmonary involvement is a less prominent part of a systemic disease. The disorders in which this is most commonly seen are anaphylactoid purpura, essential mixed cryoglobulinemia, and the vasculitis associated with malignancy, infection, or drugs.

Pulmonary Infiltrates with Eosinophilia (PIE)

The combination of pulmonary infiltrates and peripheral eosinophilia occurs in six relatively well characterized disorders. Löffler's syndrome is a benign condition characterized by fleeting pulmonary infiltrates and eosinophilia, probably related to an immune response to some external agent. Chronic eosinophilic pneumonia is a more symptomatic form of PIE. Because of its tendency to involve the periphery of the lung, its roentgenographic appearance is called the inverse of pulmonary edema. The chest radiograph in idiopathic acute eosinophilic pneumonia shows diffuse parenchymal alveolar infiltrates, pleural effusion, and pronounced septal markings. All three syndromes respond to corticosteroid therapy. PIE in asthma

is most commonly due to allergic bronchopulmonary aspergillosis. Many parasites can cause pulmonary infiltrates with blood and/or alveolar eosinophilia. These include *Strongyloides, Ascaris, Toxocara,* and *Ancylostoma* in the United States. Tropical eosinophilia consists of symptoms of wheeze, fever, and a diffuse reticulonodular pattern on the radiograph that is thought to result from an infestation with microfilariae of *Wuchereria bancrofti.* Finally, it may be associated with a collagen vascular disease, in which case the underlying disorder determines the overall presentation.

Sarcoidosis

Sarcoidosis is a systemic disease of unknown etiology characterized by noncaseating granulomas found diffusely throughout the body. It occurs most commonly in the 20s and 30s, is slightly more prevalent in women, and is roughly 10 times more frequent in black people in the United States.

Increasing evidence suggests that T cell activation is an integral factor in the pathogenesis of sarcoidosis, although the inciting agent(s) remain unknown. An increased percentage of lymphocytes in bronchoalveolar lavage (BAL) fluid is a marker of alveolitis in sarcoidosis. However, attempts to predict disease progression and need for treatment based on BAL findings have been disappointing. Other immunologic abnormalities include cutaneous anergy with decreased circulating T cells, autoantibodies to T cells, polyclonal gammopathy, and decreased B cell numbers.

Most of the dysfunction associated with sarcoidosis results from the physical presence of the granulomas in the tissues, although systemic signs of inflammation may also be present. Organs commonly involved include the lungs, skin, lymph nodes, liver, spleen, eyes, joints, central nervous system, and muscles (Table 17–5). The pre-

TABLE 17–5	Clinical Manifestations of Sarcoidosis

Pulmonary

Asymptomatic with abnormal chest x-ray
Gradually progressive cough and shortness of breath
Pulmonary fibrosis with pulmonary insufficiency
Laryngeal and endobronchial obstruction

Extrapulmonary

Löfgren's syndrome—fever, arthralgias, bilateral hilar adenopathy, erythema nodosum
Heerfordt's syndrome (uveoparotid fever)—fever, swelling of parotid gland and uveal tracts, nerve VII palsy
Skin—lupus pernio or skin plaques
Central nervous system—cranial nerve palsies, subacute meningitis, diabetes insipidus
Joints—polyarticular and monoarticular arthritis
Erythema nodosum
Punched-out cystic lesions in phalangeal and metacarpal bones
Peripheral lymphadenopathy and/or splenomegaly
Heart—paroxysmal arrhythmias, conduction disturbances
Eye—chorioretinitis, anterior uveitis, keratoconjunctivitis
Hypercalcemia with nephrocalcinosis or nephrolithiasis
Granulomatous hepatitis

senting symptoms are quite variable, although in the United States 50% of patients present with pulmonary disease, 25% with constitutional symptoms, and 7% with extrapulmonary involvement; the remainder are asymptomatic and are discovered during routine examination. Common respiratory complaints include cough and dyspnea. Erythema nodosum, often seen concomitantly with bilateral hilar adenopathy, indicates acute sarcoidosis and is associated with a good prognosis.

Diagnosis depends on the finding of noncaseating granuloma in the setting of a characteristic clinical picture with typical radiographic findings, in the absence of another specific cause of granulomatous disease, such as tuberculosis, fungal disease, carcinoma, and lymphoma. Histologic confirmation is most commonly obtained by a transbronchial biopsy during bronchoscopy. Conventional chest radiographic staging is as follows: stage 0, normal film; stage 1, bilateral hilar adenopathy; stage 2, adenopathy plus pulmonary infiltrates; and stage 3, pulmonary infiltrates alone. There is no evidence that staging has any relationship to the natural progression of disease. Rarely, the radiograph may show multiple nodules similar to those seen with metastatic tumor. Other laboratory abnormalities include hypercalcemia and hypercalciuria (up to 20% of patients), which can lead to renal calculi, and anemia. Angiotensin-converting enzyme levels may be elevated, but this is also seen in other diffuse lung disease. Pulmonary function tests usually reveal a restrictive defect with decreased diffusion capacity and are the most useful studies in assessing response to treatment.

Corticosteroids are quite effective in ameliorating the acute granulomatous inflammation, but their efficacy in altering the long-term prognosis is unproven. The usual indications for corticosteroid therapy are listed in Table 17–6. Other agents, such as chloroquine, indomethacin, azathioprine, and methotrexate, are occasionally employed, especially for symptomatic skin involvement; satisfactory studies of their efficacy have not been undertaken. Recently, ketoconazole has been demonstrated to be effective in treating hypercalcemia associated with sarcoidosis by inhibiting formation of 1,25-dihydroxycholecalciferol.

The disorder is usually self-limited with complete resolution of symptoms and chest radiographic changes within 1 to 2 years. A minority have a persistent mild abnormality with some fibrotic changes visible on chest radiography. Approximately 10% develop severe progressive disease with progressive pulmonary fibrosis or significant extrapulmonary involvement.

Pulmonary Hemorrhagic Disorder

The combination of hemoptysis, anemia, and diffuse pulmonary infiltrates along with the development of glomerulonephritis is known as Goodpasture's syndrome. This is predominantly a disease of young white men. The etiology is unknown, but the presence of anti–glomerular basement membrane antibodies lining both the glomerulus and the alveolus suggests an autoimmune mechanism. Although the lung disease may be intermittent, the kidney disease rapidly progresses to renal failure. On occasion,

TABLE 17–6	Indications for Use of Corticosteroids in Sarcoidosis
Disorder	**Treatment**
Iridocyclitis	Corticosteroid eye drops Local subconjunctival deposit of cortisone
Posterior uveitis	Oral prednisone
Pulmonary involvement	Steroids rarely recommended for stage I; usually employed if infiltrate remains static or worsens over 3-month period or the patient is symptomatic
Upper airway obstruction	Rare indication for intravenous steroids
Lupus pernio	Oral prednisone shrinks the disfiguring lesions
Hypercalcemia	Responds well to corticosteroids
Cardiac involvement	Corticosteroids usually recommended if patient has arrhythmias or conduction disturbances
CNS involvement	Response is best in patients with acute symptoms
Lacrimal/salivary gland involvement	Corticosteroids recommended for disordered function, *not* gland swelling
Bone cysts	Corticosteroids recommended if symptomatic

CNS = Central nervous system.

hemoptysis by itself may be life threatening. Bilateral nephrectomy results in cessation of the hemoptysis, but present therapy is directed at the presumed immunologic basis for the disease. Plasmapheresis is used to remove the antibodies, immunosuppressive drugs are used to decrease antibody production, and steroids are given empirically to decrease the pulmonary hemorrhage. Untreated patients usually die within 2 years.

Idiopathic pulmonary hemosiderosis can present similarly to Goodpasture's syndrome, although it predominantly affects young girls and does not involve the kidneys. The etiology is unknown, and there are no clear-cut immunologic markers. Despite this, treatment similar to that for Goodpasture's syndrome is usually attempted, although the efficacy in this disease is much less clear, and average survival is about 2 to 3 years.

Finally, pulmonary hemorrhage, with or without renal disease, may accompany one of the collagen vascular diseases, particularly SLE and periarteritis nodosa. It may also be seen with systemic vasculitis, in particular, Wegener's granulomatosis; hypersensitivity vasculitis; mixed cryoglobulinemia; and Behçet's syndrome.

Miscellaneous

Pulmonary histiocytosis X, or eosinophilic granuloma of the lung, is a relatively benign disease presenting with dyspnea and radiographic evidence of diffuse nodular or reticulonodular infiltrates with relative sparing of the lung bases. It should be suspected in patients in their 20s and 30s presenting with diffusely abnormal chest radiographs. It is easy to confuse with sarcoidosis, although pneumothorax or honeycombing on the chest radiograph and the rarity of hilar adenopathy favor histiocytosis X. Diagnosis is made pathologically, treatment is uncertain, and spontaneous remissions are common.

The lymphocytic infiltrative disorders include lymphocytic interstitial pneumonia and immunoblastic lymphadenopathy, among other specific entities. They differ from other interstitial lung diseases in their common association with dysproteinemia and frequent progression to lymphoid malignancy.

Pulmonary alveolar proteinosis is a rare, idiopathic disease in which the alveoli become filled with a proteinaceous material rich in lipids. Most patients recover spontaneously, but total lung lavage is necessary when diffuse involvement causes severe hypoxemia. These patients are particularly prone to infection with *Nocardia,* and less so to *Aspergillus* and *Cryptococcus.*

Idiopathic Pulmonary Fibrosis

A large number of patients with diffuse interstitial lung disease do not fit into any of the previously mentioned categories. These patients, usually middle-aged with no sex predominance, present with dyspnea and radiographic evidence of interstitial disease. Rarely, the disease progresses very rapidly from respiratory failure to death within 6 months of the onset of symptoms (Hamman-Rich syndrome). When the disease is more slowly progressive, it is termed idiopathic pulmonary fibrosis or cryptogenic fibrosing alveolitis. Open lung biopsy is usually necessary for definitive diagnosis because interstitial fibrosis may accompany many inflammatory processes, and a large tissue specimen, preferably from moderately involved lung regions rather than end-stage fibrotic areas, is necessary to eliminate other disorders.

Bronchiolitis Obliterans with Organizing Pneumonia

Another nonspecific manifestation of pulmonary injury is the proliferation of fibrous and inflammatory tissue in distal bronchioles and the adjacent alveolar regions, termed bronchiolitis obliterans with organizing pneumonia (BOOP). This pattern of injury may result from viral infections and toxic inhalation as well as other unknown factors. The chest radiograph reveals patchy air space opacities, and the clinical history is of continuous nonproductive cough following a flulike illness. The importance of recognizing this disorder and making the diagnosis with open lung biopsy is that most patients demonstrate a significant response to corticosteroids without subsequent progressive pulmonary fibrosis.

TREATMENT

Although the treatment of these disorders depends on the particular one being discussed, certain general statements can be made. The most rational decisions can be made only if a clear diagnosis has been obtained. If the offending substance is identified, as in the pneumoconioses and hypersensitivity pneumonitis, avoidance is the best solution. When there is an active alveolitis component, corticosteroids may be of benefit. The dose should be high (60 to 100 mg prednisone) initially and then reduced to the lowest possible dose that successfully suppresses the inflammatory response. If there is no objective evidence of improvement, the steroids should be stopped. Immunosuppressive agents are added to effect remission in certain types of vasculitis, such as Wegener's granulomatosis, but are of questionable value in Goodpasture's syndrome and have little efficacy in idiopathic pulmonary fibrosis. Plasmapheresis should be reserved for illnesses in which circulating antibody is known to be the etiologic factor, as in Goodpasture's syndrome. In selected patients with end-stage pulmonary fibrosis, single lung transplantation has been demonstrated to be effective, with significant improvement in pulmonary function and exercise tolerance.

REFERENCES

Cooper JAD (ed.): Drug induced pulmonary disease. Clin Chest Med 1990; 11(1):1–189.

Hunninghake GW, Fauci AS: Pulmonary involvement in the collagen vascular diseases, state of the art. Am Rev Respir Dis 1979; 119: 471–501.

Kelly PT, Haponik EF: Goodpasture syndrome: Molecular and clinical advances. Medicine 1994; 73:171–185.

Morgan WKC, Seaton A: Occupational Lung Disease. 2nd ed. Philadelphia, WB Saunders, 1984.

Raghu G: Interstitial lung disease: A diagnostic approach: Are CT scan and lung biopsy indicated in every patient? Am J Respir Crit Care Med 1995; 151:909–914.

Schwartz ML, King TE: Interstitial Lung Disease. Toronto, BC Decker, 1988.

Sneller MC: Wegener's granulomatosis. JAMA 1995; 273:1288–1291.

18

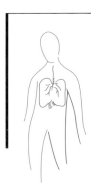

Pulmonary Vascular Disease

The pulmonary vascular bed is normally a low-pressure, low resistance system (Table 18-1). In disease states that cause the loss of cross-sectional area or an increase in vascular tone, the resulting pulmonary hypertension and redistribution of pulmonary blood flow lead to profound changes in cardiac function and pulmonary gas exchange.

PHYSIOLOGIC EFFECTS OF PULMONARY HYPERTENSION

Cardiac Function

The right and left sides of the heart are functionally integrated by their anatomic contiguity. There is continuity between their free walls, they share a common wall (the interventricular septum), and they are covered by the pericardium. When pulmonary vascular resistance is normal, the right ventricle serves as a capacitance chamber, performing only minimal contractile work. It compensates ineffectually for acute rises in pulmonary artery pressure and acutely can only generate a mean pressure of 40 mm Hg. Acute elevations of right ventricular pressure also interfere with left ventricular performance, presumably owing to a shift in the interventricular septum to the left, which decreases left ventricular compliance and impedes left ventricular filling. Chronic elevations of pulmonary artery pressure cause gradual hypertrophy of the right ventricle, which eventually allows it to generate pressures equal to those in the left ventricle.

Pulmonary Function

Abnormalities of pulmonary function in patients with pulmonary vascular disease are usually a consequence of the underlying lung disease rather than an intrinsic effect of the pulmonary vascular disease. An exception is the decreased diffusing capacity due to capillary obliteration. Pulmonary vascular occlusion and obliteration can cause shunt and ventilation-perfusion inequality by undefined mechanisms and thus may alter pulmonary gas exchange. The resulting hypoxemia is further exaggerated by the associated reduction of cardiac output and low mixed venous PO_2.

CAUSES OF PULMONARY HYPERTENSION

Table 18-2 categorizes the causes of pulmonary hypertension by the underlying pathophysiologic mechanism. In postcapillary pulmonary hypertension, the elevated pulmonary pressures are a reflection of elevated left atrial pressure or, rarely, of venous obliteration. In hyperkinetic pulmonary hypertension, the disorder is a reflection of the increased flow. Reactive pulmonary hypertension is due predominantly to hypoxic vasoconstriction. The most common etiology is chronic obstructive lung disease, discussed in Chapter 16. This chapter focuses on two disorders that typify primary involvement of the pulmonary vessels—one acute, pulmonary embolism, and one chronic, primary pulmonary hypertension.

PULMONARY EMBOLISM

A great variety of substances may embolize to the pulmonary vascular bed, with the resulting clinical presentation dependent on the composition of the embolic material. Talc granules and cotton fibers injected along with illicit drugs, sickled red blood cells, and blood-borne parasites like schistosomes lead to slowly progressive disease clinically similar to primary pulmonary hypertension. Embolization of fat, air, or amniotic fluid, however, presents as the adult respiratory distress syndrome (see Chapter 23). The consequences of the most common embolic material, thromboemboli, depend on the amount of clot reaching the lung and the cardiopulmonary status of the patient. They may vary from a persistent tachycardia or mild dyspnea to cardiopulmonary arrest. Thromboemboli directly or indirectly cause 200,000 deaths per year.

Most thromboemboli originate in the deep veins of the thigh. Less common sources include the vessels below the knee, pelvic veins, upper extremities, and mural thrombi in the right side of the heart. Stasis, intimal injury, and a hypercoagulable state are important factors in the development of thrombosis. The clinical diagnosis of deep venous thrombosis (DVT) is highly inaccurate, as physical examination is often misleading. Specialized diagnostic techniques should therefore be utilized whenever DVT is suspected (Table 18-3).

The diagnosis of pulmonary embolism is often missed in sick hospitalized patients, whereas in the

TABLE 18–1	Normal Adult Pulmonary Vascular Pressures		
Pulmonary artery pressure (mm Hg)		Systolic	30
		Diastolic	10
		Mean	15
Pulmonary wedge pressure (mm Hg)		Mean	10
Pulmonary vascular resistance (mm Hg/L/min)			1–2

TABLE 18–3	Methods of Diagnosing Deep Venous Thrombosis
Method	**Usefulness**
Contrast venography	The "gold standard"; low incidence of poststudy phlebitis
Impedance plethysmography (IPG) and Doppler ultrasonography	Highly specific and sensitive noninvasive techniques for detecting thrombi above the knee; less sensitive for thrombi confined to calf veins; false-positive studies with heart failure, ascites, and prior deep venous thrombosis
Nuclide venography	Functional study; high incidence of false-positive studies

healthy outpatient population it is overdiagnosed. Of the predisposing factors listed in Table 18–4, immobilization is the most common. Clinical findings suggestive of pulmonary embolism are nonspecific and are often more commonly indicative of other acute cardiopulmonary disorders. Typical symptoms include dyspnea (80%), pleuritic chest pain (70%), and hemoptysis (20 to 30%). Physical findings include tachypnea (70%), obvious thrombophlebitis (unusual), acute right ventricular strain (right ventricular heave, increased P_2, gallop) in less than 40% of cases, and occasionally rubs, crackles, or wheezing. A low-grade fever is common, but persistent high fever and marked leukocytosis are unusual in embolic disease and suggest, as a more likely diagnosis, an infectious etiology such as pneumonia or pleurisy. Patients who present without dyspnea, pleuritic chest pain, or tachypnea are unlikely to have acute pulmonary embolism, as 97% of patients present with some combination of these characteristics.

Abnormal chest radiographic findings are common but nonspecific and include atelectasis, infiltrates, pleural effusions, and an elevated diaphragm. Clear-cut hypovascularity is difficult to detect. The chest roentgenogram is most useful in ruling out other causes of dyspnea and chest pain such as pneumothorax and lung abscess. Electrocardiography (ECG) may be normal, but nonspecific abnormalities are common and include nonspecific ST and T wave changes, sinus tachycardia rhythm disturbances, or right ventricular strain. Hypoxemia and hypo-

capnia are typical, but arterial PO_2 is >80 mm Hg in 26% of patients without prior cardiopulmonary disease. In summary, the clinical presentation and routine laboratory studies may suggest diagnosis, but confirmation requires specific investigations (ventilation-perfusion scanning or pulmonary angiography).

A perfusion lung scan, which visualizes the gross distribution of blood flow in the lung, excludes pulmonary embolism when it is normal. A ventilation scan helps to differentiate anatomic from functional blockage of blood flow. Delayed washout of the radioactive gas suggests that airway disease may have caused the decreased perfusion secondary to hypoxic vasoconstriction. A normal ventilation scan with a perfusion scan showing segmental or larger defects is considered a high-probability ventilation-perfusion scan and is highly specific at diagnosing pulmonary embolism (87%). Specificity is even greater when there is a high degree of clinical suspicion (96%). Anything other than normal or high-probability ventilation-perfusion scan is an indeterminate scan and is nondiagnostic and cannot confirm or exclude pulmo-

TABLE 18–2	Pulmonary Hypertension

Hyperkinetic pulmonary hypertension
  Atrial and ventricular septal defects
  Patent ductus arteriosus
  Peripheral arteriovenous shunts
Postcapillary pulmonary hypertension
  Left ventricular failure
  Mitral valve disease
Obliterative or obstructive hypertension
  Embolic
  Parenchymal lung disease
  Arteritis
  Pulmonary artery stenosis
  Primary
Reactive hypertension
  High altitude
  Chronic obstructive lung disease
  Persistent or intermittent hypoventilation
    Neuromuscular disease
    Sleep apnea syndrome

TABLE 18–4	Factors Predisposing to Pulmonary Thromboemboli

Medical
  Cancer
  Stroke
  Myocardial infarction
  Congestive heart failure
  Sepsis
  Pregnancy
Surgical
  Orthopedic surgery and lower extremity fractures
  Major surgical procedures (general anesthesia > 30 min)
  Urologic, gynecologic, and neurosurgic procedures
Acquired
  Lupus anticoagulant
  Paroxysmal nocturnal hemoglobinuria
  Nephrotic syndrome
  Polycythemia vera
Inherited
  Antithrombin III, protein S, and protein C deficiency
  Dysfibrinogenemia
  Plasminogen and plasminogen activation disorders

nary embolism. The designation of low-probability scan does not necessarily exclude pulmonary emboli because approximately 14% of these patients have evidence of emboli by angiography.

If the lung scan is indeterminate, the diagnostic work-up must be extended. Two options exist. The simplest approach is to demonstrate the presence of deep venous thrombosis. Unfortunately, in as many as 30 to 40% of patients with acute pulmonary embolism, these studies may be negative because the clot has already embolized. A pulmonary angiogram is then the logical next step, especially in the precarious patient or one who is at high risk if anticoagulated. An alternative approach in patients with stable cardiopulmonary function is repetitive, noninvasive studies of the legs over a 10-day period to watch for the development of thrombosis. If the studies remain negative, treatment is unnecessary because anticoagulation is directed at preventing the formation of additional thrombi and not at treating the embolism. Definitive diagnosis of pulmonary emboli is vital, as both missed diagnosis and unwarranted anticoagulation result in high morbidity and mortality rates. A diagnostic decision tree is shown in Figure 18–1.

Acute treatment of DVT and pulmonary embolism consists of anticoagulation with heparin by continuous infusion at a dosage to prolong the partial thromboplastin time (PTT) 1.5 to 2 times the control value. A bolus dose of heparin is administered with initiation of the continuous infusion to more quickly achieve a therapeutic PTT level. Adequate heparinization in the first 24 hours is imperative since failure to do so is one of the most common causes of progression for venous thromboem-

TABLE 18–5	Treatment of Pulmonary Emboli
Treatment	**Indication**
Anticoagulation with heparin and warfarin	All patients with pulmonary emboli unless risk of bleeding is unacceptable
Fibrinolytic drugs—streptokinase, urokinase, tissue plasminogen activator	Patients with massive emboli and hemodynamic instability
Vena caval interruption with vena cava filters	When anticoagulants are contraindicated or have failed
Acute embolectomy	Rarely, if ever, useful because of high mortality

bolic disease and treatment failure. Recent studies have shown that a therapeutic PTT level is best achieved in the first 24 hours when a dosing nomogram is used to guide heparin therapy. Once therapy has been initiated, the platelet count should be monitored for the development of heparin-induced thrombocytopenia. Oral anticoagulation (warfarin) is used in conjunction with heparin therapy and can be started on the first day of treatment. Therapy with warfarin is now monitored by the international normalized ratio (INR), a measure developed to standardize the reporting of the prothrombin time (PT). The INR range recommended for treatment of venous thromboembolic disease is 2.0 to 3.0. Because the PT may become prolonged before a full anticoagulant effect is achieved, overlap therapy with heparin for 4 to 5 days is generally recommended. Warfarin may be injurious to the fetus and is contraindicated during pregnancy. If anticoagulation is indicated during pregnancy, then heparin at a dose adjusted to prolong the PTT to 1.5 times the baseline value can be used as an alternative for long-term maintenance therapy. Long-term anticoagulation should be continued for 3 months in patients whose risk has resolved, or indefinitely if the predisposing condition persists. Patients who have recurrence of thromboembolic disease may also require prolonged therapy. Most emboli completely resolve, and chronic persistent pulmonary hypertension develops in fewer than 2% of patients.

Rarely, additional therapy may be required (Table 18–5), but it should be undertaken only when clear indications are present because of significant added risks. Thrombolytic drugs (streptokinase, urokinase, or tissue plasminogen activator) are capable of augmenting the dissolution of fresh emboli and have been shown to increase resolution of pulmonary perfusion abnormalities in the first 24 hours when compared with heparin. On this basis, it is often recommended that they be used in patients with marked hemodynamic instability following acute pulmonary embolization. Thrombolytics have not, however, been demonstrated to alter overall mortality or morbidity, and because their use is accompanied by a significantly increased incidence of bleeding, routine use is unwarranted. Fragmentation of massive pulmonary emboli by catheter tip devices has shown potential in animal studies and may prove to be a useful modality.

Vena caval interruption should be considered when the thrombus originates in the lower extremities and there has been proven recurrence while receiving adequate anticoagulation therapy. It should also be used when antico-

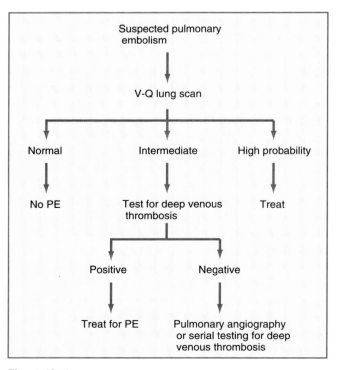

Figure 18–1

Diagnostic approach to pulmonary embolism (PE).

agulation is contraindicated. The preferred technique is the transvenous placement of a Greenfield or "bird's-nest" vena caval filter.

The best treatment for thromboembolic disease is prevention. Appropriate prophylaxis of high-risk patients is safe and efficacious. Most can be treated with low-dose subcutaneous heparin, 5000 units every 12 hours. Patients undergoing orthopedic procedures on the lower extremity, especially the hip, may not be protected by this regimen, and present recommendations suggest the use of either heparin adjusted to the therapeutic PTT levels, or low molecular weight heparin (LMWH). In patients in whom postoperative bleeding represents an unacceptable risk, as in neurosurgical procedures, intermittent pneumatic compression of the lower extremities is effective.

PRIMARY PULMONARY HYPERTENSION

Primary pulmonary hypertension (PPH) is characteristically a disease of young adult women. It can occur at any age but is most common in the 20s and 30s. In children, there is no apparent gender predominance, but the female-male ratio is about 2 : 1 in adults. Current evidence suggests that PPH occurs in predisposed individuals who develop the disease after exposure to some intrinsic or extrinsic stimulus. This hypothesis is evidenced by a familial form of PPH that accounts for 5 to 10% of all cases. PPH has been associated with drug exposure (anorexic agents, L-tryptophan, crack cocaine, chemotherapeutic agents), chronic portal hypertension, and human immunodeficiency virus infection. However, the majority of patients with these exposures or conditions do not develop PPH, lending further support to the concept of an underlying predisposition.

The pathogenesis of PPH remains speculative, but one possibility is that inflammatory or immunologic injury to the pulmonary endothelium results in an imbalance of locally produced vasoconstrictor (thromboxane, endothelin) and vasodilator (prostacyclin) factors. An abnormally high ratio of thromboxane to prostacyclin, as well as elevated endothelin expression, has been observed in some patients with PPH. Because thromboxane additionally promotes platelet aggregation, an effect that is opposed by prostacylin, an imbalance between the two could shift the pulmonary vascular bed from an anticoagulant to procoagulant state, thus contributing to the development of pulmonary thrombosis *in situ,* a pathologic feature of PPH. Release of chemotactant factors by injured endothelial cells may also promote the abnormal proliferation of vascular smooth muscle cells.

Patients with PPH typically present with progressive dyspnea and marked exercise limitation (60%). Syncopal episodes that occur during exertion or postexertion may be another early symptom (8%). With time, fatigue, chest pain, cor pulmonale, and syncopal episodes on exertion (decreased left ventricular output) develop. Physical examination may be normal or may reveal evidence of pulmonary hypertension. The chest radiograph shows an enlarged right ventricle and main pulmonary arteries, with oligemia in the outer lung fields. ECG evidence of right ventricular hypertrophy is invariable when the mean pulmonary artery pressures are chronically elevated above 40 mm Hg. Pulmonary function studies are often normal except for a small reduction in total lung capacity and diffusing capacity. Mild hypoxemia and hypocapnia are almost always found. Diagnosis is made by right heart catheterization and by excluding other causes of pulmonary hypertension. Prognosis is dismal, with only 20% surviving 3 years.

Drug therapy is actively being investigated. Chronic anticoagulation is generally recommended in all patients with primary pulmonary hypertension because thrombosis in the small pulmonary arteries is thought to contribute to progressive deterioration of right heart function. High doses of calcium channel blockers may be beneficial in patients who respond acutely to a vasodilator challenge during hemodynamic testing. Prostacyclin may reduce pulmonary vascular resistance in some patients unresponsive to conventional therapy but requires continuous intravenous administration. Inhaled nitric oxide (NO) has recently shown promise in preliminary studies. Combined heart-lung transplantation has been used successfully over the past decade in patients with progressive disease unresponsive to medical therapy. Single and double lung transplantations have been performed more recently with good results and may be the procedure of choice in patients without irreversible right-sided heart failure.

REFERENCES

Hull RD, Raskob GE, Rosenbloom DR, et al: Optimal therapeutic level of heparin therapy in patients with venous thrombosis. Arch Intern Med 1992; 152:1589–1595.

Raschke RA, Reilly BM, Guidry JR, et al: The weight-based heparin dosing nomogram compared with a "standard care" nomogram: A randomized controlled trial. Ann Intern Med 1993; 119:874–881.

Rubin LJ, et al: Primary pulmonary hypertension: ACCP Consensus Statement. Chest 1993; 104:236–250.

Stein PD: Acute pulmonary embolism. Disease-a-Month 1994; 40(9):467–523.

Tapson VF, Fulkerson WJ, Saltzman HA: Venous thromboembolism. Clin Chest Med 1995; 16(2):229–392.

19

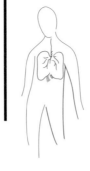

Disorders of the Pleural Space, Mediastinum, and Chest Wall

PLEURAL DISEASE

The pleural spaces are defined by the visceral pleura of the lungs and the parietal pleura of the rib cage, diaphragm, and mediastinum. The spaces themselves are potential rather than real, since the visceral and parietal pleurae are normally separated by only a thin film of fluid.

The lung's elastic recoil pulls the visceral pleura inward, and the chest wall's recoil pulls the parietal pleura outward. The net pressure in the pleural space at functional residual capacity is below atmospheric pressure. In the pleural space, fluid flows from the parietal surface into the pleural space, with subsequent reabsorption by the capillaries of the visceral pleura (Fig. 19–1). This system is remarkably well balanced and ordinarily prevents the collection of significant amounts of fluid, despite the formation and absorption of 5 to 10 L of pleural fluid each day. In addition, fluid and leakage of protein are drained by lymphatics, which can increase their absorptive capacity several-fold.

Fluid accumulates with abnormalities in the hydrostatic and osmotic pressures, increased permeability of the capillaries, or lymphatic dysfunction. Pleural inflammation, either infectious or noninfectious, increases permeability and results in the collection of a high-protein pleural fluid. Alterations in the pulmonary venous pressures, as in heart failure, increase fluid transudation from the parietal capillaries and decrease reabsorption on the visceral side. Decreasing the osmotic pressure (hypoalbuminemia) may also result in more rapid fluid transudation. Finally, lymphatic dysfunction due to anatomic or functional obstruction also facilitates the accumulation of pleural fluid.

Pleural Effusions

The causes of pleural effusions are best considered in terms of the underlying pathophysiology: transudates due to abnormalities of hydrostatic or osmotic pressure and exudates resulting from increased permeability or trauma (Table 19–1).

Patients usually present with dyspnea or nonspecific discomfort, occasionally accompanied by pleuritic chest pain—a sharp, stabbing pain exacerbated by coughing or breathing. Such pain must be carefully differentiated from pericardial or musculoskeletal pain. Rarely, the effusion is asymptomatic and discovered only on chest radiograph.

Physical examination reveals decreased vocal fremitus, dullness on percussion, and decreased breath sounds over the effusion, with bronchial breathing and egophony at its upper limit. The first radiographic sign of pleural effusion is an apparent elevation of the hemidiaphragm; when the volume of fluid reaches 250 ml, a minimal blunting of the costophrenic angle can be noted. Increasing amounts cause dense opacification of the lung fields with a concave meniscus. In certain situations, the initial radiograph is misleading and further studies are required. These situations are (1) when a subpulmonic effusion presenting as an elevated hemidiaphragm can be confirmed on lateral decubitus radiograph; (2) when a hazy diffuse density on the supine film in a seriously ill patient disappears on an upright radiograph; and (3) when a loculated effusion, especially with coexisting parenchymal disease, may require ultrasound or computed tomographic (CT) scan for diagnosis.

Thoracentesis is essential in the differential diagnosis. The gross appearance of the fluid is rarely helpful except when frank blood or the milky fluid of a chylous effusion is encountered. A pleural effusion associated with an anaerobic lung infection may have a putrid odor. The criteria for separation of the fluid into transudate and exudate (Table 19–2) are not rigid, and an effusion due to congestive heart failure may occasionally be exudative, whereas a transudate may occur with malignancy. Pleural fluid glucose concentrations <10 to 20 mg/dl are usually diagnostic of rheumatoid arthritis but may be seen in cancer and infection. Pleural fluid amylase is about twice the normal value in effusions due to pancreatitis and esophageal perforation, whereas smaller elevations may be seen with malignancy. The presence of a high rheumatoid factor or lupus erythematosus (LE) cells in the fluid is strong evidence that the effusion is due to rheumatoid arthritis and systemic LE, respectively. Measurement of pleural fluid pH in the diagnosis and management of

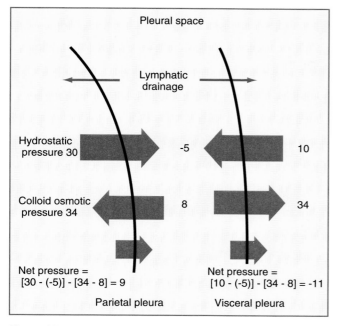

Figure 19–1

Factors affecting fluid and solute movement in the pleural space. The blood supply of the parietal pleura is from the intercostal arteries (branches of the systemic circulation), whereas the visceral pleura is predominantly supplied by the pulmonary circulation, a low-pressure system. If the osmotic pressures in the parietal and visceral vessels, which are roughly equal, as well as the changes in intrapleural pressure, are taken into account, fluid flows from the parietal surface into the pleural space and is subsequently reabsorbed by the visceral pleura (indicated pressures are in cm H_2O).

TABLE 19–2	Differentiation of Exudative and Transudative Pleural Effusion	
	Exudate	**Transudate**
Protein	>3 g/dl	<3 g/dl
Pleural/serum protein	>0.5	<0.5
LDH	>200 IU/L	<200 IU/L
Pleural/serum LDH	>0.6	<0.6

LDH = Lactate dehydrogenase.

parapneumonic effusions usually does not add to other, more routine measurements.

Surprisingly few red blood cells are required to impart a red color to the fluid; a hemothorax can be diagnosed best by measuring the pleural fluid hematocrit. Bloody fluid should arouse suspicion of malignancy, trauma, or pulmonary embolus, but it may also occur with other disease entities. The number of polymorphonuclear neutrophils is of little or no specific diagnostic value, but when the cell count is $\geq 1 \times 10^4$ cells/μl, an empyema is probably present. A high eosinophil count is usually due to air or blood in the pleural space. Cytologic examinations for malignant cells are positive in about 60% of patients on first thoracentesis, rising to about 80% if three separate samples are obtained. Gram's stain and routine culture should always be obtained and special stains and cultures added when tuberculosis or fungal disease is suspected.

Transcutaneous needle biopsy of the pleura at the bedside with subsequent histology and culture is positive in more than 50% of tuberculous effusions, whereas fluid culture is positive in only 25%. Although less frequently positive (40%) than cytologic examination, biopsy occasionally makes a diagnosis of malignant effusions when cytology is negative.

Treatment depends on the underlying cause and the degree of physiologic impairment. Specific therapy to control the underlying cause is the only successful approach. Although removal of fluid results in symptomatic improvement, lung volumes and gas exchange improve very little. Parapneumonic effusions resolve with antibiotic therapy (90%), but empyemas, that is, fluid with positive smear or culture, should be drained by repeated aspirations or tube thoracostomy; otherwise the fluid may spontaneously drain through the chest wall *(empyema necessitans)* or may lead to subpleural lung necrosis with resultant bronchopleural fistula and endobronchial spread of infection. Palliative therapy should be considered for a malignant effusion only if the patient is symptomatic and displays benefit from thoracentesis. Repeated thoracentesis should be avoided, as significant protein loss results. Pleurodesis, a procedure in which an irritant is injected into the pleural space and results in its obliteration, is useful in ~ 80% of malignant effusions.

TABLE 19–1	Pleural Effusions

Transudates

Congestive heart failure
Hypoalbuminemia—nephrotic syndrome, starvation, cirrhosis
Abdominal fluid collection—ascites, peritoneal dialysis

Exudates

Infection
  Empyema
  Bacterial—gram-positive and -negative, *Actinomyces, Mycobacterium tuberculosis*
  Viral—coxsackievirus, *Mycoplasma*
  Fungal—*Nocardia, Coccidioides* (rarely)
  Parasitic—*Amoeba, Echinococcus*
  Parapneumonic
Malignancy—bronchogenic cancer, mesothelioma, lymphoma; metastatic cancer (breast, ovary, kidney, pancreas, gastrointestinal tract)
Pulmonary embolism and infarction
Collagen vascular disease—systemic lupus erythematosus, rheumatoid arthritis
Intra-abdominal processes—pancreatitis, subphrenic abscess, Meigs' syndrome, post abdominal surgery
Trauma—hemothorax, chylothorax, ruptured esophagus
Miscellaneous—myxedema, uremia, asbestosis, lymphedema (yellow nail syndrome), drug sensitivity, Dressler's syndrome

Pneumothorax

The most common causes of air in the pleural space are listed in Table 19–3. Idiopathic spontaneous pneumo-

TABLE 19-3	Causes of Pneumothorax

Spontaneous
Idiopathic
Emphysema
Interstitial lung disease
Eosinophilic granuloma/histiocytosis X
Cystic fibrosis
Asthma
Malignancy

Traumatic
Penetrating and nonpenetrating chest trauma
Transbronchoscopic or transthoracic lung biopsy
Thoracentesis
Mechanical ventilation
Esophageal perforation

thorax typically causes dyspnea, chest pain, and few abnormalities on physical examination. On chest radiographs, the two-dimensional view grossly underestimates its true volume. Without surgery, 50% of patients develop a recurrence, usually within 2 years. Under certain circumstances, particularly in patients on mechanical ventilators, the rent in the pleura forms a one-way valve that permits air to enter but not to escape, causing positive pressure to build up in the chest (tension pneumothorax).

Treatment depends on the amount of air and the underlying status of the patient. Spontaneous pneumothorax in a healthy, asymptomatic patient may require no treatment, whereas treatment is needed for a pneumothorax of the same size in a patient with cardiopulmonary insufficiency. Treatment is almost always required for pneumothoraces greater than 50% in size or for a pneumothorax of any size in patients on mechanical ventilation or in those with diffuse lung disease. Drainage by tube thoracostomy is successful in most instances. Open thoracotomy with partial pleurectomy and oversewing of apical blebs or abrasion of the pleural surface is required with recurrent episodes.

Tumors of the Pleural Space

Mesotheliomas may be localized benign growths curable by surgical resection or aggressive, untreatable malignancies spreading extensively in the pleural space and beyond. Malignant mesotheliomas are almost always associated with asbestos exposure. More commonly, neoplasms of the pleural space are due to adjacent spread (bronchogenic carcinoma) or metastatic disease (carcinoma of the breast, ovary, and kidney and lymphoma). They produce bloody pleural effusions, although chylous effusions resulting from lymphatic obstruction are also seen.

MEDIASTINAL DISEASE

The mediastinum (literally, "middle septum") can be conveniently divided into three compartments based on the lateral chest radiograph. The anterior compartment, which lies between the sternum and the heart shadow, contains the thymus gland, the aortic arch and its branches, lymphatic tissue, and errant thyroid or parathyroid glands. The posterior compartment, lying anterior to the vertebral bodies, contains the esophagus, the descending aorta, the azygous system, the sympathetic chain, the thoracic duct, and lymph nodes. Between lies the middle mediastinum, containing the pericardial sac, the lung hila, and associated lymph nodes. Knowledge of these normal structures is critical in the assessment of mediastinal masses.

Symptoms of mediastinal disease are varied (Table 19–4), although most patients are asymptomatic with a mediastinal mass found on routine radiography. CT is invaluable because it distinguishes vascular from nonvascular lesions and cystic from solid structures and identifies local invasion. Definitive diagnosis often depends on obtaining tissue. Fine-needle cytologic samples are inadequate when lymphoma is in question, as histology is required. Markers for germ cell tumors should also be looked for in both serum and tissue.

Mediastinitis

Acute mediastinitis, formerly a rare but dramatic syndrome, is more often today a "disease of medical progress." It is, to a large extent, a complication of endoscopic procedures of the esophagus and airways. Fever, prostration, and substernal chest pain with tachypnea and tachycardia are noted. Hamman's sign, signifying pneumomediastinum, may be auscultated as a "crunch" in time with cardiac systole. Other signs of mediastinal compression may be seen (see Table 19–4). Treatment consists of antibiotics, drainage, and closure of perforated structures. A less dramatic but increasingly important form of mediastinitis is seen after cardiac surgery, either early in the postoperative course or as long as 6 months later. Classic findings are unusual in this form of the disease. Rarely, because the mediastinum is continuous with the fascial planes of the neck, oropharyngeal infections may spread there. It is a devastating complication that carries a high morbidity and mortality.

Chronic mediastinitis is usually a granulomatous process, most often caused by histoplasmosis and less frequently other fungal infections, tuberculosis, and syphilis.

TABLE 19-4	Symptoms and Signs of Mediastinal Disease

Asymptomatic
Compression or invasion of nearby structures
  Superior vena cava syndrome
  Cough
  Postobstructive pneumonia
  Hoarseness
  Horner's syndrome
Systemic symptoms
  Fever
  Weight loss
  Paraneoplastic syndromes (hypercalcemia, Cushing's syndrome, etc.)

Noninfectious causes include sarcoidosis and, in the past, the use of methysergide. An idiopathic cause should be considered only when specific disorders are ruled out. Treatment other than that specifically directed at the underlying disorder, such as surgery, is usually unsuccessful.

Mediastinal Masses

Mediastinal masses are mostly tumors but also include glandular lesions, vascular abnormalities, and esophageal disease. They are conveniently divided by anatomic location (Fig. 19–2).

CHEST WALL DISEASE

Adequate ventilation depends on efficient movement of the chest wall in response to neural stimulation. Interference with this may result in increased work of breathing, restricted lung volumes, exercise limitation, and gradual progression to respiratory failure. Total lung capacity and vital capacity are decreased, but the residual volume in chest wall disease, unlike that in parenchymal restrictive lung disease, is usually normal or even increased. Hypoventilation is the predominant mechanism of abnormal gas exchange, and thus hypercapnia is found at much higher levels of arterial PO_2 than in parenchymal lung disease. In addition, progressive ventilation-perforation in-

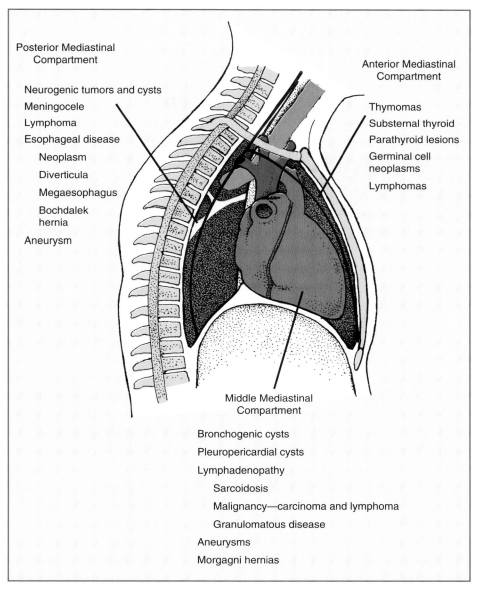

Posterior Mediastinal
Compartment

Neurogenic tumors and cysts
Meningocele
Lymphoma
Esophageal disease
 Neoplasm
 Diverticula
 Megaesophagus
 Bochdalek hernia
Aneurysm

Anterior Mediastinal
Compartment

Thymomas
Substernal thyroid
Parathyroid lesions
Germinal cell neoplasms
Lymphomas

Middle Mediastinal
Compartment

Bronchogenic cysts
Pleuropericardial cysts
Lymphadenopathy
 Sarcoidosis
 Malignancy—carcinoma and lymphoma
 Granulomatous disease
Aneurysms
Morgagni hernias

Figure 19–2
Masses of the mediastinum indicated by their anatomic location.

equality, resulting from basilar atelectasis, causes gradual widening of the alveolar-arterial gradient. Continued, prolonged hypoxemia eventually causes cor pulmonale.

Specific Disorders

Kyphoscoliosis

Kyphoscoliosis is usually idiopathic or may be associated with Marfan's syndrome or poliomyelitis. The severity of scoliosis is quantitated by measuring the angle between the upper and lower limbs of the spinal curve. Mild scoliosis (angle > 35 degrees) is common (incidence, 1 in 1000); respiratory dysfunction becomes detectable only when the angle is > 70 degrees (incidence, 1 in 10,000), and early cardiopulmonary failure is expected when the angle is > 120 degrees. Surgical correction of the deformity in adults does not influence the incidence of respiratory complications.

Obesity

Obese patients have a small expiratory reserve volume (ERV) and thus breathe close to residual volume. This condition leads to decreased ventilation of the lung bases and hypoxemia. This decrease in ventilation is magnified in the supine position, which further reduces the ERV. These abnormalities may be further complicated by disorders of ventilatory control and upper airway obstruction (see Chapter 21).

Diaphragmatic Paralysis

Unilateral diaphragmatic paralysis is usually in and of itself asymptomatic. In fact, most patients have relatively preserved pulmonary function, with about 75% of normal vital capacity. The abnormalities are greater when the patient is supine than when he or she is erect, and recumbent hypoxemia may be noted. Causes include tumor invasion, herpes zoster, and "cold cardioplegia" of cardiac surgery.

Fluoroscopy during a "sniff" maneuver is diagnostic in most cases, showing paradoxical motion of the affected side. Definitive diagnosis is made by nerve conduction studies.

In contrast, bilateral paralysis is rarely subtle; patients are profoundly dyspneic and often cannot sleep while recumbent. Paradoxical inward motion of the abdominal wall during inspiration is the classic physical finding, and the diagnosis can be confirmed by nerve conduction studies. In many cases, it is a manifestation of a generalized myopathy or neuropathy, or it may be idiopathic.

Respiratory Muscle Fatigue

Respiratory muscle dysfunction may arise as a result of excessive demands (increased work of breathing or ventilatory requirements) or decreased energy supplies (malnutrition, metabolic disturbance, decreased oxygen supply). Unfortunately, none of the techniques used to investigate fatigue in experimental settings is satisfactory for the clinical diagnosis of fatigue. In addition, although many disease states affect respiratory muscle function, the importance of respiratory muscle fatigue as a primary determinant of ventilatory failure has not been established.

Treatment

Treatment is directed at correcting reversible abnormalities and minimizing the development of parenchymal lung disease. Respiratory failure develops in some patients, and mechanical ventilation is required. Initially, this is particularly valuable during sleep at night; in many patients, it may be possible to deliver mechanical ventilation via a nose mask, circumventing the need for tracheostomy. Eventually, mechanical ventilation may be required on a continuous basis.

REFERENCES

Heitzman ER: The Mediastinum, Radiologic Correlations with Anatomy and Pathology. St. Louis, CV Mosby, 1977.
Lighe RW: Pleural Diseases. 3rd ed. Baltimore, Williams & Wilkins, 1995.
Roussos C, Macklem PT: The Thorax (Parts A and B). New York, Marcel Dekker, 1985.
Sahn SA: The pleura. Am Rev Respir Dis 1988;138:184.

20

Neoplastic Diseases of the Lung

Lung cancer causes more than 120,000 deaths per year in the United States and is the leading cause of cancer deaths in both men and women. Carcinoma of the lung is most common in the 40s and 50s and is rarely seen before the age of 35.

Cigarette smoking is the most important causative factor, estimated to be responsible for up to 90% of cases. Lung cancer is 10 to 30 times more common among smokers; approximately 4% of those who have smoked for 40 years develop lung cancer. Most studies demonstrate a small but significant risk of lung cancer from environmental smoke exposure. For example, recent investigation of environmental smoke exposure in childhood has demonstrated a doubling of lung cancer risk in later years when exposure is 25 or more smoker-years (number of household smokers times years of exposure). It has been estimated that 2% of new lung cancer cases each year are due to passive smoking exposure. All cell types except bronchoalveolar carcinoma are associated with smoking. Of the other causative agents, asbestos is the most important, especially when combined with cigarette smoking. The risk for lung cancer in heavy smokers with heavy asbestos exposure is greater than 50 times that of the nonsmoking, non–asbestos exposed population; up to 14% of smokers with asbestosis develop lung cancer. Although asbestos has been estimated to cause 5% of lung cancers, it should be noted that nonoccupational exposure poses no significant public health risk.

Other industrial risks include uranium, arsenic, chromium, chloromethyl, methylethers, polycyclic aromatic hydrocarbons, nickel, and possibly beryllium. Radon gas, a decay product of naturally occurring uranium in the earth, is associated with a dose-related increase in risk of developing bronchogenic carcinoma. Lung cancer may rarely develop in pre-existing scars due to old granulomatous disease, diffuse interstitial fibrosis, or scleroderma.

LUNG TUMOR BIOLOGY

The biology of lung carcinoma has received much attention recently, particularly regarding the role of oncogenes (*jun, ras, myc, c-erb* B-2), tumor suppressor genes (p53) and growth factors (bombesin, gastrin-releasing peptide), and other mechanisms of tumor development. Amplification or mutation of oncogenes may play a role in unregu-

lated cell growth. Recent studies have suggested that increased expression of the *myc* genes in small cell lung cancer and the *ras* and *c-erb* B-2 genes in non–small cell cancer are associated with a poor patient response and decreased survival. However, further confirmation of these studies is needed before these markers are used routinely for diagnostic and prognostic use. Other genetic factors associated with lung carcinoma may include the variable expression of certain cytochrome P-450 enzymes. This enzymatic activity is inducible by cigarette smoke and may produce carcinogenic metabolites of polycyclic aromatic hydrocarbons present in cigarette smoke. One factor possibly contributing to lung cancer risk may be the genetically regulated activity of these or related enzymes.

PATHOLOGY

Benign tumors, composing 5% of the total, are usually diagnosed on routine chest radiographs, and symptoms, if present, are usually related to bronchial obstruction. The most common central tumor is the bronchial adenoma, which usually appears benign but is potentially malignant and rarely produces features of the carcinoid syndrome. The most common peripheral tumor is the pulmonary hamartoma, which has a characteristic "popcorn" pattern of calcification.

Primary malignant neoplasms in the lung have classically been divided into four cell types, as summarized in Table 20–1. Clinically, though, one speaks of small cell and "non–small cell" lung cancer, as their behavior is so different. Small cell lung cancer has the greatest tendency to metastasize early and is almost always disseminated on presentation. The non–small cell types spread to a greater or lesser extent in the chest prior to metastasis. In addition, the non–small cell tumors may contain elements of all these cell types, making the distinction between them of little clinical use.

Metastatic spread of neoplasms to the lung is common, involving the parenchyma, endobronchial mucosa, chest wall, pleural space, or mediastinum. Direct extension is the least common mode of spread, occurring with breast, liver, and pancreatic tumors. Hematogenous spread is common with renal, thyroid, and testicular tumors and bone sarcomas and presents with asymptomatic discrete

TABLE 20–1	Features of Malignant Neoplasms	
Cell Type	**Pathologic Features**	**Common Chest X-ray Findings**
Squamous cell carcinoma	Keratin production, intercellular bridges	Central lesion with hilar involvement, cavitation frequent
Adenocarcinoma	Gland formation, mucin production	Peripheral lesion, cavitation may occur
Bronchoalveolar carcinoma	Distinction from adenocarcinoma imprecise	Usually peripheral lesion, pneumonic-like infiltrate, occasionally multifocal
Large cell carcinoma	Probably represents poorly differentiated adenocarcinoma	Usually peripheral lesion, larger than adenocarcinoma with tendency to cavitate
Small cell carcinoma	Involvement by cells twice the size of lymphocytes	Central lesion, hilar mass common, early mediastinal involvement, no cavitation

nodules on chest radiography. Lymphangitic spread presents as an infiltrate or diffuse reticulonodular pattern on chest radiography and causes severe dyspnea, usually out of proportion to the radiographic findings. This pattern is typical of spread from adenocarcinoma of the breast, stomach, pancreas, ovary, prostate, and lung.

CLINICAL PRESENTATION

Clinical presentation may be related to tumor location within the chest, metastatic spread, or extrapulmonary paraneoplastic manifestations. Most patients present with weight loss and symptoms related to local involvement, such as cough (75%) that has changed in character, hemoptysis (50%) that is rarely life threatening, dyspnea (60%), and chest pain (40%). A marked increase in sputum production (bronchorrhea) occasionally occurs with bronchoalveolar carcinoma. Pancoast's syndrome refers to

TABLE 20–2	Common Paraneoplastic Syndromes Associated with Bronchogenic Carcinoma	
Syndrome	**Cell Type Usually Implicated**	**Mechanism**
Hypertrophic pulmonary osteoarthropathy	All types except small cell	Unknown
Gynecomastia	Large cell	Chronic gonadotropin production
Syndrome of inappropriate ADH (SIADH) secretion	Usually small cell (may be associated with any cell type)	Inappropriate ADH release
Hypercalcemia	Usually squamous cell	Direct involvement of bone, prostaglandins, osteoclast-activating factor, PTH-like action
Cushing's syndrome	Usually small cell	Ectopic ACTH production
Eaton-Lambert myasthenic syndrome	Usually small cell	Unknown
Other neuromyopathic disorders (see Chapter 122)	Frequently small cell but reported with most types	Unknown
Thrombophlebitis	All types	Unknown

ACTH = Adrenocorticotropic hormone; ADH = antidiuretic hormone; PTH = parathyroid hormone.

apical tumors that involve the brachial plexus and often lead to Horner's syndrome, resulting from invasion of the inferior cervical ganglion. Compression and obstruction of the superior vena cava, usually by small cell tumor, cause facial and upper extremity edema, dyspnea, stridor, and symptoms related to increased intracranial pressure. Partial obstruction of a bronchus may lead to unilateral, persistent wheezing, whereas complete obstruction causes postobstructive pneumonia. Recurrent laryngeal nerve involvement, typical of a left hilar mass, causes hoarseness. Phrenic nerve entrapment by a mediastinal mass causes diaphragmatic paralysis. Finally, direct spread of the tumor to the pleural or pericardial space results in effusions. Bronchogenic carcinoma is frequently discovered only after it metastasizes to other organs. The brain, liver, bone, and lymph nodes are common sites, and the evaluation of tumor found in these locations, in a smoker, should include a search for a primary lung neoplasm. In 10 to 50% of patients, bronchogenic carcinoma produces one or more paraneoplastic syndromes. These may manifest as neuromuscular, skeletal, endocrine, hematologic, cutaneous, or cardiovascular abnormalities (Table 20–2).

DIAGNOSIS AND EVALUATION

A careful history and physical examination are crucial in patient evaluation, and availability of a previous chest radiograph is of tremendous value, especially when a solitary pulmonary nodule is present. Routine laboratory studies are rarely helpful in the diagnosis of bronchogenic carcinoma but can be invaluable in evaluating extrathoracic spread of the disease, especially liver function studies and serum calcium and alkaline phosphatase, which screen for bone metastases.

Therapeutic decisions are based on a correct tissue diagnosis. Cytologic examination of expectorated sputum is the easiest and least invasive approach. False-positive results are rare, but false-negative results are relatively common (40 to 50%), especially with peripheral lesions. When cytologic examination of expectorated sputum is negative, bronchoscopy should be the next procedure in patients with central lesions, lung infiltrates, hoarseness, or hemoptysis. Positive yield ranges from 90% for central, endobronchially visible tumors to 50% for peripheral lesions. Small peripheral lung nodules may be approached by percutaneous needle aspiration performed under computed tomographic (CT) guidance, which primarily provides material for cytologic examination. Diagnostic accuracy is greater than 80% for malignant disease but is disturbingly less accurate with benign lesions. Therefore, in a smoker who has a newly diagnosed lung nodule without benign radiographic characteristics and without evidence of metastatic disease and who is a good surgical candidate, proceeding directly to diagnostic and therapeutic thoracotomy is a reasonable approach (see Fig. 20–2).

Once the tumor is diagnosed, the only chance for cure is surgical. Most patients with lung cancer have underlying lung disease as a result of smoking. Therefore, it must be determined if a patient is an operative candidate, meaning being capable of withstanding the loss of lung parenchyma. Operability should be investigated first. Patients with hypercapnia generally are not surgical candidates. Hypoxemia, though, may improve if the tumor is causing physiologic obstruction or compression. In the absence of hypercapnia, simple spirometry is used to guide the physiologic assessment (Fig. 20–1A). In some patients with marginal pulmonary function indices, exercise testing may provide additional information regarding resectability.

If the patient is considered to be an operative candidate, determination of anatomic resectability is the next step (Fig. 20–1B). Endobronchial lesions within 2 cm of the carina on bronchoscopy are inoperable. Intrathoracic spread to the lungs and to the hilar or mediastinal lymph nodes can often be determined from the plain radiograph, but chest CT is an integral part of presurgical evaluation in patients with potentially resectable tumors. The sensitivity and specificity for detecting mediastinal lymph node metastases on CT depend on lymph node size criteria. Generally, lymph node diameter >1.5 cm detects metastatic spread with sensitivity and specificity approaching 80%. However, when mediastinal adenopathy is demonstrated by CT, nonresectability should be proved by biopsy.

Once intrathoracic spread is excluded, negative findings on the history and physical examination, combined with a normal routine laboratory evaluation, are usually adequate to exclude metastatic spread. Multiple imaging techniques in the absence of symptoms or signs suggesting specific organ involvement are cost inefficient and are frequently misleading.

SOLITARY PULMONARY NODULE

A solitary pulmonary nodule is defined as a rounded lesion with well-demarcated margins, up to 3 cm in diameter. Between 5 and 40% are malignant. Benign lesions are usually smaller (<2 cm), have sharp borders and no satellite lesions, and are present in younger people (younger than 40 years old). Nodules >3 cm are likely to be malignant. Other characteristics that help to distinguish benign from malignant nodules include rate of growth and the presence and pattern of calcification. Nodules with doubling times of <10 to 20 or >450 days are most likely benign. The presence of calcification with a central, speckled, diffuse, laminar, or "popcorn" pattern, but not eccentric calcification, is also evidence of its benign nature. When calcification is not evident on plain

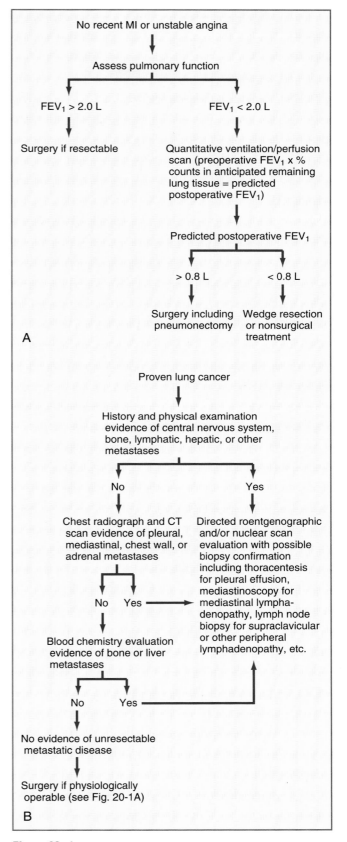

Figure 20–1

Decision regarding operability *(A)* and resectability *(B)* in the presence of proven lung cancer. CT = computed tomography; FEV_1 = forced expiratory volume in 1 second; MI = Myocardial infarction.

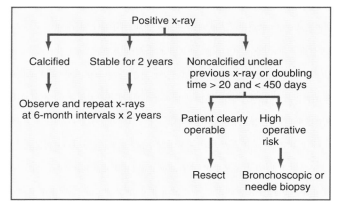

Figure 20–2
Decision tree for management of a solitary pulmonary nodule.

chest radiographs, it may possibly be demonstrated by CT, particularly thin-section CT. On rare occasions, the clinical picture is clearly benign, such as in a patient with a previously normal chest radiograph who develops well-documented histoplasmosis that resolves, leaving a single histoplasmoma. A suggested decision tree for the approach to the solitary nodule is shown in Figure 20–2.

TREATMENT AND PROGNOSIS

Surgery is the therapy of choice for patients with non–small cell carcinoma who meet both physiologic and anatomic criteria and have no evidence of extrathoracic spread. Recently, complete surgical resection of localized ipsilateral mediastinal and hilar lymph node metastases has been possible, with encouraging 5-year survival results at some centers. In addition, limited extrapulmonary invasion, particularly peripheral tumors invading the chest wall or minimal involvement of the mediastinal pleura and pericardium, no longer precludes an aggressive surgical approach. Contralateral lymph node involvement, extracapsular lymph node spread, and massive ipsilateral disease remain contraindications for surgery. There has been renewed interest in the surgical treatment of limited small cell carcinoma, but proof of efficacy has not yet been established. Although there is no evidence that postoperative radiation therapy or chemotherapy improves survival in patients who have had resection of non–small cell carcinoma, the use of tumor markers may eventually help detect specific subsets of patients in whom such therapy could be beneficial.

For those patients with small cell carcinoma or nonoperable non–small cell tumors, radiation therapy and chemotherapy are the only other modalities. Chemotherapy in various combinations has improved the median survival of patients with small cell carcinoma limited to the thorax from 3 months in untreated patients to 16 to 17 months in those receiving chemotherapy. For non–small cell carcinoma, chemotherapy has not significantly altered the outcome, and because of the significant toxicity involved, it should not be used except in controlled experimental settings.

Radiation therapy is often used in small cell carcinoma, both to treat the primary lung lesion and as prophylaxis against cerebral metastases. In general, patients with limited-stage small cell carcinoma should be treated with combination chemotherapy and chest radiotherapy. For patients with extensive-stage small cell carcinoma, radiation therapy should be reserved for palliation of specific sites. Prophylactic cranial irradiation does decrease the risk of developing brain metastasis but does not improve overall survival. Radiation therapy is generally not beneficial in non–small cell carcinoma except in some patients with small localized peripheral tumors who cannot or will not undergo resection. It is therefore limited to the palliative management of pain, recurrent hemoptysis, effusions, or obstruction of airways or the superior vena cava. With airway obstruction, radiation may be delivered by an external beam or endobronchial catheter (brachytherapy). Endobronchial laser therapy and endobronchial prostheses (stents) are additional measures used to treat airway obstruction.

The 5-year survival rate for all patients with bronchogenic carcinoma is 8 to 12% and has improved only slightly over the past few years, despite the introduction of multiple new chemotherapeutic agents. Large trials of routine screening of high-risk people with sputum cytology and chest roentgenographs have not improved survival.

REFERENCES

Filderman AE, Shaw C, Matthay RA: Lung cancer. Invest Radiol 1986; 21;80–90, 173–185.
Iannuzzi MC, Scoggin CH: Small cell lung cancer. Am Rev Respir Dis 1986;134:593–608.
Matthay RA (ed.): Lung cancer. Clin Chest Med 1993;14(1):1–203.

21

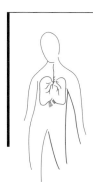

Control of Breathing in Disease States

SLEEP APNEA SYNDROME

Normal, uninterrupted sleep has a cyclic pattern alternating between rapid eye movement (REM) sleep and non–rapid eye movement sleep (non-REM). REM sleep is also called dream sleep, and in this stage there is a marked decline in chin skeletal muscle activity, the onset of rapid eye movement, irregular respiration, and generalized skeletal muscle atonia except for the diaphragm. With onset of normal sleep, ventilation declines, arterial carbon dioxide increases, and the pharynx narrows due to muscle relaxation. This partial pharyngeal collapse places an added "resistive load" on the respiratory system, and incomplete compensation for the added resistance contributes to the decreased ventilation seen in normal sleep.

Apnea is defined as complete cessation of airflow for 10 or more seconds. Hypopnea occurs when airflow decreases significantly but does not stop. Apneas and hypopneas may occur in any sleep stage, but they are most often noted during REM sleep. Many normal people have apneas and hypopneas during sleep, and these features increase with age, especially in men. When these normal events become too frequent and prolonged, they lead to unfavorable consequences that establish the sleep apnea syndrome manifest by chronically disrupted sleep and excessive daytime sleepiness. Obstructive sleep apnea (OSA) is the most common sleep disorder and must be distinguished from the less commonly observed central sleep apnea (CSA).

Central sleep apnea is caused by a fluctuating central drive of the respiratory muscles. Congestive heart failure is the most common cause, followed by neurologic disorders involving the brain stem and respiratory control centers. If oxyhemoglobin desaturation occurs in these patients, they will benefit from supplemental oxygen or respiratory assist devices during sleep (Fig. 21–1A).

Obstructive sleep apnea is common; it is estimated that 4% of middle-aged men have it. Women are affected much less frequently. Obesity is a major risk factor, but not all patients are overweight. The mechanism by which obesity predisposes to sleep apnea is not known. OSA is due to a complete collapse of the upper airway during sleep that often requires arousal for termination. There is a sequence of cyclic events. At first the pharyngeal airway collapses and airflow is impeded, despite increasing ventilatory effort. Progressive hypoxemia results, and then

arousal follows. With arousal, the upper airway opens and ventilation is restored. Sleep returns, pharyngeal muscle activity declines allowing pharyngeal occlusion, and the cycle repeats. This series of events may be repeated hundreds of times each night, resulting in marked disruption of sleep (Fig. 21–1B).

The cardiovascular response to asphyxia is to increase sympathetic nervous system activity, producing systemic vasoconstriction and hypertension. If hypoxemia occurs, there may be bradycardia and significant arrhythmias. It is not clear whether these acute cardiovascular changes that occur with each episode of apnea have an impact on the increased incidence of hypertension, stroke, and coronary artery disease noted in these subjects. Systemic hypertension has been reported to be present in 30 to 50% of patients with OSA, and many patients who have hypertension have undiagnosed OSA. A causal relationship between OSA and systemic hypertension has been difficult to establish because of shared risk factors such as age, male sex, and obesity. A long history of snoring is almost always noted with OSA, and some consider snoring as a marker for this syndrome, with a span extending from asymptomatic continuous snoring to fully developed complete obstruction.

The diagnosis of sleep apnea should be considered when patients complain of excessive daytime sleepiness. This may be associated with inability to concentrate, depression, irritability, and personality changes. The patient may not be aware of the disrupted sleep, but the sleeping partner may report loud snoring, snorting, gasping, and restlessness. The physical examination usually, but not always, reveals obesity and abundant soft tissue in the neck and oral pharynx. There may be systemic hypertension and, in advanced states, right-sided heart failure and left ventricular dysfunction. Usually the standard laboratory tests are normal; only a minority show hypoxemia and hypercarbia. If there is a reasonable clinical suspicion of OSA, polysomnography, which involves recording eye movements, submental muscle tone, and electroencephalogram and an electrocardiogram together with respiratory monitoring that includes measurements of respiratory movements, nasal and oral airflow, and arterial oxyhemoglobin saturation, is indicated. If OSA is found, the patient may then be fitted with a nasal continuous positive airway pressure (CPAP) system and evaluated for improvement. Patient accommodation to CPAP may require

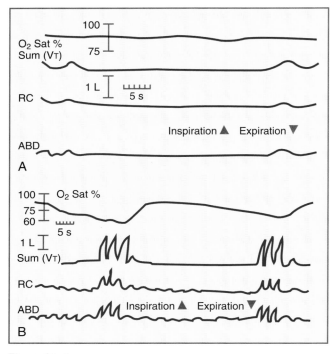

Figure 21-1

A, Central sleep apnea. There is absence of abdominal (ABD) and rib cage (RC) movement, and their sum (VT) during central apnea is associated with a small fall in arterial oxygen saturation (O₂ Sat %), measured by ear oximetry. *B,* Obstructive sleep apnea. This depicts obstructive apnea terminated by deep breaths. Apnea in the midportion of the recording is marked by absence of sum movements (VT) despite respiratory efforts indicated by paradoxical movement of RC (movement downward) and ABD (movement upward) compartments; this apnea is associated with a marked fall in arterial oxygen saturation (O₂ Sat%), measured by ear oximetry. (Modified with permission from Tobin MJ, Cohn MA, Sackner MA: Breathing abnormalities during sleep. Arch Intern Med 143:1221–1228, 1983. Copyright 1983, American Medical Association.)

time and titration of the pressure levels to obtain a good result.

Additional management considerations are to advise the patient to eliminate sedatives and alcohol. If obesity is present, weight loss may significantly improve breathing. These patients have less difficulty when sleeping in the lateral decubitus position as compared with sleeping supine. Hypothyroidism and acromegaly should be excluded. Upper airway surgery should be offered for specific structural abnormalities such as nasal polyps, deviated nasal septum, or large tonsils. Uvulopalatopharyngoplasty, the surgical removal of the uvula, redundant soft palate tissue, tonsils, and adenoids is used to relieve upper airway obstruction, but the value of this procedure for most patients is in doubt. Tracheostomy is highly effective therapy but should be used only when more conservative measures fail.

A primary abnormality of ventilatory control causing alveolar hypoventilation is rare. When it occurs, it is usually due to brain stem involvement by tumor, ische-

mia, or inflammatory disease; a primary, idiopathic form has also been described. Patients display decreased chemosensitivity, often with resting hypercapnia and cor pulmonale. Rarely, the impairment of chemosensitivity may be so severe that the patient breathes adequately only when stimulated by wakefulness but hypoventilates or becomes apneic during sleep, when rostral neural influences are removed. More frequently, ventilatory control system abnormalities interact with other disease states, modifying the overall level of ventilation and possibly contributing to the development of dyspnea and hypercapnia. For example, patients with physiologically significant chronic obstructive pulmonary disease (COPD) have a reduced ventilatory response to hypoxia and hypercapnia. This was formerly thought to be due entirely to decreased chemosensitivity of the respiratory centers; however, most of these patients actually display an increased resting respiratory center drive. In hypercapnic patients, this heightened respiratory drive fails to translate into a sufficiently increased minute ventilation to maintain a normal PCO₂ owing to the increased work of breathing and marked ventilation-perfusion mismatch. Although some relation exists between the degree of hypercapnia and the severity of airway obstruction, abnormalities of lung mechanics do not fully account for the magnitude of the change (Fig. 21–2). Development of chronic hypercapnia may, in fact, depend on complex interactions between inherent characteristics of the ventilatory control system, perception of and ability to compensate for increased ventilatory loads (such as elevated airways resistance), and pattern of breathing.

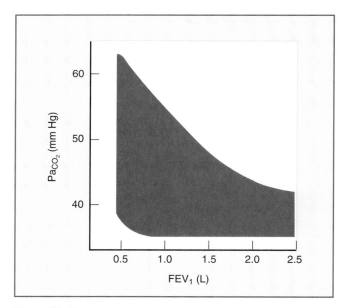

Figure 21-2

The increase in Pa₍CO2₎ as airway obstruction becomes more severe, as reflected by decreasing 1-second forced expiratory volume (FEV₁). Note the large scatter of PCO₂ values for any level of obstruction.

BREATHING PATTERN ABNORMALITIES ASSOCIATED WITH NEUROLOGIC DISEASE

Central neurogenic hyperventilation has been considered a characteristic feature of lower brain stem and upper pontine disease. Rarely, it is an isolated finding, as most patients display associated pulmonary complications that could reflexively stimulate the respiratory center through hypoxia or activation of intrapulmonary sensory receptors. Patients with advanced hepatic cirrhosis usually show alveolar hyperventilation, and on occasion the degree of respiratory alkalosis that results is extreme. Presumably, the hyperventilation results from an increased central respiratory drive. Apneustic breathing consists of sustained inspiratory pauses localizing damage to the midpons, most commonly due to a basilar artery infarct. Biot's or ataxic breathing, a haphazard random distribution of deep and shallow breaths, is caused by disruption of the respiratory rhythm generator in the medulla.

Cheyne-Stokes respiration is characterized by regular cycles of crescendo-decrescendo changes in tidal volume separated by apneic or hypopneic pauses. Many affected patients have evidence of cardiac or neurologic disease. In patients with congestive heart failure, the disturbance arises because of prolongation of the circulation time, which delays transmission of information concerning arterial PO_2 and PCO_2 to the respiratory centers, thus leading to system instability with resulting oscillations in tidal volume. It has no localizing value in patients with neurologic disease but has generally been considered to indicate an ominous prognosis, although this is sometimes not the case.

NEUROMUSCULAR DISEASE

Respiratory center function is poorly defined in neuromuscular disease. Decreased ventilatory capacity may result from impaired neural output or poor translation of this neural output into respiratory muscle contraction. Typically, the patients display an increased respiratory rate and inability to take deep breaths, with consequent tendency to atelectasis. Characteristic changes in lung volume result from an inability to adequately inspire above or expire below functional residual capacity (see Table 16–2). Paradoxical motion of the rib cage and abdomen is commonly observed. Hypoventilation may be particularly severe during sleep. Sleep disruption with resultant daytime somnolence is common and may be a result of nocturnal respiratory abnormalities. Typical causes include inflammatory polyneuropathy, amyotrophic lateral sclerosis, myasthenia gravis, poliomyelitis, and severe kyphoscoliosis. These patients may require long-term mechanical ventilatory support, particularly during sleep.

REFERENCES

Bates DV: Basic pulmonary physiology. *In* Bates DV: Respiratory Function in Disease. 3rd ed. Philadelphia, WB Saunders, 1989, pp 23–66.

Pack, AI: Obstructive sleep apnea. Adv Intern Med 1994;39:517–567.

22

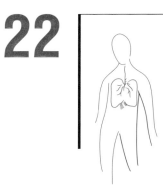

Inhalational and Environmental Injury

DROWNING AND NEAR-DROWNING

The human body is naturally buoyant; however, so much as raising a hand out of the water tips the balance to negative buoyancy. This, combined with the natural tendency for people to overestimate their swimming ability, makes drowning an unfortunately common occurrence; it is the most common cause of death in those under 25 years old. The term *drowning* generally refers to episodes resulting in immediate death, whereas the term *near-drowning* applies to all other victims, whether they survive or not.

Once immersed, the normal person can breathhold for a short time, usually limited by the rising arterial P_{CO_2}. Most drowning victims inhale some water, but in about 10% of cases, laryngeal spasm results in the aspiration of virtually no fluid. This scenario, known as "dry" drowning, results in minimal lung injury, and recovery is rapid if respiration and circulation are restored before permanent neurologic damage occurs.

In the past, a great deal of emphasis had been placed on the relative importance of freshwater and saltwater drowning in terms of their ensuing complications because of the differential effect on electrolytes and volume status. In fact, most of these are second-order effects and transient at best. The complications of near-drowning fall into two categories. The first is acute lung injury from aspirated fluids. This may be due to effects on surfactant by hypotonic freshwater or the osmolar action of hypertonic seawater. A significant percentage of patients who initially appear well after resuscitation may develop adult respiratory distress syndrome (ARDS) as a late complication. The second category comprises the effects of prolonged anoxia on end-organs such as the brain and kidney. These latter complications, which are far less reversible, often determine the ultimate prognosis. Neurologic injury is the most serious and least reversible complication in those successfully resuscitated. Cerebral edema results in elevated intracranial pressure and decreased cerebral perfusion. Little, if anything, has been shown to help, and it carries a grave prognosis.

Treatment of the near-drowning victim is simple: restore ventilation and circulation as soon as possible. No other interventions, such as draining the lungs of aspirated water, should be attempted, as they only waste time and increase mortality. In contrast to other arrest scenarios, prolonged efforts are often worthwhile, perhaps because of the protective effects of bradycardia and shunting of blood to the heart and brain ("diving reflex"), as well as the hypothermia that often accompanies near-drowning. Patients have survived as long as 70 minutes of immersion with complete recovery.

DISEASES OF ALTITUDE

Trekking and mountain climbing have become more popular, resulting in an increasing incidence of the complications of high altitude: acute mountain sickness (AMS), high-altitude cerebral edema, and high-altitude pulmonary edema.

Both the rate and height of ascent contribute to the degree of illness. Given enough time, climbers can adapt quite well even to heights that would be lethal to the unacclimated. Adaptation occurs at multiple levels, including hyperventilation, polycythemia, increased cardiac output, and changes in the hemoglobin (Hb)-oxygen (O_2) affinity. Failure to allow time for adaptation results in illness.

Acute mountain sickness and cerebral edema probably represent a spectrum of the same condition. Clinical manifestations of AMS include headache, nausea, vomiting, and signs of fluid retention, such as facial and hand swelling. Symptoms are often worse after a night's sleep at altitude, and periodic breathing may be noted. Simple rest and mild analgesics can alleviate the symptoms of AMS as the patient acclimates, or the patient may need to descend. Dexamethasone may also be useful as symptomatic treatment. Acetazolamide may be helpful as a prophylactic agent or as therapy.

If the patient does not descend, or worse, if he or she continues to ascend, the full picture of high-altitude cerebral edema may supervene. This syndrome of severe headache, confusion, and ataxia may be fatal and should be treated aggressively with O_2, dexamethasone, and descent as soon as possible.

High-altitude pulmonary edema is noncardiogenic. There may be an increase in permeability accounting for the edema fluid. An uneven distribution of hypoxic pulmonary vasoconstriction complicates matters by imposing an elevated pulmonary artery pressure on the microvessels distal to unconstricted arteries.

SMOKE INHALATION INJURY

Three of the mechanisms of noxious gas injury combine in the smoke inhalation syndrome: direct mucosal injury secondary to hot gases, tissue anoxia due to combustion products, and asphyxia as O_2 is consumed by fire.

The clinical presentation depends on the predominant form of injury. Facial burns and singed nasal hairs should arouse suspicion of lung injury, although pulmonary involvement occurs in only a small proportion of such patients. Thermal injury may produce upper airway obstruction with stridor, hoarseness, and phonation difficulties, necessitating further evaluation (with possible bronchoscopy) and intubation to maintain a patent airway. Lower airway involvement may be associated with the production of carbonaceous sputum, wheezes, and crackles. The chest radiograph is insensitive in the early stages, although pulmonary infiltrates or edema may subsequently develop.

Thermal injury is most commonly seen in the upper airway, manifesting as upper airway edema and obstruction. This injury may extend to the tracheobronchial tree, particularly if steam heat is the cause, as moist air has a high thermal content and may overwhelm the cooling system in the pharynx. Direct lung injury is rare, but pulmonary edema secondary to inadvertent fluid overload or due to sepsis is not an uncommon late complication.

Incomplete combustion, particularly of industrial compounds, produces a number of both irritant and toxic compounds. Ammonia, acrolein, sulfur dioxide, and others are encountered in today's fires. Cyanide poisoning is increasingly recognized and, in fact, may be an important cause of mortality even in residential fires.

Carbon monoxide (CO) poisoning can also complicate acute smoke inhalation injury. CO is an odorless, tasteless, and colorless gas that does not produce lung injury but has a dual effect on tissue oxygenation. Its marked affinity for Hb (210 times that of O_2) limits the O_2 carrying capacity of blood. In addition, it shifts the O_2 dissociation curve to the left, which impairs O_2 release to the tissues. Symptoms of CO intoxication include headache, nausea, fatigue, behavioral change, and ataxia, followed by mental confusion and coma. Cherry-red coloration of the lips is usually absent unless the carboxyhemoglobin (COHb) concentration is above 40%. An intoxicated patient displays a normal Pa_{O_2} and *calculated* O_2 saturation, but there is a severe reduction in *measured* O_2 saturation. Despite the severe O_2 desaturation, minute ventilation is not increased in CO intoxication, since the carotid body responds to Pa_{O_2}. Confirmation is made by measurement of blood COHb: less than 2% in healthy subjects, 5 to 10% in cigarette smokers, and 30 to 50% in fire injury victims.

Administration of supplemental O_2 relieves hypoxemia and enhances the dissociation of CO from Hb, decreasing the half-time for elimination from 300 minutes on room air to 60 minutes, with an Fi_{O_2} of 1.0. To achieve an adequate Fi_{O_2}, intubation and mechanical ventilation may be required. Hyperbaric O_2 is no longer recommended in the management of CO poisoning. Management includes removing the victim from exposure, checking vital signs, and establishing a patent airway.

Corticosteroids are no longer recommended in the management of smoke inhalation injury. Antibiotics should be prescribed only if there is evidence of infection. In the rare cases in which ARDS supervenes, the management is identical to that described in Chapter 23. Patients surviving the acute clinical course usually recover completely. Long-term complications of tracheal stenosis, bronchiolitis obliterans, or bronchiectasis are rare.

NOXIOUS GASES AND FUMES

Exposure to toxic gases and fumes is an increasing problem in modern industrial society and may cause harm by different mechanisms (Table 22–1). Simple asphyxia occurs by replacement of the O_2 in the air with another nontoxic agent. This requires very high concentrations and usually occurs in an enclosed setting, such as methane exposure in a coal mine. Tissue asphyxia, by contrast, is due to an inability of the body to use available O_2, either secondary to an increase in Hb-O_2 affinity, such as with CO, or by interfering with the cytochrome chain, as in cyanide toxicity.

The most common mechanism of injury is local irritation, the form and extent of which depend on the concentration, solubility, and duration of exposure to the toxic gas. Highly soluble gases, such as *ammonia,* rapidly

TABLE 22–1	Toxic Gases and Fumes	
Mechanism of Injury	**Agent**	**Occupational Exposure**
Simple asphyxia	Carbon dioxide	Mining, foundry work
	Nitrogen	Mining, underwater work
	Methane	Mining
Tissue asphyxia	Carbon dioxide	Mining, petroleum refining, pollution
	Cyanide	Smoke inhalation
Upper airway injury	Ammonia	Fertilizer, refrigeration, cleaning agents
	Hydrogen fluoride	Etching, refining
	Chlorine	Bleaches, swimming pools
Pulmonary edema	Nitrogen dioxide	Farming, fertilizer, silo welding
	Phosgene	Welding, paint removal
Systemic toxicity	Cadmium (renal failure)	Electroplating
	"Metal fume fever"	Welding, galvanizing
	Benzene	Petroleum refining
Allergy	Isocyanates	Plastics, paint
	Platinum	Electroplating, photography
	Formalin	Insulation, textiles, manufacturing

injure the mucous membranes of the eye and upper airway, causing an intense burning pain in the eyes, nose, and throat, with lacrimation, rhinorrhea, and a sense of suffocation. This, combined with the strong, pungent odor of ammonia, causes the victim to flee from the site of exposure. Lower airway injury is not observed unless the victim is trapped or a massive spill occurs, in which case laryngeal or pulmonary edema may ensue.

In contrast, insoluble gases, such as nitrogen dioxide, are distributed to the peripheral airways and usually cause a diffuse lung injury. Exposure to *nitrogen dioxide* is classically encountered in farmers, as large quantities of this gas are formed by fermentation during the first week after filling a silo. The victim typically presents with cough, dyspnea, bronchospasm, and weakness, with little evidence of ocular or upper airway irritation. After a period of 1 or more hours, there may be progression to frank pulmonary edema. Following recovery from the acute illness, the patient may develop bronchiolitis obliterans, characterized by progressive dyspnea. Metal fume fever is a systemic response to inhalation of certain metal oxides, such as zinc oxide. Symptoms include fever, myalgias, and malaise. Long-term sequelae are not seen. Exposure to isocyanate, platinum compounds, or formalin vapors may cause asthma, either immediate or delayed in onset; asthma is more fully discussed in Chapter 16.

Management of exposure to a toxic gas is generally supportive in nature. The victim should be removed from the source of exposure and a patent airway with adequate ventilation ensured. Correction of hypoxemia may be possible with supplemental O_2, or intubation and mechanical ventilation may be necessary. The patient should be carefully monitored for a delayed reaction to the agent. Additional measures that may be required include bronchodilators and correction of acid-base disturbance or shock. The role of prophylactic antibiotics or steroids remains undetermined.

REFERENCES

Haponik EF, Summer WR: Respiratory complications in burned patients: Pathogenesis and spectrum of inhalation injury. J Crit Care 1987;2:49–74.

Loke J: Pathophysiology and Treatment of Inhalation Injuries. New York, Marcel Dekker, 1988.

Modell JW: Drowning. N Engl J Med 1993;328:253–256.

Morgan WKC, Seaton A: Occupational Lung Diseases. 2nd ed. Philadelphia, WB Saunders, 1984.

Schoene RB, Hornbein TF: Respiratory adaptation to high altitude. *In* Murray JF, Nadel JA (eds.): Textbook of Respiratory Medicine. Philadelphia, WB Saunders, 1988.

Shaw KN, Briede CA: Submersion injuries: Drowning and near-drowning. Emerg Med Clin North Am 1989;7:355–370.

Pulmonary Critical Care

Section III

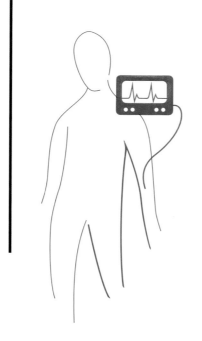

23   ESSENTIALS OF PULMONARY CRITICAL CARE MEDICINE

23

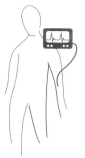

Essentials of Pulmonary Critical Care Medicine

The concept of the intensive care unit (ICU) began with continuous cardiac telemetry for acute myocardial infarction. Over time, the ICU has evolved and differentiated into specialized units to support patients who are suffering from or who are at high risk for either cardiovascular or respiratory collapse resulting from a variety of insults, including extensive surgery, trauma, neurologic injury or disease, cardiac disease, or any number of medical conditions affecting the endocrine, gastrointestinal, renal, pulmonary, and hematologic systems. This chapter focuses on the diagnosis and treatment of respiratory and circulatory collapse, the mechanical support of ventilation, and the multiple organ dysfunction syndrome (MODS).

SHOCK

Shock is best defined as "the state in which profound and widespread reduction of effective tissue perfusion leads first to reversible, and then, if prolonged, to irreversible cellular injury." Shock is classified into four etiologic categories: 1) hypovolemic, 2) cardiogenic, 3) extracardiac obstructive, and 4) distributive.

Most of the physical findings seen in shock are common to all forms, and in certain disease states, two forms of shock may be present (Table 23–1). Therefore, it is often difficult to determine the etiology of shock in a given patient. In the severest form of all types of shock, hypotension is the predominant abnormality in physical examination. Abnormal mental status, poor peripheral perfusion, and renal insufficiency are other common manifestations of shock.

A right heart catheter can be used to help diagnose and treat patients in shock. The right heart catheter can be thought of as a flexible tube with a balloon at its tip. The balloon is inflated, and the catheter is passed through the vena cava and right heart into the pulmonary artery to the point that it occludes the pulmonary artery. When the balloon is inflated, it allows for the measurement of the pressure in the pulmonary artery distal to the balloon (called the pulmonary artery occlusion pressure or the "wedge pressure"), which is an indirect measurement of the end diastolic pressure in the left ventricle. When the balloon is deflated, the catheter can be used to obtain a sample of mixed venous blood for determining the mixed venous oxygen count (MVO_2). The catheter can be used

to measure the cardiac output, a value used in calculating the systemic vascular resistance index (SVRI). These values are useful in classifying shock, and these parameters can be followed to monitor clinical attempts to optimize cardiac performance and regulate tissue oxygen delivery (Table 23–2).

Hypovolemic shock may be related to dehydration or hemorrhage. Clinical characteristics include pale, cool, clammy skin (often mottled), tachycardia, tachypnea, flat, nondistended peripheral veins, collapsed jugular veins, decreased urine output, and altered mental status. Hemodynamically, hypovolemic shock is characterized by a decreased preload resulting in decreased ventricular diastolic pressure and volume. Cardiac index is typically reduced. In addition to hypotension, a decreased pulse pressure may be noted. Metabolic demand is constant or increased, and the MVO_2 is decreased.

In cardiogenic shock, signs of congestive heart failure are typically present. The jugular and peripheral veins may be distended, and a mid-diastolic gallop sound and pulmonary edema are usually found. Hemodynamically, cardiogenic shock is characterized by an increased ventricular preload (the ventricular volume, pulmonary capillary wedge pressure, and central venous pressure are all increased), decreased cardiac index, and increased systemic vascular resistance. MVO_2 is substantially reduced, and the arterial-venous oxygen content difference is increased. Ischemic myocardial injury is the most common cause of cardiogenic shock. Acute valve dysfunction from endocarditis or blunt chest trauma may also cause acute cardiogenic shock, as can acute myocarditis, end-stage cardiomyopathy, rapid and slow cardiac rhythms, hypertrophic cardiomyopathy with obstruction, and traumatic myocardial contusion.

Extracardiac obstructive shock results from obstruction to flow in the cardiovascular circuit. Pericardial tamponade and constrictive pericarditis directly impair diastolic filling of the right ventricle. Tension pneumothorax and intrathoracic tumors impair right ventricular filling by obstructing venous return. Massive pulmonary emboli, nonembolic acute pulmonary hypertension, and aortic dissection may result in shock as a result of increased ventricular afterload. The characteristic hemodynamic patterns are similar to other low-output shock states. The cardiac index is usually decreased. The MVO_2 is low, and the arterial-venous oxygen content differences increase

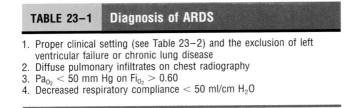

Diagnosis of ARDS

1. Proper clinical setting (see Table 23–2) and the exclusion of left ventricular failure or chronic lung disease
2. Diffuse pulmonary infiltrates on chest radiography
3. $Pa_{O_2} < 50$ mm Hg on $Fi_{O_2} > 0.60$
4. Decreased respiratory compliance < 50 ml/cm H_2O

and serum lactate is elevated. Other hemodynamic variables are dependent on the site of obstruction. Cardiac tamponade typically causes increased and equalized right and left ventricular diastolic pressures, pulmonary artery diastolic pressure, central venous pressure, and pulmonary wedge pressure.

In distributive shock, hypotension results from loss of peripheral resistance. Etiologies include anaphylaxis, spinal injury, adrenal insufficiency, and sepsis. The usual nonspecific signs of shock are present, including tachycardia and tachypnea. In contrast to other forms of shock, the extremities are warm and well perfused. Hemodynamically, distributive shock is characterized by a decrease in systemic vascular resistance.

ACUTE RESPIRATORY FAILURE

The primary function of the respiratory system is to provide a means by which oxygen can be provided to and carbon dioxide (CO_2) removed from the body. Failure of the respiratory system invariably leads to hypoxemia, which is clinically defined as an abnormally low oxygen tension in arterial blood. Hypoxemia can be attributed to any of the following five basic conditions: (1) delivery of a low partial pressure of oxygen to the alveolar space, (2) alveolar hypoventilation, (3) ventilation-perfusion (VQ) mismatch, (4) right-to-left shunting, and (5) diffusion impairments.

Respiratory failure can occur with or without an increase in arterial carbon dioxide tension. Thus, there are two types of respiratory failure. Type 1 is characterized

by an abnormally low PaO_2 with a $PaCO_2$ that is either low or normal. Type 1 respiratory failure is usually caused by a disease process that involves the lung itself (e.g., adult respiratory distress syndrome). In type 2 respiratory failure, hypoxemia occurs in the presence of hypercapnia. Type 2 failure results from decreased alveolar ventilation, either as a result of a decreased minute ventilation (e.g., central nervous system depression) or an increase in dead space ventilation (e.g., chronic obstructive pulmonary disease exacerbation). There are many diseases that may present with either type 1 or 2 respiratory failure. Therefore, classification of the type of respiratory failure in a given patient provides little useful diagnostic or prognostic information, but this classification does indicate which therapeutic modality is appropriate for the patient.

OXYGEN THERAPY AND MECHANICAL VENTILATION

The purpose of administration of oxygen and mechanical ventilation is to support the patient so that an adequate oxygen saturation ($>88\%$) in arterial blood is maintained, while measures are taken to correct the underlying cause of the respiratory failure. Because of the risk and discomfort associated with intubation and mechanical ventilation, oxygen therapy alone should be undertaken in all but the most severe cases of respiratory failure.

In patients with respiratory failure and normal or low CO_2, tensions in the arterial blood, VQ mismatch, and right-to-left shunting are the usual mechanisms for the hypoxemia. The hypoxemia caused by VQ mismatch can be corrected with the administration of relatively low amounts of oxygen. This can usually be administered via nasal cannula. When right-to-left shunting is the mechanism of hypoxemia, large amounts of oxygen are required to maintain an adequate oxygen saturation (Fig. 23–1). One problem associated with oxygen therapy is the risk for oxygen toxicity; the threshold begins when the fraction of inspired oxygen is $>50\%$.

The major focus of treatment for hypoxemic-hypercapnic respiratory failure is the judicious use of oxygen. The primary risk of using high concentrations of inspired oxygen for patients with hypercapnic respiratory failure is the precipitation of progressive hypercapnia (due to removal of the hypoxic drive to breathe). The proper oxygen concentration to use is that which produces an adequate, but not excessively high arterial oxygen tension (50 to 60 mm Hg). Even when oxygen is used judiciously, these patients may develop worsening hypercapnia, which requires mechanical ventilation for support.

The goal of ventilatory therapy may not be the normalization of arterial PCO_2 when chronic CO_2 retention has been present before the onset of the acute illness. Decreasing the arterial $PaCO_2$ to normal levels in a rapid way will cause alkalosis, and this can make it more difficult to wean the patient from the ventilator. Therefore, provision of oxygen to achieve an arterial $PaCO_2$ level that leads to a normal pH is the goal for initial treatment.

TABLE 23–2	Hemodynamic Variables in the Four Types of Shock		
Type of Shock	Pulmonary Wedge Pressure (PCWP)	Cardiac Index (CI)	Systemic Vascular Resistance Index (SVRI)
Hypovolemic	Low	Low	High
Cardiogenic	High	Low	High
Extracardiac obstructive	Normal or low (high in tamponade)	Low	High
Distributive	Normal or low	High (rarely low)	Low

Figure 23-1

The effect of changing the inspired O_2 concentration on the arterial PO_2 and O_2 content for lungs having shunts of 10 to 50%. When the shunt is small, as may be seen early in the course of adult respiratory distress syndrome (ARDS), increasing the inspired oxygen to 40 to 50% effectively increases the PaO_2. As the shunt increases and approaches 30 to 50%, the levels commonly seen in ARDS, only small increases in arterial PO_2 are achieved even when 100% O_2 is administered. Although PO_2 increases very little *(left panel),* this occurs at a steep portion of the O_2 dissociation curve so that O_2 saturation increases disproportionately, resulting in a considerable increase in O_2 content *(right panel).* (From Dantzker D: Gas exchange in the adult respiratory distress syndrome. Clin Chest Med 1982; 3:57–67.

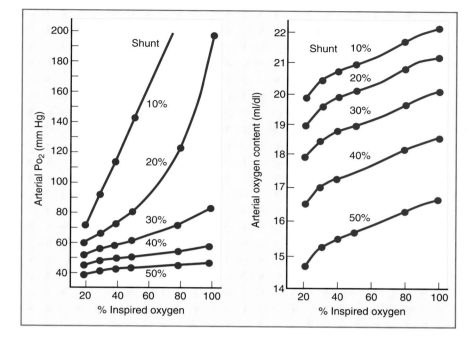

Any changes relative to baseline arterial $PaCO_2$ or pH should be made gradually since rapid changes may cause alkalosis and may lead to cardiac arrhythmias and/or convulsions.

The mechanical respiratory cycle can be broken into four parts. *Inspiration* is the phase during which the exhalation valve of the ventilator is closed and the ventilator uses pressurized air to cause gas to flow into the patient's lungs. *Cycling* is the point where changeover from inspiration to expiration occurs. During *expiration,* the main ventilatory flow is interrupted and the exhalation valve is opened to allow gas to escape from the lungs. *Triggering* is the changeover from expiration to inspiration.

Mechanical ventilators are classified on the basis of what factor terminates inspiratory flow. Pressure-cycled ventilators terminate flow when a preset pressure is reached in the airway. These ventilators are used sparingly because minute ventilation varies with changes in lung mechanics. Volume-cycled ventilators provide a preset volume to the patient over a range of airway pressures. A maximum pressure limit is set to prevent trauma to the lung in the event of a sudden change in pulmonary mechanics that could cause airway pressure increases as the machine delivers a set tidal volume. Although the precise volume delivered to the patient may vary somewhat, volume-cycled ventilators allow for greater control of the patient's ventilation. Time-cycled ventilators set tidal volume by fixing the inspiratory time and flow rate. They accomplish the same goal as volume ventilators but are smaller and more easily manufactured. In some of the newer modes of ventilation, the ventilator is flow cycled (i.e., inspiratory flow is terminated when the inspiratory flow rate drops below a preset level).

The most common modes of mechanical ventilation are assist control (AC) and synchronized intermittent mandatory ventilation (SIMV). These two modes can be used alone or in concert with continuous positive airway pressure (CPAP), positive end-expiratory pressure (PEEP), or pressure support ventilation (PSV). The majority of patients who are initially supported on mechanical ventilation usually receive AC.

In both AC and SIMV, a certain number of mechanical breaths are delivered per unit time. The difference between these two modes is the presence of triggering in the AC mode. That is to say that when the patient makes an effort to take a breath, the ventilator is triggered and gives the patient a full mechanical breath. If the patient does not make an inspiratory effort, then the machine reverses to set rate. In the SIMV mode, the machine allows the patient to take additional breaths over the set rate, but the extra breaths are not mechanically supported. Therefore, the volume of the extra breaths is determined entirely by the patient's ability and effort (Fig. 23–2).

The CPAP system uses a high-pressure reservoir and a constant flow of gas that exceeds the patient's inspiratory peak flow demands. Consequently, the patient breathes at a pressure that is constantly above ambient. This mode of ventilation is rarely used as a primary source of ventilatory support but is most commonly employed at the end of a weaning trial to determine whether a patient will tolerate extubation.

Combining PEEP with other ventilatory modes provides for a positive pressure at the end of expiration (Fig. 23–3). This increases residual reserve capacity and allows for many alveoli and small airways that would otherwise be closed at end expiration to remain open. PEEP is indicated in conditions that result in diffuse infiltrative lung disease that leads to severe hypoxemia and reduced compliance.

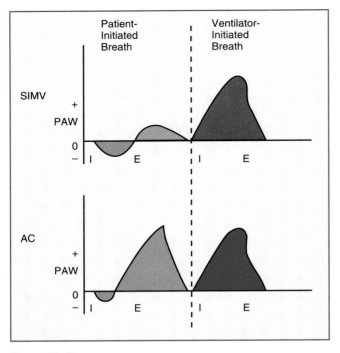

Figure 23-2
Changes in airway pressure (PAW) during patient-initiated and ventilator-initiated breaths in assist control (AC) and intermittent mandatory ventilation (SIMV). E = Expiration; I = inspiration.

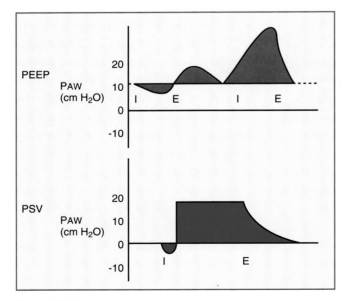

Figure 23-3
Changes in airway pressure (PAW) when positive end-expiratory pressure (PEEP) is added to intermittent mandatory ventilation *(upper panel)* and with a spontaneous breath provided with 15 cm H$_2$O of pressure support (PSV, *lower panel*). E = Expiration; I = inspiration.

Pressure support ventilation (PSV) was originally introduced to reduce the work of spontaneous breathing in the SIMV mode. With PSV, as a patient inhales, the ventilator automatically adjusts the flow to provide and maintain a preset inspiratory support pressure (see Fig. 23-3). The inspiratory phase ends after a certain minimum inspiratory flow rate is reached, whenever excessive airway pressure is detected, or after a present time interval. PSV can be used alone or in combination with SIMV. PSV compensates for the inherent impedances of the ventilator circuit and endotracheal tube. It is most commonly used for patients during the weaning phase of mechanical ventilation.

Most complications of intratracheal intubation can be divided into those that occur as a result of the endotracheal tube placement itself and those efforts resulting from prolonged intubation. During initial intubation, risks include tooth avulsion, pharyngeal injury, aspiration, right mainstem bronchus intubation, esophageal intubation, and laryngeal spasm. Prolonged intubation can result in lip or nasal ulceration, laryngeal trauma, paranasal sinusitis, and tracheal stenosis. Thus, at most institutions, patients who require intubation over 21 days usually undergo tracheostomy placement.

The trachea and major bronchi of virtually all patients in the ICU who are intubated become colonized with prevalent organisms within the first 48 hours. In a large number of these patients, this colonization progresses to diseases manifested as paranasal sinusitis, purulent bronchitis, or pneumonia. In most instances, the offending agent is a gram-negative organism, but *Staphylococcus aureus* is also a frequent pathogen.

The positive pressure required to inflate the lung during mechanical ventilation may produce complications. Barotrauma refers to the rupture of alveolar sacs followed by the accumulation of air in the pleural space or mediastinum. The resulting pneumothorax almost always requires chest tube placement. Air dissecting into the mediastinum may move up into the soft tissues of the neck and result in subcutaneous emphysema. Subcutaneous emphysema can be quite extensive, with air migrating via tissue planes into the head and down through the abdomen into the groin. When the air leak stops, the air will gradually resorb without any intervention.

Positive pressure ventilation can also result in reduction of cardiac output. This occurs by decreasing venous return, which decreases diastolic filling. This problem can be compounded by the addition of PEEP.

MULTIPLE ORGAN DYSFUNCTION SYNDROME, SYSTEMIC INFLAMMATORY RESPONSE SYNDROME, SEPSIS, AND ADULT RESPIRATORY DISTRESS SYNDROME

The MODS is defined as the presence of altered organ function in an acutely ill patient such that homeostasis cannot be maintained without intervention. MODS is a systemic process whereby the microcirculation is the primary target of injury. MODS can be primary (a result of

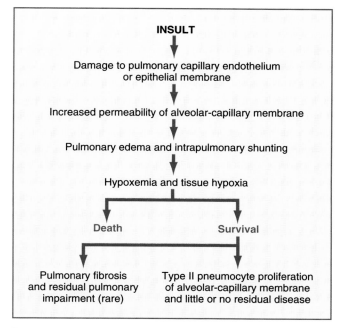

INSULT

↓

Damage to pulmonary capillary endothelium
or epithelial membrane

↓

Increased permeability of alveolar-capillary membrane

↓

Pulmonary edema and intrapulmonary shunting

↓

Hypoxemia and tissue hypoxia

Death   Survival

Pulmonary fibrosis and residual pulmonary impairment (rare)   Type II pneumocyte proliferation of alveolar-capillary membrane and little or no residual disease

Figure 23–4
Pathogenesis and outcome of the adult respiratory distress syndrome (ARDS).

a well-defined insult) or secondary (i.e., a result of the host response to an insult). The host response that leads to secondary MODS is called the systemic inflammatory response syndrome (SIRS). This response is manifested by two or more of the following conditions: (1) temperature $> 38°C$ or $< 36°C$; (2) heart rate > 90 beats/min; (3) respiratory rate > 20 beats/min or $PaCO_2$ < 32 mm Hg; (4) white blood cell count $> 12,000$ 4/cu mm, < 4000 4/cu mm, or $> 10\%$ immature (band) forms.

When SIRS develops in response to infection, the patient has sepsis syndrome. Evidence indicates that tumor necrosis factor alpha (TNF-alpha) is a proximal mediator of the host's altered septic response that leads to MODS. The cytokines (interleukins 1, 2, and 6) and gamma interferon may also contribute to the development of MODS.

The adult respiratory distress syndrome (ARDS) is present when the following three criteria are met: (1) the PaO_2 to FiO_2 ratio is ≤ 200, (2) bilateral pulmonary infiltrates are present on a frontal chest radiograph, and (3) the pulmonary artery occlusion pressure (wedge pressure) is ≤ 18. ARDS can occur as the result of direct lung injury (e.g., following aspiration of acid gastric contents or viral pneumonia) or as part of MODS. MODS is most obvious when the lung is involved. ARDS develops when the pulmonary capillary endothelium is damaged. This leads to increased permeability of alveolar capillary membrane, which is followed by the development of noncardiogenic pulmonary edema. As the air spaces fill with fluid, the gas exchange and mechanical properties of the lung deteriorate (Fig. 23–4).

Treatment of MODS, SIRS, sepsis, and ARDS should be focused toward the underlying disease process. Supportive therapy for failing organs is frequently indicated. Early administration of appropriate antibiotics is crucial in the treatment of sepsis, but these agents are not indicated in patients who have ARDS from aspiration of gastric contents. Virtually all persons with ARDS require a course of mechanical ventilation.

REFERENCES

Bone RC: Acute respiratory failure: Definition and overview. *In* Bone RC, Dantzker DR, George RB, Natthay RA, Reynolds HY (eds.): Pulmonary and Critical Care Medicine. St. Louis, Mosby, 1994.

Bone RC, Balk RA, Cerra FB, et al: Definitions for sepsis and organ failure and guidelines for the use of innovative therapies in sepsis. Chest 1992; 101:1644–1655.

Gluck E, Eubanks DH: Mechanical ventilation. *In* Parrillo JE, Bone RC (eds.): Critical Care Medicine, Principles of Diagnosis and Management. St. Louis, Mosby, 1995.

Kollef MH, Schuster DP: The acute respiratory distress syndrome. N Engl J Med 1995; 332:22–37.

Kumar A, Parrillo JE: Shock: Classification, pathophysiology and approach to management. *In* Parrillo JE, Bone RC (eds.): Critical Care Medicine, Principles of Diagnosis and Management. St. Louis, Mosby, 1995.

Ogniben FP: Arterial blood gases. *In* Parrillo JE (ed.): Current Therapy in Critical Care Medicine. 2nd ed. Philadelphia, BC Decker, 1991.

Wibbald WJ, Maring CM: The multiple organ dysfunction syndrome. *In* Bone RC, Dantzker DR, George RB, Natthay RA, Reynolds HY (eds.): Pulmonary and Critical Care Medicine. St. Louis, Mosby, 1994.

Renal Disease

Section IV

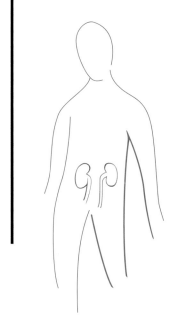

24

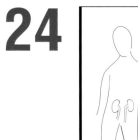

Elements of Renal Structure and Function

ELEMENTS OF RENAL STRUCTURE

The human kidneys are positioned in the retroperitoneal space at the level of the lower thoracic and upper lumbar vertebrae. Each adult kidney weighs approximately 150 gm and measures about 12 by 6 by 3 cm. A coronal section of the kidney reveals two distinct regions (Fig. 24–1A). The outer region, the cortex, is about 1 cm in thickness. The inner region is the medulla and is made up of several conical structures. The bases of these pyramidal structures are located at the corticomedullary junction, and the apices extend into the hilum of the kidney as the papillae. Each papilla is enclosed by a minor calyx; these calyces collectively communicate with major calyces, forming the renal pelvis. Urine that flows from the papillae is collected in the renal pelvis and passes to the bladder through the ureters.

Blood is delivered to each kidney from a main renal artery branching from the aorta (Fig. 24–1B). The main artery usually divides into two main segmental branches, which are further subdivided into lobar arteries supplying the upper, middle, and lower regions of the kidney. These vessels subdivide further as they enter the renal parenchyma and create interlobar arteries that course toward the renal cortex. The smaller arteries provide perpendicular branches, the arcuate arteries, at the corticomedullary junction. Interlobular arteries arising from the arcuates extend into the cortex. The glomerular capillaries receive blood through afferent arterioles that originate from these terminal interlobular arteries. The glomerular capillary bed is drained by a second muscular vessel, the efferent arteriole. This arteriole leaves the glomerulus and supplies a network of vessels that surround tubular structures in the medulla. This network, the vasa recta, includes capillaries that drain into venules. The venous drainage of the kidney is provided by interlobular, arcuate, lobular, and, ultimately, renal veins. Each renal vein drains into the inferior vena cava.

Kidneys have a rich sympathetic innervation. Sympathetic nerve endings are present on renal vasculature, tubules, and the juxtaglomerular (JG) apparatus. Stimulation of sympathetic nervous system causes renin release from the JG cells, resulting in angiotensin and aldosterone production. Although the sympathetic nervous system does not seem to play a major role in day-to-day regulation of glomerular filtration rate, it becomes important in pathologic states.

Histologically, the kidney is composed of a basic structural unit known as the nephron (Fig. 24–2). Each human kidney contains approximately 1 million nephrons. The nephron is composed of two major components: a filtering element composed of an enclosed capillary network (the glomerulus) and an attached tubule. The tubule contains several distinct anatomic and functional segments.

The Glomerulus

The glomerulus (Fig. 24–3) is a unique network of capillaries suspended between the afferent and efferent arterioles enclosed within an epithelial structure (Bowman's capsule). The capillaries are arranged into lobular structures or tufts.

The components of glomerular capillary wall are as follows:

1. Endothelial cells: These cells line the capillary lumen and are fenestrated with pores. Based on the known endothelial cell interactions in other vascular beds, the glomerular endothelial cells are likely to play an important role in glomerular pathophysiology.
2. Glomerular basement membrane: The glomerular epithelial cells and mesangial cells appear to be important in maintaining the integrity of the glomerular basement membrane. The glomerular basement membrane, a layer of hydrated gel composed of glycoproteins containing interwoven collagen fibers, is the main barrier to the filtration of plasma proteins. It functions as a filtration barrier because of the pore size and negative charge on the basement membrane, so that for a given molecular size, negatively charged particles are filtered less easily than positively charged particles. Although the largest pores in the glomerular basement membrane are 80 A° in diameter, albumin, which is 60 A° is not filtered because of the negative surface charge.
3. Epithelial cells: The visceral epithelial cells extend foot processes over the basement membrane. These cells also have a negative surface charge due to the presence of sialoproteins, thus contributing to the fil-

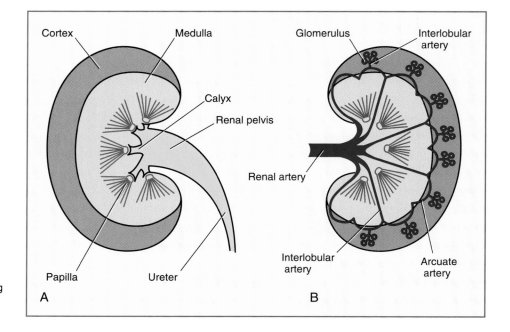

Figure 24–1
Basic renal structure. Urinary collecting structures are depicted in *A,* and the arterial supply is depicted in *B.*

tration barrier. There is evidence to suggest that glomerular epithelial cells may be the major site of injury in various noninflammatory glomerulopathies. The barrier created by these three layers allows free entry of water and low molecular weight solutes into the uri-

nary space, yet totally excludes the passage of cells and large proteins.

4. Mesangium: The glomerular tufts are suspended within the urinary space of Bowman's capsule on a lattice known as the mesangium. Mesangial cells are enclosed by a matrix of homogeneous fibrillary material containing mucopolysaccharides and glycoprotein. There is no basement membrane between the capillary endothelium and mesangial cells (see Fig. 24–3). This arrangement allows for easy entry of plasma products and an interaction with the inflammatory cells. Mesangial cells have actin-myosin elements in the cytoplasm, which accounts for their contractile property, and mesangial cell contraction alters the surface area for filtration, leading to decreased glomerular filtration rate. Mesangial cells have receptors for various vasoconstrictor hormones, e.g., antidiuretic hormone (ADH) and angiotensin II (AII). Hence, in addition to the effects on renal blood flow, these hormones alter the glomerular filtration rate through mesangial cell contraction. Another important function of mesangial cells is the production and remodeling of the extracellular matrix composed of collagen and glycoproteins. In response to growth factors like transforming growth factor β (TGF β), and platelet-derived growth factor (PDGF), the mesangial cells secrete extracellular matrix. This process results in glomerular basement membrane thickening and is an important factor in the pathogenesis of various glomerular diseases, especially diabetes. Mesangial cells also have phagocytic properties.

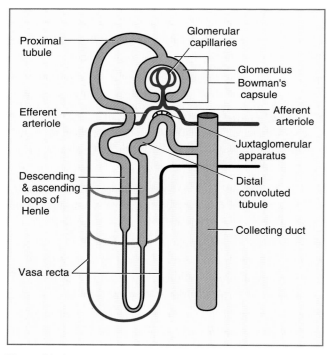

Figure 24–2
The nephron with the basic vascular structures. The glomerular capillaries are supplied by the afferent arteriole and drain into the efferent arterioles. Blood then flows through the vasa recta and is returned to the venous circulation.

The Tubule

The glomerular capsule funnels ultrafiltrate into the renal tubules. The initial portion, the proximal convoluted tu-

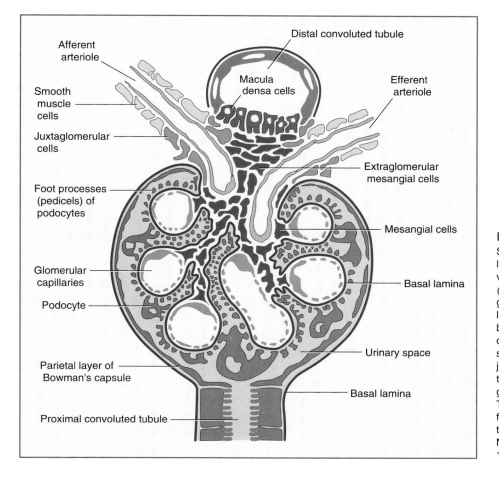

Figure 24-3
Schematic diagram of a renal glomerulus and the structures associated at the vascular pole *(top)* and urinary pole *(bottom)* (not drawn to scale). Mesangial cells are associated with the capillary endothelium and the glomerular basement membrane. The macula densa cells of the distal tubule are shown intimately associated with the juxtaglomerular cells of the afferent arteriole and the extraglomerular mesangial cells. (Modified from Kriz W, Sakai T: Morphological aspects of glomerular function. *In* Nephrology: Proceedings of the Tenth International Congress of Nephrology. London, Bailliere-Tindall, 1987; with permission.)

bule, is located in the cortex. The proximal straight tubule enters the medulla and delivers fluid to the loop of Henle. The loop forms a hairpin turn in the medulla and returns toward the cortex, forming the distal tubule. The tubule finally is directed again into the medullary tissues as the collecting duct, emptying into the renal pelvis at the ducts of Bellini located at the tips of the renal papillae.

The structural arrangement of the tubule allows the distal tubule to come into close approximation with the vascular pole of the glomerulus. The distal tubular cells in this region are taller and more numerous. This distinct region of the distal tubule is known as the *macula densa* and, together with cells originating from the adjacent afferent arteriole, it creates a specialized structure known as the *juxtaglomerular apparatus.* This structure is the site of renin formation and is important in coordinating the function of the glomerulus and tubule. The interstitium contains lymphatics and nerves.

ELEMENTS OF RENAL PHYSIOLOGY

The kidney contributes to body fluid homeostasis by excreting excess solute and water in the urine. This is accomplished by creating an ultrafiltrate of the blood at the glomerulus. This fluid, which is relatively free of cellular elements and proteins, flows through the various tubular segments, which absorb solutes and water.

Renal Blood Flow (RBF)

The kidneys receive approximately 20% of the cardiac output, which amounts to a blood flow rate of approximately 1200 ml/min, or a renal plasma flow (RPF) rate of about 600 ml/min. The renal blood supply is not proportional to the oxygen consumption; i.e., only 15% of the blood goes to the medulla, a region with high oxygen consumption, because of active sodium transport by the ascending limb of the loop of Henle. This accounts for the susceptibility of the thick ascending limb to hypoxic damage due to renal ischemia. There are several circulatory hormones and autocrine factors that modulate renal blood flow (Table 24-1).

TABLE 24-1	Factors Modulating Renal Blood Flow
Increased Flow	**Decreased FLow**
Prostaglandins (PGI_2, PGE_2)	Thromboxanes
Nitric oxide	Endothelin
Dopamine	Norepinephrine, epinephrine
Bradykinin	Leukotrines
Serotonin	Angiotensin I, II
Histamine	Adenosine
	Neuropeptide Y

Glomerular Filtration Rate (GFR)

Normal GFR is approximately 120 ml/min. Hence, the *filtration fraction,* which is defined as percent of renal plasma flow that is filtered, or mathematically expressed as GFR/RPF, is 0.2 or 20%. Glomerular filtration is a net result of an outwardly directed net pressure that moves fluid across the semipermeable capillary wall:

$$GFR = K_f(\Delta P - \Delta \Pi)$$

The factor K_f expresses both the permeability of the glomerular capillary wall and the surface area of the capillary bed available for ultrafiltration. ΔP is the difference between hydrostatic pressure in the glomerular capillary and hydrostatic pressure in the Bowman's space. $\Delta \Pi$ is the difference between colloid oncotic pressure in the glomerular capillary and the colloid oncotic pressure in the Bowman's space. Since the oncotic pressure in Bowman's space is negligible because of the absence of protein, $\Delta \Pi$ equals the colloid oncotic pressure in the glomerular capillary.

The usual urine volume is about 1.5 L per day. This means that with a normal GFR of about 180 L per day, 178.5 L of fluid is reabsorbed after filtration. If there is a 25% increase in renal perfusion pressure, this could lead to an increase in the GFR by 45 L resulting in 46.5 L of urine output per day. However, as described later, regulatory mechanisms exist in the kidney that prevent major alterations in salt and fluid balance. These regulations occur both at the level of filtration and tubular reabsorption. These mechanisms remain operative in an isolated kidney which is devoid of any contact with the circulatory factors or renal nerves, suggesting that these adaptations are intrinsic to the kidney.

Autoregulation of RBF and GFR

Over a wide range of arterial pressures between 70 and 180 mm Hg, the RBF and GFR are maintained constant. The mechanisms involved are as follows:

1. Tubuloglomerular feedback: In response to increased arterial pressure, there is an initial increase in GFR, resulting in increased sodium chloride delivery to the macula densa of the distal tubule. The macula densa senses and sends a signal to the afferent arteriole, resulting in renal vasoconstriction. In addition, there is a decrease in renin release from the JG apparatus. The opposite response occurs when there is decreased GFR and decreased sodium chloride delivery to the macular densa. These alterations protect and maintain renal blood flow and the glomerular filtration rate nearly constant over a wide range of systemic arterial pressures.
2. Myogenic theory: Alterations in the renal perfusion pressure may result in the direct or pressure- or flow-mediated release of vasoactive factors from the arteriolar endothelium, thus maintaining a constant glomerular perfusion pressure.

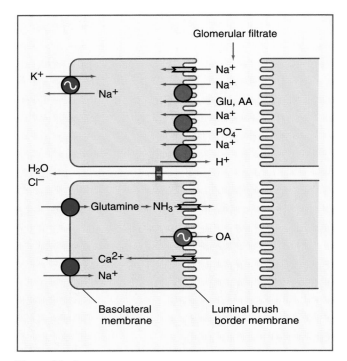

Figure 24-4

The major transport processes of the proximal tubular cells. Sodium can be reabsorbed alone; in cotransport with amino acids (AA), glucose (Glu), or anionic compounds such as phosphate; or by antitransport with hydrogen ions. The proximal nephron is also responsible for reabsorption of calcium, secretion of organic acids (OA), and formation of ammonia, which is important for the secretion of hydrogen ions in the distal nephron. Water and chloride absorption occurs primarily through paracellular pathways.

3. Glomerulotubular balance: This mechanism operates in the proximal tubules, whereby the fractional rate of the proximal absorption remains constant, at about 60%, when the GFR is varied. This balance is modulated by alterations in the effective circulating volume. In empirical terms, this modulation includes, respectively, down-setting and up-setting of the glomerulotubular balance in the volume-expanded and volume-depleted states. These alterations occur without changes in the GFR. Thus, changes in the effective circulating volume, by altering glomerulotubular balance, have a profound effect on the volume of fluid delivered to the loop of Henle.

The Proximal Tubule

The primary function of the proximal tubule is bulk isosmotic reabsorption of ultrafiltrate. Sodium is the most prevalent compound in the glomerular filtrate, and many of the transport processes in the proximal tubule involve sodium transport (Fig. 24-4).

The majority of sodium reabsorption in the proximal tubule involves active transport mechanisms. Sodium is pumped from the tubular cell across the basolateral membrane by the Na-K-ATPase transporter, thus generating an electrochemical gradient for movement of sodium across the luminal membrane. In general, the movement of sodium across the luminal membrane occurs by combined processes involving other solutes. A countertransport mechanism involving hydrogen ions (H^+) results in the reclamation of the vast majority of the filtered bicarbonate. The absorption of glucose and amino acids involves cotransport with sodium. Phosphate is substantially reclaimed in this segment by a mechanism coupled to active sodium absorption. Calcium is absorbed in parallel with sodium in the proximal tubule. Other electrolytes are absorbed in the proximal tubule by mechanisms unrelated to sodium transport. The bulk of filtered potassium is reabsorbed in this segment.

In the straight portion of the proximal tubule, organic acids, including uric acid and drugs, such as penicillin, are secreted. Most pharmacologic diuretics are also secreted in this nephron segment. This secretory process is important for the efficacy of these compounds because their activity is mediated through effect on luminal solute transport mechanisms. Ammonia synthesis, an important step in renal acid excretion, also occurs in the proximal tubule.

The removal of solutes, principally sodium salts, from the glomerular filtrate creates a slight osmotic gradient for water movement from the proximal tubular lumen to the peritubular space. This slight osmotic gradient is adequate to account for proximal isotonic water absorption because the water permeability is rather high.

The solute and water reabsorption in proximal tubules is also governed by the physical forces surrounding the tubule. For example, a high peritubular capillary hydrostatic pressure impairs water and sodium reabsorption from the proximal tubule, and a high colloid oncotic pressure in the peritubular capillary favors the absorption of water and electrolytes from the proximal tubule. Peritubular capillary oncotic pressure is determined mainly by the filtration fraction, and the hydrostatic pressure in the peritubular capillary is determined by the glomerular capillary hydrostatic pressure.

The Loop of Henle

The loop of Henle begins at the corticomedullary junction as the thin descending limb, continues around a hairpin turn as the thin ascending limb, becomes the thick ascending limb in the outer medulla, and ends in the macula densa at the level of the glomerulus from which it originated. Each segment of the loop has different permeabilities to sodium chloride and water, so that about 15% of the volume of the isosmotic ultrafiltrate is absorbed, but about 25% of the sodium chloride is absorbed. This differential absorption converts the isotonic fluid entering from the proximal tubule into a dilute fluid delivered to the distal tubule (Fig. 24–5).

Passive water absorption in the descending and salt absorption in the ascending thin limbs of the loop occur as a result of the selective permeability of these segments.

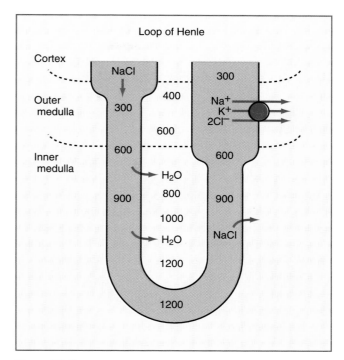

Figure 24–5

The loop of Henle is responsible for additional absorption of filtrate. Water is absorbed in the solute-impermeable descending limb. The concentrated medullary interstitium, established by solute transport at the water-impermeable ascending limb, drives water absorption from the descending limb. The hyperosmolar interstitium also provides the driving force for urinary concentration at the collecting duct. The relative osmolarity of the tubular fluid and interstitium is demonstrated by the numerals.

The thick ascending limb absorbs sodium chloride by an active, energy-dependent process. Specifically, luminal transport involves a furosemide-inhibitable $Na^+/K^+/2\,Cl^-$ cotransporter. Because this segment is impermeable to water, the luminal fluid leaving the thick ascending limb is made hypotonic with respect to plasma by active salt absorption, a vital step in urinary dilution. The addition of sodium chloride to the medullary interstitium is the primary step that allows a multiplication process to build and maintain the interstitial hypertonicity necessary to absorb water from thin descending limbs and from collecting ducts during antidiuresis.

The hairpin arrangement and countercurrent flow of the loop minimize the work needed to maintain a papillary osmolality of 1200 mOsm/kg H_2O, compared with the 300 mOsm/kg H_2O osmolality of the cortex. A similar organization of the vasa recta allows the sodium chloride absorbed from the loop of Henle and urea absorbed from the papillary collecting duct to be trapped within the interstitium at increasing concentrations. The integrity of these anatomic relationships is essential to the concentrating ability of the kidney.

A major portion of calcium absorption also occurs within the loop of Henle. Calcium absorption in the medullary portion of the thick ascending limb varies with the magnitude of the positive luminal transepithelial voltage that accompanies active salt absorption and is not regulated by PTH. In contrast, PTH stimulates the rate of calcium absorption in the cortical thick ascending limb, but sodium absorption is not changed by the hormone. The thick ascending limb of the loop of Henle is also the major site of magnesium reabsorption.

The Distal Nephron

The distal convoluted tubule is a water-impermeable cortical structure that continues the dilution of luminal fluid through active sodium chloride absorption. Sodium absorption in the distal nephron occurs primarily by a thiazide diuretic–sensitive, chloride-coupled transport process. The cortical collecting duct can reabsorb sodium by a mineralocorticoid-sensitive process. In states of volume depletion and maximal aldosterone production, the urine can be rendered virtually free of sodium. Because the cortical interstitium remains isotonic to plasma, salt absorption from these segments affects urinary dilution but not urinary concentration.

Potassium secretion begins in the late distal convoluted tubule and continues through the collecting ducts. Virtually all of the filtered potassium is reabsorbed in more proximal nephron segments so that the potassium appearing in the urine is secreted distally. Potassium secretion proceeds by diffusion of the intracellular cation down both concentration and electrical gradients into the tubular lumen. The *principal cell* in the collecting duct is the major site of potassium secretions (Fig. 24–6). The basolateral (Na^+/K^+)-ATPase establishes the concentration gradient by maintaining a high intracellular potassium concentration. The potassium is then secreted into the tubular lumen down its concentration gradient through a potassium channel. Although some potassium may leak back across the basolateral membrane, two factors favor the movement of potassium into the luminal fluid. First, the concentration of potassium in the luminal fluid is low. Enhanced distal tubular flow thus results in the maintenance of low intraluminal potassium concentrations and stimulates potassium secretion. Second, the principal cells also have a sodium channel on the apical side, which results in sodium reabsorption from the tubular lumen. This results in a negative electrical potential in the tubular lumen that favors the movement of potassium from the cell into the tubular lumen. Aldosterone stimulates potassium secretion by enhancing the activity of the basolateral (Na^+/K^+)-ATPase transporter and by increasing the permeability of the luminal cell membrane to sodium.

Proton secretion in the distal nephron allows absorption of any bicarbonate present in these segments, thereby completing reclamation of filtered bicarbonate. The major contribution of the distal nephron to acid-base homeostasis, however, is new bicarbonate generation, mediated by proton secretion into tubular fluid by a proton ATPase. The secreted H^+ can be either buffered by phosphate or excreted as ammonium ions. The secretory process in the collecting duct generates an intraluminal free H^+ concentration 1000 times greater than that of blood. The secretory process allows for the generation within the cell of bicarbonate, which is transported into the blood to replen-

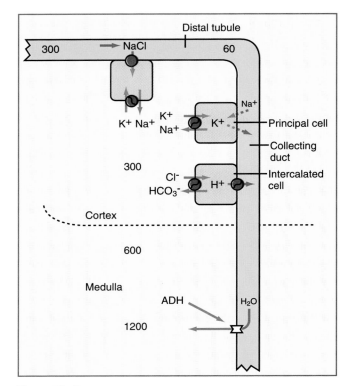

Figure 24–6

The distal nephron is responsible for fine adjustment of the final urinary constituents. Solute absorption in the water-impermeable cortical segments results in a dilute urine. Cortical collecting segments provide secretion of potassium and hydrogen ions. The medullary collecting duct is the site of urinary concentration as water is absorbed across a membrane made permeable by antidiuretic hormone (ADH) down a concentration gradient into the hypertonic interstitial compartment.

ish bicarbonate consumed during buffering of nonvolatile acids. The quantity of new bicarbonate added to body fluids is equal to the daily H^+ generation from dietary protein and is roughly 1 mEq/kg body weight daily. The same factors that determine the rate of distal potassium secretion—namely, the luminal delivery of sodium and the presence of aldosterone—also promote secretion of H^+ in the distal tubule.

The collecting ducts (cortical, medullary, and papillary) are the primary sites of ADH action. They are minimally permeable to water in the absence of ADH and, in that circumstance, can deliver the hypotonic (50 to 100 mOsm/kg H_2O) fluid issuing from the distal convoluted tubule unchanged into the urine. When ADH is present, water passes across the tubule wall readily, and the luminal fluid tonicity approaches that of the interstitium at any level. Maximal urinary concentrating ability thus depends on the availability of ADH plus the degree of the medullary hypertonicity generated from thick ascending limb NaCl absorption and trapping of salt and urea. Intrinsic renal prostaglandins impair distal water reabsorption by several mechanisms, including blockade of ADH action in the collecting duct. Thus, nonsteroidal anti-inflammatory drugs, by blocking prostaglandins, may impair renal water excretion.

TABLE 24–2	**Renal Homeostatic Functions**	
Function	**Mechanism**	**Affected Elements**
Waste excretion	Glomerular filtration	Urea, creatinine
	Tubular secretion	Urate, lactate, drugs (diuretics)
	Tubular catabolism	Pituitary hormones, insulin
Electrolyte balance	Tubular NaCl absorption	Volume status, osmolar balance
	Tubular K$^+$ secretion	Potassium concentration
	Tubular H$^+$ secretion	Acid-base balance
	Tubular water absorption	Osmolar balance
	Tubular Ca, Phos, Mg, transport	Ca, Phos, Mg homeostasis
Hormonal regulation	Erythropoietin production	Red blood cell mass
	Vitamin D activation	Calcium homeostasis
Blood pressure regulation	Altered sodium excretion	Extracellular volume
	Renin production	Vascular resistance
Glucose homeostasis	Gluconeogenesis	Maintains glucose supply in prolonged starvation

Ca = Calcium; Mg = magnesium; NaCl = sodium chloride; Phos = phosphate.

RENAL HOMEOSTATIC FUNCTIONS (Table 24–2)

Regulation of Water, Acid-Base, and Electrolyte Balance

The kidney is responsible for eliminating any excess fluid and solute that are ingested. The most commonly encountered abnormalities in fluid and electrolyte balance are referable to sodium, potassium, water, and acid-base physiology. The renal contribution to these abnormalities is discussed thoroughly in Chapter 26.

The kidney also plays a major role in the balance of other electrolytes. Calcium reabsorption from the glomerular ultrafiltrate helps to regulate body calcium balance. The bulk of filtered calcium (approximately 60%) is reabsorbed in the proximal tubule in parallel with sodium. Factors that alter fractional proximal tubular reabsorption greatly influence calcium excretion. PTH, through its action in the cortical thick ascending limb and the distal convoluted tubule, enhances calcium reabsorption.

In situations of hypocalcemia, the serum PTH is increased, and the renal conservation of filtered calcium is maximized. Concomitantly, when the serum calcium concentration is elevated, PTH is suppressed and renal tubular calcium absorption is decreased. Unfortunately, the symptoms of hypercalcemia often lead to volume depletion, which stimulates sodium and calcium conservation by the nephron. Hypercalcemia also leads to a decrease in the GFR, further limiting the urinary excretion of calcium.

Magnesium is absorbed in the proximal tubule at a rate less than that of sodium. The majority of magnesium absorption occurs in the loop of Henle. Decreases in

fractional proximal tubular absorption (extracellular fluid expansion) and decreases in sodium chloride absorption in the loop of Henle (diuretics) increase the excretion of magnesium. Renal loss of magnesium is a common cause of hypomagnesemia, and hypermagnesemia is almost always the result of a severely diminished GFR.

Waste Excretion

The kidney is responsible for elimination of nitrogenous products of protein catabolism. This is accomplished primarily by filtration at the glomerulus. Because homeostatic requirements necessitate the maintenance of low concentrations of these compounds, large volumes of ultrafiltrate formation are necessary to excrete the absolute quantity of material. The normal daily GFR of 180 L makes such mass elimination possible.

A second mechanism of solute entry into the urine is tubular secretion. Organic acids (such as urate and lactate) and organic bases (such as creatinine) are excreted in this manner. The secretory process is the major route of elimination for substances that are protein-bound. A large number of drugs, including antibiotics and diuretics, are thus excreted by this mechanism.

The kidney contributes to the metabolic degradation of a number of peptide hormones, including most pituitary hormones, glucagon, and insulin. This is accomplished by filtration of these substances at the glomerulus and catabolism by renal tubular cells. Decreased renal catabolism of insulin in diabetics with renal insufficiency may be manifest as a prolongation of the effect of exogenous insulin.

Regulation of Blood Pressure

It has been proposed that the kidney plays a major role in the genesis of hypertension. In certain forms of essential hypertension, the primary defect may be impaired sodium excretion by the kidney, leading to expanded intravascular volume. Natriuretic factors released in response to sodium retention cause vasoconstriction and promote hypertension. The blood pressure is further modulated by the release of renin which results in AII production.

Renal Hormonal Regulation

The kidney is the major site of *erythropoietin* production. This hormone is a highly glycosylated protein of 39,000 daltons. It is produced in the renal cortex, either by peritubular capillary cells or peritubular fibroblasts. Erythropoietin stimulates red blood cell production by its effect on the bone marrow. Erythropoietin production increases in states of decreased tissue oxygen delivery. This may occur as a result of chronic hypoxemia, as seen in persons living at high altitudes or in patients with lung disease, or as a result of decreased oxygen-carrying capacity of blood, as is seen in anemic individuals.

The kidney contributes to calcium homeostasis not only by directly regulating excretion but also by affecting hormonal production. *Vitamin D* requires two *in vivo* hydroxylations to become the potent hormone that regulates intestinal calcium absorption. After hydroxylation in the liver at the 25 position, renal proximal tubular cells add a second hydroxyl ion at the 1 or 24 position of the molecule. This hydroxylation step is controlled and stimulated by PTH and low phosphate.

As noted previously, the JG cells produce and secrete *renin*. Renin promotes the formation of AII, a potent vasoconstrictor that is a stimulus to aldosterone secretion. Aldosterone stimulates renal sodium absorption and excretion of potassium and hydrogen ions.

Glucose Homeostasis

The kidney participates in the regulation of plasma glucose by its ability to synthesize glucose by the gluconeogenetic pathway. Lactate, pyruvate, and amino acids are utilized by the kidney for gluconeogenesis. This function becomes important in prolonged starvation states in which up to 40% of plasma glucose is contributed by the kidney. In addition to decreased clearance and degradation of insulin, absence of this gluconeogenetic pathway in patients with severe renal dysfunction contributes to hypoglycemia.

REFERENCES

Guyton AC, Hall JE: Urine formation by the kidney: Glomerular filtration, renal blood flow, and their control. *In* Guyton AC, Hall JE (eds.): Textbook of Medical Physiology. 9th ed. Philadelphia, WB Saunders, 1996, pp 315–330.

Klahr S: Structure and function of the kidneys. *In* Wyngaarden JB, Smith LH Jr, Bennett JC (eds.): Cecil Textbook of Medicine. 19th ed. Philadelphia, WB Saunders, 1992, pp 482–492.

Tisher CC, Madsen KM: Anatomy of the kidney. *In* Brenner BM, Rector FC Jr (eds.): The Kidney. 4th ed. Philadelphia, WB Saunders, 1991, pp 3–75.

25

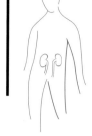

Approach to the Patient with Renal Disease

This chapter consists of three main sections: (1) Clinical Assessment of the Patient with Renal Disease, which includes the clinical assessment of renal function; (2) The Major Renal Syndromes; and (3) Anatomic Imaging of the Urinary Tract, which describes the radiologic tests that are useful in assessment of renal function and structure.

CLINICAL ASSESSMENT OF THE PATIENT WITH RENAL DISEASE

History and Physical Examination

Patients with renal disease may have no symptoms or may have only nonspecific complaints such as fatigue, malaise, or anorexia. Because of this, it is not unusual for patients to present with advanced renal disease. More specific symptoms may include back pain, edema, polyuria, nocturia, hematuria, or dark-colored ("cola"-colored) urine. A history of recurrent urinary tract infections, a history of renal stones, or a family history of renal disease should be determined. The patient should be asked about a history of hypertension, arthalgias, skin rashes, weight loss, or fever. Whether the patient has used prescription or over-the-counter medications, particularly nonsteroidal anti-inflammatory drugs (NSAIDs), and illicit drugs is an important question to be answered.

The physical examination may show signs of a systemic illness that is responsible for the patient's renal disease. Specifically, careful examination of the retina may suggest the presence of diabetes, hypertension, systemic lupus erythematosus, or bacterial endocarditis. In addition, examination of the skin for the presence of a rash, purpura, or excoriations and a joint examination for signs of arthritis are important. A rectal examination in the male patient and a pelvic examination in the female patient are crucial to exclude processes that can cause urinary tract obstruction.

Urinalysis

A complete analysis of the urine is a simple, noninvasive and inexpensive means of detecting renal pathology. A clean catch voided urine specimen should be examined promptly by both chemical and microscopic means.

Normal urine color ranges from almost colorless to deep yellow, depending on the concentration of the urochrome pigment. Abnormal urine colors may be a sign of disease or may indicate the presence of a pigment, drug, or dye. The presence of red blood cells or myoglobin often results in red or smoke-colored urine. Cloudiness of the urine may occur when a high concentration of white blood cells is present (pyuria) or when amorphous phosphates precipitate in alkaline urine.

A chemical assessment of the urine is performed with the "dipstick," a plastic strip impregnated with various reagents that detect the presence of protein, occult blood, glucose, and ketones in the urine. These assays are semiquantitative and are graded on the basis of color changes in the various reagent strips. The dipstick method for the detection of urinary protein is sensitive for albumin but does not detect immunoglobulins or tubular proteins (Tamm Horsfall mucoprotein). The urine sulfosalicylic acid test is an alternate test that detects all urinary proteins by a process of precipitation. A very concentrated urine may show trace to 1+ protein (10 to 30 mg/dl) in a normal individual. The finding of blood in the urine is abnormal and generally indicates the presence of intact red blood cells. The presence of blood detected by a dipstick that cannot be accounted for by red blood cells in the urine sediment is due to either hemoglobin or myoglobin.

Microscopic examination of the urine sediment is used to detect cellular elements, casts, crystals, and microorganisms (Table 25–1). *Microscopic hematuria* is defined as more than two red blood cells per high-power field on a centrifuged urine specimen in the absence of contamination by menstrual blood. *Pyuria* is defined as the presence of more than four white blood cells per high-power field. Epithelial cells are commonly found in the urinary sediment and may derive from any site along the urinary tract from the renal pelvis to the urethra. Renal tubular cells that contain absorbed lipids are termed *oval fat bodies*. Free fat droplets composed primarily of cholesterol esters may also be observed in the urine, particularly in association with heavy proteinuria. Both the oval fat bodies and free fat droplets have doubly refractile characteristics under the polarizing microscope and share the characteristic *"Maltese cross"* appearance.

TABLE 25–1	Microscopic Examination of the Urine
Finding	**Associations**
Casts	
Red blood cell	Glomerulonephritis, vasculitis
White blood cell	Interstitial nephritis, pyelonephritis
Epithelial cell	Acute tubular necrosis, interstitial nephritis, glomerulonephritis
Granular	Renal parenchymal disease (nonspecific)
Waxy, broad	Advanced renal failure
Hyaline	Normal finding in concentrated urine
Fatty	Heavy proteinuria
Cells	
Red blood cell	Urinary tract infection, urinary tract inflammation
White blood cell	Urinary tract infection, urinary tract inflammation
Eosinophil	Drug-induced interstitial nephritis
(Squamous) epithelial cell	Contaminants
Crystals	
Uric acid	Acid urine, acute uric acid nephropathy, hyperuricosuria
Calcium phosphate	Alkaline urine
Calcium oxalate	Acid urine, hyperoxaluria, ethylene glycol poisoning
Cystine	Cystinuria
Sulfur	Sulfadiazine antibiotics

Urinary casts are cylindric structures derived from the intratubular precipitation of Tamm Horsfall protein. The presence of red or white blood cells in the casts provides presumptive evidence of inflammatory parenchymal renal disease. *Red blood cell casts* most frequently indicate the presence of a proliferative glomerular lesion but, on occasion, may also be seen in patients with acute interstitial nephritis. Red cell casts are not present in the absence of hematuria. *Renal tubular cell casts* (often with dirty brown, coarse granular casts) in a patient with acute renal failure help to make the diagnosis of acute tubular necrosis. The presence of *leukocyte casts* in a patient with urinary tract infection indicates a diagnosis of pyelonephritis rather than a lower urinary tract infection.

In the absence of specific symptoms, crystals of calcium oxalate (envelope shaped) and uric acid (rhomboid) often identified in acidic urine are of little clinical significance. The presence of cystine crystals (benzene ring shaped) in the urine indicates the rare disease, cystinuria. Triple phosphate crystals ("coffin-lid" shaped) may be identified in alkaline urine. Bacteria in the urine are almost always recognized in a centrifuged specimen but do not necessarily imply significant bacteriuria. The presence of bacteria in an unspun specimen, however, is significant and provides presumptive evidence for a urinary tract infection.

Renal Function Tests

An approximate assessment of glomerular filtration rate (GFR) is most easily obtained by the measurement of the concentration of creatinine and urea nitrogen in the se-

rum. Creatinine is a metabolite of creatine, a major muscle constituent. In a given individual, the daily rate of production of creatinine is constant and is determined by the mass of skeletal muscle. Because body creatinine is disposed of almost entirely by glomerular filtration, its steady state concentration in the serum has been used as a marker of glomerular function. The "normal" range for serum creatinine concentration is 0.5 to 1.5 mg/dl. However, a value in this range does not necessarily imply normal renal function. For example, in a patient whose creatinine increases from 0.6 to 1.2 mg/dl, a 50% decrease in glomerular filtration rate has occurred, despite creatinine remaining in the "normal" range. A more accurate assessment of renal function is obtained by determining the creatinine clearance. However, once the relation between the serum creatinine and the creatinine clearance is established for a given patient, the serum creatinine can be followed as a reliable indicator of GFR.

The blood urea nitrogen (BUN) concentration is often used in conjunction with the serum creatinine concentration as a measure of renal excretory function. Urea is the major end product of protein metabolism, and its production reflects the dietary intake of protein as well as the protein catabolic rate. Urea is excreted by glomerular filtration, but significant amounts of urea are reabsorbed along the tubule, particularly in sodium-avid states such as extracellular volume contraction. Consequently, the BUN may vary in relation to the extracellular fluid volume, whereas, the serum concentration of creatinine is much less dependent on volume status. The usual ratio of urea nitrogen to creatinine concentration in the serum is 10:1. This ratio is increased in a number of clinical settings (such as volume depletion), catabolic states (such as infection- and catabolic drug [corticosteroid]-increased dietary protein intake), gastrointestinal hemorrhage, and obstructive uropathy.

Determination of the clearance of endogenous creatinine is a convenient test and provides a reasonable estimate of the GFR. Because 10% of creatinine is excreted by the process of tubular secretion, creatinine clearance overestimates the true GFR, particularly in azotemic patients. The creatinine clearance (C_{cr}) is calculated, as shown in Table 25–2. The daily excretion of creatinine in the urine is relatively constant and averages 10 to 20 mg/kg a day. If in a 24-hour urine collection the creatinine excretion deviates significantly from these values, the collection may not be accurate. The creatinine clearance is elevated 30% to 50% over normal values in pregnancy.

Renal tubular function is evaluated by tests that examine the ability of the kidney to maintain salt and water

TABLE 25–2	Calculation of the Creatinine Clearance

$C_{cr} = U_{cr} \times V/P_{cr}$
C_{cr} = clearance of creatinine (ml/min)
U_{cr} = urine creatinine (mg/dl)
  V = volume of urine (ml/min) (for 24-hr volume: divide by 1440)
P_{cr} = plasma creatinine (mg/dl)
    Normal range: 95 to 105 ml/min/1.75 m^2

TABLE 25–3	Calculation of the Fractional Excretion of Sodium

Fractional excretion of sodium (FE_{Na}) = fraction of sodium filtered at the glomerulus that is ultimately excreted in the urine

$$Fe_{Na} = \frac{\text{clearance of sodium}}{\text{clearance of creatinine}}$$

$$Fe_{Na} = \frac{\dfrac{UNaV}{PNa}}{\dfrac{UcrV}{Pcr}} = \frac{UNa}{PNa} \times \frac{Pcr}{Ucr}$$

P_{Na} = plasma sodium (mEq/L)

P_{cr} = plasma creatinine (mg/dl)

U_{Na} = urine sodium (mEq/L)

U_{cr} = urine creatinine (mg/dl)

balance as well as acid-base homeostasis. Maximal urinary concentrating ability can be assessed by restricting fluid intake for 18 to 24 hours. In the polyuric patient suspected of having a defect in urinary concentrating ability, the administration of five units of aqueous vasopressin once the urinary osmolality reaches steady state distinguishes patients with either central or nephrogenic diabetes insipidus. Whereas the patient with central diabetes insipidus has a doubling of the urinary osmolality with aqueous vasopressin, the individual with nephrogenic diabetes insipidus does not respond with further urinary concentration.

The fractional excretion of various solutes in the urine provides useful information about the tubular handling of a solute relative to its GFR. The fractional excretion of sodium (Fe_{Na}) is the fraction of sodium filtered at the glomerulus, which is ultimately excreted in the urine (Table 25–3). Determination of the Fe_{Na} is most useful in the differential diagnosis of acute oliguria. Note that the Fe_{Na} can be calculated on a spot specimen since the volume terms in the numerator and denominator cancel each other.

Acidification of the urine is an important tubular function that can be assessed by the measurement of the urine pH. In the presence of systemic acidosis (arterial pH <7.3), the urine pH should be ≤5.3. Failure to acidify urine in the presence of systemic acidosis suggests distal renal tubular acidosis.

A normal individual excretes <150 mg/day of protein. The glomerular basement membrane serves as an effective barrier to the passage of high–molecular weight proteins such as albumin, and the renal tubules have the capacity to reabsorb the small amount of protein that is filtered. Abnormal proteinuria may occur as a transient phenomenon in individuals with febrile illnesses or congestive heart failure or after vigorous exercise. Persistent proteinuria almost always indicates renal disease. On all timed urine samples for protein, a simultaneous determination of urine creatinine is useful as a means of assess-ing the accuracy of the collection. Patients who excrete >3.5 gm of protein have, with rare exceptions, glomerular disease. Less than 3.5 gm of urinary protein can be found in both glomerular and tubular diseases.

THE MAJOR RENAL SYNDROMES

Renal disorders are often nonspecific in their manifestations. However, certain groups of findings may be used to classify some of the more common syndromes and disorders affecting the kidneys and the urinary tract. The division of clinical manifestations into separate clinical syndromes is arbitrary, and overlap exists; however, classification of the expression of renal injury into common themes serves a useful purpose—namely, consideration of specific clinicopathologic entities (Table 25–4).

The *acute nephritic syndrome* is a clinical syndrome characterized by relatively abrupt onset of renal dysfunction accompanied by hematuria that is nephronal in origin. The presence of red blood cell casts and dysmorphic erythrocytes in the urine sediment, as well as significant degrees of proteinuria, provides highly suggestive evidence that the hematuria is nephronal in origin as compared with other sources in the urinary tract. For reasons that are not well understood, sodium avidity in the acute nephritic syndrome is considerably greater than what would be expected solely from the reduction in the GFR. Plasma albumin is generally normal, so that a significant fraction of the retained sodium remains in the vascular compartment and may result in hypertension, plasma volume dilution, circulatory overload, and congestive heart failure.

Although acute poststreptococcal glomerulonephritis is the prototype for the acute nephritic syndrome, other infections may also lead to this syndrome. Likewise, this syndrome may be due to other primary glomerular diseases, such as mesangioproliferative glomerulonephritis, and multisystem diseases, such as systemic lupus erythematosus, Henoch-Schonlein syndrome, and essential mixed cryoglobulinemia.

The *nephrotic syndrome* is characterized by increased glomerular permeability, manifested by massive proteinuria usually in excess of 3.5 gm/day/1.73 m^2 body surface area. There is a variable tendency toward edema, hypoalbuminemia, and hyperlipidemia. The urinary protein loss is necessary and sufficient to produce the rest of the abnormalities, so that from a practical point of view, the presence of massive proteinuria is sufficient to define the nephrotic syndrome.

An important step in classifying and therefore determining the type of glomerular involvement present is the urinalysis. On the basis of the urinalysis, a patient with massive proteinuria may be classified as having a nephrotic form or a nephritic form. Patients with a nephrotic form, in addition to proteinuria, may demonstrate oval fat bodies, coarse granular casts, and occasional cellular elements but lack the "active" sediment characteristic of the nephritic form. The differential diagnosis includes glomerular diseases such as minimal change disease, membranous nephropathy, diabetic nephropathy, and amyloidosis. In patients with the nephrotic syndrome

TABLE 25–4	Major Renal Syndromes	
Syndrome	**Definition**	**Example**
Acute nephritic syndrome	Abrupt onset of renal insufficiency accompanied by hematuria that is glomerular or tubular in origin	Poststreptococcal glomerulonephritis
Nephrotic syndrome	Increased glomerular permeability manifested by massive proteinuria ($>$3.5 gm/day/1.73 m^2)	
With "bland" urine sediment (pure nephrotic)	Oval fat bodies, coarse granular casts	Minimal change disease
With "active" urine sediment ("mixed" nephrotic/nephritic)	Oval fat bodies, coarse granular casts, RBCs, or RBC casts	Membranoproliferative glomerulopathy
Asymptomatic urinary abnormalities	Isolated proteinuria ($<$2.0 gm/day/1.73 m^2) or hematuria (with or without proteinuria)	IgA nephropathy
Tubulointerstitial nephropathy	Renal insufficiency associated with non–nephrotic-range proteinuria and functional tubular defects	Analgesic nephropathy
Acute renal failure	An abrupt decline in renal function sufficient to result in retention of nitrogenous waste (e.g., BUN and creatinine)	Acute tubular necrosis
Rapidly progressive renal failure	Rapid deterioration of renal function over a period of weeks to months	Rapidly progressive glomerulonephritis
Renal calculus syndrome	Renal stones	Calcium stones
Tubular defects	Isolated or multiple tubular transport defects	Renal tubular acidosis

BUN = Blood urea nitrogen; RBC = red blood cell.

and an active urinary sediment that has glomerular hematuria (by virtue of dysmorphic red blood cells and/or red blood cell casts) along with moderate to heavy proteinuria (nephrotic/nephritic syndromes), membranoproliferative nephritis, systemic lupus erythematosus, and mixed essential cryoglobulinemia would be important diagnostic considerations.

The term *rapidly progressive renal failure (RPRF)* is applied to patients who have a rapid deterioration in renal function over weeks to months. This contrasts with patients with *acute renal failure,* who have an abrupt decline in renal function over several days, and with patients with *chronic renal failure,* who have a decline in renal function that is measurable over years. The differential diagnosis of a patient who presents with RPRF is shown in Table 25–5. It should be noted that one of the important but uncommon causes of RPRF is rapidly progressive glomerulonephritis (RPGN). This is a clinical syndrome of rapid and progressive decline in renal function (usually at least a 50% decline in GFR over 3 months) associated with extensive glomerular crescent formation (usually more than 50%) as the principal histologic finding on renal biopsy. Dysmorphic erythrocytes, red blood cell casts, and heavy proteinuria are characteristic in RPGN, as in other nephritic syndromes.

TABLE 25–5	Causes of Rapidly Progressive Renal Failure

Obstructive uropathy
Malignant hypertension
Rapidly progressive glomerulonephritis
Thrombotic thrombocytopenic purpura/hemolytic uremic syndrome
Atheromatous embolic disease
Bilateral renal artery stenosis
Scleroderma
Multiple myeloma

Acute renal failure is a syndrome that can be broadly defined as an abrupt decline in renal function sufficient to result in azotemia over days to a few weeks. Acute renal failure can result from a decrease in renal blood flow (prerenal azotemia), intrinsic parenchymal disease (renal azotemia), or obstruction to urine flow (post renal azotemia). The general approach for evaluating acute renal failure is detailed in Chapter 30.

Tubulointerstitial nephropathy designates a group of clinical disorders that affect the renal tubules and interstitium principally with relative sparing of the glomeruli and renal vasculature. In the majority of cases, it is possible to classify the disease into acute interstitial nephritis or chronic interstitial nephropathy on the basis of the rate of progression of azotemia. Chronic tubulointerstitial nephropathy is characterized clinically by renal insufficiency, non-nephrotic range proteinuria, and tubular damage disproportionately severe relative to the degree of azotemia. Thus, patients with chronic tubulointerstitial disease often have modest degrees of sodium wasting, hyperkalemia, and a normal anion gap metabolic acidosis even when azotemia is modest. Acute interstitial nephritis, often caused by a drug, is characterized by sudden onset of clinical signs of renal dysfunction associated with a prominent inflammatory cell infiltrate within the renal interstitium and is often important in the differential diagnosis of patients with acute renal failure.

ANATOMIC IMAGING OF THE URINARY TRACT
(Table 25–6)

The plain film of the abdomen or *KUB (kidney, ureter, bladder)* is a simple way of determining renal size and shape. The normal kidney shadow approximates the length of 3.5 vertebral bodies or about 12 cm. In a patient with advanced renal failure, the presence of bilaterally small kidneys implies a chronic, irreversible process,

TABLE 25–6 **Imaging Studies of the Urinary Tract: Comparative Aspects**

Study	Information	Considerations
KUB	Renal size, opaque calculi	Inexpensive
Ultrasonography	Renal size, cysts, hydrone-phrosis, renal arterial/ve-nous flow by Doppler	Noninvasive
Renal scan	Renal blood flow, tubular function	Functional study
Intravenous (IV) contrast uro-gram	Renal size, shape, cysts, tu-mors, stones, obstruction	Requires IV
Computed contrast tomography (CT)	Renal size, shape, cysts, tu-mors, stones, obstruc-tion, retroperitoneal space	Requires IV
Retrograde pyelog-raphy	Ureteral obstruction	Invasive
Renal arteriography	Renal vasculature, tumors	Invasive
Renal venography	Renal vein thrombosis, renal vein blood sampling	Invasive

KUB = Kidney, ureter, bladder.

whereas, the presence of normal-sized kidneys indicates acute renal failure or chronic renal failure due to diseases such as diabetes, amyloid, or multiple myeloma. Radio-paque renal calculi composed of calcium, magnesium ammonium phosphate (struvite), or cystine are often apparent in a plain film of the abdomen.

Renal ultrasonography is another noninvasive method of obtaining an anatomic image of the kidney and the collecting system. This technique is particularly useful for the detection of renal masses, cysts, and dilatation of portions of the collecting system (hydronephrosis). Renal ultrasonography may serve as the primary imaging proce-dure for patients with unexplained renal failure to assess renal size and determine whether a patient has obstructive uropathy. Duplex ultrasonography in which B-mode ultra-sonography has been combined with pulsed Doppler im-aging may be useful in detecting disease of the major renal arteries or veins.

The *intravenous urogram* involves the intravenous administration of iodinated radiographic contrast medium that is excreted through the kidney by glomerular filtra-tion. The contrast medium concentrates in the renal tu-bules and produces a nephrogram image within the first few minutes after injection. As the medium passes into the collecting system, the calyces, renal pelvis, ureters, and bladder are visualized. The *computed tomography (CT)* scan of the kidney provides more precise informa-tion regarding renal masses as well as a definition of the perinephric space and other retroperitoneal structures. The risk of contrast medium–induced nephrotoxicity limits the utility of these studies in certain high-risk patients. In selected cases, CT scanning of the kidney can be per-formed without intravenous contrast material.

Retrograde pyelography is performed by injection of radiocontrast material directly into the ureters at the time of cystoscopy. This technique is useful in the definition

of obstructing lesions within the ureter or renal pelvis, particularly in the setting of a nonvisualizing kidney on intravenous pyelography.

The *radioisotopic renal scan* provides important noninvasive information about renal blood flow. The test involves the intravenous administration of radiolabeled compounds that are excreted by the kidney. An external scintillation camera provides an image of the kidneys and calculates the rate of uptake and excretion of the labeled compound. Technetium 99 (^{99}Tc) diethylenetriamine penta-acetic acid (DTPA) and technetium-labeled mercap-toacetyl triglycine (^{99}Tc^m Mag3) are two compounds used to assess renal vascular perfusion qualitatively. Impaired renal perfusion, as in unilateral renal artery stenosis or renal infarction, is characterized by asymmetric uptake of technetium.

Renal arteriography involves the direct injection of radiographic contrast medium into the aorta and renal arteries and is used to assess renal vasculature. Renal arteriography is particularly useful in the evaluation of patients with suspected renal artery stenosis or thrombosis and in those with a renal mass. Renal arteriography is generally limited to situations in which a strong clinical indication exists and the patient is considered a candidate for surgical intervention. Renal vein catheterization is used to confirm the diagnosis of renal vein thrombosis or to obtain blood samples from the renal vein, particularly when renovascular hypertension is suspected.

Magnetic resonance imaging (MRI) represents a new and emerging diagnostic technology that uses high mag-netic fields and radiofrequencies to construct images. The method avoids the use of ionizing radiation and the ad-ministration of contrast material. MRI provides images in a tomographic format similar to that of CT. The tech-nique is very sensitive to blood flow and represents an excellent method for evaluation of major vascular struc-tures for patency or tumor involvement.

Renal Biopsy

Most renal biopsies are performed when a glomerular lesion is suspected and less commonly in patients with unexplained acute renal failure. The percutaneous biopsy is the most commonly used technique and is a relatively safe procedure. An open renal biopsy is considered in the patient with a solitary functioning kidney or a bleeding diathesis. Potential complications of a closed renal biopsy include hematuria, renal hematoma, vascular laceration with the development of arteriovenous fistula, and the inadvertent biopsy of liver, spleen, or bowel.

REFERENCE

Andreoli TE: Approach to the patient with renal disease. *In* Wyngaar-den JB, Smith LH, Bennett JC (eds.): Cecil Textbook of Medicine. 19th ed. Philadelphia, WB Saunders, 1992, pp 477–482.

26

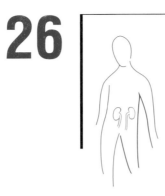

Fluid and Electrolyte Disorders

The concentrations of fluid and electrolytes in the cells and fluid compartments of the body are maintained remarkably constant despite a widely varying intake. This equilibrium is maintained by fluid and solute shifts across the cells of the body following well-defined mechanisms and by the capacity of the kidney to regulate the urinary excretion of water, electrolytes, and solutes in response to the needs of the body.

VOLUME DISORDERS

Water is the most abundant molecular component of living matter and constitutes approximately 60% of total body weight in humans (Fig. 26–1). Total body water is inversely proportional to the amount of body fat, which varies with age, sex, and nutritional status. Approximately two thirds of the total body water is contained in the intracellular compartment. Three fourths of the extracellular water is in the interstitial space, and one fourth is in the plasma. Potassium and magnesium constitute the major cations of the intracellular space, whereas sodium is the major cation of the extracellular space. Phosphate and protein are the major anions of the intracellular space, whereas chloride and bicarbonate are the major anions of extracellular space. A low protein concentration distinguishes the composition of interstitial fluid from that of plasma. The cell membrane represents the barrier between the intracellular and extracellular fluid compartments. Because membranes are relatively permeable to water, the movement of fluid across the cell membrane is determined by the osmotic gradient. Thus, except for transient changes, the intracellular and extracellular fluid compartments are in *osmotic equilibrium*. The transfer of fluid between the vascular and interstitial compartments occurs across the capillary wall and is governed by the balance between hydrostatic pressure gradients and plasma oncotic pressure gradients, as related in the *Starling equation*.

$$J_v = K_f \{\Delta P - \Delta \pi\}$$

where J_v is the rate of fluid transfer between vascular and interstitial compartments, K_f is the water permeability of the capillary bed, ΔP is the hydrostatic pressure difference between capillary and interstitium, and $\Delta \pi$ is the oncotic pressure difference between capillary and intersti-

tial fluids. Thus, an increase in the driving force for fluid movement into the interstitial compartment may result from a decrease in the colloid oncotic pressure of plasma, as may occur in hypoalbuminemia, and/or an increase in the capillary hydrostatic pressure.

Normal Volume Homeostasis

Protection of extracellular fluid volume is a fundamental characteristic of fluid and electrolyte homeostasis. The homeostatic mechanisms sense changes in the *"effective circulating volume"* (ECV). ECV is difficult to define since it is not a measurable and distinct body fluid compartment. ECV relates to the "fullness" and pressure within the arterial tree. Since only 15% of total blood volume is in the arterial compartment, it is possible for arterial blood volume to be decreased in relation to the holding capacity of the arterial tree. In a majority of circumstances, ECV correlates with the total extracellular fluid volume, except in certain disorders where ECV is decreased in the presence of an increased total extracellular fluid volume (Table 26–1). In these disorders, the ECV is decreased due to either a decreased cardiac output or arterial vasodilatation, which results in decreased fullness and pressure in the arterial circulation. Only a small subgroup of patients with nephrotic syndrome have a decreased ECV.

The afferent mechanisms sense alterations in the ECV and activate a series of effectors that create an *integrated volume response* (Fig. 26–2). Two cardinal mechanisms protect the extracellular fluid volume: alterations in systemic hemodynamics and alterations in the external sodium and water balance. Hemodynamic alterations occur within minutes of a perceived volume reduction and are characterized by tachycardia, increased peripheral resistance due to arterial vasoconstriction, and decreased venous capacitance due to venoconstriction. Renal conservation of salt and water lags behind by 12 to 24 hours and involves release of various hormones (see Fig. 26–2). Stimulation of the extrarenal baroreceptors also results in the release of antidiuretic hormone (ADH), which promotes water retention in the kidney. Vasoconstrictive factors, such as endothelins, produced and released by vascular endothelial cells, also play a role in modulating systemic hemodynamics. Alterations in the

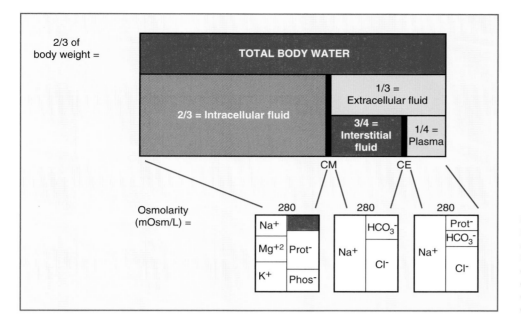

Figure 26–1

Composition of body fluid compartments. The compartments are anatomically defined by the cell membrane (CM) and capillary endothelium (CE). The osmolar concentration among compartments is equivalent despite wide variation in cation and anion composition.

glomerular hemodynamics, through changes in the peritubular Starling forces, directly modulate sodium and water reabsorption in the proximal tubules. Furthermore, vasodilator prostaglandins, such as PGE_2, maintain the glomerular filtration rate by enhancing the renal blood flow in states associated with ECV depletion. Thus, the use of nonsteroidal anti-inflammatory agents is associated with deterioration of renal function under these circumstances. In response to volume expansion, the renal excretion of salt and water is increased due to the suppression of the aforementioned pathways. The release of atrial natriuretic peptide (ANP) is a major factor promoting natriuresis in volume expanded states. ANP is released from the atrial myocytes in response to atrial stretch associated with volume expansion. It promotes natriuresis through direct effects on the filtration fraction and collecting duct sodium reabsorption and has an indirect inhibitory effect on the renin-angiotensin system.

Since the afferent sensors respond to ECV rather than the total extracellular fluid volume, in disease states like congestive heart failure and liver cirrhosis there is continued activation of the integrated volume response, thus promoting further salt and water retention.

TABLE 26–1	Disorders in Which There Is Decreased Effective Circulating Volume with Increased Total ECF Volume

Congestive heart failure
Liver disease
Sepsis
Nephrotic syndrome (minority)
Pregnancy
Anaphylaxis

ECF = Extracellular fluid.

Volume Depletion

Disorders of extracellular volume occur due to alterations in sodium balance. The causes of true volume depletion, i.e., decreased ECV and total extracellular fluid volume, are illustrated in Table 26–2. The clinical findings in states of true volume depletion are referable to an underfilling of the arterial tree and to the renal and hemodynamic responses to this underfilling. Mild volume depletion may be associated with orthostatic dizziness and tachycardia. As the intracellular compartment becomes further depleted, a recumbent tachycardia becomes evident and urine output diminishes. With severe volume depletion, the patient may present with vasoconstriction, hypotension, mental obtundation, cool extremities, and negligible urine output. Many of these clinical features can be explained on the basis of effects of vasoconstrictor hormones, such as catecholamine and AII, that are released in response to hypovolemia.

Volume depletion can occur in the absence of classical clinical findings. States of volume depletion in patients receiving cardiovascular drugs and excess renal sodium loss due to intrinsic renal disease or diuretics represent examples of clinical circumstances in which an assessment of the state of hydration may be difficult. An appropriate clinical history is always mandatory. If there is doubt about the state of hydration, particularly if the patient appears to be critically ill, measurement of the pulmonary capillary wedge pressure by means of invasive right-sided heart catheterization permits a valid assessment of the intravascular volume status.

The absolute quantity and rate of fluid replacement depends on the severity of volume depletion, which is estimated by the clinical presentation. If fluid repletion is to involve parenteral infusions, it is important to consider the distribution of the infused fluid. Solutions containing 0.9% sodium chloride and colloid solutions, which are

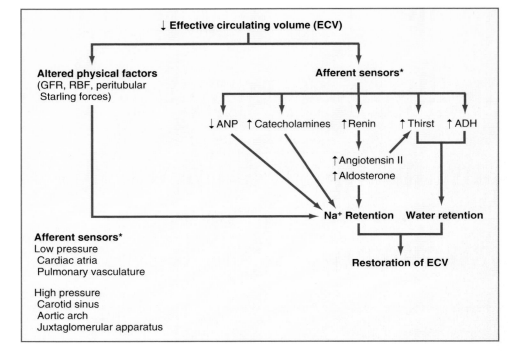

Figure 26–2
Volume repletion reaction. ADH = Antidiuretic hormone; ANP = atriopeptin; GFR = glomerular filtration rate; RBF = renal blood flow.

retained in the extracellular space, are the preferred parenteral solutions for the treatment of hypovolemia. In contrast, only one third of infused 5% glucose (D_5W) remains in the extracellular compartment.

Volume Excess

Volume expansion occurs when salt and water intake exceeds renal and extrarenal losses. The causes are listed in Table 26–3. The underlying disturbance common to these disorders is sodium and water retention by the kidney. The sodium and water retention may be primary (increased ECV) or secondary in response to a decreased ECV. The net result of renal sodium and water retention is an alteration of Starling forces, leading to increased capillary hydrostatic pressure and favoring fluid shifts from the intravascular to interstitial space. In nephrotic syndrome, the majority of patients have increased effective circulating volume due to primary renal sodium retention, whereas in a subgroup of nephrotic syndrome with minimal change disease, there is secondary renal sodium retention due to a decreased ECV. In advanced liver disease, the ECV is decreased due to arterial underfilling from vasodilatation, resulting in secondary renal sodium retention. However, in early liver disease, the volume excess may be due to primary renal sodium retention. Severe hypoalbuminemia associated with liver disease, nephrotic syndrome, or severe malnutrition, may overwhelm the local capillary homeostatic mechanisms, leading to edema formation.

The mainstay in treating volume excess is dietary sodium restriction and the use of diuretic agents (Table 26–4). Diuretics enhance natriuresis by inhibiting the reabsorption of sodium at various sites along the nephron. The cardinal example of a proximal tubular diuretic is acetazolamide, a *carbonic anhydrase inhibitor*, that blocks

TABLE 26–2	Causes of Volume Depletion

Gastrointestinal losses
  Upper GI: bleeding, nasogastric suction, vomiting
  Lower GI: bleeding, diarrhea, enteric or pancreatic fistula, tube drainage
Renal losses
  Salt and water: diuretics, osmotic diuresis, postobstructive diuresis, acute tubular necrosis (recovery phase), salt-losing nephropathy, adrenal insufficiency, renal tubular acidosis
  Water loss: diabetes insipidus
Skin and respiratory losses
  Sweat, burns, insensible losses
Sequestration without external fluid loss
  Intestinal obstruction, peritonitis, pancreatitis, rhabdomyolysis, internal bleeding

GI = Gastrointestinal.

TABLE 26–3	Causes of Volume Excess

Primary renal sodium retention (↑ effective circulating volume)
  Acute renal failure
  Acute glomerulonephritis
  Severe chronic renal failure
  Nephrotic syndrome
  Primary hyperaldosteronism
  Cushing syndrome
  Liver disease
Secondary renal sodium retention (↓ effective circulating volume)
  Heart failure
  Liver disease
  Nephrotic syndrome (minimal change disease)
  Pregnancy

TABLE 26-4	Characteristics of Commonly Used Diuretics		
Agent	**Site**	**Primary Effect**	**Secondary Effect**
Carbonic anhydrase inhibitors (acetazolamide)	Proximal tubule	Block Na^+/H^+ exchange	K^+, HCO_3^- loss
Loop diuretics (furosemide, bumetanide ethacrynic acid)	Thick ascending limb of loop of Henle	↓ $Na^+/K^+/2Cl^-$ transport	K^+ loss ↑ H^+ secretion ↑ Ca^{2+} excretion
Thiazide diuretics			
Thiazides	Distal convoluted tubule	↓ NaCl cotransport	K^+ loss, ↑ H^+ secretion ↓ Ca^{2+} excretion
Metolazone	Distal tubule, proximal tubule	↓ NaCl reabsorption	
Aldosterone antagonists (spironolactone)	Cortical collecting duct	↓ Na reabsorption	↓ K^+ loss ↓ H^+ secretion
Primary sodium channel blockers (triamterene, amiloride)	Cortical collecting duct	↓ Na reabsorption	↓ K^+ loss ↓ H^+ secretion

proximal reabsorption of sodium bicarbonate. Consequently, prolonged use of acetazolamide may lead to hyperchloremic acidosis. Metolazone, a congener of the thiazide class of diuretics, in addition to blocking sodium reabsorption in distal tubule, also exerts its natriuretic effect in the proximal tubule. Since the proximal tubule is the major site for phosphate reabsorption, profound phosphaturia may accompany the use of metolazone. *Loop diuretics* such as furosemide and bumetanide inhibit the coupled entry of sodium, chloride, and potassium across the apical membranes in the thick ascending limb of the loop of Henle. *Thiazide diuretics* inhibit coupled entry of sodium and chloride across the apical membrane of the distal tubule. The loop diuretics promote calcium excretion and thiazide diuretics decrease calcium excretion. Thus, the former are useful in the management of hypercalcemia, while the latter are useful in preventing calcium stone formation. Spironolactone, an *aldosterone antagonist,* decreases sodium reabsorption in the cortical collecting duct. Primary *sodium channel blockers,* such as amiloride, also block sodium reabsorption in the cortical collecting duct by an aldosterone-independent mechanism. The last two groups of diuretics do not cause hypokalemia, which is a common complication associated with the use of other diuretics. In states of severe sodium retention and edema formation, such as severe congestive heart failure or nephrotic syndrome, a combination of diuretics working at different sites in the nephron may be more effective than the use of a single class of diuretics. Moreover, potassium and magnesium deficits can be minimized by using potassium-sparing diuretics in combination with a potassium-wasting diuretic. In patients with cirrhosis and ascites, abdominal paracentesis with albumin infusion has been used as a good therapeutic alternative to diuretics.

OSMOLALITY DISORDERS

Body fluid osmolality, the ratio of solute to water in all fluid compartments, is maintained within a very narrow range. Because water moves freely across most cell membranes, changes in the extracellular fluid osmolality cause reciprocal changes in the intracellular volume. The extracellular fluid osmolality can be approximated by calculating the serum osmolality based upon the major solutes in that compartment:

$$\textbf{Calculated Osmolality} = 2[Na^+] + \frac{[glucose]}{18} + \frac{[BUN]}{2.8}$$

where the glucose and blood urea nitrogen (BUN) concentrations are expressed as milligrams per deciliters, and the serum sodium concentration is expressed as milliequivalents per liter.

Measured osmolality usually equals the calculated osmolality. However, in the presence of osmotically active substances, such as ethanol, methanol, or ethylene glycol, the measured osmolality is higher than the calculated osmolality. Under these circumstances, the *osmolar gap* (measured calculated osmolality) provides a clue to the presence of toxins and gives an estimated concentration of these solutes. It is important to understand that calculated or measured osmolality differs from the *effective osmolality* ($2[Na^+]$). Because urea freely distributes across cell membranes, it does not contribute to the effective osmolality. Since sodium is the major cation in the extracellular fluid, disorders of osmolality are generally reflected by an abnormal sodium concentration in the extracellular fluid. The osmoregulatory mechanisms are activated in response to changes in cell volume rather than the osmolality per se. It is important to understand that disorders of osmolality are primarily due to disturbances in water balance and not sodium balance. Disorders of sodium balance, as noted earlier, cause alterations in the extracellular fluid volume rather than in the osmolality.

Regulation of osmolality involves alteration in renal water excretion, and the sodium excretion is not affected by osmoregulatory factors unless there is a concomitant ECV depletion. Extracellular fluid osmolality is regulated

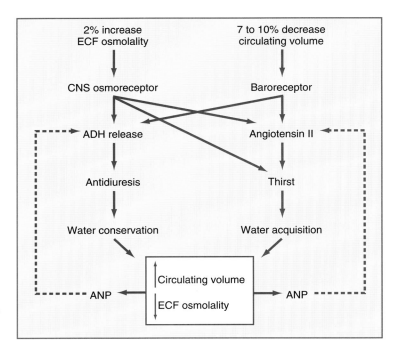

Figure 26–3

Water regulatory mechanisms. Alterations in extracellular fluid osmolality or volume stimulate *(solid lines)* thirst and release of antidiuretic hormone (ADH). The net result is a positive water balance. Counterregulation is provided by the inhibitory effects *(dashed lines)* of atriopeptins (ANPs). CNS = Central nervous system; ECF = extracellular fluid.

by dual pathways in the *water repletion reaction* (Fig. 26–3). Osmoreceptor cells in the central nervous system (CNS), located in the wall of the third ventricle, sense minor changes in the osmolality of blood in the internal carotid circulation. Neuronal signals from osmoreceptors stimulate the release of antidiuretic hormone (ADH) from the posterior pituitary gland and simultaneously stimulate the sensation of thirst. ADH causes renal water conservation by increasing water permeability and water reabsorption in the collecting ducts. Thirst leads to an increase in water intake. When the extracellular fluid volume is reduced by about 10%, water repletion is activated as a means of replenishing extracellular fluid volume irrespective of osmolality. In this case, baroreceptors in the venous and arterial circulation stimulate ADH release through neuronal pathways. This *nonosmotic* stimulation of ADH release occurs independently of osmoreceptor function. The volume stimulus to ADH secretion can override osmotic stimuli, so that significant volume contraction is a cardinal cause of hyponatremia. Water repletion activates mechanisms that counterregulate water conservation. Suppression of thirst and inhibition of ADH release leads to decreased water intake and increased renal water excretion.

HYPONATREMIA

A diagnostic approach to hyponatremia is outlined in Figure 26–4. It is evident from the causes that hyponatremia can be associated with normal, high, or low total body sodium content. In some hyponatremic disorders the serum osmolality is elevated, thus, the intracellular water content is not increased and there is no risk of brain edema. Hyperglycemia and the use of hypertonic mannitol may result in hyponatremia due to water shift from the intracellular to extracellular space. Hyponatremia associated with normal serum osmolality may be seen in patients with extreme hyperlipidemia and hyperproteinemia, due to methodologic errors in techniques to measure serum electrolyte concentration. The increasing use of ion-selective electrodes for these measurements is making these causes of "pseudohyponatremia" uncommon. Hyponatremia may also be seen in patients who undergo transurethral resection of the prostate or hysteroscopy because of the absorption of large amounts of hypo-osmolar glycine or sorbitol irrigating solutions.

The majority of hyponatremic disorders are associated with hypo-osmolality. In principle, hypo-osmolality can result from an increase in water intake and/or a decrease in renal water excretion. Under normal circumstances, the kidneys can excrete 16 to 20 L of water per day. Thus, it is unusual to develop hyponatremia solely due to excess water intake. In *primary polydipsia,* the hyponatremia is due to large water intake in the presence of impaired water excretion. Hyponatremia may also occur with modestly increased water intake in the presence of impaired glomerular filtration rate (GFR) or decreased solute intake. In the presence of decreased GFR, the renal water excretion is impaired due to decreased delivery of filtrate to the distal nephron. The patients with chronic starvation or beer potomania have poor oral intake. Since renal water excretion is dependent on the osmolar intake, these patients may develop hyponatremia at a modestly increased level of water intake.

More commonly, hyponatremia occurs as a result of the inability to dilute urine maximally because of reduction in the rate of salt absorption by the diluting segment, sustained nonosmotic release of ADH, or a combination of these two factors. In the disorders associated with decreased ECV, there is nonosmotic ADH release, which promotes water retention by the kidney. In addition, there is enhanced proximal sodium chloride reabsorption with diminished distal delivery. These disorders may be associ-

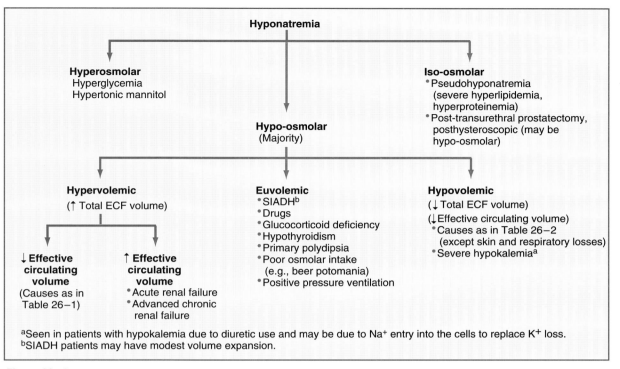

Figure 26–4

Diagnostic approach to hyponatremia. ECF = Extracellular fluid; SIADH = syndrome of inappropriate antidiuretic hormone.

ated with signs of either volume expansion or volume depletion.

The *syndrome of inappropriate ADH release (SIADH)* is the prototype of the primary release of ADH

TABLE 26–5	Causes of SIADH

Central nervous system disorders
 Trauma
 Infection
 Tumors
 Porphyria
Pulmonary disorders
 Tuberculosis
 Pneumonia
 Positive-pressure ventilation
Neoplasia
 Carcinoma: bronchogenic, pancreatic, ureteral, prostatic, bladder
 Lymphoma and leukemia
 Thymoma and mesothelioma
Drugs
 Increased ADH release
  Chlorpropamide
  Clofibrate
  Carbamazepine
  Vincristine
 Potentiate ADH action
  Chlorpropamide
  Cyclophosphamide
  Nonsteroidal anti-inflammatory agents

ADH = Antidiuretic hormone; SIADH = syndrome of inappropriate antidiuretic hormone.
Modified from Andreoli TE: Disorders of fluid volume, electrolyte, and acid-base balance. *In* Wyngaarden JB, Smith LH Jr, Bennett JC (eds.): Cecil Textbook of Medicine. 19th ed. Philadelphia, WB Saunders, 1992, p 509.

or ADH-like substances. It occurs most often in association with pathologic processes within the cranium or thorax or with the administration of certain drugs (Table 26–5). The circulating ADH allows excessive water absorption in the collecting duct with a modest expansion of the extracellular fluid volume. With the increase in volume, renal perfusion is increased and the kidney subsequently decreases sodium reabsorption in an attempt to re-establish euvolemia. A subgroup of patients with hyponatremia have a *reset osmostat,* which means simply that they are able to dilute urine but at serum sodium levels that are appreciably lower than in normal individuals. It is difficult to treat hyponatremia in this subgroup of patients.

Diagnosis and Treatment of Hyponatremic Disorders

The signs and symptoms of hyponatremia, per se, are related to brain cell swelling caused by an increase in the brain water content due to water shift from a hypo-osmolar extracellular environment. Hence, hyponatremic disorders should be considered in any patient who has acute mental status changes. An assessment of the volume status by physical examination is the most important initial step in the diagnostic approach to patients with hyponatremia. The most difficult differential diagnosis among hyponatremic disorders involves the distinction between patients who are modestly volume contracted and those who have SIADH. In both instances, the urine osmolality may be inappropriately concentrated relative to the serum osmolality. If the volume depletion is secondary to extrarenal losses, the urine sodium concentration is negligible, whereas it is usually > 30 mEq/l in patients with SIADH.

A baseline body weight, serum electrolytes, serum osmolality, urine electrolytes, and urine osmolality should be obtained, and frequent measurement of serum and urine electrolytes, intake, and urine output should be performed during the treatment of hyponatremia. As a general rule, administration of solutions with a tonicity ($[Na^+] + [K^+]$) greater than urine sodium and potassium concentration will raise serum sodium. The treatment should depend on the underlying clinical disease and volume status of the patient. Sodium and water intake should be restricted in the volume-expanded patient. In patients with decreased ECV and hypovolemia, the treatment should include isotonic sodium chloride.

In patients with SIADH, restriction of water intake is the mainstay of therapy. Demeclocycline is also useful in the treatment of this syndrome. Hypertonic saline, often in combination with furosemide, should be reserved solely for the treatment of acute symptomatic hyponatremia with circulatory collapse.

The rate of correction of serum sodium depends on the symptoms and duration of hyponatremia. Initial symptoms may include nausea, anorexia, muscle weakness, and cramps. As the hyponatremia worsens, the patient may become irritable, confused, and hostile. With extreme hyponatremia, gait disturbances, stupor, and seizures may occur. In acute hyponatremia (under 48 hours) the main risk is due to brain edema from hyponatremia, and the correction of serum sodium may be achieved rapidly up to 2.5 mEq/L/hour until the CNS symptoms and seizures subside. Even under these circumstances, an absolute change of serum sodium > 20 mEq/L/day should be avoided. In patients with chronic hyponatremia (> 48 hours), because of the risk of central pontine myelinolysis associated with rapid correction, the serum sodium concentration should be corrected at a rate of 0.5 mEq/L/hour until it reaches 120 mEq/L. Patients with asymptomatic hyponatremia (acute or chronic) do not need aggressive therapy.

HYPERNATREMIC DISORDERS

In the majority of cases, hypernatremia is due to excess water loss rather than sodium gain. Hypertonicity of the plasma is a powerful stimulus for thirst. Patients unable to sense thirst owing to diseases of the brain or those physically unable to obtain water may develop hypernatremia. The majority of hypernatremic patients, however, manifest a primary defect in urinary concentrating ability along with insufficient administration of free water (Fig. 26–5).

Water can be obligated in the urine, in excess of electrolytes, in conditions characterized by the presence of large quantities of osmotically active solutes in the filtrate. This type of *osmotic diuresis* can occur in patients with hyperglycemia, following the infusion of mannitol, or in patients excreting excessive amounts of amino acids or urea. The latter situation occurs in patients on high-protein tube feedings or total parenteral nutrition. Failure to concentrate the urine can take place otherwise only if the collecting duct is impermeable to water. *Diabetes insipidus* is a disorder in which the collecting tubule does not become water permeable. There may be a central defect in the release of ADH or a defect in renal responsiveness to the hormone (nephrogenic). Diabetes insipidus is classified as a variant of euvolemic hypernatremia, since a majority of patients with this disease do not develop ECV depletion because the water losses are primarily from the intracellular compartment.

In the diagnosis and therapy of hypernatremia, as with hyponatremia, baseline body weight, serum and urine electrolytes, and urine osmolality should be obtained. In central diabetes insipidus, the urine osmolality is usually < 100 mOsm/kg H_2O. In other disorders of renal water loss, urine osmolality is also lower than plasma osmolality. Determination of urine osmolality following the administration of ADH may help distinguish central from nephrogenic diabetes insipidus. In contrast to central diabetes insipidus, urine osmolality does not rise in patients with nephrogenic diabetes insipidus. In hypernatremia due to osmotic diuresis, urine osmolality may be

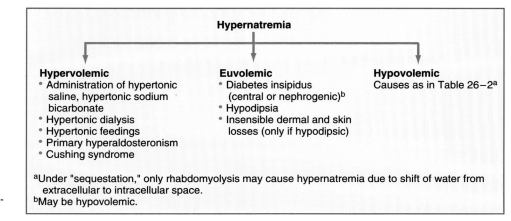

Figure 26–5
Diagnostic approach to hypernatremia.

Hypernatremia

Hypervolemic
* Administration of hypertonic saline, hypertonic sodium bicarbonate
* Hypertonic dialysis
* Hypertonic feedings
* Primary hyperaldosteronism
* Cushing syndrome

Euvolemic
* Diabetes insipidus (central or nephrogenic)[b]
* Hypodipsia
* Insensible dermal and skin losses (only if hypodipsic)

Hypovolemic
Causes as in Table 26–2[a]

[a]Under "sequestration," only rhabdomyolysis may cause hypernatremia due to shift of water from extracellular to intracellular space.
[b]May be hypovolemic.

higher than serum osmolality because of the presence of solutes, such as glucose, mannitol, or urea in the urine. In these patients, the urine osmolality due to the presence of electrolytes $(2 \times [Na^+ + K^+])$ is lower than effective plasma osmolality $(2 \times [Na^+])$.

Treatment

Hypernatremia that is associated with hypovolemia implies a sodium deficit in addition to the water deficit and may require isotonic saline infusion. In other patients, hypotonic intravenous solutions (D_5W, half-normal saline, quarter-normal saline) should be administered to correct hypernatremia. It is important to understand that the water content of these fluids varies according to the electrolyte concentration. For example, 1 L of D_5W essentially equals 1 L of free water, since all glucose is eventually metabolized. However, 1 L of half-normal saline or quarter-normal saline contains 500 ml or 750 ml, respectively, of free water. In addition, if other solutes, such as potassium or magnesium, are added to the intravenous fluids, their contribution to the tonicity of the administered fluid should be taken into account. Administration of solutions that are hypotonic relative to the urine will correct hypernatremia.

In patients with central diabetes insipidus, exogenous ADH may be provided. Chlorpropamide and clofibrate are beneficial in patients with partial central diabetes insipidus. In patients with nephrogenic diabetes insipidus, a reduction in sodium intake and administration of a thiazide diuretic may induce a degree of volume depletion resulting in a decreased urine volume. In addition, use of nonsteroidal anti-inflammatory drugs may be of therapeutic benefit in patients with nephrogenic diabetes insipidus.

As is the case in hyponatremic patients, the rate of correction of hypernatremia is important. With chronic hypernatremia (longer than 36 to 48 hours), the brain generates compounds that raise the intracellular osmolality, minimizing cell shrinkage. Thus, rapid correction of plasma osmolality may lead to a shift of water to the relatively hypertonic intracellular compartment and result in brain edema. As a general rule, hypernatremia should be corrected over 48 hours at a rate not exceeding 1 mEq/L/hour.

DISTURBANCES IN POTASSIUM BALANCE

The human body contains approximately 3500 mEq of potassium (K^+). With a normal concentration of 3.5 to 5.0 mEq/L, the ECF contains approximately 70 mEq of K^+, or only 2% of total body stores. In response to a dietary K^+ load, rapid removal of K^+ from the extracellular space is necessary to prevent life-threatening hyperkalemia. For example, in the absence of a homeostatic mechanism, if a person ingests 50 mEq of dietary K^+ in a single meal (the average daily American diet contains 100 to 120 mEq K^+ per day), the serum K^+ could rise to 7 mEq/L (assuming an extracellular volume of 14 L with a baseline serum K^+ of 4 mEq/L). Thus, the initial adaptation to a K^+ load is the rapid redistribution of K^+ from

the extracellular to the intracellular space. Various hormones including insulin, aldosterone, and catecholamines cause movement of K^+ into cells. The acid-base status of the patient is another determinant of the serum K^+ concentration, presumably due to an exchange of K^+ for hydrogen (H^+) across the cells. The greatest effect on the serum K^+ concentration is associated with metabolic acidosis involving mineral acids. The cellular permeability to the anions of the mineral acids is low, so that H^+ moves relatively unaccompanied into the cell. By contrast, metabolic acidosis caused by organic acids, such as lactic acid and ketoacids, does not cause hyperkalemia. The anions of these acids are relatively permeable and accompany H^+ into the cell. This diminishes the electrochemical gradient favoring K^+ efflux.

Although these mechanisms affect the distribution of K^+ between the fluid compartments, other mechanisms are necessary to maintain overall K^+ balance. Humans ingest approximately 100 mEq K^+ daily, the bulk of which is eliminated by the kidney. The basic mechanism involved in the distal tubular secretion is the movement of intracellular K^+ from the principal cell into the tubular lumen down an electrochemical gradient. Factors that enhance this gradient promote K^+ secretion. These factors include the rate of distal tubular flow, the distal delivery of sodium, the presence of poorly reabsorbable anions in the tubular fluid, and stimulation by aldosterone.

The ratio of extracellular to intracellular K^+ establishes the resting membrane potential of the cell. Hence, hyper- or hypokalemia is associated with alteration of the resting membrane potential, which accounts for the majority of the symptoms and findings of these disorders.

Diagnostic Approach to K+ Disorders

A careful history with emphasis on the diet and use of medications and laxatives should be obtained. Spurious hyper- and hypokalemia must be excluded. In addition to the serum electrolytes, serum magnesium, urine electrolytes, and urine osmolality should be obtained. The next step should be to determine whether an abnormal renal K^+ handling is involved in the genesis of the disorder. This may be determined by measuring the 24-hour urine K^+ excretion. With extrarenal hyperkalemia, renal K^+ excretion should be > 200 mEq/day, and if hypokalemia is due to extrarenal losses, the renal K^+ excretion should be < 20 mEq/day. An alternative method to estimate distal tubule K^+ secretion, the major determinant of final urine K^+ is *TTKG (transtubular K+ gradient)*. This is expressed as

$$TTKG = \frac{Urine\ K \times Serum\ Osm.}{Urine\ Osm. \times Serum\ K}$$

In hyperkalemia, the appropriate renal response is reflected in a TTKG > 8 to 10, and in hypokalemia with appropriate renal K^+ conservation, TTKG is generally < 2. Any deviation from these values suggests that renal defect in K^+ handling is contributing to the K^+ disorder.

This formula is not useful in the states where urine is hypo-osmolar to plasma.

Hyperkalemia

The ratio of the intracellular to extracellular K^+ concentration is the major determinant of the resting potential of the cell membrane. As the extracellular K^+ concentration increases, the cell membrane is partially depolarized, the sodium permeability is diminished, and the ability to generate action potentials is decreased. In muscle tissue, this accounts for muscle weakness and paralysis. In the heart, hyperkalemia is manifest as changes in the electrocardiogram (ECG). These changes include peaked T waves, decreased amplitude or the absence of P waves, wide QRS complex, sinus bradycardia, and conduction defects.

A pathophysiologic approach to the causes of hyperkalemia is outlined in Figures 26–6 and 26–7. Vigorous phlebotomy techniques can result in lysis of red blood cells, releasing intracellular K^+ into the serum sample. Thrombocytosis ($> 1 \times 10^6/mm^3$) and leukocytosis ($> 60,000/mm^3$) may also be associated with "spurious hyperkalemia." These disorders can be diagnosed rapidly by determining the plasma and serum concentrations of K^+. True hyperkalemia is present if these values differ by ≤ 0.2 mEq/L.

Chronic renal insufficiency, per se, does not cause hyperkalemia unless it is fairly advanced, with a GFR < 10 to 15 ml/minute. Thus, hyperkalemia in chronic renal insufficiency is usually due to a distal tubular defect in K^+ secretion rather than the impaired glomerular filtration rate, as shown in Figure 26–7. Failure to increase plasma aldosterone by the administration of corticotropin or furosemide confirms the diagnosis of *hyporeninemic hypoaldosteronism*. Prostaglandin deficiency may play a role in the pathogenesis of this disorder. Determination of the urine K^+ in response to a single dose of an oral mineralocorticoid (such as 9α-fludrocortisone) may help to differentiate hypoaldosteronism from aldosterone resistance. With aldosterone resistance, there will be no increase in urine K^+ excretion in response to the mineralocorticoid.

Treatment of hyperkalemia depends on the urgency of clinical findings. If cardiac standstill is imminent, the most rapid method of reversing the effects of hyperkalemia is to re-establish the normal membrane potential. Calcium antagonizes the membrane effects of hyperkalemia and can provide rapid protection of the cardiac conduction system. This protection, however, is short lived and must be accompanied by other therapies to decrease the extracellular K^+ concentration. The distribution of K^+ into the intracellular compartment by administration of sodium bicarbonate, β_2-adrenergic agonists, or insulin, rapidly decreases the serum concentration of K^+. The ultimate goal of the treatment is the net removal of K^+ from the body. Exchange resins, such as sodium polystyrene sulfonate, can enhance the K^+ excretion from the gastrointestinal tract. Attempts can be made to enhance renal excretion by improving the distal delivery of sodium utilizing sodium bicarbonate and administration of loop diuretics. Finally, dialysis can be used to remove excess extracellular K^+. For long-term chronic management of patients with an aldosterone deficiency, an oral preparation of a mineralocorticoid can be used. It is important to identify and discontinue any offending drug that may contribute to the hyperkalemia.

Hypokalemia

Since K^+ is the most abundant intracellular cation, its deficiency results in a wide variety of defects. For example, rhabdomyolysis and adynamic ileus have been associ-

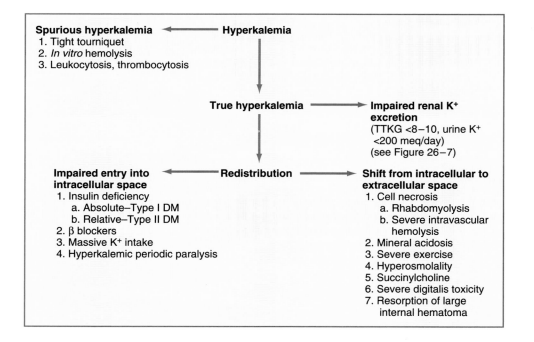

Figure 26–6

Diagnostic approach to hyperkalemia. DM = Diabetes mellitus; TTKG = transtubular potassium gradient.

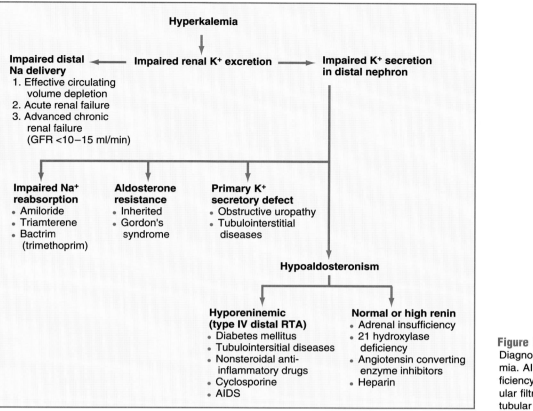

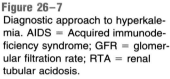

Figure 26–7
Diagnostic approach to hyperkalemia. AIDS = Acquired immunodeficiency syndrome; GFR = glomerular filtration rate; RTA = renal tubular acidosis.

ated with hypokalemia. Chronic hypokalemia stimulates thirst and may cause nephrogenic diabetes insipidus. However, the most prominent abnormalities relate to the cardiovascular system. Typically, hypokalemia is associated with flattening of the T waves and development of U waves. The most urgent abnormality is an association with arrhythmias, particularly in patients receiving digitalis. Hypokalemia, through a stimulation of renal ammo-

nia synthesis, may worsen the hepatic encephalopathy in patients with liver cirrhosis.

A diagnostic approach to hypokalemia is outlined in Figures 26–8 and 26–9. Like hyperkalemia, spurious hypokalemia can also occur with leukocytosis (>60,000 cells/mm³) due to active uptake of K⁺ by white cells from the serum. True hypokalemia is caused by redistribution, extrarenal K⁺ loss, poor intake, or renal K⁺

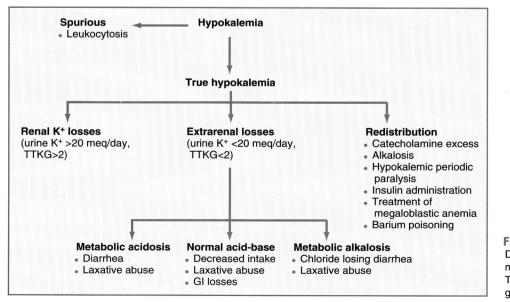

Figure 26–8
Diagnostic approach to hypokalemia. GI = Gastrointestinal; TTKG = transtubular potassium gradient.

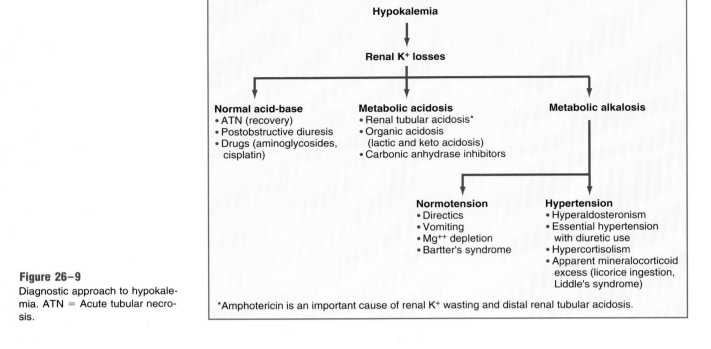

Figure 26–9
Diagnostic approach to hypokalemia. ATN = Acute tubular necrosis.

losses. Since only 2% of total-body K$^+$ is distributed in the extracellular compartment, serum K$^+$ measurements may not accurately reflect the total-body stores. In fact, hypokalemia can occur in the presence of normal total-body K$^+$ stores. This occurs when there is a shift of K$^+$ from the extracellular to the intracellular space. Excess circulating catecholamines, insulin administration, and alkalosis are the major causes of redistribution of K$^+$ from the extracellular to the intracellular space. Redistribution hypokalemia is particularly important in the clinical setting of myocardial infarction and exacerbation of chronic obstructive pulmonary disease. These patients are particularly prone to arrhythmias, since excess catecholamines (stress, inhaled β_2-agonists) cause K$^+$ shifts in the setting of total-body K$^+$ depletion due to frequent diuretic usage.

In patients with hypokalemia, acid-base status, presence or absence of hypertension, urinary chloride, and urinary potassium are very helpful in narrowing down the diagnostic possibilities. In patients with diuretic abuse (patients with eating disorders), the urine sodium and chloride are high in the presence of metabolic alkalosis, a profile similar to that of *Bartter's syndrome,* which is a rare defect of primary renal tubular sodium chloride reabsorption. In this setting, a urine screen for diuretics may be necessary to make the diagnosis. In comparison, patients with surreptitious vomiting have a low urinary chloride. Patients who abuse laxatives have a low urine sodium and chloride, with metabolic acidosis or normal acid-base status. Glycyrrhizic acid, the active ingredient in licorice, blocks 11β-dehydrogenase, an enzyme that normally protects the mineralocorticoid receptor from the glucocorticoids, resulting in an unregulated activation of the mineralocorticoid receptors in the distal nephron.

Determination of serum magnesium should always be performed in a patient with hypokalemia. Hypokalemia that is associated with hypomagnesemia is resistant to therapy unless concomitant magnesium deficiency is corrected. Given the factors that determine transmembrane K$^+$ shifts, it may be difficult to determine the net potassium deficit. An estimate for a 70-kg man based on the serum concentration is 100 to 200 mEq deficit in total-body K$^+$ when the serum concentration decreases from 4 to 3 mEq/L. Below 3 mEq/L, every 1 mEq/L decrease in the serum concentration of K$^+$ reflects an additional 200 to 400 mEq deficit in total-body K$^+$. Hypokalemia should be treated with oral K$^+$ supplementation. Intravenous K$^+$ administration should only be used in urgent situations such as arrhythmias, digitalis toxicity, and intolerance to oral form in patients with adynamic ileus. The rate of intravenous K$^+$ administration generally should not exceed 10 mEq/hour, and, only under ECG monitoring, the K$^+$ administration rate can be increased up to 20 mEq/hour. Hypokalemia associated with chronic diuretic therapy may be treated with the addition of a K$^+$-sparing diuretic.

DISTURBANCES IN ACID-BASE BALANCE

Most metabolic processes occurring in the body result in the production of acid. The largest source of endogenous acid production is from the catabolism of glucose and fatty acids to carbon dioxide and water or effectively carbonic acid. The average daily production of water by this metabolic process is approximately 400 ml, or 22,000 mmol. Thus, the rate of volatile acid production is about 22,000 mEq of H$^+$ daily. Cellular metabolism of sulfur-containing amino acids, the oxidation of phosphoproteins and phospholipids, nucleoprotein degradation, and the incomplete combustion of carbohydrates and fatty acids, also result in the formation of a number of nonvolatile acids. Approximately 1 mEq/kg body weight of H⁺ is produced by these processes daily.

The normal concentration of H⁺ in arterial blood is 40 mEq/L, equating to a pH of 7.40. This concentration is maintained relatively constant despite variations in the endogenous and exogenous acid input. An acid load is acutely neutralized by circulating and intracellular buffers. The capacity of these buffering systems is limited, however, and would be quickly depleted by the normal endogenous acid production. Mechanisms for excreting acid must therefore be effective to maintain acid-base homeostasis.

Volatile acid is effectively eliminated by the lungs. Pulmonary ventilation excretes the carbon dioxide formed by cellular respiration. The primary factors regulating alteration in the rate of minute ventilation are subtle changes in cerebrospinal fluid pH, or arterial pH. Nonvolatile acid excretion is affected through the kidneys.

Renal Hydrogen Ion Excretion

The kidney contributes to acid-base homeostasis by the reclaimation of 4500 mEq of bicarbonate filtered at the glomerulus daily and by the generation of new bicarbonate that replenishes the body buffer stores. These functions are accomplished by the secretion of H⁺ by various nephron segments (Fig. 26–10). The bulk of filtered bicarbonate is reabsorbed in the proximal tubule. In contrast to the distal tubule, the proximal tubule is a high-capacity bicarbonate reabsorption system due to the presence of carbonic anhydrase in the luminal membrane. Carbonic anhydrase in the luminal membrane rapidly catalyzes the dehydration of carbonic acid to carbon dioxide and water, thus maintaining the gradient for H⁺ secretion in the proximal tubule. Distal tubule lacks a luminal carbonic anhydrase and has only a cytoplasmic carbonic anhydrase,

which limits its capacity to reclaim bicarbonate. The rate of proximal bicarbonate reabsorption is increased by volume depletion; by an elevation in the P_{CO_2}, as seen in chronic respiratory acidosis; and by hypokalemia. Conversely, volume expansion or the reduction of the P_{CO_2} lowers the proximal tubular resorptive rate for bicarbonate.

The distal tubule is responsible for reclaiming the remainder of the filtered bicarbonate. This segment must also eliminate H⁺ quantitatively equivalent to the nonvolatile acid production. The H⁺ excretion is accomplished by secretion into the tubular fluid. The inorganic bases of nonvolatile acid production, such as phosphates, are filtered at the glomerulus and are poorly reabsorbed by the nephron. These "fixed" bases, as well as ammonia produced by proximal tubular cells, can effectively trap the secreted H⁺ in the tubular fluid for elimination in the urine. Aldosterone and the P_{CO_2} affect the distal secretion of H⁺.

Assessment of Acid-Base Status

The initial step in evaluating acid-base problems is to obtain an arterial blood gas measurement and serum electrolyte concentrations (Fig. 26–11). The arterial blood gas measures the pH, P_{O_2}, and P_{CO_2}. The bicarbonate concentration is then calculated using the Henderson-Hasselbalch equation, which relates the pH directly to the bicarbonate concentration and inversely to the P_{CO_2}. Because there is little soluble CO_2 in serum, the total CO_2 obtained with the serum electrolytes is effectively a measure of the serum bicarbonate concentration. This measured value should differ from that calculated on a concomitant blood gas determination by no more than 2 mEq/L. The validity of the blood gas determination can be estimated further by applying the bicarbonate concen-

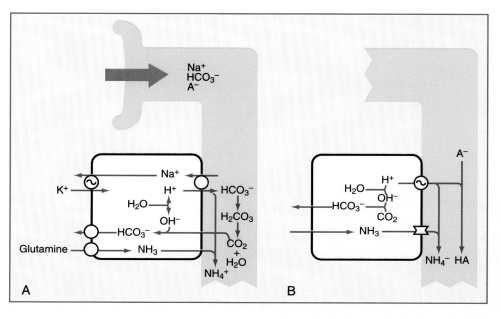

Figure 26–10
Renal mechanisms for hydrogen ion secretion. The proximal tubule *(A)* is responsible for the bulk reabsorption of filtered bicarbonate. The distal nephron hydrogen ion secretion *(B)* is responsible for reclaiming additional bicarbonate as well as titrating inorganic anions (A⁻).

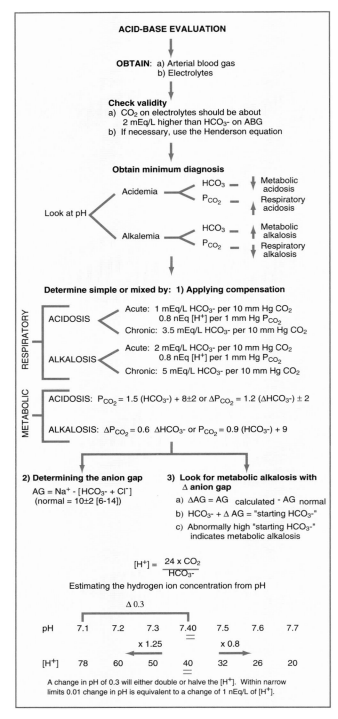

Figure 26–11
Scheme for assessing acid-base homeostasis.

minimum diagnosis should be established, as shown in Figure 26–11. Next, a measurement of the compensatory response and the anion gap should be performed. If the compensation of a primary acid-base defect is inappropriate, a mixed acid-base disorder is considered. The presence of a normal serum pH in combination with abnormal PCO_2 and serum bicarbonate provides another clue to a mixed acid-base disorder. The anion gap is useful in the diagnostic approach to metabolic acidosis. When an organic acid (such as lactic acid) is added to the extracellular fluid compartment, the bicarbonate concentration falls as the acid is buffered. The anion gap increases as the organic base is accumulated. Quantitatively, the increase in anion gap should be equivalent to the decrease in bicarbonate concentration. Thus, by adding the difference between the calculated and normal anion gap to the prevailing bicarbonate concentration, an estimate of the "starting" bicarbonate concentration can be made. An abnormally elevated initial bicarbonate indicates a concomitant metabolic alkalosis.

Metabolic Acidosis

Metabolic acidosis is characterized by a decrease in the serum bicarbonate concentration. This occurs either by excretion of bicarbonate-containing fluids or by utilization of bicarbonate as a buffer of acids. In the latter instance, the nature of the base may affect the electrolyte composition. It is thus convenient to consider the metabolic acidosis by means of the anion gap (Table 26–6).

Metabolic acidoses have a normal anion gap whenever there are abnormally large net bicarbonate losses. This may occur because the kidneys fail to reabsorb or regenerate bicarbonate, there are extrarenal losses of bicarbonate, or excessive amounts of substances yielding hydrochloric acid have been administered. Thus, gastrointestinal bicarbonate loss and renal tubular acidosis are the major causes of normal anion gap acidosis.

The urinary anion gap is defined as follows:

Urinary anion gap = unmeasured anions − unmeasured cations = $[Na^+ + K^+] - Cl^-$

It is useful in evaluating patients with normal anion gap acidosis. The test provides an approximate index of urinary ammonia excretion, as measured by a negative urinary anion gap. Thus, a normal renal response would be a negative urinary anion gap, generally in the range of 30 to 50 mEq/L. In such an instance, it is likely that the acidosis is due to gastrointestinal losses, rather than a renal lesion.

A classification scheme and diagnostic features of the renal tubular acidosis (RTA) syndromes is outlined in Table 26–7. In proximal RTA, the primary defect is an impairment of bicarbonate reabsorption in the proximal tubule and may be associated with defective phosphate, glucose, urate, and amino acid reabsorption. Type I distal RTA is characterized by the inability to acidify maximally urine. Patients with type IV distal RTA have impaired urinary acidification due to hypoaldosteronism. A large subset of these patients has diabetes mellitus.

tration and the measured PCO_2 to the Henderson-Hasselbalch equation:

$$[H^+] = \frac{24 \times PCO_2}{[HCO_3^-]}$$

Based on the pH, PCO_2, and serum bicarbonate, a

TABLE 26–6	Causes of Metabolic Acidosis

Normal anion gap
  Bicarbonate losses
    Extrarenal
      Small bowel drainage
      Diarrhea
    Renal
      Proximal renal tubular acidosis
      Carbonic anhydrase inhibitors
      Primary hyperparathyroidism
  Failure of bicarbonate regeneration
  Distal renal tubular acidosis
  Aldosterone deficiency
    Addison's disease
    Hyporeninemic hypoaldosteronism
  Aldosterone insensitivity
    Interstitial renal disease
    Aldosterone antagonists
  Ureteroileostomy (ileal bladder)
  Acidifying salts
    Ammonium chloride
    Lysine or arginine hydrochloride
  Diabetes mellitus (recovery phase)
Wide anion gap
  Reduced excretion of acids
    Renal failure
  Overproduction of acids
    Ketoacidosis
      Diabetic
      Alcoholic
      Starvation
    Lactic acidosis
    Toxin ingestion
      Methanol
      Ethylene glycol
      Salicylates
      Paraldehyde
      Isopropyl alcohol

Modified from Andreoli TE: Disorders of fluid volume, electrolyte, and acid-base balance. *In* Wyngaarden JB, Smith LH Jr, Bennett JC (eds.): Cecil Textbook of Medicine. 19th ed. Philadelphia, WB Saunders, 1992, p 523.

The causes of wide anion gap acidosis are listed in Table 26–6. In renal failure, inorganic compounds, such as phosphates and sulfates, are the major contributors to the increased anion gap. Organic compounds also accumulate with diminished renal function. Ketoacidosis results from accelerated lipolysis, and ketogenesis, due to a relative insulin deficiency. This can occur in the diabetic

TABLE 26–7	Characteristics of Renal Tubular Acidosis (RTA) Syndromes

Condition	Urine pH*	Serum Potassium
Type I distal RTA†	>5.5	NL or ↓
Proximal RTA (type II)	<5.5	↓
Type IV distal RTA (Hyporeninemic hypoaldosteronism)	<5.5	↑
Voltage-dependent RTA‡	>5.5	↑

* Urine pH assessed during acidemia
† May be seen with amphotericin use
‡ Described in patients with obstructive uropathy
NL = Normal.

who has an absolute deficiency of insulin production. Alcoholic ketoacidosis and starvation ketoacidosis result from the suppression of endogenous insulin secretion due to inadequate carbohydrate ingestion. In addition, in alcoholic ketoacidosis, insulin resistance contributes to ketone formation. The syndrome of lactic acidosis results from impaired cellular respiration. Lactate is produced from the reduction of pyruvate in muscle, red blood cells, and other tissues as a consequence of anaerobic glycolysis. In situations of diminished oxidative metabolism, excess lactic acid is produced. This anaerobic state also favors a shift of ketoacids to the reduced form, beta-hydroxybutyrate. The nitroprusside reaction, which is catalyzed by the ketoacids acetoacetate and acetone, is thus nonreactive in the setting of lactic acidosis. Lactic acidosis occurs most commonly in disorders characterized by inadequate oxygen delivery to tissues, such as shock, septicemia, and profound hypoxemia. Certain toxins may also sufficiently alter mitochondrial function, establishing an effective anaerobic state. Some of these toxins may undergo metabolism into organic acids that can contribute to the generation of large anion gap acidosis. Methanol is metabolized by alcohol dehydrogenase to formic acid. Ethylene glycol is metabolized to glycolic and oxalic acids. Salicylates are themselves acidic compounds and can cause a wide anion gap acidosis.

The treatment of metabolic acidosis depends on the underlying cause and the severity of the manifestations. The rapid administration of parenteral sodium bicarbonate is generally indicated when the pH is less than 7.1, and hemodynamic instability is evident. Oral bicarbonate supplementation may be sufficient if the acidosis is due to gastrointestinal bicarbonate loss or RTA.

Although bicarbonate supplementation is beneficial in proximal RTA, it is difficult to achieve a normal serum bicarbonate concentration. This is a result of bicarbonaturia, which accompanies the rise in serum bicarbonate. In contrast, in type I distal RTA, adequate bicarbonate supplementation may completely correct the acidosis. Furthermore, the treatment of acidosis also corrects hypercalciuria and nephrocalcinosis, which are commonly seen with type I distal RTA. Therapy of type IV distal RTA involves correction of hyperkalemia and bicarbonate supplementation.

The treatment of organic acidosis should be directed at the underlying disorder. If the generation of the organic acid can be interrupted, the organic base pair may be metabolized, effectively regenerating bicarbonate. The acidemia of diabetic ketoacidosis, for example, can be effectively treated by administration of insulin, thereby inhibiting further ketogenesis. In lactate acidosis, therapy should be directed toward improving tissue perfusion. In alcoholic and starvation ketoacidosis, administration of dextrose-containing intravenous fluids corrects the acidosis.

Metabolic Alkalosis

The administration of base or the effective removal of H^+ increases the bicarbonate concentration of the extracellular fluid. Normally, an elevation of the serum bicarbonate concentration is corrected by excretion of the excess bicarbonate. The maintenance of a metabolic alkalosis, therefore, implies a defect in the renal mechanism regulating bicarbonate excretion, mainly the proximal tubular bicarbonate absorption. Elevation of the PCO_2, hypokalemia, or volume depletion increases the proximal tubular bicarbonate absorption and can sustain a metabolic alkalosis.

The most common cause of metabolic alkalosis is gastric loss of hydrochloric acid by vomiting or mechanical drainage. Diuretic (thiazide and loop) use is commonly associated with metabolic alkalosis. Volume depletion associated with vomiting and diuretic use enhances proximal bicarbonate reabsorption. Volume depletion also leads to aldosterone secretion, which stimulates distal tubular H^+ secretion. K^+ secretion is likewise stimulated. Endogenous or exogenous mineralocorticoid excess (see Fig. 26–9) is another important cause of metabolic alkalosis. In all these disorders, concomitant hypokalemia promotes the maintenance of metabolic alkalosis.

The renal compensation for sustained hypercapnia results in an increase in the serum bicarbonate concentration. If the ventilatory rate acutely increases, the PCO_2 falls rapidly but the bicarbonate concentration remains transiently elevated, resulting in a posthypercapnic alkalosis. Furthermore, the elevated PCO_2 stimulates proximal tubular bicarbonate absorption. As noted before, administration of bicarbonate in a setting of organic acidosis may result in alkalosis when the organic anion is metabolized. Excessive alkali ingestion (e.g., milk-alkali syndrome) is an uncommon cause of metabolic alkalosis. It results from impaired renal bicarbonate excretion due to renal failure, in the setting of excess alkali intake.

A history and physical examination should be performed, and urinary chloride should be measured. The determination of urinary chloride is helpful in formulating a rational approach to the diagnosis and treatment of metabolic alkalosis (Table 26–8). Volume expansion with sodium chloride is the mainstay of therapy in patients with vomiting-induced, diuretic-induced, and posthypercapnic metabolic alkalosis (chloride-responsive alkalosis). K^+ chloride repletion also aids in the therapy. However, volume expansion may be harmful in diuretic-induced alkalosis associated with congestive heart failure. The use of carbonic anhydrase inhibitors may be beneficial in this setting. Metabolic alkalosis associated with primary mineralocorticoid excess, Bartter's syndrome, and milk-alkali syndrome is unresponsive to volume expansion (chloride-resistant alkalosis). Treatment of underlying cause is the mainstay of therapy in primary mineralocorticoid excess states. In Bartter's syndrome, K^+ chloride supplements and K^+-sparing diuretics are required.

Respiratory Acidosis

Respiratory acidosis occurs with any impairment in the rate of alveolar ventilation. Acute respiratory acidosis occurs with a sudden depression of the medullary respiratory center (narcotic overdose), with paralysis of the respiratory muscles, and with airway obstruction. Chronic respiratory acidosis generally occurs in individuals with chronic airway disease (emphysema), with extreme kyphoscoliosis, and with extreme obesity (Pickwickian syndrome).

The serum bicarbonate concentration is increased, the magnitude of which depends on the acuity and the severity of respiratory disorder. Acute increases in the PCO_2 result in somnolence, confusion, and, ultimately, CO_2 narcosis. Asterixis may be present. Because CO_2 is a cerebral vasodilator, the blood vessels in the optic fundi are often dilated, engorged, and tortuous. Frank papilledema may be present in severe hypercapnic states.

The only practical treatment for acute respiratory acidosis involves treatment of the underlying disorder and ventilatory support. In patients with chronic hypercapnia who develop an acute increase in the PCO_2, attention should be directed toward identifying factors that may have aggravated the chronic disorder. Alkalinizing salts should be avoided in patients with chronic respiratory acidosis.

Respiratory Alkalosis

Respiratory alkalosis occurs when hyperventilation reduces the arterial PCO_2 and consequently increases the arterial pH. Acute respiratory alkalosis is most commonly a result of the hyperventilation syndrome. It may also occur in damage to the respiratory centers, in acute salicylism, in fever and septic states, and in association with various pulmonary processes (pneumonia, pulmonary emboli, or congestive heart failure). The disorder may be produced iatrogenically by injudicious mechanical ventilatory support. Chronic hyperventilation occurs in the acclimatization response to high altitudes (a low ambient oxygen tension), in advanced hepatic insufficiency, and in pregnancy.

Acute hyperventilation is characterized by lightheadedness, paresthesias, circumoral numbness, and tingling of the extremities. Tetany occurs in severe cases. When anxiety provokes hyperventilation, air rebreathing with a paper bag generally terminates the acute attack.

TABLE 26–8	Causes of Metabolic Alkalosis

Chloride-sensitive alkalosis (urinary chloride <20 mEq/L)
  Vomiting
  Nasogastric suction
  Diuretic use
  Posthypercapnic
Chloride-resistant alkalosis (urinary chloride >20 mEq/L)
  mineralocorticoid excess
    Diuretic use*
    Bartter's syndrome
    Potassium depletion
    Milk-alkali syndrome

* Active diuretic use may be associated with high urinary chloride.

REFERENCES

Andreoli TE: Disorders of fluid volume, electrolyte, and acid-base balance. *In* Wyngaarden JB, Smith LH Jr, Bennett JC (eds.): Cecil Textbook of Medicine. 19th ed. Philadelphia, WB Saunders, 1992, pp 499–528.

Bichet DG, Schrier RW: Cardiac failure, liver disease, and nephrotic syndrome. *In* Schrier RW, Gottschalk CW (eds.): Diseases of the Kidney. 5th ed. Boston, Little, Brown & Co, 1992, pp 2453–2493.

Narins RG, Emmett M: Simple and mixed acid-base disorders. Medicine 1980; 59(3):161.

27

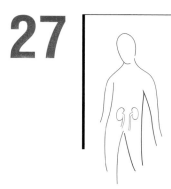

Glomerular Diseases

THE GLOMERULUS

The glomerulus consists of a capillary bed that receives blood from the afferent arteriole and is drained by the efferent arteriole and contains four different cell types: the glomerular (visceral) epithelial cell (podocyte), the endothelial cell, the mesangial cell, and the parietal epithelial cell (Fig. 27–1). The podocyte supports the delicate glomerular basement membrane (GBM) by means of an extensive trabecular network. The mesangium provides a skeletal framework for the entire capillary network and, owing to its contractile capability, can control blood flow along the glomerular capillaries in response to a host of mediators. The endothelial cells line the capillary lumen, and the parietal epithelial cells cover Bowman's capsule.

MECHANISMS OF GLOMERULAR INJURY

Immunologic mechanisms play a major role in glomerular injury and consist primarily of two types (Fig. 27–2). Occasionally, antibodies to the GBM develop, resulting in a glomerulonephritis (GN) characterized by linear deposition of IgG along the capillary walls. Much more frequently, discrete deposition of granular deposits of immunoglobulins and complement is seen. These immunoglobulins, together with their respective circulating antigens, may be deposited in the GBM. Alternatively, antigens may localize individually to the GBM, and there may occur *in situ* activation of antigen-antibody complexes. In both instances, the antigen-antibody complex localization in the GBM initiates the cascade of glomerular injury. Such deposits may be seen in the mesangium, along the subendothelial surface of the GBM, or within the outer region of the capillary wall in the subepithelial space.

Other glomerular diseases occur in which immunologic mechanisms are thought to play a role but no deposits are detectable. Minimal change nephrotic syndrome, now thought to be a disorder of the glomerular epithelial cell, may be due to non–complement-fixing anti–glomerular epithelial cell antibodies. Idiopathic crescentic GN (anti-GBM antibodies are absent) is possibly mediated by either mononuclear cell–mediated immune reactions, induction of endothelial leukocyte adhesion molecules (ELAM) on endothelium, or anti-neutrophil cytoplasmic antibody (ANCA)–mediated local neutrophil activation.

Neutrophil infiltration in response to immune complex–complement interaction, ELAM induction, or the presence of ANCA can lead to glomerular injury through the release of proteolytic enzymes and/or reactive oxygen metabolites. Other circulating cells have been suggested to play a role in glomerular injury. Platelets may be important in various forms of glomerular injury and are particularly important in mesangial proliferative lesions. Macrophages in concert with activated lymphocytes are likely important in antibody-independent, cell-mediated glomerular injury. The glomerular cells themselves may be activated to produce oxidants and/or proteases with subsequent damage to either the GBM or the mesangium. Finally, in other disorders such as diabetes or amyloidosis, the glomerular injury may be secondary to metabolic imbalances.

CLINICAL MANIFESTATIONS OF GLOMERULAR DISEASE

The usual initial manifestations of glomerular disease are often nonspecific generalized complaints (hypertension, edema, malaise) or urinary abnormalities (proteinuria, hematuria). Altered glomerular function, either proteinuria consequent to changes in GBM permeability or decreased glomerular filtration rate (GFR) secondary to abnormal ultrafiltration, characterizes glomerular disease.

The glomerular capillaries provide a filtration barrier that prevents the passage of proteins into the urine on the basis of protein size, shape, and electrical charge. Normally, < 150 mg of protein is excreted in the urine per day. Nephrotic-range proteinuria (> 3.5 gm/day in adults) represents diffuse glomerular injury with loss of the net negative charge on the capillary wall and/or structural defects in the filtration barrier. The presence of either red blood cell (RBC) casts or dysmorphic RBCs in the urine characterizes nephronal bleeding indicative of either proliferative GN or acute interstitial nephritis. Dysmorphic RBCs are best seen using phase contrast microscopy and consist of red cells of varying size, shape, and hemoglobin content.

Renal salt retention is a common feature of glomerular disease and may be expressed as edema, volume over-

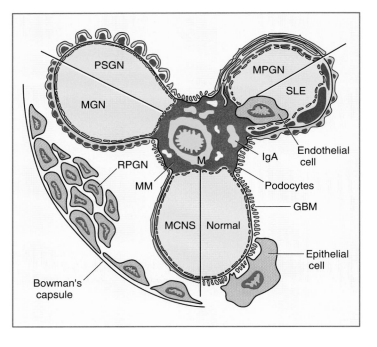

Figure 27-1

Schematic drawing of a glomerulus illustrating the normal features as well as several diseases. GBM = Glomerular basement membrane; IgA = IgA deposits in IgA nephropathy; M = mesangial cell; MCNS = minimal change nephrotic syndrome; MGN = membranous glomerulopathy; MM = mesangial matrix; MPGN = membranoproliferative glomerulopathy; PSGN = poststreptococcal glomerulonephritis; RPGN = rapidly progressive glomerulonephritis; SLE = systemic lupus erythematosus.

load, congestive heart failure, and hypertension. Although the mechanisms responsible for reduced salt excretion are poorly understood, sodium acquisitiveness is considerably greater than that expected solely from the reduction in GFR.

The renal function in glomerular disease depends on the type and varies from normal renal function (e.g., minimal change disease) to relentless progressive end-stage renal disease (e.g., rapidly progressive GN).

APPROACH TO THE PATIENT WITH GLOMERULAR DISEASE

Glomerular diseases have been classified in numerous ways. Here they are organized and discussed as they relate to the four major glomerular syndromes: acute nephritic syndrome, rapidly progressive GN, nephrotic syndrome (with either "bland" or "active" urine sediment), and asymptomatic urinary abnormalities (Table 27-1).

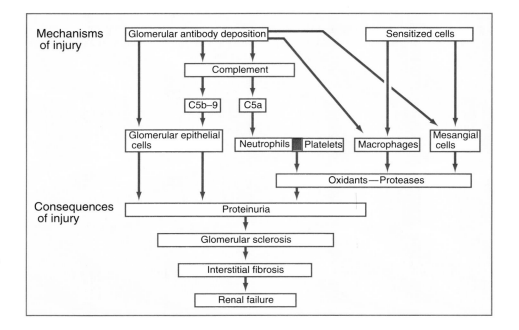

Figure 27-2

Schematic depiction of the mechanisms that mediate glomerular injury *(top)* and the consequences of those processes *(bottom)* leading to renal failure. (From Shah SV [ed.]: Mechanisms of glomerular injury. Semin Nephrol 1991;11:253-372.)

TABLE 27–1	Glomerular Syndromes
Acute nephritic syndrome	Nephronal hematuria (RBC casts and/or dysmorphic RBCs) temporally associated with acute renal failure
Rapidly progressive glomerulonephritis	Nephronal hematuria (RBC casts and/or dysmorphic RBCs) with renal failure developing over weeks to months and diffuse glomerular crescent formation
Nephrotic syndrome	Massive proteinuria ($>$3.5 gm/day/1.73 m²) with variable edema, hypoalbuminemia, hyperlipidemia, and hyperlipiduria
With "bland" sediment	"Pure" nephrotic syndrome
With "active" sediment	"Mixed" nephrotic/nephritic syndrome
Asymptomatic urinary abnormalities	Isolated proteinuria (usually $<$2.0 gm/day/1.73 m²) or hematuria (with or without proteinuria)

RBC = Red blood cell.

The diagnosis of glomerular diseases is based on pathologic features related to glomerular alterations. Definitions of some of the more commonly used terms are given in Table 27–2.

ACUTE NEPHRITIC SYNDROME

This syndrome is characterized by the abrupt onset (days) of hematuria with RBC casts or dysmorphic RBCs and proteinuria (usually nonnephrotic range) temporally associated with impairment of renal function. The manifestation of altered renal function may be oliguria, impairment of renal function as measured by rise in blood urea nitrogen (BUN), and creatinine or retention of salt and water resulting in the development of hypertension. Acute nephritic syndrome is most commonly due to proliferative GN, of which poststreptococcal GN is a prototype, and less commonly from acute interstitial nephritis. Table 27–3 lists the diseases commonly associated with this

TABLE 27–2	Pathologic Features of Glomerular Disease
Focal	Some (but not all) glomeruli contain the lesion
Diffuse (global)	Most glomeruli ($>$75%) contain the lesion
Segmental	Only a part of the glomerulus is affected by the lesion (most focal lesions are also segmental, e.g., focal segmental glomerulosclerosis)
Proliferation	An increase in cell number due to hyperplasia of one or more of the resident glomerular cells with or without inflammatory cell infiltration
Membrane alterations	Capillary wall thickening due to deposition of immune deposits or alterations in basement membrane
Crescent formation	Epithelial cell proliferation and mononuclear cell infiltration in Bowman's space

condition. The measurement of complement levels is useful in narrowing down the diagnostic possibilities.

Poststreptococcal glomerulonephritis (PSGN) occurs as a postinfectious complication of nephritogenic strains of group A, beta-hemolytic streptococcal infection. Pharyngitis (strep throat) is a common antecedent infection in northern states, but PSGN occurs in fewer than 5% of those infected, usually within a 5- to 20-day latent period. Streptococcal pyoderma more commonly occurs in the southern United States and may also lead to PSGN in as many as 50% of infected individuals. PSGN is the hallmark disease for the acute nephritic syndrome and is typically seen in children aged 3 to 12, although it can occur in adults. Both sexes are equally affected with PSGN, which occurs more frequently in the summer and autumn in North America. The patient presents with typical acute nephritic syndrome associated with malaise, cola-colored urine, mild hypertension, periorbital edema, and non–nephrotic-range proteinuria.

Laboratory findings include RBCs and RBC casts, white blood cells, and proteinuria on urinalysis, an elevated antistreptolysis O titer, a low serum complement (usually returning to normal at 6 to 12 weeks), and azotemia. Histologically, PSGN is a diffuse proliferative (mesangial and endothelial cells) and exudative (neutrophils and monocytes) GN with coarsely granular capillary loop deposits of IgG and C3 and subepithelial electron-dense humplike deposits by electron microscopy (Fig. 27–3).

The differential diagnosis is that of an acute GN with hypocomplementemia and includes other forms of postinfectious GN (e.g., bacterial endocarditis, shunt nephritis), systemic lupus erythematosus (SLE), and membranoproliferative GN. The diagnosis can usually be based on the typical renal presentation following a streptococcal infection, hypocomplementemia, and serologic evidence. Because the diagnosis is most often straightforward, a renal biopsy is indicated only if the disease follows an atypical course in children. Most adults with acute nephritic syndrome require a kidney biopsy to establish the diagnosis.

There is no specific therapy for PSGN, although antibiotics should be administered if cultures are positive for *Streptococcus*. Salt restriction and, in some cases, diuretics and antihypertensive agents may be required to

TABLE 27–3	Differential Diagnosis of Acute Nephritic Syndrome	
Low Serum Complement Level	**Normal Serum Complement Level**	
Acute postinfectious glomerulonephritis	IgA nephropathy	
Membranoproliferative glomerulonephritis	Idiopathic rapidly progressive glomerulonephritis	
Type I	Anti-GBM disease	
Type II	Polyarteritis nodosa	
Systemic lupus erythematosus	Wegener's granulomatosis	
Subacute bacterial endocarditis	Henoch-Schönlein purpura	
Visceral abscess	Goodpasture's syndrome	
"Shunt" nephritis		
Cryoglobulinemia		

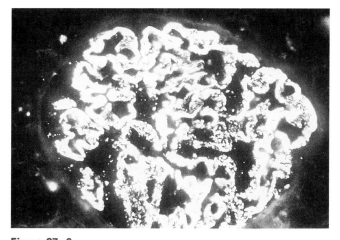

Figure 27–3
Immunofluorescence demonstrating coarsely granular capillary loop deposits of IgG.

manage sodium retention (manifested by hypertension, edema, congestive heart failure, and other signs). Complete recovery occurs in at least 85 to 90% of all patients. However, minor urinary sediment abnormalities may continue for several years in some patients (<2%), but progression to chronic renal failure is exceedingly rare, typically occurring only in older adults who contract the disease. Fewer than 5% of patients have oliguria for more than 7 to 9 days, and the prognosis in these patients is less favorable.

Nonstreptococcal postinfectious glomerulonephritis may occur after bacterial infections (e.g., staphylococcal, pneumococcal), viral infections (e.g., mumps, hepatitis B, varicella, coxsackie, infectious mononucleosis), protozoal infection (e.g., malaria, toxoplasmosis), and a host of others (e.g., schistosomiasis, syphilis). The clinical and histologic manifestations may vary somewhat, depending on the infecting agent. Still, most have features similar to those of PSGN and an equally good prognosis if the underlying infection is eradicated.

Glomerulonephritis associated with infective endocarditis commonly occurs in patients with chronic right-sided cardiac involvement and negative blood cultures. It usually manifests itself as a mild form of the acute nephritic syndrome (hematuria and proteinuria with a mild decrease in renal function). A similar pattern may occur in patients with infected ventriculoatrial shunts *(shunt nephritis)*. The histologic and immunofluorescent picture is similar to that of PSGN, although the lesions are usually more focal and segmental. Rarely, crescentic GN develops and is manifested by acute renal failure. Elimination of infection with appropriate antibiotic therapy usually results in a return of renal function to normal.

Glomerulonephritis associated with visceral abscess has been reported more frequently in patients with pulmonary abscesses. However, numerous other sites have also been reported. These patients develop the acute nephritic syndrome with a proliferative GN often showing many crescents. In contrast to PSGN, the complement levels are usually not depressed, and immune deposits are usually lacking. Successful antibiotic therapy results in recovery of renal function in only 50% of patients.

Systemic lupus erythematosus, Henoch-Schönlein purpura, and mixed essential cryoglobulinemia may present as an acute GN, but more typically they are associated with other glomerular syndromes and are therefore discussed later.

RAPIDLY PROGRESSIVE GLOMERULONEPHRITIS (RPGN)

Rapidly progressive glomerulonephritis is a syndrome characterized by nephronal hematuria (RBC casts and/or dysmorphic RBCs) with renal failure developing over weeks to months and diffuse glomerular crescent formation on renal biopsy (Fig. 27–4). Classification is complicated by the fact that RPGN can occur with immune deposits (either anti-GBM or immune complex type) or without immune deposits. In addition, it can be an idiopathic primary glomerular disease or can be superimposed on other glomerular diseases either primary or secondary. The classification scheme used here is based on the immunofluorescence information obtained from renal biopsy (Table 27–4).

Anti-GBM GN, characterized by linear capillary loop staining with IgG and C3 (Fig. 27–5), and extensive crescent formation, accounts for 15 to 20% of all cases of RPGN, although overall it accounts for less than 5% of all forms of GN. About two thirds of these patients have Goodpasture's syndrome with associated pulmonary hemorrhage. The remainder have an idiopathic form of anti-GBM GN. Goodpasture's syndrome affects young men six times more frequently than women and usually presents with hemoptysis and dyspnea. Idiopathic anti-GBM GN is seen in older patients (above 50 years) and affects both sexes equally. Anti-GBM antibodies are present in serum (detectable using indirect immunofluorescence on normal kidney); serum C3 is normal. Therapy consists of

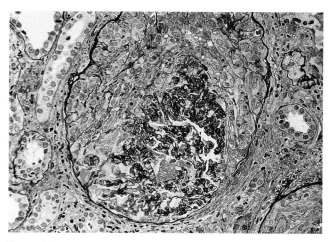

Figure 27–4
Glomerulus demonstrating crescent formation.

TABLE 27–4	Types of Rapidly Progressive Glomerulonephritis (RPGN)

Anti-GBM Antibody–Mediated RPGN (Linear Immunofluorescent Pattern)

Idiopathic anti-GBM antibody–mediated RPGN
Goodpasture's syndrome
Associated with other primary glomerular diseases
    Membranous glomerulopathy

Immune Complex–Mediated RPGN (Granular Immunofluorescent Pattern)

Idiopathic immune complex–mediated RPGN
Associated with other primary glomerular diseases
    Membranoproliferative glomerulopathy (type II > type I)
    IgA nephropathy
Associated with secondary glomerular diseases
    Postinfectious glomerulonephritides
    Systemic lupus erythematosus
    Mixed essential cryoglobulinemia
    Henoch-Schönlein purpura

Non–Immune-Mediated RPGN (Negative Immunofluorescent Pattern)

Idiopathic pauci-immune RPGN (ANCA-associated)
Systemic vasculitides

high-dose oral prednisone in concert with plasma exchange. A high index of suspicion resulting in earlier diagnosis and vigorous treatment has increased survival to more than 50%, as opposed to 10 to 15% a decade ago.

Immune complex RPGN is almost always associated with another underlying disease, and the correct diagnosis can usually be made by seeking the other clinical and laboratory features of these conditions. About 40% of all cases of RPGN are of this type (granular deposits of immunoglobulins and complement). Prognosis of the underlying condition declines dramatically in the presence of immune complex RPGN, and prompt diagnosis and treatment (as described previously) are required if renal function is to be preserved.

Non–immune-mediated RPGN (also referred to as pauci-immune GN), is found in about 40% of patients

with crescentic GN and is seen in association with one of the systemic vasculitides such as polyarteritis nodosa, Wegener's granulomatosis, or as an idiopathic form that is thought to represent a vasculitis limited to the glomerular capillaries. The idiopathic form is usually found in patients in their 50s or 60s, and as many as 25% require dialysis at presentation. A helpful diagnostic feature is the presence of ANCA, found in approximately 80% of patients with pauci-immune GN. When ANCA is detected by indirect immunofluorescence, two major patterns are observed: cytoplasmic staining (C-ANCA) and perinuclear staining (P-ANCA). P-ANCA is most common in pauci-immune necrotizing and crescentic GN and in patients with microscopic polyarteritis nodosa. Patients with sinus involvement (Wegener's granulomatosis) commonly have C-ANCA, although there is a great deal of overlap. Because of the success in treatment of Wegener's granulomatosis with cytotoxic agents such as cyclophosphamide and steroids, many patients with ANCA-positive pauci-immune GN receive a similar type of treatment, although the duration of treatment with cyclophosphamide has been subject to considerable debate.

NEPHROTIC SYNDROME

The nephrotic syndrome is characterized by the presence of proteinuria, hypoalbuminemia, edema, hyperlipiduria, and hyperlipidemia. However, the finding of proteinuria of > 3.5 gm/24 hr/1.73 m², so-called nephrotic-range proteinuria, is sufficient for the designation of nephrotic syndrome. Table 27–5 includes the renal lesions commonly associated with the nephrotic syndrome. They are divided into diseases with or without RBC casts ("bland" or "active" urine sediment). Each of these entities may occur as a primary renal lesion or as a secondary component of a systemic disease.

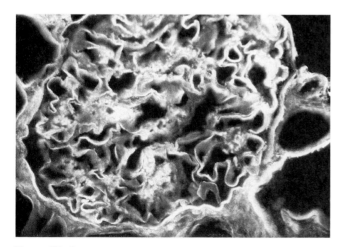

Figure 27–5
Immunofluorescence demonstrating a linear pattern of IgG.

TABLE 27–5	Glomerulopathies Associated with Nephrotic Syndrome

Nephrotic-Range Proteinuria with "Bland" Urine Sediment (Pure Nephrotic)

Primary glomerular disease
    Minimal change nephrotic syndrome (nil lesion, lipoid nephrosis)
    Membranous glomerulopathy
    Focal glomerulosclerosis
Secondary glomerular disease
    Diabetic nephropathy (Kimmelsteil-Wilson glomerulosclerosis)
    Amyloidosis

Nephrotic-Range Proteinuria with "Active" Urine Sediment ("Mixed," Nephrotic/Nephritic)

Primary glomerular disease
    Membranoproliferative glomerulopathy, types I, II, III
Secondary glomerular disease
    Membranoproliferative glomerulopathy
    Systemic lupus erythematosus
    Henoch-Schönlein purpura
    Mixed essential cryoglobulinemia

Nephrotic Syndrome with "Bland" Urine Sediment

Minimal Change Nephrotic Syndrome (MCNS)

This disorder is also known as nil lesion or lipoid nephrosis; more than 85 to 90% of all children with nephrotic syndrome have this condition. It almost always presents as the sudden onset of the nephrotic syndrome in children aged 2 to 6 years with a male-female ratio of 2:1. In adults, MCNS accounts for only 15 to 20%, with a more equal male-female ratio. As children approach teenage years and early adulthood, the incidence of MCNS as a cause of nephrotic syndrome diminishes, unless an associated hematologic neoplasm is present. Some adults with malignant neoplasms have developed MCNS, most commonly in association with Hodgkin's disease.

Laboratory features include those of the typical nephrotic syndrome with bland urinary sediment, normal renal function (unless there is severe volume contraction), and normal complement levels. Histologically, the light microscopy is normal (hence the term *nil lesion*) and no immunoglobulins or complement deposition is seen. Electron microscopy reveals effacement (fusion) of the foot processes, which is the result of the proteinuria (see Fig. 27–1).

The natural course of MCNS in children includes a spontaneous remission rate in more than 40 to 50% of cases. However, owing to the sensitivity of the proteinuria to steroid therapy, many patients are given a trial of 60 mg/m²/day in children and 1.5 to 2 mg/kg/day in adults. At 4 weeks (or sooner, if remission occurs), alternate-day therapy with 35 mg/m² in children and 0.9 mg/kg in adults is begun and continued for 4 more weeks, with a tapering regimen given over the next 4 to 6 months. Eighty-five to 90% of all patients with MCNS respond to this protocol (usually by the fourth week in children and the eighth week in adults). Adults older than 40 may require 16 to 20 weeks of steroid therapy before a complete remission occurs. Following development of a complete remission, 40 to 50% remain free of proteinuria or have infrequent relapses. The remainder become "frequent" relapsers (more than twice a year) or steroid dependent. These patients may benefit from adjunctive therapy with cytotoxic alkylating agents such as chlorambucil (0.15 to 0.2 mg/kg/day) or cyclophosphamide (2.0 mg/kg/day) for 8 to 12 weeks. However, there are significant risks associated with the use of these agents, including gonadal failure and carcinogenesis, particularly with long-term use or in combination with corticosteroids. Recent studies indicate that cyclosporine therapy is of value in selected patients and may induce prolonged remissions in steroid-resistant patients.

About three fourths of individuals are disease free at 10 years, with a 10-year survival rate of 95%. Patients show an increased risk of infection (particularly pneumococcus and *Haemophilus* infection) and thrombosis of renal and peripheral veins. The development of chronic renal failure due to MCNS is essentially nonexistent. Patients failing to respond to steroids are generally found to have another glomerulopathy, most often focal glomerulosclerosis.

Focal Glomerulosclerosis (FGS)

Focal glomerulosclerosis accounts for 10 to 15% of children and 15 to 20% of adults with idiopathic nephrotic syndrome (Table 27–6). Although heavy proteinuria and edema are usually present at onset, some patients have asymptomatic proteinuria and hematuria. Hypertension, azotemia, and microscopic hematuria are commonly found at the time of diagnosis. Serum complement levels are normal.

Light microscopy reveals focal and segmental collapse of capillary loops and mesangial sclerosis sometimes associated with hyalin insudation at the edge of the sclerotic focus. Proliferation or infiltration is absent. Focal mild tubular drop-out with interstitial fibrosis is often present. Patchy deposition of IgM, C3, and occasionally other immunoreactants is seen in the segmental sclerotic foci, but the etiologic significance of these findings is unknown. Electron-dense deposits are typically absent by electron microscopy. Patients with acquired immunodeficiency syndrome (AIDS)–related FGS often show numerous tuboreticular structures within the endothelial cytoplasm—collections of microtubules that apparently form in response to elevated serum levels of interferon. Such structures are also very common in biopsies of patients with SLE.

Approximately 30% of patients respond to steroid therapy with a lasting remission and good long-term renal function. But most (60 to 70%), particularly those with persistent nephrotic syndrome, progress to chronic renal failure (55% by 10 years). The remainder follow a long-term course with relapses and remissions and late onset of renal failure. Recurrence of FGS in transplants occurs in as many as 40% of patients.

Heroin abusers and patients with AIDS may develop the nephrotic syndrome and the histologic lesion of FGS. These patients typically follow a much more rapid downhill course, often with progression to ESRF in less than 1 year. A variant of FGS known as "collapsing glomerulopathy" is a distinct entity characterized by black racial predominance, massive proteinuria, relatively rapidly progressive renal insufficiency, and distinctive pathologic findings. Although collapsing glomerulopathy resembles hu-

TABLE 27–6	Features of Focal Segmental Glomerulosclerosis

Nephrotic-range proteinuria with "bland" urinary sediment
Focal, segmental collapse of capillary loops and mesangial sclerosis with hyaline droplets
Etiology
   Idiopathic
      "Collapsing" glomerulonephritis
     Secondary
        Heroin
        Acquired immunodeficiency syndrome (AIDS)
        Reflux nephropathy

man immunodeficiency virus (HIV) nephropathy both pathologically and clinically, it differs clinically by having no evidence for associated-HIV infection and differs pathologically by lacking endothelial, tubuloreticular inclusions.

Membranous Glomerulopathy (MGN) (Table 27–7)

Membranous glomerulopathy typically follows a slowly progressive course with intermittent remissions and exacerbations. Spontaneous complete remissions occur in as many as 25% of patients, with another 20 to 25% experiencing a partial remission (proteinuria <2 gm but >200 mg/day). These patients may maintain a stable GFR for decades. The remaining 50% progress to end-stage renal failure (ESRF) by 5 to 10 years.

Treatment of membranous nephropathy is controversial. At this time, it is reasonable to suggest or recommend that patients with a favorable long-term prognosis (e.g., children, adults with non–nephrotic-range proteinuria) need not receive specific treatment. Similarly, adult patients, particularly women younger than 40 years old with nephrotic syndrome but with normal renal function and modest degree of proteinuria (<9 gm/day), could be managed conservatively, without steroids or cytotoxic agents, and observed for either spontaneous remission or progression. Patients with persisting severe proteinuria (>9 gm/day), particularly men older than 40 years, with symptomatic nephrotic syndrome or progressive renal failure, may be treated best by a combination of cytotoxic drugs, such as oral methylprednisone and chlorambucil used sequentially over a 6-month period. This treatment may improve the likelihood of remission and decrease the incidence of chronic renal failure.

Diabetic Nephropathy

Diabetic nephropathy is the single most important cause of end-stage renal disease (ESRD) in the United States, with diabetic patients accounting for approximately 35% of all patients enrolled in the ESRD program. The cumulative incidence of nephropathy is 30 to 50% in insulin-dependent diabetes mellitus (IDDM) and 10 to 15%

TABLE 27–7	Features of Membranous Glomerulopathy

Nephrotic-range proteinuria with "bland" urinary sediment
GBM thickening with "spike" formation, granular deposits of IgG and complement, subepithelial electron-dense deposits
Etiology
  Idiopathic
  Secondary
    Infections: syphilis, hepatitis B
    Neoplasms: carcinoma of the lung, stomach, breast
    Drugs: gold, D-penicillamine, captopril
    Collagen vascular diseases: systemic lupus erythematosus, rheumatoid arthritis, mixed connective tissue disease

GBM = Glomerular basement membrane.

in non–insulin-dependent diabetes mellitus (NIDDM), although certain populations of patients with NIDDM (for example, Pima Indians) have a higher incidence of nephropathy. Because of the high prevalence of NIDDM, it contributes a significant portion of patients with ESRD. Currently available data strongly support the concept that diabetic nephropathy is a direct result of the metabolic derangements seen in diabetics and that normalization of carbohydrate metabolism would be protective against the development of renal disease. In early diabetes, some of the biochemical alterations can lead to hyperfiltration with the GFR elevated above normal by 20 to 30%.

Diabetic nephropathy is a clinical syndrome characterized by persistent albuminuria (>300 mg/24 hr), a relentless decline in GFR, and raised arterial blood pressure. Nephropathy is rare during the first 5 years of diabetes, after which the incidence increases until it reaches a peak at approximately 15 years of diabetes. Several studies have suggested that microalbuminuria, being defined as a urinary albumin excretion rate >30 mg/24 hr (20 μg/min) and ≤300 mg/24 hr (200 μg/min), strongly predicts the development of diabetic nephropathy in both IDDM and NIDDM. Approximately 1 to 5 years after the onset of microalbuminuria, proteinuria increases and can be detected by protein dipstick measurement on routine urinalysis. This increment in proteinuria is associated with a significant risk for the development or worsening of existing hypertension and progressive decline in renal function. The rate at which patients with proteinuria progress is highly variable, but untreated, the GFR may decrease at an average rate of 1 ml/min/mo. It should be noted that a high percentage of patients with NIDDM (in contrast to IDDM) have modest proteinuria and hypertension when initially seen, indicating that other diseases may be responsible for the renal damage. Indeed, renal biopsy studies have shown that about one third of the patients with NIDDM have nephropathy that is not related to their diabetes. In addition, whereas diabetic retinopathy is found in >90% of patients with IDDM, nearly one third of the patients with proven diabetic nephropathy have no evidence of retinopathy. Regardless, the absence of retinopathy and/or renal insufficiency without proteinuria, presence of RBC casts, and low levels of complement should lead to a search for other causes of renal disease.

Kimmelstiel-Wilson nodular glomerulosclerosis, although the classic diabetic glomerular lesion, is found in only 15 to 20% of patients with diabetic nephropathy. It consists of a nodular increase in hyaline material massively expanding the mesangial areas surrounded by dilated and uniformly thickened capillary loops. The nodular foci have a focal and segmental distribution. The more common lesion is that of diffuse glomerulosclerosis, a uniform increase in hyaline material within the mesangial areas associated with capillary loop changes described previously. Hyaline arteriolosclerosis involving both the afferent and efferent arterioles, as well as tubulointerstitial atrophy and fibrosis, accompanies both the nodular and the diffuse forms of diabetic glomerulosclerosis. The insudative lesions—capsular drops and fibrin caps—consist of small, eosinophilic droplets on the parietal side of Bowman's capsule or the inner surface of a capillary loop, respectively. The presence of linear deposition of IgG along the capillary walls, as well as focal, segmental deposition of IgM and C3, is nonspecific and is thought to represent passive trapping.

The major therapeutic interventions in diabetic nephropathy include vigorous control of blood sugar, antihypertensive treatment, and restriction of dietary proteins. Strict control of blood glucose prevents diabetic microangiopathic lesions in experimental animals, and evidence is accumulating that euglycemia in humans with early diabetes has similar effects. Meticulous control of hypertension slows the rate of decline in GFR. In addition, a growing body of evidence suggests that angiotensin-converting enzyme (ACE) inhibitors have a more marked antiproteinuric effect than other antihypertensive agents. Studies are currently under way to determine whether they also uniquely or disproportionately spare glomerular function. Thus, the current practice seems to be the use of ACE inhibitors in patients with either incipient or overt diabetic nephropathy. Their use has also been recommended, although not proven, in patients who have microalbuminuria, even in the face of normal blood pressure. There is suggestive evidence that in patients with diabetic nephropathy, protein restriction reduces the progression of kidney disease.

Amyloidosis

Systemic amyloidosis is classified into four types according to the chemical composition of fibrillar deposits, which correspond to clinical patterns termed primary, secondary, hereditary, and dialysis associated. The most common form in the United States is primary or AL, which is a plasma cell dyscrasia. Secondary amyloidosis, which develops after chronic inflammatory or infectious disease has deposits composed of AA proteins. There are several autosomal dominant hereditary forms of which the most well known is familial amyloidotic polyneuropathy. The fourth form occurs in chronic hemodialysis patients, where the amyloid fibril is a beta$_2$-microglobulin. Up to 80% of patients with AL or AA forms of amyloidosis have renal involvement. Nephrotic syndrome is the initial feature in 75% of patients with secondary amyloidosis and in approximately 25% of patients with primary amyloidosis and is a rare complication of familial amyloidosis. Diagnosis is often not suspected on clinical grounds and is made when a patient undergoes renal biopsy for nephrotic syndrome (Fig. 27–6).

There are no reliable biochemical tests for diagnosis, and definitive diagnosis must be made by tissue biopsy. Most patients with primary and 65% of patients with secondary amyloidosis have a positive abdominal fat aspirate. It is positive in only a minority of patients with dialysis-associated amyloidosis. Even when amyloid is known to be present, a kidney biopsy may be necessary to make a definitive diagnosis and to rule out other diseases. There are no specific treatments for amyloidosis. In patients with primary amyloidosis, colchicine, melphalan, and prednisone have been used. Colchicine is the drug of choice in patients with amyloidosis secondary to familial Mediterranean fever.

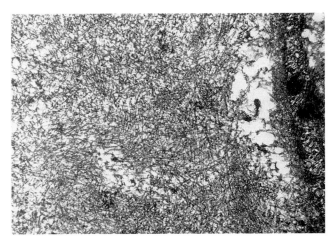

Figure 27–6
Electron micrograph demonstrating the nonbranching fibrils characteristic of amyloidosis.

Nephrotic Syndrome with "Active" Urine Sediment

Many patients present with pure nephrotic syndrome. However, a variety of patients with glomerular diseases present with a "mixed" pattern of nephrotic/nephritic syndrome, including the various forms of membranoproliferative glomerulopathy as well as SLE, Henoch-Schönlein purpura, and mixed essential cryoglobulinemia.

Types of Membranoproliferative Glomerulopathy (MPGN)

Membranoproliferative glomerulopathy is a disease of young people, with most cases diagnosed in those between the ages of 5 and 30 years. Overall, MPGN accounts for 10 to 15% of all cases of idiopathic nephrotic syndrome. The clinical manifestations are variable, with around 50% presenting with nephrotic syndrome, 25 to 30% with asymptomatic proteinuria, and 15 to 20% with acute nephritic syndrome. Regardless of the major pattern, concurrent hematuria and proteinuria are almost always present. Serum C3 levels are depressed in more than 70% of patients at disease onset. Thus, MPGN must be differentiated from other forms of GN showing hypocomplementemia (Table 27–8).

Membranoproliferative glomerulopathy is characterized overall by thickening of capillary loops and mesangial hypercellularity, often with lobular accentuation. Several subtypes exist. Type I MPGN has subendothelial deposits with mesangial interposition producing capillary loop splitting (see Fig. 27–1). Type II (dense deposit disease, DDD) has characteristic broad, very electron-dense deposits widening the GBM. Immunofluorescence examination of both types I and II reveals extensive granular C3 deposition in the capillary loops, usually with absence of immunoglobulins. There are several different morphologic variants with features similar to either type I or II MPGN that have been reported as type III MPGN.

The pathogenesis is unknown, although the associa-

TABLE 27-8 Features of Membranoproliferative Glomerulopathy

Nephrotic-range proteinuria with "active" urinary sediment
  Idiopathic
    Type I: Mesangial hypercellularity and capillary loop "splitting"
    Type II: Mesangial hypercellularity with GBM "dense deposits"
    Type III: Morphologic variants
      Type I changes plus subepithelial deposits
      Changes intermediate between type I and type II
  Associated with other diseases (secondary)
    Hepatitis C and B
    Systemic lupus erythematosus
    Essential mixed cryoglobulinemia
    Sickle cell disease
    Partial lipodystrophy (type II)

GBM = Glomerular basement membrane.

tion of MPGN with alterations in complement activation suggests a pathogenetic link. The presence of C3 nephritic factor is most likely an associated event rather than a cause of MPGN, and its presence does not appear to alter the prognosis.

Membranoproliferative glomerulopathy is a slow but progressive disease, with approximately 30% of patients in chronic renal failure at the end of 10 years. Poor prognostic indicators include the presence of nephrotic syndrome or azotemia at the time of diagnosis. Spontaneous remission of proteinuria occasionally occurs but does not usually affect the long-term outcome. There is currently no consensus on any given therapeutic regimen that is both safe and effective in MPGN, although a combination of steroid and cytotoxic drug therapy or antiplatelet agents have been used.

Type II MPGN recurs in virtually 100% of renal transplants, but recurrence is far less common in type I MPGN (about 25%). However, recurrence does not interfere with long-term graft survival.

Systemic Lupus Erythematosus (SLE) GN

Systemic lupus erythematosus is primarily a disease of young women, although it may occur in both sexes at any age. It accounts for approximately 5 to 10% of patients with nephrotic syndrome, and it can be the presenting manifestation of a patient with SLE without any other systemic manifestations. It should be suspected in any individual, especially a young woman, who presents with proteinuria accompanied by hematuria, especially when accompanied by low levels of complement. Renal disease may be the presenting feature of a patient with SLE. Diagnosis rests on serologic evidence of antinuclear antibody production in the presence of inflammation of multiple organs. Clinical evidence of renal disease is present in as many as 85 to 90% of SLE patients, varying from minimal changes to nephritic and/or nephrotic syndrome. Virtually all patients are found to have renal injury if a kidney biopsy is performed. The nephrotic syndrome with a "nephritic" sediment is most common, and 10 to 15% of patients also have azotemia. Serum complement levels are usually low during periods of active renal disease. A small number of patients present with RPGN. Renal function deteriorates over a matter of weeks, and numerous cellular crescents are seen on renal biopsy.

The clinical presentation and the severity of renal disease correlate with the underlying histopathology, best classified using the World Health Organization scheme (Table 27–9). Essentially, these categories can be grouped as proliferative (types II, III, IV) or membranous (type V) glomerulopathies, with greater proliferation (type IV) associated with poorer prognosis. Multiple immunoglobulins and various components of complement are almost invariably present within the glomeruli and may involve all levels of the GBM as well as the mesangium (Fig. 27–7; also see Fig. 27–1). It has been suggested that the presence and amount of subendothelial deposits seen by electron microscopy are good predictors of progression.

The treatment of lupus nephritis is controversial, but patients with class I and II disease do not need any treatment directed at the renal lesions. Therapy should be dictated by the extrarenal manifestations. Patients with definite but mild to moderate renal disease accompanied by focal glomerular lesions detected by light microscopy may be managed by the lowest possible dose of steroids and observed carefully for the development of more diffuse renal disease. Several long-range studies of patients with diffuse proliferative GN (class IV) have suggested that the addition of cytotoxic drugs to a regimen of pred-

TABLE 27-9 Histologic Class, Clinical Presentation, and Prognosis in SLE Nephritis

Histologic Type	WHO Class	Frequency (%)*	Proteinuria (%)	Nephrotic Syndrome (%)†	Azotemia (%)‡
Normal	I	<5			
Mesangial	II	15	70	0	~10
Focal proliferative	III	20	100	15	~20
Diffuse proliferative	IV	50	100	~90	75
Membranous	V	15	100	~90	20

* Percent of patients with SLE who show this lesion on biopsy.
† Proteinuria exceeding 3.0 gm/24 hr.
‡ Serum creatinine exceeding 1.2 mg/dl or BUN exceeding 25 mg/dl.
BUN = Blood urea nitrogen; SLE = systemic lupus erythematosus; WHO = World Health Organization.
Adapted from Couser WG: Glomerular disorders. *In* Wyngaarden JB, Smith LH Jr (eds.): Cecil Textbook of Medicine. 19th ed., Philadelphia, WB Saunders, 1992, p 566.

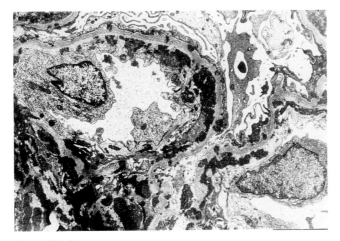

Figure 27–7

Electron micrograph from a patient with SLE with *(a)* massive subendothelial deposits, *(b)* a few subepithelial deposits, and *(c)* mesangial deposits.

nisone may offer benefit in these patients with SLE by providing a better preservation of renal function.

Patients with SLE tolerate dialysis about as well as patients with non-SLE renal failure. Indeed, for reasons that are not yet understood, SLE patients who are placed on chronic dialysis often note dramatic amelioration of other manifestations of SLE. Renal transplantation is also as well tolerated, with recurrence of SLE GN being relatively rare.

Henoch-Schönlein Purpura (HSP)

Henoch-Schönlein purpura is seen most often in children (boys more than girls) and is characterized by purpuric lesions on the buttocks and legs, episodic abdominal pain, arthralgias, fever, malaise, and proteinuria (often nephrotic range) with hematuria and RBC casts. Serum C3 levels are typically normal, although CH_{50} may be low.

The glomeruli reveal varying degrees of mesangial hypercellularity and crescent formation, with the prognosis declining as the proliferation increases. Uncommonly, exuberant crescent formation occurs associated with a rapid progression to renal failure. IgA and C3 staining of the mesangium is prominent with numerous mesangial electron-dense deposits seen by electron microscopy. Immunofluorescence examination of lesions or of unaffected skin shows IgA and C3 within dermal capillaries.

Henoch-Schönlein purpura tends toward a benign, self-limited course of remission and relapse, usually disappearing after a few months to years. More than half of the patients recover completely from their renal injury, but about 10% progress to ESRD. Persistent nephrotic syndrome, acute nephritic syndrome at onset, and older age suggest a poor prognosis. Therapy is ineffective against the renal manifestations of HSP, although patients with extensive crescent formation should be managed aggressively. Recurrence is uncommon in renal transplants.

Essential Mixed Cryoglobulinemia

Mixed cryoglobulins composed of monoclonal IgM rheumatoid factor and polyclonal IgG are characteristic of a disorder called essential mixed cryoglobulinemia. It occurs usually in middle age, affecting women slightly more than men, and presents with purpura, fever, Raynaud's phenomenon, arthralgias, and weakness. Renal manifestations are seen in 40 to 50% of patients and vary from proteinuria and/or hematuria to acute nephritic syndrome. Many patients are hypocomplementemic with a decrease in early complement components such as C4 and normal levels of C3. Thus, the presence of palpable purpura in a patient with proteinuria and hematuria with high titers of rheumatoid factor with or without low levels of C4 is highly suggestive of the diagnosis of essential mixed cryoglobinemia. The glomeruli show a diffuse proliferative glomerulonephritis with intraluminal hyaline thrombi. IgG, IgM, and C3 are usually present in subendothelial areas and the mesangium.

It has been estimated that about 50% of patients with essential mixed IgG-IgM cryoglobinemia have underlying chronic hepatitis C virus infection. Anti–hepatitis C viral antibody, hepatitis C viral core antigens, and hepatitis C RNA can be found in the cryoglobulins and in the renal deposits of patients with hepatitis C virus infection associated with mixed cryoglobinemia. All patients should be screened for the presence of hepatitis C, and in those patients who demonstrate the presence of hepatitis C, alpha-interferon therapy should be considered. Patients with renal insufficiency or acute nephritic syndrome usually progress to ESRF. However, the overall survival rate in HSP patients with renal manifestations is about 75%. Plasmapheresis to decrease the circulating cryoprecipitates may improve the prognosis of patients with severe renal HSP.

ASYMPTOMATIC URINARY ABNORMALITIES

A variety of renal lesions may present as either isolated proteinuria or hematuria, with or without proteinuria (Table 27–10). Isolated proteinuria without hematuria is usually an incidental finding in an asymptomatic patient. These patients generally excrete less than 2 gm of protein per day with a bland urine sediment and have normal renal function. About 60% of these patients have so-

TABLE 27–10	Asymptomatic Urinary Abnormalities

Isolated Proteinuria

Proteinuria without hematuria
Postural proteinuria

Isolated Hematuria (with or Without Proteinuria)

IgA nephropathy (Berger's disease)
Hereditary nephritis
   Alport's syndrome
   Thin basement membrane disease
Benign recurrent hematuria

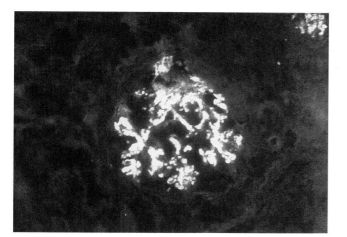

Figure 27–8
Immunofluorescence demonstrating the mesangial distribution of IgA.

called postural proteinuria, with absence of proteinuria while lying flat and return of proteinuria upon standing. The long-term outcome of isolated proteinuria (postural or nonpostural) is excellent, with the majority of patients experiencing a steady decline in protein excretion. However, in some patients, this condition represents a very early manifestation of a more serious glomerular disease such as MGN, IgA nephropathy, focal glomerulosclerosis, diabetic nephropathy, or amyloidosis. Finally, it should be noted that mild proteinuria may accompany a febrile illness, congestive heart failure, or infectious diseases.

Hematuria with or without proteinuria in an otherwise asymptomatic patient may represent the fortuitous early discovery of another glomerular disease such as SLE, Henoch-Schönlein purpura, postinfectious GN, or idiopathic hypercalciuria in children. However, asymptomatic hematuria is also the primary presenting manifestation of a number of specific glomerular diseases discussed later.

IgA Nephropathy (Berger's Disease)

This disease, characterized by mesangial IgA deposits (Fig. 27–8), is the final diagnosis in as many as 50% of patients with asymptomatic hematuria. It has become the most common cause of primary glomerular disease in the United States and Europe. The typical presentation is gross hematuria following a viral illness, with men affected two to three times more frequently than women and whites much more commonly affected than blacks. Most other patients present with asymptomatic hematuria discovered on an incidental examination, accompanied by mild to moderate proteinuria. Most patients are between the ages of 15 and 35. Microscopic hematuria usually remains after the gross hematuria resolves. Mild proteinuria of less than 1 gm/day is common, but nephrotic-range proteinuria may be seen in as many as 10% of patients. Serum complement is normal.

Light microscopic changes vary from normal glomeruli (grade I), through mesangial hypercellularity (grade II), to a mixed group of abnormalities including segmental sclerosis, crescent formation, tubular atrophy, and interstitial fibrosis (grade III). Mesangial deposits of IgA, even in glomeruli unaffected when judged by light microscopy, are characteristic of this disease (see Fig. 27–1); some patients also have IgG and C3 deposition.

Progressive renal insufficiency develops in 20 to 30% of patients after 20 years. Some have a more rapid progression, with renal failure in as little as 4 years. Poor prognostic indicators include nephrotic-range proteinuria, hypertension, and the higher-grade renal biopsy changes. No effective therapy is currently available. Mesangial IgA deposits recur frequently in renal transplants but with minimal long-term effects on function.

Hereditary Nephritis (Alport's Syndrome)

This disorder usually presents in childhood with recurrent gross hematuria, with or without vague lower back or abdominal pain. Mild proteinuria is often present, but nephrotic syndrome is rare. Sensorineural deafness is present in about 50% of the patients. Family history may reveal any of the number of different patterns, although most pedigrees show some X linkage. Males are usually more affected than females and often develop renal failure by age 30. Light microscopy reveals nonspecific interstitial foam cells, and immunofluorescence is negative for immunoglobulins and complement. The diagnostic ultrastructural abnormalities include alternating areas of thinned and thickened capillary loops with lamination and splitting of the GBM.

No effective treatment is currently available. It has been demonstrated that the GBM in patients with Alport's syndrome does not react with anti-GBM antibody, implying a lack of certain GBM antigens. Therefore, although Alport's syndrome does not recur in renal transplants, allografts may develop anti-GBM antibody GN owing to the presence of GBM antigens for which the recipient lacks immune "tolerance."

Thin Basement Membrane Disease

This condition affects both sexes equally and often occurs in families without an X-linked pattern. The disease usually presents as microscopic hematuria without proteinuria in an otherwise asymptomatic young adult. Light and immunofluorescence examination are normal, whereas ultrastructural examination demonstrates the markedly thinned GBM. Prognosis is excellent, although a few patients with progressive renal failure have been reported.

Benign Recurrent Hematuria

This diagnosis is given to those with asymptomatic hematuria when the other possibilities are excluded. The majority of these patients are young adults found to have microscopic hematuria on routine examination or with gross hematuria associated with a febrile illness, exercise, or immunization. Renal biopsy is normal in most but may show focal or diffuse mesangial proliferation. Immunofluorescence is sometimes negative but may show mesangial deposits of IgM or IgG with C3 or C3 alone. Ultrastructural studies are equally variable, with many reports of normal glomeruli, although electron-dense deposits have been seen in GBM and/or mesangium in some patients. Overall the prognosis is excellent, with as many as 50% in complete remission at 5 years and only a few with declining renal function.

CHRONIC GLOMERULONEPHRITIS (CGN)

Chronic glomerulonephritis is the culmination of many different glomerular diseases associated with the progressive loss of functioning nephrons. At the earliest time points, only mild proteinuria with a slight decrease in GFR and minimal hypertension may be seen. Inevitably, these patients generally progress to ESRD (see Chapter 31). The differentiation of these patients from those with nonglomerular disorders such as hypertensive nephrosclerosis is usually difficult. The presence of heavy proteinuria and/or glomerular bleeding suggests glomerulonephritis. Unfortunately, these patients usually present in a more advanced stage, and the correct diagnosis is never ascertained.

REFERENCES

Couser WG: Glomerular disorders. *In* Wyngaarden JB, Smith LH Jr (eds.): Cecil Textbook of Medicine. 19th ed. Philadelphia, WB Saunders, 1992, pp 551–568.

Couser WG: Glomerular and vascular diseases. *In* Jacobson HR, Striker GE, Klahr S (eds.): The Principles and Practice of Nephrology. 2nd ed. St. Louis, Mosby–Year Book Inc., 1995, pp 102–200.

Glassock RJ, Cohen AH, Adler SG: Primary glomerular diseases. *In* Brenner BM (ed.): The Kidney. 5th ed. Philadelphia, WB Saunders, 1996, pp 1392–1497.

Glassock RJ, Cohen AH, Adler SG: Secondary glomerular diseases. *In* Brenner BM (ed.): The Kidney. 5th ed. Philadelphia, WB Saunders, 1996, pp 1498–1596.

Shah SV (ed.): Mechanisms of glomerular injury. Semin Nephrol 1991; 11:253–372.

28

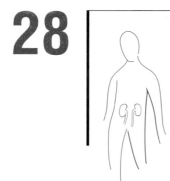

Major Nonglomerular Disorders

TUBULOINTERSTITIAL NEPHROPATHY

Tubulointerstitial nephropathy encompasses a group of clinical disorders that affect the renal tubules and interstitium principally, with relative sparing of the glomeruli and renal vasculature. In the majority of cases of interstitial nephropathy, the disease can be placed into one of two categories on the basis of the rate of progression of the azotemia: (1) acute interstitial nephritis (AIN), causing a rapid (days to weeks) decline in renal function and characterized histologically by an acute inflammatory infiltrate, or (2) chronic interstitial nephropathy, causing a slowly progressive (years) azotemia characterized histologically by predominantly interstitial scarring and fibrosis with a variable but less impressive amount of round-cell infiltration.

AIN

Acute interstitial nephritis is a clinicopathologic syndrome that is characterized by the sudden onset of clinical signs of renal dysfunction associated with a prominent inflammatory cell infiltrate within the renal interstitium. It is an important cause of acute renal failure (ARF) and may account for as many as 10 to 20% of ARF cases.

Etiology

The most common causes of AIN are listed in Table 28–1. Recently the best-documented cases of AIN have resulted from complication of therapy with a wide variety of drugs, especially antibiotics and nonsteroidal anti-inflammatory drugs. Septicemia of any cause can result in AIN, but certain infectious agents such as leptospirosis, legionnaires' disease, and mononucleosis appear to have a particular predilection for causing AIN.

Acute pyelonephritis is classified in histologic grounds as a form of AIN. The mechanism for the nephritis is direct bacterial invasion of the renal medulla, in contrast to the allergic forms of AIN described previously. The clinical manifestations are predominantly those of infection, fever, chills, and flank pain, and acute pyelonephritis only rarely causes ARF.

Severe glomerulonephritis, although sometimes ac-

companied by an interstitial inflammatory infiltrate, is generally excluded from classifications of AIN. In some patients, such as those with systemic lupus erythematosus (SLE), interstitial inflammation may be out of proportion to the degree of glomerular injury, and interstitial nephritis is the predominant finding.

Clinical Features

The major clinical manifestation of AIN is the development of acute renal insufficiency. Many patients develop some combination of fever, skin rash, peripheral eosinophilia, and arthralgias, particularly in the course of AIN due to drugs. The absence of any or all of these features is common and therefore does not preclude the diagnosis of AIN. Hypertension and edema, important features of acute glomerulonephritis, are uncommon in AIN.

Acute interstitial nephritis is often accompanied by signs of renal inflammation, and urinary abnormalities often provide the first clue to the diagnosis of AIN in a patient with ARF. Hematuria, often macroscopic, is common when AIN is caused by drugs, as are sterile pyuria and leukocyte casts. Eosinophiluria is highly suggestive of AIN but is not often observed. Wright's stain test of the urine is necessary to demonstrate eosinophils. Red blood cell (RBC) casts have been found on rare occasions to be associated with AIN and may make the presentation indistinguishable from that of glomerulonephritis. Mild to moderate proteinuria is present in the majority of patients.

Drug-induced AIN is treated by discontinuing the offending drug. Another appropriate drug can be substituted in cases of underlying infection. In the majority of cases, this results in restoration of renal function within several weeks. A short course of high-dose corticosteroids (1 mg/kg/day of prednisone for 1 to 2 weeks) may accelerate recovery, but the added risk in patients with underlying infections must be weighed against possible benefits, especially because the latter have not been established unambiguously.

Chronic Tubulointerstitial Nephropathy

Chronic tubulointerstitial nephropathy is a clinicopathologic entity characterized clinically by slowly progressive

TABLE 28-1	Causes of Acute Interstitial Nephritis
Drug related	Antimicrobial drugs
	Penicillins (especially methicillin)
	Rifampin
	Sulfonamides
	Ciprofloxacin
	Cephalosporins
	Nonsteroidal anti-inflammatory drugs
	Allopurinol
	Sulfonamide diuretics
Systemic infections	Legionnaires' disease
	Leptospirosis
	Streptococcal infections
	Cytomegalovirus
	Infectious mononucleosis
Primary renal infections	Acute bacterial pyelonephritis
Immune disorders	Transplant rejection
	Systemic lupus erythematosus
Idiopathic	

renal insufficiency, non–nephrotic-range proteinuria, and functional tubular defects and pathologically by interstitial fibrosis with atrophy and loss of renal tubules. Chronic interstitial nephropathy is an important cause of chronic renal failure and appears to be responsible for 15 to 30% of all end-stage renal disease (ESRD).

Diagnosis and Clinical Features

Chronic tubulointerstitial nephropathy is characterized by tubular defects disproportionately severe relative to the degree of azotemia, as well as the absence of manifestations (RBC casts or the nephrotic syndrome) characteristic of glomerular disease (Table 28–2). Most patients with chronic interstitial nephropathy have little or no clinical evidence of active renal inflammation. The urinalysis may show modest pyuria and minimal hematuria, but in most cases there are no cellular casts.

Certain causes of chronic interstitial nephritis dam-

TABLE 28-2	Clinical Findings that Suggest Chronic Tubulointerstitial Disease

Hyperchloremic metabolic acidosis (out of proportion to the degree of renal insufficiency)
Hyperkalemia (out of proportion to the degree of renal insufficiency)
Reduced maximal urinary concentrating ability (polyuria, nocturia)
Partial or complete Fanconi's syndrome
  Phosphaturia
  Bicarbonaturia
  Aminoaciduria
  Uricosuria
  Glycosuria
Urinalysis
  May be normal but may contain cellular elements; absence of RBC casts
  Modest proteinuria (<2.0 gm/day); absence of nephrotic range proteinuria

RBC = Red blood cell.

age principally a specific segment of the nephron and thereby alter only those tubular functions that are normally ascribed to that segment. Conditions such as multiple myeloma or heavy metal toxicity, which affect primarily proximal tubule structures, may present with proximal renal tubular acidosis (RTA), glycosuria, aminoaciduria, and uricosuria. Distal RTA, salt wasting, and hyperkalemia are seen in patients with isolated distal tubular damage, as may occur with chronic obstruction or amyloidosis. Alternatively, patients with analgesic nephropathy, sickle cell disease, or polycystic kidney disease may present with a concentrating defect secondary to medullary involvement.

Specific Causes of Chronic Tubulointerstitial Disease (Table 28–3)

Urinary Tract Obstruction

Urinary tract obstruction is the single most important cause of chronic tubulointerstitial nephropathy and is discussed later in this chapter.

Chronic Pyelonephritis and Reflux Nephropathy

The term *chronic pyelonephritis* was used previously to describe what we currently call chronic tubulointerstitial nephropathy. The term is now specifically reserved for radiologic findings that demonstrate deformity of the pelvis and calyces typically most pronounced in the upper and lower poles. It is now generally accepted that bacteriuria alone is unlikely to result in chronic renal injury. The lesion of chronic pyelonephritis results from vesicoureteral reflux or urinary tract infection in association with obstruction. The development of heavy proteinuria is usually due to focal segmental sclerosis seen in association with reflux and is a poor prognostic sign.

Drugs

ANALGESIC NEPHROPATHY. Excessive consumption of certain analgesic agents such as phenacetin or acetaminophen (phenacetin is largely converted to acetaminophen), usually in combination with aspirin, may result in chronic interstitial nephritis. Analgesic nephropathy occurs more frequently in women (usually middle aged) who have ingested large quantities (>3 kg) of antipyretic-analgesic mixtures. Patients frequently do not report taking analgesics, so when the diagnosis is suspected, the possibility of analgesic nephropathy should be vigorously pursued. Emotional stress, neuropsychiatric disturbances, and gastrointestinal disturbances are commonly associated with analgesic nephropathy. Anemia is present in most patients and is frequently more severe than can be attributed to their degree of renal insufficiency, in part because of gastrointestinal blood loss. Sloughing of a necrotic papilla into the urinary tract may be associated with gross hema-

TABLE 28–3	Conditions Associated with Chronic Tubulointerstitial Nephropathy

Urinary tract obstuction
Drugs
    Analgesics/NSAIDs
    Nitrosurea
    Cisplatin
    Cyclosporin
    Lithium
Vascular diseases
    Nephrosclerosis
    Atheroembolic disease
Heavy metals
    Lead
    Cadmium
Metabolic disorders
    Hyperuricemia/hyperuricosuria
    Hypercalcemia/hypercalciuria
    Hyperoxaluria
    Potassium depletion
    Cystinosis
Hereditary diseases
    Medullary cystic disease
    Hereditary nephritis
    Polycystic kidney disease
    Sickle hemoglobinopathies
Malignancies and granulomatous diseases
    Multiple myeloma
    Sarcoidosis
    Tuberculosis
    Wegener's granulomatosis
Immunologic diseases
    Systemic lupus erythematosus
    Sjögren's syndrome
    Cryoglobulinemia
    Goodpasture's syndrome
    Vasculitis
    Amyloidosis
Other diseases
    Balkan nephropathy
    Radiation nephritis

NSAID = Nonsteroidal anti-inflammatory drug.

turia, flank pain (ureteral colic), passage of tissue in the urine, and an abrupt decline in renal function.

A variety of findings on intravenous urography or retrograde pyelography, including calyceal filling defects due to the presence of a sloughed papilla (ring sign), may suggest the diagnosis. Demonstration of papillary necrosis in the absence of other common causes (e.g., diabetes mellitus, urinary tract obstruction, often with infection, or sickle cell disease) should suggest analgesic nephropathy. Patients with analgesic nephropathy are at increased risk for development of transitional cell carcinoma of the urinary tract, particularly of the renal pelvis. The appearance of hematuria should lead to prompt evaluation to exclude a uroepithelial neoplasm. With cessation of analgesic use, renal function generally stabilizes or improves.

CYTOTOXIC AND IMMUNOSUPPRESSIVE AGENTS. Several agents such as cyclosporine, cisplatin, and nitrosoureas, which are more often associated with ARF, may also sometimes cause chronic tubulointerstitial nephropathy.

Vascular Diseases

HYPERTENSIVE NEPHROSCLEROSIS. The pathologic hallmark of benign nephrosclerosis is an arteriolopathy that is most pronounced in the interlobular and afferent arterioles. Interstitial and glomerular changes appear to result from the subsequent ischemia. Tubular atrophy and interstitial scarring may precede signs of glomerular injury in arteriolar nephrosclerosis.

RADIATION NEPHRITIS. Clinically evident renal injury is uncommon with less than 1000 to 2000 cGy but develops in approximately 50% of patients receiving higher doses. In the early stage of radiation nephritis, tubular necrosis, medial and intimal thickening of the small renal arteries, and damage to the glomerular endothelium are present. Later, glomerulosclerosis, collagenous thickening of the small renal arteries, and interstitial fibrosis are prominent. Evidence of renal damage occurs several months to years after renal irradiation. Manifestations range from mild proteinuria, urinary concentrating defects, and benign hypertension with a reduced glomerular filtration rate (GFR) to malignant hypertension with end-stage renal failure (ESRF).

Heavy Metals

LEAD. Although occupational lead exposure has declined over the past several decades, environmental exposure to lead aerosols has markedly increased. Lead accumulates in tubule cells and causes proximal convoluted tubule cell injury, which may result in glycosuria and aminoaciduria and chronic interstitial disease. The presence of hypertension, gout ("saturnine" gout), and renal insufficiency in a patient should suggest the possibility of lead nephropathy. Disodium ethylenediaminetetra-acetic acid (EDTA) administration may be used to test for a lead burden.

Metabolic Abnormalities

Although prolonged hyperuricemia is associated with renal dysfunction, the role of chronic hyperuricemia in producing renal insufficiency is not clear. It has been suggested that the nephropathy seen in association with saturnine gout may actually be secondary to lead exposure, based on greater mobilization of lead following EDTA administration, or to the hypertension that often accompanies primary or secondary hyperuricemia.

Primary hyperoxaluria, enteric hyperoxaluria, and cystinosis, a recessively inherited disease, may result in ESRF from chronic interstitial nephritis. The major renal complication of chronic hypokalemia and hypercalcemia is nephrogenic (vasopressin-resistant) diabetes insipidus, which results in mild polyuria. Chronic hypercalcemia may result in nephrocalcinosis and chronic interstitial nephritis with reduced GFR that may be only slowly and incompletely reversible.

TABLE 28-4	Characteristics of Renal Cystic Disorders					
Feature	**Simple Cysts**	**ADPKD**	**ARPKD**	**ACKD**	**MCD**	**MSK**
Inheritance pattern	None	Autosomal dominant	Autosomal recessive	None	Often present, variable pattern	None
Incidence or prevalence	Common, increasing with age	1/200–1/1000	Rare	40% in dialysis patients	Rare	Common
Age of onset	Adult	Usually adults	Neonates, children	Older adults	Adolescents, young adults	Adults
Presenting symptoms	Incidental finding, hematuria	Pain, hematuria, infection, family screening	Abdominal mass, renal failure, failure to thrive	Hematuria	Polyuria, polydipsia, enuresis, renal failure, failure to thrive	Incidental, urinary tract infections, hematuria, renal calculi
Hematuria	Occurs	Common	Occurs	Occurs	Rare	Common
Recurrent infections	Rare	Common	Occurs	No	Rare	Common
Renal calculi	No	Common	No	No	No	Common
Hypertension	Rare	Common	Common	Present from underlying disease	Rare	No
Method of diagnosis	Ultrasound	Ultrasound, gene linkage analysis	Ultrasound	CT scan	None reliable	Excretory urogram
Renal size	Normal	Normal to very large	Large initially	Small to normal, occasionally large	Small	Normal

ACKD = acquired cystic kidney disease; ADPKD = autosomal dominant polycystic kidney disease; ARPKD = autosomal recessive polycystic kidney disease; CT = computed tomography; MCD = medullary cystic disease; MSK = medullary sponge kidney.
From Gabow PA: Cystic diseases of the kidney. *In* Wyngaarden JB, Smith LH Jr, Bennett JC (eds.): Cecil Textbook of Medicine. 19th ed. Philadelphia, WB Saunders, 1992, p 609.

Malignancies

Renal involvement is common in patients with multiple myeloma, with progressive renal insufficiency seen in more than two thirds of patients. The so-called myeloma kidney (cast nephropathy) is characterized by laminated refractile tubular casts (surrounded by inflammatory cells and multinucleated giant cells) and by tubular atrophy and interstitial fibrosis. In those with kappa light chain disease, Fanconi's syndrome may precede the diagnosis of myeloma or the onset of renal insufficiency by many months. In 5 to 15% of cases of myeloma, patients develop nephrotic syndrome as a result of glomerular lesions (amyloidosis). In patients with lymphomas and leukemias, particularly acute lymphoblastic leukemia, neoplastic cells may infiltrate the renal interstitium and cause renal enlargement, but renal function is rarely compromised.

Immune Disorders

A variety of immune disorders may be associated with both acute and chronic interstitial nephritis, including several types of glomerulonephritis, chronic renal transplant rejection, and SLE. Renal involvement in Sjögren's syndrome is usually in the form of chronic interstitial nephritis. The most common functional abnormalities are distal RTA and urinary concentrating defects.

CYSTIC DISEASES OF THE KIDNEY

Renal cyst diseases are characterized by epithelium-lined cavities filled with fluid or semisolid debris within the kidneys. Certain clinical settings suggest specific cystic disorders (Table 28–4). An abdominal mass in a neonate or infant should suggest the possibility of either autosomal dominant polycystic kidney disease (ADPKD) or autosomal recessive polycystic kidney disease (ARPKD). Renal failure in adolescence suggests ARPKD or medullary cystic disease. The finding of a solitary cyst in a 50-year-old person is most compatible with a simple cyst. A history of renal disease in a family raises the possibility of ADPKD, ARPKD, or medullary cystic disease. Recurrent renal stones can occur in ADPKD or medullary sponge kidney. The onset of hematuria in a patient undergoing chronic hemodialysis may possibly indicate acquired cystic disease.

Simple Cysts

Simple renal cysts increase in frequency with age, being present in up to 50% of the population over 50 years of age. Simple cysts are most often asymptomatic and are usually discovered as an incidental finding during imaging studies. Renal ultrasonography, together with computed tomography (CT), permits accurate differentiation of benign from malignant lesions in most instances.

Polycystic Kidney Disease (PKD)

Polycystic kidney diseases include ADPKD, usually referred to as adult PKD, and ARPKD, often referred to as infantile or childhood PKD. ARPKD occurs in association with congenital hepatic fibrosis and causes death from renal failure in the first year of life.

Autosomal Dominant Polycystic Kidney Disease

Autosomal dominant PKD is the most common hereditary disease in the United States, affecting 500,000 people. The clinical disorder can be caused by at least two different genes. The most common type, ADPKD1, is carried on chromosome 16. The location of the other gene has not been determined. Complete penetrance of the gene is estimated to occur by 90 years of age.

Clinical manifestations of ADPKD rarely occur before the age of 20 to 25 years. This accounts for the frequent passage of the genetic trait to offspring by asymptomatic yet affected individuals of childbearing age. Patients usually present either for screening because of a family history of the disease or for evaluation of symptoms. Pain and hematuria are the most common clinical manifestations. Nonspecific, dull lumbar pain is a frequent symptom and usually occurs when the kidneys are sufficiently enlarged to be palpable on examination of the abdomen. Sharp, localized pain may result from cyst rupture or infection or from passage of a renal calculus. Microhematuria is frequently the initial sign of PKD; gross hematuria may also occur.

Hypertension, the most common cardiovascular manifestation of ADPKD, occurs in 60% of patients before the onset of renal insufficiency. Nocturia due to a urinary concentrating defect is often present at the time of diagnosis, and most patients show impaired salt conservation on a restricted salt intake. Urinary tract infection and pyelonephritis are common complications. Up to one third of patients with PKD have multiple, asymptomatic hepatic cysts; about 10% of the patients have cerebral aneurysms; and about 25% of all patients have mitral valve prolapse. The natural history of renal functional impairment with ADPKD is variable. The disease progresses to ESRF in about 25% of individuals by age 50 and in almost 50% by age 70.

The diagnosis of PKD is made on the basis of radiographic evidence of multiple cysts distributed throughout the renal parenchyma, in association with renal enlargement, increased cortical thickness, and elongation and splaying of the renal calyces. The demonstration of the characteristic bilateral renal cystic involvement is best accomplished by renal ultrasonography. In adults, CT scan with contrast medium occasionally reveals more cystic involvement than is apparent by ultrasonography. Imaging studies that reveal only a few cysts require differentiation of early ADPKD from multiple simple cysts. The presence of extrarenal involvement, particularly hepatic cysts, lends support to the diagnosis of ADPKD. The information on gene location now permits identification of presymptomatic carriers of ADPKD1 through gene linkage analysis. If there is a need for definitive diagnosis, this technique can be used in many families and can predict gene status with 99:1 likelihood. Because gene linkage is expensive, requires the cooperation of other family members, and supplies no anatomic information, it is probably best reserved for patients with nondiagnostic imaging studies.

The treatment for patients with ADPKD is aimed at preventing complications of the disease and preserving renal function. Patients and family members should be educated about the inheritance and manifestations of the disease. Therapy for PKD is directed toward control of hypertension and prevention and early treatment of urinary tract infections. ESRF is managed by either dialysis or transplantation. Bilateral nephrectomy may be required prior to transplantation in patients with inordinately large kidneys or those with a history of frequent or persistent urinary tract infection.

Acquired Cystic Kidney Disease

Acquired cystic kidney disease refers to the development of cysts in a large number of patients with ESRD undergoing dialysis. Occasionally, carcinomas complicate this disorder. Although the diagnosis can be established with ultrasonography, CT scan is the diagnostic method of choice in acquired cystic kidney disease because the kidneys and cysts are often small.

Medullary Cystic Disorders

Medullary cystic disease (nephrophthisis) occurs as a rare, autosomal recessive disease, sometimes accompanied by retinitis pigmentosa. Prolonged enuresis in childhood due to a urinary concentrating defect and anemia are early indications of the renal disease. Neither radiography nor renal biopsy has a high rate of success in demonstrating the small medullary cysts. Medullary cystic disease regularly results in ESRF during adolescence or early adulthood.

Medullary sponge kidney is a more common, benign disorder that is often detected incidentally on abdominal radiographs. Medullary sponge kidney is relatively common and often presents as a result of passage of a renal calculus. It is estimated that about 10% of patients who present with renal stones may have medullary sponge kidney. Nephrocalcinosis occurs in about half the patients and accounts for identification of asymptomatic patients on routine abdominal radiography. The diagnosis is made on intravenous pyelography (IVP) by the characteristic radial pattern ("bouquet of flowers," "paint brush") of contrast-filled medullary cysts. Treatment for urinary tract infection and renal calculus formation is indicated. Renal failure does not occur as part of the basic disease.

URINARY TRACT OBSTRUCTION

Obstruction to urine flow may occur at any point from the renal pelvis to the urethral meatus. The causes of obstruction are manifold but may be classified into the few general groups given in Table 28–5. The age and sex of the patient obviously influence the likelihood of a given pairing of etiology and site. Unilateral ureteral obstruction usually causes no detectable change in urinary flow or total renal function. Azotemia or renal failure occurs only if the drainage of both kidneys is significantly compromised. Total urinary tract obstruction is a significant cause of ESRF.

A change in urinary habits is often the presenting

TABLE 28-5	Causes of Urinary Tract Obstruction
Congenital urinary tract malformation	Meatal stenosis
	Ureterocele
	Posterior urethral valves
Intraluminal obstruction	Calculi
	Blood clots
	Sloughed papillary tissue
Extrinsic compression	Pelvic tumors
	Prostatic hypertrophy
	Retroperitoneal fibrosis
Acquired anomalies	Urethral strictures
	Neurogenic bladder
	Intratubular precipitates

sign of urinary tract obstruction. Complete obstruction is the most common cause of true anuria. However, polyuria, especially nocturia, is not uncommon in partial obstruction and may occur as a consequence of defective urinary concentration.

Urinary tract obstruction as a cause of renal failure must be sought in any patient who presents with renal failure of unknown etiology, especially in the absence of proteinuria. In addition, total anuria in a setting of acute renal failure or widely varying urine output is highly suggestive of urinary tract infection. Renal sonography is the preferred means of diagnosing urinary tract obstruction and depends on identification of hydronephrosis. Dilation of the urinary tract may not be evident within the first 24 hours of obstruction, in which case an IVP showing a prolonged nephrogram phase with delayed filling can provide valuable diagnostic information. A 24- or 48-hour film may show contrast medium concentrated either in dilated calyces or in the renal pelvis. Retrograde examination of the ureters is rarely required to make the diagnosis but may be necessary to define the anatomy of the obstruction before surgical intervention.

Management of urinary tract obstruction is directed toward identification of the site and cause of obstruction and relief of the obstruction, usually through surgical intervention. Elimination of obstruction is at times associated with a postobstructive diuresis, due partially to a solute diuresis from salt and urea retained during obstruction and partially to the renal concentrating defect. In some cases, definitive relief of obstruction is not possible and urinary diversion may be required. This may be as simple as an indwelling urethral catheter or more complex, such as an ileal conduit. In all cases, control of urinary tract infection is of paramount concern. Urinary tract infection in an obstructed kidney constitutes a urologic emergency and requires prompt relief of the obstruction.

NEPHROLITHIASIS

Nephrolithiasis is a common cause of morbidity in the United States, accounting for hospitalization of 1 in 1000 of the population each year. The peak incidence is in the age group of 18 to 45 years, with 5 to 10 times more males affected than females. A high incidence is found in whites with more affluent socioeconomic status, perhaps because of a low-fiber diet.

Depending on stone composition, five types of renal calculi are recognized (Table 28-6). Calcium stones are the most common, accounting for 75% of all stone types. The majority of these are calcium oxalate stones, which contribute to more than 50% of all diagnosed renal calculi. Calcium phosphate stones require an alkaline pH for their precipitation and therefore are less common except in patients with RTA.

Patients with nephrolithiasis usually present with gross hematuria and acute excruciating colicky type pain located in the flank and radiating to the groin on the same side. Initial evaluation of the patient with nephrolithiasis should include past history of hematuria or passing a stone, urinary infections, family history, and detailed dietary history. Initial serologic screening should include electrolytes, creatinine, serum calcium, phosphate, and uric acid. Management of patients with nephrolithiasis requires identification of the specific type of stone. Urinalysis is helpful in determining the pH, identifying hematuria, ruling out infection, and, most importantly, identifying the type of crystals. Intravenous pyelogram with

| TABLE 28-6 | Frequency Distribution, Risk Factors, and Radiologic Appearance of Renal Calculi |

Type of Stone	Percent of All Stones	Risk Factors	Radiologic Appearance
Calcium oxalate/phosphate	75	Hypercalciuria (40–50%) Hypocitraturia (20–40%) Hyperuricosuria (15–25%) Hyperoxaluria (<5%) Decreased urine volume (5–10%)	Opaque, round, multiple calculi
Magnesium-ammonium-phosphate (triple phosphate/struvite)	10–15	Anatomic urologic abnormality Infection with urease-producing organism Hypercalciuria Hyperuricosuria	Opaque, staghorn
Uric acid	10–15	Hyperuricosuria Urine pH <5.0 Decreased urine volume	Radiolucent
Cystine	1	Hypercystinuria Decreased urine volume	Radiopaque, may be staghorn

tomographic cuts can identify many of the stone types. Uric acid stones are easily identifiable since they are the only radiolucent stones. Cystine stones are less radiopaque than radiocontrast and may have staghorn appearance. Also, triple phosphate stones assume the calyceal shape and can be identified radiologically. The most reliable method of identifying stones is by crystallographic studies when the stone is identified through straining of urine.

Forty percent of patients with a first episode of nephrolithiasis have a second episode within 2 to 3 years, and 75% have a recurrence in 7 to 10 years. After 20 years of follow-up, less than 10% of the patients remain stone free. Based on these figures, all patients presenting with first episode of nephrolithiasis should be advised to take in approximately 3 L of fluid per day to maintain at least 2 L of urinary volume per day. Eight to ten ounces should be taken during the night, because this is the period of maximum urinary concentration. The evidence for dietary modifications in lowering the risk of recurrent nephrolithiasis is available only for protein and salt intake. Accordingly, patients should be advised to restrict their intake of protein to 1 to 1.5 gm/kg and to use salt in moderation. A comprehensive metabolic work-up may be initiated 6 to 8 weeks after passing the first stone, especially in patients with high occupational or dietary risk of recurrence. This should include two 24-hour urine collections for volume, creatinine, urea, sodium, calcium, phosphate, urate, oxalate, and citrate excretion, together with serum parathyroid hormone (PTH) determination (Fig. 28–1).

Calcium Stones

As mentioned previously, calcium stones can be either calcium oxalate or calcium phosphate. Only a minority of patients with calcium stones have identifiable systemic disease such as hyperparathyroidism, sarcoidosis, hypervitaminosis D, RTA, or gastrointestinal disease responsible for hyperoxaluria. About 50% of patients have hypercalciuria in absence of any of the diseases described here with normal serum calcium and PTH.

Several risk factors are identified in patients with calcium stones. Hypercalciuria can result from hypercalcemia secondary to hyperparathyroidim, sarcoidosis, malignancy, and immobilization. RTA, volume overload, and loop diuretics can increase calcium concentration in the urine. Ninety percent of patients with hypercalciuria are idiopathic. In these patients, the presence of hypercalciuria of more than 4 mg/kg per 24 hours in absence of the causes described here is usual. Hypercalciuria tends to be familial, with hyperabsorption at the gut level, normal or low PTH, increased 1,25 vitamin D, and mild hypophosphatemia.

Hyperuricosuria is a risk factor because urate crystals increase the precipitability of calcium oxalate and calcium phosphate. Hypocitraturia is a well-known risk factor since citrate in urine binds calcium and prevents its precipitation. Normally citrate is reabsorbed in the proximal tubule. This reabsorption is enhanced in the presence of acidosis. Accordingly, conditions such as RTA, renal failure, severe hypokalemia, or treatment with acetazolamide can result in hypocitraturia and increase risk for calcium

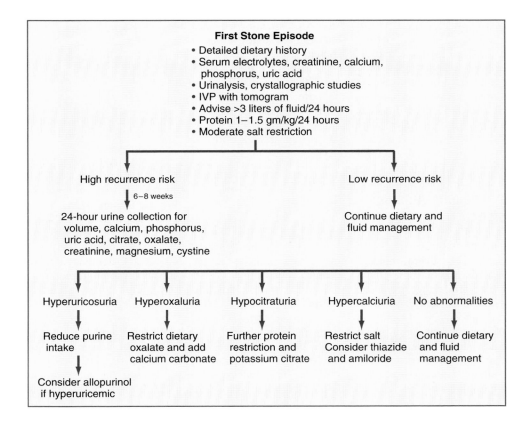

Figure 28–1
Management protocol for patients with idiopathic nephrolithiasis.

stones. A proportion of patients with hypocitraturia have none of the risk factors described here and are said to have idiopathic hypocitraturia.

Hyperoxaluria can result from increased production in patients with primary oxalosis, which is an extremely rare condition and usually results in renal failure with multisystem dysfunction. More commonly, hyperoxaluria is a result of increased gastrointestinal absorption in patients with small bowel dysfunction, such as inflammatory bowel disease.

Medical management of the patients with calcium stones depends on identification of a metabolic disorder contributing to the stone formation. Stones 4 to 7 mm in diameter have a 50% chance of passing spontaneously. Surgical intervention is indicated when a stone is unlikely to pass spontaneously or when there is loss of renal function or increasing hydronephrosis on serial studies, infection, and intractable pain.

Uric Acid Stones

Uric acid stones are caused by the precipitation of uric acid in the urine. The main risk factors are dehydration, hyperuricosuria due to overproduction with hyperuricemia, or increased secretion associated with RTA. Ten to fifteen percent of patients have abnormal serum uric acid, while 80% of those forming uric acid stones have no definable abnormality of either serum uric acid or urinary uric acid excretion. More than 75% of patients with recurrent uric acid stones have hyperacidic urine, which accelerates the precipitation of uric acid.

The mainstay of treatment of uric acid stones is to increase volume and alkalinization of urine in an effort to reduce precipitation of uric acid. Alkalinization of urine (with a goal urinary pH of 6 to 7) can be achieved during the day with oral sodium bicarbonate. To achieve alkalinization at night when the urine is most acidic, acetazolamide may be used as an evening dose. In a very small number of patients with hyperuricosuria, allopurinol may be indicated. The majority of uric acid stones dissolve with effective urinary alkalinization within a few weeks. Patients who fail such treatment can be treated with extracorporeal shock wave lithotripsy.

Magnesium-Ammonium-Phosphate (Struvite) Stones

Patients with struvite stones usually have a past medical history of several episodes of urinary tract infections treated with multiple courses of antibiotics. Infection with urease-producing organisms leads to urea accumulation, which is metabolized to ammonium. Ammonium precipitates phosphate. Ammonium phosphate later traps calcium and magnesium, resulting in magnesium ammonium phosphate stones. Radiologically, triple phosphate stones appear as radiopaque stones, usually filling the collecting system of the involved kidney. Although infection is an important factor in producing triple phosphate stones, often there is a nidus responsible for initiation of infection. Forty percent of patients with struvite stones have hypercalciuria, and approximately 15% have hyperuricosuria. Patients with metabolic abnormalities resulting in either hypercalciuria or hyperuricosuria should be treated as are patients with calcium or uric acid stones. Management of patients with triple phosphate stones should focus on treating risk factors and on evaluation for anatomic abnormalities. The goal of treatment is to eradicate infection, which is difficult to achieve. Percutaneous nephrolithotomy is currently the primary surgical intervention of choice.

Cystine Stones

Cystine crystals are classic six-sided crystals. When present in urine, they indicate that patients have excess cystine excretion to form cystine stones. The normal solubility of cystine is 240 to 480 mg/L. Patients with cystine stones have an excretion rate of 480 to 3600 mg per 24 hours. Solubility is achieved by alkalinization or urine. Fluid management depends on measurement of cystine excretion and calculating the minimum volume to minimize solubility and to avoid overnight dehydration. Goal alkalinization of urine is to achieve a pH of more than 7. Penicillamine may be added to the therapy of those who fail fluid management. Recently, evidence for captopril reduction of cystine excretion has become available, and its use in management of patients with cystine stones who fail medical treatment is with percutaneous ultrasound lithotripsy.

RENAL TUMORS

Most renal tumors appear to originate from the tubulointerstitial components of the kidney. Renal cell carcinoma, for instance, is thought to be of proximal tubular origin. The evaluation of a patient for any renal mass may proceed according to the scheme given in Figure 28–2. This plan attempts to differentiate benign cystic lesions from solid masses and to identify malignant characteristics in solid renal masses. Multiple modalities exist for the accurate diagnostic study of renal masses, and because of their sensitivity, an increasing number of incidental renal masses are being identified in asymptomatic patients. A systematic algorithmic approach should result in fewer than 10% of renal masses being indeterminate prior to management.

A demonstrated renal mass by IVP with or without nephrotomography requires renal ultrasonography to determine more accurately whether the mass is cystic or solid. About two thirds of renal masses fulfill all ultrasonography criteria for a simple cyst and require no further work-up. When a mass is suspected on IVP but is not confirmed on ultrasonography (15% of cases), renal CT is required, particularly in symptomatic patients.

If the mass on ultrasonography is solid or complex (20% of cases), a renal CT scan (both with and without

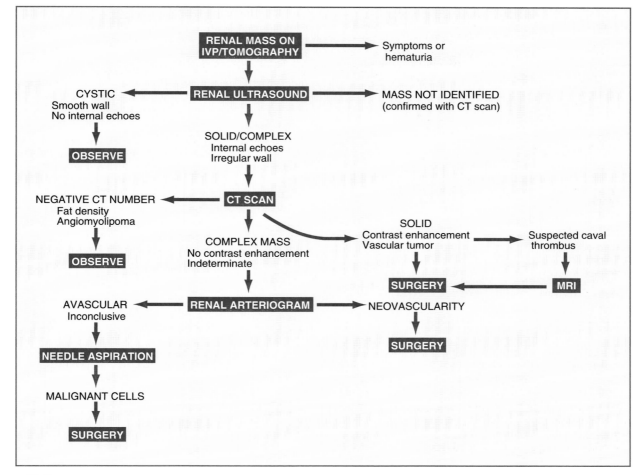

Figure 28–2

Scheme for the evaluation of a patient with a renal mass. (Adapted from Williams RD: Tumors of the kidney, ureter, and bladder. *In* Wyngaarden JB, Smith JL Jr, Bennett JC [eds.]: Cecil Textbook of Medicine. 19th ed. Philadelphia, WB Saunders, 1992, p. 615.)

intravenous injection of iodine contrast) has replaced renal arteriography as the next diagnostic step. CT is as accurate as, and obviates the potential morbidity of, angiography in defining renal masses. In addition, CT can usually give sufficient local staging information to allow definitive surgical management. When contrast enhancement on CT is coupled with areas of a negative CT number (relative tissue density in Hounsfield units) typical of fat, a diagnosis of angiomyolipoma is appropriate and no further work-up is required. In indeterminate cases, arteriography or needle aspiration cytology or both may be needed to define the diagnosis further; however, in these unusual cases, final definition is likely to require surgery.

Benign tumors of the kidney include cortical adenomas and angiomyolipomas (hamartomas). The former are more common in older men and frequently harbor nests of malignant cells. Therefore, adenomas are usually diagnosed after surgical evaluation of a solid renal mass. Angiomyolipomas are highly vascular fatty tumors that mimic renal cell carcinomas in both presentation and angiographic appearance. Significantly, over half of these

tumors are seen in patients with tuberous sclerosis. Surgical exploration may be necessary for differentiating angiomyolipoma from renal cell carcinoma in patients without tuberous sclerosis, especially if CT scan results are equivocal.

Renal cell carcinoma, or hypernephroma, is the most frequent malignant renal neoplasm in adults and accounts for about 2% of cancer deaths in both sexes. The term *hypernephroma* originated from the gross appearance of most of these tumors, which, because of their high lipid content, resemble adrenal tissue. The classic clinical presentation of renal cell carcinoma, a triad of hematuria, flank pain, and palpable flank mass, is seen in only about 10% of patients. However, any one of these features is present in well over half of all patients as an initial manifestation of the tumor.

Renal cell carcinoma is notable for the large number of systemic, extrarenal manifestations of the tumor (Table 28–7). Fever is seen in about one fifth of cases, and an elevated erythrocyte sedimentation rate is seen in half the patients. Anemia is seen in about one third of patients, but polycythemia is a striking finding in some cases.

TABLE 28–7	Manifestations of Renal Cell Carcinoma: Approximate Incidence at Presentation

Manifestation	Percent of Total
Local	
Hematuria	60
Abdominal mass	45
Pain	40
"Classic triad"—hematuria/mass/pain	10
Systemic	
Common	
Weight loss	30
Anemia	20
Fever	10
Uncommon	
Erythrocytosis	<5
Leukemoid reaction	<5
Varicocele	<5
Hepatopathy	<5
Hypercalcemia	<5
Cushing syndrome	<5
Galactorrhea	<5

The tumors are highly vascular, supplied by vessels with thin, amuscular walls. Extension of the tumor into normal renal veins and even into the vena cava is not uncommon. Metastatic spread is chiefly via vascular routes, and the lungs, bone, and liver are most frequently sites of metastasis. The tumors often undergo cystic, internal degeneration, thus mimicking benign renal cysts. Calcification within a renal mass, the result of internal necrosis, is a significant radiographic indicator of malignancy.

Treatment of renal cell carcinoma requires surgical excision of the tumor, usually by radical nephrectomy. A small, localized tumor may be removed by heminephrectomy, or even *ex vivo* dissection, when preservation of renal functional mass is critical. The tumors respond poorly to radiation and chemotherapy. Vena caval angiography may be valuable preoperatively to ascertain the presence of venous tumor thrombus. Survival is related to cellular morphology, local extension, and distant metastases and ranges from about 10 to 50% for a 10-year survival based on these factors.

Reversible hepatic dysfunction has been described, as has peripheral neuropathy. Ectopic hormone syndromes associated with renal cell carcinoma include hypercalcemia from osteoclast-stimulating factors and Cushing's syndrome from tumor production of an adrenocorticotropic hormone (ACTH)–like factor. Hypercalcemia in renal cell carcinoma is frequently associated with bone metastasis of the tumor.

The tumors usually have three cell types: clear cells, granular cells, and spindle cells; the last-named cell type and extensive nuclear anaplasia carry a poor prognosis.

REFERENCES

Fick GM, Gabow PA: Hereditary and acquired cystic disease of the kidney. Kidney Int 1994; 46(4):951–964.

Kelly CJ, Neilson EG: Tubulointerstitial diseases. *In* Brenner BM (ed.): The Kidney. 5th ed. Philadelphia, WB Saunders, 1995, pp 1655–1679.

McKinney TD: Tubulointerstitial diseases and toxic nephropathies. *In* Wyngaarden JB, Smith LH Jr, Bennett JC (eds.): Cecil Textbook of Medicine. 19th ed. Philadelphia, WB Saunders, 1992, pp 568–579.

Pak CYC: Renal calculi. *In* Wyngaarden JB, Smith LH Jr, Bennett JC (eds.): Cecil Textbook of Medicine. 19th ed. Philadelphia, WB Saunders, 1992, pp 603–608.

Williams RD: Tumors of the kidney, ureter, and bladder. *In* Wyngaarden JB, Smith LH Jr, Bennett JC (eds.): Cecil Textbook of Medicine. 19th ed. Philadelphia, WB Saunders, 1992, pp 614–619.

29

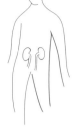

Hypertension and Vascular Disorders of the Kidney

In this chapter we review the pathophysiology and management of hypertension, which affects approximately 20% of the population in the United States. In addition, we consider several vascular disorders that affect the kidney.

ARTERIAL HYPERTENSION

Despite understanding the mechanisms of normal regulation of blood pressure, the cause of primary hypertension (not secondary to another disease process) is not discernible in most instances. Disorders that lead to excess activity of any of the regulatory factors can result in hypertension. The development of hypertension has a strong genetic component. The control of blood pressure is felt to be influenced by several different genetic loci. Recently, alterations in the gene coding for angiotensinogen have been described in hypertensive populations. In addition, environmental factors such as obesity, alcohol consumption, sedentary lifestyle, and sodium intake have an impact on blood pressure.

The blood pressure of the general population demonstrates extreme variance, with a unimodal distribution. There is a strong correlation of mortality and morbidity with increasing levels of systolic and diastolic blood pressure. This correlation provides the basis for the arbitrary definition of abnormal blood pressure (Table 29–1). A diagnosis of hypertension is made in an adult over 18 years of age if the average of two or more blood pressure measurements on at least two subsequent visits is 90 mm Hg or higher diastolic or 140 mm Hg systolic. The blood pressure in healthy children and pregnant women is typically lower, so that readings in excess of 120/80 may be considered abnormal. Isolated systolic hypertension (ISH) is described when the systolic blood pressure is greater than 160 mm Hg in association with a diastolic blood pressure less than 90 mm Hg. ISH is correlated with enhanced morbidity. Hypertension is typically classified as mild, moderate, severe or very severe, depending upon the level of the diastolic blood pressure (Table 29–1).

Hypertension occurs in more than 60 million Americans. The prevalence in whites is approximately 15% but is over 25% in the black population. This marked racial difference in the rates of hypertension remains unexplained. The prevalence of hypertension also increases with advancing age. Hypertension is more common in men than in women up to approximately age 50. The rate thereafter is higher in women.

Clinical Assessment of Hypertension

The history and physical examination can be useful in discerning primary from secondary hypertension as well as elucidating the potential end-organ effects of established hypertension. The medical history should include a determination of factors that may predispose to the development of hypertension, including the dietary intake of sodium and alcohol, concomitant medical therapy (particularly oral contraceptives or other estrogen preparations), and a positive family history of hypertension. A history of weakness, muscle cramps, and polyuria suggests hypokalemia and possible hyperaldosteronism. The presence of headaches, palpitations, or hyperhidrosis suggests catecholamine excess. The end-organ effects of hypertension are usually manifested in the heart, brain, and kidneys, so that the history should include symptoms of coronary artery disease, congestive heart failure, cerebrovascular disease, and uremia.

The physical examination should focus on potential end-organ damage. The optic fundi should be carefully observed for evidence of arteriolar sclerosis. The presence of hemorrhages and exudates (grade III retinopathy) or papilledema (grade IV retinopathy) indicates severe, life-threatening hypertension. Signs of congestive heart failure or peripheral vascular disease should be determined. The abdomen should be auscultated for the presence of a bruit. A careful neurologic examination should be performed to determine possible deficits related to a stroke.

Routine laboratory screening prior to initiating pharmacologic therapy should include serum electrolytes to determine potential metabolic disorders that may be associated with secondary causes of hypertension. The serum creatinine and a urinalysis should be obtained to determine potential renal dysfunction, which could be related as either a cause or an effect of hypertension. The serum glucose, cholesterol, and uric acid levels are helpful in assessing other cardiovascular risk factors and can be used as a baseline for monitoring the effects of antihypertensive therapy. Serial electrocardiograms and echocardi-

TABLE 29-1	Classification of Blood Pressure for Adults Aged 18 Years or Older

Category	Systolic (mm Hg)	Diastolic (mm Hg)
Normal	<130	<85
High normal	130–139	85–89
Hypertension		
Stage 1 (mild)	140–159	90–99
Stage 2 (moderate)	160–179	100–109
Stage 3 (severe)	180–209	110–119
Stage 4 (very severe)	≥210	≥120

From the fifth report of the Joint National Committee on Detection, Evaluation, and Treatment of High Blood Pressure (JNC V). Arch Intern Med 1993; 153:164.

ograms may be useful in assessing the effects of hypertension and antihypertensive treatment on the heart.

Extreme elevations of the blood pressure (diastolic >120 mm Hg) may be observed in asymptomatic patients and are considered to represent accelerated hypertension. When accelerated hypertension is associated with acute cardiovascular sequelae, the patient is considered to be suffering from hypertensive crisis or malignant hypertension. These patients often present with encephalopathy characterized by the rapid onset of confusion, headache, visual disturbances, and seizures. Papilledema occurs as a result of increased intracranial pressure. Death from a cerebrovascular accident frequently occurs if the hypertension is untreated. Renal damage due to necrotizing arteriolitis results in proteinuria, hematuria, and acute renal failure. Acute left ventricular failure or unstable angina may be the presenting feature of malignant hypertension. All of these end-organ sequelae may be reversed by successful treatment of the elevated blood pressure.

Causes of Secondary Hypertension

In approximately 5% of adults with hypertension, the disease can be found to have a specific cause. Certain features of the patient may assist in identifying those who should undergo evaluation of a potential reversible cause. Patients younger than 30 years or older than age 55 have the greatest prevalence of correctable secondary hypertension. Patients with blood pressure that is difficult to manage pharmacologically or with an abrupt increase in the blood pressure after years of adequate control should be considered for evaluation. Certain features of the initial screening history, physical examination, and laboratory evaluation may suggest a specific secondary cause (Table 29–2).

Renovascular Hypertension

An obstruction of the renal vasculature prevents adequate perfusion of the kidney and leads to stimulation of renin production. The subsequent activation of angiotensin induces vasoconstriction and leads to the development of hypertension. Secondary hyperaldosteronism occurs and promotes an increase in renal sodium reabsorption, which aids in sustaining hypertension.

Atherosclerotic lesions account for approximately two thirds of the cases of reversible renovascular hypertension. This disorder is most often observed in older individuals with evidence of extensive atherosclerotic disease. The lesion most often occurs at the aortic ostia. The other major lesion causing renal arterial occlusion is fibromuscular hyperplasia. It typically occurs in young white women and involves either the renal arteries, generally not at the aortic ostia, or intrarenal segmental branches. Fibromuscular hyperplasia can affect one or both renal arteries.

Renovascular hypertension should be suspected in any individual with abrupt onset of hypertension, particularly patients who are younger than 30 or older than 55. The presence of an upper abdominal bruit that is systolic-diastolic and high pitched and radiates laterally from the midepigastrium is strongly suggestive of functionally significant renal artery stenosis but is present in only about 20% of patients with proven renal vascular hypertension.

TABLE 29-2	Causes of Secondary Hypertension

Cause	Symptoms/Signs	Manifestations	Confirmation
Renovascular	Flank bruit, diffuse atherosclerosis	↓ K$^+$, ↑ creatinine	Arteriogram, ↑ renal vein renin, captopril renal scan
Renal disease	Edema	Acute or chronic renal failure	↑ Creatinine, BUN
Steroid excess			
Aldosterone	Weakness, cramps	↓ K$^+$, alkalosis	↓ Renin, ↑ aldosterone, CT scan
Dexamethasone suppressible	Hypertension in childhood	↓ K$^+$, alkalosis	Hypertension suppressed by dexamethasone
Glucocorticoid	Cushingoid appearance	Hyperglycemia	↑ Cortisol
Pheochromocytoma	Paroxysmal, orthostatic	↑ Urine VMA, catecholamines	CT scan, angiography
Hyperparathyroidism	Peptic ulcers, bone pain, kidney stones	↑ Ca$^+$	↑ Parathyroid hormone
Oral contraceptives	None	Patient taking oral contraceptives	↑ Angiotensinogen

BUN = Blood urea nitrogen; CT = computed tomography; VMA = vanillylmandelic acid; ↓ = decrease; ↑ = increase.

Hypokalemic metabolic alkalosis may be caused by secondary hyperaldosteronism. Renal dysfunction manifested by an elevated serum creatinine may be present.

Renal ultrasonography may demonstrate asymmetry in renal size if lesions are unilateral. Duplex Doppler studies also provide a noninvasive method of assessing a possible vascular occlusion. A significant decrease in renal blood flow, as demonstrated by nuclear renography after a dose of an angiotensin-converting enzyme (ACE) inhibitor, is an excellent screening test for renal artery stenosis. The diagnosis of an obstructing lesion is made definitively by angiography.

The functional significance of an obstructing lesion, however, is best determined from measurements of the plasma renin activity (PRA) in the renal veins after stimulation of renin production with the ACE inhibitor captopril. Systemic venous PRA may be elevated but is not specific for renal vascular hypertension. In the setting of a unilateral lesion, selective renal vein PRA is elevated on the affected side and suppressed on the contralateral side.

Syndromes of Steroid Excess

The autonomous production of aldosterone causes excessive absorption of sodium in the nephron. The resultant increase in the intravascular volume elevates the blood pressure. Renal perfusion is enhanced and renin production is suppressed. The effects of aldosterone on the nephron also lead to excessive renal secretion of potassium and hydrogen ions, resulting in hypokalemia and a metabolic alkalosis.

Excessive aldosterone production is most often described in the setting of a mineralocorticoid-producing adrenal adenoma or bilateral adrenal hyperplasia. Rarely, adrenal carcinoma may also be associated with primary aldosteronism. A simple screening test is to determine the plasma renin level, which is low in primary aldosteronism. A definite diagnosis is made by detecting elevated levels of aldosterone in the plasma that do not suppress with saline volume expansion or converting-enzyme inhibition. Computed tomography (CT) of the adrenal glands should be performed to determine the presence of an adenoma or bilateral hyperplasia. Use of an iodinated cholesterol scintiscan may be useful in detecting small adenomas. Direct adrenal venous sampling of aldosterone may help differentiate adenoma from bilateral hyperplasia.

Dexamethasone-suppressible hyperaldosteronism is a rare disorder typically presenting as mineralocorticoid-induced hypertension in young individuals. The genetic alteration in this syndrome has been described. This condition involves a chimeric gene in which the promoter region belongs to the 11β-hydroxylase gene and the structural portion to the aldosterone synthase gene. This results in adrenocorticotropic hormone (ACTH) being able to stimulate the release of aldosterone. This condition can be specifically diagnosed by the use of polymerase chain reaction techniques. Dexamethasone ameliorates the disorder by suppressing ACTH synthesis. Glucocorticoid excess (Cushing syndrome) can lead to findings consistent with hyperaldosteronism owing to the effects of glucocorticoid on aldosterone receptors.

Pheochromocytoma

Pheochromocytoma is a rare tumor of the chromaffin cells of the neural crest. The tumor occurs most often in the adrenal medulla but can be located anywhere along the sympathetic ganglia in the abdomen or chest. The medullary tumors usually produce norepinephrine and epinephrine, whereas the peripheral tumors usually produce only norepinephrine. Hypertension occurs secondary to the increased cardiac output and increased peripheral vascular resistance stimulated by the adrenocorticoids.

The release of the catecholamines from these tumors may be intermittent, so that patients usually describe paroxysms of headaches, flushing, hyperhidrosis, and palpitations in association with hypertension. The diagnosis of pheochromocytoma may be suggested by the demonstration of elevated plasma epinephrine or norepinephrine or elevated urinary excretion of catecholamines or their metabolites, vanillylmandelic acid or metanephrine. The inability to suppress elevated plasma catecholamines by a single dose of clonidine provides additional evidence of the tumor. The localization of the tumor can most often be made by CT of the abdomen (particularly the adrenals) or the chest. The localization by scintigraphy of the guanethidine analogue ^{131}I-metaiodobenzylguanidine (MIBG) may be useful in locating small or extra-adrenal tumors. Selective arteriography or differential venous catecholamine sampling may be required for confirmation of the tumor location.

Treatment of Hypertension

The goal of treating hypertension is to reduce the risk of morbidity and mortality due to the cardiovascular consequences of the disorder. Antihypertensive treatment is indicated in patients with systolic blood pressures in excess of 140 mm Hg and diastolic pressures greater than 90 mm Hg. The treatment of ISH reduces the morbidity and mortality in that population of hypertensive patients.

The initial therapy of hypertension should be directed at nonpharmacologic alterations in the patient's lifestyle. Such therapy should include dietary modifications to reduce sodium and alcohol intake and for the patient to eat a balanced diet meeting recommended daily adult (RDA) requirements for minerals, vitamins, and other nutrients. Weight reduction should be recommended to the obese individual. Exercise should be encouraged, and behavior modification should be considered to reduce stressful lifestyles. Occasionally, blood pressure can be reduced adequately by these nonpharmacologic strategies, but more often the patient requires pharmacologic intervention.

The most commonly prescribed antihypertensive agents are described in Table 29–3. The recent recommendation from the Joint National Committee on Detection, Evaluation, and Treatment of High Blood Pressure

TABLE 29–3	Commonly Prescribed Oral Antihypertensive Drugs			
Class	Protype Drug	Mechanism	Side Effects	Precautions
Diuretics	Thiazide, furosemide	Inhibit tubular NaCl absorption	Hypokalemia, hyperuricemia, hyperglycemia	Furosemide is more useful in chronic renal failure
	Spironolactone	Aldosterone antagonist	Hyperkalemia	Avoid with marked renal failure
Adrenergic inhibitors Central	Clonidine, methyldopa	Decreased CNS sympathetic outflow	Drowsiness, fatigue, dry mouth, sexual dysfunction	Rapid clonidine withdrawal may lead to rebound hypertension
Peripheral	Guanethidine	Vasodilation	Orthostasis, sexual dysfunction	Use with caution in elderly
Beta	Propranolol	↓ Heart rate and contractility	Bradycardia, fatigue, insomnia	Avoid in obstructive airway disease, CHF, heart block
Alpha$_1$	Prazosin	Vasodilation	Orthostasis, "first-dose" hypotension, tachycardia	Tachyphylaxis to drug effect often noted
Combined alpha, beta	Labetalol	↓ Heart rate and contractility, vasodilation	Dizziness, fatigue, headache	Avoid in obstructive airway disease, CHF, heart block
Vasodilators	Hydralazine, minoxidil	Vasodilation	Tachycardia, fluid retention	Positive antinuclear antibody, lupus syndrome with hydralazine, hypertrichosis with minoxidil
Calcium channel blockers	Nifedipine, diltiazem, verapamil	Vasodilation	Tachycardia, fluid retention	Useful in patients with concomitant coronary disease
ACE inhibitors	Captopril	Inhibition of AII production	Rash, neutropenia, cough, hyperkalemia, angioedema	May cause worsening of renal function with chronic renal disease
Angiotensin receptor blockers	Losartan	Inhibits binding of AII to AT$_1$	Rash, hyperkalemia	May cause worsening of renal function with chronic renal disease

AII = Angiotensin II; AT$_1$ = angiotensin II receptor; CHF = congestive heart failure; CNS = central nervous system; NaCl = sodium chloride.

(JNC V) is to use diuretics and beta blockers as preferred first-line therapy for mild to moderate hypertension (Fig. 29–1). This recommendation was made due to the availability of long-term clinical trials with these agents. The JNC V pointed out that the ACE inhibitors, calcium channel antagonists, alpha$_1$-receptor blockers, and alpha-beta blockers were effective in lowering blood pressure. The decision to choose diuretics and beta blockers as the first-line therapy is due to the lack of long-term follow-up with the other antihypertensive classes.

The JNC V guidelines do not preclude an individualized approach to the treatment of hypertension. A consideration to the efficacy of the various agents in different populations must be taken into account. For example, black subjects respond better to diuretics, calcium channel blockers, and alpha-beta blockers than to beta blockers. Subjects with angina and hypertension would be better treated with beta blockers or calcium channel blockers. An ACE inhibitor might be considered as therapy for diabetics with hypertension. In the elderly, a diuretic or a calcium channel blocker would be a good choice for antihypertensive therapy. A consideration of the patient's tolerance for side effects should also be included in the choice of an agent. For example, a healthy, active patient with hypertension may not tolerate the decrease in exercise tolerance that a beta blocker may produce, and patients with bronchospastic disease should not receive beta

blockers. Finally, the issue of cost must be taken into consideration when selecting antihypertensive agents.

Hypertensive emergencies require a more aggressive approach to treatment (Table 29–4). Parenterally administered therapy such as sodium nitroprusside, labetalol, hydralazine, and diazoxide are often indicated to minimize the end-organ damage. Such therapy should be administered in a critical care setting with intensive monitoring of the blood pressure and organ function. Accelerated hypertension without manifestations of acute end-organ dysfunction can be treated with oral agents that acutely lower the blood pressure, such as clonidine or calcium channel blockers.

The treatment of secondary hypertension should obviously be directed at eliminating the primary disorder. The goal of treating renovascular hypertension should be the removal of an obstructing lesion in the renal arterial system by transluminal angioplasty or surgical revascularization. The treatment of choice for patients with a single adrenal adenoma is unilateral adrenalectomy. In patients who are poor surgical candidates or who have bilateral adrenal hyperplasia, pharmacologic therapy with an aldosterone antagonist should be used. Treatment of pheochromocytoma is surgical unless the tumor is metastatic or the patient is inoperable for other reasons. Patients should be prepared for 1 to 2 weeks before surgery with both alpha- and beta-adrenergic blocking agents and vol-

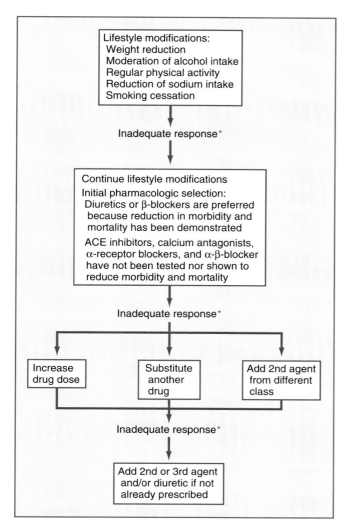

Figure 29–1

Treatment algorithm. *Asterisk* indicates that response means the patient achieved goal blood pressure or is making considerable progress toward this goal. ACE = Angiotensin-converting enzyme. (From the fifth report of the Joint National Committee on Detection, Evaluation, and Treatment of High Blood Pressure [JNC V]. Arch Intern Med 1993; 153:164.)

Vascular Biology

Endothelial cells form the inner lining of all vascular tissue and are the elements in direct contact with the blood components. The endothelium plays three major regulatory functions with regard to maintenance of blood flow. First, it is a regulator of vascular tone. Vascular relaxation is mediated by endothelium-derived prostacyclin and the endothelium-relaxing factor nitric oxide. The endothelins, potent vasoconstrictors, are peptides produced and released by endothelial cells. Second, the endothelium acts as a regulator of the coagulation cascade. Various circulating stimuli allow the endothelial surface expression of tissue factor that can activate the coagulation cascade. Alternatively, coagulation is inhibited by the production of prostacyclin, which diminishes platelet adherence. The endothelium also metabolizes some factors responsible for clot formation, such as adenosine diphosphate released from platelets. In established thrombi, the endothelium plays a major role in fibrinolysis by forming plasminogen activators. Finally, the endothelium regulates cell growth, which has important implications regarding tissue injury as well as determining normal vascular architecture. The growth of adjacent smooth muscle cells is regulated by platelet-derived growth factor, which is in part produced by endothelial tissue.

Although endothelial cells might be considered regulators, the smooth muscle cells that underlie the endothelium can be considered the effectors of the vascular tissue. These cells constrict in response to the endothelins and dilate in response to relaxing factor. This dilation is

ume expansion to avert marked hemodynamic alterations that can occur perioperatively. Alpha blockade must be complete before beta-blocking agents are used. Otherwise, particularly in tumors secreting both epinephrine and norepinephrine, beta blockade without antecedent alpha blockade may result in a hypertensive crisis.

VASCULAR DISORDERS OF THE KIDNEY

The understanding of the normal vascular responses to circulating and physical stresses exerted by blood flow has led to a better understanding of the pathophysiology of many vascular disorders (Fig. 29–2). The renal vasculature exhibits these physiologic responses and demonstrates a wide spectrum of disorders similar to those observed in the vascular tissues throughout the body.

TABLE 29–4	Parenteral Drugs for Hypertensive Emergencies	
Drug	**Advantages**	**Precautions**
Vasodilators		
Nitroprusside	Rapid onset, allows effective titration, no sedation	Requires intensive care monitoring, thiocyanate toxicity with prolonged use
Diazoxide	Rapid onset	Large boluses may cause severe hypotension, prolonged effect, sodium retention, reflex tachycardia, angina
Hydralazine	IM preparation	Reflex tachycardia, angina
Nitroglycerin	Dilates coronary vessels	Requires intensive care monitoring; flushing, headache
Enalapril	Longer duration of action	May cause rapid decrease of renal function, hyperkalemia
Adrenergic Inhibitors		
Methyldopa	Gradual decline in blood pressure, safe in pregnancy	Inconsistent effect, sedation
Labetalol	Little reflex tachycardia, prolonged duration	Bronchospasm, bradyarrhythmias; avoid with left ventricular failure

IM = Intramuscular.

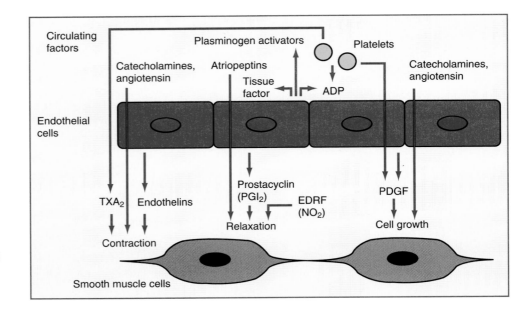

Figure 29–2
Principles of vascular biology. Systemic and locally produced factors modulate vascular tone, tissue growth, and platelet activity. EDRF = Endothelium-derived relaxing factor; PDGF = platelet-derived growth factor; TxA$_2$ = thromboxane A$_2$.

mediated through a mechanism that may also be stimulated by atriopeptins. Although the transient architecture of vascular lumen may be mediated by constriction or relaxation of the smooth muscle layer, proliferation of these cells may lead to a chronic alteration in the structure of the vessel. The growth of the smooth muscle cells depends upon local factors derived from the endothelium or platelets. Circulating factors such as angiotensin II and catecholamines are also promoters of vascular smooth muscle cell growth. The smooth muscle cells may also indirectly affect the vascular architecture by regulating the production of extracellular matrix constituents.

It is evident that vascular tissue contains the capability either to promote or to inhibit the basic processes of vascular tone, intravascular coagulation, and cell growth. Although this complex array may not be active in normal intact vessels, it is essential in the setting of disruption of the vascular architecture. These mechanisms create a balance that allows injured vascular tissue to heal while allowing adequate flow distal to the site of injury. Any imbalance of these systems promotes vascular pathology. These pathologic changes can occur in the major arterial or venous vessels or their branches.

Renal Arterial Occlusion

Partial obstruction of the renal arterial system by atheromatous plaque or fibromuscular dysplasia leads to renovascular hypertension, as discussed previously. Occasionally, complete occlusion of the major renal artery or its main branches occurs. Thrombosis of renal arteries is most often seen in cases of severe blunt abdominal trauma. Thrombosis can also occur rarely after surgical manipulation or during angiographic study of the renal artery and in association with aneurysms of the aorta or main renal arteries. Occlusion of renal arteries may also occur as an embolic phenomenon, often in patients with underlying atherosclerotic vascular disease. The emboli

usually originate from the heart during atrial fibrillation or after myocardial infarction. Valvular vegetations of bacterial endocarditis sometimes embolize to and obstruct renal arteries. Simultaneous embolization to other organs may provide evidence of the nature of the occlusive disease in the kidney.

Nuclear renography is useful in the initial evaluation of suspected renal infarction. The absence of blood flow in a dynamic study or defects in activity on static images are strongly suggestive of arterial occlusion. Renal arteriography is necessary to determine the location and extent of the occlusion. Successful revascularization of the main artery or segmental branches usually requires surgical embolectomy or bypass grafting. Thrombolytic agents or transluminal angioplasty followed by anticoagulation may be useful in selected instances. Conservative management may be adequate in most instances of unilateral or segmental occlusion.

Arterioles and Microvasculature

Disorders of the main renal vessels are usually unilateral. The processes that involve the smaller vessels of the kidney, however, are diffuse, involving both kidneys (Table 29–5). Most diseases of the renal arterioles are systemic and involve several organ systems. These disorders are usually initiated by vascular injury and advance because of the vascular responses to the injury. Clinically, the arteriolar disorders are usually associated with hypertension due to activation of the renin-angiotensin-aldosterone axis. Renal failure may occur acutely but is usually progressive over a period of weeks to months.

Atheromatous embolization from aortic plaque usually follows manipulation of an atherosclerotic aorta and affects multiple small vessels. There may be evidence of embolization to other tissues, particularly the optic fundi or lower extremities. Pathologic examination of the kidney reveals the presence of cholesterol clefts surrounded

TABLE 29–5	**Renal Vascular Disorders**	
Vessel	**Disorder**	**Manifestation**
Arteries	Thrombosis	Acute renal failure
	Embolization	Hypertension
Arterioles and microvasculature	Atheroembolization	Rapidly progressive renal failure, systemic signs of embolization
	Hypertensive nephrosclerosis	Slowly progressive renal failure
	Malignant hypertension	Acute renal failure, proteinuria
	Scleroderma	Malignant crisis wih hypertension and rapidly progressive renal failure
	HUS/TTP	Rapidly progressive renal failure, thrombocytopenia, hemolytic anemia
Renal vein	Thrombosis	Acute renal failure, proteinuria, pulmonary embolism

HUS = Hemolytic-uremic syndrome; TTP = thrombotic thrombocytopenic purpura.

by tissue reaction in small to medium-sized renal arteries. There is no treatment for this disorder, and the prognosis is very poor, reflecting the severity of the primary atheromatous disease.

Benign nephrosclerosis is a misnomer used to describe a slow process of intrarenal vascular sclerosis and ischemic change that complicates the course of chronic essential hypertension. Although the intrarenal arteries show signs of sclerotic thickening, the dominant lesion is at the level of the afferent arteriole, where hyaline thickening leads to a homogeneous, eosinophilic appearance of the vessel. The glomeruli have ischemic wrinkling of the basement membranes and become progressively sclerotic, whereas the tubules undergo atrophy and are replaced by fibrotic tissue.

Clinically, there may be mild proteinuria, but the urinary sediment is unremarkable. Radiography shows a progressive decrease in kidney size. The glomerular filtration rate (GFR) slowly diminishes, eventually reaching the stage of symptomatic renal failure. Treatment is directed at control of the blood pressure, which has been shown to slow the progression to end-stage renal failure.

Malignant nephrosclerosis is a generalized necrotizing arteritis seen in conjunction with accelerated hypertension. The kidneys are generally contracted in size and have petechial hemorrhages on the surface. Fibrinoid necrosis without inflammation in the renal arterioles and sometimes extending into the glomerular tufts is the characteristic lesion. A second prominent lesion is the "onion skin" endothelial proliferation in small arteries produced by concentric layers of collagen and proliferating endothelial cells.

The patient usually presents with extreme elevation of the diastolic blood pressure—in excess of 120 mm Hg. Hypertensive encephalopathy often occurs concomitantly. Proteinuria and hematuria occur in association with acute renal failure. The goal of therapy is to rapidly lower the diastolic blood pressure to about 100 mm Hg, with a more gradual lowering to about 80 mm Hg over the course of a few days. The renal function frequently decreases further during the initial phase of blood pressure control but recovers as the vascular lesions heal and autoregulation of renal blood flow is re-established. If the vascular injury is quite severe, the healing may occur over several weeks or months as normal blood pressure is maintained.

Scleroderma is a progressive connective tissue disease of uncertain etiology. The disease affects the vasculature of several organs, including the kidney. The renal arterioles usually demonstrate intimal proliferation with progressive luminal occlusion. An accelerated process may occur and is associated with the necrotic arteriolar and glomerular changes observed in malignant hypertension. The clinical course of renal involvement reflects the pathologic changes. The initial arteriolar changes may be associated with a normal GFR and urinalysis. The development of proteinuria or mild hypertension often heralds the onset of the accelerated scleroderma renal crisis. This phase is similar to the presentation of malignant hypertension. Therapy is directed at control of the blood pressure. ACE inhibitors initiated at the onset of renal involvement may avert a renal crisis.

The *hemolytic-uremic syndrome* (HUS) and *thrombotic thrombocytopenic purpura* (TTP) are two disorders characterized by thrombotic microangiopathy. The clinical features, pathogenesis, and therapy of these two disorders are similar so that they are often considered one entity with variable presentations. The renal lesion varies in severity and is characterized by fibrin thrombi in the glomerular capillary loops. The arterioles may likewise demonstrate thrombi with fibrinoid necrosis. The disorders are associated with a microangiopathic hemolytic anemia with thrombocytopenia.

Hemolytic-uremic syndrome is generally observed in children following a nonspecific gastrointestinal or influenzal syndrome. Verotoxin-producing strains of *Escherichia coli* have been reported to be associated with hemorrhagic colitis and HUS. An adult form is observed most often in young women in association with the use of oral contraceptives or in the peripartum period. Some antineoplastic agents have also been associated with HUS. The clinical syndrome in TTP is dominated by neurologic manifestations. The clinical course of renal involvement may be either acute or rapidly progressive renal failure. The rate of spontaneous recovery in children with HUS is high, so that only supportive therapy is necessary. The prognosis in adults is not as good, so additional therapy is indicated. Evidence suggests that plasma exchange in association with fresh plasma and corticosteroids may induce remissions.

Renal Vein Occlusion

Renal vein occlusion is a thrombotic event. The incidence of renal vein thrombosis may be as high as 30% in nephrotic glomerulopathies, especially membranous nephropathy. It may occur in infants who develop severe volume depletion accompanying gastroenteritis or sepsis.

The venous occlusion is usually asymptomatic. The thrombus can embolize, however, and the patient may present with an acute pulmonary embolism or infarction. The renal function may decline acutely, particularly in children or adults with the nephrotic syndrome.

Renal ultrasonography may demonstrate a thrombus in the renal vein. Renal venography is usually required for a definitive diagnosis. Anticoagulation is indicated in patients with proven or threatened pulmonary embolism. Fibrinolytic therapy may be considered in patients with acute renal failure or severe flank pain. Renal function generally improves with resolution of the thrombus. Prophylactic anticoagulation is not recommended for the patient with nephrotic syndrome who is at risk for developing thrombosis.

REFERENCES

Albers FJ: Clinical characteristics of atherosclerotic renovascular disease. Am J Kid Dis 1994; 24(4):636–641.

Alderman MH: Non-pharmacological treatment of hypertension. Lancet 1994; 344:307.

Calhoun DA, Oparil S: Treatment of hypertensive crisis. N Engl J Med 1990; 323:1177.

The fifth report of the Joint National Committee on Detection, Evaluation, and Treatment of High Blood Pressure (JNC V). Arch Intern Med 1993; 153:154.

Lifton RP, Dluhy RG, Powers M, et al: A chimaeric 11 B-hydroxylase/aldosterone synthase gene causes glucocorticoid-remediable aldosteronism and human hypertension. Nature 1992; 355:262.

Mann SJ, Pickering TG: Detection of renovascular hypertension: State of the Art: 1992. Ann Intern Med 1992; 117:845–853.

Remuzzi G, Ruggenenti P: The hemolytic uremic syndrome. Kid Intern 1995; 47:2–19.

Vane JR, Angaard EE, Botting RM: Regulatory functions of the vascular endothelium. N Engl J Med 1990; 323:27.

Werbel SS, Ober KP: Pheochromocytoma: Update on diagnosis, localization and management. Med Clin North Am 1995; 79(1):131.

30

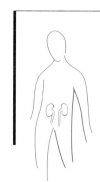

Acute Renal Failure

DEFINITION AND ETIOLOGY

Acute renal failure (ARF) is a syndrome that can be broadly defined as an abrupt decrease in renal function sufficient to result in retention of nitrogenous waste (e.g., blood urea nitrogen [BUN] and creatinine) in the body. ARF can result from a decrease of renal blood flow (prerenal azotemia), intrinsic renal parenchymal diseases (renal azotemia), or obstruction of urine flow (postrenal azotemia) (Fig. 30–1).

The most common intrinsic renal disease that leads to ARF is an entity referred to as acute tubular necrosis (ATN), which designates a clinical syndrome in which there is an abrupt and sustained decline in glomerular filtration rate (GFR) occurring within minutes to days in response to an acute ischemic or nephrotoxic insult. Its clinical recognition is largely predicated upon exclusion of prerenal and postrenal causes of sudden azotemia, followed by exclusion of other causes of intrinsic ARF (i.e., glomerulonephritis, acute interstitial nephritis, vasculitis). Said in another way, it is necessary to exclude carefully the other defined renal syndromes before concluding that ATN is present. Although the name *acute tubular necrosis* is not an entirely valid histologic description of this syndrome, the term is ingrained in clinical medicine and is therefore used in this chapter.

DIFFERENTIAL DIAGNOSIS AND DIAGNOSTIC EVALUATION OF THE PATIENT

Acute Azotemia During Hospitalization

Despite the exhaustive list of conditions that can cause acute azotemia in hospitalized patients, a careful history and physical examination and simple laboratory tests often suffice for diagnosis. In hospitalized adults, prerenal azotemia is the single most common cause of acute azotemia, and ATN is the most common intrinsic renal disease that leads to ARF. Thus, the most important differential diagnosis is between prerenal azotemia (e.g., volume depletion) and ATN (secondary to ischemia or nephrotoxins). In the elderly male patient, bladder outlet obstruction must also be excluded. In addition, depending on the clinical setting, other diagnoses to be considered are acute interstitial nephritis (e.g., secondary to methicillin), ather-

omatous emboli (prior aortic surgery and/or aortogram), ureteral obstruction (pelvic or colon surgery), or intrarenal obstruction (e.g., acute uric acid nephropathy).

Chart Review, History, and Physical Examination

Determination of the cause of ARF depends on a systematic approach, as depicted in Table 30–1. The difficulty in arriving at a correct diagnosis in a hospitalized patient is not the failure to identify a possible etiology for the ARF; the problem is often just the opposite, that is, there are several possible causes of ARF. Correct diagnosis depends on careful analysis of available data on the clinical course of each patient with ARF and examining the sequence of deterioration in renal function in relation to chronology of the potential etiologies of ARF. Correct diagnosis also requires a knowledge of the natural history of the different causes of ARF. Some of the important data that should be sought from chart review are presented in Table 30–2.

Reduced body weight, postural changes in blood pressure and pulse, and decreased jugular venous pulse all suggest a reduction in extracellular fluid volume. Prerenal azotemia may also develop in states in which extracellular fluids are expanded (e.g., cardiac failure, cirrhosis, nephrotic syndrome) but the "effective" blood volume is decreased. Careful abdominal examination may uncover a distended, tender bladder, indicating lower urinary tract obstruction. In any case in which lower tract obstruction is suspected as a cause of acute azotemia, examination of the prostate and a sterile "in-and-out" diagnostic post-void bladder catheterization should be performed as a part of the physical examination. The urine volume should be recorded and a specimen saved for studies described later.

Additional findings that may be helpful are the occurrence of fever and rash in some patients with acute interstitial nephritis. A history of a recent aortic catheterization and the finding of livedo reticularis are diagnostic clues for cholesterol or atheromatous emboli.

Differentiating prerenal azotemia from ATN may be difficult, partly because evaluation of volume status in a critically ill patient is not easy, and any cause of prerenal azotemia, if severe enough, may lead to ATN. Evaluation of the urine volume and urine sediment and a number of

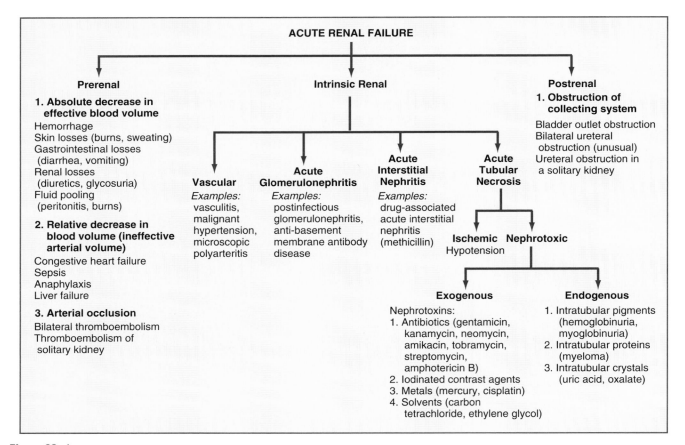

Figure 30–1
Causes of acute renal failure.

urinary indices are particularly helpful in making the correct diagnosis.

Urine Volume

The urine volume is often less than 400 ml/day in oliguric ATN. Normal urine output does not exclude the diagnosis of ATN because a substantial number of patients with ATN have urine outputs as high as 1.5 to 2.0 L/day. This nonoliguric ATN is frequently associated with nephrotoxic antibiotic-induced ARF. On the other hand, total anuria (0 urine output) should suggest a diagnosis other than ATN, the most important being obstruction. Widely varying daily urine outputs also suggest obstruction.

Urine Sediment

In prerenal failure, a moderate number of hyaline and finely granular casts may be seen, but coarsely granular and cellular casts are infrequent. In ATN, the sediment is usually quite characteristic: "dirty" brown granular casts and renal tubular epithelial cells, free and in casts, are the most striking elements and are present in 70 to 80% of patients with ATN. A "benign" sediment containing few

formed elements should alert the physician to the possibility that obstruction is present. In ARF associated with intratubular oxalate (e.g., methoxyflurane anesthesia) or uric acid deposition (associated with acute hyperuricemia after chemotherapy of neoplastic disease), the sediment contains abundant oxalate or uric acid crystals.

The "Urinary Indices"

An important series of diagnostic tests relates to an assessment of renal tubular function. The most widely used and convenient tests are measurements of sodium and creatinine simultaneously obtained from plasma and urine serum samples. The rationale for the use of these indices is as follows: the ratio of urine to plasma creatinine (U/P_{cr}) provides an index of the fraction of filtered water excreted. If it is assumed that all of the creatinine filtered at the glomerulus is excreted into the urine and that relatively little is added by secretion (an oversimplification but an acceptable one), any increment in the concentration of creatinine in urine over that in plasma must be due to the removal of water.

In prerenal azotemia, owing to the reduction in the amount of glomerular filtrate entering each nephron and to an added stimulus to salt and water retention, U/P_{cr} typically is considerably greater than it is in ATN, and

TABLE 30–1	Diagnostic Approach to Acute Renal Failure

1. Record review (see Table 30–2); special attention to evidence for recent reduction in GFR and sequence of events leading to deterioration of renal function to determine possible causative factors
2. Physical examination, including evaluation of hemodynamic status
3. Urinalysis, including careful sediment examination
4. Determination of urinary indices
5. Bladder catheterization
6. Fluid-diuretic challenge
7. Radiologic studies, particular procedure being dictated by clinical setting, e.g., ultrasonography to look for obstruction
8. Renal biopsy

GFR = Glomerular filtration rate.

urinary sodium concentrations characteristically are low (Table 30–3). In contrast, in the ATN variety of ARF, the nephrons excrete a large fraction of their filtered sodium and water, resulting in lower U/P_{cr} and a higher fractional excretion of sodium. Interpretations of these tests, however, must be made in conjunction with other assessments of the patient because there are clinically important exceptions to these generalizations. For example, certain types of ATN, such as radiographic dye–induced renal injury, may present with all the clinical characteristics of ATN but with fractional excretions of sodium less than 1%.

Indications for Other Diagnostic Tests and Renal Biopsy

If the diagnosis of prerenal azotemia or ATN is reasonably certain and the clinical setting does not require the exclusion of other causes of acute azotemia, generally no further diagnostic evaluation is necessary. Further diagnostic evaluation is indicated when (1) the diagnosis is uncertain, especially if the clinical setting suggests other possibilities (e.g., obstruction, vascular accident); (2) clinical findings make the diagnosis of prerenal azotemia or ATN unlikely (e.g., total anuria); and/or (3) the oliguria persists beyond 4 weeks.

Sonography provides a noninvasive method of determining the presence or absence of dilatation of the collecting system. It is, therefore, an important and safe screening test to rule out obstruction. Radionuclide methods are available to assess renal blood flow and excretory (secretory) function. Blood flow studies can easily discriminate between the presence or absence of renal blood flow and the symmetry of flow to the two kidneys but are less accurate in quantitating absolute rates of flow. Renal biopsy is rarely required for ARF occurring in the hospital setting, in contrast to ARF occurring outside the hospital, for which renal biopsy is often indicated.

Evaluation of a Patient Who Presents with Renal Failure

Azotemia first discovered outside the hospital may be either chronic or acute in origin. Useful points in decid-

ing whether the renal failure is acute or chronic are summarized in Table 30–4. The majority of those who present with advanced azotemia have chronic renal failure. Before a detailed evaluation is carried out, priority should be given to identifying complications of renal failure that may be lethal unless treated promptly. Some of these, such as marked fluid overload and pericardial tamponade, may be detected on clinical examination. However, life-threatening complications such as severe hyperkalemia or extreme metabolic acidosis require laboratory evaluation. As mentioned in Section I, the electrocardiogram (ECG) is valuable in assessing the effects of hyperkalemia on the heart.

Even before the nature of the underlying disease causing azotemia is known, often a decision to initiate dialysis has to be made. Dialysis should be instituted promptly in patients with severe hyperkalemia, acidosis, marked fluid overload, or uremic manifestations. Many

TABLE 30–2	Record Review in a Hospitalized Patient Who Develops Acute Renal Failure

	Comments
1. Prior renal function	Determine whether the azotemia is acute
	Patients with prior renal insufficiency are particularly susceptible to ARF, secondary to contrast dyes
2. Presence of infection	Sepsis may cause ARF, even in the absence of hypotension
3. Nephrotoxic agents	Aminoglycosides (e.g., gentamicin) are an important cause of ATN in hospitalized patients; typically causes nonoliguric ATN during first 2 weeks of therapy
	Methicillin may cause acute interstitial nephritis
	Cytotoxic drugs, e.g., cisplatin, may cause ARF
4. Contrast studies including oral cholecystogram, intravenous pyelography, angiography	An important cause of ATN in hospitalized patients; typically causes oliguric ATN within 24–48 hr after study
5. Episodes of hypotension	Suggests prerenal azotemia or ischemic ATN
6. History of blood transfusions	Incompatible blood transfusion is an unusual cause of ATN
7. Review of chart for history of loss or sequestration of extracellular fluid volume, intake-output and serial weights	Provide important clues to the possibility of prerenal azotemia
8. Type of surgery	Patients who have had cardiac or vascular surgery or with obstructive jaundice are particularly susceptible to ATN
9. Type of anesthesia	Methoxyflurane and the related less-toxic enflurane are causes of nonoliguric ATN
10. Amount of blood loss during surgery and whether associated with hypotension	Suggests prerenal azotemia or ischemic ATN

ARF = Acute renal failure; ATN = acute tubular necrosis.

TABLE 30–3	Urinary Diagnostic Indices		
Index		Prerenal Azotemia	Acute Tubular Necrosis
Urine sodium U_{Na} (mEq/L)		<20	>40
U_{Cr} (mg/dl)/P_{Cr} mg/dl		>40	<20
U_{OSM} (mOsm/kg H_2O)		>500	<350
Renal failure index			
$RFI = \dfrac{U_{Na}}{U_{Cr}/P_{Cr}}$		<1	>1
Fractional excretion of filtered sodium			
$FeNa = \dfrac{U_{Na} \times P_{Cr}}{P_{Na} \times U_{Cr}} \times 100$		<1	>1

uremic manifestations are nonspecific. However, a pericardial rub or neurologic manifestations such as asterixis are indications for prompt dialysis.

Laboratory Evaluation

In hospitalized adults in whom prerenal and postrenal azotemia have been excluded, ARF is usually due to ATN. By contrast, in an outpatient setting in which prerenal and postrenal causes have been excluded, ARF is more often due to other renal parenchymal diseases. Examination of the urine for blood and protein and of the urine sediment can give valuable information that often helps to narrow considerably the diagnostic possibilities and to suggest further appropriate laboratory evaluation.

1. Presence of 3^+ to 4^+ protein, 2^+ to 3^+ blood, and active sediment with red blood cells (RBCs) and RBC casts is characteristic of proliferative glomerulonephri-

TABLE 30–4	Useful Features that Suggest Acute or Chronic Renal Failure	
Feature	Acute Renal Failure	Chronic Renal Failure
Previous history	Normal renal function	Prior history of elevated blood urea nitrogen or creatinine
Kidney size	Normal	Small with exception of multiple myeloma, diabetes, amyloid, polycystic kidney disease
Bone film	No evidence of renal osteodystrophy	May show evidence of renal osteodystrophy
Hemoglobin/hematocrit	Anemia may be present, but a normal hemoglobin level in a patient with advanced azotemia is presumptive evidence of ARF	Anemia frequently is present

ARF = Acute renal failure.

tis. Evaluation of history and physical examination (suggesting, for example, systemic lupus erythematosus), complement levels, antinuclear factor, and kidney biopsy (if the kidney size is normal) generally helps to clarify the diagnosis.

2. Presence of only a few RBCs in the urine sediment with a strongly heme-positive urine or a heme-positive supernatant (having removed the RBCs by centrifugation) is most commonly due to myoglobinuria or hemoglobinuria. Patients with rhabdomyolysis have marked increase in the muscle enzymes such as creatinine phosphokinase. The urine sediment in patients with myoglobinuria may show RBCs, pigmented casts, granular casts, and numerous uric acid crystals.

Kidney size gives important clues as to whether the renal failure is acute or chronic and whether obstruction is present. Renal ultrasonography is the initial procedure of choice because it is noninvasive and reliable. Normal-sized kidneys in a patient with advanced azotemia generally suggest that the patient has acute rather than chronic renal failure; however, several important causes of chronic renal failure, including diabetes mellitus, multiple myeloma, and amyloidosis, may be associated with normal-sized kidneys. The renal ultrasound examination is also helpful in (1) making a diagnosis of polycystic kidney disease; (2) determining whether one or two kidneys are present; and (3) localizing the kidney for renal biopsy.

Normal kidney size in a patient who presents with renal failure is often an indication for renal biopsy. Before a renal biopsy is carried out, the blood pressure must be controlled, bleeding and coagulation parameters checked, and the presence of two kidneys confirmed.

CLINICAL PRESENTATION, COMPLICATIONS, AND MANAGEMENT OF ACUTE TUBULAR NECROSIS

Acute renal failure results in signs and symptoms that reflect loss of the regulatory, excretory, and endocrine functions of the kidney. The loss of excretory ability of the kidney is expressed by a rise in the plasma concentration of specific substances normally excreted by the kidney. The most widely monitored indices are the concentrations of BUN and creatinine in the serum. In patients without complications, the BUN rises by about 10 to 20 mg/dl/day, and the HCO_3^- falls to a steady-state level of 17 to 18 mEq/L. The serum K^+ need not rise appreciably unless there is a hypercatabolic state, gastrointestinal bleeding, or extensive tissue trauma.

Because ATN is inherently a catabolic disorder, patients with ATN generally lose about 0.5 pound per day. Further weight loss can be minimized by providing adequate calories (1800 to 2500 kcal) and about 40 gm of protein per day. The use of hyperalimentation with 50% dextrose and essential amino acids has had little effect on minimizing mortality and morbidity in patients with ATN, except in patients who also have significant burns.

Hyperkalemia is a life-threatening complication of ARF and often necessitates urgent intervention. The elec-

TABLE 30–5	Major Complications of Acute Renal Failure

Metabolic

Hyperkalemia
Hypocalcemia, hyperphosphatemia
Hypermagnesemia
Hyperuricemia

Cardiovascular

Pericarditis
Arrhythmias

Neurologic

Asterixis
Neuromuscular irritability
Somnolence
Coma
Seizures

Hematologic

Anemia
Coagulopathies
Hemorrhagic diathesis

Gastrointestinal

Vomiting
Nausea

Infectious

Pneumonia
Urinary tract infection
Wound infection
Septicemia

tromechanical effects of hyperkalemia on the heart are potentiated by hypocalcemia, acidosis, and hyponatremia. Thus, the ECG, which measures the summation of these effects, is a better guide to therapy than a single K^+ determination. The cardiac effects of hyperkalemia are primarily referable to blunting the magnitude of the action potential in response to a depolarizing stimulus. The sequential ECG changes observed in hyperkalemia are peaked T waves, prolongation of the PR interval, widening of the QRS complex, and a sine wave pattern and are mandatory indications for prompt treatment. It must be emphasized that the most common biochemical abnormality responsible for death in patients with ATN is hyperkalemia.

Moderate acidosis is generally well tolerated and does not need treatment unless it is used as an adjunct to controlling hyperkalemia or when plasma bicarbonate falls below 15 mEq/L. Hyperkalemia and acidosis not easily controlled by medical therapy are indications for initiating dialysis.

In most patients, hypocalcemia is asymptomatic and does not require treatment. Phosphate-binding gels may be used in patients with significant hyperphosphatemia. Anemia regularly develops in patients with ATN and does not require treatment unless symptomatic or contributing to heart failure.

In a well-managed patient (with use of early dialysis), many of the uremic manifestations outlined in Table 30–5 either do not develop or are minimal. However, infection remains the main cause of death despite vigorous dialysis. Thus, meticulous aseptic care of intravenous catheters and wounds and avoidance of the use of indwelling urinary catheters are important in the management of such patients.

The indications for initiating dialysis are severe hyperkalemia and/or acidosis not easily controlled by medical treatment, fluid overload, and a rate of rise of the BUN in excess of 20 mg/dl/24 hr. In the absence of any of the above, most nephrologists advocate dialysis when the BUN reaches about 100 mg/dl because the goal of modern therapy is to avoid the occurrence of uremic symptoms. Therefore, the patient is dialyzed as frequently as necessary to keep the BUN < 100 mg/dl. When this approach is used, most patients do not develop uremic symptoms, the diet and fluid intake can be liberalized, and the overall management of the patient is easier. Finally, it is critical to review carefully the indications for and the doses of all drugs administered to patients with ATN. Monitoring of blood concentrations of drugs is an important adjunct to effective treatment.

Outcome and Prognosis

The oliguric phase of ATN typically lasts for 1 to 2 weeks and is followed by the diuretic phase. It is important to remember that about one fourth to one third of the deaths occur in the diuretic phase. This is not surprising because, with the availability of dialysis, the most important determinant of the outcome is not the uremia per se but rather the underlying disease that causes the ATN.

As noted previously, infection continues to be the most important cause of death in patients with ATN. In modern acute care hospitals, the outcome of patients who develop ATN is highly variable and, depending on the nature of the underlying disease, mortality rates may be in excess of 50%. In patients who survive the acute episode, the renal function returns essentially to normal, with the only residual findings being a modest reduction in GFR and inability to maximally concentrate and acidify urine.

Prevention

The first principle of good management is prophylaxis. This requires recognition of the clinical settings in which ATN normally occurs (e.g., in patients undergoing cardiac or aortic surgery) and recognition of patients particularly susceptible to ATN. Correcting fluid deficiencies before surgery and keeping patients particularly at risk adequately hydrated prior to radiocontrast studies are some useful measures. Nephrotoxic drugs should be used only when essential and then only with careful monitoring of the patient. Finally, pretreatment with allopurinol before chemotherapy of massive tumors diminishes uric acid excretion.

Pathogenesis of Acute Tubular Necrosis

Despite the common use of the term *acute tubular necrosis,* necrosis of the tubules may not be observed, and the

TABLE 30–6	Spectrum of Renal Toxicity Associated with Nonsteroidal Anti-Inflammatory Drugs (NSAIDs)		
Type	**Pathophysiology**	**Features**	**Associated Conditions**
Acute renal failure	↓ Renal blood flow	Prerenal azotemia, sodium retention	Congestive heart failure, cirrhosis, volume depletion, renal insufficiency
Hyperchloremic metabolic acidosis	↓ Renin/aldosterone production	↑ K^+, ↑ Cl^-, ↓ CO_2	Interstitial renal disease
Acute interstitial nephritis	Lymphocytic infiltration of renal interstitium	Acute renal failure, ± heavy proteinuria	Unknown

CO_2 = Carbon dioxide.

histologic picture is often nondiagnostic. The vast majority of patients with ATN have as their initiating event either a decrease in renal plasma flow or exposure to a nephrotoxic agent. Specific forms of toxic nephropathy are discussed in the following section.

Although an initial decrease in renal blood flow appears to be a requisite for the development of ischemic ATN, blood flow returns nearly to normal within 24 to 48 hours after the initial insult. Despite adequate renal blood flow, tubular dysfunction persists and the GFR remains depressed. Leakage of glomerular ultrafiltrate from the tubular lumen into the renal interstitium across the damaged renal tubular cells, obstruction to flow due to debris or crystals in the lumen of the tubules, and a decrease in the glomerular capillary ultrafiltration coefficient (K_f) have all been proposed to play a pathophysiologic role in sustaining the clinical picture of ATN.

A variety of biochemical changes have been suggested as being responsible for cell injury in ARF. These include mitochondrial dysfunction, ATP depletion, phospholipid degradation, elevation in cytosolic free calcium, decrease in (Na^+/K^+)-ATPase activity, alterations in substrate metabolism, lysosomal changes, and the production of oxygen free radicals. It is not yet clear which changes are causative and which may simply be by-products of advanced cell injury.

SPECIFIC CAUSES OF ACUTE RENAL FAILURE

Exogenous Nephrotoxins

Radiographic Contrast Agents

Radiocontrast-induced ARF is one of the most common causes of nephrotoxic ARF. Nonionic agents do not appear to be any less nephrotoxic than ionic ones. The most important risk factor appears to be underlying renal insufficiency, although dehydration and concomitant exposure to other nephrotoxins are also important. The individuals at highest risk are diabetic patients with serum creatinine greater than 5 mg/dl. In the absence of other risk factors, diabetes per se does not appear to pose a major risk.

Aminoglycosides

The most important manifestation of aminoglycoside (e.g., tobramycin, gentamicin, amikacin) nephrotoxicity is

ARF, accounting for 10 to 15% of all cases of this disorder in the United States. Up to 10% of patients receiving aminoglycosides develop some degree of renal dysfunction, even though the blood levels may be maintained in the therapeutic range. ARF is usually mild and nonoliguric and is manifested by a rise in the serum creatinine level after several days of therapy with one of the aminoglycosides. However, oliguria and severe renal failure requiring dialysis may be seen. The prognosis for recovery of renal function after several days is excellent.

The Nonsteroidal Anti-Inflammatory Drugs (NSAIDs)

Renal toxicity related to NSAIDs has emerged as a very common form of drug-induced nephrotoxicity. NSAIDs are potent inhibitors of prostaglandin synthesis, a property that contributes to their nephrotoxic potential in certain high-risk patients in whom renal vasodilatation depends on prostaglandins. Several distinct patterns of nephrotoxicity have been associated with these agents (Table 30–6). The most frequent pattern of injury related to NSAIDs is a prerenal azotemia, particularly in patients who either are volume contracted or have a reduced effective circulating volume. Susceptible individuals include those with congestive heart failure, cirrhosis, chronic renal disease, and volume depletion. A hyperchloremic metabolic acidosis, often associated with hyperkalemia, has also been recognized as an effect of the NSAIDs, particularly in individuals with pre-existing chronic interstitial renal disease. Hyporeninemic hypoaldosteronism occurs in these individuals in states of renal prostaglandin inhibition. Hyponatremia is occasionally identified in patients taking NSAIDs and is the result of an impairment in the ability of the kidney to generate a maximally dilute urine when renal prostaglandin production is inhibited. Finally, NSAIDs have been associated with the development of an acute interstitial nephritis, often associated with renal insufficiency and nephrotic-range proteinuria. Discontinuation of the offending agent usually results in a resolution of this disorder.

Cisplatin

Renal injury is a well-recognized and dose-dependent complication of cisplatin use in the management of many carcinomas. Hypomagnesemia due to renal losses of magnesium may be severe and can occur in as many as 50% of patients. Patients should be well hydrated prior to administration of cisplatin, and known nephrotoxins should be avoided whenever possible. The usual lesion is that of ATN, but with severe damage or recurrent administration of the drug, chronic interstitial disease may ensue.

Ethylene Glycol Toxicity

Ingestion of ethylene glycol, usually in the form of antifreeze, produces a characteristic syndrome of severe high anion gap metabolic acidosis and a large osmolal gap. ARF generally manifests after 48 to 72 hours. Patients exhibit disorientation and agitation initially, progressing to central nervous system depression, stupor, and coma. Cardiovascular collapse is a terminal event.

The Angiotensin-Converting Enzyme (ACE) Inhibitors

Angiotensin-converting enzyme inhibitor–associated ARF is thought to be hemodynamic in origin from loss of autoregulation of renal blood flow and GFR and has been typically reported when these drugs are given to patients with bilateral renal artery stenosis or with moderately advanced azotemia. Allergic acute interstitial nephritis similar to that observed with methicillin has also been reported.

Endogenous Nephrotoxins

Rhabdomyolysis

Since the first description of the causative association between rhabdomyolysis and ARF during the crush injuries of World War II, the spectrum of causes of rhabdomyolysis, myoglobinuria, and renal failure has markedly broadened. The most frequent causes are (in order) alcohol abuse, muscle compression, seizures, metabolic derangements, drugs, and infections. Muscle pain and dark brown orthotoluidine-positive urine without RBCs are important diagnostic clues but must be confirmed by elevations of creatine phosphokinase and myoglobin. About one third of patients with rhabdomyolysis develop ARF, frequently associated with hyperkalemia, hyperuricemia, hyperphosphatemia, early hypocalcemia, and a reduced BUN/creatinine ratio because of excessive creatinine release from muscle. Late hypercalcemia is also a typical feature of the disease.

Hyperuricemic Acute Renal Failure

Acute renal failure may occur in patients with "high turnover" malignancies (acute lymphoblastic leukemia and poorly differentiated lymphomas) who either spontaneously or, more frequently, after cytotoxic therapy, release massive amounts of purine uric acid precursors, leading to uric acid precipitation in the renal tubules. During massive cell lysis, phosphate and potassium are also released in large amounts, resulting in hyperphosphatemia and hyperkalemia. The peak uric acid level is often > 20 mg/dl, and a ratio of urinary uric acid–creatinine concentrations greater than 1 : 1 suggests the diagnosis of acute uric acid nephropathy. Prevention of ARF includes establishing a urinary output of ≥ 3 L per 24 hours and treatment with allopurinol prior to institution of cytotoxic therapy.

Hepatorenal Syndrome

The hepatorenal syndrome is defined as kidney failure in patients with severely compromised liver function in the absence of clinical, laboratory, or anatomic evidence of other known causes of renal failure. It closely resembles prerenal failure except that it does not respond to conventional volume replacement. In the United States and Europe, the great majority of cases of hepatorenal syndrome occur in patients with advanced alcoholic cirrhosis. Hepatorenal syndrome may begin insidiously over a period of weeks to months or appear suddenly and cause severe azotemia within days. The common precipitating causes are deterioration of liver function, sepsis, the use of nephrotoxic antibiotics or NSAIDs, overzealous use of diuretics, diarrhea, or gastrointestinal bleeding. It can, however, occur without any apparent precipitating cause. The hallmark of hepatorenal syndrome is oliguria with urine osmolality two to three times the concentration of plasma, and urine that is virtually sodium free, similar to that of patients with prerenal azotemia.

The initial step in management is to search diligently for and treat correctable causes of azotemia. An important step in the management is to exclude reversible prerenal azotemia. Because hepatorenal syndrome and prerenal azotemia have similar urinary diagnostic indices, one must often use a functional maneuver, i.e., administration of volume expanders to differentiate between these two entities. Once a diagnosis of hepatorenal syndrome is established, there is no specific treatment, and the management is conservative.

ARF Related to Pregnancy

Acute renal failure is presently a rare occurrence in industrialized nations, occurring in < 1 in 10,000 deliveries. In the first trimester, septic abortion accounts for the majority of patients with ARF. In late pregnancy, ARF is a complication of pre-eclampsia or uterine bleeding in abruptio placentae. ATN is an uncommon complication of pre-eclampsia, occurring in about 1 to 2% of the cases; however, it does occur in a larger percentage, approximately 5% of patients with hemolysis, elevated liver enzymes, low platelets (HELLP) syndrome. Abruptio placentae can also cause ATN but is also the most common cause of renal cortical necrosis.

Postpartum ARF, also known as postpartum hemolytic uremic syndrome, is characterized by hypertension and microangiopathic hemolytic anemia (75%) and occurs anywhere from 1 to 2 days to several months after delivery, the most common time frame being from 2 to 5 weeks postpartum. Glomerular lesions resemble those found in adult hemolytic uremic syndrome with fibrin deposition, thickened capillary walls, and subendothelial swelling with large granular subendothelial deposits. Overall, prognosis is poor, with a chance of recovery of renal function in only a minority of the patients.

REFERENCES

Chapman AB, Schrier RW: Acute renal failure in pregnancy. *In* The Principles & Practice of Nephrology. 2nd ed. Jacobson HR, Striker GE, Klahr S (eds.). St. Louis, Mosby–Year Book, 1995, pp 445–453.

Lazarus JM, Brenner BM: Acute Renal Failure. 3rd ed. New York, Churchill Livingstone, 1993.

Paller MS, Ferris TF: The kidney and hypertension in pregnancy. *In* The Kidney. 5th ed. Brenner BM (ed.). Philadelphia, WB Saunders, 1996, pp 1731–1763.

Shah SV: Acute renal failure. *In* The Principles & Practice of Nephrology. 2nd ed. Jacobson HR, Striker GE, Klahr S (eds.). St. Louis, Mosby–Year Book, 1995, pp 544–594.

31

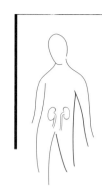

Chronic Renal Failure

Chronic renal failure is defined as progressive and irreversible loss of renal function. The most common etiologies of renal insufficiency ultimately leading to end-stage renal disease (ESRD) are listed in Table 31–1. Loss of <75% of glomerular filtration rate (GFR) does not usually result in pronounced symptoms, as the remaining glomeruli adapt with hyperfiltration, and the surviving tubules adjust by maintaining adequate acid-base, fluid, and electrolyte balance. For example, the doubling of serum creatinine from 0.7 mg/dl to 1.4 mg/dl signifies a loss of approximately 50% GFR, emphasizing the importance of early recognition and intervention at this early stage. When patients present with elevated serum creatinine, acute renal failure must be differentiated from chronic renal failure, as discussed in Chapter 30. Every attempt should be made to arrive at the specific etiology of chronic renal failure. Biopsy is the most specific tool to reach definitive diagnosis. This allows specific treatment of the underlying etiology, assessment of the prognosis, and suitability of kidney transplantation. If the biopsy is not performed because of small kidney size, diagnosis is made based on present, past, and family history, serologic evaluation, examination of the urine sediment, and ultrasound evaluation. Although most chronic kidney diseases are associated with progressive decrease in kidney size, few systemic diseases are characterized by presentation of normal kidney size despite advanced renal failure. These are diabetes mellitus, multiple myeloma, polycystic kidney disease, and amyloidosis.

ADAPTATION TO NEPHRON LOSS

To ensure adequate solute, water, and acid-base balance, the surviving nephrons in the diseased kidney must adjust by increasing their filtration and excretion rates. Without such adjustments, patients with chronic renal failure are vulnerable to edema formation and severe volume overload, hyperkalemia, and hyponatremia. Thus, during progressive renal disease, sodium balance is maintained by increasing its fractional excretion per nephron. Acid excretion is usually maintained until late stages in chronic renal failure when the GFR falls below 15 ml/min. Initially, increased tubular ammonia synthesis provides an adequate buffer of hydrogen in the distal nephron. Later, significant decrease in distal bicarbonate regeneration re-

sults in hyperchloremic metabolic acidosis. Further loss in remaining nephrons leads to retention of organic ions such as sulfates, resulting in anion gap acidosis and titration of bone bicarbonate stores.

Once renal insufficiency is established, there is a tendency for renal disease to progress regardless of the initial insult. This suggests a maladaptive process in the surviving nephrons to be the likely mechanism/s responsible for progressive renal insufficiency. Figure 31–1 illustrates different pathways through which these maladaptive mechanisms can result in progression of renal insufficiency and, ultimately, ESRD. Glomerular hypertrophy and glomerular capillary hypertension leading to glomerulosclerosis have been implicated as important factors in the development of progressive renal insufficiency. For example, decreased glomerular capillary pressure with angiotensin-converting enzyme (ACE) inhibitors has been found in animal and human studies to retard such progression in renal failure.

Compensatory glomerular hypertrophy is invariably associated with tubular hypertrophy in the remaining nephrons. Although this adaptive mechanism can be beneficial in maintaining fluid, electrolyte, and acid-base balance, the long-term consequence is perpetuation of tubulointerstitial damage. Tubular hypertrophy is usually associated with increased energy expenditure, a metabolic event associated with generation of reactive oxygen metabolites. These have been proposed as mechanisms of tubulointerstitial damage in animal models of renal diseases. Also, hyperlipidemia has been implicated in progressive renal insufficiency through mesangial proliferation and sclerosis.

Conservative Management of Chronic Renal Failure

Diet

In the past, dietary protein restriction has been advocated to reduce uremic symptoms. Recent evidence suggests the role of high protein intake in glomerular hyperfiltration and the role of hyperlipidemia in mesangial proliferation and sclerosis. These data suggest the use of dietary restrictions to slow the progression of renal disease. Protein restriction also results in reduction in phosphate load, the

TABLE 31-1	Percent Distribution of Incidence of ESRD by Primary Diagnosis, 1990–1992

Primary Etiology	Incidence (%)
Diabetes	36.0
Hypertension	30.0
Glomerulonephritis	12.0
Cystic kidney	3.0
Interstitial nephritis	3.0
Obstruction	2.0
Collagen vascular disease	2.0
AIDS-related	0.5

AIDS = Acquired immunodeficiency syndrome.

major stimulus for adaptive hyperparathyroidism. Although the evidence from human studies is less certain, strong evidence of the beneficial effect of dietary protein restriction has been provided by several animal studies. The National Study of Dietary Modification in Renal Disease suggests a beneficial effect of protein restriction at the level of 0.75 mg/kg/day in patients with GFR of 25 to 50 ml/min. At present, it seems prudent to advise aggressive dietary management in patients with renal insufficiency, with proper restriction of sodium, potassium, phosphorus, and protein intake. Sodium should be restricted, especially in hypertensive and edematous patients. The high prevalence of atherogenic cardiovascular disease in patients with renal insufficiency justifies dietary restriction of cholesterol and fat.

Hypertension

Several controlled trials have conclusively confirmed that aggressive management of hypertension attenuates the rate of progression of renal failure. Significant benefit has been demonstrated in patients with diabetic nephropathy, as well as in patients with other chronic renal diseases. In addition, a recent trial convincingly demonstrated the nephroprotective effect of captopril above and beyond control of hypertension in patients with nephropathy and type 1 diabetes mellitus. In addition, the use of calcium channel blockers may be beneficial by blocking the deleterious effect of angiotensin II on progression of renal insufficiency. Thus, it may be beneficial to combine ACE inhibitors and calcium channel blockers in patients who require more than one drug for control of hypertension.

Management of Reversible Causes of Acute Deterioration in Renal Function

The rate of decline in GFR for individual patients is log linear. Accordingly, plotting 1 over the serum creatinine against time usually predicts the rate at which a specific patient will reach ESRD, as shown in Figure 31–2. When such a patient suddenly demonstrates acceleration of renal failure, the differential diagnosis for such acceleration should be considered, as presented in Table 31–2.

Avoiding Toxic Drug Effects

Many drugs that are excreted by the kidney should be avoided or adjusted in renal insufficiency, as shown in

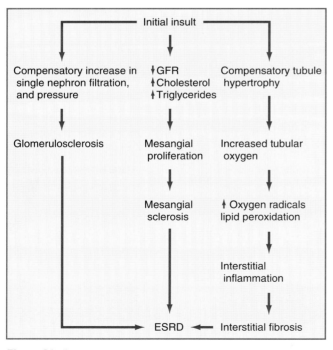

Figure 31–1
Factors responsible for the progression of renal disease. ESRD = End-stage renal disease; GFR = glomerular filtration rate.

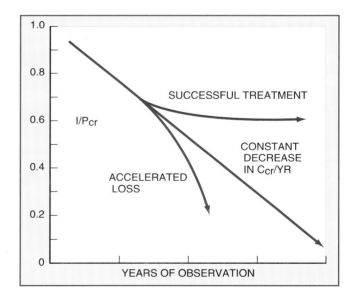

Figure 31–2
Use of the reciprocal of plasma creatinine concentration, $1/P_{cr}$, to follow the progress of glomerular disease in a patient. (From Sullivan LP, Grantham JJ: Physiology of the Kidney. 2nd ed. Philadelphia, Lea & Febiger, 1982.)

TABLE 31-2	Reversible Causes of Acute Deterioration in Renal Function

Decreased renal perfusion
    Overdiuresis, gastrointestinal losses
    Heart failure
    Third spacing
Obstruction
Infection
    Urinary tract
    Sepsis
Nephrotoxins
    Endogenous—myoglobulin, hemoglobin, uric acid, calcium, phosphorus
    Exogenous—contrast, drugs
Poorly controlled hypertension

Table 31–3, to avoid toxicity. In addition, patients with renal insufficiency are more susceptible to the nephrotoxic effects of over-the-counter medications such as nonsteroidal anti-inflammatory drugs (NSAIDs).

CLINICAL MANIFESTATIONS OF RENAL FAILURE

The Uremic Syndrome

Patients with renal insufficiency usually become symptomatic when GFR is <10 ml/min. Diabetics with renal insufficiency usually demonstrate symptoms at a higher GFR. Uremia is a syndrome that affects every organ system. Uremia is likely the consequence of combined effects of several retained molecules and the deficiency of important hormones and factors, rather than the effect of a single uremic toxin (Fig. 31–3). Urea, in addition to being the most commonly used measure of renal failure and adequacy of dialysis, can cause symptoms of fatigue, nausea, vomiting, and headaches. Its breakdown product (cyanate) can result in carbamylation of lipoproteins and peptides with possible adverse effects leading to multiple organ dysfunctions.

Guanidines, by-products of exogenous or indigenous protein metabolism, are increased in renal failure. They could inhibit 1-alpha hydroxylase activity within the kidney, leading to deficient calcitriol production and secondary hyperparathyroidism. High parathyroid hormone level has been implicated in various manifestations of uremia, especially in cardiomyopathy and metastatic calcifications. Beta-2 microglobulin accumulation in patients with renal failure has been associated with neuropathy, carpal tunnel syndrome, and amyloid infiltration of the joints.

Specific Manifestations of Uremia (Fig. 31–4)

CARDIOVASCULAR EFFECTS. Mortality from cardiovascular disease in renal failure patients is three and a half times that of an age-matched population. Hypertension is common in renal failure and is usually aggravated by fluid

TABLE 31-3	Drug Dosage in Chronic Renal Failure		
Major Dosage Reduction	**Minor or No Reduction**	**Avoid Usage**
Antibiotics		
Aminoglycosides	Erythromycin	NSAIDs
Penicillin	Nafcillin	Nitrofurantoin
Cephalosporins	Clindamycin	Nalidixic acid
Sulfonamides	Chloramphenicol	Tetracycline
Vancomycin	Isoniazid/rifampin	
Quinolones	Amphotericin B	
Fluconozole	Aztereonam/tazobactam	
Acyclovir/gancyclovir	Doxycycline	
Foscarnet		
Imipenem		
Others		
Digoxin	Antihypertensives	Aspirin
Procainamide	Benzodiazepines	Sulfonylureas
H₂ antagonists	Quinidine	Lithium carbonate
Meperidine	Lidocaine	Acetazolamide
Codeine	Spironolactone	
Propoxyphene	Triamterene	

NSAID = Nonsteroidal anti-inflammatory drug.

retention. More than 60% of patients starting dialysis have echocardiographic manifestations of left ventricular hypertrophy, dilation, and systolic or diastolic dysfunction. Accelerated atherogenesis is responsible for the high prevalence of coronary artery disease in this population and the high rate of recurrent coronary artery stenosis postangioplasty. Pericarditis can occur in uremic patients before initiating dialysis and in patients already on dialysis. Initiation of dialysis or intensifying dialytic therapy usually results in resolution of pericarditis in patients receiving inadequate dialysis therapy. Pericarditis occurring in the setting of adequate dialysis may not respond to a further increase in dialysis therapy and may require surgical drainage.

GASTROINTESTINAL DISEASE. Gastrointestinal disturbances are among the earliest and most common signs of the uremic syndrome. Patients with renal failure usually de-

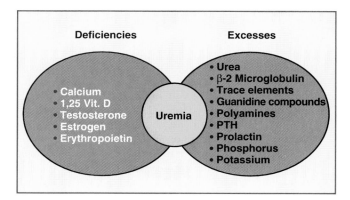

Figure 31–3
Etiologic factors of uremia. PTH = Parathyroid hormone.

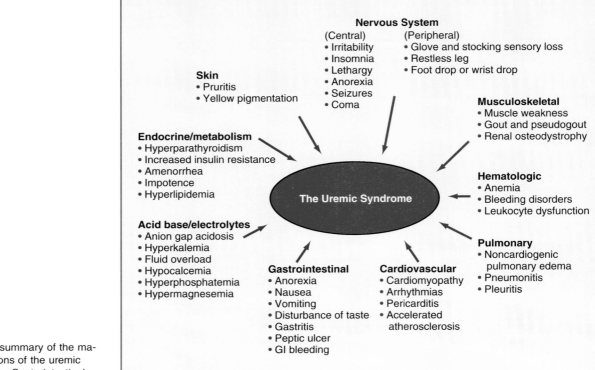

Figure 31–4
Diagrammatic summary of the major manifestations of the uremic syndrome. GI = Gastrointestinal.

scribe a metallic taste and loss of appetite. Later, nausea and vomiting become intractable and improve after starting dialysis. Several pathologic processes can lead to gastrointestinal bleeding. Among these, gastritis, peptic ulceration, and arteriovenous malformations are the most common.

NEUROLOGIC MANIFESTATIONS. Central nervous system manifestations are frequent and present early, often with subtle changes in cognitive function, and memory and sleep disorders. Lethargy, irritability, frank encephalopathy, asterixis, and seizures are late manifestations of uremia and are usually avoided by early start of dialysis therapy. Peripheral neurologic manifestations present as a symmetric sensory neuropathy in a glove and stocking distribution. Peripheral motor impairment can result in restless legs and foot or wrist drop, which may respond to dialysis.

MUSCULOSKELETAL MANIFESTATIONS. Alterations in calcium and phosphate homeostasis and renal osteodystrophy are common manifestations of uremia. Hyperparathyroidism and disturbance of vitamin D metabolism are commonly found. Hypocalcemia and secondary hyperparathyroidism are the result of phosphate retention and lack of 1-alpha hydroxylase activity in the failing kidney, which results in deficiency of the most active form of vitamin D. Over time, the adaptive parathyroid hypertrophy becomes maladaptive, leading to severe bone disease and tissue calcinosis. Calcium and phosphate homeostasis in the setting of renal failure is demonstrated in Figure 31–5. Excess parathyroid hormone contributes to the neuro-

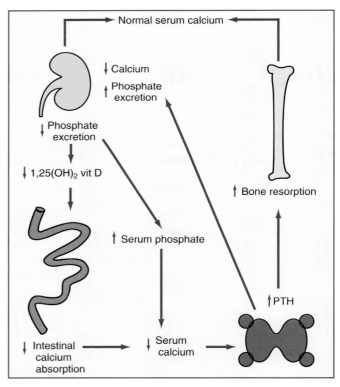

Figure 31–5
Calcium and phosphate homeostasis in the setting of renal failure. The decreased excretion of phosphate initiates the cycle directed at normalization of the serum calcium concentration. PTH = Parathyroid hormone.

toxicity and proximal myopathy of uremia. Control of hyperparathyroidism with phosphate binders, calcium supplementation, and 1, 25 Vitamin D together with dialysis therapy is now achievable. This aggressive management has resulted in significant reduction in renal osteodystrophy in dialysis patients.

HEMATOLOGIC EFFECTS. Erythropoietin, a hormone produced by the kidney that regulates the production of erythrocytes by the bone marrow becomes progressively deficient as renal mass declines. This is the most common cause of anemia in chronic renal failure. Routine administration of erythropoietin to patients with ESRD results in correction of anemia, improved quality of life, and decreased dependence on blood transfusions. Bleeding disorders are common in uremia. Defective platelet aggregation has been demonstrated in these patients and is partially corrected by dialysis.

ENDOCRINE ABNORMALITIES. Symptoms of hypothyroidism and the uremic syndrome may overlap, but hypothyroidism is not part of the uremic syndrome. Alterations in thyroid function testing may contribute to the difficulty of diagnosing thyroid dysfunction in the uremic patient. While T_3 resin uptake may be increased, T_3 and T_4 are usually normal or low, and thyroid-stimulating hormone (TSH) is usually normal or low but occasionally increased. On occasion, the use of a thyrotropin-releasing hormone (TRH) stimulation test may be needed for diagnosis of thyroid disorders in uremia. Deranged pituitary gonadal axis can result in impotence, amenorrhea, sterility, and uterine bleeding. Hyperprolactinemia may be responsible for some of these abnormalities of the pituitary gonadal axis. There are decreased plasma levels of testosterone, estrogen, and progesterone, with normal or increased levels of follicle-stimulating hormone (FSH) and luteinizing hormones.

METABOLIC DISORDERS IN UREMIA. As renal function diminishes, many diabetic patients have a decrease in their insulin requirements. This is partly due to the increased half-life of exogenously administered insulin. At the same time, increased peripheral insulin resistance in uremic patients has been recognized. Increased glucagon production and decreased renal metabolism may be responsible for uremic hypermetabolism. Lipid abnormalities are common findings in the early course of renal failure. They are most consistent with type IV hyperlipoproteinemia with marked increase in plasma triglycerides and less of an increase in total cholesterol. These abnormalities of lipid metabolism are considered major contributors to accelerated atherosclerosis in the renal failure population in addition to their role in mesangial proliferation and progressive renal failure.

DERMATOLOGIC MANIFESTATIONS. The uremic hue is likely the result of retained urochrome and other pigmented substances. Pruritus is a common complaint of patients with renal failure, and the exact etiology is not certain. It usually responds to dialysis, control of hyperparathyroidism, improved calcium and phosphate balance, and, occasionally, ultraviolet rays. Calciphylaxis is a rare occurrence in well-managed patients. It results from painful skin calcification in patients with calcium × phosphorus products that exceed 70 in the presence of severe hyperparathyroidism.

Treatment of End-Stage Renal Failure

A plan for a modality of renal replacement therapy should be discussed with the patient early in the course of renal failure and before the appearance of uremic symptoms. The current criteria for initiation of dialysis is GFR ≥ 15 ml/min for diabetics and < 10 ml/min for nondiabetics. Creatinine clearance overestimates GFR in advanced renal failure because of tubular secretion of creatinine. More accurate estimation of GFR can be calculated from the average of creatinine and urea clearances. Patients with volume overload resistant to diuretics, acidosis, persistent hyperkalemia, intractable gastrointestinal symptoms, or encephalopathy should be started on dialysis even though their creatinine clearance may exceed the previously set criteria. The choice of replacement therapy largely depends on the patient's physical and sociodemographic characteristics. Most patients are initiated either on hemodialysis or peritoneal dialysis. In general, transplantation is encouraged because of a better quality of life and a greater chance for rehabilitation.

Hemodialysis

More than 100,000 patients with ESRD are maintained on chronic hemodialysis. It continues to be the form of treatment for the great majority of patients in the United States. As illustrated in Figure 31–6, blood obtained through a temporary or permanent vascular access that ensures blood flows of ≥ 300 ml/min is pumped through a large number of capillaries manufactured from semisynthetic membranes. In an opposite direction, a dialysate that contains sodium chloride, acetate, or bicarbonate and varying concentrations of potassium is circulated. Diffusion through the membrane allows low–molecular-weight substances such as urea to leave the blood side and move to the dialysate side according to the concentration gradient. Similarly, bicarbonate, which is usually at a concentration of 35 mEq/L, diffuses to the plasma side. Removal of excess water and sodium chloride is achieved by ultrafiltration, which is dependent on the hydrostatic pressure across the membrane. The average patient on hemodialysis requires 3.5 hours of dialysis three times a week to achieve creatinine clearance > 140 L/week. Such low clearance can support good patient survival only when aggressive dietary modification is followed. Residual renal function is lost more rapidly on hemodialysis than on peritoneal dialysis. Patients on hemodialysis are at high risk of development of volume overload, pulmonary edema, hyperkalemia, hyperphosphatemia, and metabolic bone disease if compliance with restricted diet and fluid intake is not optimal. Cellulose-based dialysis membranes are complement activating and potentially have a role for increased susceptibility to infection, which is seen in this population.

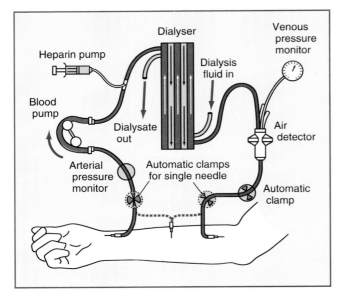

Figure 31–6
Essential components of a dialysis delivery system, which, together with the dialyzer, make up an "artificial kidney." In isolated ultrafiltration, no dialysis fluid is used (bypass mode). Also shown is the apparatus for using a single needle for inflow and outflow of blood from the patient. (From Keshaviah PR, Shaldon S: In Drukker W, Parsons FM, Maher JF (eds.): Replacement of Renal Function by Dialysis. 3rd ed. Boston, Martinus Nijhoff Publishers, 1988. Reprinted by permission of Kluwer Academic Publishers.)

Peritoneal Dialysis

In this modality, the peritoneum acts as a semipermeable membrane like a hemodialysis filter. This technique has several advantages: it allows independence from the long time spent in dialysis units, it does not require stringent dietary restrictions as in hemodialysis, and rehabilitation rates are somewhat better than those observed in hemodialysis. With either continuous ambulatory peritoneal dialysis (CAPD) or continuous cyclic peritoneal dialysis (CCPD), there is enough flexibility to allow full-time employment. In CAPD, dialysate of 1.5- to 2.5-L volumes are left in the peritoneal cavity for varying amounts of time to be exchanged four to six times daily. In CCPD, the patient is connected to a cycler machine that allows inflow of smaller-volume dialysate with shorter dwell time through the night, with the patient free from dialysis during the day. Several modifications in this regimen can be made to fit the specific patient to achieve adequate clearance. In peritoneal dialysis, larger-size molecules are removed more efficiently than smaller-size molecules, and ultrafiltration is achieved through higher dextrose concentration in the dialysate. In spite of lower weekly creatinine clearance in patients on peritoneal dialysis, residual renal function is preserved longer, and their survival matches those observed in hemodialysis. The two major drawbacks of peritoneal dialysis are infection of the percutaneous catheter placed into the peritoneal cavity and difficulty in achieving adequate clearance in patients with large body mass. Peritonitis in peritoneal dialysis patients can be treated with intraperitoneal administration of anti-

biotics. Fungal peritonitis and infection in the tunnel around the dialysis catheter are indications for catheter removal.

KIDNEY TRANSPLANTATION

Renal transplantation is one of several modalities for renal replacement therapy, with hemodialysis or peritoneal dialysis often required before, during, or after transplantation. Successful transplantation is probably the most satisfactory treatment for ESRD. When cyclosporine became available in 1983, the success rate improved significantly, with 85 to 90% 1-year graft survival, compared with 65% with azathioprine and steroids.

Cadaver Versus Living Donor Kidney Transplantation

Advantages and disadvantages of cadaver versus living kidney donor transplantation are listed in Table 31–4. Living-related donation contributes to about 10 to 20% of all kidney transplants. With cadaver donor organ supply failing to meet the demand, the pressure for living donation increases. Even with the advent of cyclosporine, the gap between living donor graft survival and cadaver organ survival remains. Recently, unrelated donors with a stable and close emotional relationship with the recipient, such as a spouse, have been considered in many transplant centers. Graft survival for these unrelated donors is better than cadaver graft survival, despite less histocompatibility matching of human leukocyte antigen (HLA). Living or cadaver donation should only be performed

TABLE 31–4	Comparison of Donor Sources for Kidney Transplantation
Advantages	**Disadvantages**
Living Donor	
Better tissue match with less likelihood of rejection	Small potential risk of operation to donor
Smaller doses of drugs for immunosuppression	Requires willing, medically suitable family member
Waiting time for transplant reduced	
Avoid sequelae of chronic dialysis	
Elective surgical procedure	
Better early graft function with shorter hospitalization	
Better short- and long-term success	
Cadaver Donor	
Available to any recipient	Tissue match not as similar
Other organs available for combined transplants (i.e., kidney-pancreas transplant)	Waiting time variable
	Operation must be performed urgently
Vascular conduits available for complex vascular reconstruction	Early graft function may be compromised
	Short- and long-term success not as good as from living donor

between ABO blood group–compatible donors. A major advantage of a living-related transplant is histocompatibility matching. As demonstrated in Figure 31–7, a potential recipient can share one haplotype match with both parents and one in four of his or her siblings or share two haplotype matches with one in four of the siblings, with the last possibility of sharing none of the histocompatibility antigens with the remaining sibling. HLA-identical matches consistently demonstrate superior graft survival and less chance for rejection than either one-haplo or cadaveric transplants.

Immunosuppressant Drug Therapy

Prophylaxis against and the treatment of rejection is at the heart of success of kidney transplantation. Over the course of the past three decades, the immunosuppressive protocols for renal transplantation have undergone remarkable evolution. All the protocols for immunosuppression aim at disruption of the lymphocyte cell cycle. Azathioprine and steroids, with or without antilymphocyte preparations, were the mainstay of clinical immunosuppression in the 1960s and 1970s. Since the introduction of cyclosporine in the early 1980s, the number of drugs capable of suppressing the immune system has increased steadily. These agents, by virtue of their specific mode of action, have succeeded in preventing most patients from having early and irreversible rejections without severe toxic effects. The mechanism of action of some of the most commonly used immunosuppressants is illustrated in Figure 31–8.

Cyclosporine

The addition of cyclosporine to immunosuppressive protocols since the early 1980s has favorably affected graft survival, with a 20% increase in cadaveric kidney survival in the first year. Cyclosporine is extracted from the fungus *Tolypocladium inflatum*. The original preparation was extremely hydrophobic with erratic absorption, which

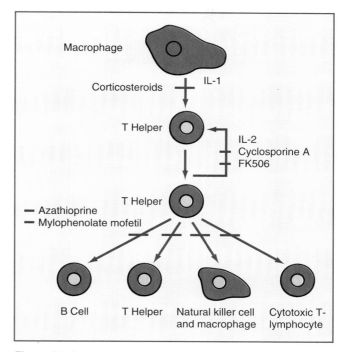

Figure 31–8
Site of action of immunosuppressive agents. IL = Interleukin.

resulted in highly fluctuating plasma levels. A new microimmulsion preparation, which results in more predictable levels and less dependence on bile for absorption, has recently been introduced. The hepatic cytochrome oxidase P-450 system is essential for cyclosporine metabolism. It is important to recognize that several drugs that induce or inhibit this system would significantly interfere with cyclosporine level and may result in inadequate levels, resulting in rejection or high levels, leading to toxicity. Examples of medications that lead to high cyclosporine levels are ketoconazole, verapamil, diltiazem, ciprofloxacin, and erythromycin. Other medications that can lower cyclosporine levels by inducing the P-450 cytochrome system are rifampin and the antiseizure medications dilantin, valproic acid, and phenobarbital.

Cyclosporine exerts its specific immunosuppressive activity by interfering with several cytokines, the most important of which is interleukin (IL)-2, by the activated lymphocytes. Some of the most important side effects of cyclosporine are listed in Table 31–5 and respond to appropriate reduction in the dose. The most significant of these is nephrotoxicity. This is usually related to decreased glomerular blood flow and usually responds well to dose reduction.

Acute Rejection

T lymphocytes survey the human body and are capable of recognizing foreign antigens when presented in association with HLA antigens, especially class 2 histocompatibility antigens. When the recipient T helper cells identify those foreign HLA class 2 antigens presented by dendritic

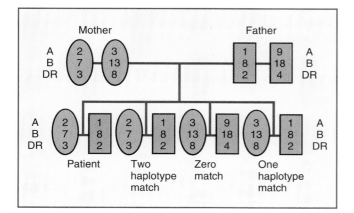

Figure 31–7
Diagrammatic respresentation of inheritance of human leukocyte antigen (HLA) tissue types in a family with four siblings.

TABLE 31–5	Side Effects of Commonly Used Immunosuppressive Drugs			
	Corticosteroids	**Azathioprine**	**Cyclosporine**	**Mylophenolate Mofetil**
Renal	Fluid retention		Preglomerular vasoconstriction Striped interstitial fibrosis Hyperkalemia	
Cardiovascular	Hypertension		Hypertension	
Hematologic		Bone marrow suppression Macrocytosis	Hemolytic uremic syndrome	Leukopenia Anemia
Neurologic	Proximal muscle weakness Mood changes Depression		Tremor Seizures	
Gastrointestinal	Gastritis	Acute pancreatitis	Cholestasis	Vomiting Diarrhea Abdominal pain
Metabolic	Glucose intolerance Dislipidemia		Dislipidemia ↓ Glucose tolerance	
Dermatologic	Acne Easy bruisability	Hair loss	Hypertrichosis Brittle fingernails	
Miscellaneous	Osteoporosis Aseptic necrosis Obesity Accelerated cataracts		Gingival hypertrophy	

or other antigen-presenting cells in the transplanted kidney, lymphocyte activation results. Activated cytotoxic lymphocytes invade the tubular interstitial region of the transplanted kidney, resulting in tubulitis and deterioration in function. Clinically, acute rejection is detected by graft tenderness, rise in serum creatinine, oliguria, and sometimes fever. Frequent monitoring of renal function has allowed early detection of acute rejection based on rising serum creatinine before any clinical signs or symptoms manifest. The incidence of acute rejection is high between the second and twelfth weeks post-transplantation. Severe forms of acute rejection, carrying a poor prognosis, usually involve the intrarenal arteries with vasculitis and are usually resistant to steroid therapy, necessitating antilymphocyte therapy. Kidney function may be lost in the first few hours after transplantation from hyperacute rejection, which results from preformed antibodies to the donor kidney at the time of transplantation.

Post-Transplant Infection

Until recently, infection was the leading cause of mortality in kidney transplant recipients. Now infection is preceded by mortality from myocardial infarction and other cardiac causes. In addition to common community-ac-

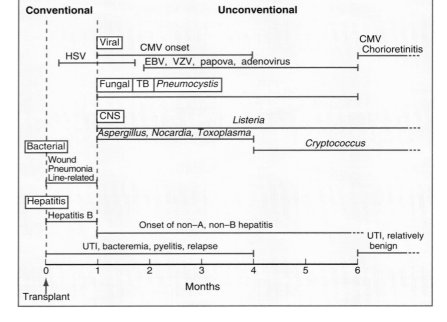

Figure 31–9

Timetable for the occurrence of infection in the renal transplant patient. Exceptions to this timetable should initiate a search for an unusual hazard. CMV = Cytomegalovirus; CNS = central nervous system; EBV = Epstein-Barr virus; HSV = herpes simplex virus; UTI = urinary tract infection; VZV = varicella-zoster virus. (Reprinted by permission of Excerpta Medica from Rubin RH, Wolfson JS, Cosimi AB, Tolkoff-Rubin NE: Infection in the renal transplant recipient. Am J Med, 1981; 70:405–411. Copyright 1981 by Excerpta Medica Inc.)

quired bacterial and viral infections, kidney transplant recipients are also susceptible to numerous viral, fungal, and other opportunistic infections, which normally do not cause severe illness in the immunocompetent host. Fortunately, the timetable of these infections is predictable, and an educated guess based on the time of infection post-transplantation, together with the specific set of syndromes associated with each infection, can help early recognition and prompt treatment of these infections. Figure 31–9 illustrates the temporal relationship between transplantation and these infections.

Post-Transplant Malignancy

It is well known that immunosuppression increases the risk of developing malignancy. Fortunately, skin malignancy is the one malignancy with the highest incidence in the transplant population. Sun exposure is the most significant risk factor, and protection provides excellent primary prevention. With such awareness and aggressive management, metastasis from skin malignancies is rare.

Transplant recipients are also at high risk of developing Kaposi's sarcoma and post-transplant lymphoproliferative disease, a rare occurrence in the immunocompetent host. Cancer surveillance should be an essential part of post-transplant follow-up, with patient education to recognize and report early changes in bowel habits, respiratory symptoms, hematuria, musculoskeletal symptoms, or weight changes.

REFERENCES

Drukker W, Parsons FM, Maher JF: Replacement of Renal Function by Dialysis. 2nd ed. Boston, Martinus Nijhoff Publishers, 1988.

Lewis EJ, Hunnsicker LG, Bain RP, Rhode RD: The effect of angiotensin-converting enzyme inhibitor on diabetic nephropathy. N Engl J Med 1993; 329:1456–1462.

Rubin RH: Infection in the organ transplant recipient. *In* Rubin RH, Young LS (eds.): Clinical Approach to Infection in the Compromised Host. 3rd ed. New York, Plenum, 1994, pp 629–705.

Warnock DG: Chronic renal failure. *In* Wyngaarden JB, Smith LH Jr, Bennett JC (eds.): Cecil Textbook of Medicine. 19th ed. Philadelphia, WB Saunders, 1992, pp 533–541.

Gastrointestinal Disease

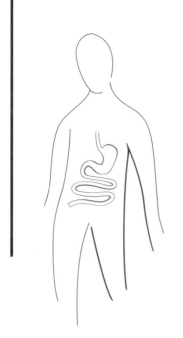

32

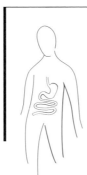

The Common Clinical Manifestations of Gastrointestinal Disease

A. Abdominal Pain

Abdominal pain often heralds gastrointestinal (GI) disease and brings the patient to the attention of the internist, gastroenterologist, or surgeon. Abdominal pain is subjective and can therefore be confusing or helpful in establishing a diagnosis. For example, acute appendicitis may be more readily diagnosed by history and physical examination than by sophisticated imaging techniques. In this section, the etiology, characteristics, and patterns of abdominal pain are reviewed, and an approach to the problem of acute abdominal pain is discussed.

ORIGIN

Sensory information regarding pain travels in sympathetic pathways to spinal sensory neurons. The afferent endings are located in the smooth muscle layers of the hollow organs, in organ capsules, in the peritoneum, and in the walls of intra-abdominal blood vessels. Several of the pain sensations that are readily identified with skin injury, such as cutting, tearing, and burning, are absent in the intestines. However, there are three types of sensation that produce pain in the gut:

1. Stretching the wall of a hollow organ or the capsule of a solid organ can produce abdominal pain. This type of stretching usually occurs because there is forceful muscle contraction, muscle spasms, distention, or traction.
2. Inflammatory responses associated with the release of mediators such as prostaglandins, histamine, and serotonin or bradykinin may stimulate sensory nerve endings.
3. Ischemia may produce pain owing to the release of tissue metabolites.

CHARACTERISTICS

The position, quality, timing, and pace of abdominal pain are critical to differential diagnosis. Abdominal pain fre-

quently exhibits one of the following three patterns:

1. Visceral pain is usually dull and difficult to localize. Patients may describe it as being in the midline and having a crampy or gnawing quality.
2. Parietal pain is usually severe and is easily localized.
3. Referred pain is any pain remote from the diseased viscus.

While visceral pain is difficult for patients to localize, specific patterns may give clues to the involved part of the GI tract that is involved. Esophageal pain is usually substernal but may localize to a specific region of the chest. It may also masquerade as cardiac pain by radiating to the left arm or back. Pain from disease of the stomach, duodenum, or pancreas is generally epigastric and may radiate to the back, especially if the posterior duodenum or pancreas is involved. Pain from the liver, gallbladder, and biliary drainage system may be epigastric but frequently localizes to the right upper quadrant. Gallbladder or biliary pain may also refer to the scapula, especially on the right. Pain due to abscesses under the diaphragm (subphrenic) or in the liver may be referred to the shoulder. Jejunal and ileal pain is generally periumbilical and vague. The exception is that pain from the terminal ileum may localize to the right lower quadrant and mimic appendiceal pain. Colonic pain localizes poorly but is usually felt in the lower half of the abdomen unless the surrounding parietal peritoneum is inflamed. Rectal pain may be felt in the region of the anus but may also be felt over the sacrum posteriorly. Unusual patterns of abdominal pain include angina-like syndromes from esophageal spasm or meat impaction and from left upper quadrant discomfort from the transverse colon. Pain from the transverse or descending colon can also resemble pain from the left side of the back or left hip. Finally, pain from the posterior appendix—either ruptured or unruptured—may produce flank and back pain.

The qualities that patients ascribe to pain and its progression may be very helpful diagnostically. Pain due to esophageal reflux (heartburn) is often described as burning; pain from peptic ulcer disease may also burn but is frequently described as more "achy" and relieved with food or antacids. Pain that is caused by intestinal obstruction recurs persistently in a severe and crampy (colicky) manner, but between episodes of obstruction these patients usually have no pain. The pain associated with cystic duct obstruction is usually steady rather than colicky despite its name—biliary colic. Pain due to inflammation of the parietal peritoneum is generally steady, may be well localized, and often helps identify the offending organ owing to proximity of the pain to the diseased tissue. Peritoneal irritation forces patients to lie very still to avoid worsening pain. Irritation of the peritoneum may be accompanied by percussion tenderness, voluntary guarding, and rigidity of the overlying muscles. Ischemic disease of the intestine usually produces severe, poorly localized pain without tenderness. Abdominal aortic aneurysms cause sudden, severe, and "ripping" or "tearing" pain.

The character of some types of abdominal pain changes with time. For example, appendicitis may begin with vague, poorly localized pain that shifts to the right lower quadrant. If the appendix ruptures, the patient will have pain typical of diffuse peritoneal irritation. Typical pain patterns are catalogued in Table 32–1.

NAUSEA AND VOMITING

Nausea and vomiting may or may not be associated with abdominal pain. Vomiting is controlled through a center in the medulla and can be provoked by stimulation of either cholinergic neurons from the intestine or dopaminergic neurons in the chemoreceptor trigger zone surrounding the vomiting center. Obstruction and distention of any of the hollow viscera can produce vomiting; this is particularly so with more proximal obstruction. Any disease that irritates or inflames the peritoneum may also induce vomiting. Severe motility disturbances of the stomach, such as in diabetic gastroparesis, frequently produce vomiting. In these intestinal disorders, vagal afferents stimulate the vomiting center, producing nausea and vomiting. Drugs and gastric mucosal irritants may also induce vomiting via this pathway or through the surrounding chemoreceptor trigger zone. Other situations associated with vomiting include increased intracranial pressure, psychogenic vomiting, hypersecretion of gastric acid (Zollinger-Ellison syndrome), pregnancy, uremia, and early morning emesis of alcoholics.

APPROACH TO THE PATIENT WITH ACUTE ABDOMINAL PAIN

Abdominal pain often presents with a great disparity between the severity of the patient's symptoms and disease. Thus, the evaluation and care of patients with severe acute abdominal pain ("acute abdomen") present one of the most difficult challenges in clinical medicine. Some causes of the acute abdomen are emergencies, yet may present with minimal findings. In contrast, people with benign self-limited illnesses may present dramatically. The differential diagnosis of the acute abdomen includes acute appendicitis, cholecystitis, pancreatitis, intestinal obstruction, intestinal perforation, intestinal infarction, strangulated viscus, acute diverticulitis, ruptured ectopic pregnancy, and ruptured aortic aneurysm. It is essential to remember that diseases of the lung (pneumonia), kidney (kidney stone), pelvic organs, liver, hematopoietic system (sickle cell crisis), and metabolic disorders (acute porphyria) may also cause acute abdominal pain.

The diagnosis of acute abdominal pain requires a careful, accurate, and detailed history. The history should focus on the onset, quality, and radiation of the pain and the pace of the illness. Symptoms such as fever, nausea, constipation, diarrhea, and bleeding may also give important clues. The past medical history may be extremely valuable as well. In particular, prior abdominal surgery or peptic ulcer disease might suggest that the patient has an obstruction due to adhesions or a newly perforated ulcer. During the physical examination, it is important to observe the patient for the immobility associated with diffuse peritonitis or the restlessness associated with intestinal colic. Also, it is essential to rule out pulmonary causes of abdominal pain such as pneumonia, right-sided heart failure, and pulmonary thromboembolism. The abdominal examination must address the following items in particular: (1) the nature, quality, and frequency of bowel sounds; (2) the presence of localized or diffuse tenderness and whether it can be elicited by percussion alone; (3) the presence of any masses or hernias; (4) the presence or absence of fluid in the abdomen; and (5) the presence or absence of enlargement of the liver and spleen. Examination for peritoneal irritation is best sought by light percussion. Percussion tenderness that refers to a different location in the abdomen is valuable diagnostically. Aggressive attempts to demonstrate rebound tenderness are contraindicated. Thorough rectal and pelvic examinations are absolutely essential because they provide the best clues to genitourinary, colonic, and appendiceal disease.

Useful laboratory data include hematocrit, white blood cell count and differential, urinalysis, and stool examination for blood and pus. Serum tests for lipase, amylase, bilirubin, transaminases, and lipids may also be helpful. The diagnosis of acute pancreatitis relies on a combination of clinical and laboratory findings because other diseases such as intestinal ischemia or ruptured ectopic pregnancy can elevate the serum amylase level.

Certain radiographic procedures may also be useful. These include the chest, upright abdominal, and supine abdominal films. These help identify specific gas patterns that have differential diagnostic value and also enhance the search for free intra-abdominal air commonly seen with a perforated viscus. Obstruction or perforation may also be diagnosed by meglumine diatrizoate (Gastrografin), sodium diatrizoate (Hypaque), or barium studies of the small bowel or colon. Additional helpful imaging studies include computed tomography (CT) scans, techne-

TABLE 32–1 Pain Patterns of Abdominal Disease

	Substernal	Epigastric					
Onset	**Chronic**	**Acute**			**Chronic**		
Disease/diagnosis	Reflux esophagitis	Perforated duodenal ulcer	Cholecystitis	Pancreatitis	Duodenal ulcer	Gastric ulcer	Nonulcer dyspepsia
Pain quality	Burning; after meals/at night	Severe; ±history of chronic ulcer pain	Steady/biliary colic	Steady, boring	Gnawing, burning before meals/at night	Gnawing, worsened by food	Same as duodenal ulcer ±bloating
Pain referral	Left arm	±Back	Tip of scapula	Back	±Back	Occasionally to the back	None
Pain progression	Upper chest	Rapid, over entire abdomen	Intensity increases steadily over hours to right upper quadrant	±Peritoneal signs	None	None	None
Associated findings	Water brash in mouth	Guarding; free peritoneal air	Fever, gallstones on sonography, and failure to visualize on ^{99m}Tc-HIDA scan	Nausea and vomiting	Temporary relief with food or antacids	±Relief by antacids	±Relief with food or antacids

Periumbilical					Lower Quadrants			
Acute			**Chronic**		**Acute**		**Chronic**	
Appendicitis	Small bowel obstruction	Intestinal infarction	Inflammatory bowel disease	Intestinal angina	Diverticulitis	Colon obstruction	Dissecting aortic aneurysm	Irritable bowel syndrome
Cramping, steady	Cramping	Severe, aching, diffuse	Cramping, aching, may be in lower quadrants	Colicky, aching, diffuse	Steady, aching, left lower quadrant	Crampy	Sudden, severe, tearing; may be periumbilical	Cramping, steady or intermittent
±Back or groin	Back	None	None	None	Back	Back	Flank, inguinal regions	None
Localization to right lower quadrant	None	If treatment is delayed, peritonitis	None	Pain relief from 1–2 hours	None	None	None	None
Referred percussion tenderness to right lower quadrant	Hyperactive bowel sounds, nausea and vomiting; dilated bowel loops on x-ray	Unimpressive clinical presentation, occult blood in stool, absent bowel sounds	Diarrhea, blood and pus in stools, urgency, tenesmus	Weight loss	Palpable inflammatory mass, constipation, fever, leukocytosis	Vomiting, constipation, distention, hyperactive bowel sounds	Shock, abdominal bruit, abdominal mass	Alternating constipation and diarrhea, bloating

^{99m}Tc-HIDA = Technetium-labeled iminodiacetic acid.

tium-labeled iminodiacetic acid (^{99m}Tc-HIDA) scans, ultrasonography, and endoscopic procedures.

All patients with severe abdominal pain deserve adequate pain relief while diagnostic studies are being completed. The outcome, of course, depends on recognizing and treating the underlying disease process. It is frequently important to obtain surgical consultation early because intervention may be required. Occasionally, the final diagnosis must be reached by exploratory laparotomy.

IRRITABLE BOWEL SYNDROME

Irritable bowel syndrome (IBS) is a very common disorder associated with abdominal pain and alternating constipation and diarrhea that has no recognized organic cause. Up to 12% of the general population has IBS, and 40% of referrals to gastroenterologists in the United States are for IBS. Symptoms of IBS usually begin in young adulthood and last for many years. Women with this disorder are much more likely than men to be seen by physicians. The etiology and pathogenesis of IBS are completely obscure; the syndrome may include some diseases that are not yet characterized. For example, patients with adult-type hypolactasia (lactose intolerance) were previously classified as having IBS. The two major factors that contribute to the pathogenesis of this disease are (1) increased and abnormal colonic motility, particularly segmental contractions stimulated by meals, emotion, mechanical distention, or drugs; and (2) enhanced sensitivity to discomfort produced by normal intestinal gas or pressure in the sigmoid colon.

The abdominal pain of IBS varies greatly in both severity and pattern. The pain may be described as dull in the lower abdomen or sharp in the hypogastrium. It is common for the pain to be meal related and relieved by passing flatus or stool and quite uncommon for the pain to awaken the patient at night. Almost all patients have disturbed bowel habits—either constipation or diarrhea or both. Bleeding is not a feature of IBS except possibly from irrelevant hemorrhoids. IBS should never be considered an adequate explanation for occult blood in the stool. Certain unpleasant personality characteristics have been attributed to IBS but are more properly associated with the subset of patients who have IBS and seek frequent care from multiple physicians.

Evaluation of patients suspected of having IBS must include a thorough history, physical examination, stool analysis, routine laboratory tests, and probably a proctosigmoidoscopy and barium enema to rule out organic disease of the colon.

Patients with IBS have a need for education and understanding from their physician to cope with the confusing symptoms. Patients who come to the doctor frequently may also need psychological counseling. No drug has been shown to be of great value in IBS, and narcotics must be assiduously avoided. Some patients describe considerable diminution in their symptoms, particularly constipation, with the use of bulk-forming agents such as Metamucil. Anticholinergics or low doses of tricyclic antidepressants may help relieve pain in selected patients. Dietary manipulation has not been shown to be generally helpful.

REFERENCES

Schuster MM: Irritable bowel syndrome. *In* Sleisenger MH, Fordtran JS (eds.): Gastrointestinal Disease. 5th ed. Philadelphia, WB Saunders, 1993, pp 917–933.

Silen W (ed.): Cope's Early Diagnosis of the Acute Abdomen. 16th ed. Oxford, England, Oxford University Press, 1983.

Wyngaarden JB, Smith LH Jr, Bennett JC (eds.): Cecil Textbook of Medicine. 19th ed. Philadelphia, WB Saunders, 1992, pp 656–662, 721–723.

B. Gastrointestinal Hemorrhage

DEFINITION

Gastrointestinal bleeding is a common clinical problem, but a small number of lesions actually bleed. Blood loss ranges from occult to massive. About 80% of acute GI bleeding stops without intervention, but some recurrent bleeding becomes a life-threatening emergency.

Management of patients with GI bleeding revolves around three major issues: (1) most important, correcting hypovolemia; (2) stopping bleeding by the least invasive means; and (3) preventing recurrent bleeding. The second and third goals cannot be readily attained until the bleeding source is identified. Prompt and adequate resuscitation takes priority over all other measures.

PRESENTATION OF GASTROINTESTINAL HEMORRHAGE

Blood loss from the GI tract may be either (1) acute—it is sudden or massive and may present with obvious hypovolemia; or (2) chronic—often the patient is completely unaware of the bleeding. Acute bleeding may present in one of several ways:

Hematemesis: Vomiting bright red blood or blood that looks like coffee grounds is called hematemesis. This clinical finding shows the bleeding source to be proximal to the ligament of Treitz.

Melena: Black, tarry, usually foul-smelling stools that are passed after a bleed of more than 500 ml between the pharynx and the right colon are called melena. Melena is usually a sign of bleeding from an upper intestinal tract lesion.

Hematochezia: The passage of bright red or maroon stool is termed hematochezia and is usually due to a GI tract lesion distal to the ligament of Treitz or massive bleeding from a proximal lesion.

The patient with chronic GI blood loss may present with fatigue, dyspnea, syncope, angina, or a positive test for fecal occult blood. Patients with iron deficiency usually give no history of overt blood loss.

ETIOLOGY OF GASTROINTESTINAL BLEEDING

While many lesions in the GI tract bleed, most bleeding episodes are caused by a small number of diagnoses (Table 32–2).

Upper Gastrointestinal Bleeding

More than 90% of upper GI bleeding cases are caused by peptic ulcer, erosive gastritis, Mallory-Weiss tears, and esophagogastric varices.

TABLE 32–2	Causes of GI Bleeding	
Upper GI	**Upper or Lower GI**	**Lower GI**
Duodenal ulcer	Neoplasms	Hemorrhoids
Gastric ulcer	Arterial-enteric fistulas	Anal fissure
Anastomotic ulcer	Vascular anomalies	Diverticulosis
Esophagitis	Angiodysplasia	Ischemic bowel
Gastritis	Arteriovenous	disease
Mallory-Weiss tear	malformations	Inflammatory bowel
Esophageal varices	Hematologic disease	disease
Hematobilia	Elastic tissue diseases	Meckel's diverticulum
	Pseudoxanthoma	Solitary colonic ulcer
	elasticum	Intussusception
	Ehlers-Danlos	
	syndrome	
	Vasculitis syndrome	

GI = Gastrointestinal.

Peptic Ulcer

Ulcerations of the duodenum, stomach (gastric), and regions of surgical anastomoses may bleed. Bleeding may be the presenting symptom of the peptic ulcer disease without a history of pain.

Gastritis

Erosive gastritis that leads to bleeding may be caused by ingestion of alcohol or nonsteroidal anti-inflammatory drugs (NSAIDs) such as aspirin and ibuprofen. Gastric erosions are also common in severely ill patients with major trauma or systemic illness, burns, or head injury. Severe forms of erosive gastritis with significant bleeding are also commonly seen in patients with portal hypertension. In the seriously ill, the gastric pH must be kept above 4 using H_2-receptor antagonists or antacids.

Mallory-Weiss Tears

Mallory-Weiss tears occur in the mucosa near the junction of the esophagus and stomach and can present with mild to massive hematemesis. Fifty percent of these patients give a history of vomiting that precedes emesis of a large amount of blood, but they often have no other history to guide the diagnosis. Definitive diagnosis is made on endoscopy, and the tears are treated with adjunctive H_2-receptor antagonists.

Esophagogastric Varices

Bleeding from esophageal varices is usually massive and occurs without warning. Portal hypertension causes the development of collaterals such as esophageal varices. Hepatic cirrhosis due to alcohol consumption is the most common cause of variceal bleeding in the United States, although any cause of portal hypertension, including portal vein thrombosis and schistosomiasis, may produce the same syndrome. Bleeding from esophagogastric varices is

complicated in patients with cirrhosis for the following reasons:

1. Patients with varices frequently bleed from other causes such as gastritis or peptic ulceration.
2. If portal hypertension is treated with portosystemic shunting, the patient may suffer considerable morbidity without improved survival. Therefore, obliteration of esophageal varices by sclerosis or ligation has become standard therapy.
3. Cirrhosis may also lead to encephalopathy, which frequently worsens during episodes of bleeding.
4. Bleeding may be exacerbated by the liver's inability to make adequate clotting factors and secondary hypersplenism that results in thrombocytopenia.

Several other lesions of the upper GI tract may lead to bleeding, including carcinoma of the esophagus, carcinoma of the stomach, esophagitis, and catastrophic erosion of synthetic arterial grafts into the upper intestine, particularly the duodenum.

Lower Gastrointestinal Bleeding

Lower GI bleeding is generally caused by lesions of the anorectum and colon.

Non-Neoplastic Anorectal Lesions

Small amounts of bright red blood on the surface of the feces and toilet tissue are most commonly caused by hemorrhoids, anal fissures, or fistulas. Inflammation of the rectum (proctitis) from infectious diseases is seen more commonly in male homosexuals and may cause hematochezia.

Neoplastic Lesions of the Colon and Rectum

Carcinoma of the colon and colonic polyps usually present with occult blood loss; however, they may ulcerate and thereby present with acute lower GI bleeding.

Ulcerative, Bacterial, and Ischemic Colitis

Bleeding may accompany inflammatory diarrheas as seen in ulcerative colitis, but it may also occur in infectious diarrheas caused by *Shigella, Campylobacter, Entamoeba histolytica,* and occasionally *Salmonella.* Usually these patients present with diarrhea and have mucus and white blood cells in the stool. Ischemic colitis may also present with bloody diarrhea, particularly in elderly patients.

Colonic Diverticula

Sigmoid diverticulae are common in the United States. Most bleeding diverticulae are in the more right colon and are the most common cause of severe lower GI bleeding. Diverticulitis may produce abdominal pain but usually does not cause bleeding.

Angiodysplastic Lesions

Many patients acquire submucosal malformations of the arteriovenous system called angiodysplasia. These lesions may produce either acute or occult bleeding, and they are often difficult to visualize by endoscopy or angiography. They tend to develop with aging and long-term renal failure and may be associated with calcific aortic stenosis.

Small Intestinal Lesions

Significant intestinal bleeding is usually not caused by lesions in the small intestine distal to the ligament of Treitz. A major exception is Meckel's diverticulum, which may cause discrete ulceration and bleeding.

Bleeding Diatheses

Blood dyscrasias (leukemia, thrombocytopenia), disorders of coagulation (disseminated intravascular coagulation), vascular malformations (Osler-Weber-Rendu syndrome), vasculitides (Henoch-Schönlein purpura), and connective tissue disorders (pseudoxanthoma elasticum) may cause GI blood loss from either upper or lower tract lesions.

APPROACH TO THE PATIENT WITH GASTROINTESTINAL HEMORRHAGE

Patients who present with GI bleeding must be approached in a systemic and orderly manner (Fig. 32–1), i.e., (1) initial assessment, (2) resuscitation, (3) definitive diagnosis, and (4) treatment. The management of GI bleeding must be adapted to the nature and pace of bleeding. Massive, continuous bleeding demands immediate diagnostic and therapeutic intervention, especially when transfusions fail to keep up with the rapid rate of blood loss.

Initial Assessment

If it is suspected that a patient has bled acutely from the GI tract, vital signs are noted and intravenous infusion of crystalloid, such as normal saline, is begun before any further investigation. Blood is sent for typing and cross-matching, a complete blood count, prothrombin and partial thromboplastin times, and platelet count. The last three tests identify a bleeding diathesis that may worsen with massive transfusion. Serum is sent for routine electrolytes, blood urea nitrogen (BUN), creatinine, and liver enzymes to help evaluate renal and hepatic function.

The vital signs, including an assessment of orthostatic changes in blood pressure and pulse, determine volume loss. An orthostatic fall in blood pressure greater

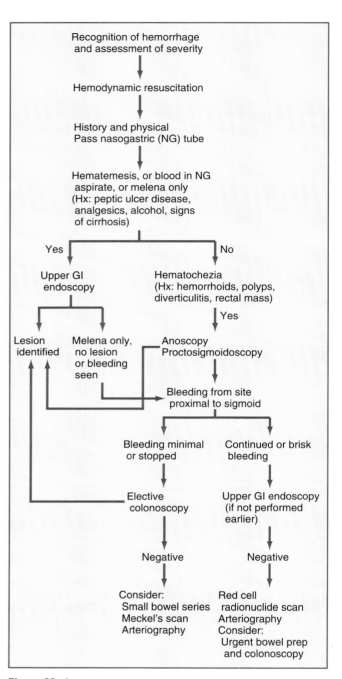

Figure 32–1

Diagnostic approach to the patient with gastrointestinal hemorrhage. GI = Gastrointestinal.

than 10 mm Hg usually signifies a 20% or greater loss of blood volume. Some patients, however, exhibit only a marked increase in heart rate upon standing without the concomitant fall in blood pressure. Resting tachycardia almost always accompanies hypotension, but heart rate alone is not a reliable indicator. As blood loss worsens to 40% of blood volume, the signs of shock, including pallor, cool limbs, marked tachycardia, and hypotension, are usually apparent. The amount of hematemesis or melena cannot be used to predict the degree of bleeding or risk to the patient. If the bleeding is close to the mouth or anus, the physician may overestimate its importance, and if it is a distance from any orifice, its importance may be underestimated. The hematocrit is completely unreliable for assessing blood loss in its early stages because even massive bleeding does not drop the hematocrit until volume re-expansion has occurred; this equilibration takes place over several hours. Initially low hematocrits suggest chronic or subacute blood loss and may be associated with a low mean corpuscular volume.

Resuscitation

The potential for catastrophic complications mandates the placement of patients with acute GI bleeding in an intensive care unit. GI bleeding is generally managed initially by internists, but early surgical consultation is indicated because surgery may be urgently required later. Resuscitation is the primary goal of early management and mandates maintenance of intravascular volume and tissue oxygenation. Nasal oxygen may be a useful adjunct in the elderly patient or in those with heart or lung disease. Vital signs, orthostatic blood pressure changes, and urine output are the most valuable clinical indicators, and they may be supplemented with measures of central venous or wedge pressure as needed.

Volume resuscitation is accomplished with crystalloid solutions given through large-bore intravenous lines. Actively bleeding patients may require packed red cells to replace volume losses. Fresh frozen plasma is an excellent volume expander but is usually reserved for patients with a correctable coagulopathy.

The amount of blood given to a patient is determined by an assessment of continued bleeding, the degree of pre-existing anemia, and other conditions that may impair tolerance of blood loss. Massive bleeding may require whole blood administration under pressure. In contrast, a healthy young person with hemodynamic stability who has stopped bleeding from a duodenal ulcer may tolerate a very low hematocrit (20 to 25%) and may be treated with oral iron and no transfusion. The decision to transfuse is therefore based on the presence of hypotension, evidence of decreased tissue perfusion, ongoing bleeding, and balancing the risk of transfusion versus no transfusion.

Diagnosis

The first step in assessing GI bleeding is to determine whether the bleeding source is upper or lower tract. The history can be extremely helpful in this situation. Hematemesis is diagnostic of bleeding proximal to the ligament of Treitz. Recent ingestion of NSAIDs or alcohol may suggest gastritis. A classic history of peptic ulcer pain or a prior or family history of GI bleeding may be informa-

tive; half the patients with Mallory-Weiss tears give a history of vomiting. A change in bowel habits, especially constipation, may suggest colon cancer. In a smoker or in elderly patients, abrupt onset of acute abdominal pain with bleeding may suggest ischemic disease of the colon. Patients who have had an abdominal aortic bypass are at risk for development of aortoenteric fistulas.

Physical examination may suggest chronic liver disease and raise the specter of esophageal varices as a bleeding source. Examination of the skin may show telangiectasias that suggest either chronic liver disease or Osler-Weber-Rendu syndrome. The rectal examination is essential to rule out a mass and to detect the presence of melenic stool. The presence of melena suggests bleeding in the upper tract or the right colon.

Upper tract bleeding is usually confirmed by passing a nasogastric tube. Gastric aspirates with no "coffee grounds" or gross blood make upper GI bleeding proximal to the pylorus much less likely. Hemoccult testing is not informative. This test may miss active bleeding from duodenal ulcers or from aortoenteric fistulae. The combination of hypovolemia and a protein load from bleeding increases the BUN in many cases.

Upper GI endoscopy is the most rapid, safe, and definitive means for diagnosing the site of blood loss in upper tract lesions and is also useful therapeutically. If bleeding has stopped, a double-contrast barium upper GI series detects most malignancies and peptic ulcers, but it misses gastritis and Mallory-Weiss tears. Potential malignancies and gastric ulcers require a biopsy, making endoscopy the procedure of choice because of its high sensitivity and specificity for diagnosis, capacity for biopsy, and potential for therapeutic intervention in the bleeding patient.

Lower GI tract bleeding is first evaluated by rectal examination, anoscopy, and proctosigmoidoscopy, which detects lesions in the distal 20 to 30 cm of colon, including hemorrhoids, cancer, inflammatory bowel disease, and polyps. Colonoscopy can detect bleeding lesions proximal to 20 cm after thorough colonic purging. If bleeding is sufficiently brisk, colonoscopy is likely to be futile and angiography more useful. If suspected lower GI bleeding has occurred and no diagnosis in the lower tract is forthcoming, an upper GI source must be sought, usually with upper GI endoscopy. Lesions of the small bowel distal to the ligament of Treitz are difficult to detect but are fortunately uncommon. They may be detected with small bowel series, enteroclysis, or, in rare cases, a Meckel scan.

Evaluation of chronic GI blood loss can be undertaken with either an endoscopic or a radiographic approach. The latter includes a barium enema, proctosigmoidoscopy, and an upper GI series. Endoscopic evaluations of chronic GI blood loss usually begin with a full colonoscopy and, if negative, an upper GI endoscopy. If all of these studies are negative, small bowel studies with barium are performed. Angiography may be used to search for vascular lesions.

Despite the many diagnostic tools available today, the source of bleeding sometimes cannot be determined. In many patients the lesions may be subtle or inaccessible, and some patients have so many lesions that it is impossible to single out the one that is bleeding. Fortunately, few patients are repeatedly hospitalized for bleeding from undiagnosed lesions.

Treatment

About 80% of patients with GI bleeding stop bleeding spontaneously. Management is focused on preventing further bleeding and identifying the bleeding source. For example, bleeding due to peptic ulcer disease is treated with antacids, H_2-receptor blockers, sucralfate or omeprazole. Expectant management is the rule for gastritis, Mallory-Weiss tears, angiodysplasia, and diverticulosis when bleeding has ceased spontaneously. In contrast, malignant lesions and polyps must be removed endoscopically or surgically. If bleeding does not recur in the hospital, long-term management depends on the site and type of lesions as well as the patient's ability to tolerate surgery. For example, a patient with a peptic ulcer that fails to stop bleeding usually requires therapeutic endoscopic intervention or surgery.

Several nonsurgical techniques have become standards of care for management of GI hemorrhage recently, but proof of efficacy is limited. Endoscopic treatment of bleeding lesions includes electrocoagulation, thermocoagulation, submucosal injection of epinephrine, laser photocoagulation, sclerosis, and variceal ligation. Other nonsurgical procedures include radiologic techniques such as administering intra-arterial vasopressin and selective embolization of arteries supplying bleeding lesions.

The treatment of bleeding esophageal varices requires separate consideration. Patients with these lesions are frequently not good operative candidates because they have poor health status, liver disease, and a bleeding diathesis due to prolonged prothrombin time and/or low platelet counts. They frequently rebleed and require considerable in-hospital support. Volume replacement is the first priority in patients with bleeding varices, but overexpansion of blood volume may precipitate rebleeding; infusion of crystalloid tends to worsen edema and ascites in these patients as well. GI bleeding in patients with severe liver disease may provoke hepatic encephalopathy and deterioration in renal function (see Chapter 42). Purging the bowel of blood and treatment with lactulose may help decrease the risk and severity of encephalopathy. Noninvasive efforts to diminish bleeding include intravenous vasopressin and replacing clotting factors with fresh frozen plasma and platelets. The use of a Minnesota tube to tamponade bleeding varices with a balloon may be required but serves only to temporize. The most accepted treatment of acutely bleeding esophageal varices is endoscopic injection of sclerosant solutions directly into the varices (sclerotherapy). Studies have shown that this procedure arrests bleeding in up to 90% of cases. Emergency decompression of the entire portal system with a portosystemic shunt operation may be necessary to stop a massive variceal hemorrhage. Recently, some institutions are performing transjugular intrahepatic portosystemic shunt (TIPS) procedures in radiology suites. Prevention of re-

current bleeding by obliterating varices through sclerotherapy or elective shunt surgery is preferred to emergency shunt surgery. The advantages and disadvantages of these procedures are discussed in Chapter 43.

REFERENCES

Cello JP: Gastrointestinal hemorrhage. *In* Wyngaarden JB, Smith LH Jr, Bennett JC (eds.): Cecil Textbook of Medicine. 19th ed. Philadelphia, WB Saunders, 1992, pp 742–745.

Cello JP, Crass RA, Grendell JH, Trunkey DD: Management of the patient with hemorrhaging esophageal varices. JAMA 1986; 256: 1480.

Steer ML, Silen W: Diagnostic procedures in gastrointestinal hemorrhage. N Engl J Med 1983; 309:646.

C. Malabsorption

The purpose of the GI tract is to digest and absorb nutrients and eliminate everything else. These nutrients include macronutrients, such as carbohydrates, proteins, and fat, and micronutrients, including vitamins and trace elements. The GI tract may digest, solubilize, transport, and resynthesize up to 80 gm of fat per day, whereas the terminal ileum needs to absorb only 1 μg of vitamin B_{12} per day. In addition to absorption, the gut circulates water, electrolytes, bile salts, pancreatic juice, and intestinal secretions that are reabsorbed in the small intestine and colon. Food is a complex mixture of nutrients and nonnutrients that must be separated as it passes through the GI tract. The preparation for digestion begins with (1) the controlled release of food that has been fragmented by the stomach into the intestine; (2) the secretion of pancreatic juice, bile, and water into the lumen of the intestine to allow digestion of food into an isotonic mixture of simple molecules; and (3) terminal digestion of peptides and disaccharides by the brush border enzymes of the small intestine enterocyte. All of these steps occur prior to absorption of nutrients.

Nutrients are absorbed at the brush border surface of the enterocytes. The surface area of the enterocytes is expanded by complex folding of the small bowel surface into valvulae conniventes, intestinal villi, and microvilli of the individual enterocyte. The various portions of this surface are exposed to the nutrient mixture during the 1.5 to 2.0 hours required to pass from the stomach to the colon. Colonic absorption focuses primarily on salvage of water and electrolytes. Some molecules may be absorbed throughout the length of the small intestine, and some must be absorbed in a very limited region (e.g., vitamin B_{12} and bile acids in the terminal ileum). The extraordinary complexity of the digestive and absorptive processes lends itself to a large number of disorders that may lead to maldigestion or malabsorption. In this section, a general classification of both of these disorders and a rational approach to diagnosis are discussed.

NORMAL ABSORPTION

Malabsorption cannot be understood without a thorough understanding of normal absorption. The absorption of only three of the major classes of nutrients (fat, protein, and carbohydrates) is discussed in this section; the absorption of water and electrolytes is discussed in Section D of this chapter because malabsorption of water and electrolytes produces diarrhea.

Digestion and Absorption of Fat (Fig. 32–2)

Dietary fat is ingested predominantly in the form of triglycerides with long-chain fatty acids that include saturated (palmitic and stearic) and unsaturated (oleic and linoleic) varieties. Triglycerides leave the stomach and enter the duodenum emulsified and therefore not subject to absorption. Long-chain fatty acids and peptides in the duodenum stimulate bile flow via cholecystokinin. Lipase secreted by the pancreas and bound to the surface by colipase in the presence of bile salts releases the fatty acids from positions 1 and 3, leaving a 2-monoglyceride. These products of lipolysis are then incorporated into mixed micelles, with the bile salts enhancing their solubility and allowing them to traverse the unstirred water layer that overlies the intestinal epithelium. The fatty acids released from lipolysis and 2-monoglycerides diffuse from the micelles into the cell cytoplasm, where they are, for the most part, resynthesized into triglycerides and packaged into chylomicrons and very low density lipoproteins (VLDL) and exported to the lymphatics. Bile salts remain in the intestinal lumen, are reutilized in new micelles, and are finally reabsorbed in the terminal ileum. More than 95% of ingested neutral fat is efficiently absorbed from the intestine; the fat-soluble vitamins (A, D, E, K) are absorbed in tandem with fat.

Digestion and Absorption of Proteins

Proteins are much simpler to digest and absorb than fat because they are water soluble. The hydrolysis of proteins to amino acids and oligopeptides is initiated in the stomach with pepsin but is completed by trypsin, elastase, chymotrypsin, and carboxypeptidase in the proximal small intestine. There are several distinct transport systems for amino acids based on their chemical characteristics: (1) the dibasic amino acid system, which may be abnormal in cystinuria; (2) a neutral amino acid system, which is abnormal in Hartnup disease; (3) the imino acid–glycine system; and (4) the dicarboxylic acid system. Amino acids are absorbed in tandem with sodium ions in the jejunum.

Digestion and Absorption of Carbohydrates

The major dietary carbohydrates are starch and the disaccharides sucrose and lactose. Oligosaccharides and disaccharides cannot be absorbed, forcing complete digestion before absorption. Salivary and pancreatic amylases hydrolyze glucose from starch, a glucose polymer. Brush border amylases and limit dextrinases complete the digestion of starch. The terminal digestion of disaccharides is accomplished by sucrase, lactase, and maltase activities. The constituent monosaccharides, glucose and galactose, are absorbed in conjunction with sodium in a mechanism similar to peptide absorption, and fructose is absorbed by facilitated diffusion.

CLASSIFICATION OF THE MALABSORPTION SYNDROMES (Table 32–3)

Multiple disorders cause malabsorption, including genetic defects and diffuse mucosal diseases. It is most helpful

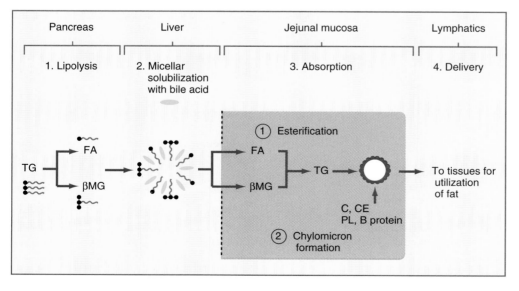

Figure 32–2
Schematic of intestinal absorption, showing the participation of pancreas, liver, and intestinal mucosal cells in fat absorption. βMG = Beta-monoglyceride; C = cholesterol; CE = cholesterol esters; FA = fatty acids; PL = phospholipids; TG = triglycerides. (From Wilson FA, Dietschy JM: Gastroenterology 61:911, 1971, © by The American College of Gastroenterology.)

TABLE 32–3	Classification of the Malabsorption Syndromes

Inadequate Digestion

Pancreatic exocrine deficiency
    Primary—e.g., chronic pancreatitis, cystic fibrosis, carcinoma of the pancreas
    Secondary—gastrinoma with acid inactivation of pancreatic lipase
Intraluminal bile salt deficiency
    Liver disease—especially biliary cirrhosis
    Disease or bypass of the terminal ileum—impaired recycling mechanism
    Bacterial overgrowth syndrome—increased deconjugation of bile salts
Specific abnormalities—disaccharidase deficiencies

Inadequate Absorption

Inadequate absorptive surface—e.g., short bowel syndrome, bypass fistulas, extensive Crohn's disease
Specific mucosal cell defects
    Genetic—abetalipoproteinemia, Hartnup disease, cystinuria, monosaccharide absorptive defects
    Acquired—hypovitaminosis D
Diffuse disease of the small intestine
    Immunologic or allergic injury—celiac disease (gluten-sensitive enteropathy), ? eosinophilic enteritis, ? Crohn's disease
    Infections and infestations—Whipple's disease, giardiasis, tropical sprue, bacterial overgrowth syndrome
    Infiltrative disorders—lymphoma, mastocytosis, amyloidosis
    Fibrosis—systemic sclerosis, radiation enteritis

Lymphatic Obstruction

Lymphangiectasia
Whipple's disease
Lymphoma

Multiple Mechanisms

Postgastrectomy steatorrhea
Bacterial overgrowth syndrome
Disease or bypass of the distal ileum
Scleroderma, lymphoma, Whipple's disease
Diabetes mellitus

Drug-Induced Malabsorption

Neomycin, cholestyramine, antacids, ethanol, chronic ingestion of laxatives, biguanides

Hyperabsorptive "Malabsorption"

Hemochromatosis, hypervitaminosis D
Enteric hyperoxaluria

---

to think of maldigestion and malabsorption syndromes in the context of abnormalities of one or more of the normal processes discussed in the previous section of this chapter.

Inadequate Digestion

Ingested food must be broken down for absorption to take place at the intestinal border. Digestion is accomplished largely by pancreatic enzymes secreted into the intestinal lumen. Of particular importance are lipase and colipase and the proteases, particularly trypsin. Chronic diseases of the pancreas, such as chronic pancreatitis or cystic fibrosis, may lead to malabsorption due to maldigestion. Even Zollinger-Ellison syndrome may lower the

duodenal pH enough to impair lipase activity and cause fat malabsorption.

For pancreatic enzymes to digest fat, an adequate concentration of luminal bile salts to solubilize the neutral fats must be present. Bile salt deficiency can be caused by (1) decreased hepatic synthesis and transport, although this is rare; (2) cholestasis (biliary cirrhosis); (3) deconjugation of bile salts due to bacterial overgrowth; or (4) interference in ileal reabsorption due to ileal disease or surgery.

In addition to disorders of digestion associated with pancreatic enzymes or bile salts, highly specific defects in digestion may occur as well. The digestion and absorption of lactose, the dominant sugar in milk, depends upon an adequate supply of the enzyme lactase. Failure to absorb ingested lactose leads to flatulence, distention, cramps, and diarrhea. Adult-type lactose intolerance may be inherited, as in African blacks and Asians, or may be secondary to any type of diffuse mucosal injury; these include celiac disease and viral gastroenteritides.

Inadequate Absorption

In this condition, food products are fully digested but are not adequately absorbed. This results from a decreased amount of otherwise normal absorptive surface. The simplest example is short bowel syndrome due to surgical removal of most of the small intestine. Inadequate absorption most commonly occurs after mesenteric infarction, Crohn's disease, and bypass surgery for morbid obesity.

It is also possible for the absorptive surface to have a normal area but not function normally. This problem occurs frequently within the mucosal cell and may be highly specific owing to a gene defect. Examples of selective absorption defects include cystinuria and Hartnup disease for certain amino acids and abetalipoproteinemia, which leads to fat malabsorption due to defective intracellular synthesis of apolipoproteins. Selective defects can also be acquired, such as reduced calcium absorption in the absence of adequate 1,25-dihydroxycholecalciferol or a drop in lactase production due to gastroenteritis.

More commonly, malabsorption is seen with diffuse disease processes involving the mucosa or submucosa of the small intestine. Several causes of diffuse injury have been identified, although in many cases the mechanisms are complicated or undefined.

Immunologic or Allergic Injury

Gluten-sensitive enteropathy (celiac sprue) and the rare disorder eosinophilic gastroenteritis dominate this category.

Infections and Infestations

Whipple's disease is a systemic disorder caused by a bacterium that has recently been identified as an actinomycete, *Tropheryma whippelii*. This disorder is marked by dramatic malabsorption and packing of the small intestinal submucosa with macrophages that stain positively with periodic acid–Schiff (PAS). Patients with this disease may have a complex presentation that includes fever, adenopathy, pigmentation changes, arthralgias, and occasionally severe neurologic manifestations. Whipple's disease is rare but is potentially curable. Infestation with *Giardia lamblia* may also cause malabsorption; however, its clinical presentation is dominated by cramps, flatulence, and diarrhea. Bacterial overgrowth syndromes may also produce diffuse mucosal injury.

Infiltrative Disorders

The mucosa and/or submucosa may be infiltrated to an extent sufficient to impair absorption. Examples include intestinal lymphoma, amyloidosis, and mastocytosis.

Fibrosis

The intestinal wall may be thickened in fibrotic diseases such as progressive systemic sclerosis and radiation injury. The cause of malabsorption in these conditions is complex, but it may result in part from a motility disturbance that leads to bacterial overgrowth.

Lymphatic Obstruction

Obstructive lesions of the mesenteric lymphatics may impair fat absorption. This may contribute to malabsorption syndromes in diffuse intestinal lymphomas and is also seen in Whipple's disease and congenital lymphangiectasia. In general, lymphangiectasia is more likely to present as a protein-losing enteropathy with secondary hypoalbuminemia.

Multiple Mechanisms

Because the digestive and absorptive processes are complex and interrelated, many disorders may impair multiple processes. For example, subtotal gastrectomy with a Billroth II–type gastroenterostomy may lead to a modest degree of malabsorption. This problem is caused by rapid gastric emptying and intestinal transit, leading to inadequate mixing of pancreatic and biliary secretions from the blind loop of the duodenum. Because the food does not pass through the proximal duodenum, release of secretin and cholecystokinin is decreased, and bacterial overgrowth may occur in the afferent blind duodenal loop. Bacterial overgrowth can lead to deconjugation of bile salts and may also injure the intestinal epithelium. All of these events, alone or in concert, may lead to a malabsorptive state. Diabetes mellitus may also cause multiple defects because exocrine deficiency of the pancreas or motility disorders in the small intestine may supervene, producing bacterial overgrowth due to stasis.

TABLE 32–4	Some Drug-Induced Absorptive Defects
Drug	**Substance Malabsorbed**
Ethanol	Folates, vitamin B_{12}
Antacids	Phosphate
Phenytoin	Folates
Neomycin	Fatty acids, vitamin B_{12}
Cholestyramine	Bile acids, thyroxine
Tetracycline	Iron

Drug-Induced Malabsorption

Drugs can induce malabsorption of specific nutrients. Some of them are listed in Table 32–4.

Hyperabsorptive "Malabsorption"

Malabsorption is normally thought of as too little absorption, but there are also disorders in which too much nutrient is absorbed. For example, hemochromatosis is a genetic disorder that leads to hyperabsorption of iron, and hypervitaminosis D leads to excessive absorption of calcium. Enteric hyperoxaluria is an acquired disorder associated with excess oxalate absorption caused by fat and calcium malabsorption.

CLINICAL MANIFESTATIONS OF MALABSORPTION

The clinical presentation of the large number of diseases listed in Table 32–3 is varied. Some of these diseases present with features that seem unrelated to the malabsorption; others present in highly specific ways, such as pernicious anemia with a selective malabsorption of vitamin B_{12} or rickets due to poor absorption of calcium. This brief discussion focuses on the signs and symptoms of malabsorption, particularly the malabsorption of fat.

Early Manifestations

The early manifestations of malabsorption are difficult to detect by patient and physician. A change in bowel habits may occur; the patient may report producing bulky stools with visible oil that can be difficult to flush. More commonly, the patient suffers weight loss, fatigue, depression, and bloating. Nocturia may be caused by nocturnal reabsorption of intestinal fluids.

Late Manifestations

The major late manifestations of malabsorption are summarized in Table 32–5. They generally relate to nutritional deficiencies that are secondary to the malabsorption. These patients frequently appear wasted owing to

TABLE 32–5	Correlation of Data in Maldigestion and Malabsorption	
Clinical Features	**Laboratory Findings**	**Pathophysiology**
Wasting edema	↓ Serum albumin	↑ Albumin loss (gut), ↓ protein ingestion, ↓ protein absorption
Weight loss, oily bulky stools	↑ Stool fat excretion, ↓ serum carotene	↓ Ingestion and absorption fat, CHO, protein
Paresthesias, tetany	↓ Serum Ca^{2+}, ↑ alkaline phosphatase, ↓ mineralization bones (x-ray), ↓ serum Mg^{2+}	↓ Absorption Ca^{2+}, vitamin D, Mg^{2+}
Ecchymoses, petechiae, hematuria	↑ Prothrombin time	↓ Absorption vitamin K
Anemia	Macrocytosis, ↓ serum vitamin B_{12}, ↓ absorption vitamin B_{12} and/or folic acid, microcytosis, hypochromia, ↓ serum iron, no iron in marrow	↓ Absorption vitamin B_{12} and/or folic acid, ↓ absorption iron
Glossitis	↓ Serum vitamin B_{12}, folic acid	↓ Aborption B vitamins
Abdominal distention, borborygmi, flatulence, watery stools	↓ Xylose absorption, ↓ disaccharidases in intestinal biopsy, fluid levels, small intestine (x-ray)	↓ Hydrolysis, disaccharides and ↓ absorption, monosaccharides and amino acids

CHO = Carbohydrate.
From Gray GM: Maldigestion and malabsorption: Clinical manifestations and specific diagnosis. *In* Sleisenger MH, Fordtran JS (eds.): Gastrointestinal Disease. 3rd ed. Philadelphia, WB Saunders, 1983, p 230.

diminished muscle mass, but they may have abdominal distention with active bowel sounds. Blood pressure tends to be low, and the patient may exhibit increased skin pigmentation. Abdominal pain is uncommon unless the specific disorder causing the malabsorption causes pain, as in chronic pancreatitis or intestinal lymphoma. At this late stage, clinical diagnosis is much easier, but determining a specific cause of malabsorption may be difficult.

CLINICAL TESTS OF DIGESTION AND ABSORPTION

Many tests are available that help in diagnosing maldigestion and malabsorption. A brief discussion of the more useful tests follows.

Fecal Fat Analysis

Identification of steatorrhea (fat in the stool) is essential in any assessment of maldigestion or malabsorption. The simplest test to detect stool fat is a Sudan III–stained stool smear. This test is qualitatively useful but has no quantitative capacity. The gold standard is to measure quantitatively the total fat in a 3-day stool specimen while the patient is on a diet consisting of 80 to 100 gm of fat per day. Normal fat excretion should be less than 6 gm/day and is usually less than 2.5 gm. Values higher than 6 gm/day clearly indicate steatorrhea (fat malabsorption) but do not help identify the pathogenesis of the steatorrhea.

Tests of Pancreatic Exocrine Function

Some of the tests of pancreatic exocrine function are described in Chapter 38. The bentiromide test determines the split of an orally administered synthetic peptide by pancreatic chymotrypsin. Excretion in 6 hours of less than 50% of a 500-mg dose of bentiromide in the form of urinary arylamines is diagnostic of pancreatic exocrine insufficiency. Pancreatic disease may also be suspected when diffuse calcification is seen in the region of the pancreas on plain abdominal films or a CT scan. A new test that measures stool chymotrypsin is gaining favor.

Xylose Absorption-Excretion Test

The capacity of the mucosa to absorb sugars can be assessed by absorption of D-xylose. D-Xylose is a poorly metabolized 5-carbon sugar that is absorbed well in the intestine, but it is not degraded or concentrated in any tissue and is largely excreted in the urine. The test is performed by having the patient ingest 25 gm of D-xylose and then collecting the urine for 5 hours thereafter. Normal subjects excrete more than 4.5 gm of D-xylose in 5 hours, but this normal value can be reduced somewhat by age, poor renal function, the presence of large amounts of edema or ascites, and bacterial overgrowth. In patients who have bacterial overgrowth, the D-xylose test should return to normal with the use of antibiotics.

Radiographic Studies

Radiographic studies of the stomach and small intestine in malabsorption are nonspecific, although thickening of mucosal folds, modest dilatation of the intestinal lumen, and occasional clumping and segmentation of the barium in a moulage pattern may be observed. On rare occasions, barium studies may provide a definitive diagnosis by identifying a "blind loop," a diverticulum, or an unexpected fistula.

Small Intestinal (Jejunal) Biopsy

Biopsy of the small intestinal mucosa is frequently necessary to identify mucosal defects leading to the malabsorption syndrome. The utility of this procedure is summarized in Table 32–6.

Vitamin B₁₂ Absorption (the Schilling Test)

Vitamin B_{12} is absorbed in a complex process. It is first conjugated by R-factor proteins in the saliva, which are subsequently degraded in the duodenum under the influence of pancreatic trypsin. After the release of the R factors, vitamin B_{12} is complexed to intrinsic factor, a protein secreted by the stomach. The vitamin B_{12}–intrinsic factor complex passes through the intestine and is absorbed by a specific receptor in the distal ileum. Defects in pancreatic enzymes required in the degradation of R proteins, secretion of intrinsic factor, or ileal absorption of vitamin B_{12}–intrinsic factor complexes may lead to vitamin B_{12} deficiency. The Schilling test identifies the source of the malabsorption. In stage 1 of the Schilling test, the patient ingests radiolabeled vitamin B_{12} after a parenteral dose of 1 mg of vitamin B_{12} to prevent hepatic storage, thereby enhancing excretion of the label. In stage 2, vitamin B_{12} plus intrinsic factor is administered. Stage 3 involves repeating stage 1 after antibiotics are administered. Gastric disease leading to inadequate production of intrinsic factor leads to malabsorption of vitamin B_{12} in all stages of the Schilling test except stage 2, when intrinsic factor is provided. Disease of the pancreas leading to incomplete degradation of R factors causes low excretion of vitamin B_{12} in stage 1 because vitamin B_{12} is permanently complexed to the R factors but normal absorption in stage 2 because the vitamin B_{12} was already bound to intrinsic factor. Ileal disease leading to vitamin B_{12} malabsorption produces decreased absorption in all three stages of the Schilling test.

TABLE 32–6	Utility of Small Bowel Biopsy Specimens in Malabsorption

Often Diagnostic

Whipple's disease
Amyloidosis
Eosinophilic enteritis
Lymphangiectasia
Primary intestinal lymphoma
Giardiasis
Abetalipoproteinemia
Agammaglobulinemia
Mastocytosis

Abnormal But Not Diagnostic

Celiac sprue
Systemic sclerosis
Radiation enteritis
Bacterial overgrowth syndrome
Tropical sprue
Crohn's disease

Breath Tests

Several tests detect the presence of compounds produced by intraluminal bacteria by examining the breath. The ^{14}C-xylose test measures $^{14}CO_2$ produced in the breath at 30 and 60 minutes after ingestion of the radioactive sugar; it is elevated in the presence of bacterial overgrowth in the small intestine. A related test detects free hydrogen in the breath after ingestion of any of a variety of sugars. Glucose ingestion should lead to H_2 production via fermentation because it is fully absorbed in the small intestine. In the presence of bacterial overgrowth, breath hydrogen tends to increase early after ingestion. This test can also be used to detect specific carbohydrate maldigestion syndromes such as sucrase or lactase deficiency, in which expired H_2 is increased after a 50-gm dose of the sugar. The increase in breath hydrogen occurs in these cases after undigested sugar reaches the colon.

Miscellaneous Tests

Other important but nonspecific tests that may provide clues to the degree and cause of malabsorption include body weight, serum albumin, prothrombin time (indirectly assesses vitamin K), cholesterol, carotene, folic acid, calcium, and magnesium. These tests are used primarily as adjuncts and to assess the severity of malabsorption but do not aid the differential diagnosis.

APPROACH TO THE PATIENT WITH SUSPECTED MALDIGESTION AND/OR MALABSORPTION

Because of the large number of diagnostic tests, a rational algorithm for the use of the various tests is necessary (Fig. 32–3). The best test for fat malabsorption is the 72-hour fecal fat analysis; however, this test is difficult to obtain in practice, so it may be necessary to establish steatorrhea with qualitative stool fat examination and serum carotene. If the stool fat is normal, the patient may have selective abnormalities for absorption of a specific carbohydrate. This condition must be suspected if the symptoms are primarily cramps, flatulence, and diarrhea. The most common cause of carbohydrate malabsorption is lactose intolerance; specific tests include oral tolerance tests, but measurement of breath hydrogen is more sensitive and specific. An osmotic gap in fecal material suggests an osmotic cause of the diarrhea due to short-chain fatty acids or carbohydrates. The osmotic gap is calculated by the following formula; plasma osmolality $- 2$ ($Na^+ + K^+$) (fecal sodium plus fecal potassium). Osmotic gap is not calculated by measuring stool osmolality because (1) it increases with time in the specimen container; and (2) true osmolality is equal to serum osmolality because the colon cannot maintain a gradient for the concentration of water.

When fat malabsorption is demonstrated (> 6 gm/24 hours or increased qualitative stool fat and decreased serum carotene), a xylose absorption-excretion test should

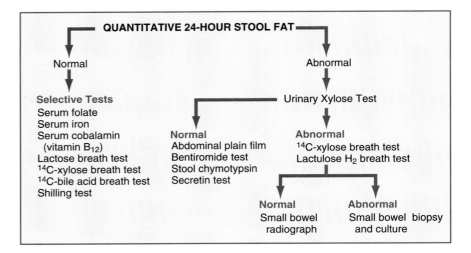

Figure 32-3
Approach to the patient with suspected maldigestion or malabsorption. (Adapted from Toskes PP: Malabsorption: *In* Wyngaarden JB, Smith LH Jr [eds]: Cecil Textbook of Medicine. 18th ed. Philadelphia, WB Saunders, 1988, p 740.)

be performed next. A normal xylose test rules out diffuse mucosal disease and suggests that the patient's disorder is digestive, such as pancreatic or bile salt deficiency. Specific tests for pancreatic insufficiency should then be performed. These may include plain abdominal films, bentiromide test, secretin test, or stool chymotrypsin. If the urinary xylose excretion is abnormal, breath hydrogen testing may be used to diagnose bacterial overgrowth using glucose. When no bacterial overgrowth is present, mucosal biopsy should be performed. Small bowel radiographs may also be helpful.

Most cases of malabsorption can be diagnosed through appropriate combinations of the above tests. Occasionally, clinical trials for treatable conditions should be instituted, such as a gluten-free diet for celiac disease, pancreatic enzyme replacement for pancreatic exocrine function, metronidazole for *Giardia lamblia* infection, or broad-spectrum antibiotics for suspected bacterial overgrowth.

TREATMENT

The treatment of malabsorption is too complex to cover completely here. Various treatments include H_2-receptor antagonists or H^+-K^+-ATPase inhibitors for gastrinoma; the daily use of pancreatic enzymes; antibiotics for bacterial overgrowth or Whipple's disease; a gluten-free diet for celiac sprue; the use of medium-chain fatty acids, which are more easily absorbed; surgical repair of intestinal or biliary obstruction; repair of blind loops or fistulas; and chemotherapy for lymphoma. Replacement therapy for the loss of specific nutrients or vitamins may also be required. In the case of the short bowel syndrome, total parenteral nutrition may be the only feasible treatment option.

ASSOCIATED DISORDERS

A large number of conditions may lead to nutrient malabsorption. A sample of these conditions is listed in Table 32-3. Two of these entities, celiac sprue and bacterial overgrowth syndrome, are discussed in this section. Several other specific disorders are discussed elsewhere in this book and appended references.

Celiac Sprue (Gluten-Sensitive Enteropathy, Nontropical Sprue)

Celiac sprue is a chronic, familial disorder associated with lifelong sensitivity to dietary gluten. Gluten is a complex of proteins found in wheat and wheat products. In these patients, diffuse mucosal injury results from the ingestion of gluten. The injury produces flattening of the villi, leading to a significant decrease in gut absorptive surface. The crypts are hyperplastic, and lymphocytes infiltrate the lamina propria.

Pathogenesis

The mechanism by which gluten causes injury is not definitively known, but it appears to be immunologic in origin. Celiac sprue is associated with the human leukocyte antigens HLA-B8 and HLA-Dw3, suggesting a linkage on chromosome 6, which supports the immunologic hypothesis. As many as 10% of first-degree relatives of patients with celiac sprue are concordant for the disorder. Another hypothesis suggests that incomplete hydrolysis of gluten peptides leads to toxic intermediates that directly injure the intestinal epithelium. Although the cause is not known, it is clear that the lesion is produced locally because the intestine can fully recover when gluten is removed; the syndrome promptly reappears with reintroduction of gluten. Therefore, the pathogenesis of the malabsorption is a diffuse mucosal abnormality. This loss of functional mucosa may also lead to reduced secretion of cholecystokinin and secretin, which exacerbates the malabsorption by diminishing pancreatic and biliary function.

Signs and Symptoms

The signs and symptoms of celiac sprue are essentially the same as for other malabsorption syndromes. They are often more severe in childhood and diminish in adolescence and adulthood. The GI symptoms may be very mild, but the patient may have severe anemia due to iron deficiency and even a bleeding diathesis due to vitamin K deficiency. Metabolic bone disease due to calcium malabsorption has also been seen.

Diagnosis

Patients with celiac sprue normally have impaired fat absorption, an abnormal xylose test, and an abnormal mucosal pattern on small bowel series. The Schilling test is usually normal, but if the disorder extends to the ileum, it may also be abnormal. Jejunal biopsy suggests the diagnosis, but response to a gluten-free diet proves it.

Treatment and Prognosis

Treatment requires strict, lifelong adherence to a gluten-free diet. Food starch made from wheat, barley, and oats must be replaced with corn and rice products. The clinical response usually requires a few weeks and may proceed over a period of months. However, reversion to the symptoms can occur within days of reinstitution of a regular diet. The long-term prognosis for this syndrome is excellent, although there may be a slightly higher incidence of non-Hodgkin's lymphoma in adult life.

Bacterial Overgrowth Syndrome

The small intestine normally harbors fewer than 10^4 colony-forming units per milliliter of fluid and is considered relatively sterile as a result of the motility of the intestine, gastric acid, and intestinal immunoglobulins. Overgrowth of bacteria in the small intestine frequently results in malabsorption. This can be due to decreased motility, surgically created blind loops, or decreased gastric acid secretion.

Pathogenesis

The malabsorption seen in bacterial overgrowth syndrome may result from three mechanisms: (1) deconjugation of bile salts leading to impaired micelle formation and fat malabsorption; (2) patchy direct injury to mucosal cells due to bacteria or bacterial products; and (3) direct utilization of nutrients by bacteria, best established for vitamin B_{12}.

Conditions Associated with Bacterial Overgrowth

A large number of disorders are associated with bacterial overgrowth. These include gross structural derangements, such as diverticula, fistulas, blind loops, strictures, and obstruction, and also diseases that impair intestinal motility, most commonly diabetes, amyloidosis, progressive systemic sclerosis, and intestinal pseudo-obstruction. Bacterial overgrowth has also been seen in pancreatic insufficiency and hypogammaglobulinemia. Surgical damage to the ileocecal valve leading to reflux of colonic contents may also predispose to small intestinal bacterial overgrowth.

Diagnosis

An approach to the patient with malabsorption is shown in Figure 32–3. When bacterial overgrowth is suspected because of an abnormal D-xylose test, a definitive diagnosis can be obtained by the ^{14}C-xylose, lactulose, or glucose breath hydrogen test. Other approaches include (1) a positive three-stage Schilling test; (2) direct culture of jejunal fluid (usually $> 10^7$ colony-forming units/ml with a mixed culture is required for diagnosis); and (3) a 10- to 14-day therapeutic trial of a broad-spectrum antibiotic.

Treatment

Treatment depends upon the cause of the overgrowth syndrome. Surgery may be required for structural abnormalities. More commonly, patients are treated indefinitely with intermittent antibiotics such as metronidazole, trimethoprim-sulfamethoxazole, and tetracycline. Cephalosporins in combination with metronidazole may be required, and in severe cases, total parenteral nutrition is necessary.

REFERENCES

Toskes PP: Malabsorption. *In* Wyngaarden JB, Smith LH Jr, Bennett JC (eds.): Cecil Textbook of Medicine. 19th ed. Philadelphia, WB Saunders, 1992, pp 687–698.
Wright TL, Heyworth MF: Maldigestion and malabsorption. *In* Sleisenger MH, Fordtran JS (eds.): Gastrointestinal Disease. 4th ed. Philadelphia, WB Saunders, 1989, pp 263–282.

D. Diarrhea

DEFINITION

Diarrhea is defined as an increase in stool weight (> 200 gm/day) that may be associated with increased liquidity, stool frequency, perianal discomfort, and urgency, with or without fecal incontinence. This section discusses normal water and solute handling by the intestine and the pathophysiology and evaluation of diarrhea. Other specific clinical entities have already been discussed in Section C and are further discussed in Chapter 36. Infectious causes are covered in Chapter 103.

NORMAL INTESTINAL PHYSIOLOGY

The intestine is normally presented with approximately 10 L/day of fluid, 1.5 to 2 L from ingested food and liquids and the remainder from salivary, gastric, biliary, pancreatic, and small intestinal secretions. The small bowel absorbs all but 1 L of this fluid, with the colon absorbing 90% of the remaining fluid, leading to fecal output of 100 to 150 ml per day.

The mechanisms that control fluid and solute absorption differ in different regions of the gut. A single general principle, however, governs all absorption: solutes are absorbed by specific mechanisms, with water following passively. The energy source for transport of most intestinal solutes is the sodium gradient generated by the (Na^+/K^+)-ATPase pump at the basolateral surface. This gradient is the driving force for transport of protons, sodium chloride, glucose, amino acids, and bile acids across cell membranes. Bicarbonate transport drives and accounts for the relatively alkaline nature of ileal and colonic contents as well as the fluid immediately adjacent to the enterocytes and under the mucous layer. Jejunal and ileal fluids typically have the following solute concentrations: Na^+, 140 mM; K^+, 6.0 mM; Cl^-, 100 mM; and HCO_3^-, 30 mM.

Colonic solute transport is restricted to electrolytes and proceeds by a mechanism different from that of the small bowel. The colon has a specific sodium channel that generates an electrical potential across the colon wall and drives chloride and potassium secretion, leading to the high potassium concentration seen in colonic contents. Organic acids produced by colonic bacteria may react with bicarbonate and produce organic anions and CO_2. Thus, colonic fluid has a different concentration profile for the electrolytes outlined above for the small bowel. These include Na^+, 40 mM; K^+, 90 mM; Cl^-, 15 mM; HCO_2^-, 30 mM; and organic anions, 85 mM.

The small bowel and the colon are both capable of secreting electrolytes in water. In the small bowel, crypt cells are responsible for most secretion. They appear to use sodium-coupled entry of chloride anions across the basolateral membrane to support secretion of chloride across the luminal cell membrane. Sodium and water follow the chloride passively owing to electrical and osmotic gradients (Fig. 32–4). Colonocytes probably secrete chloride by a similar mechanism, in which chloride uptake across the basolateral membrane is coupled to sodium and potassium entry.

The movement of water across intestinal membranes is passive but prodigious. Water absorption is linked to solute absorption, and therefore the presence of any osmotically active solutes such as magnesium, phosphate, sulfate, or nonabsorbable carbohydrates impairs water absorption or leads to water secretion.

CLASSIFICATION AND PATHOPHYSIOLOGY

Any of the following abnormalities may lead to diarrhea: (1) a decrease in the normal absorption of solutes in water; (2) increased secretion of electrolytes obligating

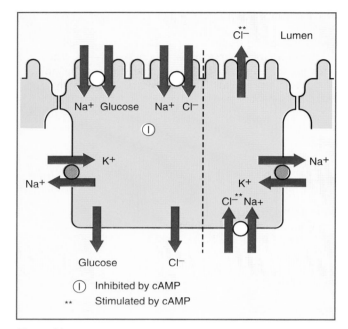

Figure 32–4

Schematic representation of electrolyte and glucose transport mechanisms in the small intestine. Absorptive mechanisms (shown on the left) and secretory mechanisms (shown on the right) are driven by (Na^+/K^+)-ATPase (shown in closed circles). Cyclic AMP produces a secretory diarrhea by both inhibiting absorption and stimulating secretion of sodium and chloride. Coupled absorption of sodium and glucose is unaffected, and this is the basis for current oral rehydration formulas. cAMP = Cyclic adenosine monophosphate.

water to the intestinal lumen; (3) the presence of poorly absorbed, osmotically active solutes in the gut lumen; (4) increased intestinal motility; and (5) inflammatory disease producing blood, pus, or mucus (Table 32–7).

Secretory Diarrhea

Secretory diarrhea is usually due to abnormalities in both absorption and secretion of electrolytes. Cholera is the prototypic disease characterized by secretory diarrhea. The cholera organism attaches to the enterocyte surface and elaborates a series of toxins. The major cholera toxin binds to a glycolipid on the cell surface. This interaction leads to virtually irreversible activation of a guanosine triphosphate (GTP) binding protein (G-protein) that stimulates adenyl cyclase to make cyclic adenosine phosphate (cAMP). The rise in intracellular cAMP has two separate effects that both cause diarrhea. First, it inhibits the Na^+/Cl^- cotransporter, blocking NaCl absorption. Second, it activates the chloride channel, prompting massive Cl^- secretion. All of these events occur without any physical damage to the cell. Cholera toxin induces specific abnormalities so the cell can still absorb large amounts of Na^+ if coupled to glucose absorption. Thus, cholera and all other secretory diarrheas are best treated with oral solutions containing sodium and glucose.

Secretory diarrhea has other causes, but most of

TABLE 32–7	Classification of Diarrhea*		
Type	**Mechanism**	**Examples**	**Characteristics**
1. Secretory	Increased secretion and/or decreased absorption of Na^+ and Cl^-	Cholera VIP-secreting tumor Bile salt enteropathy Fatty acid–induced diarrhea	Large volume, watery diarrhea No blood or pus No solute gap Little or no response to fasting
2. Osmotic	Nonabsorbable molecules in gut lumen	Lactose intolerance (lactase deficiency) Generalized malabsorption (particularly carbohydrates) Mg^{2+}-containing laxatives	Watery stool, no blood or pus Improves with fasting Stool may contain fat globules or meat fibers and may have an increased solute gap
3. Inflammatory	Destruction of mucosa Impaired absorption Outpouring of blood, mucus	Ulcerative colitis Shigellosis Amebiasis	Small frequent stools with blood and pus Fever
4. Decreased absorptive surface	Impaired reabsorption of electrolytes	Bowel resection Enteric fistula	Variable
5. Motility disorder	Increased motility with decreased time for absorption of electrolytes and/or nutrients	Hyperthyroidism Irritable bowel syndrome	Variable
	Decreased motility with bacterial overgrowth	Scleroderma Diabetic diarrhea	Malabsorption

VIP = Vasoactive intestinal polypeptide.
* Diarrhea is, in many instances, due to a combination of mechanisms. The diarrhea of generalized malabsorption, for example, is attributable to osmotic and secretory diarrhea as well as decreased absorptive surface.

them are poorly understood. Increases in cyclic guanosine monophosphate (cGMP) or intracellular calcium may also lead to secretion. Small bowel disorders that produce atrophic villi, such as celiac sprue, are often associated with electrolyte secretion abnormalities as well. Presumably, this is due to inadequate absorptive surface in the face of normal crypt secretion. Disorders associated with malabsorption in osmotic diarrheas are sometimes associated with secretory components, but the mechanism is not well understood. Nonabsorbed bile acids and fatty acids may stimulate ion secretion in the colon, leading to a non–small-bowel secretory diarrhea.

Secretory diarrhea frequently presents as massive watery diarrhea that continues despite fasting. Because the diarrhea is primarily water and electrolytes, fecal osmolality can be entirely accounted for by the measurement of Na^+, K^+, Cl^-, and HCO_3^-, with the fecal solute gap [plasma osmolality $- 2(Na^+ + K^+)$] near zero.

Osmotic Diarrhea

Osmotic diarrhea is caused by the accumulation or generation of poorly absorbed solutes in the lumen of the intestine. The diarrhea occurs because the intestine *cannot* maintain a water gradient. Thus, excess luminal solute obligates water losses. This can occur by three mechanisms: (1) ingestion of poorly absorbed solutes such as lactulose, SO_4^{2-}, PO_4^{3-}, or Mg^{2+}; (2) generalized malabsorption; and (3) failure to absorb a specific dietary component such as lactose. Examples of osmotic diarrhea are listed in Table 32–8.

Osmotic diarrhea is completely preventable by fasting. Osmotically active molecules obligate luminal water, diluting the sodium and potassium (Fig. 32–5). Fecal fluid osmolality is assumed to be equal to serum osmolality (290 mOsm/kg) since the colon cannot generate or maintain a water gradient. The difference between serum osmolality (calculated or measured) and $2[Na^+ + K^+]$ in stool should be less than 10. The progressive changes in luminal electrolytes during processing of a normal meal and a meal destined to proceed to osmotic diarrhea are depicted in Figure 32–5.

Abnormal Intestinal Motility

At least three types of motility disturbances may result in diarrhea: (1) diminished peristalsis, leading to bacterial overgrowth (see Section C of this chapter); (2) increased small bowel motility, leading to maldigestion and absorption; and (3) rapid colonic emptying, preventing desiccation of the stool associated with increased stool liquidity.

TABLE 32–8	Some Causes of Osmotic Diarrhea

Disaccharidase deficiencies
Glucose-galactose or fructose malabsorption
Lactulose, mannitol, sorbitol ("chewing gum diarrhea") ingestion
Magnesium ingestion (antacids, laxatives)
Sulfate, phosphate ingestion (laxatives)
Sodium citrate ingestion
Steatorrhea (pancreatic insufficiency)
Generalized malabsorption
    Small bowel mucosal disease (celiac disease)
    Bacterial overgrowth (bile acid deconjugation, villous atrophy)

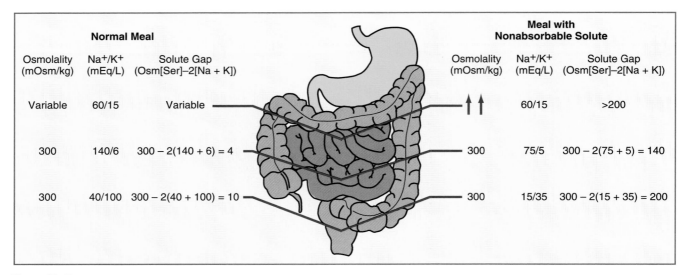

Figure 32–5

Changes in luminal electrolytes during a normal meal and a meal causing osmotic diarrhea. Each row of data shows a comparison of osmolality, sodium/potassium concentration, and solute gaps at a given level of the intestine for normal meals *(left)* and in meals producing osmotic diarrhea *(right)*. Note that the osmolality of luminal contents stabilizes equal to serum in the small intestine. Osmotically active molecules obligate water in the intestine but *do not* elevate the osmolality.

Diarrhea due to motility disturbances may be associated with irritable bowel syndrome, postgastrectomy and postvagotomy syndromes, both nephropathic and enteropathic diabetes, progressive systemic sclerosis, and thyrotoxicosis.

EVALUATION OF DIARRHEA

As with all clinical problems, evaluating diarrhea requires a detailed history and physical examination and prudent selection and interpretation of laboratory tests.

History and Physical Examination

The patient's description, or better, the physician's observation of abnormal stool can be quite informative. Voluminous stools suggest a source in the small bowel or proximal colon, whereas small stools associated with urgency suggest disease of the left colon or rectum. Blood in the stool suggests mucosal damage or inflammation, whereas frothy stools and flatus suggest carbohydrate malabsorption. Stools that are foul smelling or greasy or have visible oil or fat are uncommon but indicate severe steatorrhea. Obtaining a thorough history of drug exposure, with particular attention to over-the-counter drugs is essential and must include antibiotics, antacids, antihypertensives, thyroxine, digitalis, propranolol, quinidine, colchicine, lactulose, sugar-free gum, ethanol, and especially laxatives. It is essential to determine the pace of the patient's present illness, that is, its duration and its rate of change; prior history of surgery; systemic complaints; history of travel inside or outside the country; family his-

TABLE 32–9	Tests That May Be Useful in the Work-Up of Diarrhea

Stool	Gastric analysis
Consistency	X-ray studies
Frequency/24 hr	Upper GI, small bowel, barium
Volume/24 hr	enema
WBCs by Wright's stain	Abdominal and pelvic sono-
Blood	gram, CT scan
Sudan stain for fat	Abdominal angiogram
Quantitative fat/24 hr	Small bowel studies
NaOH for phenolphthalein and	Aspirate (O and P, colony
other laxatives	count cultures)
Cultures for enteric pathogens	Biopsy
Ova and parasites	Mucosal disaccharidase assay
Clostridium difficile toxin	D-Xylose absorption test
Osmolality	Schilling test with intrinsic
Na, K, Cl	factor
pH	^{14}C-bile acid absorption
Reducing substances	Carbohydrate breath tests
Mg, SO_4, PO_4	Exocrine pancreatic function
Proctoscopy	Upper endoscopy
Mucosal appearance	Colonoscopy
Biopsy	Urine
Blood	5-Hydroxyindoleacetic acid
Electrolytes	(5-HIAA)
Immunoglobulins, albumin	Metanephrines, vanillylman-
T_3, T_4	delic acid (VMA)
Ameba serology	NaOH (for phenolphthalein)
Folate, vitamin B_{12}	Heavy metals, drug screen
Ca, Mg, PO_4	Room search for drugs
Erythrocyte sedimentation rate	Intestinal perfusion studies
Eosinophil count	Therapeutic trials
Special assays	
Vasoactive intestinal polypeptide	
Calcitonin	
Gastrin	
Prostaglandins	
Other	

CT = Computed tomography; GI = gastrointestinal; WBC = white blood cell.
From Fine KD, Krejs GJ, Fordtran JS: Diarrhea. *In* Sleisenger MH, Fordtran JS (eds.): Gastrointestinal Disease. 5th ed. Philadelphia, WB Saunders, 1993, pp 1043–1072.

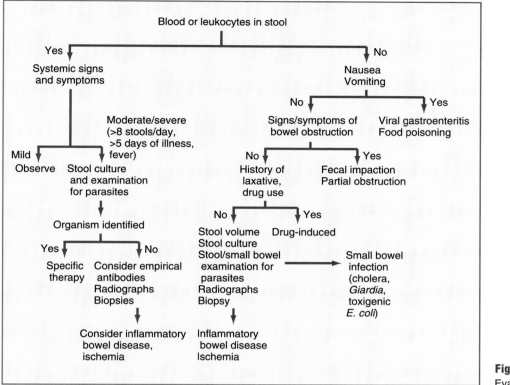

Figure 32–6
Evaluation of acute diarrhea.

tory; and sexual orientation. Acute diarrheas are usually caused by infectious agents or toxins such as staphylococcal food poisoning, whereas chronic diarrheas are usually not infectious.

The physical examination may lead to the diagnosis of diarrhea. Important signs to look for include evidence of weight loss, suggesting malabsorption; systemic signs of rheumatic diseases, such as fever or arthritis; adenopathy that might suggest lymphoma; neuropathy; autonomic neuropathy; orthostatic hypotension (with a pulse rate of 100); or flush, as seen in malignant carcinoid syndrome.

Laboratory Tests

Even when the cause of diarrhea is obvious from the history or physical examination, laboratory tests may be helpful in defining the pathophysiology of a patient's illness. Table 32–9 is a compendium of tests useful in evaluating diarrhea, but of course only a subset should be performed on any given patient. Selecting the most appropriate test is facilitated by grouping the patients into categories:

1. Acute diarrhea is usually associated with toxins, as in food poisoning, infections, drugs, or occasionally fecal impaction. Inflammatory bowel disease (IBD) and intestinal ischemia are not commonly implicated in acute diarrhea. So-called traveler's diarrhea usually occurs within 2 weeks of travel to a tropical or developing area and is self-limited.

2. Chronic diarrhea can be subdivided into multiple categories:
   a. Secretory diarrhea, usually caused by drugs, hormones, bile acids, fatty acids, or microscopic/collagenous colitis
   b. Osmotic diarrhea, generally caused by drugs, laxatives, malabsorption, or sugar-free gum
   c. Inflammatory diarrhea due to ischemic colitis, parasitic infection such as that caused by amebae, or IBD (ulcerative colitis, Crohn's disease)
   d. Motility disorders such as IBS, progressive systemic sclerosis, and the autonomic neuropathy of diabetes
   e. Disorders of lost absorptive surface, as is seen in postsurgical diarrhea syndromes

General algorithms for the evaluation of acute and chronic diarrhea are shown in Figures 32–6 and 32–7.

All patients with diarrhea should have their stools examined for consistency, blood, and white blood cells by Wright's stain. Fecal leukocytes in acute diarrheas strongly suggest invasive microorganisms such as *Shigella, Entamoeba histolytica, Campylobacter, Escherichia coli,* and occasionally gonococci or antibiotic-associated colitis. In patients with chronic diarrhea, fecal leukocytes suggest ulcerative colitis, Crohn's disease, or ischemia. Toxin-induced secretory diarrheas, malabsorption syndromes, laxative abuse, and giardiasis do not produce fecal leukocytes. The presence of fecal blood indicates inflammation and has a significance similar to pus.

Additional examinations are performed depending on the clinical presentation and progress. Stools should be examined for ova and parasites and cultured for bacterial pathogens. Proctoscopy is helpful in these cases, primarily when pseudomembranous colitis is present. Blood cultures and white blood count and differential may be helpful in patients with evidence of systemic illness, particularly salmonellosis. Serologic tests for amebiasis can help diagnose this readily treatable disease.

In evaluating chronic diarrhea, the initial selection of tests is designed to answer the following questions:

1. Does the patient exhibit the signs of inflammation of the mucosa? If so, imaging studies of the intestine such as endoscopy (upper and lower), barium enema, and possibly enteroclysis, are required with biopsy.
2. Is malabsorption present? In this case, stool fat and the D-xylose absorption test should be performed.
3. Is there evidence of structural, mucosal, or motility disturbance? Radiographic or endoscopic methods and biopsies should be obtained if appropriate.

More specialized tests are then selected on the basis of the observations made on the foregoing examinations.

Stool culture and examination must always be performed prior to purging for endoscopic procedures or radiographic studies because the preparation for the diagnostic studies may interfere with these tests. However, proctosigmoidoscopy can be performed without any special preparation of the bowel. Biopsies of the rectum can be diagnostic of Whipple's disease, schistosomiasis, amyloidosis, and inflammation.

Quantitative fecal fat determination is the most definitive diagnostic procedure for detecting steatorrhea, and if steatorrhea is present, it must be thoroughly evaluated. Interpretation of fecal fat excretion requires knowledge of dietary fat intake, which is generally standardized at 100 gm/day for the duration of the test.

Specialized assays for drug-related hormones such as vasoactive intestinal polypeptide (VIP), prostaglandins,

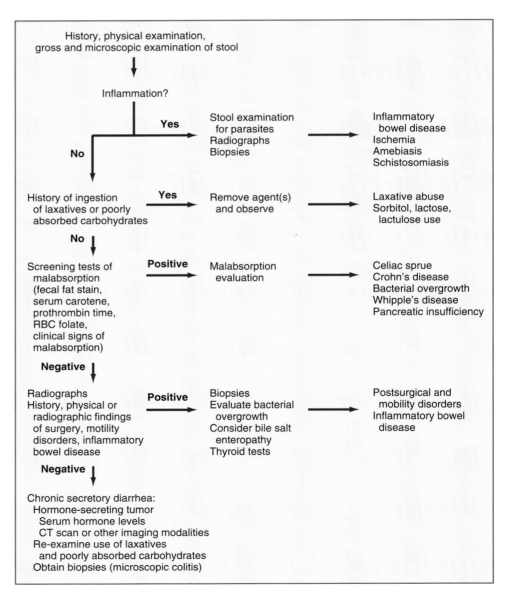

Figure 32–7

Evaluation of chronic diarrhea. CT = Computed tomography; RBC = red blood cell.

calcitonin, gastrin, and several others are helpful only in the rare patient who has more than 1 L/day of secretory diarrhea. Interpretation is difficult because most positives are false positives. It is also helpful to alkalinize the patient's stool, watching for the characteristic pink color associated with phenolphthalein (laxative) use.

Ignorance of diagnosis and the need to treat often force us to use empiric trials in individual cases, such as antibiotics for bacterial overgrowth, metronidazole for giardiasis, lactose-free diet for lactose malabsorption, cholestyramine for bile acid malabsorption, and pancreatic enzymes for pancreatic exocrine insufficiency.

Therapy

The ideal therapy should cure the underlying disorder. When this is not possible, drugs may be used to diminish symptoms, such as corticosteroids in the treatment of IBD or nonspecific diarrhea treatment. Specific antisecretory drugs are being explored, and in some patients, the somatostatic analogue has been dramatically effective. The most important aspect of diarrhea therapy is the replacement of fluid and electrolytes, particularly in patients with other diseases, the very young, and the very old. Oral volume replacement is best achieved with sodium glucose solutions because sodium and glucose are easily absorbed together. Opiates such as diphenoxylate, loperamide, and codeine may reduce the frequency and volume of diarrhea stool, probably owing to increased contact time in the colon. Avoid opiates in patients with IBD because they may aggravate or precipitate toxic megacolon. Opiates relieve symptoms of chronic diarrhea but may prolong acute illnesses such as shigellosis.

Antibiotics are not usually necessary for acute diarrheas because the illnesses are too brief to need therapy. Detailed discussion of the use of antibiotics and antiparasitic agents is included in Chapter 94.

SPECIFIC CLINICAL DISORDERS

Patients with acquired immunodeficiency syndrome (AIDS) and early symptomatic human immunodeficiency virus (HIV) disease are susceptible to multiple infections and malignant diseases of the intestine. These are discussed in some detail in Chapters 37, 103, 108, and 109. *Cryptosporidium* infestation has proved to be a very difficult diarrheal illness to manage in AIDS patients. There are no efficacious drugs that eliminate the infestation; management revolves around fluid, electrolytes, and opiates to diminish the diarrheal volume. Patients with AIDS are susceptible to multiple other organisms causing diarrhea. The management of these is largely symptomatic.

REFERENCES

Fedorak RN, Field M: Antidiarrheal therapy. Dig Dis Sci 1987; 32:195.

Field M, Fordtran JS, Schultz SG (eds.): Secretory Diarrhea. Bethesda, MD, American Physiological Society, 1980.

Fine KD, Krejs GJ, Fordtran JS: Diarrhea. *In* Sleisenger MH, Fordtran JS (eds.): Gastrointestinal Disease. Pathophysiology, Diagnosis, and Management. 5th ed. Philadelphia, WB Saunders 1993, pp 1043–1072.

Krejs GJ: Diarrhea. *In* Wyngaarden JB, Smith LH Jr, Bennett JC (eds.): Cecil Textbook of Medicine. 19th ed. Philadelphia, WB Saunders, 1992, pp 680–686.

Wilberts B, Bray D, Lewis J, Laff M, Roberts K, Watson JD (eds.): Cell signaling. *In* Molecular Biology of the Cell. 2nd ed. New York, Garland Publishing, 1989.

33

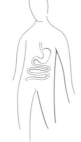

Radiographic and Endoscopic Procedures in Gastroenterology

In the past, barium radiography and fluoroscopy of the luminal gastrointestinal (GI) tract were the only diagnostic methods available for evaluating potential GI lesions. Over the last decade, newer techniques and refinements of older methods have increased our ability to image the GI tract noninvasively. In addition, endoscopic examination of the luminal GI tract and the pancreaticobiliary tree has revolutionized our approach to many disorders. One can actually visualize the GI tract and in some cases direct definitive therapy to identified abnormalities without resorting to surgery.

Radiography and endoscopy can be complementary, with each technique having distinct advantages and disadvantages. This may result in confusion as to the most appropriate diagnostic test in various clinical settings. This chapter briefly reviews the radiographic and endoscopic procedures currently available and their optimal use.

RADIOGRAPHIC PROCEDURES

Table 33–1 summarizes the radiographic and endoscopic procedures in general use.

Plain Radiographs and Barium Contrast Studies

Plain radiographs of the abdomen in the supine, upright, and lateral decubitus positions are simple to obtain and relatively inexpensive, but their usefulness is limited. These tests are most valuable for diseases that cause abnormalities in the bowel gas pattern, such as small bowel or colonic obstruction, perforation of a hollow viscus (represented by free intraperitoneal air), and pneumatosis intestinalis. Abnormalities of the bowel wall may also occasionally be identified (e.g., thumb-printing with colonic or small bowel ischemia). Plain abdominal radiographs are also useful in detecting diseases associated with intra-abdominal calcifications such as cholelithiasis, nephrolithiasis, and chronic pancreatitis.

Contrast studies using barium sulfate or water-soluble iodinated agents (Gastrografin [meglumine diatri-zoate], Hypaque [sodium diatrizoate]) provide information about the anatomy of the luminal GI tract. Single-contrast studies are performed using a bolus of contrast material and may detect obstruction or large lesions, but they may not detect small mucosal abnormalities. Double-contrast studies, in which barium is administered first followed by a radiolucent substance such as air that results in a thin barium coating in the mucosa, has a much greater sensitivity and may detect tumors, obstructions, and small lesions confined to the mucosa.

In the esophagus, single- and double-contrast barium swallows detect esophageal strictures and masses that produce luminal narrowing and, when severe, proximal dilation. Double-contrast studies may improve the sensitivity for detecting subtle mucosal abnormalities such as reflux esophagitis, esophageal ulcerations, or varices; endoscopy is more sensitive in the detection of these mucosal lesions. The use of fluoroscopy during a barium swallow, particularly when combined with video recordings, demonstrates swallowing disorders in the hypopharynx as well as esophageal motility disorders.

The standard single- or double-contrast examination of the upper GI tract (upper GI series) is commonly used to detect peptic ulcer disease or gastric neoplasms. In addition, motility disorders can be demonstrated by visualizing abnormal or decreased gastric emptying. Most gastric ulcerations (benign and malignant) may be identified radiographically; however, it is not always possible to correctly identify an ulcer as benign or malignant based on the radiographic appearance alone. Therefore, endoscopic mucosal biopsy is recommended. In many clinical situations the lesion may simply be followed radiographically until complete healing is documented. The use of the double-contrast technique increases the yield for the detection of erosive lesions associated with aspirin or nonsteroidal anti-inflammatory drug (NSAID) use or lesions at the anastomosis of prior gastric surgery. As with the esophagus, endoscopy is more sensitive for detecting shallow mucosal abnormalities.

Radiographic examination of the small bowel is limited by the pooling and dilution of barium. In addition, overlapping loops of bowel segments may obscure pathology. The standard small bowel follow-through examina-

TABLE 33–1	Radiographic and Endoscopic Procedures	

Procedure	Advantages	Disadvantages
Plain film of the abdomen	Identifies gas (intramural, intraperitoneal, as well as luminal) and calcifications	Few specific features
Barium swallow	Shows mass lesions and motility disorders well	Misses many superficial mucosal lesions
Double-contrast barium examination of the upper gastrointestinal tract ("UGI series")	Delineates ulcers and tumors well	Misses some superficial mucosal lesions Misclassifies ~5% of malignant gastric ulcers
Small bowel series	Simpler to perform Evaluates transit time, caliber, and proximal mucosa and often shows mass lesions	May miss distal or subtle lesions
Enteroclysis (small bowel enema)	Improved definition of mucosa and bowel wall of entire small bowel	Requires oral intubation
Double-contrast barium enema ("pneumocolon")	Shows polyps, tumors, fistulas, diverticula, and other structural changes (e.g., inflammatory bowel disease) well	Uncomfortable for some patients Impossible in those with lax anal sphincter May miss superficial mucosal and rectal lesions Misses vascular lesions
Percutaneous transhepatic cholangiography	Excellent definition of intrahepatic bile ducts Option for therapeutic intervention	Extrahepatic bile ducts may not be well visualized Nondilated ducts may be missed
Angiography	Demonstration of acutely bleeding lesions Definition of vascularity of mass lesions	Invasive Large contrast load Bleeding lesions visualized only if blood loss exceeds 0.5 ml/min Expensive
Ultrasonography	No radiation exposure Real-time examination Best for fluid-filled lesions, gallstones, and bile ducts	Gas obscures examination Bowel poorly visualized
Computed tomography	Excellent anatomic definition Visualizes bowel wall thickness, mesentery, retroperitoneum, aorta well Density changes may indicate nature of diffuse parenchymal disease	Expensive Radiation exposure Bowel sometimes not well visualized Possible reactions to iodinated intravenous contrast media
MRI of the abdomen	Excellent anatomic definition Identifies patency of vessels Sensitive detection of hepatic tumors No radiation	Expensive Patient must be cooperative No contrast agents available Operator dependent
Liver-spleen scan	Demonstrates mass lesions (>1–2 cm) Increased bone marrow uptake suggests portal hypertension	Limited anatomic definition
99mTc-HIDA liver scan	Best test for cystic duct obstruction	Will not visualize if bilirubin >6 mg/dl Poor anatomic definition
99mTc-RBC scan	Approximate localization of intermittently bleeding lesion	Poor anatomic definition
Esophagogastroduodenoscopy	Direct visualization of upper GI tract Identifies virtually all mucosal lesions Permits biopsy, electrocautery	Expensive Invasive May miss motility and compressive lesions
Flexible sigmoidoscopy (to 25 cm)	Direct visualization of rectum, sigmoid, and distal descending colon Permits biopsy and polypectomy Useful for monitoring of inflammatory bowel disease	Invasive Misses lesions in more proximal colon
Colonoscopy	Direct visualization of large bowel Permits biopsy and polypectomy, electrocautery, and laser treatment of bleeding	Expensive Invasive Higher rate of complications than barium enema
Endoscopic retrograde cholangiopancreatography	Only method for visualizing pancreatic ducts; permits biopsy of ampullary lesions and sphincterotomy for common duct stones	Requires considerable skill Expensive

GI = Gastrointestinal; MRI = magnetic resonance imaging; 99mTc-HIDA = technetium-labeled iminodiacetic acid; 99mTc-RBC = technetium-labeled red blood cell.

tion, in which barium is ingested orally, can evaluate the caliber of the small bowel, provide information about gross mucosal abnormalities, and determine transit time. Small lesions of the more distal small bowel are difficult to detect, whereas large mass lesions, obstruction, and Crohn's disease (CD) can usually be demonstrated easily. A more recent technique for evaluating the entire small bowel is the small bowel enema (enteroclysis), in which barium followed by a radiolucent methylcellulose solution is delivered directly into the jejunum through a special tube placed orally. This method of imaging is operator dependent, time consuming, and not widely available and involves more radiation than the standard small bowel follow-through, but it is very sensitive in detecting small lesions or a Meckel's diverticulum. The terminal ileum may be identified by enteroclysis or pneumocolon, in which air is introduced into the rectum (introduced rectally) after opacification of the terminal ileum by barium (introduced orally). Radiographic evaluation of the small bowel may be indicated when evaluating malabsorption, inflammatory bowel disease (CD), or obstruction. Newer small bowel endoscopes can reliably evaluate the distal duodenum and proximal jejunum, although consistent evaluation of the more distal small bowel is not yet available. These endoscopes also have the potential for mucosal biopsy as well as coagulation of bleeding lesions.

Single- and double-contrast (air-contrast) radiographs of the colon have long been the standard for colonic evaluation. The double-contrast technique can detect mucosal lesions such as small polyps or early inflammatory bowel disease, which may not be seen with the single-contrast technique. Colonoscopy more reliably identifies these mucosal abnormalities. The clinical problem being investigated (e.g., fecal occult blood loss, inflammatory bowel disease, neoplasm, diarrhea, or obstruction) determines the choice of either double-contrast barium enema or colonoscopy. Importantly, the need for tissue examination may favor initial colonoscopic evaluation. In contrast to barium, water-soluble iodinated compounds are particularly useful when a perforation is suspected (e.g., perforation of a diverticulum or a duodenal ulcer) because these compounds are less toxic to the peritoneum than barium. However, they should not be used in the upper GI tract when aspiration is likely or a fistula to the bronchial tree is present because they are quite toxic to the lungs. Although they demonstrate less mucosal detail, water-soluble contrast agents may be particularly useful when distal colonic obstruction is anticipated (e.g., carcinoma, volvulus). Significant amounts of barium above a colonic ob-

struction may be problematic if surgery becomes necessary. This is less of a concern with small bowel obstruction due to dilution of the barium.

Ultrasonography and Computed Tomography

Ultrasonography (US) and computed tomography (CT) have revolutionized both the diagnosis and management of many abdominal diseases. US and CT can examine organs such as the pancreas that cannot be directly visualized by barium studies. US and CT are most useful in imaging solid abdominal organs (liver, spleen, pancreas, kidney, retroperitoneal lymph nodes), as well as the gallbladder and bile ducts. Table 33–2 outlines the relative merits of US and CT.

Ultrasound, which uses high-frequency sound waves rather than x-rays, can examine both solid and fluid-filled structures noninvasively. With the development of real-time images and Doppler techniques, US can now evaluate both dynamic and static abdominal processes. US images, like those of CT, are displayed in cross-section. US has the ability to (1) detect abdominal masses as small as 2 cm in diameter; (2) differentiate fluid-filled cysts from solid masses; (3) identify gallstones more rapidly and with greater sensitivity than can oral cholecystography or CT; (4) evaluate for dilated bile ducts (intra- and extrahepatic); and (5) detect ascites and some vascular abnormalities such as abdominal aortic aneurysms. Air or gas obscures the US beam, so structures under gas-filled loops of bowel may not be visualized reliably.

Computed tomography uses multiple x-ray beams and detectors in conjunction with computer analysis to identify and display small differences in tissue density. CT provides a more precise anatomic definition than US,

TABLE 33–2	Comparison of Ultrasonography and Computed Tomography	
	Ultrasonography	**Computed Tomography**
Organs best visualized	Kidney Gallbladdder Liver and bile ducts Pancreas Spleen Blood vessels	Liver and dilated bile ducts Retroperitoneal lymph nodes Mesentery Gallbladder Aorta Spleen Pancreas Kidney Pelvic organs
Lesions best visualized	Fluid-filled masses/cysts Gallstones Dilated bile ducts Aortic aneurysms Ascites	Tumors/cysts/abscesses Lymphadenopathy Mass lesions Pancreatic tumor Abdominal aortic aneurysm Trauma or parenchymal hematoma of liver, spleen, and kidney Fatty liver
Advantages	Real-time examination Noninvasive Guided needle aspiration Assess blood flow	Less dependent upon a skilled operator Guided needle aspiration
Disadvantages	Skilled operator necessary Gas obscures deeper organs	Absence of fat makes examination more difficult Expensive

and the imaging quality is not affected by bowel gas. Current scanners obtain images of very high quality within seconds. CT is used primarily for the detection and characterization of abdominal mass lesions (tumors, cysts, abscesses) and pancreatic disease. In addition, it may detect biliary dilation, calcified gallstones, and intra-abdominal hemorrhage. CT is also useful in demonstrating increased thickness of the intestinal or colonic wall due to processes such as ischemia, Crohn's disease, appendicitis, and diverticulitis. With this method, mesenteric abnormalities such as parenchymal liver diseases (cirrhosis, tumor, abscess, vascular lesion, fatty infiltration) may be well delineated. Finally, lesions and parenchymal abnormalities such as rupture or hematoma of the liver, spleen, kidneys, aortoenteric fistulas, and retroperitoneal adenopathy are also well characterized by CT.

Both US and CT also aid in the placement of drainage catheters (e.g., abscess) and direct thin-needle aspiration biopsy of lesions virtually anywhere in the abdomen.

Radionuclide Imaging

The traditional liver-spleen scan, using technetium 99m (^{99m}Tc)-sulfur colloid, which undergoes phagocytosis by reticuloendothelial cells, has largely been supplanted by US or CT, although it still remains useful for the evaluation of some benign hepatic neoplasms (see Chapter 44). Recently developed agents, such as ^{99m}Tc-HIDA (technetium-labeled iminodiacetic acid), which are taken up directly by hepatic parenchymal cells and excreted in bile, have improved sensitivity for the diagnosis of acute cholecystitis (see Chapter 45) and biliary atresia in infants. Although common bile duct obstruction may be suggested by these scans, they are generally not useful for other biliary tract disorders because their anatomic definition is poor. There is also a lack of specificity in certain conditions. The affinity of ^{99m}Tc-pertechnetate for gastric mucosa makes this agent useful for the detection of Meckel's diverticula, 85% of which contain ectopic gastric mucosa. Radiolabeled foods are currently used to measure the gastric emptying of both liquids and solids in disorders such as diabetic gastroparesis. Indium 111 (^{111}In)-labeled leukocytes injected intravenously may be helpful in localizing intra-abdominal abscesses or detecting the inflammatory activity of CD. ^{99m}Tc-sulfur colloid and ^{99m}Tc-labeled red blood cells are commonly used for localizing the site of lower GI bleeding or when small bowel bleeding is suspected.

Visceral Angiography

Angiography is a highly specialized procedure with a small but definite morbidity. To demonstrate the vasculature of an organ, a catheter is inserted into an appropriate artery or vein that is subsequently injected with contrast. At present, angiography is most often employed for the evaluation of acute severe GI bleeding, primarily of the colon or small bowel, that cannot be visualized endoscopically. If a bleeding site is identified, intra-arterial vasopressin may be infused or the vessels may be occluded with embolized material (coils, Gelfoam). Less commonly, angiography can be used to evaluate vascular lesions (e.g., hepatoma, angioma, angiosarcoma) as well as to demonstrate metastatic liver disease not detected by routine imaging studies.

Magnetic Resonance Imaging (MRI)

Cross-sectional images of the body can also be obtained without x-rays by using magnetic field and radiofrequency radiation combined with computer analysis. This imaging study displays organs by their chemical composition rather than x-ray density. In some situations MRI provides better resolution than does CT and may also offer the opportunity to follow *in situ* chemical reactions. MRI may be particularly useful for evaluating intrahepatic tumors. It also visualizes patent blood vessels well and may be useful for assessing patency of grafts, shunts, or veins. It is currently undergoing evaluation for use in detecting many abdominal processes, but it does not yet have a well-established role.

Visualization of the Biliary Tree

Oral cholecystography (OCG) was used for many years to detect gallbladder stones. OCG involves the oral intake of an iodinated compound that concentrates in the gallbladder; radiographs taken 12 hours after ingestion show filling in the gallbladder. The technique identifies gallstones only in those patients with a functioning gallbladder and a patent cystic duct. US has supplanted OCG for the detection of gallbladder stones, given its greater sensitivity (>95%), lack of radiation, and rapidity.

Bile ducts are identified only when filled with contrast material. Contrast material may be injected percutaneously through the liver into the biliary tree with a small, 23-gauge needle (percutaneous transhepatic cholangiography [PTC]) or at the level of the ampulla with a small catheter placed endoscopically (endoscopic retrograde cholangiopancreatography [ERCP]). Table 33–3 compares these two procedures; both provide excellent detail of the biliary tree. The choice between PTC and ERCP depends on a number of specific circumstances.

ENDOSCOPIC PROCEDURES

An endoscope is a multichanneled tool that permits the passage of air and water and contains one or more channels for aspiration. Through the aspirating channel, one can pass a variety of instruments including cytology brushes, biopsy forceps, injection needles, electrocautery snares, wire baskets, and thermal probes that control hemorrhage.

Endoscopy has important advantages over routine barium contrast studies of the luminal GI tract: (1) greater

TABLE 33–3	Comparison of Percutaneous Transhepatic Cholangiography and Endoscopic Retrograde Cholangiopancreatography	
	Percutaneous Transhepatic Cholangiography (PIC)	**Endoscopic Retrograde Cholangiopancreatography (ERCP)**
Lesions best visualized	Intrahepatic ductal lesions Multiple lesions in a single duct system Several punctures may be made to examine ducts in all lobes	Extrahepatic ductal lesions Pancreatic duct Ampulla of Vater
Therapeutic implications	Temporary external drainage of bile Placement of stents through bile duct obstructions Balloon dilatation of biliary stricture	Sphincterotomy for removal of common duct stones Placement of stents Balloon dilatation of strictures Biopsy of ampullary lesions
Success rate		
Dilated ducts	100%	>90%
Nondilated ducts	60–80%	>90%
Disadvantages	Experienced operator required May miss additional lesions in left lobe	Experienced operator required May not visualize ducts proximal to a lesion
Complications	Bleeding Biliary infection/sepsis Hemobilia	Pancreatitis Biliary infections/sepsis

sensitivity for mucosal lesions (e.g., small peptic ulcer, erosive lesions, esophagitis); (2) greater specificity in certain circumstances (e.g., a small lesion identified at barium enema could be retained stool rather than a polyp); (3) the ability to perform mucosal biopsies as well as cytology to exclude malignancy; and (4) the ability to perform therapy at the time of diagnosis (e.g., injection sclerosis of bleeding esophageal varices). The primary disadvantages of endoscopy are that it is an invasive procedure with potential for morbidity and mortality, although extremely rare (less than 1 death in 10,000 for upper endoscopy), and is costly. Further, it cannot detect motility disturbances of the esophagus or small symptomatic rings of the distal esophagus.

The choice of endoscopy versus radiographic imaging depends on the specific question one wishes to answer (e.g., etiology of significant GI bleeding versus vague abdominal pain), the likely diagnosis, the possible need for therapeutic intervention, locally available skill, and cost. In some circumstances, radiographic and endoscopic procedures complement one another.

Esophagogastroduodenoscopy (EGD)

The upper GI tract to the second portion of the duodenum may be evaluated with standard upper endoscopes. EGD is usually performed in the patient with upper GI hemorrhage as well as in suspected upper GI malignancy. Endoscopy has become the diagnostic procedure of choice in most instances of upper GI hemorrhage, especially when the bleeding is brisk and therapeutic intervention is probable. In evaluating malignancy, endoscopic biopsy supplemented by brush cytology has almost 100% sensitivity, although the accuracy may be reduced for submucosal or infiltrative lesions. Other common indications for EGD include the evaluation of abdominal complaints when the upper GI series is nondiagnostic or the patient is refractory to standard antiulcer therapy, abdomi-

nal pain, esophageal symptoms, injection of esophageal varices, and removal of foreign bodies.

Endoscopic Retrograde Cholangiopancreatography

Cannulation of the ampulla of Vater in the second portion of the duodenum can be accomplished using a special side-viewing endoscope. This highly technical procedure allows for selective cannulation of either the pancreatic duct or the common bile duct, followed by injection of a radiographic contrast medium that highlights the ductal systems. Standard radiographs can then be taken of the contrast-outlined ducts. The primary indications for ERCP include the diagnosis and treatment of pancreatic cancer and obstructive jaundice, the placement of biliary as well as pancreatic endoprostheses (stent), and sphincterotomy. In obstructive jaundice, ERCP is preferred to PTC when ductal dilation is absent but the possibility of biliary disease remains, if there is associated pancreatic or duodenal pathology, or if a coagulation defect is present. In specialized centers, motility measurements of the sphincter of Oddi, located in the ampulla, are used to diagnose sphincter dysfunction. A detailed comparison of ERCP and PTC is outlined in Table 33–3.

Endoscopic sphincterotomy involves an electrocautery incision into the duodenal papilla with a special catheter. Once the papilla is opened, direct access to the biliary tree is established. This is most useful in patients with common bile duct stones who have previously undergone a cholecystectomy and in those considered a poor surgical risk. Sphincterotomy may also be used for treatment of obstructing ampullary tumors, papillary stenosis, sphincter of Oddi dysfunction, and, in some cases, before insertion of an endoprosthesis. When performed by the experienced endoscopist, sphincterotomy has a morbidity (bleeding, pancreatitis) of 5 to 10%, with a mortality of approximately 0.5%.

Sigmoidoscopy and Colonoscopy

Evaluation of the distal colorectum can be performed with rigid sigmoidoscopy. This is a rapid, inexpensive procedure that is somewhat poorly tolerated by patients. However, this procedure may be useful for the initial evaluation of patients with lower GI bleeding when an anorectal source is suspected (hemorrhoid, fissure, tumor). Sigmoidoscopy, using either the 30- or 60-cm flexible instrument, may be used to evaluate more of the distal colon and rectum with a greater degree of sensitivity. Sigmoidoscopy is commonly used in the evaluation of bloody diarrhea, chronic diarrhea, distal colorectal disease, and occult blood in the stool after a normal barium enema and as a screening tool for colon cancer. Ulcerative colitis may be reliably diagnosed by sigmoidoscopy and mucosal biopsy; CD, however, may not involve the distal colon, thus requiring colonoscopy, barium enema, or small bowel follow-through for diagnosis. Colonoscopy allows visualization of the entire colon to the level of the cecum and even into the terminal ileum in most patients. Colonoscopy is commonly performed in the evaluation of suspected colonic neoplasm (e.g., fecal occult blood, iron deficiency anemia), in evaluation of lower GI bleeding, in surveillance for the development of malignancy in ulcerative colitis and polyposis syndromes, and in diagnosis and evaluation of the extent of inflammatory bowel disease. Diagnostic colonoscopy has a perforation rate of 2 to 4 per 1000 and increases with polypectomy to 1 per 100 to 3 per 1000.

Removal of colonic polyps at the time of colonoscopy is an important therapeutic application. In patients with lower GI bleeding, colonoscopy may be used as a therapeutic alternative because the colonoscopist gains the ability to coagulate lesions such as vascular ectasias. In contrast to patients with active upper GI bleeding, colonoscopy in those with lower GI bleeding is a more difficult procedure because the lumen is obscured by blood. In the patient with brisk bleeding, ^{99m}Tc-labeled red cell scanning or angiography may be preferable as the initial diagnostic test.

Laparoscopy

With the widespread use and documented sensitivity of US and CT, laparoscopy is less commonly used to evaluate the peritoneum and liver. At present, it is used primarily to biopsy suspected malignancies of the peritoneum or hepatic surface.

REFERENCES

LaBerge JM, Ostroff JW: Endoscopic and radiologic treatment of biliary disease. *In* Sleisenger MH, Fordtran JS (eds.). Gastrointestinal Disease: Pathophysiology, Diagnosis, and Management. 5th ed. Philadelphia, WB Saunders, 1993, pp 1902–1926.

Sleisenger MH, Fordtran JS (eds.): Gastrointestinal Disease: Pathophysiology, Diagnosis, and Management. 5th ed. Philadelphia, WB Saunders, 1993.

Vennes JA: Gastrointestinal endoscopy. *In* Bennett JC, Plum F (eds.): Cecil Textbook of Medicine. 20th ed. Philadelphia, WB Saunders Co, 1996.

Wall SW: Diagnostic imaging procedures in gastroenterology. *In* Bennett JC, Plum F (eds.): Cecil Textbook of Medicine. 20th ed. Philadelphia, WB Saunders Co, 1996.

34

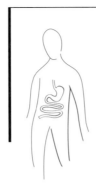

Diseases of the Esophagus

Although the esophagus appears to be a simple organ, esophageal diseases are common and range from trivial complaints of heartburn to major clinical problems of aspiration, obstruction, and hemorrhage. This chapter briefly outlines normal esophageal function and describes a group of unique symptoms characteristic of esophageal disorders. The major benign categories of esophageal diseases, gastroesophageal reflux disease, and motility disorders, are discussed, followed by a brief review of other common esophageal diseases. Malignant diseases of the esophagus are discussed in Chapter 37.

NORMAL ESOPHAGEAL PHYSIOLOGY

The esophagus is a hollow tube bordered at each end by high-pressure valves, or sphincters. The esophagus serves a single but very important function: conveying solids and liquids from the mouth to the stomach. The upper esophageal sphincter (UES) prevents aspiration and swallowing of excessive amounts of air, and the lower esophageal sphincter (LES) prevents the movement of gastric contents in the opposite direction (i.e., gastroesophageal reflux). Swallowing is a complex and well-coordinated motor activity that involves many muscle groups and five cranial nerves (V, VII, IX, X, XII). Swallowing can be divided into three stages: the oral stage, which is voluntary, and the pharyngeal and esophageal stages, which are involuntary. The oral stage involves chewing food and forming it into an oral bolus while propelling it by the tongue into the posterior pharynx. In the pharyngeal stage, food is passed from the pharynx across the UES into the proximal esophagus. This entire process occurs in about 1 second and involves five important steps: (1) the soft palate is elevated and retracted to prevent nasopharyngeal regurgitation; (2) the vocal cords are closed and the epiglottis swings backward to close the larynx and prevent aspiration; (3) the UES relaxes; (4) the larynx is pulled upward, thereby stretching the opening of the esophagus and upper sphincter; and (5) contractions of the pharyngeal muscles provide a driving force to propel food into the esophagus. In the esophageal stage, ingested food is transported from the UES to the stomach while the LES is relaxed. This is accomplished primarily by an orderly stripping wave initiated by swallowing and progressing along the esophagus (i.e., primary peristalsis).

After the food bolus passes, the LES re-establishes a tonic contraction, thereby preventing regurgitation of gastric contents.

CLINICAL SYMPTOMS OF ESOPHAGEAL DISEASE

Dysphagia is the sensation of food being hindered ("sticking") in its normal passage from the mouth to the stomach. Dysphagia is divided into two distinct syndromes (Fig. 34–1): that due to abnormalities affecting the pharynx and UES (oropharyngeal dysphagia) and that due to any of a variety of disorders affecting the esophagus itself (esophageal dysphagia). Oropharyngeal dysphagia is usually described as the inability to initiate the act of swallowing. It is a "transfer" problem of impaired ability to move food from the mouth into the upper esophagus. Esophageal dysphagia results from difficulty in "transporting" food down the esophagus and may be caused by motility disorders or mechanical obstructing lesions. Patients most often report that their food hangs up somewhere behind the sternum. If this symptom is localized to the lower part of the sternum, the lesion is most likely in the distal esophagus, although the patient may also refer the feeling of blockage to the lower part of the neck. To classify the symptom of esophageal dysphagia, three questions are crucial: (1) What type of food causes symptoms? (2) Is the dysphagia intermittent or progressive? and (3) Does the patient have heartburn? An algorithm for approaching patients with dysphagia is shown in Figure 34–1.

Heartburn (pyrosis) is the most common of all esophageal symptoms, resulting from the reflux of gastric contents into the stomach. It is usually described as a burning pain that radiates up behind the sternum. It has many synonyms, including "indigestion," "acid regurgitation," "sour stomach," and "bitter belching." Heartburn is predictably aggravated by several factors, including certain foods (high fat, chocolate, or spicy products), bending over or lying down, alcohol (especially red wines), caffeine, smoking, and emotions. Heartburn is usually relieved by ingesting antacids, baking soda, or milk, albeit only transiently. Heartburn may be accompanied by regurgitation, or water brash. Regurgitation is a sour or bitter fluid in the mouth that comes from the stomach and

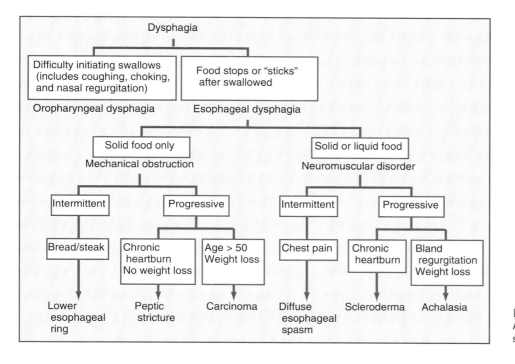

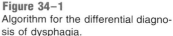

Algorithm for the differential diagnosis of dysphagia.

often occurs at night or when bending over. Water brash describes the sudden filling of the mouth with clear, slightly salty fluid. This fluid is not regurgitated material but rather secretions from the salivary glands as part of a protective, vagally mediated reflex from the distal esophagus.

Odynophagia, or pain on swallowing, is usually associated with caustic ingestion, pill-induced esophagitis, infectious esophagitis caused by viral or fungal agents, and, very rarely, severe gastroesophageal reflux disease or obstructing tumors.

Severe substernal chest pain that is often indistinguishable from angina pectoris may be esophageal in origin. Although once commonly thought to be secondary to esophageal motility disorders, such as diffuse esophageal spasm, more recent studies suggest that gastroesophageal reflux is more likely a cause.

GASTROESOPHAGEAL REFLUX DISEASE

Definition

Gastroesophageal reflux disease (GERD) refers to a spectrum of clinical manifestations due to reflux of stomach and duodenal contents into the esophagus. Many otherwise healthy individuals have occasional heartburn or regurgitation. However, this becomes a disease when the symptoms are severe and frequent or associated esophageal mucosal damage occurs.

Etiology and Pathogenesis

The common denominator for gastroesophageal reflux is the creation of a common cavity phenomenon represent-

ing equalization of intragastric and esophageal pressures. The LES is the major barrier against GERD, with a secondary component from the crural diaphragm during inspiration. Acid refluxing into the esophagus is normally cleared by a two-step process: peristaltic esophageal motor contractions rapidly clear fluid volume from the esophagus, and residual acid is neutralized by swallowed saliva. Patients with symptomatic GERD usually exhibit one or more of the following (Fig. 34–2): decreased or absent tone in the LES, inappropriate relaxation of the lower esophageal sphincter unassociated with swallowing, and decreased acid clearance due to impaired peristalsis. Other factors such as abnormal saliva, excessive acid production, delayed gastric emptying, and reflux of bile salts and pancreatic enzymes may be implicated in some patients. Patients with moderate to severe GERD have a sliding hiatal hernia that interferes with normal esophageal clearance by acting as a fluid trap.

Clinical Manifestations

Heartburn, ranging in degree from mild to severe, is the most common symptom of GERD, with associated complaints including dysphagia, odynophagia, regurgitation, water brash, and belching. Dysphagia for solids is usually secondary to a peptic stricture. Other causes may include esophageal inflammation alone, peristaltic dysfunction seen with severe esophagitis, and esophageal cancer arising from a Barrett's esophagus. GERD may present with symptoms not immediately referable to the gastrointestinal (GI) tract, including chest pain, respiratory, and ear, nose, and throat problems. Respiratory complaints include chronic cough, recurrent aspiration, and asthma. Associated complaints related to the ear, nose, and throat include hoarseness, sore throat, throat clearing and a full

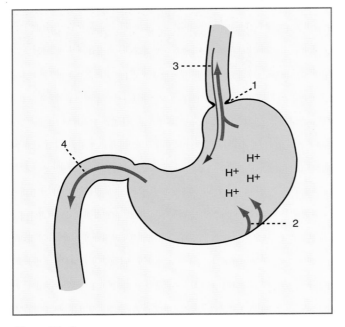

Figure 34-2
Pathogenesis of gastroesophageal reflux disease. 1, Impaired lower esophageal sphincter—low pressures or frequent transient lower esophageal sphincter relaxation. 2, Hypersecretion of acid. 3, Decreased acid clearance due to impaired peristalsis or abnormal saliva production. 4, Delayed gastric emptying and/or duodenogastric reflux of bile salts and pancreatic enzymes.

sensation in the neck (globus sensation). Bleeding from esophageal erosions and ulcerations may be brisk but most commonly is chronic in nature.

Diagnosis

The diagnosis of GERD is best made by the history. Objective tests are useful to quantify the severity of disease and to address three questions: (1) Does reflux exist? (2) Is acid reflux responsible for the patient's symptoms? and (3) Has reflux led to esophageal damage? Reflux may be demonstrated during a barium swallow or by radionuclide scintigraphy after placing technetium 99 (^{99m}Tc)-sulfur colloid in the stomach. Esophageal manometry is useful for demonstrating abnormal peristalsis and poor LES tone but does not show reflux. The most sensitive and physiologic test for the presence of acid reflux is prolonged esophageal pH monitoring. This is done by placing a pH probe in the distal esophagus and monitoring acid exposure in an ambulatory state in the patient's home or work environment. The presence of reflux does not necessarily mean that it is responsible for the patient's symptoms. The acid perfusion (Bernstein) test may be used to identify atypical symptoms secondary to acid sensitivity. In this study, symptoms should be reproduced by dripping acid, but not saline, via a nasogastric tube into the distal esophagus. More helpful is the correlation of a patient's symptoms with the actual recording of acid reflux episodes during prolonged esophageal pH monitoring. Finally, symptoms due to acid reflux do not always

correlate with the extent of damage to the esophageal mucosa. This is important to identify because patients with esophagitis tend to be more difficult to treat and are more likely to develop severe esophageal complications. Esophageal erosions, ulcerations, and strictures can be assessed by barium swallow. To bring out subtle narrowings, it may be necessary to give a solid bolus challenge such as a tablet, marshmallow, or even an aggravating food product. However, the barium swallow misses mild grades of esophagitis; therefore, endoscopy with biopsies is the most sensitive test for reflux-induced mucosal damage. Endoscopic changes range from very shallow linear erosions associated with friability to confluent ulcerations to complete mucosal denudation. A few patients exhibit Barrett's epithelium, columnar epithelium in the esophagus produced by severe chronic reflux and associated with an increased risk of transformation to adenocarcinoma.

Treatment and Prognosis

Gastroesophageal reflux disease is a chronic problem that may wax and wane in intensity, and relapses are common. In patients without esophagitis, the therapeutic goal is simply to relieve the acid-related symptoms. In patients with esophagitis, the ultimate goal is to heal or minimize the esophagitis while attempting to prevent further complications. As shown in Table 34-1, lifestyle modifications remain the cornerstone of effective antireflux treatment and may be curative in patients with mild

TABLE 34-1	Treatment of Gastroesophageal Reflux Disease

Simple (Lifestyle) Measures
Elevation of the head of the bed
Avoidance of food or liquids 2-3 hr before bedtime
Avoidance of fatty or spicy foods
Avoidance of cigarettes, alcohol
Weight loss
Liquid antacid (aluminum hydroxide–magnesium hydroxide) 30 ml 30 min after meals and at bedtime

Persistent Symptoms
Without Esophagitis
  Alginic acid antacids (Gaviscon), 10 ml 30 min after meals and at bedtime
  Promotility drugs
    Cisapride, 10 mg four times a day
    Metoclopramide, 10 mg four times a day
  H_2-receptor blockers
    Cimetidine, 400 mg twice a day
    Ranitidine, 150 mg twice a day
    Famotidine, 20 mg twice a day
    Nizatidine, 150 mg twice a day
With Esophagitis
  H_2-receptor blockers—regular or double dose depending on severity
  H_2-receptor blocker and promotility agent
  Proton pump inhibitor
    Omeprazole, 20 mg every morning
    Lansoprazole, 30 mg every morning
Antireflux surgery

symptoms. Patients with more severe symptoms without esophagitis generally respond to alginic acid, promotility drugs, or H_2-receptor blockers. Promotility drugs, such as cisapride, act by increasing LES pressure, improving esophageal contractions, and increasing gastric emptying when delayed. H_2-receptor blockers act solely by decreasing acid secretion. Patients with esophagitis generally need an H_2 blocker, usually in a twice-daily dose, to heal their mucosal injury. Patients with intractable symptoms or ulcerative esophagitis may need a proton pump inhibitor to control their disease by markedly turning off acid secretion. Chronic therapy is necessary in patients with severe reflux symptoms and those with esophagitis. Surgical management is reserved for those younger and healthier patients requiring constant high-dose and powerful medications to control their reflux disease. Several procedures are available, but all generally consist of returning the hiatal hernia and esophageal gastric junction into the abdomen and restoring LES function by wrapping the lower esophagus with a cuff of gastric fundal muscle.

Complications

Gastroesophageal reflux disease complications include esophageal (peptic) stricture, esophageal ulcer, Barrett's esophagus, pulmonary aspiration, and upper GI hemorrhage.

MOTILITY DISORDERS OF THE OROPHARYNX AND ESOPHAGUS

Oropharyngeal Disorders

Definition and Pathogenesis

Oropharyngeal motility problems may arise from dysfunction of the UES, neurologic disorders (cerebrovascular accidents are most common), skeletal muscle disorders, or local structural lesions (Table 34–2). It is a common problem in the elderly population and frequently associated with poor prognosis owing to a high incidence of aspiration pneumonia.

Clinical Manifestations

Symptoms may occur gradually or have a rapid onset. Patients present with a variety of complaints, including food sticking in the throat, difficulty initiating a swallow, nasal regurgitation, and coughing when swallowing. They also may complain of dysarthria or display nasal speech because of associated muscle weakness.

Diagnosis

The clinical history is often characteristic, and associated neurologic and muscular abnormalities discovered on physical examination may help in making a correct etio-

TABLE 34–2	Clinical Disorders Associated with Oropharyngeal Dysphagia*

Motility Disorders of the Upper Esophageal Sphincter
Zenker's diverticulum
Cricopharyngeal bar

Neurologic Disorders
Cerebrovascular disease
Poliomyelitis
Amyotrophic lateral sclerosis
Multiple sclerosis
Brain stem tumors

Skeletal Muscle Disorders
Polymyositis
Muscular dystrophies
Myasthenia gravis
Metabolic myopathy (thyrotoxicosis, myxedema, steroid myopathy)

Local Structural Lesions
Neoplasms
Extrinsic compression (thyromegaly, cervical spur)
Surgical resection of the oropharynx

*Only a listing of major causes under each subheading.

logic diagnosis. Rapid-sequence cine-esophagography is required to adequately assess the abnormalities occurring in swallowing over less than a 1-second period. Esophageal manometry and endoscopy have ancillary diagnostic roles.

Treatment and Prognosis

Treatment consists of correcting recognizable reversible causes, including Parkinson's disease, myasthenia gravis, hyper- or hypothyroidism, and polymyositis. Unfortunately, the majority of cases are not amenable to medical or surgical therapy. Some cases may improve or resolve with time. For example, many patients with oropharyngeal dysphagia secondary to cerebrovascular accidents improve over a 3- to 6-month period. Other patients require retraining and use of various swallowing maneuvers and techniques to achieve an adequate and safe swallow. This rehabilitation can be managed by a speech and swallowing therapist using cine-esophagography with various types of foods to help plan and evaluate therapy. Rare patients may be helped by a cricopharyngeal myotomy, which cuts the UES.

Esophageal Disorders

Definition and Pathogenesis

Motility disorders of the esophageal body may arise from diseases of smooth muscle (e.g., scleroderma) or the intrinsic nervous system (e.g., achalasia, Chagas' disease). In achalasia, loss of the ganglion cells in Auerbach's plexus leads to increased tone and impaired relaxation of the LES, which is also associated with absent peristalsis.

TABLE 34–3	Esophageal Motor Disorders		
	Achalasia	**Scleroderma**	**Diffuse Esophageal Spasm**
Symptoms	Dysphagia Regurgitation of nonacidic material	Gastroesophageal reflux disease Dysphagia	Substernal chest pain (angina-like) Dysphagia with pain
X-ray appearance	Dilated, fluid-filled esophagus Distal "bird beak" stricture	Aperistaltic esophagus Free reflux Peptic stricture	Simultaneous noncoordinated contractions
Manometric findings			
Lower esophageal sphincter	High resting pressure Incomplete or abnormal relaxation with swallow	Low resting pressure	Normal pressure
Body	Low-amplitude, simultaneous contractions after swallow	Low-amplitude peristaltic contractions or no peristalsis	Some peristalsis Diffuse and simultaneous nonperistaltic contractions, occasionally high amplitude

The cause of the other motility disorders, such as diffuse esophageal spasm and its variants, is uncertain.

Clinical Manifestations

The three most common motility disorders are achalasia, scleroderma, and diffuse esophageal spasm, each of which exhibits a unique pattern of symptoms (Table 34–3).

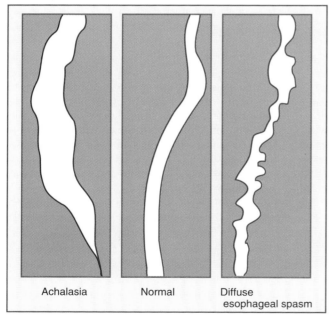

Achalasia   Normal   Diffuse esophageal spasm

Figure 34–3

Radiologic appearance of achalasia *(left)* and diffuse esophageal spasm *(right)*. In achalasia the esophageal body is dilated and terminates in a narrowed segment or "bird beak." The appearance of numerous simultaneous contractions is typical of diffuse esophageal spasm. (Courtesy of Dr. EE Templeton and Dr. CA Rohrmann. From Pope CE II: *In* Sleisenger MH, Fordtran JS [eds.]: Gastrointestinal Disease. 3rd ed. Philadelphia, WB Saunders, 1983.)

Diagnoses

The clinical history is often very suggestive and cineesophagography (Fig. 34–3) combined with esophageal manometry (see Table 34–3) confirms the diagnosis in most cases. An infiltrating carcinoma of the gastric cardia can mimic achalasia; thus, endoscopy with biopsies is an important part of the evaluation.

Treatment and Prognosis

Achalasia usually responds to brisk dilatation of the LES with a pneumatic bag, a procedure that ruptures some of the sphincter muscle fibers. Surgical myotomy (the Heller procedure) is beneficial for those few patients who do not respond to pneumatic dilatation. Therapy for scleroderma includes aggressive treatment of GERD because more than half of these patients have esophagitis. Patients with diffuse esophageal spasm and its variants may respond to nitroglycerin and anticholinergic agents or calcium channel–blocking drugs, although results are often disappointing. Occasionally, these patients, especially if they have severe dysphagia and weight loss, may improve with pneumatic dilatation or a long esophageal myotomy.

OTHER ESOPHAGEAL DISORDERS

Carcinoma of the esophagus is discussed in Chapter 37.

Rings and Webs

These may occur in the proximal or distal (Schatzki's ring) esophagus. The cause is uncertain but may be congenital or secondary to GERD. The Plummer-Vinson syndrome consists of an upper esophageal web, dysphagia, and iron deficiency anemia, usually in middle-aged women. Many rings and webs are asymptomatic, but dysphagia is the rule if the luminal diameter is < 13 mm but unlikely if ring diameter is > 20 mm. Patients complain of intermittent dysphagia for solid foods such as bread and steak. Occasionally, they can present with sudden, total esophageal obstruction caused by a meat impaction—"steak house syndrome." Rings and webs can easily be disrupted mechanically with peroral dilators.

Iatrogenic Esophagitis

Iatrogenic esophageal injury may be caused by ingested pills or caustic material. More than half the cases of pill-induced esophagitis result from tetracycline and its derivatives, particularly doxycycline. Other commonly prescribed medications causing esophageal injury include slow-release potassium chloride, iron sulfate, quinidine, steroids, and nonsteroidal anti-inflammatory agents. A common factor is a history of improper pill ingestion, including taking the pills with too little or no fluids or taking them just prior to bedtime and lying down. Patients usually present with odynophagia and dysphagia. A careful history can make the diagnosis, and endoscopy confirms the mucosal erosions or ulcerations. Symptoms usually resolve when the drug is stopped. It is important to educate these people about the proper techniques for ingesting medications. Caustic ingestion of either strong acid or alkali (Drano) agents is generally accidental in children or results from suicide attempts in adults. These agents cause severe esophageal injury, leading to necrosis and eventual stricture formation. Patients with caustic ingestion present with dysphagia, odynophagia, oral pain and burns, and excessive salivation. Steroids and broad-spectrum antibiotics are often used to treat caustic injuries, although their efficacy is uncertain. Severe injuries may produce long strictures that may be difficult to treat even with peroral dilatation.

Infection

The most common infections causing esophagitis are fungal *(Candida)* and viral (herpes, cytomegalovirus). These usually occur in patients with acquired immunodeficiency syndrome (AIDS) or patients on immunosuppressant therapy. However, these infections also occur in patients with less severe immune defects (diabetic, malnourished elderly, postoperative, and antibiotic- and steroid-treated patients) and occasionally occur in otherwise healthy individuals. Severe odynophagia and dysphagia are the common symptoms resulting from mucosal inflammation and ulceration. Diagnosis is best made by endoscopic visualization with biopsies and brushings.

REFERENCES

Baron TH, Richter JE: The use of esophageal function tests. Adv Intern Med 1993; 38:3661.

Castell DO, Donner MW: Evaluation of dysphagia: A careful history is crucial. Dysphagia 1987; 2:65.

DeVault KR, Castel DO: Current diagnosis and treatment of gastroesophageal reflux disease. Mayo Clin Proc 1994; 69:867.

Richter JE: Motility disorders of the esophagus. *In* Yamada T (ed.): Textbook of Gastroenterology. Philadelphia, JB Lippincott, 1996.

Wilcox CM, Karowe MW: Esophageal infections: Etiology, diagnosis, and management. Gastroenterology 1994; 2:188.

35

Diseases of the Stomach and Duodenum

The stomach is a capacious organ between the esophagus and intestines that functions (1) as a reservoir in which food is stored, mixed, and then expelled into the duodenum and (2) as the primary site of acid secretion, which is important in the digestion of food and in protecting the body from ingested toxins and bacteria. This chapter reviews the common medical problems associated with disturbed gastroduodenal physiology. Specifically, acid-peptic diseases, including gastric and duodenal ulcers, Zollinger-Ellison syndrome, and gastritis, and abnormalities of gastric emptying associated with nausea and vomiting are discussed.

NORMAL GASTRIC PHYSIOLOGY

Gastric Emptying

As food enters the proximal stomach, a vagally mediated inhibition of fundic tone (receptive relaxation) permits storage of food without a rise in intragastric pressure. Ingested liquids are dispersed throughout the stomach in rapid fashion and then emptied primarily by low-level tonic contractions that generate a pressure gradient from the proximal stomach to the duodenum. Solids, on the other hand, require peristalsis to move them from stomach to duodenum. After an initial storage period in the proximal stomach (approximately 30 minutes), solids are redistributed to the antrum, where they are mixed by segmental contractions. These contractions occur up to three times per minute and originate in a pacemaker situated in the midbody along the greater curvature. The mixed food is pushed toward the pylorus. This valve narrows, expelling into the duodenum only particles of food that have been reduced to ≤ 1 mm while forcing larger particles backward for further processing. Local mechanisms, including low pH, high osmolarity, fatty acids, and caloric density, control liquid and solid emptying via the vagus nerve and hormones such as secretin, cholecystokinin, gastric inhibitory polypeptide, and glucagon. Nondigestible solids are emptied differently. Particles > 1 mm^3 cannot be emptied by contraction waves in the fed state but rather are emptied by the interdigestive migrating motor complex. This pattern occurs in the fasting state every 90 to 120 minutes and consists of a series of contractions beginning in the stomach and sweeping through the small bowel.

Gastric Secretion

Both hydrochloric acid (HCl), secreted by the parietal cells, and pepsinogen, secreted primarily by the chief cells, are found in the gastric mucosa, predominantly in the body and fundus of the stomach. These two agents are secreted in parallel; no condition is known in which there is selective secretion of either HCl or pepsinogen. Three endogenous chemicals stimulate the secretion of acid: acetylcholine, gastrin, and histamine (Fig. 35–1). Acetylcholine is released locally from vagal (cholinergic) nerve terminals in the stomach, stimulated by stretch reflexes within the stomach or by the cephalic phase of gastric secretion (the sight, smell, taste, or thought of food). Vagal stimulation also elicits a modest release of gastrin. Gastrin is released from chief cells in the gastric antrum by the presence of food (particularly amino acids) in the gastric lumen, alkalinization of the gastric lumen, and neural release of gastrin-releasing peptide (GRP). The release of gastrin is turned off by low pH levels and the hormone somatostatin. Histamine is found in mast cells in the gastric wall in close proximity to the chief cells. The role and control of local histamine release are unknown, but histamine and its structural analogues are powerful gastric secretagogues when administered systemically; the use of H$_2$-receptor antagonists markedly inhibits HCl secretion by the stomach.

Acid secretion in the resting, unfed stomach does not correlate with serum gastrin concentrations and is primarily related to vagal tone and the presence or absence of the bacterium *Helicobacter pylori*. A high vagal tone may lead to basal hypersecretion, whereas *H. pylori* infection can lower basal acid output. Basal secretion of acid averages about 1 to 2 mEq/hr in men and less in women, but the normal range varies considerably. In response to a meal, acid secretion is stimulated in three phases: the cephalic phase via primarily the vagus nerve, the gastric phase via the release of gastrin stimulated by amino acids and gastric alkalinization, and the intestinal phase via further release of gastrin and other nongastrin secretagogues by digested food products. Maximally stimulated

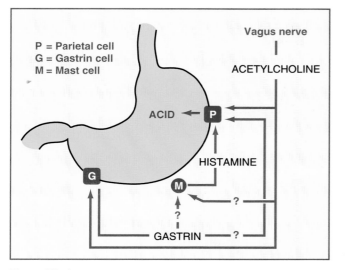

Figure 35–1

The parietal cell with three receptors—histamine, gastrin, and acetylcholine. All act to stimulate a K^+, H^+-ATPase (the hydrogen pump at the luminal side of the cell). However, the characteristics of each compound differ enough to suggest that each acts at a different receptor. Histamine causes increases in intracellular adenyl cyclase and cyclic AMP, which in turn activate or increase the amount of the K^+, H^+-ATPase. Cholinergic drugs and gastrin cause influx of Ca^{2+}, which in turn activates the K^+, H^+-ATPase. (From Richardson CT: Peptic ulcer: Pathogenesis. *In* Wyngaarden JB, Smith LH Jr, Bennett JC: [eds.]: Cecil Textbook of Medicine. 19th ed. Philadelphia, WB Saunders, 1992, p 653.)

by a meal or secretagogue (pentagastrin), the acid secretory rate may rise as high as 50 mEq/hr for men and 30 mEq/hr for women. The ratio of basal to maximal acid output (MAO), which is usually much <50%, is sometimes determined in the study of patients with suspected abnormal secretory drives.

Secretion of pepsinogen is largely under vagal control. Pepsinogen is converted to pepsin in the gastric lumen by acid. Relatively little digestion takes place in the stomach, but release of peptides and amino acids by pepsin helps trigger the release of other digestive hormones such as gastrin and cholecystokinin. Intrinsic factor, a glycoprotein whose primary role is to facilitate vitamin B_{12} absorption, is secreted by parietal cells under the same stimulatory conditions as HCl.

Normal Mucosal Defense

The stomach and duodenum have developed several defense mechanisms to protect the mucosa from the acid-pepsin mix of gastric juice (Fig. 35–2). A thin coat of mucus is formed continuously and spreads out protectively over the mucosal cells. This activity diminishes the exposure of these cells to luminal gastric acid. Sodium bicarbonate is secreted from surface epithelial cells of the stomach and duodenum in response to a pH <3. Bicarbonate neutralizes the HCl that diffuses back from the lumen. The epithelial cells are constantly being shed and renewed so that damaged cells are promptly replaced. Epithelial cells also migrate to cover denuded areas and in this way contribute to epithelial restitution. Prostaglandins play an important role in protecting gastroduodenal mucosa by stimulating the secretion of mucus and bicarbonate, maintaining blood flow during periods of potential injury, and possibly suppressing acid secretion. Tissue prostaglandins decrease with age and are inhibited by commonly ingested drugs such as nonsteroidal anti-inflammatory agents (NSAIDs).

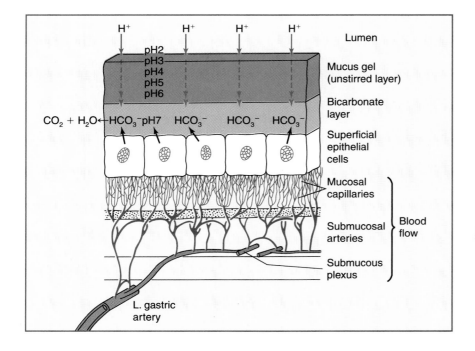

Figure 35–2

Model illustrating mechanisms maintaining mucosal integrity. Superficial epithelial cells secrete mucus and bicarbonate that aid in maintaining a pH gradient between lumen and mucosa and protect the underlying epithelial cells from damage by acid and pepsin. Mucosal blood flow is also believed to be a mechanism important in maintaining mucosal integrity. (From Richardson CT: Peptic ulcer: Pathogenesis. *In* Wyngaarden JB, Smith LH Jr, Bennett JC [eds.]: Cecil Textbook of Medicine, 19th ed. Philadelphia, WB Saunders, 1992, p 654.)

GASTRITIS

Gastritis can be defined by its gross appearance, histopathology, or clinical presentation, but none of these definitions is perfect. The term *gastritis,* which implies inflammation, is a misnomer because some of the entities considered lack appreciable inflammatory changes, e.g., erosions due to aspirin or NSAIDs. Gastritis may be associated with visible disruption of the gastric mucosa (erosions) or a grossly normal appearing mucosa. It is often blamed for chronic abdominal pain, but the link between symptoms and gastritis is poorly established. For example, NSAIDs produce both gastric damage and symptoms, yet neither is predictive of the other. The diagnosis of gastritis may be suspected if a careful history is taken; however, endoscopy coupled with biopsies is the best way to make the diagnosis.

Erosive or Hemorrhagic Gastric Disease

In these forms of gastritis, infiltration of the lamina propria by inflammatory cells accompanies superficial erosions that may be diffuse or localized. Unlike ulcers, erosions are superficial breaks that do not extend deeper than the mucosa itself and therefore do not cause perforation or severe bleeding. The mechanism of mucosal injury is often unclear and probably multifactorial. Certain drugs, especially aspirin, NSAIDs, and ethanol, cause mucosal injury by suppressing endogenous prostaglandins and producing local damage. Stress-related mucosal disease represents acute erosive injury to the stomach in many severe surgical or medical conditions with bleeding as a complicating factor. The etiology is multifactorial, resulting from a compromise in mucosal blood flow or in other elements of mucosal defense in the presence of back-diffusion of acid. Gastritis can also sometimes by attributed to specific events, such as radiation, ingestion of alkali, and, rarely, bacterial infection (phlegmonous gastritis). Following surgery, reflux of bile salts and/or pancreatic enzymes may produce acute gastritis.

Many cases of erosive gastritis are probably mild and escape diagnosis. An important complication is bleeding from the superficial erosions. This usually responds to conservative management and removal of the precipitating agents if known. Antacids or H_2-receptor antagonists are used as well but have not been shown to affect healing. Severe bleeding, if caused by isolated lesions, may be amenable to endoscopic therapy. Diffusely bleeding lesions may respond to vasopressin, administered intravenously or intra-arterially into an angiographically placed catheter. Stress-related gastritis can generally be decreased or prevented if the gastric pH is maintained above 3.5, a pH level at which pepsin activity is markedly reduced. This can be facilitated by antacid drip or hourly antacids (15 to 30 ml) via nasogastric tube. H_2-receptor antagonists are approved for intravenous use; a slow bolus infusion is effective in increasing gastric pH (cimetidine, 300 mg every 8 hours; ranitidine, 50 mg every 12 hours; famotidine, 20 mg every 12 hours). Continuous infusion may provide smoother control of pH; for example, an infusion of cimetidine (300 mg priming dose, 37.5 mg/hr) produces effective gastric neutralization. Sucralfate in a dose of 1 gm every 4 to 6 hours is also effective in reducing stress-related bleeding. Prophylactic therapy for gastrointestinal bleeding should be reserved for patients in the intensive care unit (ICU) with coagulopathy, multisystem organ failure (especially respiratory failure), head injury, or burns.

Nonerosive Gastritis

This form of gastritis involves inflammatory changes in the mucosa that are often grossly normal and lacks, as the name implies, erosive changes. Nonerosive gastritis can be classified by whether the fundus (type A) or antrum (type B) is primarily involved and by whether the inflammation is superficial, deep, or atrophic, with decreased or absent glandular elements and mucosal thinning.

In fundal or type A gastritis, the maximal inflammatory changes occur along the greater curvature in the fundus and body, with minimal or no inflammation in the antrum. Parietal cell antibodies appear in most patients, and pernicious anemia may develop, suggesting an immunologic mechanism. Hyposecretion of acid results from fundic gland atrophy. The relative absence of damage to the antrum accounts for the ability of many of these patients to develop marked hypergastrinemia as the feedback inhibition of acid on gastrin release is lost. This type of gastritis may be a normal component of aging, but only a small portion of affected individuals go on to develop pernicious anemia. These patients have an increased risk of gastric carcinoids and adenocarcinoma. No specific therapy exists for fundal gastritis.

In antral or type B gastritis, the predominant inflammatory component is confined to the antrum, and it does not progress to atrophic gastritis; there is also a striking association with both peptic ulcers and *H. pylori.* A gram-negative microaerophilic organism, *H. pylori* may be the most common human infective agent worldwide. It is found primarily in the stomach but may occasionally be found in areas of gastric metaplasia (e.g., duodenal bulb). The organism lives in the gastric crypts, producing a histologic gastritis characterized by a dense neutrophilic infiltration. The mechanism by which the inflammatory response is produced is unknown, but the organism does have the ability to produce a variety of virulence factors. In addition to causing gastritis, *H. pylori* can suppress basal acid output and enhance serum gastrin release, especially in response to a meal. *H. pylori* is detected by biopsies with tissue staining, culture, or determination of the presence of urease, which the organism produces in abundance. Although *H. pylori* is clearly associated with antral gastritis, the relationship to symptoms is poor, and no clinical benefit seems to occur from eradication of the organism in the absence of ulcer disease. *H. pylori* is commonly associated with gastric and duodenal ulcers, and recent studies suggest that it may be an important cofactor in the development of gastric adenocarcinoma and primary gastric antral B-cell lymphomas, also known as mucosa-associated lymphoid tissue (MALT) lymphoma. Complete regression of these lesions has been documented following eradication of *H. pylori* using antibiotic therapy.

PEPTIC ULCER DISEASE OF THE STOMACH AND DUODENUM

Epidemiology

The lifetime prevalence of peptic ulcer disease is approximately 10%, with about equal prevalence in men and women. Duodenal ulcers are more frequent than gastric ulcers. The incidence of ulcer disease increases with age, which may be explained by the increased use of NSAIDs in the elderly and the reduction in tissue prostaglandins with age. Genetic factors seem to be important in some patients with peptic ulcers. There is an increased incidence in first-degree relatives of patients with duodenal ulcers and a positive association with high levels of serum pepsinogen I, which appears to be inherited as a dominant trait and may reflect total chief cell mass. Other factors predisposing to ulcer disease include smoking (possibly due to diminished bicarbonate secretion by the pancreas), ethnic background (blacks may develop ulcers at an earlier age), and certain diseases (chronic lung disease, cirrhosis, hyperparathyroidism, chronic renal failure—especially after transplantation—and polycythemia vera). Regardless of age, the use of NSAIDs increases the incidence of superficial gastric mucosal erosions and gastric ulcers. Duodenal ulcers also occur as a result of NSAID use but to a lesser degree than gastric ulcers. The ulcer risk does not appear to depend upon the type of NSAID used. The evidence that glucocorticoids cause ulcers is controversial but is probably caused by concomitant NSAID use. The possible role of psychological factors is unclear, but emotional distress may increase gastric secretion, particularly in the basal state. Although it has been suggested that the overall incidence of ulcer disease is decreasing, this probably does not reflect a true change in the natural history of the disease. Over the last three decades, the mortality rates, surgical rates, and office visits for ulcer disease have decreased by more than 50%.

Pathophysiology

Peptic ulcers occur whenever the normal balance between acid-pepsin and mucosal defense factors is disrupted (Fig. 35–3). The presence of acid is obligatory for the formation of a peptic ulcer; a large majority of patients have acid secretion well within normal limits. Therefore, the primary event in the formation of an ulcer is disruption of normal mucosal defense factors. Unfortunately, how this occurs remains poorly understood. It is now believed that *H. pylori*, NSAIDs, and acid are the most important factors in the development of peptic ulcers. NSAIDs probably act by inhibiting gastroduodenal mucosal defensive factors. Idiopathic ulcers now account for ≤ 10% of

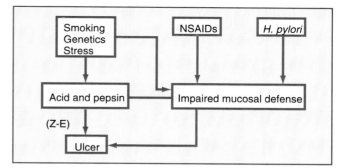

Figure 35–3

Acid and peptic activity overpower mucosal defense to produce ulcers most commonly when mucosal defense is impaired by exogenous factors. Two factors, nonsteroidal antiinflammatory drugs (NSAIDs) and *Helicobacter pylori* infection, appear to be linked to the impairment of mucosal defense. The hypersecretion of gastric acid in the Zollinger–Ellison syndrome (Z–E) is one exception in which ulcers occur in the absence of *H. pylori* infection. In ordinary peptic ulcer disease, other risk factors are also important (smoking, genetic factors, and psychological stress), but the evidence is conflicting about whether these factors impair mucosal defense, modulate the secretion of acid, or both. (Adapted from Sull AH: Pathogenesis of peptic ulcer and implications for therapy. N Engl J Med 322:910, 1990. Copyright 1990. Massachusetts Medical Society. All rights reserved.)

all gastric ulcers and almost no duodenal ulcers. *H. pylori* predisposes to ulceration, either in the stomach or in areas of inflamed gastric metaplasia in the duodenal bulb. Virtually 100% of patients with duodenal ulcer are infected with *H. pylori*, whereas about 70 to 80% of patients with gastric ulcers are so infected. Gastric ulcers in patients who are not infected with *H. pylori* are usually associated with the use of NSAIDs or the Zollinger-Ellison syndrome. Antibiotic therapy to eradicate *H. pylori* markedly decreases the recurrence rate of duodenal ulcers. On the other hand, *H. pylori* is found in substantial proportions of normal healthy subjects, increasing in prevalence from < 10% in subjects under age 30 to > 60% in subjects over age 60. Thus, most patients with *H. pylori* never develop an ulcer regardless of acid secretory levels, suggesting that other cofactors must be important in the genesis of ulcer disease.

Clinical Manifestations

Although many ulcers may be asymptomatic, especially in the elderly, the majority of patients with peptic ulcers present with epigastric pain. The pain, frequently described as burning or gnawing, most typically occurs 1 to 3 hours after eating, is relieved with food or antacids, and may awaken the patient from sleep. The cause of the pain is unknown, but the concept of acid bathing an "open wound" and producing pain is overly simplistic. The pain tends to occur in clusters, perhaps over several weeks, with subsequent periods of remission of varying duration. Ulcer pain generally subsides before the complete healing of the ulcer itself. In addition to pain, patients with peptic ulcers tend to have a variety of symptoms that can best be described as "dyspepsia"—bloating, nausea, anorexia, excessive eructations, and epigastric discomfort.

In the absence of complications, the physical examination is rarely helpful in diagnosing peptic ulcer disease. Frequently there is a moderate amount of epigastric tenderness, but this finding does not reliably point to the presence of an active ulcer. Physical examination may also give evidence of one of the other diseases associated with an ulcer diathesis.

Complications

Complications are not infrequent in peptic ulcer disease. In fact, it has been estimated that one third of patients with a diagnosis of ulcer have one or more complications in their lifetime. These complications are the main indication for peptic ulcer disease surgery.

Bleeding

Bleeding from peptic ulcer disease is the most common cause of upper gastrointestinal (GI) bleeding. It occurs in 15% of ulcer patients, may be the first manifestation of the disease, and carries an overall mortality rate of about 7%. Ulcer bleeding is particularly common in elderly patients and is probably related to their use of NSAIDs, which are not only ulcerogenic but may predispose an ulcer to bleed. Factors associated with a poor outcome from a bleeding ulcer include age (>60), hemodynamic instability following the bleed, an excessive number of blood transfusions (greater than six units total), the presence of concomitant diseases, and continuation or recurrence of bleeding in the hospital. Patients who have bled once from a peptic ulcer have an increased chance of bleeding again (30 to 50% chance).

Ulcers bleed when the crater breaches one wall of a vessel. Large, deep ulcers high on the lesser gastric curve or posterior duodenal bulb are more likely to erode major vessels and result in substantial bleeding. Although bleeding from these large vessels does not cease spontaneously and requires urgent therapy, most ulcers (approximately 85%) stop bleeding at least temporarily. The treatment of a patient who has bled from a peptic ulcer is determined at the time of diagnostic endoscopy. If the ulcer is actively bleeding, it can be treated with a contact thermal probe (e.g., BICAP or heater probe), injection of a vasoconstrictor agent (e.g., epinephrine), or emergency surgery. No pharmacologic therapy has been shown to be effective in stopping active bleeding. Endoscopic therapy succeeds in $>90\%$ of cases, but if it is unsuccessful or if bleeding recurs, then surgery should be considered for all patients but those identified as a poor risk. In these latter patients, angiographic embolization of the bleeding vessel may be an effective alternative. If the ulcer is not bleeding, it usually should be left alone. The exception is the presence of an ulcer with a visible vessel. This rebleeds about 50% of the time in the hospital and should therefore undergo prophylactic endoscopic therapy. Bleeding ulcers are as likely to heal as nonbleeding ulcers, and

follow-up endoscopy is usually not necessary. Eradication of *H. pylori* or maintenance therapy using acid suppression medications reduces the risk of rebleeding.

Perforation

A peptic ulcer may erode through the entire wall of the duodenum or stomach. Sometimes this leads to penetration of an adjacent organ such as the pancreas, with resulting pancreatitis and intractable pain. More frequently, especially with anterior duodenal ulcers and lesser curvature gastric ulcers, there is free perforation into the peritoneal cavity. This complication occurs in 5 to 10% of patients with duodenal ulcers and 2 to 5% with gastric ulcers. Factors that predispose to perforation are NSAIDs and, perhaps, stress. Not infrequently, especially in the elderly, perforation is the first symptom of a peptic ulcer. The presentation is typically that of an acute abdomen, with the sudden onset of severe abdominal pain, peritoneal signs (abdominal muscle rigidity, rebound tenderness), and hypotension with tachycardia. Free air in the abdominal cavity can usually be demonstrated by an upright radiograph. In most patients with free perforation, emergency surgery is indicated to repair the site and to wash out the peritoneal cavity. Because these patients have a high risk of future problems with ulcer disease, a definitive surgical procedure may be carried out at the same operation. In some poor-risk patients, the perforation is allowed to seal spontaneously while the patient is maintained on nasogastric suction, fluids, antibiotics, and H_2-receptor antagonist therapy.

Obstruction

Today the least common manifestation (5%) of ulcer disease is obstruction leading to symptoms of delayed gastric emptying with nausea, vomiting, epigastric pain, fullness, and early satiety. This complication is most frequent in ulcers involving the pyloric channel. Whereas edema surrounding an acute ulcer may produce transient obstructive symptoms that resolve with ulcer healing, chronic obstruction is the result of repeated bouts of acute ulceration leading to the formation of scar tissue. On physical examination the patient may present with a succussion splash and signs of dehydration. Laboratory studies may show metabolic alkalosis and hypokalemia from intractable vomiting. Obstruction can be readily demonstrated by an upper GI series or a positive saline load test (>400 ml of gastric juice recovered 30 minutes after instilling 750 ml of saline via nasogastric tube into an empty stomach). The specific cause of obstruction can be best demonstrated by endoscopy. An attempt should be made to treat all patients with gastric obstruction initially by medical means—nasogastric tube drainage, repair of fluid and electrolyte deficits, H_2-receptor antagonist therapy, and possibly parenteral nutrition. At least half of the patients so treated, presumably those with edema as the cause, respond to therapy, usually within 7 days. On the other hand, if obstruction persists, resectional surgery with va-

TABLE 35–1	Diagnostic Tests for *Helicobacter pylori*				
Test	Sensitivity (%)	Specificity (%)	Cost*	Follow-Up Use?	
Invasive tests (each requires endoscopy)					
Histology	93–99	95–99†	+++	Yes	
Culture	77–92	100†	+++	Yes	
Biopsy urease test	89–98	93–98	+	Yes	
Noninvasive tests					
^{13}C-urea breath test	90–100	98–100	++	Yes	
^{14}C-urea breath test	90–97	89–100	++	Yes	
Serology	88–99	86–95	+	Not for short-term use	

* Excluding cost of endoscopy if required.
† Estimated.
From Graham DY: Diagnosis of *Helicobacter pylori* infection. *In* Graham DY (ed.): *Helicobacter pylori* Diagnosis and Treatment. Deerfield, IL, Discovery International, 1995, p 3.

gotomy or possibly balloon dilatation of the pylorus is required.

Intractable Pain

The pain of a peptic ulcer is rarely intractable if the patient is compliant with a treatment regimen. With the more powerful H_2-receptor antagonists and proton pump inhibitors, most ulcers heal and pain resolves. The persistence of pain with an unhealed ulcer should raise questions about noncompliance with medical therapy, surreptitious use of NSAIDs, or possibly a hypergastrinemia state. A nonhealing ulcer may also represent penetration posteriorly or into an adjacent viscus.

Diagnosis

The definitive diagnosis of a peptic ulcer depends on visualizing the ulcer crater by direct inspection endoscopically (the most sensitive and specific method) or indirectly by radiographic studies (upper GI series). In young patients with dyspepsia, an empiric trial of antiulcer therapy is warranted. If prompt and long-lasting relief is achieved, no further evaluation is necessary. Patients older than 50, with weight loss, anorexia, or suspicion of malignancy, should have endoscopy performed initially. Endoscopy is the preferred initial diagnostic test because of its availability and sensitivity and because it allows for biopsy of gastric ulcers and the obtaining of tissue for the presence of *H. pylori* should an ulcer be discovered. If a gastric ulcer is found radiographically, it is imperative to demonstrate that it is benign rather than malignant. Malignancy should be suspected from the radiograph if (1) the ulcer is located completely within the gastric wall or a mass, (2) there is nodularity of the ulcer mass or the adjacent gastric mucosa, (3) there are no folds radiating to the ulcer margin, or (4) the ulcer is very large. Nevertheless, endoscopy should be performed in all patients with gastric ulcers to obtain brush cytology specimens and a minimum of six to eight pinch biopsies to adequately rule out malignancy.

When the presence of a typical peptic ulcer has been established radiographically or endoscopically, it is imper-

ative to define whether *H. pylori* is present, since antibiotic therapy and eradication of the bacteria significantly decrease the recurrence rate of peptic ulcer disease. The diagnosis can be established endoscopically by staining biopsy material taken from the gastric antrum or by placing the biopsy specimen into a medium, allowing rapid identification of urease. Noninvasive testing can be used in patients when a duodenal ulcer is detected radiographically, in patients with a remote ulcer who have not received *H. pylori* treatment, or to document eradication of *H. pylori* (Table 35–1). In only a few clinical situations is the measurement of serum gastrin or the basal and peak acid output of the stomach indicated (Table 35–2), primarily for the suspicion of a gastrinoma (to be discussed subsequently). In the patient with recurrent or intractable ulcer disease (5 to 10% of all ulcers); medical noncompliance; surreptitious or continued NSAID, aspirin, or tobacco use; gastric hypersecretion; malignancy; or unusual causes of ulcer disease such as Crohn's disease, lymphoma or infection should be suspected. It may also be important to diagnose the presence of *H. pylori* infection (see previous section).

Many common diseases may produce epigastric pain simulating peptic ulcer disease. These include functional dyspepsia, gastric cancer, biliary tract disease, pancreati-

TABLE 35–2	Clinical Situations in Which Measurement of Serum Gastrin Levels Is Indicated

Family history of peptic ulcer
Ulcer associated with hypercalcemia or other manifestations of multiple endocrine neoplasia type I
Multiple ulcers
Peptic ulceration of postbulbar duodenum or jejunum
Peptic ulceration associated with diarrhea*
Chronic unexplained diarrhea*
Enlarged gastric folds on upper gastrointestinal x-ray
Before surgery for "intractable" ulcer
Recurrent ulcer after ulcer surgery

* Not due to antacid ingestion.
Adapted from Schiller LR: Peptic ulcer: Epidemiology, clinical manifestations, and diagnosis. *In* Wyngaarden JB, Smith LH Jr, Bennett JC (eds.): *Cecil Textbook of Medicine.* 19th ed. Philadelphia, WB Saunders, 1992, p 657.

tis, esophagitis, pleurisy, pericarditis, and, rarely, an inferior myocardial infarction.

Treatment

Most patients with peptic ulcers can be treated successfully by medical methods. Surgery is usually required only for the complications of ulcer disease. In addition to the specific measures to be described, all patients with peptic ulcer disease should discontinue cigarette smoking, drink alcohol only in moderation, and discontinue using aspirin and NSAIDs. Although diet was once considered of great importance in the treatment of peptic ulcer, there is no good evidence that changes in diet influence the rate of healing.

Medical Management

The medical treatment of ulcer disease is directed at eradicating *H. pylori* and healing the ulcer. Ulcer healing can be achieved by decreasing acid secretion or by reducing mucosal damage.

Reduction of Gastric Acid

A number of agents can reduce the rate of secretion of acid by acting at various sites in the normal or hyperstimulated parietal cell (Fig. 35–4). Antimuscarinic drugs (e.g., atropine) reduce fasting and food-stimulated acid secretion but are not frequently used today because of unwanted side effects. H_2-receptor antagonists are the most popular and extensively studied drugs for the treatment of ulcer disease. Four products are commercially available for the acute treatment of duodenal or gastric ulcers. These include cimetidine used in a dose of 300 mg four times a day, 400 mg twice a day, or 800 mg at bedtime; ranitidine, 150 mg twice a day or 300 mg at bedtime; famotidine, 20 mg twice a day or 40 mg at bedtime; and nizatidine, 150 mg twice a day or 300 mg at

bedtime. Single nighttime dosing is as effective as multiple-dose regimens, with improved compliance. At these doses, all H_2-receptor antagonists are equal, with no clinical advantage of any one over the other three. Treatment of *H. pylori* as well as maintenance therapy with a half-dose at bedtime also reduces the incidence of recurrent ulcerations. These drugs are remarkably safe but do have some side effects. Most reports cite the effects of cimetidine and ranitidine because these two drugs have been available the longest. The central nervous system side effects (e.g., headache, mental confusion) are rare, reversible, and seen most often in patients with liver and renal failure. Gynecomastia and impotence have been reported with cimetidine because of its antiandrogenic effect. The H_2-receptor antagonists, particularly cimetidine, may also inhibit the metabolism of certain other drugs (e.g., theophylline, warfarin, and phenytoin) by the liver. The substituted benzimidazoles are extremely potent inhibitors of acid secretion because they block the H^+,K^+-ATPase enzyme found at the secretory surface of parietal cells that mediates the final common pathway into the gastric lumen. The two available drugs in this class are omeprazole and lansoprazole. Omeprazole at doses of 20 mg once daily, or lansoprazole, 30 mg daily, produce ulcer healings slightly better than do H_2-receptor antagonists when the latter are given in standard doses. Because of the more rapid healing of peptic ulcers using proton pump inhibitors, they are the initial drugs of choice in patients with large ulcers (> 1.5 to 2.0 cm diameter), ulcers complicated by bleeding or perforation, and significant underlying medical problems in whom complications such as bleeding would be fatal. The sustained hypochlorhydria produced by omeprazole results in hypergastrinemia, which in rats has led to the development of carcinoid tumors. The hypergastrinemia is reversible, however, and no such drug-related tumors have been documented in humans. Recently, omeprazole has received Food and Drug Administration (FDA) approval for long-term use in reflux esophagitis.

Aluminum and magnesium hydroxide–containing antacids are highly effective in healing gastric and duodenal ulcers and are as effective as H_2-receptor antagonists. Low-dose antacids (e.g., one tablet, 25 mmol neutralizing capacity, four times daily) are as effective as high-dose regimens. Even low doses of magnesium hydroxide–containing antacids have side effects (constipation for aluminum and mild diarrhea for magnesium). Because of their low cost, antacids are generally reserved for patients with limited funds who must purchase medications.

Improvement of Mucosal Defense (Fig. 35–5)

Sucralfate is effective for the acute therapy of duodenal ulcers in doses of 1 gm four times a day or 2 gm twice a day and as a maintenance therapy in a dose of 1 gm twice a day. Results with gastric ulcers are less well studied. Sucralfate's mechanism of action is unknown, but theories include that it forms a viscous shield over the ulcer crater, preventing acid from reaching regenerating tissue; adsorbs pepsin; stimulates endogenous prostaglandins; destroys oxygen radicals; and recruits epidermal

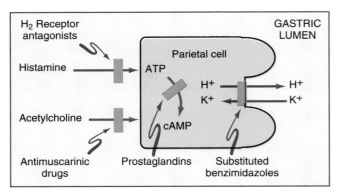

Figure 35–4
Sites of action of drugs employed to inhibit acid secretion. ATP = Adenosine triphosphate; cAMP = cyclic adenosine monophosphate. (From Peterson WL: Peptic ulcer: Medical therapy. *In* Wyngaarden JB, Smith LH Jr, Bennett JC [eds.]: Cecil Textbook of Medicine. 19th ed. Philadelphia, WB Saunders, 1992, p 659.)

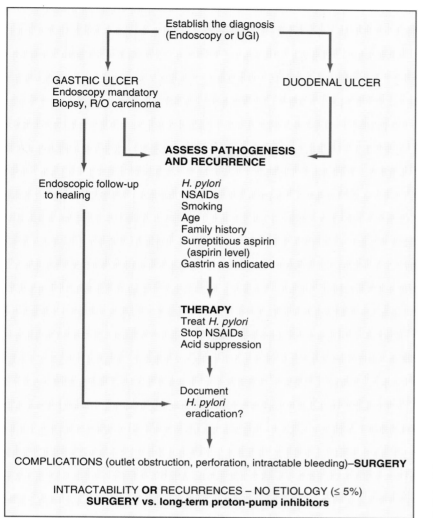

Establish the diagnosis
(Endoscopy or UGI)

GASTRIC ULCER
Endoscopy mandatory
Biopsy, R/O carcinoma

DUODENAL ULCER

**ASSESS PATHOGENESIS
AND RECURRENCE**

Endoscopic follow-up
to healing

H. pylori
NSAIDs
Smoking
Age
Family history
Surreptitious aspirin
(aspirin level)
Gastrin as indicated

THERAPY
Treat *H. pylori*
Stop NSAIDs
Acid suppression

Document
H. pylori
eradication?

COMPLICATIONS (outlet obstruction, perforation, intractable bleeding)–**SURGERY**

INTRACTABILITY **OR** RECURRENCES – NO ETIOLOGY (≤ 5%)
SURGERY vs. long-term proton-pump inhibitors

Figure 35–5
Algorithm for approach and treatment of the patient with peptic ulcer disease. *H. pylori = Helicobacter pylori;* NSAID = nonsteroidal anti-inflammatory drug; R/O = rule out; UGI = upper gastrointestinal.

growth factor to the ulcer site. The agent is minimally absorbed and virtually without side effects. Exogenous prostaglandins, such as PGE_1, conceivably promote ulcer healing either at low doses by mucosal protective effects or at higher doses by inhibiting acid secretion. Only misoprostol, a prostaglandin E_1 analog, is commercially available; it is approved in doses of 200 μg four times a day, only for the prevention of NSAID-induced gastric ulcers in patients at high risk of ulcer complications. (previous ulcer disease, the elderly). It significantly decreases the incidence of both NSAID-induced gastric *and* duodenal ulcer.

More than 80% of duodenal ulcers heal after 6 to 8 weeks of treatment with either H_2-receptor antagonists or sucralfate (4 weeks with proton pump inhibitors). If this initial approach is not successful, care should be taken to determine patient compliance and the actual presence of an unhealed ulcer (by endoscopy). These patients should be switched to a proton pump inhibitor, the rationale being that hypersecretion of acid may not have been adequately reduced with standard therapy. Patients should also be carefully questioned about the use of NSAIDs,

and one should always consider the Zollinger-Ellison syndrome. Gastric ulcers require special consideration because of the possibility of carcinoma (about 4% of gastric ulcers) and should be carefully followed until healing. Gastric ulcers are usually treated for 8 weeks, at which time assessment of healing is done, preferably with endoscopy or an upper GI series. Biopsies and cytologic specimens are taken any time an unhealed gastric ulcer is noted. If these studies prove negative, gastric ulcers are usually treated longer with the same regimen because these ulcers seem to be larger than duodenal ulcers and therefore take longer to heal. If healing still does not occur, the dose of the H_2-receptor antagonist may be increased or therapy changed to a proton pump inhibitor. If intense medical therapy still fails to heal the ulcer, surgery should be considered.

Both gastric and duodenal ulcers have a high recurrence rate after effective medical therapy, with rates being reported as high as 70 to 80% in 1 year. Eradicating *H. pylori* reduces the recurrence rate of peptic ulcer from ≥75% annually using standard acid suppression to as low as 10% using a variety of antibiotic regimens. Most of these regimens use two to three drugs and consist of a combination of proton pump inhibitors (omeprazole, 20 mg *twice* daily) and bismuth subsalicylate, metronidazole, tetracycline, amoxicillin, or newer macrolide antibiotics for 2 to 4 weeks. These regimens continue to evolve, and no single regimen is clearly superior. Alternatively, long-term acid suppression therapy may be used in patients with risk factors for recurrence such as smoking, NSAID use, or possible alcohol use. Some patients with recurrent peptic ulcers can be managed satisfactorily by initiating another 4- to 6-week course of therapy (i.e., "on demand therapy"). Treatment is with H_2-receptor antagonists at half-doses in the evening or, for duodenal ulcers, sucralfate in doses of 1 gm twice daily.

Surgical Management

Today, surgery for peptic ulcer disease is indicated only for complications because failure of healing on medical therapy is rare. The surgical procedures most frequently employed are shown in Figure 35–6. In various combinations, they are devised to decrease acid secretion by reducing the cephalic phase (vagotomy) or the gastric phase (antrectomy) by removing a major source of gastrin. Various drainage procedures are then used to maintain gastric emptying in the postvagotomy state. Increasingly proximal ("superselective") vagotomy rather than truncal vagotomy may be used to reduce acid secretion more selectively without adverse effects on gastric motility and

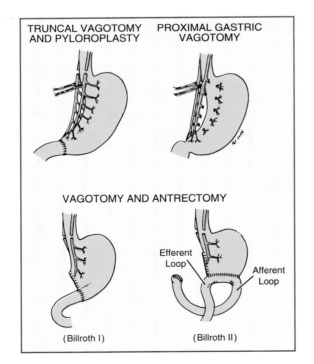

Figure 35–6
Surgical procedures for peptic ulcer disease. (From Thirlby RC: Peptic ulcer: Surgical therapy. *In* Wyngaarden JB, Smith LH Jr, Bennett JC [eds.]: Cecil Textbook of Medicine. 19th ed. Philadelphia, WB Saunders, 1992, p 661.)

emptying. However, the trade-off has been a higher rate of recurrent ulcer disease (i.e., 10% with proximal gastric vagotomy versus 1% with truncal vagotomy and antrectomy). In patients with intractable, benign gastric ulcers, vagotomy may not be required because acid production is usually normal or low. Antrectomy or subtotal gastrectomy may be the treatment of choice.

Although surgical treatment of peptic ulcer disease is usually successful in relieving symptoms and preventing recurrence, some infrequent complications may be distressing to the patient. The most common of these is the dumping syndrome, which results from disruption of the normal storage function of the stomach. Ingested food is dumped prematurely into the duodenum, leading to nausea, vomiting, weakness, abdominal pain, and diarrhea. These symptoms appear soon after eating. More rarely there are late symptoms (1 to 3 hours after eating), which probably result from reactive hypoglycemia due to rapid and excessive carbohydrate absorption followed by an overshoot of insulin release. Other postsurgery problems include weight loss usually related to early satiety, postvagotomy diarrhea, anemia as a result of iron, vitamin B_{12}, and/or folate deficiency, and alkaline reflux gastritis and esophagitis, and the afferent loop syndrome. The latter problem occurs in patients who have a Billroth II type of gastroenterostomy. Symptoms occur when pancreatic and biliary secretions collect in a partially obstructed afferent loop, causing distention and pain. Eventually, the fluid bypasses the partial obstruction, rushes into the stomach, and provokes vomiting. This complication may require reconstructive surgery.

THE ZOLLINGER-ELLISON SYNDROME

The Zollinger-Ellison syndrome, caused by a functioning islet cell tumor that secretes gastrin (gastrinoma), accounts for well under 1% of clinically diagnosed peptic ulcers. The possibility of this rare entity should be considered in several circumstances: (1) ulcers are located in unusual sites such as the second or third portion of the duodenum or the jejunum; (2) there is unusually severe peptic ulcer disease that is refractory to treatment or recurrent after surgery; (3) there is ulcer disease accompanied by diarrhea and sometimes malabsorption (see Chapter 32); and (4) a strong family history of ulcer disease exists, especially if there is evidence of other endocrine tumors.

Pathogenesis

Single, or often multiple, gastrinomas secrete excessive amounts of gastrin, which drives acid secretion by the parietal cell. In addition, gastrinomas have a trophic effect on the parietal cells, increasing their number by as much as three to five times. These tumors are generally found in the pancreas or duodenal bulb but, rarely, can be found outside this area. Although slow growing, most gastrinomas are histologically and biologically malignant, with early metastases regionally and to the liver. In approximately one fourth of patients, the gastrinoma is associated with other endocrine adenomas, most commonly in the pattern known as the multiple endocrine neoplasia type I (MEN I) syndrome, in which adenomas may involve the islet cells, the parathyroid glands, the thyroid, and the pituitary.

Clinical Manifestations

The clinical manifestations are usually those of severe peptic ulcer disease, as noted previously. Diarrhea may precede peptic ulcer formation or be a prominent symptom. Approximately 50% of patients have gastroesophageal reflux disease, which can be severe.

Diagnosis

The diagnosis of the Zollinger-Ellison syndrome is usually not difficult. Generally, it depends on the demonstration of an elevated serum gastrin and the presence of increased basal secretion of gastric acid (i.e., basal acid output [BAO] > 15 mmol/hr or a BAO/maximum acid output [MAO] ratio of $\geq 50\%$). A markedly elevated serum gastrin without hypersecretion is usually the result of hypochlorhydria. Intravenous secretin (1 unit/kg) produces a marked increase in serum gastrin level in most patients with gastrinoma but not in patients with ordinary duodenal ulcers.

Treatment

An attempt should be made to find and remove a resectable tumor, although this can be considered curative in only about one quarter of patients. If surgery is not successful, the patient should be treated with proton pump inhibitors or alternatively high dose H_2-antagonists to maintain the BAO at < 10 mmol/hr. Total gastrectomy may still be required for the rare patient who does not respond or is not compliant with medical therapy.

ABNORMALITIES OF GASTRIC EMPTYING

Abnormal gastric motility can cause rapid or delayed stomach emptying. Rapid emptying is usually secondary to gastric surgery. Delayed stomach emptying is much more common and may be secondary to mechanical obstruction or the inability of the stomach to generate effective propulsive forces (i.e., functional obstruction, or gastroparesis).

Pathogenesis and Clinical Manifestations

Rapid emptying may produce a number of symptoms, including lightheadedness, diaphoresis, palpitations, abdominal pain, and diarrhea. This constellation of symptoms has been referred to as "the dumping syndrome." Potential causes include the postgastrectomy and postvagotomy states, Zollinger-Ellison syndrome, pancreatic in-

TABLE 35–3	Causes of Delayed Gastric Emptying

Mechanical obstruction
  Duodenal or pyloric channel ulcer
  Pyloric stricture
  Tumor of the distal stomach
Functional obstruction (gastroparesis)
  Drugs
    Anticholinergics
    β-Adrenergics
    Opiates
  Electrolyte imbalance
    Hypokalemia
    Hypocalcemia
    Hypomagnesemia
  Metabolic disorders
    Diabetes mellitus
    Hypoparathyroidism
    Hypothyroidism
    Pregnancy
  Vagotomy
  Viral infections
  Neuromuscular disorders
    Myotonic dystrophy
    Diabetes mellitus (autonomic neuropathy)
    Scleroderma
    Polymyositis
    Aberrant gastric pacemaker (i.e., tachygastria)
  Brain stem tumors
  Gastroesophageal reflux
  Psychiatric disorders
    Anorexia nervosa
    Psychogenic vomiting
  Idiopathic

sufficiency, and celiac sprue. Symptoms may be mediated by the release of active agents, such as serotonin, prostaglandins, vasoactive intestinal polypeptides, insulin, opiates, and others. Delayed stomach emptying is much more common and has multiple causes (Table 35–3). Ulcers, strictures, and tumors all decrease the size of the gastric outlet, thereby impeding gastric emptying. Functional causes of gastroparesis interfere with emptying by transiently or permanently disrupting the neural or muscular function of the stomach. Symptoms of delayed gastric emptying include nausea, vomiting, abdominal fullness and bloating, early satiety, anorexia, and weight loss. It is impossible to determine from the presenting symptoms whether delayed emptying is caused by mechanical obstruction or functional gastroparesis.

Diagnosis

The best clues to abnormalities of gastric emptying are a good history and precipitating factors. An audible succussion splash over the abdomen may provide a clue to delayed emptying of the stomach. Patients with rapid gastric emptying and diarrhea may have hyperactive bowel sounds, but these findings are nonspecific. Delayed gastric emptying is suggested by a dilated stomach on an abdominal flat plate film or by obtaining food and a large amount of secretions after nasogastric intubation. After the stomach has been decompressed and cleaned out, upper GI endoscopy should be performed to exclude a mechanical cause of obstruction. If this study is negative, a radionuclide scintigraphic study can be done to assess the emptying of a solid meal. If this study is abnormally slow, a diagnosis of gastroparesis is made with confidence. Likewise, rapid emptying would be consistent with a dumping syndrome.

Treatment

Rapid gastric emptying is usually treated with dietary modification and antispasmodic medications. A high-fat, high-fiber diet consumed in six small meals that excludes concentrated carbohydrates and fluids with the meals may be helpful. Antispasmodic agents can delay gastric emptying by means of their anticholinergic effects. Useful agents include propantheline bromide at a dose of 7.5 to 15 mg three to four times a day or dicyclomine at 10 to 40 mg four times a day. Reconstructive surgery aimed at slowing the transit of food through the small intestine using reversed intestinal segment or Roux-en-Y jejunal interpositions is occasionally necessary. Electrolyte abnormalities should be improved and incriminating drugs removed in patients with delayed gastric emptying. Enriched liquids are easier to empty than solids, and multiple small feedings each day are suggested. Prokinetic drugs are used in treating chronic gastroparesis, although the results vary from disease to disease and patient to patient. Most of these drugs promote gastric emptying via cholinergic pathways or the inhibition of dopamine, which slows gastric motility. Available drugs include bethanechol at a dose of 10 to 20 mg four times a day and metoclopramide at a dose of 5 to 20 mg four times a day. Central nervous system side effects (agitation, nervousness, depression) occur in 25 to 30% of patients taking metoclopramide because it crosses the blood-brain barrier. Cisapride in a dose of 10 to 20 mg three to four times a day, is a powerful prokinetic agent that works through the cholinergic nervous system and does not cross the blood-brain barrier. Additionally, the long-used antibiotic erythromycin stimulates motility by interacting with receptors for the hormone motilin. Although acute administration of intravenous erythromycin in diabetics improves gastric emptying, a marked decrease in efficacy is seen with chronic oral administration.

REFERENCES

Isenberg JI, McQuaid KR, Laine L, Walsh JH: Acid-peptic disorders. *In* Yamada T (ed.): Textbook of Gastroenterology. 2nd ed. Philadelphia, JB Lippincott, 1995, pp 1347–1430.

Lin HC, Hasler WL: Disorders of gastric emptying. *In* Yamada T (ed.): Textbook of Gastroenterology. 2nd ed. Philadelphia, JB Lippincott, 1995, pp 1318–1346.

NIH consensus development panel on *Helicobacter pylori* in peptic ulcer disease: JAMA 1994; 272:65.

Soll AH: Pathogenesis of peptic ulcer and implications for therapy. New Engl J Med 1990; 322:909.

Wolfe MM, Soll AH: The physiology of gastric acid secretion. N Engl J Med 1988; 319:1707.

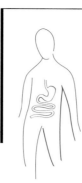

36

Inflammatory Bowel Disease

DEFINITION

Inflammatory bowel disease (IBD) is the rubric given to ulcerative colitis (UC) and Crohn's disease (CD), which are chronic inflammatory intestinal diseases of unknown etiology. UC and CD are discussed together to facilitate their comparison and highlight their differences. IBD is more common in whites than nonwhites and in Ashkenazic Jews than in Sephardic Jews and has approximately equal incidence in men and women. The incidence of UC is approximately the same as that of CD worldwide. Symptoms frequently begin in early adult life—ages 15 to 30—but may begin in the elderly. A comparison of clinical and pathologic features of CD and UC is given in Table 36–1.

ETIOLOGY AND PATHOGENESIS

Several causes have been proposed, although none has been proved. Genetic factors and immunologic dysregulation are significant in both forms of IBD. Monozygotic twins have a higher concordance than dizygotic twins.

Immunologic Origin

The presence of extraintestinal manifestations of IBD, the obvious infiltration of diseased mucosa with lymphocytes, the reports of cytotoxic T cells, and antibodies to colonic epithelial cells all suggest an immunologic basis for mucosal injury in IBD. Many investigations have focused on immune regulatory events, but definitive understanding of the pathogenesis of these diseases is yet to be achieved.

Infectious Origin

Several unsupported hypotheses suggest possible etiologic agents. While no organism has been consistently isolated or associated with IBD, studies comparing HLA-B27 transgenic rats grown in normal and germ-free environments suggest that gut flora are necessary for an experimental form of IBD.

Environmental Factors

Apparently, environmental factors trigger a series of responses that lead to the development of IBD. For example, the incidence of IBD is increasing in regions of Asia that are undergoing technologic development.

Psychological Origin

Very few gastroenterologists believe that IBD has a psychological origin, but many believe that emotional states can exacerbate symptoms in IBD. Emotional problems may further complicate longer-term management because of the debilitating nature of the disease.

PATHOLOGY

Examination of tissue in IBD often is required to make the distinction between UC and CD.

UC

Acute lesions in UC are diffuse and superficial, begin at the anal verge, and involve only the mucosa and submucosa. The lesions begin in the distal rectum and extend proximally to varying degrees. Patients with pancolitis (total colonic involvement) may have very mild ileitis, but essentially UC involves only the colon. The epithelium in UC is typically infiltrated with neutrophils and exhibits diffuse inflammation; the mucosa is friable owing to diffuse superficial ulceration. Pathologic examination usually shows multiple microabscesses around the crypts. In the presence of severe inflammation, the colon may develop marked distention with thin walls, leading to the syndrome known as "toxic megacolon" and perforation. Chronic UC can cause hyperplasia of the muscularis mucosae, shortening the colon and destroying the haustra. Endoscopic examination of the diseased mucosa in UC frequently reveals pseudopolyps, outcroppings of granulation tissue that develop between areas of inflammation. They are "pseudo" because they have no neoplastic epithelium. The colonic epithelium may develop dysplasia or

TABLE 36–1	Comparison of the Pathologic and Clinical Features of Ulcerative Colitis and Crohn's Disease		
Feature	**Ulcerative Colitis**	**Crohn's Disease**	
Pathologic			
Discontinuous involvement	0	+ +	
Transmural inflammation	0/+*	+ + +	
Deep fissures and fistulas	0	+ +	
Confluent linear ulcers	0	+ +	
Crypt abscesses	+ + +	+	
Focal granulomas	0	+ +	
Clinical			
Rectal bleeding	+ + +	+	
Malaise, fever	+	+ + +	
Abdominal pain	+	+ + +	
Abdominal mass	0	+ +	
Fistulas	0	+ + +	
Endoscopic			
Diffuse, continuous involvement	+ + +	0/+	
Friable mucosa	+ + +	0/+	
Rectal involvement	+ + +	+	
Cobblestoning	0	+ + +	
Linear ulcers	0	+ +	

*In toxic megacolon.

cancer. Carcinoma is the only complication of UC likely to produce a stricture or fistula.

CD

Crohn's disease has also been called regional enteritis because of the frequent involvement of the terminal ileum. Unlike in UC, the inflammation in CD is discontinuous and transmural. The rectum is involved in all UC patients but in fewer than half the patients with CD. CD has the capacity to involve any area of the gastrointestinal (GI) tract from the mouth to the anus, with approximately one third involving primarily the colon, one third ileum alone, and one third both ileum and colon. Rarely, the proximal small bowel, stomach, or mouth may be involved. Because the inflammatory process is transmural, nonadjacent loops of bowel may adhere to each other and develop masses, fistulas, or obstruction. The mucosa may appear relatively normal in CD or may develop a cobblestone or ulcerated appearance. Ulcers are often deep and linear, with the long axis of the ulcer parallel to the long axis of the bowel. The inflammatory infiltrate in the thickened bowel wall contains lymphocytes, macrophages, neutrophils, and, in about half of the cases, granulomas. CD is frequently complicated by fistula formation and perirectal disease, but epithelial dysplasia is not as common as in UC. CD increases the risk of colon cancer but much less than UC does.

CLINICAL MANIFESTATIONS

The clinical manifestations of IBD may be intestinal or extraintestinal.

Intestinal Manifestations

The primary manifestations of acute UC are rectal bleeding, diarrhea, urgency, fever, weight loss, and sometimes abdominal pain. The disease may be quite mild, with only a slight increase in stooling when the disease is limited to the rectum (ulcerative proctitis). In contrast, 10 to 15% of patients with UC present with an acute illness requiring immediate hospitalization to prevent or treat complications such as hypokalemia, toxic megacolon, shock, or colonic perforation. The severity of the diarrhea and extent of inflammatory disease determine whether the patient exhibits additional findings such as leukocytosis, anemia, hypokalemia, fever, weakness, anorexia, tachycardia, or hypotension. The abdomen may be normal on physical examination but may also be distended and tender. Most patients with UC have a remitting-relapsing course, with remissions lasting for weeks, months, or years punctuated by severe exacerbations.

The onset of CD is usually more subtle than that of UC, probably because the lesions are not as close to the rectum in CD. When the ileum is primarily involved, patients may present with evidence of low-grade intestinal obstruction with colicky pain, with or without diarrhea, and occasionally with a mass in the lower right quadrant. Dramatic rectal bleeding seen in UC is usually not seen in CD, although occult blood is common. Because the ileum is in the right lower quadrant and CD causes an inflammatory response, patients may present with symptoms mimicking those of acute appendicitis. When CD involves the colon, diarrhea is much more common than when it involves only the small bowel. Colonic involvement also predisposes to perirectal fistulas, abscesses, and fissures. CD is associated with more frequent extraintestinal manifestations, discussed later. Toxic megacolon is less common than in UC because most patients with CD do not have pancolitis. Perforation of the bowel into the peritoneum is uncommon in CD. As one would expect from the pathologic lesions, CD is much more likely to produce enterocutaneous, enterourinary, or enterovaginal fistulas and less likely to produce hemorrhage or perforation than is UC. Any part of the intestinal tract may be involved, even the buccal mucosa.

Extraintestinal Manifestations

Both UC and CD of the colon have been associated with the extraintestinal manifestations listed in Table 36–2. Nutritional deficiencies occasionally occur but are usually secondary to the anorexia, fever, diarrhea, blood loss, and malabsorption that may be present, especially in CD.

Inflammatory bowel disease is associated with two distinct forms of arthritis, sometimes termed enteropathic arthritis: (1) a nondeforming acute inflammatory arthritis of unknown cause that affects large joints and (2) a sacroiliitis of the ankylosing spondylitis type in patients who have HLA-B27. The former arthritides parallel the colonic disease, although they may precede the clinical onset of IBD. This process is generally oligoarticular and asymmetric and tends to involve the knees and ankles.

TABLE 36–2	Extraintestinal Manifestations of Inflammatory Bowel Disease

1. Nutritional abnormalities
     Weight loss, hypoalbuminemia, vitamin deficiencies, deficiencies of calcium, zinc, magnesium, phosphate
2. Hematologic abnormalities
     Anemia (iron loss, folate deficiency), leukocytosis, thrombocytosis
3. Skin manifestations
     Pyoderma gangrenosum, erythema nodosum
4. Arthritis
     Ankylosing spondylitis and sacroiliitis (B27-associated), peripheral large joint involvement
5. Hepatic and biliary abnormalities
     Fatty liver, pericholangitis, sclerosing cholangitis, gallstones, carcinoma of the bile ducts
6. Renal abnormalities
     Kidney stone diathesis (calcium oxalate, urid acid), obstructive uropathy, fistulas to urinary tract
7. Eye abnormalities
     Iritis, conjunctivitis, episcleritis
8. Miscellaneous
     Fever, increased thrombophlebitis, osteoporosis, osteomalacia

Modified from Rosenberg IH: Crohn's disease. *In* Wyngaarden JB, Smith LH Jr (eds.): Cecil Textbook of Medicine. 18th ed. Philadelphia, WB Saunders, 1988, p 745.

The latter arthritides persist and progress even after colectomy for UC, while the former generally resolve with colectomy. The clinical and radiographic findings in the HLA-B27–associated arthritis of IBD are largely indistinguishable from those seen in idiopathic ankylosing spondylitis.

Diverse abnormalities of the hepatobiliary system also occur in patients with IBD. Investigators have described the development of fatty liver and mild pericholangitis that may not be detected without noting an increased alkaline phosphatase. A rare but more severe complication called sclerosing cholangitis may supervene. This syndrome is characterized by progressive stricture of intrahepatic and extrahepatic ducts, leading to obstructive jaundice and secondary biliary cirrhosis. Sclerosing cholangitis is seen more commonly in UC than in CD, but an increased incidence of cholelithiasis due to inadequate absorption of bile salts by the diseased ileum is seen primarily in CD. Primary carcinoma of the bile duct has also been described but is rare. Ocular manifestations of IBD include iritis, uveitis, and episcleritis. Erythema nodosum occurs in approximately 5% of patients and is more common in women. One to 2% of patients with active UC also have pyoderma gangrenosum, a rare indolent, necrotic skin lesion. Patients with IBD may develop renal lesions: (1) kidney stones, especially calcium oxalate stones due to absorptive hyperoxaluria caused by malabsorption of calcium complexed to fatty acids; (2) obstructive uropathy from fibrosis in or near the urinary tract in CD; (3) kaliopenic nephropathy; or (4) rarely, amyloidosis. Patients with IBD have an increased risk for thrombophlebitis. Osteoporosis and osteomalacia may complicate the course of IBD as well (see Chapters 75 and 76).

On rare occasions, the extraintestinal manifestations present before the bowel disease and occasionally are the most important cause of morbidity. Most of these symptoms remit with improvement of the colitis or following colectomy.

DIAGNOSIS

The challenge of the diagnostic process is to determine if a patient with diarrhea, abdominal pain, rectal bleeding, and fever has IBD. In patients who appear to have IBD, it is important to distinguish between UC and CD. Other disorders that appear on the differential diagnosis vary with the clinical presentation; they include bacillary dysentery, amebiasis, ischemic colitis, pseudomembranous colitis, angiodysplasia, dysplasia, colon cancer, collagenous colitis, and microscopic colitis. No laboratory tests distinguish the IBD syndromes from each other or from non-IBD syndromes. The diagnosis depends on (1) direct visualization of the colonic or ileal mucosa with biopsy; (2) radiologic studies that may definitively demonstrate the ileal involvement of CD, in which a characteristic appearance distinguishes it from UC; and (3) exclusion of other illnesses that present similarly, including syndromes due to *Yersinia enterocolitica, Entamoeba histolytica, Campylobacter, Chlamydia,* or the toxin of *Clostridium difficile.*

The characteristic endoscopic findings in acute UC are described later. The mucosa is friable and frequently granular, and the lesions are generally diffuse. The lesions bleed easily when rubbed with a cotton swab or bumped with an endoscope. When UC has been established for years, pseudopolyps and deep ulcers may be apparent. In CD, the mucosa tends to be involved in patches and may exhibit a cobblestone appearance or linear ulcerations.

Radiographic studies are important in the diagnosis and management of IBD. Air-contrast barium enema usually demonstrates the diffuse character of the disease in UC and may even clearly identify pseudopolyps (Fig. 36–1); however, this study may be normal in early disease and is not as sensitive as endoscopy. Late in the disease, the "lead-pipe" appearance of the shortened colon with associated loss of haustra may be apparent. Radiographic studies of Crohn's colitis typically show patchy involvement, sparing of the rectum in half of the cases, longitudinal ulcers, and segmental narrowing of the bowel. Barium studies are indispensable in the detection of fistulous communications. The abnormalities of the ileal epithelium may also be diagnosed with barium enema and frequently exhibit the classic "string sign." These entities may not be easily distinguished early in the course of the disease.

TREATMENT AND PROGNOSIS

The treatment for UC and CD is similar because both disorders require long-term treatment using the same or related drugs. In addition, psychological problems, anemia, and other systemic and nutritional difficulties are treated similarly. However, the prognosis is sufficiently

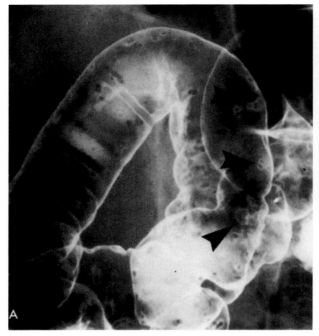
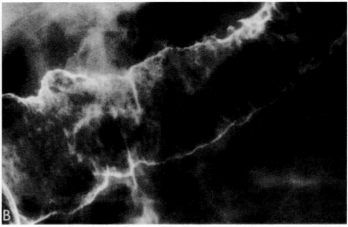

Figure 36–1

Double-contrast barium enema in a patient with ulcerative colitis demonstrating *(A)* pseudopolyps and *(B)* multiple irregular serrations in the transverse colon representing mucosal ulcerations. (From Sleisenger MH, Fordtran JS [eds.]: Gastrointestinal Disease: Pathophysiology, Diagnosis, and Management. 3rd ed. Philadelphia, WB Saunders, 1983, pp 1134–1135.)

different in these illnesses to warrant separate discussions of their management.

UC

It is critical to remember during all stages of UC treatment that this disease is completely curable with colectomy. However, most patients consider colectomy a last resort.

No single drug is curative. Sulfasalazine, related derivatives of pyridine–acetylsalicylic acid, antibacterial compounds, corticosteroids, and symptom-controlling medications such as antispasmodics and sedatives continue to be the drugs of choice. In severe cases, immunosuppressants, such as azathioprine, 6-mercaptopurine, and cyclosporine, are used under very tight control.

Mild to moderate acute colitis often responds to supportive measures supplemented by 3 to 4 gm/day of sulfasalazine alone. Sulfasalazine is hydrolyzed by bacteria in the colon to yield sulfapyridine and 5-aminosalicylate (5-ASA). The latter is considered to be the agent that improves the symptoms and the former, the potential cause of allergic reactions. Newer preparations of 5-ASA without a sulfa moiety become available in the upper small intestine. If treatment with 5-ASA derivatives is insufficient, corticosteroids are usually added. These are initially given orally in doses ranging from 20 to 60 mg/day of prednisone, then tapered if possible. Patients who exhibit only left-sided involvement may be managed successfully with corticosteroid or 5-ASA enemas. When the disease is in remission, patients are normally continued on sulfasalazine or some other 5-ASA derivative indefinitely to minimize recurrence. Severe UC can degenerate into toxic megacolon (see "Complications"). This is a medical emergency requiring immediate hospital-

ization, electrolyte monitoring, blood replacement, high-dose corticosteroids, broad-spectrum antibiotics, and surgical consultation. A patient's failure to respond clinically to treatment within 48 hours may indicate the need for colectomy.

In UC, total colectomy with either a permanent ileostomy or an ileoanal pull-through procedure to restore rectal continence is the surgical treatment of choice. This procedure prevents further episodes of IBD because UC does not involve noncolonic tissues. The indications for elective colectomy generally include the following:

1. Failure of medical management. Patients who have had acute exacerbations that fail to respond to therapy ultimately require colectomy. A subset of this group includes patients who respond well, but whose therapy requires high-dose steroids that have unacceptable long-term side effects.
2. The risk or presence of colonic carcinoma. Patients may develop dysplastic epithelium that is detected by biopsy. When severe dysplastic changes begin to develop, colectomy is indicated.

The mortality from acute exacerbations of UC is low (< 1%). More than 90% of patients respond to standard therapy, but recurrence is the rule. The lifespan of patients with UC is not significantly reduced from normal. When patients die of UC, it is usually due to acute complications such as perforated colon, bleeding, sepsis, or late development of carcinoma of the colon.

CD

Medical management of CD is quite similar to that of UC; 5-ASA and corticosteroids are the primary pharmacologic agents used. CD is usually not acute unless intestinal obstruction is the cause of the presentation, it generally responds slowly, and remissions are frequently incomplete. 5-ASA derivatives are not as effective in CD as UC and are usually reserved for patients who have extensive colonic involvement. Some gastroenterologists believe that using parenteral hyperalimentation to "put the bowel to rest" may also assist in the therapy of CD.

Surgical treatment of CD is not curative and is avoided whenever possible because the disease frequently recurs near the excision, and postoperative adhesions can be extensive. Surgery is usually reserved for resection of fistulas, treatment of abscesses, and relief of obstruction. It is critical to remove as little bowel as possible because these patients may require multiple operations and end up with short bowel syndrome.

Patients with CD do not enjoy the favorable prognosis seen in UC because their disease does not respond as well to medical management, and surgery is not a curative option. However, these patients have a normal lifespan, and when they die of their disease, it is usually due to sepsis rather than bleeding or cancer.

COMPLICATIONS

Complications associated with IBD have been discussed as the extraintestinal and clinical manifestations of these diseases. One must also be concerned about long-term problems such as growth retardation in children, malnutrition, weakness, lassitude, recurrent pain, and depression. These, of course, are complications associated with any chronic debilitating illness; however, two special complications are discussed in more detail.

Toxic Dilatation of the Colon (Toxic Megacolon)

This complication is more typically seen in UC than in CD and is characterized by an atonic and distended colon with a very thin wall. Patients with this complication are frequently toxic, have an explosive onset of illness, and exhibit tachycardia, fever, and leukocytosis. Diarrhea is generally decreased because of a loss of propulsive activity in the colon. Patients frequently have hypokalemia and hypoalbuminemia. Toxic megacolon may occur spontaneously, but it also has occurred after initiation of opiates and anticholinergics and in preparation for colonoscopic or barium enema examinations. The diagnosis is usually suggested by diffuse dilatation of the colon (>6 cm), particularly the transverse colon. There is an impending danger of perforation until the dilatation is reversed, and medical reversal in less than 48 hours is essential or surgery is indicated.

Carcinoma of the Colon

A general discussion of carcinoma of the colon is found in Chapter 37. There is an increased risk of colon carcinoma in IBD but more so in UC than CD. The incidence of carcinoma in UC relates to two variables: (1) pancolitis, that is, the presence of complete colonic involvement

with inflammation, and (2) the duration of active colitis. The incidence of cancer begins to increase significantly after 10 years of active disease. The carcinoma typical of UC patients is somewhat different from colon cancer in the general population: (1) its distribution is more even in the colon; (2) it is frequently multifocal; (3) it is typically discovered at a more advanced stage and therefore has a worse prognosis; (4) it is quite difficult to diagnose because the associated symptoms are masked by the underlying disease; and (5) it occurs on a base of very abnormal mucosa. For these reasons, detailed follow-up protocols exist for patients with chronic pancolitis involving repeated colonoscopy and screening biopsies. The biopsies are used to guide the timing of preventive colectomy.

ISCHEMIC COLITIS

In elderly patients, ischemic injury to the colon may mimic IBD. Ischemic injury, whether acute or chronic, is usually caused by progressive atherosclerosis. It may also occur from vascular injury due to an aneurysmal dissection, surgery, congestive heart failure, or vasculitis, or from hypercoagulable states. The ischemia occurs most commonly in "watershed areas" between distributions of major vessels and is usually caused by low-perfusion states rather than complete vascular occlusion. Because of extensive collateral supply, the rectum is almost always spared. Presentation may be chronic, acute, or both.

Acute Ischemic Colitis

This usually presents with sudden local abdominal pain associated with tenderness and rectal bleeding. These symptoms may be accompanied by hypotension, tachycardia, fever, and, in severe cases, peritoneal irritation. Colonoscopy may reveal a normal pericolonic mucosa but more typically shows multiple ulcerations and/or submucosal hemorrhage. Barium enema is somewhat dangerous during the acute period but exhibits classic findings of narrowing and "thumb-printing" subsequently. In the acute phase, ischemic colitis may appear very much like IBD or diverticulitis. The symptoms from acute ischemic episodes involving the colon are generally self-limited and resolve within several weeks. Angiography is rarely needed, and surgery is usually reserved for patients with frank infarction or perforation. After patients recover from the acute episode, they may remain symptom-free for life, or they may develop chronic symptoms.

Subacute or Chronic Ischemic Colitis

This is characterized by diarrhea and long periods of mild to moderate abdominal pain that is vague in character and may be accompanied by fear of eating, weight loss, or significant bleeding. Chronic ischemic colitis may resemble IBD clinically as well as endoscopically. Fibrosis frequently develops in the region of ischemic injury, leading to narrowing of the colon and, occasionally, strictures requiring surgical revision. Revascularization is usually not indicated.

DIVERTICULITIS

Colonic diverticula are saccules of mucosa covered by serosa but do not include the muscular layer. They develop commonly in later life, particularly in Western societies, and occur at the site of arterioles or penetrations of the muscular wall. The formation of diverticulae is believed to be caused by any condition that chronically increases local intraluminal pressures, such as low-fiber diets. The majority of diverticulae are located in the sigmoid colon and produce no symptoms. They may become clinically important if they bleed or become infected. The vessels in or around diverticula may produce arterial bleeding that must be differentiated from other causes such as angiodysplasia or carcinoma. The differential diagnosis of lower GI bleeding is discussed in Chapter 32. Inflammatory diverticulitis is a region of localized infection but may lead to microabscess formation. Occasionally, large abscesses involve an adjacent organ. Clinically, acute diverticulitis presents similarly to appendicitis except that symptoms are localized to the left lower quadrant. The left lower quadrant pain is often associated with localized tenderness, leukocytosis, fever, and occasionally a palpable inflammatory mass. Bleeding from the inflamed region is rare. A tender mass is occasionally detectable by rectal examination but is more typically seen on sigmoidoscopy as a narrow lumen and inflamed mucosa. During the acute phase, barium enema should be considered a hazardous procedure.

Diverticulitis is managed by withholding solid food and treating with broad-spectrum antibiotics and intravenous fluids. Surgical intervention is usually not required but may be necessary when perforation, fistulas, or large abscesses complicate the presentation. Many physicians recommend diets high in indigestible fiber to promote large-volume daily bowel movements to prevent the development of diverticulosis.

REFERENCES

Brandt LJ, Boley SJ: Ischemic and vascular lesions of the bowel. *In* Sleisenger MH, Fordtran JS (eds.): Gastrointestinal Disease: Pathophysiology, Diagnosis, and Management. 5th ed. Philadelphia, WB Saunders, 1993, pp 1927–1961.

Danzi JT: Extraintestinal manifestations of idiopathic inflammatory bowel diseases. Arch Intern Med 1988; 148:297.

Hanauer SB: Inflammatory bowel disease. *In* Wyngaarden JB, Smith LH Jr, Bennett JC (eds.): Cecil Textbook of Medicine. 19th ed. Philadelphia, WB Saunders, 1992, p 699.

Jewell DP: Ulcerative colitis. *In* Sleisenger MH, Fordtran JS (eds.): Gastrointestinal Disease: Pathophysiology, Diagnosis, and Management. 5th ed. Philadelphia, WB Saunders, 1993, pp 1305–1330.

Kirsner JB, Shorter RG: Inflammatory Bowel Disease. 3rd ed. Philadelphia, Lea & Febiger, 1988.

Kornbluth A, Salomon P, Sachar DB: Crohn's disease. *In* Sleisenger MH, Fordtran JS (eds.): Gastrointestinal Disease: Pathophysiology, Diagnosis, and Management. 5th ed. Philadelphia, WB Saunders, 1993, pp 1270–1304.

37

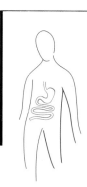

Neoplasms of the Gastrointestinal Tract

Neoplasms of the gastrointestinal (GI) tract continue to be the most common malignant tumors. The more frequent neoplasms—those of the esophagus, stomach, and colon—are discussed in this chapter. Neoplasms of the pancreas and liver are discussed in Chapters 38 and 44, respectively.

CARCINOMA OF THE ESOPHAGUS

More than 95% of esophageal neoplasms are squamous cell in origin. Adenocarcinomas, which arise from tumors at the gastroesophageal junction, comprise approximately 5%. Benign neoplasms are unusual, with leiomyomas being the most frequent.

Incidence

The incidence of esophageal carcinoma has dropped in the last two decades to approximately 5 per 100,000. Blacks, particularly men, are four to five times more commonly affected than whites, whereas white females have the lowest incidence. Dramatic regional differences exist in the world; in certain areas of China, the incidence exceeds 1 per 1000 people.

Etiology and Pathogenesis

The cause of squamous cell esophageal carcinoma is unknown, although many associations exist. Environmental factors are most commonly implicated, particularly in those areas of the world having the highest incidence. In the United States, tobacco and alcohol abuse are considered primary risk factors not only for esophageal cancer, but for squamous cell tumors of the head and neck as well. Esophageal injury due to lye ingestion, radiation, or long-term stasis (achalasia) also increases the incidence. Adenocarcinoma is strongly identified with Barrett's epithelium, a metaplasia of the distal esophagus in which gastric mucosa and intestinal epithelium appear in association with long-term gastroesophageal reflux. The incidence of esophageal carcinoma is also increased in patients with the rare inherited disorder associated with thickened skin of the palms and soles (tylosis).

Clinical Manifestations

Dysphagia is the most frequent and important symptom of esophageal carcinoma. Initially, patients report difficulty in swallowing solid foods, which progresses to difficulty in swallowing liquids; anorexia and weight loss commonly accompany dysphagia. With complete obstruction, regurgitation and aspiration with secondary pneumonia may result. Pneumonia may also occur with a tracheoesophageal fistula. Less common manifestations are related primarily to the involvement of adjacent structures in the mediastinum and include substernal pain and hoarseness due to impingement on the recurrent laryngeal nerve. GI bleeding is often occult in nature, although it may be massive and fatal when the tumor erodes the aorta. Clubbing of the nails and, rarely, paraneoplastic endocrine abnormalities (hypercalcemia, Cushing syndrome) have been noted.

Complications

Esophageal cancer tends to be a "silent" malignancy until late in the course owing to the distensibility of the esophagus; therefore, the tumor has to be large before dysphagia results. Local complications are most often related to mediastinal extension or esophageal narrowing. Because the esophagus has no serosal lining, the tumor tends to metastasize early to regional lymph nodes, the liver, and the lungs.

Diagnosis

In patients over age 40 and those with risk factors for esophageal carcinoma, new-onset dysphagia should prompt evaluation for an esophageal tumor. A double-contrast barium study of the esophagus usually shows an abnormality if carcinoma is present. Endoscopy may also be an appropriate initial test to exclude carcinoma and may be required for biopsy of any suspicious lesions. Mucosal biopsy and cytology of an identified esophageal lesion has a high degree of specificity.

Computed tomography (CT) scanning of the chest is often performed in the staging evaluation to exclude involvement of adjacent structures (bronchus, aorta), as well as to detect mediastinal lymphadenopathy or lung or liver metastases. In some centers, endoscopic ultrasonography plays a useful role in detecting extent of the tumor and thus its resectability.

Treatment and Prognosis

Because early warning signs or symptoms may be absent, esophageal cancer is often incurable at the time of diagnosis. Although approximately 10 to 50% of patients undergo surgical resection for its palliative effects, surgical resection may cure the disease in 5 to 10% of cases. However, the operative mortality for curative resection may approach 15%. In the patient who is not an operative candidate, high-dose radiation therapy may provide palliation. Other palliative therapies include placement of a plastic tube (prosthesis) or metal stent across the obstruction, coagulation of the tumor using either laser or thermal probes, or endoscopic dilation.

CARCINOMA OF THE STOMACH

Adenocarcinomas comprise >90% of the malignant tumors of the stomach. Other less common neoplasms include lymphomas or metastatic disease (melanoma, breast). Benign neoplasms include leiomyomas and adenomas. This chapter focuses on adenocarcinomas.

Incidence

As recently as the 1940s, gastric carcinoma was the most common neoplasm in the United States. There has been an unexplained decrease in incidence, and now gastric adenocarcinoma is the seventh most common neoplasm. There is marked variation in the incidence of gastric cancer throughout the world, with very high rates reported in Japan, parts of South America, and Eastern Europe. When population groups emigrate from areas of high incidence to those of low incidence, the rate drops very slowly over several generations.

Etiology and Pathogenesis

Environmental factors have long been suggested as a cause of gastric carcinoma because of the regional incidence of the disease as well as the changes that occur in migrating populations. A variety of associations have been described (Table 37–1). Gastric cancer is more common in men, the elderly, blacks as compared with whites, those with a poor socioeconomic status, and those with a positive family history. Recent evidence suggests a strong association with *Helicobacter pylori* gastritis, probably through its role in leading to atrophic gastritis. Other mucosal abnormalities (adenomatous polyps), pernicious anemia (associated with carcinoid tumors), and the postgastrectomy state also appear to be precancerous conditions. A diet high in salt and nitrates is thought to be a potential environmental factor. Although many of these

TABLE 37–1	Adenocarcinoma of the Stomach	
Associated Factors	**Clinical Manifestations**
Environment—geographic differences	Anorexia, early satiety, weight loss
Diet—? nitrosamines	Dysphagia, vomiting, weakness
Blood group A	Epigastric distress to severe, boring pain
Helicobacter pylori gastritis	
Atrophic gastritis	Anemia, occult blood in stools
Adenomatous polyps (>2 cm)	Epigastric mass, signs of metastases
Subtotal resection for benign ulcer disease	Rare—Virchow's node, Blumer's shelf, Trousseau's syndrome, acanthosis nigricans

factors have been associated with gastric cancer, the fall in incidence over the last several decades cannot be explained by any particular factor.

Clinical Manifestations

The clinical presentation of gastric carcinoma depends on a variety of factors, including the morphologic characteristics of the tumor (infiltrating versus ulcerating), size of the tumor, presence of gastric outlet obstruction, and metastatic versus nonmetastatic disease (see Table 37–1). Epigastric abdominal pain is a frequent complaint that may mimic peptic ulcer disease or may be more constant and severe in nature, with food exacerbating the pain. Nausea may occur and vomiting is frequent, especially with gastric outlet obstruction. Anorexia and weight loss are also common. Most tumors originate in the distal part of the stomach; proximal lesions may cause obstruction of the distal part of the esophagus, resulting in dysphagia. Acute or chronic blood loss that results in iron deficiency anemia may also occur. Other less frequent symptoms and signs may be related to distant metastases, direct extension in the abdominal cavity, or a paraneoplastic syndrome. Obstructive jaundice, malignant ascites, or a gastrocolic fistula may result from local spread, whereas Trousseau's syndrome (thrombophlebitis), dermatomyositis, and acanthosis nigricans represent paraneoplastic manifestations. Physical examination can reveal a healthy-appearing patient or one with apparent loss of weight. Abdominal examination may document epigastric tenderness or a mass. With metastatic disease, a Virchow node (left supraclavicular), a Blumer shelf (mass in the perirectal pouch), or a Krukenberg tumor (metastases to the ovaries) may also be found on physical examination.

Diagnosis

An upper GI series is often the first examination performed in the evaluation for gastric carcinoma. Using a double-contrast technique with multiple projections increases the sensitivity and more fully evaluates the entire stomach. The radiographic characteristics of the tumor are variable and depend on its morphologic and pathologic characteristics. For example, gastric carcinoma may present as a large polypoid mass, a benign-appearing gastric ulcer (early gastric carcinoma), or abnormal folds with a thickened, non-distensible wall (linitis plastica). Radiographic characteristics that suggest a malignant gastric ulcer include an irregular ulcer base, an ulcer within a mass, and the appearance of convergent folds. However, the true differentiation between a benign and a malignant ulcer can be made conclusively only by biopsy.

Upper endoscopic evaluation may also be appropriate as the initial diagnostic test in selected patients because mucosal abnormalities identified using this technique can be biopsied as well as supplemented by brushings for cytology; together they increase the diagnostic specificity to 95%. Gastric ulcers often have to be followed either radiographically or endoscopically until healing is complete to confirm benignancy; however, in rare cases, even malignant ulcers may heal. No serologic cancer markers are useful diagnostically or for detecting recurrence after surgery.

Treatment and Prognosis

Gastric cancer can be cured only by definitive surgical therapy. Unfortunately, fewer than one third of gastric cancers are resectable for cure at presentation. After the diagnosis is established, staging is performed to determine the presence of local spread or distant metastases. This is usually performed by liver chemistry tests, abdominal imaging studies, most commonly CT, and biopsy of any suspected nodes. Occasionally, laparoscopy may be performed. If distant metastases are identifed, palliative resection may be performed to prevent obstruction or further bleeding. For a localized tumor, the resection can be limited to the area of the tumor, which limits morbidity. The 5-year survival for most patients is <5%. In contrast, the patient with early gastric cancer, in which tumor has not spread to regional lymph nodes, can often be cured with definitive surgical therapy. Radiation therapy for gastric carcinoma is generally unsatisfactory. A variety of chemotherapeutic regimens have been used with only modest success and no cures. Endoscopic therapies offer few palliative options.

CARCINOMA OF THE COLON

Adenocarcinomas comprise >95% of all malignant tumors of the large bowel; the following discussion of colonic carcinoma also includes rectal cancer. Other rare colonic neoplasms, such as carcinoid tumor, leiomyomas, and diseases that metastasize to the colon, are not discussed here.

Incidence

The colon and rectum are now the third most common site of carcinoma in men and the second in women. Overall, colorectal cancer is the third most common cause of cancer death. Approximately 150,000 new cases are diagnosed annually, which represents 15% of all malignant tumors. Variations in incidence occur throughout the world such that in more developed regions like the United States, Western Europe, Australia, and New Zealand the frequency is much higher than in South America or Africa. People who emigrate tend to acquire the risk characteristic of their new environment.

Etiology and Pathogenesis

The cause of colon cancer is unknown, although a number of associations have been described. Environmental factors, particularly diet, have been commonly implicated, given noted regional variations and changes in incidence with migration. A diet low in fiber but high in animal fat and protein, perhaps that derived from beef, has been most frequently suggested as important and correlates with the diets of persons throughout the world where the incidence is highest. Excess fats and colonic bacteria have been postulated to interact in some way to produce metabolites such as toxic bile acids. In contrast, a diet high in fiber has been associated with a much lower incidence of the disease. Given these associations, the possible protective effects of various dietary factors, including calcium, selenium, and supplemental bran, await further studies.

A number of important risk factors other than dietary are outlined in Table 37–2. Although colon cancer not associated with familial polyposis has been identified in individuals in their teens and 20s, the incidence clearly increases above the age of 40 and doubles for each succeeding decade. Disorders associated with increased mucosal cell turnover may also lead to an increased risk; inflammatory bowel disease, especially ulcerative colitis (see Chapter 36), and certain familial polyposis syndromes (see later) are examples. A history of previous cancer or adenoma of the colon, colon cancer in one or more first-degree relatives, or the "family cancer syndrome" (multifocal cancers in other organs, especially the female sex organs) increases the risk of colonic carcinoma as well. Thus, hereditary influences may play an important role in some patients. Furthermore, there is evidence that sequential activation of several oncogenes may be of key importance in the origin of some colorectal tumors (Fig. 37–1).

TABLE 37–2	Risk Factors for Carcinoma of the Colon

Increasing age
Inflammatory bowel disease
Personal history of colon cancer or adenoma
Family history of colon cancer
Familial polyposis syndromes (adenomatous polyps)
History of breast or female genital cancer
Peutz-Jeghers syndrome (hamartomas)

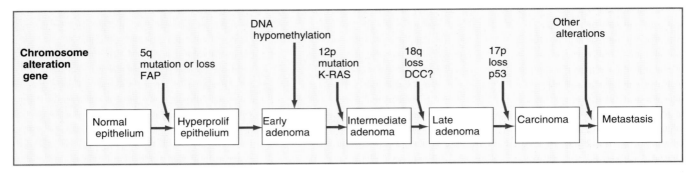

Figure 37-1

A genetic model for colorectal tumorigenesis. (Reprinted with permission from Fearon ER, Vogelstein B: A genetic model for colorectal tumorigenesis [review]. Cell 1990; 61:759–767. Copyright by Cell Press.)

Clinical Manifestations

As with cancer of the esophagus and stomach, colon carcinoma has very few early warning signs. It may be totally asymptomatic and found incidentally during abdominal surgery or at screening sigmoidoscopy. GI blood loss is the most common presenting finding and can be identified as occult blood in the stool, melena, or bright red rectal bleeding, depending on the location of the tumor. Abdominal pain is an uncommon presenting symptom, although it may be a consequence of obstruction (most commonly left-sided tumors) or bowel wall invasion. Alteration of bowel habits is an important but uncommon symptom that usually results from left-sided or distal tumors. Overflow diarrhea may occur when a distal tumor results in severe but incomplete colonic obstruction. Weight loss and anorexia are nonspecific symptoms that may occur in any malignancy, although they usually appear late in the clinical course. Other presenting symptoms and signs include perforation, malignant ascites, and liver metastases with jaundice.

Diagnosis

Carcinoma of the colon should be suspected in any patient over age 40 who presents with occult blood in the stool, iron deficiency anemia, overt rectal bleeding, or alteration in bowel habits, especially if associated with abdominal discomfort or any risk factors noted in Table 37–2. Bright red blood from the rectum found on the stool may suggest hemorrhoidal disease, although colon carcinoma must be excluded in the patient over age 40. Initial diagnostic evaluation should begin with digital rectal examination. However, the majority of colorectal tumors cannot be palpated by digital rectal examination, requiring radiographic or colonoscopic evaluation. Approximately 50% of colorectal tumors can now be identified with the 60-cm flexible sigmoidoscope (Fig. 37–2), although in the elderly, tumors tend to be located in the more proximal colon. If a double-contrast barium enema examination is performed, it should be accompanied by a flexible sigmoidoscopic examination because the barium study tends to be less sensitive in the distal colorectum. Colonoscopy may be the initial diagnostic test used in patients who have a suspicious lesion found on barium enema or in those with persistent symptoms despite a "negative" radiographic examination. Biopsy performed at colonoscopy establishes the diagnosis in almost 100% of cases. Determination of carcinoembryonic antigen (CEA) is not helpful in establishing the diagnosis of colon cancer but is useful in follow-up surgery to detect recurrence.

The differential diagnosis of colon carcinoma depends on particular clinical symptoms and signs, including diverticulitis, ischemic colitis, colonic vascular ectasias, inflammatory bowel disease, and benign polyps.

Treatment and Prognosis

The only effective therapy is to surgically remove the tumor and the adjacent colon and mesentery. Colonos-

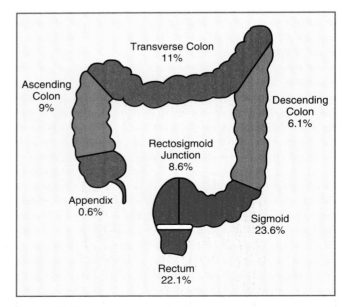

Figure 37-2

Distribution of large bowel cancer by anatomic segment according to the third national cancer survey (segment unspecified). (Data from Shottenfeld D, Fraumeni J Jr [eds.]: Cancer Epidemiology and Prevention. Philadelphia, WB Saunders, 1982, pp 703–727.)

copy and abdominal CT are usually performed preoperatively to exclude synchronous colonic neoplasms and to determine the presence of peritoneal, lung, or liver metastases. The type of surgical procedure used depends on the location of the tumor. Hemicolectomy is performed for right- and left-sided lesions, anterior resection with anastomosis to the rectal stump for sigmoid or upper rectal tumors, and a combined abdominal and perineal resection with a permanent colostomy for distal lesions of the rectum. In the patient who has metastatic disease, surgery still provides the best palliation for obstruction, bleeding, or perforation. Radiation therapy is efficacious for rectal cancer and may be done preoperatively or for painful bony metastasis. Chemotherapy with 5-fluorouracil in combination with levamisole improves survival for patients who have Duke's stage C disease at diagnosis (see later). In addition, isolated hepatic metastases may be resected to improve patients' survival.

The results of surgical treatment for carcinoma of the large bowel are excellent, with acceptable morbidity and mortality even in the elderly patient. As with all GI malignancies, the survival for colon carcinoma depends on the stage of tumor at diagnosis, commonly called the Duke's classification: Duke's A lesions (confined to the bowel wall) have a 5-year survival of >80%; Duke's B (through the bowel wall) have a 5-year survival of 60 to 80%; Duke's C (through the bowel to the serosa) have approximately 50% even when lymph nodes are involved; Duke's D (metastatic disease) have a 5-year survival of ≤25%. After surgery, routine follow-up includes surveillance colonoscopy or barium radiography to exclude missed synchronous polyps, cancers, or recurrent lesions, as well as measurements of CEA. However, detection of a "curable" recurrence by CEA elevation is very rare. In addition, recent evidence suggests that routine CEA monitoring does not prolong survival.

Screening and Prevention

The complex process of colonic carcinogenesis evolves over many years. Benign adenomatous polyps as well as early localized carcinomas can be cured either by colonoscopic polypectomy (if technically possible) or surgery. Given the link between adenomatous polyps and cancer, there is now considerable interest in screening populations for colonic polyps and carcinomas with annual testing for fecal occult blood and periodic (every 3 to 5 years) proctosigmoidoscopy beginning at age 40 to 50. If occult blood is found in the stool, radiographic or colonoscopic examination of the entire colon should be performed. It is unclear whether this screening strategy is cost effective or decreases mortality in the general population, although the tumors found as a result of occult blood testing tend to be at an earlier stage. In contrast, individuals at high risk for developing colon carcinoma, such as those having the familial polyposis syndrome, prior adenomatous colonic polyps or cancer, or long-standing ulcerative colitis involving the entire colon, should be screened periodically with examinations of the entire colon.

POLYPS OF THE GASTROINTESTINAL TRACT

A polyp is defined as an overgrowth of tissue, usually of epithelial cells, that arises from the mucosal surface and extends into the lumen of the GI tract. Polyps can be single or multiple, sporadic or familial, pedunculated (on a stalk) or sessile (flat base), neoplastic or non-neoplastic, benign or malignant. Polyps may occur anywhere throughout the GI tract, although those arising in the colon are of greatest importance, given their prevalence and malignant potential. A simplified classification of colonic polyps is given in Table 37–3. Only neoplastic polyps and benign polyps associated with the distinct polyposis syndromes are discussed here.

Incidence

Adenomatous colonic polyps are very common and increase with age, so that a 50-year-old man has a 20% chance of having an adenomatous colonic polyp, and a 70-year-old man has a 30 to 40% chance. Patients with one polyp have a higher frequency of synchronous colonic polyps and a greater potential for developing additional polyps over time.

Etiology and Pathogenesis

The cause of colonic polyps, other than that clearly associated with inherited disorders, is unknown. An indirect body of evidence suggests that most colon carcinomas arise from previously benign adenomatous polyps, usually after a period of at least 5 to 10 years. Therefore, the previously identified risk factors associated with colonic carcinoma (see Table 37–2) may also pertain to benign adenomatous polyps.

A very small percentage of benign polyps progress to malignancy, and the causative factors for this transition are unknown. Given the malignant potential of colonic polyps, it is advisable to remove any adenomatous polyp when found. The majority of colonic polyps are small (<1 cm in diameter), usually asymptomatic, and found incidentally either at autopsy or on radiographic or colonoscopic examination. When the lesions are >2 cm, GI bleeding may occur (usually occult); only very large pol-

TABLE 37–3	Polyps of the Colon

Neoplastic Polyps

Benign adenomatous polyps (tubular, mixed, or villous)
  Random occurrences
  Familial—familial polyposis of the colon, Gardner's syndrome (see Fig. 37–3), Turcot's syndrome, family cancer syndrome
  Malignant polyps—carcinomatous changes, *in situ* or invasive

Non-Neoplastic Polyps

Inflammatory "pseudopolyps"
Peutz-Jeghers syndrome—hamartomas
Mucosal polyps with normal epithelium
Juvenile polyps

yps, which often contain a focus of carcinoma, cause hematochezia. Abdominal pain or alterations in bowel habits are unusual. Very rarely, villous adenomas may produce watery diarrhea containing high concentrations of potassium, which results in symptomatic hypokalemia.

Diagnosis

The accurate diagnosis of a colonic polyp depends on the size of the polyp and is facilitated by the study performed. Single-contrast barium enemas may not reliably demonstrate polyps < 1 cm in diameter, although double-contrast techniques usually identify lesions > 5 mm. Colonoscopy identifies most but not all colonic polyps. Regardless of its size, the type of colonic polyp—benign or malignant—can be determined only by mucosal biopsy.

Treatment

Although only a small proportion of adenomatous colonic polyps undergo malignant transformation, all identified adenomas should usually be removed. Although this can be accomplished readily with the colonoscope, large ses-

sile lesions may require surgical resection. Patients with previous adenomatous polyps are at increased risk for subsequent adenomas, and thus follow-up at regular intervals is indicated.

THE FAMILIAL POLYPOSIS SYNDROMES

The familial polyposis syndromes are rare, dominantly inherited disorders in which multiple polyps can be found throughout the GI tract (see Table 37–3).

Familial Polyposis of the Colon

In this rare genetic disorder (1 in 8000 births), adenomatous polyps develop progressively throughout the colon so that by the patient's 20s, thousands of adenomatous polyps "carpet" the colon. The patient may be asymptomatic unless bleeding or symptoms associated with colorectal cancer develop. Colorectal cancer is an inevitable consequence in the natural history of this syndrome, occurring approximately 10 to 15 years after the onset of polyposis. In these patients, adenomatous polyps may also occur in the upper GI tract. In the patient with a diagnosis of

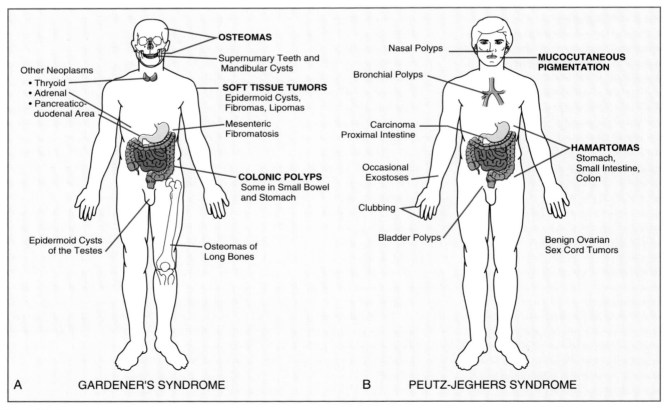

Figure 37–3

A, Schematic representation of Gardner's syndrome. The triad of colonic polyposis, bone tumors, and soft tissue tumors (heavy print) is the primary feature; other features are indicated in lighter print. *B,* Schematic presentation of the Peutz-Jeghers syndrome. Mucocutaneous pigmentation and benign gastrointestinal polyposis (heavy print) are the primary features of this syndrome. Lighter print shows the secondary features. (From Boland CR, Kim YS: *In* Sleisenger MH, Fordtran JS [eds.]: Gastrointestinal Disease: Pathophysiology, Diagnosis, and Management. 3rd ed. Philadelphia, WB Saunders, 1983.)

familial polyposis, elective complete colectomy is required (usually after full growth has been achieved). Given the dominant inheritance pattern, other family members must be screened.

Gardner's Syndrome

In this syndrome resembling familial polyposis coli, extracolonic manifestations of benign soft tissue tumors and osteomas are present (Fig. 37–3). Polyps of the upper GI tract may also occur. As with familial polyposis coli, the colonic polyps have malignant potential, and thus total colectomy is indicated.

Peutz-Jeghers Syndrome

In contrast to the polyps found in Gardner's syndrome and familial polyposis coli, these polyps are hamartomas that have no malignant potential themselves but are associated with adenocarcinomas of the small intestine. Characteristic mucocutaneous pigmentation, especially of the buccal mucosa as well as the lips and soles of the feet and dorsum of the hands, is well recognized (see Fig. 37–2). Patients with this syndrome are usually asymptomatic or may present with GI bleeding, abdominal pain, or commonly intussusception with small bowel obstruction requiring urgent surgical intervention.

REFERENCES

Boland CR, Kim YS: Gastrointestinal polyposis syndromes. *In* Sleisenger MH, Fordtran JS (eds.): Gastrointestinal Disease: Pathophysiology, Diagnosis, and Management. 5th ed. Philadelphia, WB Saunders, 1993, pp 1430–1448.

Boyce HW Jr: Tumors (of the esophagus). *In* Sleisenger MH, Fordtran JS (eds.): Gastrointestinal Disease: Pathophysiology, Diagnosis, and Management. 5th ed. Philadelphia, WB Saunders, 1993, pp 401–418.

Bresalier RS, Kim YS: Malignant neoplasms of the large intestine. *In* Sleisenger MH, Fordtran JS (eds.): Gastrointestinal Disease: Pathophysiology, Diagnosis, and Management. 5th ed. Philadelphia, WB Saunders, 1993, pp 1449–1483.

Davis GR: Neoplasms of the stomach. *In* Sleisenger MH, Fordtran JS (eds.): Gastrointestinal Disease: Pathophysiology, Diagnosis, and Management. 5th ed. Philadelphia, WB Saunders, 1993, pp 763–792.

Fearon ER, Vogelstein B: A genetic model for colorectal tumorigenesis. Cell 1990; 61:759–767.

Itzkowitz SH, Kim YS: Polyps and benign neoplasms of the colon. *In* Sleisenger MH, Fordtran JS (eds.): Gastrointestinal Disease: Pathophysiology, Diagnosis, and Management, 5th ed. Philadelphia, WB Saunders, 1993, pp 1402–1429.

Levin B: Neoplasms of the large and small intestine. *In* Wyngaarden JB, Smith LH Jr, Bennett JC (eds.): Cecil Textbook of Medicine. 19th ed. Philadelphia, WB Saunders, 1992, p 713.

38

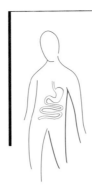

The Pancreas

NORMAL STRUCTURE AND FUNCTION

The pancreas is a relatively small (<110 gm) but versatile organ containing two specific and seemingly independent components: the endocrine pancreas and the exocrine pancreas. The endocrine pancreas consists of the islets of Langerhans, packets of endocrine cells scattered throughout the pancreas that secrete insulin, glucagon, and other polypeptide hormones. The endocrine pancreas is discussed in other chapters. The cells of the exocrine pancreas cluster into acini that are further grouped into lobules. Acinar cells are drained by ductules that converge into large ducts, which terminate in the duct of Wirsung, the main pancreatic duct. Pancreatic juice ultimately drains through the sphincter of Oddi and papilla into the second portion of the duodenum. In addition, the minor accessory duct (duct of Santorini) joins the main pancreatic duct in the head of the gland and runs a separate course through the head of the pancreas, entering the duodenum through the minor ampulla several centimeters cephalad. The minor pancreatic duct remains patent in approximately 70% of people. The head of the pancreas lies within the curvature of the second duodenum, with the body and tail extending retroperitoneally to the hilum of the spleen for a total of 12 to 15 cm (Fig. 38–1). The head of the pancreas is in close anatomic relationship to a number of important structures, including the common bile duct, inferior vena cava, aorta, and origin of the superior messenteric artery, splenic artery and vein, and right adrenal gland and kidney.

When stimulated, the normal pancreas may secrete a large volume (>7 L/day) of a characteristic fluid.

Electrolyte Composition

Pancreatic juice is isotonic with extracellular fluid at all rates of secretion. The concentrations of the two principal anions, namely bicarbonate (HCO_3^-) and chloride (Cl^-) vary reciprocally, totaling about 150 mEq/L. The centroacinar and ductular cells add HCO_3^- to the Cl^--rich juice from the acini, and at maximal flow rates the concentration of HCO_3^- approaches 130 mEq/L, resulting in an alkaline pancreatic juice. This HCO_3^--rich fluid neutralizes hydrochloric acid entering the second duodenum from the stomach and raises the intraluminal pH to levels at which the pancreatic enzymes become catalytically active (pH > 3.5 to 4.0).

Protein Content

Pancreatic juice is rich in proteins and is composed primarily of digestive enzymes and proenzymes (inactive until converted into the active form in the small intestine), which are secreted by the acinar cells. Enzymes released in an active form include lipase, amylase, and ribonuclease, whereas the inactive forms include proteases and phospholipase. Inactive enzymes secreted into the duodenum are activated in a cascade fashion: enterokinase converts trypsinogen to trypsin; trypsin then activates all other proenzymes. Colipase (which enhances the activity of lipase) and trypsin inhibitors are also secreted by the pancreas.

Control of Secretion

Pancreatic enzyme secretion is stimulated by a number of factors. Most secretion occurs in the postprandial state in response to one or more stimuli:

1. Hormones—cholecystokinin (CCK), which stimulates a fluid rich in protein (enzymes), and secretin, which stimulates an HCO_3^--rich fluid, are the two most important stimulators. Both are released from cells of the proximal intestine. CCK may also potentiate the action of secretin.
2. Vagal cholinergic stimulation—vagal stimulation is in part responsible for basal secretion. Vagal stimulation also enhances enzyme secretion as well as the response to CCK.
3. Feedback inhibition—human studies have documented a feedback loop whereby intraduodenal protease activity (i.e., trypsin) suppresses circulating CCK levels. This may be important in patients with chronic pancreatitis, in whom continued stimulation (due to loss of intraduodenal protease activity) may cause abdominal pain.

Studies of Pancreatic Structure and Function

Until the development of ultrasonography (US) and computed tomography (CT), the pancreas was a relatively "invisible" organ. Now the pancreas can be examined invasively with endosocopic retrograde cholangiopancreatography (ERCP) and noninvasively with US and CT

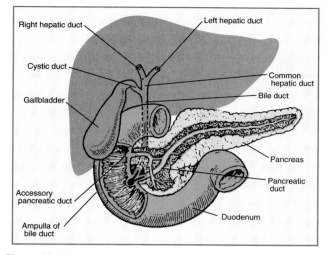

Figure 38–1
Connections of the ducts of the gallbladder, liver, and pancreas. (From Bell GH, Emslie-Smith D, Paterson CR: Textbook of Physiology and Biochemistry. 9th ed. Edinburgh. Churchill Livingstone, 1976; with permission.)

(Fig. 38–2). Pancreatic stones can be removed, pancreatic pseudocysts can be drained, and pancreatic ductal strictures can be stented nonsurgically at the time of ERCP. Percutaneous biopsy as well as drainage of infected cysts can also be accomplished using US and CT. Magnetic resonance imaging (MRI) may be a useful diagnostic tool in the future.

Pancreatic enzymes can be measured in the blood or in the gastrointestinal (GI) fluid. Acute injury to the pancreatic acini results in leakage of the enzyme amylase into the blood, which is measured clinically as an increase in the serum amylase. Approximately two thirds of normal serum amylase (25 to 125 U/L) originates from the salivary glands. In addition to amylase, lipase and trypsinogen are also released into the blood stream with pancreatic injury. Pancreatic secretion can be estimated by aspirating duodenal contents through a tube following stimulation with secretin, secretin-CCK, or a test meal. These tests are cumbersome and are performed only at specialized centers. The bentiromide test, which measures the intestinal hydrolysis of a synthetic peptide by pancreatic chymotrypsin, is described in Chapter 32C on malabsorption. This widely available test is specific but relatively insensitive. These quantitative studies of secretion are performed to determine the presence or absence of pancreatic exocrine insufficiency.

ACUTE PANCREATITIS

Definition

Acute pancreatitis is an inflammatory disorder of the pancreas associated with edema, various amounts of autodigestion, necrosis, and, in some cases, hemorrhage. Clinically, it is defined by a typical symptom complex associated with an elevated serum amylase level. Patho-

physiologically, it is a single entity with varying etiologies, degrees of severity, and the potential to progress to chronic pancreatitis.

Etiology and Pathogenesis

The risk factors associated with acute pancreatitis are listed in Table 38–1. In the United States, the two most common causes of the disease are alcoholism and common bile duct stone disease. Acute pancreatitis is thought to result from inappropriate intrapancreatic activation of proteases, which causes autodigestion of the gland (Fig. 38–3). How this occurs and how these diverse causes culminate in a common end point—namely, pancreatic inflammatory disease—is unknown. Postulated mechanisms of alcohol-induced pancreatitis include physiochemical alterations of protein resulting in plugs that block the small pancreatic ductules and free radical mechanisms. Biliary pancreatitis occurs when a stone passes through the ampulla of Vater, causing an intermittent obstruction. However, the precise mechanisms causing biliary pancreatitis are not fully understood; simply ligating the pancreatic duct or diverting bile through the pancreas does not typically result in pancreatitis. Further episodes may be prevented by removing the risk factors associated with this disorder.

Clinical Manifestations

The cardinal symptom of acute pancreatitis is abdominal pain that is usually constant, moderate to severe although occasionally mild, and located in the epigastrium, frequently radiating to the back. The pain may be relieved by leaning forward. Nausea and vomiting are prominent associated symptoms. On examination the abdomen is usually tender but without signs of peritoneal irritation. In

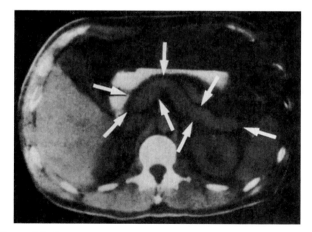

Figure 38–2
Normal pancreas demonstrated by computed tomography. (Courtesy of Dr. Eugene P. DiMagno, Mayo Medical School, Rochester, Minnesota.) (Reprinted from Grendell JH: The pancreas. *In* Smith LH Jr, Thier SO [eds.]: Pathophysiology: The Biological Principles of Disease. 2nd ed. Philadelphia, WB Saunders, 1985, p 1225.)

TABLE 38-1	Conditions Associated with Acute Pancreatitis

* Ethanol abuse
  Cholelithiasis
* Abdominal trauma
  Abdominal surgery
  Hypercalcemia
  Hyperlipidemia
  Drugs—anticonvulsant (valproic acid), antibiotics (sulfonamides, tetracycline), antimetabolite (6-mercaptopurine), diuretics (hydrochlorothiazide, furosemide)
  Viral infections—mumps, coxsackie, hepatitis, others
  Scorpion bite
  Carcinoma of the pancreas
* Pancreas divisum
  Peptic ulcer with posterior penetration
* Hereditary (familial) pancreatitis
  Endoscopic retrograde cholangiopancreatography (ERCP)
  Hypoperfusion (vasculitis)

* Associated with chronic pancreatitis.

severe cases, physical findings may include peritoneal signs, ileus, high fever, confusion, and tachycardia with impending hypovolemic shock. Uncommon manifestations resulting from the peripancreatic inflammatory processes include (1) left-sided pleural effusion; (2) discoloration of the flanks (Grey Turner's sign) or around the umbilicus (Cullen's sign) in hemorrhagic pancreatitis; (3) ascites; (4) jaundice from impingement on the common bile duct; and (5) epigastric mass from a pseudocyst. Those resulting from the systemic effects of pancreatic enzymes released into the blood stream include (1) respiratory distress syndrome; (2) renal failure; and (3) subcutaneous fat necrosis.

Diagnosis

Acute pancreatitis should be considered in any patient having an acute onset of severe continuous epigastric pain, especially when it is associated with any of the known risk factors (see Table 38–1). In the patient with moderately severe abdominal pain, the differential diagnosis includes a perforated viscus (especially peptic ulcer disease), acute cholecystitis, acute bowel infarction, and a variety of other causes of the "acute abdomen."

The gold standard for diagnosis is an elevation of the serum amylase level. However, the serum amylase may be normal in up to one third of patients having alcoholic pancreatitis and mildly elevated in those having abdominal pain as a consequence of another process (Table 38–2). Therefore, CT studies may be needed to document an enlarged pancreas to confirm the diagnosis. In acute pancreatitis, the serum amylase level usually rises

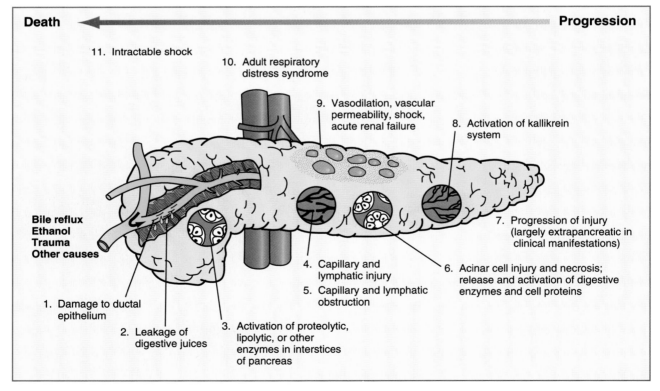

Figure 38-3
The pathophysiology of acute pancreatitis is not fully understood, but, as this schematic implies, a cascade of events seems likely, beginning with the release of toxic substances into the parenchyma and ending with shock and death. Damage to the ductal epithelium or acinar cell injury may result from bile reflux, increased intraductal pressure, alcohol, or trauma. (Modified from Grendell JH: The pancreas. *In* Smith LH Jr, Thier SO [eds.]: Pathophysiology: The Biological Principles of Disease. 2nd ed. Philadelphia, WB Saunders, 1985, p 1228.)

TABLE 38-2	Causes of Hyperamylasemia Other Than Acute Pancreatitis

Pancreatic Amylase

Pancreatic pseudocyst
Gastric, duodenal, small bowel
  perforation
Mesenteric infarction
Opiate administration
Following ERCP

Nonpancreatic Amylase

Salivary adenitis
Diabetic ketoacidosis
Lactic acidosis
Renal insufficiency
Ectopic pregnancy (ruptured)
Postoperative state

ERCP = Endoscopic retrograde cholangiopancreatography.

rapidly, as does the serum lipase, and may remain elevated for 3 to 5 days, but its absolute level of elevation does not correlate with severity. The serum lipase may occasionally be elevated even after the serum amylase has returned to normal.

Although urinary clearance of amylase rises with an attack of acute pancreatitis, measurements of this parameter yield little diagnostic information, in contrast to that obtained by measuring the serum lipase alone. In fact, measuring the urinary clearance of amylase is more helpful in the diagnosis of macroamylasemia. Other laboratory abnormalities may include hyperglycemia, hypocalcemia, and leukocytosis. Concomitant elevations of the aminotransferases, alkaline phosphatase, and bilirubin, which may be both striking and transient, suggest gallstone disease.

Treatment and Prognosis

Because the pathogenesis of pancreatitis is not completely understood, no specific therapy exists that can abort the inflammatory cascade. Treatment remains largely supportive: (1) careful monitoring of volume status because large volumes of fluid may be lost in the retroperitoneum from the "chemical burn"; (2) pain relief, preferably using meperidine; (3) nasogastric suction, which "puts the pancreas at rest" (useful primarily in the patient with associated nausea and vomiting or a severe attack); and (4) treatment of complications. Other measures such as empiric antibiotics, H₂-blocker therapy, and octreotide therapy are without proven benefit.

The patient's prognosis may be estimated at the time of admission and at 48 hours by using the Ranson criteria (Table 38–3). A patient having fewer than three criteria on admission has a mortality rate of < 1%; 40% if five or six signs are positive; and 100% if seven or more signs are positive. *In general, however, the mortality rate of acute pancreatitis is approximately 10% with approximately 90% recovery within the first 2 weeks.* In the early phases of the disease, hemodynamic instability, pulmo-

nary compromise, or renal failure results in death, whereas infection is the most common late complication causing death.

Complications

The local and systemic complications of acute pancreatitis are listed in Table 38–4. A pseudocyst is a liquefied collection of necrotic debris and pancreatic enzymes that is surrounded by either a rim of pancreatic tissue or some adjacent tissues; it contains no true epithelial lining. The spontaneous disappearance of a pseudocyst depends on a number of factors including, most importantly, the size of the cyst and whether it occurred in the setting of acute or chronic pancreatitis. The complications of a pseudocyst include infection, bleeding, and rupture into the peritoneum. A pancreatic abscess is a localized infection of the pancreas that usually occurs late in the course of a severe attack and may result in death unless surgical debridement is performed. Infection of necrotic tissue, termed infected pancreatic necrosis, may occur as early as 1 week in the course of pancreatitis. Early diagnosis and appropriate management of these infectious complications are important for improving the survival of patients with severe pancreatitis.

CHRONIC PANCREATITIS

Definition

Chronic pancreatitis represents a slowly progressive destruction of the pancreatic acini, with varying amounts of inflammation, fibrosis, and dilation and distortion of the pancreatic ducts. Chronic relapsing pancreatitis is defined as superimposed acute attacks that occur in the setting of chronic pancreatitis. Varying degrees of pancreatic destruction and exocrine/endocrine insufficiency result.

TABLE 38-3	Signs Used to Assess Severity of Acute Pancreatitis

At Time of Admission or Diagnosis

Age > 55 year
White blood cell count > 16,000/mm³
Blood glucose > 200 mg/dl
LDH > 2× normal
ALT > 6× normal

During Initial 48 Hours

Decrease in hematocrit > 10%
Serum calcium < 8 mg/dl
Increase in blood urea nitrogen > 5 mg/dl
Arterial Po₂ < 60 mm/Hg
Base deficit > 4 mEq/L
Estimated fluid sequestration > 600 mL

Modified from Ranson JH, Rifkind KM, Turner JW: Prognostic signs and nonoperative peritoneal lavage in acute pancreatitis. Surg Gynecol Obstet 1976; 43:209–219. By permission of Surgery, Gynecology and Obstetrics.

TABLE 38–4	Complications of Acute Pancreatitis

Local

Pancreatic

Phlegmon
Pancreatic fluid collection and pseudocyst complicated by
  bleeding, infection, rupture, pain, or weight loss
Pancreatic abscess and infected necrosis

Nonpancreatic

Pancreatic ascites or pleural effusion
Bile duct obstruction
Colonic obstruction or stricture

Cardiovascular

Hypotension and shock
Electrocardiographic changes
Pericardial effusion and tamponade

Pulmonary

Hypoxia
Atelectasis, pneumonia
Pleural effusion
Adult respiratory distress syndrome (ARDS)
Respiratory failure

Metabolic

Hypocalcemia
Hyperglycemia
Hypertriglyceridemia
Metabolic acidosis

Renal

Oliguria
Azotemia
Acute tubular necrosis
Renal artery or vein thrombosis

Hematologic/coagulation

Vascular thrombosis
Disseminated intravascular coagulation (DIC)

Gastrointestinal bleeding

Other

Fat necrosis
Encephalopathy
Sudden blindness

Adapted from Formark CE, Grendell JH: Complications of pancreatitis. Semin Gastrointest Dis 1991; 2:166; with permission.

Etiology and Pathogenesis

Many of the same conditions listed in Table 38–1 are associated with chronic pancreatitis. In general, biliary tract disease is not associated with chronic pancreatitis. In the United States, the most common cause of chronic pancreatitis is alcoholism in adults and cystic fibrosis in children. In developing countries, protein-calorie malnutrition is the main cause. However, in some cases of chronic pancreatitis the etiology is unknown; the pathophysiologic mechanisms underlying the persistent inflammation and destruction of the gland are poorly understood.

Clinical Manifestations

The most important symptoms and signs of chronic pancreatitis are listed in Table 38–5. In general, moderate to severe intractable abdominal pain is the most frequent finding, although the pain may be mild or even absent in some patients or episodic in relapsing pancreatitis. The pain may persist for a number of years before other manifestations such as pancreatic calcifications, diabetes, or malabsorption appear. Rarely, these later signs may be the initial manifestation in the absence of abdominal pain. The pain may be located primarily in the back or may radiate to the back, as in acute pancreatitis. Weight loss may result from anorexia or associated malabsorption (steatorrhea and azotorrhea).

Given the location of the pancreas and its adjacent structures, progressive inflammatory disease may result in encasement of the common bile duct with fibrosis leading to obstructive jaundice. GI bleeding may result from splenic vein thrombosis with formation of gastric varices and subsequent hemorrhage or a pseudoaneurysm of a large artery in the peripancreatic area, leading to massive hemorrhage. Abdominal pain and an associated abdominal mass may be present with a pseudocyst. When there is >90% destruction of the gland, malabsorption and endocrine insufficiency with diabetes mellitus result.

Diagnosis

The diagnosis of chronic pancreatitis is usually considered in the patient with chronic abdominal pain and an associated risk factor for chronic pancreatitis combined with pancreatic calcifications, exocrine insufficiency (malabsorption), and diabetes mellitus. However, the spectrum of presentations is broad; some patients present with diabetes, and others are found incidentally to have pancreatic calcification in the absence of any specific symptoms or signs. In the patient with abdominal pain and weight loss, the differential diagnosis includes abdominal malignancies, especially carcinoma of the pancreas, stomach, or colon. Other causes of persistent epigastric abdominal pain include peptic ulcer disease, mesenteric ischemic disease, and even functional abdominal complaints when the pain is mild.

In contrast to acute pancreatitis, chronic pancreatitis does not usually produce an elevated serum amylase level unless associated with a distinct attack. Thus, the diagnosis is often established by the clinical presentation in combination with imaging studies of the pancreas. Imaging studies may demonstrate (1) pancreatic calcifica-

TABLE 38–5	Symptoms and Signs of Chronic Pancreatitis

Abdominal pain
Weight loss
Diabetes mellitus
Steatorrhea
Jaundice
Palpable pseudocyst
Pancreatic ascites
Gastrointestinal bleeding

tion by plain abdominal radiography, US, or CT; (2) dilated pancreatic ducts by US or CT but best shown by ERCP; and (3) abnormal pancreatic ductal features by ERCP.

Malabsorption can be documented by fecal analysis for fat and its pancreatic origin deduced by the tests described in Chapter 32C. Pancreatic stimulation tests demonstrate reduction in pancreatic juice volume, HCO_3^- content, amylase output, and tryptic activity.

Treatment and Prognosis

The treatment of chronic pancreatitis is directed toward preventing further pancreatic injury, relieving pain, and replacing lost endocrine/exocrine function. Further injury to the pancreas may be prevented if any of the factors in Table 38–1 can be reversed, especially alcohol abuse, although changing this pattern yields inconsistent results. Despite abstinence from alcohol, most cases of acute alcoholic pancreatitis result in chronic pancreatitis. The replacement of lost exocrine function is described in Chapter 32C on malabsorption. Treatment of chronic abdominal pain in the setting of chronic pancreatitis is often frustrating and represents a difficult challenge. General approaches include the following:

1. Analgesics—attempts should be made to begin with nonaddictive analgesics before administering narcotics. However, severe pain may require narcotics that carry the potential for addiction.
2. "Putting the pancreas at rest"—large doses of supplemental pancreatic enzymes may reduce abdominal pain. This has been best established in patients with idiopathic pancreatitis, with little documented efficacy in those with alcoholic chronic pancreatitis. Avoidance of alcohol may prevent further exacerbations of abdominal pain and acute episodes of pancreatitis.
3. Surgical therapy—intractable pain may require surgical drainage of a presumed obstruction or of an associated pseudocyst, although the long-term results are variable. Partial resection of the gland itself should be based on the location of the ductal changes as assessed by ERCP.

Although the mechanism is unclear, the pain of chronic pancreatitis decreases over time in some patients. When this situation occurs, endocrine and exocrine insufficiencies become the more important management problems.

Complications

The complications associated with chronic pancreatitis are listed in Table 38–6. In contrast to those occurring in acute pancreatitis, these complications are related primarily to destruction of the gland itself and associated peripancreatic diseases rather than to systemic processes.

CARCINOMA OF THE PANCREAS

Definition

Carcinoma of the pancreas is an almost uniformly fatal malignancy. More than 90% of these tumors are adenocarcinomas arising from the ductal cells. Less common tumors include islet cell tumors, epidermoid tumors, and adenocarcinomas arising from the acinar cells. Carcinoma of the pancreas is now the fourth most common malignant tumor (after tumors of the lung, colon, and breast), accounting for approximately 5% of cancer deaths in the United States.

Etiology and Pathogenesis

The cause of pancreatic carcinoma is unknown. Epidemiologic studies have suggested the following risk factors: advanced age, smoking, diabetes mellitus, some forms of chronic pancreatitis, and certain dietary habits such as increased consumption of animal fat and protein.

Clinical Manifestations

The clinical manifestations tend to be nonspecific and often insidious in nature such that the malignancy has reached an advanced stage by the time of diagnosis. The most common presenting symptoms include epigastric abdominal pain and weight loss. The pain is usually less severe than in acute pancreatitis, is constant, and may radiate to the back. Because the most common location for pancreatic carcinoma is in the head of the gland, obstructive jaundice is a common presenting symptom, often associated with a large palpable gallbladder (Courvoisier's sign). Anorexia, nausea, and vomiting may occur, especially when the tumor obstructs the stomach or duodenum. Emotional disturbances, most commonly depression, have been recognized at the time of diagnosis. Other less common presenting symptoms and signs include migratory thrombophlebitis (Trousseau's sign), acute pancreatitis, diabetes mellitus, paraneoplastic endocrine syndromes (Cushing syndrome, hypercalcemia), GI bleeding resulting from splenic vein thrombosis or involvement of the stomach, and a palpable abdominal mass. Rarely, with adenocarcinoma, fat necrosis may produce painful subcutaneous nodules or bone pain from intramedullary involvement.

TABLE 38–6	Complications of Chronic Pancreatitis

Pseudocyst formation
Pancreatic ascites
Common bile duct obstruction
Diabetes mellitus
Splenic vein thrombosis
Exocrine insufficiency
Peptic ulcer

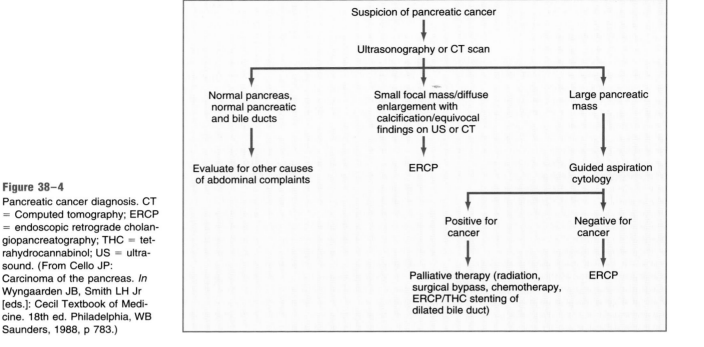

Figure 38–4
Pancreatic cancer diagnosis. CT = Computed tomography; ERCP = endoscopic retrograde cholangiopancreatography; THC = tetrahydrocannabinol; US = ultrasound. (From Cello JP: Carcinoma of the pancreas. *In* Wyngaarden JB, Smith LH Jr [eds.]: Cecil Textbook of Medicine. 18th ed. Philadelphia, WB Saunders, 1988, p 783.)

Diagnosis

Pancreatic carcinoma should always be considered in the elderly patient who presents with abdominal pain, weight loss, depression associated with weight loss, the sudden onset of diabetes mellitus or acute pancreatitis without other known risk factors, or obstructive jaundice. If the tumor is located in the head of the gland, laboratory studies may document obstructive jaundice. CA19-9 holds promise as a diagnostic tumor marker in some cases.

The diagnosis is often suggested clinically, but either invasive or noninvasive imaging studies are necessary to establish the diagnosis. When an abdominal mass is identified by CT, fine-needle aspiration biopsy may be performed. Figure 38–4 provides an algorithm for using these modalities. The sensitivity of US for the diagnosis of pancreatic carcinoma is less than that of CT (>80%). ERCP has a sensitivity of >90% because it reliably detects carcinomas arising from ductal cells. Arteriography is rarely required. Endoscopic US is emerging as the most sensitive technique to determine resectability for cure.

Treatment and Prognosis

The therapy for pancreatic carcinoma is frustrating and disappointing. The tumor is often metastatic at the time of diagnosis, and thus surgical resection for cure is unusual. Surgery is often performed for palliation, especially in the patient with intestinal or gastric outlet obstruction or biliary obstruction. Decompression of the biliary system may provide relief from jaundice, severe pruritus, or

cholangitis. ERCP with an endoprosthesis (stent) placed through the tumor-encased bile duct provides a viable alternative. Surgery and endoscopic palliation are equivalent in terms of mortality. Radiation therapy or chemotherapy may be palliative in some patients but is often ineffective. In those few patients who have the potential for a curative resection, the 5-year survival rate is >50%; in general, however, the 5-year survival rate is <5%.

Complications

The complications of carcinoma have been discussed as part of the clinical manifestations. The most common site of metastatic disease is the liver.

REFERENCES

Cello JP: Carcinoma of the pancreas. *In* Sleisenger MH, Fordtran JS (eds.): Gastrointestinal Disease: Pathophysiology, Diagnosis, and Management. 5th ed. Philadelphia, WB Saunders, 1993, pp 1682–1694.

DiMagno EP: Carcinoma of the pancreas. *In* Bennett JC, Plum F (eds.): Cecil Textbook of Medicine. 20th ed. Philadelphia, WB Saunders, 1996, p 736.

Grendell JH, Cello JP: Chronic pancreatitis. *In* Sleisenger MH, Fordtran JS (eds.): Gastrointestinal Disease: Pathophysiology, Diagnosis, and Management. 5th ed. Philadelphia, WB Saunders, 1993, pp 1654–1681.

Soergel KH: Acute pancreatitis. *In* Sleisenger MH, Fordtran JS (eds.): Gastrointestinal Disease: Pathophysiology, Diagnosis, and Management, 5th ed. Philadelphia, WB Saunders, 1993, pp 1628–1653.

Soergel KH: Pancreatitis. *In* Bennett JC, Plum F (eds.): Cecil Textbook of Medicine, 20th ed. Philadelphia, WB Saunders, 1996, p 729.

Diseases of the Liver and Biliary System

Section VI

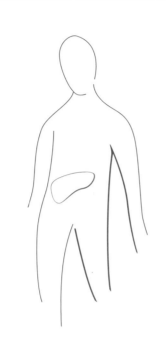

39

Laboratory Tests in Liver Disease

The liver, the largest internal organ in the body, plays a central role in many essential physiologic processes, including glucose homeostasis, plasma protein synthesis, lipid and lipoprotein synthesis, bile acid synthesis and secretion, and vitamin storage (B_{12}, A, D, E, and K), as well as biotransformation, detoxification, and excretion of a vast array of endogenous and exogenous compounds. The clinical manifestations of liver disease are, likewise, varied and may be quite subtle. Clues to the existence, severity, and etiology of liver disease may be obtained from a careful history and physical examination as well as by routine laboratory screening tests. Clinical clues to the presence of liver disease are briefly mentioned here and are discussed more fully in other chapters. This chapter focuses on the use of laboratory tests for evaluating liver disease.

CLINICAL APPROACH TO LIVER DISEASE

Table 39-1 outlines useful clinical clues to the presence of liver disease. Other important historical information to be obtained includes a history of jaundice or liver disease in family members, recent travel, exposure to individuals or animals with liver or parasitic disease, blood transfusions, sexual promiscuity, use of intravenous drugs, and exposure to alcohol, toxins, or drugs.

LABORATORY TESTS OF LIVER FUNCTION AND DISEASE

Unlike tests used to assess function of other organ systems (e.g., arterial blood gas, creatinine clearance), many so-called liver function tests do not directly measure hepatic function and may not accurately reflect etiology or severity of a disease process. Nevertheless, an understanding of the utility of different types of laboratory tests of the liver is extremely important in characterizing underlying liver disease. Tests currently available can be divided into two categories: (1) tests of hepatic function or capacity and (2) screening tests that suggest the presence and/or type of liver disease. Specific diagnostic tests such as serologic tests for viral, autoimmune, and inherited liver disease are covered in other chapters.

TESTS OF HEPATIC FUNCTION

The great variety of functions performed by the liver has made it difficult to devise a simple, cheap, reproducible, and noninvasive test that accurately reflects hepatic capacity for all functions. Instead, currently available tests of liver function are indirect, static measurements of serum levels of compounds that are synthesized, metabolized, and/or excreted by the liver. The liver has a large reserve capacity, and therefore results of "function" tests may remain relatively normal until liver dysfunction is severe.

Table 39-2 outlines the most widely available and useful liver function tests. The serum albumin level and prothrombin time (PT) both reflect the hepatic capacity for protein synthesis. The PT, which responds rapidly to altered hepatic function because of the short serum half-lives of Factors II and VII (hours), is useful as frequently as daily as a marker of hepatic function. However, coexistent vitamin K deficiency must be excluded and/or treated prior to using the PT as a measure of hepatic function. In contrast, the serum half-life of albumin is 14 to 20 days, and serum levels fall only with prolonged liver dysfunction. Malnutrition and renal or gastrointestinal losses merit consideration in the setting of significant hypoalbuminemia, especially if the PT is relatively well preserved.

A number of additional functional tests have been developed based on assessment of metabolic capabilities of the liver. The most frequently used such test is the ^{14}C-aminopyrine breath test, which measures the rate at which the liver metabolizes ^{14}C-labeled aminopyrine to $^{14}CO_2$, which is collected and measured in exhaled breath. Other similar tests, including galactose and caffeine clearance, have been developed. These tests are performed only in some academic centers.

SCREENING TESTS OF HEPATOBILIARY DISEASE

Screening tests of hepatobiliary disease (see Table 39-2) may be divided into two categories: (1) tests of biliary obstruction and/or cholestasis and (2) tests of hepatocellular damage, based on the mechanisms responsible for the abnormal test. However, none of the tests is specific for

TABLE 39-1	**Clinical Manifestations of Liver Disease**	
Sign/Symptom	**Pathogenesis**	**Liver Disease**
Constitutional		
Fatigue, anorexia, malaise, weight loss	Liver dysfunction	Acute or chronic hepatitis Cirrhosis
Fever	Hepatic inflammation or infection	Liver abscess Alcoholic hepatitis Viral hepatitis
Fetor hepaticus	Sulfur compounds, produced by intestinal bacteria, not cleared by the liver	Acute or chronic liver failure
Cutaneous		
Spider telangiectasias, palmar erythema	Altered estrogen and androgen metabolism with altered vascular physiology	Cirrhosis
Jaundice	Diminished bilirubin excretion	Biliary obstruction Severe liver disease
Pruritus	Uncertain	Biliary obstruction
Xanthomas and xanthelasma	Increased serum cholesterol	Biliary obstruction/cholestasis
Endocrine		
Gynecomastia, testicular atrophy, diminished libido	Altered estrogen and androgen metabolism	Cirrhosis
Hypoglycemia	Decreased glycogen stores and gluconeogenesis	Acute liver failure Alcohol binge with fasting
Gastrointestinal		
Right upper quadrant abdominal pain	Liver swelling, infection	Acute hepatitis Hepatocellular carcinoma Liver congestion (heart failure) Acute cholecystitis Liver abscess
Abdominal swelling	Ascites	Cirrhosis, portal hypertension
Gastrointestinal bleeding	Esophageal varices	Portal hypertension
Hematologic		
Decreased red cells, white cells, and/or platelets	Hypersplenism	Cirrhosis, portal hypertension
Ecchymoses	Decreased synthesis of clotting factors	Liver failure
Neurologic		
Altered sleep pattern, subtle behavioral changes, somnolence, confusion, ataxia, asterixis, obtundation	Hepatic encephalopathy	Liver failure, portosystemic shunting of blood

extensive list of disorders where bilirubin production (hematologic disorders), hepatic metabolism (congenital abnormalities of bilirubin, liver disease), or excretion (biliary obstruction) are altered. Hence, an elevated serum bilirubin determination is not specific for any etiology of liver disease. However, such an abnormality, especially in association with predominant elevations in other tests of biliary obstruction, should prompt an evaluation for potentially treatable biliary abnormalities. It is important to recognize that serum bilirubin levels may not return

TABLE 39-2	**Clinical Tests of Hepatic Function**	
	Property Examined	**Significance of Abnormal Results**
Tests of Hepatic Function		
(Normal values)		
Serum albumin (3.5–5.5 mg/dl)	Protein synthetic capacity (over days to weeks)	Decreased synthetic capacity Protein malnutrition Increased protein loss (nephrotic syndrome, protein-losing enteropathy) Increased extracellular fluid volume
Prothrombin time (10.5–13 sec)	Protein synthetic capacity (hours to days)	Decreased synthetic capacity (especially Factors II and VII) Vitamin K deficiency Consumptive coagulopathy
^{14}C-aminopyrine breath test (5–19.5% of dose excreted at 2 hr)	Drug-metabolizing capacity	Decreased metabolic capacity (diffuse liver disease) Severe portosystemic shunting of blood
Screening Tests of Hepatobiliary Disease		
Tests of biliary obstruction or impaired bile flow		
Serum bilirubin (0.2–1.0 mg/dl) (3.4–17.1 πmol/L)	Extraction of bilirubin from blood conjugation and excretion into bile	Hemolysis Diffuse liver disease Cholestasis Extrahepatic bile duct obstruction Congenital disorders of bilirubin metabolism
Serum alkaline phosphatase (also 5'-nucleotidase and gamma glutamyl transpeptidase) (56–176 U/L)	Increased enzyme synthesis and release	Bile duct obstruction Cholestasis Infiltrative liver disease (neoplasms, granulomas) Bone destruction/remodeling Pregnancy
Tests of hepatocellular damage		
Aspartate aminotransferase (AST:SGOT) (10–30 U/L)	Release of intracellular enzyme	Hepatocellular necrosis Cardiac or skeletal muscle necrosis
Alanine aminotransferase (ALT:SGPT) (5–30 U/L)	Release of intracellular enzyme	Same as AST: however, more specific for liver cell damage

either category, and it is the overall pattern and the relative magnitude of abnormalities in these two categories of tests that often provide diagnostic clues to the type of liver disease present.

The *serum bilirubin* level reflects a balance between bilirubin production and its conjugation and excretion into bile by the liver. The differential diagnosis for hyperbilirubinemia (see Chapter 40) requires consideration of an

TABLE 39–3	Characteristic Patterns of Liver Function Tests					
Disorder	**Bilirubin**	**Alkaline Phosphatase**	**AST**	**ALT**	**Prothrombin Time**	**Albumin**
Gilbert's syndrome (abnormal bilirubin metabolism)	↑	NL	NL	NL	NL	NL
Bile duct obstruction (pancreatic cancer)	↑↑↑	↑↑↑	↑	↑	↑–↑↑	NL
Acute hepatocellular damage (toxic, viral hepatitis)	↑–↑↑↑	↑–↑↑	↑↑↑	↑↑↑	NL–↑↑↑	NL–↓↓
Cirrhosis	NL–↑	NL–↑	NL–↑	NL–↑	NL–↑↑	NL–↓↓

ALT = Alanine aminotransferase; AST = aspartate aminotransferase; NL = normal; ↑ = increase; ↓ = decrease (arrows indicate extent of change: ↑–↑↑↑ = slight to large.

promptly to normal after relief of biliary obstruction or improvement in liver disease because some bilirubin binds covalently to albumin and is removed from the circulation only as albumin is catabolized (half-life, 14 to 20 days).

Serum alkaline phosphatase activity reflects a group of isoenzymes derived from liver, bone, intestine, and placenta. Serum levels are elevated in association with a variety of conditions including cholestasis, partial or complete bile duct obstruction, bone regeneration, pregnancy, and also with neoplastic, infiltrative, and granulomatous liver diseases. An isolated elevated alkaline phosphatase level may be the only clue to partial obstruction of the common bile duct, to obstruction of ducts in a single lobe or segment of liver, or to neoplastic or granulomatous hepatic disease. In cholestasis, serum alkaline phosphatase levels rise due to retention of bile acids in the liver, which solubilize alkaline phosphatase off the hepatocyte plasma membrane as well as stimulating its synthesis. 5′-Nucleotidase and gamma glutamyl transpeptidase, other hepatocyte plasma membrane enzymes, are similarly released into the circulation during bile duct obstruction or cholestasis and are used to confirm that an elevated alkaline phosphatase level is due to hepatobiliary disease. Many patients with elevated alkaline phosphatase levels who are suspected of having hepatobiliary disease may require endoscopic retrograde cholangiopancreatography to visualize abnormalities in the biliary system.

Aspartate (AST, SGOT) and *alanine* (ALT, SGPT) *aminotransferases* are intracellular aminotransferring enzymes present in large quantities in hepatocytes. Following injury or death of liver cells, they are released into the circulation. In general, the serum transaminases are sensitive (albeit nonspecific) tests of liver damage, and the height of the serum transaminase activity reflects the severity of hepatic necrosis, but there are important exceptions. For instance, both enzymes require pyridoxal 5′-phosphate as a cofactor, and the relatively low serum transaminase values seen in patients with severe alcoholic hepatitis (often <300 U/L) may reflect deficiency of this cofactor. Although transaminase levels are increased in a wide array of liver diseases, high levels (>15 times the upper limit of normal) infrequently indicate acute bile duct obstruction or hepatic ischemia and generally indicate acute hepatocellular necrosis from viral or toxic causes. Patients who present with isolated asymptomatic elevations of aspartate aminotransferase and alanine aminotransferase may have fatty liver (due to obesity or alcohol intake) and hepatocellular disease, such as hemochromatosis or chronic viral hepatitis, and should be screened for treatable diseases. Some patients may require liver biopsy.

Individual liver function tests frequently do not indicate the nature of the underlying liver disease. However, the overall *pattern* of liver test abnormalities and the relative magnitude of abnormalities in individual tests often provide significant insight into the nature of the liver disease. Table 39–3 outlines common patterns of liver test abnormalities.

LIVER BIOPSY

Biopsy and histologic examination of liver tissue are frequently valuable in the differential diagnosis and treatment of diffuse or localized parenchymal diseases (e.g., cirrhosis, hepatitis, hemochromatosis, tumors) or hepatomegaly. Liver biopsy is generally safe (serious complications <0.5%); however, it is contraindicated in uncooperative patients and those with significant coagulation abnormalities or thrombocytopenia.

REFERENCES

Stolz A, Kaplowitz N: Biochemical tests for liver disease. *In* Zakim D, Boyer T (eds.): Hepatology: A Textbook of Liver Disease. 2nd ed. Philadelphia, WB Saunders, 1990, pp 637–667.

Weisiger RA: Laboratory tests in liver disease. *In* Bennett JC, Plum F (eds.): Cecil Textbook of Medicine. 20th ed. Philadelphia, WB Saunders, 1996, pp 759–762.

40

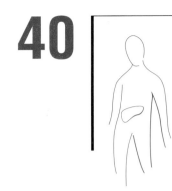

Jaundice

DEFINITION

The term *jaundice,* or *icterus,* describes the yellow pigmentation of skin, sclerae, and mucous membranes produced by increased serum bilirubin (hyperbilirubinemia). Jaundice is a common sign of a variety of liver and biliary diseases and serves as a starting point for evaluating many of these disorders. Serum bilirubin normally ranges from 0.5 to 1.0 mg/dl. Jaundice usually becomes clinically evident at levels >2.5 mg/dl and is most readily detected in the sclerae.

BILIRUBIN METABOLISM

About 4 mg/kg of bilirubin is produced each day, mainly (80 to 85%) derived from the catabolism of the hemoglobin heme group of senescent red blood cells. The heme ring is cleaved in the reticuloendothelial system to form biliverdin, which in turn is oxidized to bilirubin, a water-insoluble tetrapyrrole. A smaller proportion of bilirubin (15 to 20%) is derived from the destruction of maturing erythroid cells in the bone marrow (ineffective erythropoiesis) and from the heme groups of predominantly hepatic hemoproteins such as cytochrome P-450 and cytochrome *c* (Fig. 40–1).

This unconjugated bilirubin is liberated into the plasma and is transported to the liver bound tightly but reversibly to albumin. Unconjugated bilirubin is apolar and insoluble in water and is virtually incapable of being excreted in the bile or urine. However, it readily dissolves in lipid-rich environments and traverses the blood-brain barrier and placenta. Three phases of hepatic bilirubin metabolism are recognized: (1) uptake, (2) conjugation, and (3) excretion into the bile, the last step being overall rate limiting. Uptake is reversible and follows dissociation of bilirubin from albumin.

Unconjugated bilirubin is rendered water soluble and capable of being excreted in the aqueous bile by its conjugation with a sugar, glucuronic acid. Mono- and diglucuronides of bilirubin are formed in the hepatic endoplasmic reticulum catalyzed by the enzyme uridinediphosphate (UDP)–glucuronyl transferase. If the biliary excretion of conjugated bilirubin is impaired, the pigment regurgitates from hepatocytes into plasma. Conjugated bilirubin is both water soluble and less tightly bound to albumin than unconjugated pigment, so that it is readily filtered by the glomerulus and appears in the urine when plasma levels are increased (see Fig. 40–1). With sustained conjugated hyperbilirubinemia (e.g., obstructive jaundice), a proportion of the conjugated bilirubin becomes covalently bound to albumin and is therefore unavailable for renal or biliary excretion.

Conjugated bilirubin excreted in the bile is not reabsorbed by the intestine but is converted by bacterial action in the gut to colorless tetrapyrroles termed *urobilinogens.* Up to 20% of urobilinogen is reabsorbed and undergoes an enterohepatic circulation, a proportion being excreted in the urine. Thus, both impaired hepatocellular excretion and marked overproduction of bilirubin may lead to increased appearance of urobilinogen in the urine.

LABORATORY TESTS FOR BILIRUBIN

The van den Bergh reaction is the most commonly used test for bilirubin in biologic fluids. When carried out in an aqueous medium, the test shows a colored reaction only with water-soluble bilirubin derivatives (called the *direct* van den Bergh fraction). The addition of methanol enables a colored reaction to take place with water-insoluble bilirubin (called the *indirect* van den Bergh fraction). Direct and indirect van den Bergh fractions provide clinically useful estimations of conjugated and unconjugated bilirubin, respectively. However, the correlation between actual levels of conjugated bilirubin and levels estimated by the direct-reacting fraction is poor. Normal plasma actually contains >95% unconjugated bilirubin.

CLINICAL CLASSIFICATION OF JAUNDICE

A logical first step in studying a jaundiced patient is to determine whether there is an unconjugated or a conjugated hyperbilirubinemia. This question is usually easily resolved by serum testing.

Classification of jaundice according to this distinction is shown in Table 40–1. Mechanisms contributing to predominantly unconjugated hyperbilirubinemia include (1) overproduction, (2) decreased hepatic uptake,

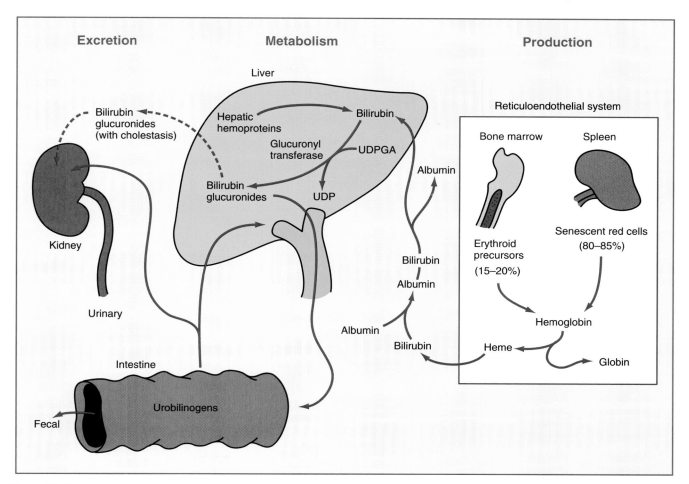

Figure 40-1

Bilirubin production, metabolism, and excretion. UDP = Uridinediphosphate; UDPGA = uridinediphosphate glucuronic acid.

and (3) decreased conjugation. Conjugated hyperbilirubinemia implies either (1) a defect in hepatocellular excretion of bilirubin or (2) mechanical obstruction to the major extrahepatic bile ducts. Occasionally, jaundice may result from a single abnormality in the pathway from bilirubin production to biliary excretion (hemolysis, inherited disorder of bilirubin metabolism), although more frequently there are multiple rather than isolated causes of jaundice (in an individual patient.) For example, the jaundice occurring in patients with hepatocellular disease (i.e., hepatitis, cirrhosis) may result from a combination of diminished red cell survival and impairment of all three stages of hepatocellular bilirubin transport and metabolism.

Unconjugated Hyperbilirubinemia

The causes of unconjugated hyperbilirubinemia are relatively easily determined. These disorders are rarely associated with significant hepatic dysfunction. Several common causes of unconjugated hyperbilirubinemia are discussed here.

Overproduction

Hemolysis from a variety of causes may lead to bilirubin production sufficient to exceed the clearing capacity of the liver, with subsequent development of jaundice. This *hemolytic jaundice* is characteristically mild; serum bilirubin levels rarely exceed 5 mg/dl in the absence of a coexistent hepatic disease. Ineffective erythropoiesis, which may be substantially increased in megaloblastic anemias, may also lead to mild jaundice.

Impaired Hepatic Uptake

Impaired uptake is very rarely encountered as an isolated cause for clinical jaundice, but it may play a role in the mild jaundice following administration of certain drugs,

TABLE 40–1	Classification of Jaundice

Predominantly Unconjugated Hyperbilirubinemia

Overproduction
    Hemolysis (spherocytosis, autoimmune disorders, etc.)
    Ineffective erythropoiesis (e.g., megaloblastic anemias)
Decreased hepatic uptake
    Gilbert's syndrome
    Drugs (e.g., rifampin, radiographic contrast agents)
    Neonatal jaundice
Decreased conjugation
    Gilbert's syndrome
    Crigler-Najjar syndrome types I and II
    Neonatal jaundice
    Hepatocellular disease
    Drug inhibition (e.g., chloramphenicol)

Predominantly Conjugated Hyperbilirubinemia

Impaired hepatic excretion
    Familial disorders (Dubin-Johnson syndrome, Rotor syndrome, benign
      recurrent cholestasis, cholestasis of pregnancy)
    Hepatocellular disease
    Drug-induced cholestasis
    Primary biliary cirrhosis
    Sepsis
    Postoperative
Extrahepatic ("mechanical") biliary obstruction
    Gallstones
    Tumors of head of pancreas
    Tumors of bile ducts
    Tumors of ampulla of Vater
    Biliary strictures (postcholecystectomy, primary sclerosing cholangitis)
    Congenital disorders (biliary atresia)

such as rifampin (competition for bilirubin uptake) and in Gilbert's syndrome (see later).

Impaired Conjugation

A genetically determined decrease or absence of UDP-glucuronyl transferase is encountered in the Crigler-Najjar syndrome, whereas mild, acquired defects in the enzyme may be produced by drugs (e.g., chloramphenicol).

Neonatal Jaundice

All steps of hepatic bilirubin metabolism are incompletely developed in the neonatal period, while production is also increased. The major defect is in conjugation, however, leading to the common finding of mild to moderate unconjugated hyperbilirubinemia between the second and fifth days of life. When significant increased production of bilirubin occurs in the neonatal period (hemolytic disease secondary to blood group incompatibility), severe unconjugated hyperbilirubinemia may occur, carrying the risk of neurologic damage (kernicterus).

Gilbert's Syndrome

This very common disorder affects up to 7% of the population, with a marked male predominance. It commonly manifests during the teens or 20s as mild unconjugated hyperbilirubinemia, exacerbated by fasting, and noted clinically or as an incidental laboratory finding. The mechanism appears to involve increased production, diminished uptake, and defective conjugation of bilirubin to varying proportions in different individuals. Nonspecific gastrointestinal symptoms and fatigue are commonly associated, but the condition is entirely benign. The diagnosis is strongly suggested by unconjugated hyperbilirubinemia with normal hepatic enzymes and the absence of overt hemolysis. Liver biopsy is generally not indicated to confirm the diagnosis.

Conjugated Hyperbilirubinemia

Conjugated hyperbilirubinemia indicates either impaired hepatic excretion or altered biliary drainage of bilirubin. This finding frequently occurs in the setting of impaired formation or excretion of all components of bile, a situation termed *cholestasis.* However, it may also occur due to hepatocellular injury independent of cholestasis. Frequently, the clinical challenge in patients with *cholestatic jaundice* is distinguishing whether hyperbilirubinemia results from an intrahepatic defect or extrahepatic biliary obstruction.

Typically in cholestatic jaundice, the alkaline phosphatase is increased to three to four times normal along with conjugated hyperbilirubinemia (see Chapter 39). When prolonged, cholestasis may lead to hypercholesterolemia, malabsorption of fat and fat-soluble vitamins, and retention of bile salts, which may lead to pruritus. Biochemical evidence of liver cell damage (elevated transaminases, prolonged prothrombin time uncorrected by administration of vitamin K) may be minimal or marked, depending upon the cause of the cholestasis. In some forms of cholestasis, bilirubin metabolism and excretion are well preserved, and these patients may have all the features of cholestasis without jaundice.

Impaired Hepatic Excretion

This pathogenetic category of jaundice, also called intrahepatic cholestasis, is applied to all disorders in the transport of conjugated bilirubin from the hepatocyte to the radiologically visible intrahepatic bile ducts. Thus it includes a wide range of conditions from drug-induced cholestasis (impaired canalicular transport) to primary biliary cirrhosis (destruction of the small intrahepatic bile ductules). The following are some important causes of intrahepatic cholestasis.

DRUG-INDUCED CHOLESTASIS. Typical cholestatic jaundice may be produced by a wide array of drugs, including phenothiazines, oral contraceptives, and methyltestosterone. Eosinophilia may accompany drug-induced jaundice.

SEPSIS. Systemic sepsis, mainly due to gram-negative organisms, may produce a predominantly conjugated hyperbilirubinemia, usually accompanied by mildly elevated serum alkaline phosphatase levels.

POSTOPERATIVE JAUNDICE. This increasingly recognized syndrome has an incidence of 15% following heart surgery and 1% following elective abdominal surgery. Occurring 1 to 10 days postoperatively and multifactorial in origin, the elevated bilirubin is predominantly of the conjugated variety with increased alkaline phosphatase and minimally abnormal transaminase levels.

HEPATOCELLULAR DISEASE. Hepatocellular disease (i.e., hepatitis and cirrhosis) from a variety of causes (see Chapters 41 and 43) may result in a typical cholestatic jaundice. Evidence of hepatocellular damage and dysfunction is usually prominent and includes elevated transaminases, prolonged prothrombin time, hypoalbuminemia, and clinical features of hepatic dysfunction (see Chapter 42). In hepatocellular disease, all three steps of hepatic bilirubin metabolism are impaired. Excretion, the rate-limiting step, is usually the most profoundly disturbed, leading to a predominantly conjugated hyperbilirubinemia. Jaundice may be profound in acute hepatitis (see Chapter 41) without adverse prognostic implications. In contrast, in chronic liver disease, persistent jaundice usually implies decompensation of hepatic function and a poor prognosis.

Extrahepatic Biliary Obstruction

Complete or partial obstruction of the extrahepatic bile ducts may result from a variety of causes, including impaction of gallstones, carcinoma of the head of the pancreas, tumors of the bile ducts, bile duct strictures, and chronic pancreatitis with bile duct compression. In complete obstruction, conjugated hyperbilirubinemia is prominent and usually plateaus at 30 to 40 mg/dl in the absence of renal failure, hepatocellular damage, or infection within the bile ducts, all of which may develop during the course of mechanical obstruction and cause a further rise in bilirubin. Stools may become clay-colored as a result of the failure of bile to enter the intestine. In partial obstruction, jaundice may be mild or even absent, becoming prominent when infection of the ducts (cholangitis) complicates the obstruction.

APPROACH TO THE DIAGNOSIS OF JAUNDICE

The differential diagnosis of hepatic causes of jaundice applies to those patients with predominately conjugated hyperbilirubinemia. A history of darkened urine invariably implies conjugated hyperbilirubinemia and should prompt evaluation. A careful history and physical examination and judicious use of laboratory studies are of paramount importance in obtaining clues to the nature of jaundice and specifically in determining whether hepatocellular injury, impaired hepatic excretion, or biliary obstruction is involved. A history of pale stools and pruritus suggests cholestasis rather than hepatocellular injury. An inquiry about the use of drugs or alcohol, risk factors for viral hepatitis, and pre-existing liver disease may also provide information regarding potential causes of cholestasis and hepatocellular injury. Recurrent abdominal pain

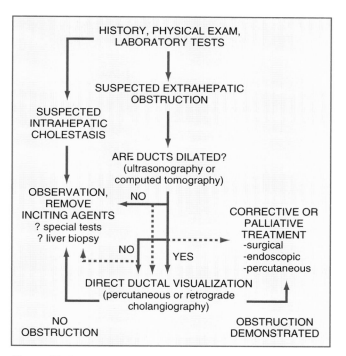

Figure 40-2
Approach to the patient with cholestatic jaundice. The algorithm demonstrates the systematic consideration of the available diagnostic options.

and nausea (gallstones) and epigastric pain radiating to the back with weight loss and gallbladder distention (carcinoma of the pancreatic head) suggest biliary obstruction. Serum transaminases are usually elevated <5- to 10-fold and the alkaline phosphatase levels are usually greater than two to three times normal in patients with biliary obstruction. Conversely, serum transaminases are often elevated >10- to 15-fold and the alkaline phosphatase levels are less than two to three times normal in hepatocellular disease. Further serologic testing for hepatitis (see Chapter 41) and autoantibody testing (antimitochondrial antibody for primary biliary cirrhosis) may also be helpful.

Once initial evaluation has established the presence of cholestatic jaundice, more sophisticated diagnostic procedures are frequently employed to distinguish intrahepatic cholestasis from biliary obstruction and to provide potential treatment in cases of biliary obstruction. A diagnostic approach is outlined in Figure 40-2. If extrahepatic obstruction is suspected, noninvasive means are used to determine whether bile ducts are dilated. In jaundiced patients, dilation of the ducts is usual when a mechanical obstruction is present but is absent in cases of intrahepatic cholestasis. Either ultrasonography or computed tomography (CT) may be used to assess bile ducts, the former preferred because of lower cost and absence of radiation. Additional definitive clues, such as the presence of stones in the common duct or gallbladder, may be obtained as well. If dilated ducts are found on noninvasive imaging, direct cholangiography provides the most reliable approach to nonoperative management and potential treatment of cholestatic jaundice. This may be accomplished by either percutaneous puncture of the intrahepatic biliary tree (percutaneous transhepatic cholangiography) or by endoscopic retrograde cholangiography.

If intrahepatic cholestasis is suspected clinically and extrahepatic obstruction is excluded by noninvasive means and/or direct cholangiography, then liver biopsy is sometimes useful in determining a cause for cholestasis. Regardless, in situations where a potential inciting agent is found, an ideal approach is to discontinue the agent and observe for resolution of jaundice.

REFERENCE

Scharschmidt BF: Bilirubin metabolism, hyperbilirubinemia and the approach to the jaundiced patient. *In* Bennett JC, Plum F (eds.): Cecil Textbook of Medicine. 20th ed. Philadelphia, WB Saunders, 1996, pp 755–759.

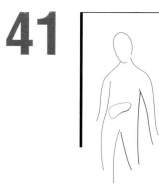

41

Acute and Chronic Hepatitis

DEFINITION

The term *hepatitis* is applied to a broad category of clinicopathologic conditions that result from the damage produced by viral, toxic, pharmacologic, or immune-mediated attack upon the liver. The common pathologic features of hepatitis are hepatocellular necrosis, which may be focal or extensive, and inflammatory cell infiltration of the liver, which may predominate in the portal areas or extend out into the parenchyma. Clinically, the liver may be enlarged and tender with or without jaundice, and laboratory evidence of hepatocellular damage is invariably found in the form of elevated transaminase levels. Independent of its cause, the clinical course of hepatitis may range from mild or inapparent to a dramatic illness with evidence of severe hepatocellular dysfunction, marked jaundice, impairment of coagulation, and disturbance of neurologic function. Hepatitis is further divided into acute and chronic types on the basis of clinical and pathologic criteria.

Acute hepatitis implies a condition lasting less than 6 months, culminating either in complete resolution of the liver damage with return to normal liver function and structure or in rapid progression of the acute injury toward extensive necrosis and a fatal outcome.

Chronic hepatitis is defined as a sustained inflammatory process in the liver lasting longer than 6 months.

It may be impossible to differentiate acute from chronic hepatitis on histologic criteria alone. Inflammatory cells extending beyond the limits of the portal tracts surrounding isolated nests of hepatocytes (piecemeal necrosis) and portal and/or central areas of the hepatic lobules connected by swaths of inflammation, necrosis, and collapse of architecture (bridging necrosis) are seen in liver biopsies taken from patients with severe forms of chronic hepatitis. However, these features may also be seen in uncomplicated acute hepatitis that will ultimately resolve completely. A purely histologic diagnosis of chronic hepatitis usually requires evidence of progression toward cirrhosis, such as significant fibrous scarring and disruption of the hepatic lobular architecture.

ACUTE HEPATITIS

Agents commonly causing acute hepatic injury are listed in Table 41–1. The mechanisms whereby these agents produce hepatic damage include direct toxin-induced necrosis (e.g., acetaminophen, *Amanita phalloides* toxin) and host immune-mediated damage, which probably plays an important, but not well understood, role in viral hepatitis and in some cases of drug-induced hepatitis. In the case of frank hepatotoxins such as *Amanita* poisoning, massive hepatic necrosis is the dominant process, and the clinical course is more aptly described as fulminant hepatic failure (see Chapter 42) rather than acute hepatitis. Such a course is less common but well recognized with all the causative agents listed in Table 41–1.

Acute Viral Hepatitis

Etiology

Viral hepatitis is now recognized to be caused by at least six viruses. Hepatitis viruses A, B, C, D, and E (Table 41–2) have been characterized at the molecular level, and a new virus, hepatitis F, which may be responsible for a significant proportion of blood-borne hepatitis not due to other agents, is presently being characterized. Cytomegalovirus and Epstein-Barr virus occasionally cause hepatitis. Hepatitis D virus, an incomplete RNA virus, causes hepatitis either simultaneously with the B virus or in individuals already chronically infected with the B virus. The hepatitis C virus accounts for the vast majority of cases of hepatitis previously designated "non-A, non-B." The B virus has been most extensively characterized. The complete B virus (Dane particle) consists of several antigenically distinct components (Fig. 41–1), including a surface coat (hepatitis B surface antigen, HBsAg) and a core of circular DNA, DNA polymerase, hepatitis B core antigen (HBcAg), and hepatitis e antigen (HBeAg). HBsAg may exist in serum either as part of the Dane particle or as free particles and rods. Surface antigen, as well as HBcAg and HBeAg, elicit distinct antibody responses from the host, which are valuable in serologic diagnosis and characterization of the state of B virus replication in the liver.

Transmission

Hepatitis A virus (HAV) is excreted in the feces during the incubation period (Fig. 41–2) and is transmitted by

TABLE 41–1	Causes of Acute Hepatitis

Viral Hepatitis

Hepatitis A virus
Hepatitis B virus
Hepatitis C virus
Hepatitis D virus ("delta agent")
Epstein-Barr virus
Cytomegalovirus

Alcohol

Toxins

Amanita phalloides mushroom poisoning
Carbon tetrachloride

Drugs

Acetaminophen
Isoniazid
Halothane
Chlorpromazine
Erythromycin

Other

Wilson's disease

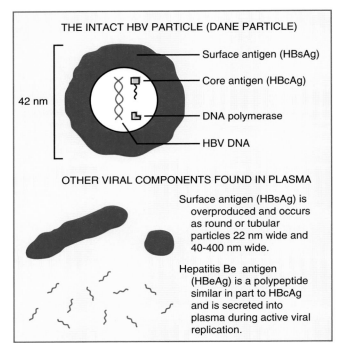

Figure 41–1
Different types of hepatitis B virus (HBV) particles in plasma.

the fecal-oral route. It is thus implicated in most instances of water-borne and food-transmitted infection and in epidemics of viral hepatitis. The hepatitis B virus (HBV) is present in virtually all body fluids and excreta of carriers and is transmitted mainly by parenteral routes. Thus, transmission occurs most commonly via blood and blood products, contaminated needles, and intimate personal contact. Persons at high risk of infection with the B virus therefore include sexual partners of acutely as well as chronically infected individuals, with male homosexuals being at particularly high risk; health professionals, particularly surgeons, dentists, and workers in clinical laboratories and dialysis units; intravenous drug abusers; and infants of infected mothers ("vertical transmission"). Pa-

tients with increased exposure to blood or blood products and/or with impaired immunity (e.g., dialysis patients, patients with leukemia or Down syndrome) are also highly susceptible to B virus infection.

Hepatitis C virus (HCV), similar to HBV, is largely parenterally transmitted. Hepatitis C is currently the main cause of post-transfusion hepatitis. HCV is also a common cause of hepatitis in intravenous drug users and accounts for at least 50% of cases of sporadic, commu-

TABLE 41–2	Characteristics of Common Causative Agents of Acute Viral Hepatitis

	Hepatitis A	Hepatitis B	Hepatitis D	Hepatitis C	Hepatitis E
Causative agent	27-nm RNA virus	42-nm DNA virus; core and surface components	36-nm hybrid particle with HBsAg coat	Flavivirus-like RNA agent	27–34 nm nonenveloped RNA virus
Transmission	Fecal-oral; water- or food-borne	Parenteral inoculation or equivalent; direct contact	Similar to HBV	Similar to HBV	Similar to HAV
Incubation period	2–6 wk	4 wk–6 mo	Similar to HBV	5–10 wk	2–9 wk
Period of infectivity	2–3 wk in late incubation and early clinical phase	During HBsAg positivity (occasionally only with anti-HBc positivity)	During HDV RNA or anti-HDV positivity	During anti-HCV positivity	Similar to HCV
Massive hepatic necrosis	Rare	Uncommon	Yes	Uncommon	Yes
Carrier state	No	Yes	Yes	Yes	No
Chronic hepatitis	No	Yes	Yes	Yes	No
Prophylaxis	Hygiene, immune serum globulin, vaccine	Hygiene, hepatitis B immune globulin, vaccine	Hygiene, HBV vaccine	Hygiene	Hygiene, sanitation

HAV = Hepatitis A virus; HBc = hepatitis B core; HBsAg = hepatitis B surface antigen; HBV = hepatitis B virus; HCV = hepatitis C virus; HDV = hepatitis D virus.

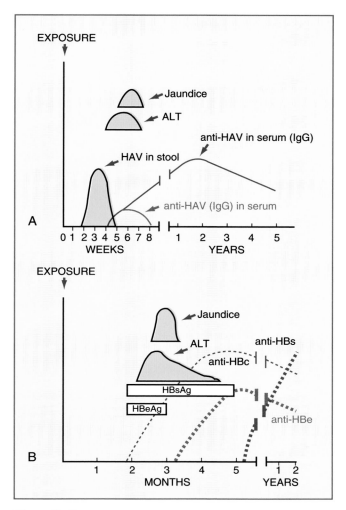

Figure 41–2

Sequence of clinical and laboratory findings in *(A)* a patient with acute hepatitis A virus (HAV) and *(B)* a patient with hepatitis B. ALT = Alanine transaminase; HBc = hepatitis B core; HBe = hepatitis e; HBeAg = hepatitis e antigen; HBs = hepatitis B surface; HBsAg = hepatitis B surface antigen.

nity-acquired hepatitis. In many such cases, the mode of transmission of the virus is unclear. The hepatitis E virus is the cause of an epidemic, water-borne hepatitis that has been associated with outbreaks, mainly in Asia and Africa.

Clinical and Laboratory Manifestations

Acute viral hepatitis typically begins with a prodromal phase lasting several days and characterized by constitutional and gastrointestinal symptoms including malaise, fatigue, anorexia, nausea, vomiting, myalgia, and headache. A mild fever may be present. Symptoms suggestive of "flu" may be prominent; arthritis and urticaria, attributed to immune complex deposition, may be present, particularly in hepatitis B. Smokers often describe an aversion to cigarettes. Jaundice soon appears with bilirubinuria and a loss of stool color, often accompanied

by an improvement in the patient's sense of well-being. Jaundice may be absent (anicteric hepatitis); in such cases—probably the majority of cases of acute viral hepatitis—medical attention is often not sought. The liver is usually tender and enlarged; splenomegaly is found in about one fifth of patients.

Transaminases (alanine transaminase [ALT] and aspartate transaminase [AST]) are released from the acutely damaged hepatocytes, and serum transaminase levels rise, often to levels >20-fold normal. Bilirubinuria and an elevated serum bilirubin are usually found, with mild elevations in serum alkaline phosphatase levels. The white cell count is normal or slightly depressed.

The icteric phase of acute viral hepatitis may last from days to weeks, followed by gradual resolution of symptoms and laboratory values.

Complications

CHOLESTATIC HEPATITIS. In some patients, most commonly during HAV infection, a prolonged, although ultimately self-limited, period of cholestatic jaundice may supervene with marked conjugated hyperbilirubinemia, elevation of alkaline phosphatase, and pruritus. Investigation may be required to differentiate this condition from mechanical obstruction of the biliary tree (see Chapter 45).

FULMINANT HEPATITIS. Massive hepatic necrosis occurs in <1% of patients with acute viral hepatitis, leading to a devastating and often fatal condition called fulminant hepatic failure. This is discussed in detail in Chapter 42.

CHRONIC HEPATITIS. This may develop following acute hepatitis B, C, or D. Hepatitis A never progresses to chronicity, although occasionally it follows a relapsing course. Persistence of transaminase elevation beyond 6 months suggests evolution to chronic hepatitis, although a slowly resolving acute hepatitis may occasionally lead to abnormal liver function tests well beyond 6 months with eventual complete resolution. Chronic hepatitis is considered in detail later in this chapter. HBV infection without evidence of any liver damage may persist, resulting in asymptomatic or "healthy" hepatitis B carriers. In Asia and Africa, many such carriers appear to have acquired the virus from infected mothers during infancy.

RARE COMPLICATIONS. Rarely, acute viral hepatitis may be followed by aplastic anemia, whereas cryoglobulinemia, glomerulonephritis, and vasculitis may complicate the course of hepatitis B. Pancreatitis with elevation of serum amylase may also occur.

Serodiagnosis

The ability to detect the presence of viral components in hepatitis B and C and antibodies to components of hepatitis A, B, C, and D has enabled considerable progress to be made in the study of the epidemiology of viral hepatitis. These so-called viral markers can be diagnostic of the cause of acute viral hepatitis (Table 41–3). An etiologic

TABLE 41–3	Serologic Markers of Viral Hepatitis		
Agent	**Marker**	**Definition**	**Significance**
Hepatitis A virus (HAV)	Anti-HAV IgM type IgG type	Antibody to HAV	Current or recent infection or convalescence Current or previous infection; confers immunity
Hepatitis B virus (HBV)	HBsAg HBeAg	HBV surface antigen e antigen; a component of the HBV core	Positive in most cases of acute or chronic infection Transiently positive in acute hepatitis B May persist in chronic infection Reflects presence of viral replication, whole Dane particles in serum, and high infectivity
	Anti-HBe	Antibody to e antigen	Transiently positive in convalescence May be persistently present in chronic cases Usually reflects low infectivity
	Anti-HBc (IgM or IgG)	Antibody to HBV core antigen	Positive in all acute and chronic cases Reliable marker of infection, past or current IgM anti-HBc reflects active viral replication Not protective
	Anti-HBs	Antibody to HBV surface antigen	Positive in late convalescence in most acute cases Confers immunity
Hepatitis C virus (HCV)	Anti-HCV	Antibodies to a group of recombinant HCV peptides (C22-3, C200)	Positive on average 15 wk after exposure; not protective Persists in chronic infection
Hepatitis D virus (HDV)	Anti-HDV (IgM or IgG)	Antibody to HDV antigen	Acute or chronic infection; not protective

diagnosis is of great importance in planning preventive and public health measures pertinent to the close contacts of infected patients and in evaluating the prognosis. The time course of appearance of these markers in acute hepatitis A and B is shown in Figure 41–2. Epstein-Barr virus and cytomegalovirus hepatitis may also be diagnosed by the appearance of specific antibodies of the IgM class. In acute hepatitis B, HBsAg and HBeAg are present in serum. Both are usually cleared within 3 months, but HBsAg may persist in some uncomplicated cases for 6 months to 1 year. Clearance of HBsAg is followed after a variable "window" period by emergence of anti-HBs, which confers long-term immunity. Anti-HBc and anti-HBe appear in the acute phase of the illness, but neither provides immunity. Uncommonly, during the serologic window period, anti-HBc may be the only evidence of hepatitis B infection, and IgM anti-HBc, a marker of active viral replication, is suggestive of recent infection. Hepatitis D infection superimposed on HBV infection may be detected by specific antibody to this agent. Acute hepatitis C is accompanied by a viremia that can be detected using a sensitive polymerase chain reaction assay for the HCV RNA. Antibodies detected by presently used second-generation tests (EIA-Z) using a group of recombinant HCV antigens develop within 15 weeks of exposure or within 6 to 7 weeks after biochemical abnormalities are discovered.

Management

There is no specific treatment for acute viral hepatitis. Management is largely supportive, including rest in proportion to the severity of symptoms, maintaining hydration, and adequate dietary intake. Most patients show a preference for a low-fat, high-carbohydrate diet. Vitamin supplementation is of no proven value, although vitamin K may be indicated if prolonged cholestasis occurs. Activity is restricted to limit fatigue. Alcohol should be avoided until liver enzymes return to normal. Measures to combat nausea can include small doses of metoclopramide and hydroxyzine. Hospitalization is indicated in patients with severe nausea and vomiting or with evidence of deteriorating liver function, such as hepatic encephalopathy (see Chapter 42) or prolongation of the prothrombin time. In general, hepatitis A may be regarded as noninfectious after 2 to 3 weeks, whereas hepatitis B is potentially infectious to intimate contacts throughout its course, although the risk is very small once HBsAg has cleared. Although hepatitis C may also be transmitted to intimate contacts, the risk of this is considered less than for hepatitis B.

Prevention

Both feces and blood from patients with hepatitis A contain virus during the prodromal and early icteric phases of the disease. Raw shellfish concentrate the virus from sewage pollution and may serve as vectors of the disease. General hygienic measures should include handwashing by contacts and careful handling, disposal, and sterilization of excreta and contaminated clothing and utensils. Close contacts of patients with hepatitis A should receive immune serum globulin (ISG) as soon as possible. Travelers to endemic areas where sanitation facilities are poor may be protected by prior administration of ISG or by using recently available hepatitis A vaccines. The use of such vaccines in other high-risk groups is presently under study.

Hepatitis B is rarely transmitted by the fecal-oral route, but it is still prudent to avoid contact with the excreta of patients. Far more important is the meticulous disposal of contaminated needles and other blood-contaminated utensils.

Efforts at preventing hepatitis B have involved the use of ISG enriched in anti-HBs (hepatitis B immune globulin [HBIG]) and the recombinant hepatitis B vaccine. Postexposure prophylaxis after blood or mucosal exposure (e.g., needlestick, eye splash, sexual contacts of acute hepatitis B patients, neonates born to mothers with acute or chronic infection) should be given as soon as possible—within 7 days with HBIG and subsequently with hepatitis B vaccine. Preventive vaccination is currently recommended for high-risk groups and individuals (health care professionals, dialysis patients, hemophiliacs, residents and staff of custodial care institutions, sexually active homosexual males) and is advocated universally for children.

No accepted prevention strategies are available for HCV. Since immune globulin does not contain HCV-neutralizing antibodies, there is little rationale or evidence to support its use for postexposure prophylaxis. However, there is evidence that early treatment of acute hepatitis C with agents such as interferon-α may significantly reduce the development of chronic infection. In addition, the advent of widespread blood product screening for anti-HCV has begun to reduce the incidence of post-transfusion hepatitis.

Alcoholic Fatty Liver and Hepatitis

Alcohol abuse is the most common cause of liver disease in the Western world. Three major pathologic lesions resulting from alcohol abuse are (1) fatty liver, (2) alcoholic hepatitis, and (3) cirrhosis. The first two lesions are potentially reversible, may sometimes be confused clinically with viral hepatitis or gallbladder and biliary tract disease, and are described in this chapter. Alcoholic cirrhosis is discussed in Chapter 43.

Mechanism of Injury

Alcohol appears to produce liver damage by several mechanisms that are still incompletely understood. Fatty liver may be related to increased nicotinamide-adenine dinucleotide phosphate (NADPH) generated during alcohol metabolism, which promotes fatty acid synthesis and triglyceride formation. Because alcohol also impairs the release of triglyceride in the form of lipoproteins, fat accumulates in hepatocytes. Acetaldehyde produced from oxidation of alcohol may be directly hepatotoxic and is implicated in the production of the more severe hepatic lesions seen in alcoholics. Immune-mediated hepatic damage may also play a role in producing the lesion of alcoholic hepatitis.

Individuals vary considerably in their ability to withstand the effects of alcohol on the liver. Nevertheless, consumption by men of 40 to 60 gm of ethanol per day (one beer or one mixed drink $\cong$ 10 gm of ethanol) for 10

to 15 years carries a substantial risk of the development of alcoholic liver disease, whereas women appear to have a lower threshold of injury. Malnutrition may potentiate the toxic effects of alcohol on the liver, and genetic factors may contribute to individual susceptibility.

Clinical and Pathologic Features

Alcoholic fatty liver may present as an incidentally discovered tender hepatomegaly. Some patients consult a physician because of right upper quadrant pain. Jaundice is very rare. Transaminase levels are usually mildly elevated (less than five times normal). Liver biopsy shows diffuse or centrilobular fat occupying most of the hepatocyte.

Alcoholic hepatitis, a much more severe and prognostically ominous lesion, is characterized by the histologic triad of (1) alcoholic hyalin (Mallory bodies), an intracellular eosinophilic aggregate of cytokeratins, usually seen near or around the cell nuclei of hepatocytes; (2) infiltration of the liver by polymorphonuclear leukocytes; and (3) a network of intralobular connective tissue surrounding hepatocytes and central veins (spider fibrosis). Patients with this histologic lesion may be asymptomatic or extremely ill with hepatic failure. Anorexia, nausea, vomiting, weight loss, and abdominal pain are common presenting symptoms. Hepatomegaly is present in 80% of patients with alcoholic hepatitis, and splenomegaly is often present. Fever is common, but bacterial infection should always be excluded, because patients with alcoholic liver disease are prone to develop pneumonia as well as infection of the urinary tract and peritoneal cavity. Jaundice is commonly present and may be pronounced with cholestatic features, requiring differentiation from biliary tract disease (see Chapter 40). Cutaneous signs of chronic liver disease may be found, including spider angiomas, palmar erythema, and gynecomastia. Parotid enlargement, testicular atrophy, and loss of body hair may be prominent (see Chapter 43). Ascites and encephalopathy may be present and indicate severe disease. The white cell count may be strikingly elevated, whereas transaminase levels are only modestly raised, an important differentiating feature from other forms of acute hepatitis. The AST/ALT ratio frequently exceeds 2, in contrast to viral hepatitis, in which the transaminase levels are usually increased in parallel. A prolonged prothrombin time, hypoalbuminemia, and hyperglobulinemia may be found.

Diagnosis

A history of excessive prolonged alcohol intake is often difficult to elicit from patients with alcoholic liver disease. However, historical, clinical, and biochemical features of alcoholic hepatitis are often sufficient to establish the diagnosis. It is important to realize that many patients suspected or found to imbibe excessively may have causes other than alcohol for liver disease (e.g., chronic viral hepatitis). Thus, when other etiologies of liver disease are suspected and alcohol intake is uncertain, a liver biopsy may be extremely helpful in establishing the diagnosis.

Complications and Prognosis

Alcoholic fatty liver reverts to complete histologic normality with cessation of alcohol intake. Alcoholic hepatitis can also revert to normal but more commonly either progresses to cirrhosis, which may already be present at the time of initial presentation, or runs a rapid course to hepatic failure and death. Not infrequently its course is complicated by the development of encephalopathy, ascites, and deteriorating renal function with increasing blood urea nitrogen (BUN) and creatinine levels (hepatorenal syndrome) or gastrointestinal bleeding from varices.

Treatment

Treatment of acute alcoholic hepatitis is supportive. Attempts should be made to treat the underlying alcoholism, although this is often unrewarding. A high-calorie diet with vitamin (particularly thiamin) supplementation is instituted and may require administration by nasogastric tube in severely anorectic patients. Protein should be included but may need to be restricted in patients with encephalopathy (see Chapter 43). Treatment with corticosteroids may be of benefit in selected patients with severe disease.

Drug- and Toxin-Induced Hepatitis

A broad spectrum of hepatic pathology may result from a variety of therapeutic drugs and nontherapeutic toxins (Table 41–4). The pathophysiologic mechanisms whereby this wide variety of hepatic lesions is produced are complex. At one end of the spectrum is a predictable, dose-dependent, direct toxic effect upon hepatocytes leading to frank hepatocellular necrosis. This is typified by the effects of acetaminophen and carbon tetrachloride, both of which produce centrilobular hepatocellular necrosis in virtually all individuals in whom a sufficient quantity is ingested. Other reactions are generally not predictable and usually occur for unknown reasons in susceptible individuals (idiosyncratic drug reaction). In some instances, genetically determined differences in pathways of hepatic drug metabolism may result in metabolites with greater toxic potential. Examples include viral hepatitis-like reactions (halothane, isoniazid), cholestatic hepatitis (chlorpromazine), granulomatous hepatitis (allopurinol), chronic hepatitis (methyldopa), and pure cholestasis without inflammatory cell infiltration or hepatocellular necrosis (estrogens, androgens). Immune-mediated hepatic damage may contribute in some, possibly resulting from the drug or its metabolites acting as a hapten on the surface of hepatocytes. A few important examples of drug-induced hepatitis are discussed here.

TABLE 41–4	Classification of Drug-Induced Liver Disease
Category	**Examples**
Predictable hepatotoxins with zonal necrosis	Acetaminophen
	Carbon tetrachloride
Nonspecific hepatitis	Aspirin
	Oxacillin
Viral hepatitis–like reactions	Halothane
	Isoniazid
	Phenytoin
Cholestasis	
	Estrogens
Noninflammatory	17α-substituted steroids
Inflammatory	Chlorpromazine
	Antithyroid agents
Fatty liver	
Large droplet	Ethanol
	Corticosteroids
Small droplet	Phenylbutazone
	Allopurinol
Chronic hepatitis	Methyldopa
	Nitrofurantoin
Tumors	Estrogens
	Vinyl chloride
Vascular lesions	6-Thioguanine
	Anabolic steriods
Fibrosis	Methotrexate
Granulomas	Allopurinol
	Sulfonamides

Acetaminophen

Acetaminophen is converted by the hepatic cytochrome P-450 drug-metabolizing system to a potentially toxic metabolite that is subsequently rendered harmless through conjugation with glutathione. When massive doses are taken (>10 to 15 gm), the formation of excess toxic metabolites depletes the available glutathione and produces necrosis. Acetaminophen overdose, commonly taken in a suicide attempt, leads to nausea and vomiting within a few hours. These symptoms subside and are followed in 24 to 48 hours by clinical and laboratory evidence of hepatocellular necrosis (raised transaminase levels) and hepatic dysfunction (prolonged prothrombin time, hepatic encephalopathy). Similar findings may occur with therapeutic doses of acetaminophen in chronic alcoholic patients. Extensive liver necrosis may lead to fulminant hepatic failure and death. Severe liver damage may be predicted on the basis of blood levels of the drug from 4 to 12 hours after ingestion. Early treatment of patients at high risk with N-acetylcysteine (within 16 hours of the ingestion), which is thought to promote hepatic glutathione synthesis, may be life saving.

Isoniazid (INH)

Isoniazid as a single-drug prophylaxis against tuberculosis commonly produces subclinical hepatic injury (20% incidence), as evidenced by raised serum transaminase levels. This appears to be transient and self-limiting in most cases. There is, however, a 1% incidence of overt hepatitis with clinical and pathologic features of viral hepatitis, which progresses to massive, fatal hepatic necrosis in one tenth of affected patients. Individual and age-related differences in hepatic acetylation of potentially toxic INH metabolites may be important in this injury. Thus, the incidence of severe hepatic damage increases with age, such that significant elevation of transaminase levels in persons over age 35 is an indication for discontinuing the drug.

Halothane

Historically, this anesthetic agent caused an uncommon acute viral hepatitis-like reaction several days after exposure in susceptible individuals. Hepatic injury was due in part to an allergic response to hepatic neoantigens produced by halothane metabolism, and the severity of this reaction increased with repeated exposure. Newer, commonly used halogenated anesthetic agents (isoflurane, enflurane) exhibit this hepatotoxic capacity in a much smaller number of patients.

Chlorpromazine

Chlorpromazine produces a cholestatic reaction, often weeks to months after the drug is begun. Fever, anorexia, and a rash may accompany jaundice and pruritus. Eosinophilia is common. Erythromycin may produce a similar picture, but right upper quadrant pain, mimicking acute cholecystitis, is often prominent.

CHRONIC HEPATITIS

An inflammatory process within the liver that fails to resolve after 6 months is in general considered chronic hepatitis.

Etiology

Many of the causes of acute hepatitis can ultimately lead to chronic hepatitis (Table 41–5). Notable exceptions are HAV and hepatitus E virus (HEV). HBV is a common cause of chronic hepatitis worldwide, and it is thought that superimposition of hepatitis D virus (HDV) infection may produce a more severe outcome. Approximately 2 to 4% of patients receiving blood transfusions develop hepatitis C, which becomes chronic in at least 70% of cases. Several drugs may produce a chronic hepatitis, the best recognized being methyldopa. In contrast to acute hepatitis, an etiologic agent is sometimes difficult to identify in cases of chronoic hepatitis. The pathogenesis of these idiopathic forms may represent quiescent autoimmune disease, undetected past drug-induced injury, antibody negative viral infections, or misdiagnosed cholestatic liver injury (e.g., primary biliary cirrhosis, primary sclerosing cholangitis).

TABLE 41–5	Causes of Chronic Hepatitis

Viral

Hepatitis B
Hepatitis B with superimposed hepatitis D
Hepatitis C

Drugs and Toxins

Methyldopa
Nitrofurantoin
Amiodarone
Isoniazid

Autoimmune

Genetic Disorders

Wilson's disease
Alpha$_1$-antitrypsin deficiency

Idiopathic

Classification, Natural History, and Treatment

The initial classification of chronic hepatitis was developed 25 years ago at a time when causes of chronic hepatitis were poorly understood. This scheme was based on hepatic histopathologic findings thought to correlate with severity and potential progression of disease. Thus, chronic persistent hepatitis, where inflammatory activity was confined to portal areas, was thought to have a uniformly good prognosis. Chronic lobular hepatitis, where inflammatory activity and necrosis was scattered throughout the lobule, similar to late-resolving acute hepatitis, was thought to have a generally good prognosis. Chronic active hepatitis, when inflammatory activity spilled out of portal areas into the lobule (periportal hepatitis, piecemeal necrosis) in association with necrosis and fibrosis, was thought to have a significant risk for progression to cirrhosis and liver failure.

Although these histologic criteria remain generally useful, the recognition of many etiologic causes of chronic hepatitis and their natural histories independent of histology and the realization that the development of progressive disease may occur regardless of histologic stage has prompted a reclassification of chronic hepatitis. This classification is based on the etiologic agent responsible for disease, the grade of injury (determined by the numbers and location of inflammatory cells), and the stage of disease (determined by the degree, location, and distortion of normal architecture by fibrosis). It allows integration of knowledge of the natural history of specific etiologies with histologic features of present and past hepatic damage to assess the severity and prognosis of the process. Thus, in general, both serologic studies and a liver biopsy are used in the diagnosis and in planning treatment for chronic hepatitis.

Hepatitis B accounts for approximately 10% of chronic hepatitis in this country, and roughly 30 to 40% of patients with chronic hepatitis B develop progression to cirrhosis and end-stage disease with the attendant risk of hepatocellular carcinoma. Hepatitis C accounts for at least 30 to 40% of chronic hepatitis in the United States and in general has a long natural history with slow progression. As many as 10% of these patients develop cirrhosis. A smaller percentage develop end-stage liver disease and hepatocellular carcinoma. Treatment of chronic hepatitis B and C with agents such as interferon-α has decreased inflammatory activity and, in a minority of patients, suppressed viral activity for prolonged periods of time. Prolonged toxin-induced injury has an extremely variable natural history, often dependent on the duration of exposure prior to recognition. This fact underscores the need for careful consideration of drug involvement in any case of chronic liver injury. Autoimmune liver disease has been subdivided into several types. However, the typical disease, characterized by significant hepatic inflammation with plasma cells and fibrosis in a young female with the presence of hypergammaglobulinemia and antinuclear and anti–smooth muscle antibodies, is most frequent. Extrahepatic manifestations including amenorrhea, rashes, acne, vasculitis, thyroiditis, and Sjögren's syndrome are common. Evidence of hepatic failure and the presence of chronic disease on biopsy at the time of diagnosis are frequent. Treatment with corticosteroids, often with azathioprine for steroid sparing, is efficacious and in many cases prolongs survival. Wilson's disease and α_1-antitrypsin deficiency generally present before age 35, and a family history of liver disease may be present. Serologic studies and special stains on liver biopsy sections are useful in the diagnosis. Specific, effective treatment is available for Wilson's disease.

REFERENCES

Bass NM: Toxic and drug-induced liver disease. *In* Bennett JC, Plum F (eds.): Cecil Textbook of Medicine. 20th ed. Philadelphia, WB Saunders, 1996, pp 772–776.

Boyer JL, Reuben A: Chronic hepatitis. *In* Schiff L, Schiff E (eds.): Diseases of the Liver. 7th ed. Philadelphia, JB Lippincott, 1993, pp 586–637.

Dasmet VJ, Gerber M, Hoofragle JH, et al: Classification of chronic hepatitis: Diagnosis, grading and staging. Hepatology 1994;19:1513.

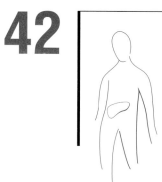

42

Fulminant Hepatic Failure

Fulminant hepatic failure (FHF) is arbitrarily defined as the onset of encephalopathy occurring within 8 weeks in a patient with acute liver disease. "Late-onset hepatic failure" is proposed for those patients who develop encephalopathy between 8 weeks and 24 weeks from the onset of jaundice. This discrimination may have prognostic and therapeutic importance in deciding which patients should undergo liver transplantation. The pathogenesis of fulminant hepatic failure involves severe widespread hepatic necrosis, commonly due to acute viral infection with B, A, D, or C viruses. It may also result from exposure to hepatotoxins such as acetaminophen, isoniazid, halothane, valproic acid, mushroom toxins (e.g., those of *Amanita phalloides*), or carbon tetrachloride. Reye's syndrome, a disease predominantly of children, and acute fatty liver of pregnancy, both of which are characterized by microvesicular fatty infiltration and little hepatocellular necrosis, often resemble FHF. In a number of patients with FHF, no cause is found, although a viral infection is usually presumed to be responsible.

DIAGNOSIS

The diagnosis rests on the combination of hepatic encephalopathy, acute liver disease (elevated serum bilirubin, transaminase levels), and liver failure, the last-named usually indicated by prolongation of the prothrombin time.

TREATMENT

Treatment of FHF remains supportive, as the underlying etiology of liver failure is rarely treatable (see Hepatic Transplantation). However, most processes that result in widespread liver cell necrosis and FHF are transient events, and liver cell regeneration with recovery of liver function often occurs if patients do not succumb to the complications of liver failure in the interim. Meticulous supportive treatment in an intensive care unit setting has been shown to improve survival. Patients with fulminant hepatic failure should be cared for in centers with experience with this disease. Numerous complications (Table 42–1) attend FHF, and careful identification and treatment of each are essential.

Hepatic encephalopathy, the *sine qua non* of FHF, is often the first and most dramatic sign of liver failure. The pathogenesis of hepatic encephalopathy, discussed in Chapter 43, remains unclear; however, most clinical observations suggest a role for protein- and gut-derived toxins that are normally taken up and detoxified by the liver. Hepatic encephalopathy that accompanies FHF differs from that associated with chronic liver disease in two important aspects: (1) it is rarely due to a reversible precipitating factor (see Table 43–6) and often responds to therapy only when liver function improves; and (2) it is frequently associated with two other potentially treatable causes of coma—hypoglycemia and cerebral edema. Therapy for hepatic encephalopathy in FHF differs slightly from the principles outlined in Chapter 43. Protein intake is limited to 20 to 40 gm/day in stages I to II encephalopathy; for stages III or IV give intravenous (IV) nitrogen 30 to 40 gm/day to maintain nitrogen balance. Lactulose should be given in the form of enemas and avoided orally or per nasogastric tube. Unfortunately, lactulose enemas are often ineffective when used for encephalopathic patients with FHF and should be discontinued if no improvement is noted after several enemas are administered. Intubation is necessary to protect the airway from aspiration and to allow ventilation in patients with advanced encephalopathy.

Cerebral edema, the pathogenesis of which is unknown, is a common complication and the leading cause of death in FHF. Clinically, it is difficult to differentiate from hepatic encephalopathy, and computed tomography (CT) scans of the head are often unreliable. Therefore, most liver centers use extradural intracranial monitoring to detect and follow intracranial pressures (ICP). The goal is to maintain an ICP < 20 mm Hg, and treatment includes controlling agitation, head elevation 20 to 30 degrees, hyperventilation, administration of mannitol, barbiturate-induced coma, and if all fails, urgent liver transplantation.

Hypoglycemia is a common complication of liver failure resulting from impaired hepatic gluconeogenesis and insulin degradation. All patients should receive 10% glucose IV infusions with frequent monitoring of blood glucose levels. Other metabolic abnormalities commonly occur, including *hyponatremia, hypokalemia, respiratory alkalosis,* and *metabolic acidosis.* Thus, frequent monitoring of blood electrolytes and pH is indicated.

Gastrointestinal hemorrhage occurs frequently and is

TABLE 42–1	Management of Selected Problems in Fulminant Hepatic Failure	
Complication	**Pathogenesis**	**Management**
Hepatic encephalopathy	Liver failure	Limit protein (20–40 mg/day) (if stage 3–4 give IV nitrogen only); lactulose enemas, consider neomycin
Cerebral edema	Unknown	Elevate bed 20–30 degrees, hyperventilate (Pco_2 25–30 mm Hg) IV mannitol; 0.5–1 gm/kg bolus over 5 min pentobarbital infusion; urgent liver transplantation
Coagulopathy and GI hemorrhage	Decreased synthesis of clotting factors Gastric erosions	Vitamin K (subcutaneously); FFP only if actively bleeding; IV H_2 antagonists prophylaxis
Hypoglycemia	↓ Gluconeogenesis Insulin degradation	IV 10% dextrose, monitor every 2 hours; 30–50% dextrose may be needed
Agitation	May be due to Encephalopathy ↑ Intracranial pressure Hypoxemia	Search for treatable causes (i.e., ↓ Po_2); treat with short-acting benzodiazepines (i.e., lorazepam) or morphine sulfate; use pancuronium bromide if violent

GI = Gastrointestinal; IV = intravenous.

commonly due to gastric erosions and impaired synthesis of clotting factors. All patients should receive vitamin K (subcutaneously) and prophylactic IV H_2-receptor antagonists to maintain gastric pH above 5. Fresh frozen plasma should be used if clinically significant bleeding occurs or if major procedures, including intracranial pressure monitoring and central line placement, are performed.

HEPATIC TRANSPLANTATION

Hepatic transplantation (see Chapter 43) has been performed with considerable success in patients with FHF and is the treatment of choice for patients who appear unlikely to recover spontaneously. Because of the need for urgent transplantation, potential candidates should be transferred to transplant centers before they develop significant complications (such as coma, cerebral edema, hemorrhage, or infection).

Transplantation is usually indicated in patients with severe encephalopathy or coagulopathy or in those whose clinical course is protracted and subacute. The cause is also important in determining prognosis. Patients with FHF due to viral hepatitis A, B, and D or acetaminophen overdose are more likely to recover spontaneously, whereas those with FHF secondary to drugs, cryptogenic FHF, or Wilson's disease rarely survive without transplantation.

Many other forms of therapy for fulminant hepatic failure have been tried, including corticosteroid administration, exchange transfusion, plasmapheresis, hemodialysis, charcoal hemoperfusion, and extracorporeal perfusion through a human cadaver or pig liver. To date, none has been shown to offer any advantage over conventional supportive therapy or liver transplantation.

PROGNOSIS

Short-term prognosis without liver transplantation is very poor, with the average reported survival being about 20%. Long-term prognosis for those who survive is excellent. Follow-up studies have shown normal liver function and histology in virtually all surviving patients, regardless of the cause of the fulminant failure. Survival in the range of 80 to 90% can be expected following liver transplantation for fulminant hepatic failure.

REFERENCES

Katelaris PH, Jones DB: Fulminant hepatic failure. Med Clin North Am 1989;73:955.
Scharschmidt BF: Acute and chronic hepatic failure and hepatic encephalopathy. *In* Bennett JC, Plum F (eds.): Cecil Textbook of Medicine. 20th ed. Philadelphia, WB Saunders, 1996, pp 797–800.

43

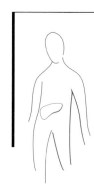

Cirrhosis of the Liver and Its Complications

DEFINITION

Cirrhosis is the irreversible end result of fibrous scarring and hepatocellular regeneration that constitute the major responses of the liver to a variety of longstanding inflammatory, toxic, metabolic, and congestive insults. In cirrhosis, the normal hepatic lobular architecture is replaced by interconnecting bands of fibrous tissue surrounding nodules derived from foci of regenerating hepatocytes.

Regenerative nodules may be small (<3 mm, micronodular cirrhosis), a typical feature of alcoholic cirrhosis, or large (>3 mm, macronodular cirrhosis). The latter, also termed postnecrotic cirrhosis, is more commonly seen as a sequel to chronic active hepatitis. The pathology of cirrhosis determines its natural history and clinical manifestations. Thus, fibrous scarring and disruption of the hepatic architecture distort the vascular bed, leading to portal hypertension and intrahepatic shunting. Normal hepatocyte function is disturbed by the resulting inadequacy of blood flow and ongoing direct toxic, inflammatory, and/or metabolic damage to the hepatocytes.

CLINICAL AND LABORATORY FEATURES

Clinical features of cirrhosis are attributable to hepatocellular dysfunction (often called "stigmata of chronic liver disease") and portal hypertension (Table 43–1). Hepatocellular dysfunction leads to impaired protein synthesis (hypoalbuminemia and prolongation of prothrombin time), hyperbilirubinemia, low blood urea nitrogen (BUN), and elevated ammonia levels. Hypersplenism, due to splenomegaly, results in thrombocytopenia and leukopenia but is usually of little clinical significance and does not warrant splenectomy.

SPECIFIC CAUSES OF CIRRHOSIS

Most of the conditions that may lead to cirrhosis (Table 43–2) are rarely encountered. Alcohol abuse and hepatitis C are by far the most common causes of cirrhosis in the Western world, whereas hepatitis B is a major cause in the Third World. Cryptogenic cirrhosis is a diagnosis of exclusion.

Alcohol

Alcoholic cirrhosis may coexist with alcoholic hepatitis (see Chapter 41). Features of hepatocellular dysfunction are thus often marked and may improve with abstinence. Micronodular cirrhosis is the rule but is not specific for alcoholic cirrhosis. Evidence of malnutrition and vitamin deficiency is frequently found, particularly in the severely alcoholic patient. Anemia of mixed etiology is common, often with macrocytic indices.

Primary Biliary Cirrhosis

Almost exclusively a disease affecting women, primary biliary cirrhosis manifests mainly between the ages of 30 and 65 and results from a progressive, probably immune-mediated destruction of the interlobular bile ducts. Cholestatic features predominate with high serum levels of alkaline phosphatase and cholesterol. Pruritus is a major early symptom, followed later in the course of the disease by xanthomas, hyperpigmentation, and bone pain due to osteoporosis or osteomalacia. Commonly associated conditions include Sjögren's syndrome, scleroderma, and the CREST syndrome (calcinosis, Raynaud's syndrome, esophageal dysfunction, sclerodactyly, telangiectasia). Antimitochondrial antibodies are present in high titer, and serum IgM levels are elevated. Liver biopsy may show characteristic destructive lesions of the bile ducts and is of value in confirming the diagnosis. Jaundice is a prominent feature late in the course of the disease. Treatment with ursodeoxycholic acid (replaces endogenous toxic bile acids) improves pruritus and appears to slow the progression of disease, although studies are ongoing to determine whether such treatment may delay the need for liver transplantation or prolong life.

Chronic Active Hepatitis

See Chapter 41.

Hemochromatosis

See Chapter 61.

TABLE 43-1	**Causes of Cirrhosis**

Alcohol
Hepatitis viruses (B and C)
Drugs and toxins
Autoimmune chronic active hepatitis
Biliary cirrhosis
    Primary biliary cirrhosis
    Secondary biliary cirrhosis
        Bile duct strictures
        Sclerosing cholangitis
        Biliary atresia
        Tumors of the bile ducts
        Cystic fibrosis
Chronic hepatic congestion
    Budd-Chiari syndrome
    Chronic right heart failure
    Constrictive pericarditis
Genetically determined metabolic diseases
    Hemochromatosis
    Wilson's disease
    Alpha$_1$-antitrypsin deficiency
    Galactosemia
Cryptogenic

Wilson's Disease

See Chapter 61.

MAJOR COMPLICATIONS OF CIRRHOSIS

The major sequelae of cirrhosis are:

1. Portal hypertension, which may result in
   a. Variceal hemorrhage
   b. Ascites, which can be further complicated by spontaneous bacterial peritonitis
   c. Hepatic encephalopathy
   d. Hepatorenal syndrome
   e. Hepatopulmonary syndrome
2. Hepatocellular carcinoma

The pathophysiologic interrelationships among these complications are shown diagrammatically in Figure 43–1.

Portal Hypertension

The distortion of hepatic architecture in cirrhosis leads to a marked increase in resistance to portal venous flow, which in turn leads to an increase in portal venous pressure.

Although cirrhosis is the most important cause of portal hypertension, any process leading to increased resistance to portal blood flow into (presinusoidal) or through the liver (sinusoidal) or to hepatic venous outflow from the liver (postsinusoidal) results in portal hypertension (Table 43–3). Because the pressure within any vascular system is proportional to both resistance and blood flow, a marked increase in blood flow alone may result in portal hypertension.

Portal hypertension leads to the formation of venous collaterals between the portal and systemic circulations. Collaterals may form at several sites, the most important clinically being those connecting the portal to the azygos vein, which form dilated, tortuous veins (varices) in the submucosa of the gastric fundus and esophagus. The normal portal pressure gradient (hepatic vein–portal vein) is 4 to 6 mm Hg. When the gradient is >12 mm Hg, esophageal varices may rupture.

Variceal Hemorrhage

Hemorrhage occurs most frequently from varices in the esophagus and is a common and serious complication of portal hypertension, with a mortality rate of 30 to 60%. Large varices bleed most commonly, and bleeding occurs when high tension in the walls of these vessels leads to rupture. Bleeding may present as hematemesis, hematochezia, melena, or any combination of these (see Chapter 32B). Bleeding may lead to shock, stop spontaneously, or recur. Impaired hepatic synthesis of coagulation factors (hepatocellular dysfunction) and thrombocytopenia (hypersplenism) may further complicate the management of variceal bleeding. The management of esophageal varices includes early medical intervention to prevent bleeding as well as the treatment of acute variceal hemorrhage (Fig. 43–2). Nonselective beta blockers (propranolol and nadolol) and mononitrates (isosorbide mononitrate) are effective in preventing variceal hemorrhage by reducing portal blood flow and pressure. Screening for varices is appropriate in cirrhotics who have clinical features of portal hypertension. Somatostatin (or its synthetic analog octreotide) and vasopressin are given intravenously to reduce splanchnic blood flow and are used in the acute setting of esophageal hemorrhage until endoscopic therapy or surgery is performed. Intravenous nitroglycerin should be given with vasopressin to minimize systemic vasoconstrictive toxicity. Endoscopic therapy includes in-

TABLE 43-2	**Clinical and Laboratory Features of Cirrhosis**

Clinical	Laboratory
Hepatocellular Dysfunction	
Jaundice	Hyperbilirubinemia
Spider angiomas	
Palmar erythema	
Gynecomastia	
Loss of body hair	
Testicular atrophy	
Dupuytren's contracture	
Muscle wasting, edema	Hypoalbuminemia, low BUN
Bruising	Prolonged prothrombin time
Signs of hepatic encephalopathy	Elevated blood ammonia
Fetor hepaticus	
Portal Hypertension	
Splenomegaly	Thrombocytopenia, leukopenia
Ascites	
Caput medusae	
Variceal bleeding	

BUN = Blood urea nitrogen.

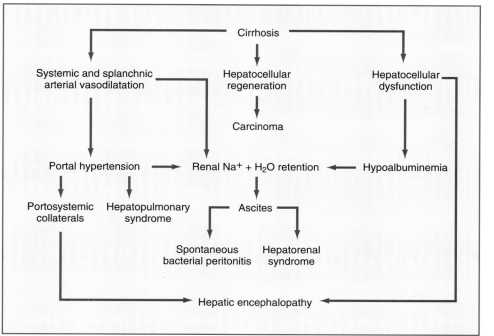

Figure 43–1
Interrelationships between the complications of cirrhosis.

jection with sclerosing solutions and/or band ligation, and both modalities are equally effective. Band ligation has less adverse effects. Repeated courses can lead to variceal obliteration. Balloon tamponade (Sengstaken-Blakemore tube) is an effective temporary measure for patients who have failed endoscopic therapy. These subjects will undergo portal decompression either by a variety of surgical procedures or by interventional radiology with a transjugular intrahepatic portosystemic shunt (TIPS). The patient's candidacy for a liver transplantation will affect which portal decompressive procedure is performed.

Hepatic Dysfunction (see Chapters 39 and 42)

The cirrhotic liver is often impaired in the synthesis of proteins by hepatocytes (hypoalbuminemia, impaired syn-

TABLE 43–3	Causes of Portal Hypertension

Increased resistance to flow
  Presinusoidal
    Portal or splenic vein occlusion (thrombosis, tumor)
    Schistosomiasis
    Congenital hepatic fibrosis
    Sarcoidosis
  Sinusoidal
    Cirrhosis (all causes)
    Alcoholic hepatitis
  Postsinusoidal
    Veno-occlusive disease
    Budd-Chiari syndrome
    Constrictive pericarditis
Increased portal blood flow
  Splenomegaly not due to liver disease
  Arterioportal fistula

thesis of coagulation factors) and in normal hepatic detoxification processes.

Ascites

Ascites is the accumulation of excess fluid in the peritoneal cavity. Although cirrhosis is the most common cause of ascites, it may result from numerous other causes (Table 43–4). The serum-ascites albumin gradient (SAAG) has replaced the exudative/transudative classification of ascites. A high SAAG (≥ 1.1 g/dl) signifies portal hypertension but does not determine its etiology. Ascites becomes clinically detectable when > 500 ml have accumulated. Shifting dullness to percussion is the most sensitive clinical sign of ascites, but ultrasonography more readily detects small fluid volumes.

Several theories explain the formation of ascites in cirrhosis. Initially, systemic arterial vasodilatation (peripheral arterial vasodilatation theory) results in excess renal reabsorption of sodium and water leading to hypervolemia and overflow of fluid into the peritoneum (overflow theory) causing ascites. Ascites causes a decreased "ineffective" intravascular volume (underflow theory) that results in enhanced production of renin, aldosterone, and antidiuretic hormone, thereby further increasing sodium and water retention and perpetuating ascites formation.

Treatment of ascites consists initially of sodium restriction. Restricted fluid intake may be necessary if hyponatremia (< 120 mEq/L) is present. The administration of spironolactone, an aldosterone antagonist, supplemented with a loop diuretic (e.g., furosemide) is often effective. Diuresis should be promoted cautiously, because aggressive diuretic therapy may result in hypokalemia and a depleted plasma volume, leading to hepatic encephalopathy and impaired renal function. Refractory

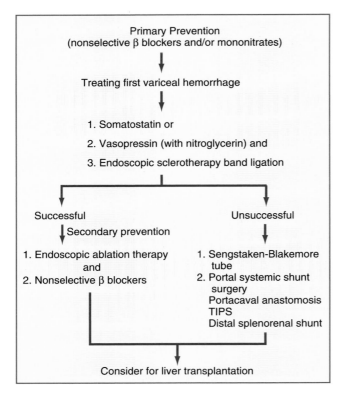

Figure 43–2
Primary prevention (nonselective beta blockers and/or mononitrates).

ascites occurs in about 10% of cirrhotics and is defined by persistent tense ascites despite Aldactone (400 mg/day) and Lasix (160 mg/day) or if azotemia develops (creatinine >2 mg/dl) using submaximal dosages. Treatment for these patients includes repeated large-volume paracentesis (most physicians simultaneously give intravenous albumin, but whether this is of any benefit is unclear), surgically implanted plastic peritoneal shunts (LeVeen or Denver), TIPS, portacaval anastomoses, or liver transplantation.

Two important complications occur in patients with cirrhotic ascites: spontaneous bacterial peritonitis and the hepatorenal syndrome.

TABLE 43–4	Causes of Ascites

Serum-Ascites Albumin Gradient	
High >1.1 gm/dl	**Low <1.1 gm/dl**
Cirrhosis	Peritoneal carcinomatosis
Chronic hepatic congestion	Tuberculosis
Right heart failure	Pancreatic and biliary
Budd-Chiari syndrome	disease
Constrictive pericarditis	Nephrotic syndrome
Nephrotic syndrome	
Massive liver metastases	
Myxedema	
Mixed ascites	

Spontaneous Bacterial Peritonitis (SBP)

Infection of ascitic fluid, usually with coliform bacteria, may occur in patients with cirrhosis. Fever, abdominal pain, and tenderness may be present, or the infection may be clinically silent. Hepatic encephalopathy may be precipitated. The diagnosis is strongly suspected if the ascitic fluid polymorphonuclear leukocyte count is $>250/mm^3$ and is confirmed by culture. Treatment with a third-generation cephalosporin for 5 to 7 days is usual, and in selected patients (i.e., liver transplant candidates) prophylaxis therapy with norfloxacillin (400 mg/day) should be given.

Hepatorenal Syndrome

Serious liver disease from any cause may be complicated by a form of functional renal failure termed the hepatorenal syndrome. It almost invariably occurs in the presence of severe ascites. Typically, the kidneys are histologically normal, with the capacity of regaining normal function in the event of recovery of liver function. Severe cortical vasoconstriction has been demonstrated angiographically, which reverses when these kidneys have been transplanted in noncirrhotic subjects. The renal dysfunction is characterized by a declining glomerular filtration rate (GFR), oliguria, low urine sodium (<10 mEq/L), and azotemia, often with a disproportionately high BUN/creatinine ratio. The decline in renal function often follows one of three events in a cirrhotic patient with ascites: sepsis, a vigorous attempt to reduce ascites with diuretics, or a large-volume paracentesis.

The hepatorenal syndrome is usually progressive and fatal. It should be diagnosed only after plasma volume depletion (a common cause of reversible, prerenal azotemia in patients with cirrhosis, particularly with diuretic use) and other forms of acute renal injury have been ruled out.

Patients should be given volume expanders to exclude prerenal azotemia. Successful reversal of hepatorenal syndrome has been documented using low-dose vasopressin, octreotide, or norepinephrine to raise the systemic vascular resistance and thereby increase renal blood flow. Liver transplantation has become an accepted treatment for hepatorenal syndrome.

Hepatic Encephalopathy

Hepatic encephalopathy (also called hepatic coma or portosystemic encephalopathy) is a complex neuropsychiatric syndrome that may complicate advanced liver disease and/or extensive portosystemic collateral formation (shunting). Two major forms of hepatic encephalopathy are recognized:

Acute hepatic encephalopathy usually occurs in the setting of fulminant hepatic failure. Cerebral edema plays a more important role in this setting: coma is common and mortality is very high (see Chapter 42).

Chronic hepatic encephalopathy usually occurs with chronic liver disease, commonly manifests as subtle disturbances of neurologic function, and is often reversible.

The pathogenesis of hepatic encephalopathy is thought to involve the inadequate hepatic removal of predominantly nitrogenous compounds or other toxins ingested or formed in the gastrointestinal tract. Inadequate hepatic removal results from impaired hepatocyte function as well as the extensive shunting of splanchnic blood directly into the systemic circulation via portosystemic collaterals. Nitrogenous and other absorbed compounds are thought to gain access to the central nervous system (CNS), leading to disturbances in neuronal function. Ammonia, derived from both amino acid deamination and bacterial hydrolysis of nitrogenous compounds in the gut, has been strongly implicated in the pathogenesis of hepatic encephalopathy, but its blood levels correlate poorly with the presence or degree of encephalopathy. Other proposed neurotoxins include gamma-aminobutyric acid, mercaptans, short-chain fatty acids, and benzodiazepine-like compounds. Mercaptans are also thought to produce the characteristic breath odor (fetor hepaticus) of patients with chronic liver failure. Another hypothesis suggests that an imbalance between plasma branched-chain and aromatic amino acids, a common consequence of severe liver disease, leads to decreased synthesis of normal neurotransmitters and to increased formation of "false neurotransmitters" from aromatic amino acids in the CNS.

The clinical features of hepatic encephalopathy include disturbances of higher neurologic function (intellectual and personality disorders, dementia, inability to copy simple diagrams [i.e., constructional apraxia], disturbance of consciousness), disturbances of neuromuscular function (asterixis, hyperreflexia, myoclonus), and rarely, a Parkinson-like syndrome and progressive paraplegia. As with other metabolic encephalopathies (which may show many of the signs of hepatic encephalopathy), asymmetric neurologic findings are unusual but can occur, and brain stem reflexes (e.g., pupillary light, oculovestibular, and oculocephalic responses) are preserved until very late. Hepatic encephalopathy is usually divided into stages according to its severity (Table 43–5). Subtle disorders of psychomotor function may exist in many patients with cirrhosis in whom conventional neurologic examination is normal. Such subclinical encephalopathy (termed stage 0 encephalopathy) is important in that it may impair work performance.

The differential diagnosis of hepatic encephalopathy includes hypoglycemia, subdural hematoma, meningitis, and sedative drug overdose, all of which are common in patients, particularly alcoholics, with liver disease.

Treatment

Treatment of hepatic encephalopathy is based on four simple principles.

IDENTIFY AND TREAT PRECIPITATING FACTORS. Table 43–6 lists several important factors that may precipitate or se-

TABLE 43–5	Stages of Hepatic Encephalopathy
Stage*	Clinical Manifestations
I	Apathy Restlessness Reversal of sleep rhythm Slowed intellect Impaired computational ability Impaired handwriting
II	Lethargy Drowsiness Disorientation Asterixis
III	Stupor (arousable) Hyperactive reflexes, extensor plantar responses
IV	Coma (response to painful stimuli only)

* Stage 0 encephalopathy is used to describe subclinical impairment of intellectual function.

verely aggravate hepatic encephalopathy in patients with severe liver disease. Gastrointestinal bleeding and increased protein intake may provide increased substrate for the bacterial or metabolic formation of nitrogenous compounds that induce encephalopathy. Patients prone to develop hepatic encephalopathy have markedly increased sensitivity to CNS-depressant drugs, and their use should be avoided in these patients.

REDUCE AND ELIMINATE SUBSTRATE FOR THE GENERATION OF NITROGENOUS COMPOUNDS

Restrict Dietary Protein. Patients in coma should receive no protein, whereas those with mild encephalopathy may benefit from restriction of protein intake to 40 to 60 gm/day. Vegetable protein diets also appear to be less encephalopathogenic.

Cleanse Bowels. This is important mainly in patients with encephalopathy precipitated by acute gastrointestinal

TABLE 43–6	Hepatic Encephalopathy: Precipitating Factors

Gastrointestinal bleeding
Increased dietary protein
Constipation
Infection
CNS-depressant drugs (benzodiazepines, opiates)
Deterioration in hepatic function
Hypokalemia ⎫
Azotemia   ⎬ Most often induced by diuretics
Alkalosis   ⎪
Hypovolemia ⎭

CNS = Central nervous system.

bleeding or constipation and is achieved by administration of enemas.

REDUCE COLONIC BACTERIA. Neomycin administered orally reduces the number of bacteria that are responsible for production of ammonia and other nitrogenous compounds.

PREVENT AMMONIA DIFFUSION FROM THE BOWEL. This is achieved by administration of lactulose, a nonabsorbable disaccharide, which, when fermented to organic acids by colonic bacteria, leads to a lower stool pH. This lowered pH traps ammonia in the colon as nondiffusible NH_4^+ ions, but other mechanisms such as inhibition of bacterial ammonia production may also be important.

Hepatopulmonary Syndrome (HPS)

Hepatopulmonary syndrome is an increasingly recognized clinical entity (10 to 15% of cirrhotics), characterized by abnormalities of arterial oxygenation in patients with chronic liver disease and/or portal hypertension. The pathophysiology of this syndrome involves intrapulmonary vascular dilatation in the absence of architectural damage. These vascular abnormalities consist of precapillary dilatation, direct arterial-venous communications, and dilated pleural vessels. Intrapulmonary vascular dilatation is detected by contrast echocardiography, which reveals delayed visualization of microbubbles in the left heart chambers. The vascular dilatation leads to impaired oxygen transfer from alveoli to the central stream of red blood cells within capillaries, resulting in a "functional" intrapulmonary right-to-left shunt which improves with 100% oxygen. Clinical features range from subclinical abnormalities in gas exchange to profound hypoxemia causing dyspnea at rest. Patients often require supplemental oxygen and have significant limitations in their performance of usual daily activities. No proven medical therapy exists at this time. As in hepatorenal syndrome, HPS is a functional disorder that reverses in the majority of cases post liver transplantation.

Hepatocellular Carcinoma

Hepatocellular carcinoma and its relationship to cirrhosis are discussed in Chapter 44.

HEPATIC TRANSPLANTATION

Liver transplantation is a highly successful procedure in patients with progressive, advanced, and otherwise untreatable liver disease. Advances in surgical techniques and supportive care, the use of cyclosporine and FK506 for immunosuppression, and careful selection of patients have all contributed to the recent encouraging results of liver transplantation. Seventy to 80% of patients undergoing liver transplantation survive at least 3 years, usually with good quality of life. The types of liver disease for which transplantation is most commonly performed include cirrhosis due to alcoholic liver disease, autoimmune hepatitis, primary biliary cirrhosis, primary sclerosing cholangitis, and hepatitis C. Hepatitis B patients undergo transplantation if they do not have hepatitis e antigen and/or hepatitis B virus DNA in their serum. Hepatitis B immunoglobulin is given post transplantation to help prevent recurrence. Excellent results have also been obtained in patients with fulminant hepatic failure (see Chapter 42). Transplantation for malignant hepatobiliary disease has been less successful owing to recurrent disease in the transplanted liver.

The timing of liver transplantation presents a particular challenge because no technology for artificial support, analogous to hemodialysis, is yet available. The survival of ambulatory patients undergoing liver transplantation electively is greater than that of those who are critically ill at the time of the operation. Thus, transplantation is usually considered when there is refractory ascites and/or SBP, recurrent variceal hemorrhage, intractable pruritus, or unacceptable quality of life.

REFERENCES

Conn HO, Attenbury CE: Cirrhosis. *In* Schiff L, Schiff L, Schiff ER (eds.): Diseases of the Liver. 7th ed. Philadelphia, JB Lippincott, 1993, pp 875–921.

Genelin P, Groszmann RJ: Portal hypertension. *In* Schiff L, Schiff ER (eds.): Diseases of the Liver. 7th ed. Philadelphia, JB Lippincott, 1993, pp 935–959.

Neuberger J, Lucey MR (eds.): Liver Transplantation: Practice and Management. London, BMJ, 1994, pp 34–100.

Scharschmidt BF: Acute and chronic hepatic failure. *In* Wyngaarden JB, Smith LH Jr, Bennett JC (eds.): Cecil Textbook of Medicine. 19th ed. Philadelphia, WB Saunders, 1992, pp 797–800.

44

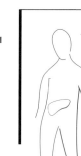

Neoplastic, Infiltrative, and Vascular Diseases of the Liver

HEPATIC NEOPLASMS

Hepatic neoplasms can be divided into three groups: (1) benign neoplasms, (2) primary malignant neoplasms, and (3) metastatic malignant neoplasms. This chapter briefly reviews all three categories of hepatic neoplasms and concludes with a brief discussion of the diagnostic approach to these lesions.

Benign Neoplasms

The group of benign neoplastic lesions includes hemangioma, hepatocellular adenoma, nodular regenerative hyperplasia, focal nodular hyperplasia, and rare mesenchymal tumors (e.g., fibromas, lipomas, leiomyomas).

Hemangiomas, the most common mesenchymal hepatic neoplasm, are often asymptomatic and incidentally discovered. Diagnosis is readily made when a hyperechoic lesion on ultrasound corresponds to a peripheral enhancing lesion that eventually completely fills during dynamic computed tomography (CT) scanning, a magnetic resonance imaging (MRI) reveals a high-intensity signal on t_2-weighted images (most sensitive test), or a technetium 99m (^{99m}Tc) red cell scan shows retention of isotope. No treatment is necessary unless lesions are very large (may spontaneously rupture) or symptomatic.

Adenomas almost exclusively occur in women, are associated with estrogens and oral contraceptives, and may enlarge during pregnancy. They are usually incidentally identified, but patients may have signs or symptoms of an abdominal mass that can spontaneously hemorrhage during menstruation, pregnancy, or post partum, causing shock and requiring surgical resection. Adenomas consist of normal hepatocytes without portal tracts and Kupffer cells. The diagnosis is suggested by the appearance of a cold spot on ^{99m}Tc sulfur colloid scans (due to absence of Kupffer cells) and as vascular lesions on angiography. Management of asymptomatic adenomas is controversial; however, due to potential rupture and malignant transformation, elective segmental liver resection is often performed. A trial period of observation may be warranted if oral contraceptives can be discontinued and regression of tumor is noted.

Hepatocellular Carcinoma

Hepatocellular carcinoma is rare in the United States (accounting for $<2.5\%$ of all malignancies). In other areas of the world, including sub-Sahara Africa, China, Japan, and Southeast Asia, it is one of the most frequent malignancies and is an important cause of mortality, particularly in middle-aged males. Hepatocellular carcinoma often arises in a cirrhotic liver and is closely associated with chronic hepatitis B or C virus infection. The advent and widespread use of vaccination to prevent infection with hepatitis B virus are expected to reduce markedly the incidence of this disease, the only disease for which effective immunization against a malignancy is currently available. The risk of hepatocellular carcinoma is low in primary biliary cirrhosis and Wilson's disease, intermediate in cirrhosis due to alcohol, and high in hemochromatosis. Other risk factors for development of hepatocellular carcinoma, as well as its clinical manifestations, are listed in Table 44–1. A tissue specimen is often necessary to confirm the diagnosis of hepatocellular carcinoma. Diagnosis of small, surgically resectable lesions in high-risk areas is possible with intensive screening programs that employ ultrasound examinations and serum α-fetoprotein levels, although the long-term outcome remains unclear. Most patients present with widespread, often multifocal disease, and the median survival from the time of diagnosis is <6 months. Systemic and intra-arterial chemotherapy, arterial embolization, intratumor ethanol injection, radiation therapy, and hepatic transplantation have yielded disappointing results.

Other primary hepatocellular malignancies include cholangiocarcinoma, angiosarcoma (related to exposure to vinyl choride, arsenic, or Thorotrast), hepatoblastoma, and cystadenocarcinoma.

Tumor Metastases to the Liver

Metastatic tumors constitute the majority of hepatic masses in this country and, in decreasing order, most commonly originate from the lung, colon, pancreas, breast, stomach, unknown primary, ovary, prostate, and gallbladder.

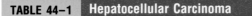

TABLE 44–1	Hepatocellular Carcinoma

Incidence

From 1–7 per 100,000 to >100 per 100,000 in high-risk areas

Sex

4:1 to 8:1 male preponderance

Associations

Chronic hepatitis B infection
Chronic hepatitis C infection
Hemochromatosis (with cirrhosis)
Cirrhosis (alcoholic, cryptogenic)
Aflatoxin ingestion
Thorotrast
α_1-Antitrypsin deficiency
Androgen administration

Common Clinical Presentations

Abdominal pain
Abdominal mass
Weight loss
Deterioration of liver function

Unusual Manifestations

Bloody ascites
Tumor emboli (lung)
Jaundice
Hepatic or portal vein obstruction
Metabolic effects
  Erythrocytosis
  Hypercalcemia
  Hypercholesterolemia
  Hypoglycemia
  Gynecomastia
  Feminization
  Acquired porphyria

Clinical/Laboratory Findings

Hepatic bruit or friction rub
Serum α-fetoprotein level >400 ng/ml

LIVER ABSCESS

Pyogenic and amebic liver abscesses are important mass lesions of the liver. Unlike hepatic neoplasms, abscesses often present as a relatively acute febrile illness associated with pain in the right upper quadrant of the abdomen. Lesions can be localized by radionuclide scan, ultrasonography, or CT. The clinical presentation, diagnosis, and treatment of these lesions are discussed in Chapter 102.

GRANULOMATOUS LIVER DISEASE

Hepatic granulomas are common, being found in 2 to 10% of all liver biopsies, often in association with an elevated serum alkaline phosphatase level. However, they are rarely a specific finding and have been reported in association with a variety of infections, systemic illnesses, hepatobiliary disorders, drugs, and toxins, some of which are listed in Table 44–2. Although granulomas are a nonspecific finding, occasionally specific features are seen, such as acid-fast bacilli in tuberculosis, ova in schistosomiasis, larvae in toxocariasis, and birefringent granules in starch, talc, or silicone granulomas. The dif-

ferential diagnosis of hepatic granulomas is one of the most extensive in medicine, and the work-up requires meticulous attention to details of the history, physical examination, and laboratory tests. Indeed, in ≥20% of patients, no cause for granulomas is found despite extensive investigation. A subset of these patients have a syndrome consisting of fever, hepatomegaly, and hepatic granulomas which responds to corticosteroids, described as "granulomatous hepatitis." These patients may possibly have a variant of sarcoidosis.

Liver biopsy (and culture, particularly of acid-fast bacteria) is of considerable value in the diagnosis of sarcoidosis, miliary tuberculosis, and histoplasmosis, as virtually all patients with these disorders have hepatic granu-

TABLE 44–2	Diseases Associated with Hepatic Granulomas

Infections

Bacterial, spirochetal
  Tuberculosis and atypical mycobacterium infections
  Tularemia
  Brucellosis
  Leprosy
  Syphilis
  Whipple's disease
  Listeriosis
Viral
  Infectious mononucleosis
  Cytomegalovirus infections
Rickettsial
  Q fever
Fungal
  Coccidioidomycosis
  Histoplasmosis
  Cryptococcal infections
  Actinomycosis
  Aspergillosis
  Nocardiosis
Parasitic
  Schistosomiasis
  Clonorchiasis
  Toxocariasis
  Ascariasis
  Toxoplasmosis
  Amebiasis

Hepatobiliary Disorders

Primary biliary cirrhosis
Granulomatous hepatitis
Jejunoileal bypass

Systemic Disorders

Sarcoidosis
Wegener's granulomatosis
Inflammatory bowel disease
Hodgkin's disease
Lymphoma

Drugs/Toxins

Beryllium
Parenteral foreign material (starch, talc, silicone, etc.)
Phenylbutazone
Alpha methyldopa
Procainamide
Allopurinol
Phenytoin
Nitrofurantoin
Hydralazine

lomas. Characteristic granulomas are seen in many patients with primary biliary cirrhosis, and granulomas may be the first clue to Hodgkin's disease.

Diagnostic Approach to Hepatic Lesions

Obviously, clinical presentation and coexisting liver disease will dictate the diagnostic approach of a liver mass. Generally, an ultrasound is the first test ordered since it is inexpensive, noninvasive, and useful for differentiating cystic from solid tumors. Once a solid tumor is identified, radionuclide scanning may be reasonable, although lesions < 3 cm are often too small to be detected. A solid lesion that exhibits uptake in a subject with cirrhosis most likely represents a regenerative nodule. If a lesion does *not* exhibit uptake, further evaluation using rapid-sequence CT, MRI, red blood cell scan, or angiography will be necessary to diagnose hemangiomas, adenomas, and/or hepatocellular carcinoma. Often these tests will be nondiagnostic, and a tissue specimen, by percutaneous liver biopsy, CT-guided fine-needle aspirate, or laparoscopy, is needed to confirm a diagnosis.

VASCULAR DISEASE OF THE LIVER

Portal vein thrombosis, hepatic vein thrombosis (Budd-Chiari syndrome), and veno-occlusive disease are uncommon disorders of hepatic vasculature; affected patients usually present with portal hypertension with or without associated liver dysfunction.

Portal vein thrombosis may develop after abdominal trauma, umbilical vein infection, sepsis, or pancreatitis, or in association with cirrhosis or hypercoagulable states; in most cases, however, particularly in children, the cause is unknown. The disease produces the manifestations of portal hypertension (see Chapter 43); however, liver histology is usually normal. The diagnosis is established by angiography. Thrombolysis may be attempted in acute portal vein thrombosis. Although controversial, long-term anticoagulation may be used in chronic thrombosis secondary to hypercoagulable states. Variceal hemorrhage is managed with endoscopic obliteration. Prophylaxis with beta blockers is not recommended because portal inflow decreases, potentially propagating the thrombus. If endoscopic treatment fails, surgical management with portosystemic shunting may be attempted, but it is often difficult due to the absence of suitable patent vessels.

The *Budd-Chiari syndrome* is associated with polycythemia vera, paroxysmal nocturnal hemoglobinuria, tumors, pregnancy, use of oral contraceptives and other hypercoagulable states, abdominal trauma, and congenital webs of the vena cava. Illness may be acute or chronic with abdominal pain, hepatomegaly, ascites, and portal hypertension as prominent features. The diagnosis is usually suspected when centrilobular necrosis is seen on liver biopsy and is established angiographically by inability to catheterize the hepatic veins. Although elevation of serum bilirubin and transaminase levels may be mild, liver function is often poor, and mortality rates of 40 to 90% are reported. Anticoagulants have not proven useful; however, side-to-side portacaval shunts, performed to relieve hepatic congestion, may improve survival, and liver transplantation may be curative.

REFERENCES

Di Bisceglie AM, Rustgi VK, Hoofnagle JH, et al: Hepatocellular carcinoma. Ann Intern Med 1988; 108:390.

Kew MC: Hepatic tumors. Semin Liver Dis 1984; 4:89.

Maddrey WC: Parasitic, bacterial, fungal, and granulomatous liver disease. *In* Bennett JC, Plum F (eds.): Cecil Textbook of Medicine. 20th ed. Philadelphia, WB Saunders, 1996, pp 781–785.

Margolis S, Homcy C: Systemic manifestations of hepatoma. Medicine 1972; 51:381.

Scharschmidt BF: Hepatic tumors. *In* Bennett JC, Plum F (eds.): Cecil Textbook of Medicine. 20th ed. Philadelphia, WB Saunders, 1996, pp 802–805.

Zakim D, Boyer T (eds.): Hepatology: A Textbook of Liver Disease. 2nd ed. Philadelphia, WB Saunders, 1990, pp 572–615, 1098–1114, 1206–1240.

45

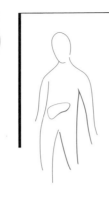

Disorders of the Gallbladder and Biliary Tract

The liver produces 500 to 1500 ml of bile per day. The major physiologic role of the biliary tract and gallbladder is to concentrate this material and to conduct it in well-timed aliquots to the intestine. In the intestine, bile acids participate in normal fat digestion, whereas cholesterol and a variety of other endogenous and exogenous compounds carried in bile are excreted in the feces. Normally unobtrusive, the gallbladder and biliary tree are the source of considerable pain and disability when they become infected or obstructed. This chapter briefly outlines the normal physiology of the biliary system and then focuses on the pathophysiology and clinical consequences of gallstones, the most important biliary tract disorder, closing with a brief discussion of neoplasms and other causes of bile duct obstruction. The reader is referred to Chapter 40 for a detailed discussion of the diagnostic approach to jaundice and biliary obstruction and to Chapter 33 for a review of the various imaging techniques used to study the biliary tract.

NORMAL BILIARY PHYSIOLOGY

Bile, a complex fluid secreted by hepatocytes, passes via the intrahepatic bile ducts into the common bile duct. Tonic contraction of the sphincter of Oddi during fasting diverts about half of hepatic bile into the gallbladder, where it is stored and concentrated. Cholecystokinin, released after food is ingested, causes the gallbladder to contract and the sphincter of Oddi to relax, allowing delivery of a timed bolus of bile, rich in bile acids, into the intestine. Bile acids, detergent molecules possessing both fat-soluble and water-soluble moieties, convey phospholipids and cholesterol from the liver to the intestine, where cholesterol undergoes fecal excretion. In the intestinal lumen, bile acids solubilize dietary fat and promote its digestion and absorption. Bile acids are, for the most part, efficiently reabsorbed by the small intestinal mucosa, particularly in the terminal ileum, and are recycled to the liver for re-excretion, a process termed *enterohepatic circulation* (Fig. 45–1).

PATHOPHYSIOLOGY OF GALLSTONE FORMATION (CHOLELITHIASIS)

Gallstones, the most common cause of biliary tract disease in the United States, occur in 20 to 35% of people by age 75 years and are of two types: 75% consist primarily of cholesterol, whereas 25%, termed pigment stones, are composed of calcium bilirubinate and other calcium salts. Cholesterol, which is insoluble in water, normally is carried in bile solubilized by bile acids and phospholipids. However, in most individuals, many of whom do not develop gallstones, bile contains more cholesterol than can be maintained in stable solution (Fig. 45–2); that is, it is supersaturated with cholesterol. In the supersaturated bile of some individuals, microscopic cholesterol crystals form. The interplay of nucleation (mucus, stasis) and "antinucleating" (apolipoprotein A-I) factors may determine whether cholesterol gallstones form in supersaturated bile. Gradual deposition of additional layers of cholesterol leads to the appearance of macroscopic cholesterol gallstones.

The gallbladder is key to gallstone formation; it constitutes an area of bile stasis in which slow crystal growth can occur and it also may provide mucus or other material to act as a nidus to initiate cholesterol crystal formation. Many of the recognized predisposing factors for cholelithiasis can be understood in terms of the pathophysiologic scheme just outlined: (1) biliary cholesterol saturation is increased by estrogens, multiparity, oral contraceptives, obesity, and terminal ileal disease (which decreases the bile acid pool); and (2) bile stasis is increased by bile duct strictures, parenteral hyperalimentation, fasting, and choledochal cysts.

The pathophysiology of pigment stones is less well understood; however, increased production of bilirubin (hemolytic states), increased biliary Ca^{2+} and CO_3^{2-}, cirrhosis, and bacterial deconjugation of bilirubin to a less soluble form are all associated with pigment stone formation.

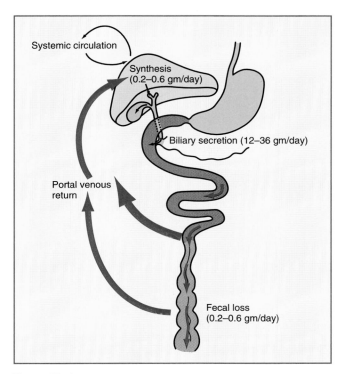

Figure 45–1
The enterohepatic circulation of bile salts in humans. The liver secretes 12 to 36 gm of bile salts per day in bile. Ninety-five percent of these bile salts are reabsorbed, with specific bile salt transporters in the terminal ileum accounting for much of the up-take. Bile salts recycle to the liver via portal blood, where they are efficiently extracted by hepatocytes and resecreted into bile. The liver also synthesizes sufficient bile salts to equal daily fecal losses (0.2 to 0.6 gm/day). Because of efficient uptake of bile salts by both intestine and liver, delivery of 12 to 36 gm of bile salts to the intestine daily is achieved by recycling a small pool (3 gm) of bile salts 4 to 12 times per day. (Modified from Carey MC: The enterohepatic circulation. *In* Arias IM, Popper H, Schacter D, et al [eds.]: The Liver: Biology and Pathobiology. New York, Raven Press, 1982.)

CLINICAL MANIFESTATIONS OF GALLSTONES

Most individuals with gallstones are asymptomatic. Duct obstruction is the underlying cause of all manifestations of gallstone disease. Obstruction of the cystic duct distends the gallbladder and produces biliary pain, while superimposed infection or inflammation leads to acute cholecystitis. Obstruction of the common duct may produce pain, jaundice, infection (cholangitis), pancreatitis, and/or hepatic damage and biliary cirrhosis. The natural history of gallstone disease is outlined in Figure 45–3.

Asymptomatic Gallstones

Approximately 60 to 80% of patients with gallstones in the United States are asymptomatic. Over a 20-year period it appears that only about 18% of these individuals develop biliary pain and only 3% require a cholecystectomy. Asymptomatic patients should be followed expec-

tantly, with prophylactic cholecystectomy considered in three high-risk groups: (1) diabetics, who have a greater mortality (10 to 15%) from acute cholecystitis; (2) persons with a calcified gallbladder, which may be associated with carcinoma of the gallbladder; and (3) persons with sickle cell anemia, in whom hepatic crises may be difficult to differentiate from acute cholecystitis. Dissolution of cholesterol gallstones by orally administered chenodeoxycholic acid or ursodeoxycholic acid is successful in some selected patients; however, a policy of expectant management followed by cholecystectomy is probably more cost-effective. Alternative methods to eliminate gallstones include (1) dissolving cholesterol stones by instilling methyl-tert-butyl ether into the gallbladder and (2) fragmenting stones by extracorporeal shockwave lithotripsy.

Chronic Cholecystitis and Biliary Pain

The term *chronic cholecystitis* has been used to denote nonacute symptoms due to the presence of gallstones. A better term is *biliary pain,* as only a loose correlation exists between the presence of symptoms and pathologic findings such as inflammation in the gallbladder wall. Gallbladders from symptomatic patients may be grossly normal with mild histologic inflammation or may exhibit shrinking, scarring, and thickening, often as a result of previous attacks of acute cholecystitis. Symptoms arise from contraction of the gallbladder during transient ob-

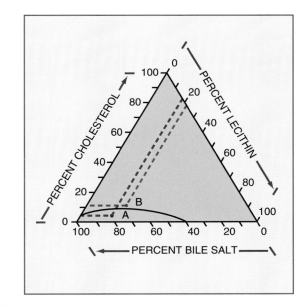

Figure 45–2
Phase diagram for plotting different mixtures of bile salt, lecithin, and cholesterol. The curved line represents the boundary of the micellar zone for aqueous solutions containing 4 to 10% solids. Any mixture, such as A, falling within this area contains cholesterol in solution. Any mixture, such as B, falling outside this area has excess cholesterol as a precipitate or supersaturated solution. The points A and B actually depict the average composition of gallbladder bile obtained from normal persons and patients with cholesterol gallstones, respectively.

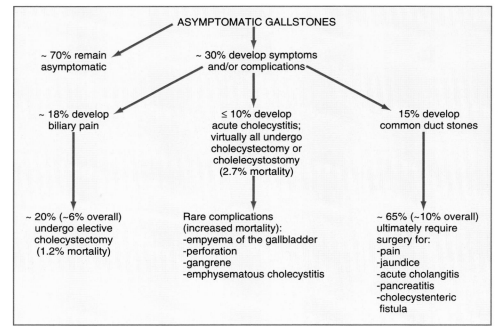

Figure 45-3
Natural history of asymptomatic gallstones. The clinical syndromes associated with gallstones are shown here, and the numbers represent the approximate percentage of adults who develop one or more of these symptoms or complications over a 15- to 20-year period. Over this period, approximately 30% of individuals with gallstones undergo surgery. (The risk of developing complications of gallstones varies considerably among series. The figures shown here represent those derived from more recent studies.)

struction of the cystic duct by gallstones. Biliary pain usually is a steady, cramplike pain in the epigastrium or right upper quadrant (RUQ), which comes on quickly, reaches a plateau of intensity over a few minutes, and begins to subside gradually over 30 minutes to several hours. Referred pain may be felt at the tip of the scapula or right shoulder. Nausea and vomiting may accompany biliary pain, whereas fever, leukocytosis, and a palpable mass (signs of acute cholecystitis) do not. Attacks occur at variable intervals (days to years). Other symptoms such as dyspepsia, fatty food intolerance, flatulence, heartburn, and belching may occur in patients with gallstones; however, they are nonspecific and frequently occur in individuals with normal gallbladders. Gallstones can be best demonstrated by ultrasonography (which demonstrates gallstones in >95% of patients). Alternatively, one can use oral cholescystography (which demonstrates stones in two thirds of patients; the gallbladder is not visualized in one third of patients, a finding taken to indicate gallbladder disease). Cholecystectomy, either laparoscopic or conventional, which carries a mortality of <0.5%, is the treatment of choice for recurrent biliary pain and may be accompanied by examination of the common duct for concomitant choledocholithiasis. Surgery relieves symptoms of biliary pain in virtually all patients and prevents development of future complications such as acute cholecystitis, choledocholithiasis, and cholangitis. Alternative approaches to eliminating gallstones, including dissolution and fragmentation, are less commonly used because gallstones may recur.

Acute Cholecystitis

Acute cholecystitis refers to acute right subcostal pain and tenderness due to obstruction of the cystic duct and sub-

sequent distention, inflammation, and secondary infection of the gallbladder. Acalculous cholecystitis, accounting for 5% of cases, is associated with prolonged fasting, as occurs with trauma, surgery, or parenteral hyperalimentation, and gallbladder bile that is viscous or "sludgelike." Acute cholecystitis usually begins with epigastric or RUQ pain that gradually increases in severity and usually localizes to the area of the gallbladder. Unlike biliary pain, the pain of acute cholecystitis does not subside spontaneously. Anorexia, nausea, vomiting, fever, and right subcostal tenderness are commonly present, as is Murphy's sign (increased subhepatic tenderness and inspiratory arrest during a deep breath). In approximately one third of patients, a tender, enlarged gallbladder may be felt. Mild jaundice occurs in about 20% of patients as a result of concomitant common duct stones or bile duct edema. Complications of acute cholecystitis include emphysematous cholecystitis (bacterial gas present in gallbladder lumen and tissues), empyema of the gallbladder, gangrene, and perforation. Approximately 10% of patients present with or develop one of these complications and require emergency surgery. The onset of severe fever, shaking chills, increased leukocytosis, increased abdominal pain or tenderness, or persistent severe symptoms, alone or in combination, indicates progression of disease and suggests development of one of these complications.

Radionuclide scanning following intravenous administration of ^{99m}Tc-DISIDA is the most accurate test with which to confirm the clinical impression of acute cholecystitis (cystic duct obstruction). If the gallbladder fills with the isotope, acute cholecystitis is unlikely, whereas if the bile duct is visualized but the gallbladder is not, the clinical diagnosis is strongly supported. An ultrasound examination that shows the presence of gallstones (or sludge in acalculous cholecystitis), along with localized tenderness over the gallbladder, also provides strong supportive evidence for acute cholecystitis. Oral cholecystograms are of no value in this clinical setting, as they are unreliable in the acutely ill patient.

Patients with acute cholecystitis may improve over 1 to 7 days with conventional expectant management, which includes nasogastric suction, intravenous fluids, and judicious antibiotics and pain medication. Because of the high risk of recurrent acute cholecystitis, most patients need to undergo cholecystectomy, often performed within the first 24 to 48 hours or, less often, 4 to 8 weeks after an acute episode, as either conventional or laparoscopic cholecystectomy (Fig. 45–4).

Emergency surgery is performed on patients with advanced disease and complications, usually associated with infection and sepsis. Cholecystostomy (either operative or percutaneous), rather than cholecystectomy, may be a useful technique in patients in whom there is a high operative risk. Patients who are good operative risks and in whom the diagnosis is certain are scheduled for prompt cholecystectomy within 24 to 48 hours. Antibiotics are used in patients with suppurative complications. Expectant management is reserved for those with uncomplicated disease who are not good operative candidates or those in whom the diagnosis is not clear.

The mortality of acute cholecystitis of 5 to 10% is almost entirely confined to patients over age 60 with serious associated diseases and to those with suppurative complications. Complications of acute cholecystitis include infectious complications already listed and gallstone ileus (intestinal obstruction due to erosion of a gallstone through the gallbladder and duodenal walls into the intestinal lumen).

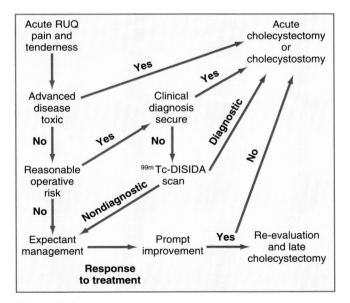

Figure 45–4
Scheme for managing patients with right upper quadrant pain and tenderness who are thought to have acute cholecystitis. This scheme is based on a policy of early operation (conventional or laparoscopic) for appropriate patients and use of cholecystostomy (operative or percutaneous) for patients who are poor operative risks.

Choledocholithiasis and Acute Cholangitis

In the United States, most gallstones in the common duct come from the gallbladder; this occurs in up to 15% of persons with cholelithiasis. Less commonly, stones may form *de novo* in the biliary tree. Ductal stones may be asymptomatic (30 to 40%) or may produce biliary colic, jaundice, cholangitis, pancreatitis, or a combination of these. Secondary hepatic effects include biliary cirrhosis and hepatic abscesses.

Intermittent cholangitis, consisting of biliary pain, jaundice, and fever plus chills (Charcot's triad), is the most common manifestation of choledocholithiasis. Biliary infection may be mild or it may be severe, with suppurative cholangitis, sepsis, and shock. Diagnosis is based on a compatible clinical picture and radiologic or endoscopic evidence of ductal stones. Treatment includes hospitalization, treatment of infection, and removal of stones. The latter may be accomplished surgically in patients with an intact gallbladder by cholecystectomy and choledochotomy. Alternatively, endoscopic sphincterotomy and stone extraction may be combined with laparoscopic cholecystectomy. In individuals with a previous cholecystectomy or those who are poor surgical candidates, endoscopic sphincterotomy, which opens the sphincter of Oddi and allows passage of gallstones up to 1 cm, is the preferred approach.

The most severe form of cholangitis, suppurative cholangitis, rapidly results in life-threatening sepsis. Initially, patients may have only mild signs of biliary obstruction, yet they require rapid evaluation and treatment, including intravenous fluids and antibiotics and emergency procedures (usually endoscopic or percutaneous) to drain the biliary tree. The high mortality of 50% for this disease reflects the age of the patients generally affected, the speed with which sepsis develops, and the frequent failure to identify the biliary tree as the source of sepsis.

Other Disorders of the Biliary Tree

A number of other processes, all of which may present as biliary obstruction, jaundice, or infection, may involve the biliary tree. The approach to evaluating these entities is outlined in Chapter 33.

Benign biliary strictures usually result from surgical injury and may cause symptoms days to years later. Early diagnosis is important, as strictures that partially obstruct and are clinically asymptomatic may cause secondary biliary cirrhosis. Biliary stricture should be suspected in anyone with a history of RUQ surgery and a persistently elevated serum alkaline phosphatase level. A similar type of benign stricture is seen in alcoholics in whom the intrapancreatic portion of the common bile duct is compressed by pancreatic fibrosis. Endoscopic balloon catheter dilatation is useful in many of these patients, and surgical repair or bypass may also be considered.

Sclerosing cholangitis is an idiopathic condition of nonmalignant, nonbacterial chronic inflammatory narrowing of the intra- and extrahepatic bile ducts. It most commonly occurs in males, often in association with ulcerative colitis. Patients frequently present with pruritus and jaundice, though asymptomatic elevations in the serum alkaline phosphatase may also be seen. Endoscopic retrograde cholangiopancreatography or percutaneous transhepatic cholangiography shows characteristic changes ("beading") of the bile ducts. Therapy includes antibiotics for bacterial cholangitis, medical treatment of cholestasis (ursodeoxycholic acid), attempts at improving biliary drainage (if a "dominant stricture" is present), and liver transplantation.

Structural abnormalities such as choledochal cysts, Caroli's disease (saccular intrahepatic bile duct dilation), and duodenal diverticuli may also cause bile duct obstruction, often with secondary choledocholithiasis. Hemobilia with intermittent bile duct obstruction by blood clots may be caused by hepatic injury, neoplasms, or hepatic artery aneurysms.

Biliary neoplasms are rare but include carcinoma of the gallbladder, scirrhous or papillary adenocarcinoma of the bile ducts, and carcinoma of the ampulla of Vater. The last two neoplasms usually present as unremitting painless jaundice, although necrosis and sloughing of tumor may cause intermittent obstruction and the appearance of occult fecal blood. Carcinoma of the gallbladder often presents as advanced disseminated disease, although symptoms also may resemble those of acute or chronic cholecystitis or bile duct obstruction. The incidence of cholangiocarcinoma is increased in patients with primary sclerosing cholangitis. Resection of most of these tumors is difficult or impossible and prognosis is poor. For patients with unresectable tumor, the goal is palliation, and for those with severe symptoms due to obstruction, percutaneous or endoscopic stenting of the biliary tree may be helpful. The use of stents for benign disease has increased as experience has been gained and therapeutic advances have occurred. However, definitive surgical repair or bypass may be useful.

Motility disorders of the biliary tree were not well recognized in the past. With the use of newer endoscopic techniques for measuring biliary pressures and motility, it has become apparent that a small group of patients with biliary-type pain have symptoms due to hypertension, dysmotility, and/or stenosis of the sphincter of Oddi, and in this select group, endoscopic or surgical sphincterotomy is of value.

REFERENCES

Gracie WA, Ransohoff DF: The natural history of silent gallstones. The innocent gallstone is not a myth. N Engl J Med 1982; 307:798.

Phillips JO, Wiesner RH, LaRusso NF: Sclerosing cholangitis. *In* Kirsner JB (ed.): The Growth of Gastroenterologic Knowledge During the Twentieth Century. Baltimore, Williams & Wilkins, 1994.

Sleisenger MH, Fordtran JS (eds.): Gastrointestinal Disease: Pathophysiology, Diagnosis and Management. 5th ed. Philadelphia, WB Saunders, 1993.

Thistle JL, Cleary PA, Lachin JM, et al: The natural history of cholelithiasis: The national cooperative gallstone study. Ann Intern Med 1984; 101:171.

Vlahcevic ZR, Heuman DM: Diseases of the gallbladder and bile ducts. *In* Bennett JC, Plum F (eds.): Cecil Textbook of Medicine. 20th ed. Philadelphia, WB Saunders, 1996, pp 805–816.

Hematologic Disease

Section VII

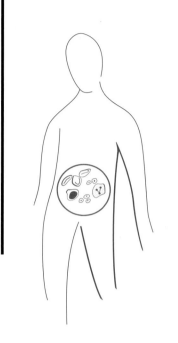

46

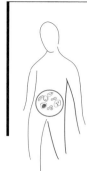

The Blood and Bone Marrow

Hematology is the study of the blood and bone marrow and their disorders. These diseases can best be understood by understanding the origin and function of the blood and blood cells and bone marrow and noting the effects when the normal physiology goes awry.

THE BLOOD

The blood consists of a liquid phase containing a great variety of substances and cellular elements of three main varieties: erythrocytes, leukocytes, and platelets. The red cells may be distinguished by supravital staining as reticulocytes (which are the newly produced cells) and mature red cells; the morphology of the red cells (size and shape) is important in delineating abnormalities. Platelets are not divided morphologically into different classes, but their morphology is also observed in stained preparations to detect abnormalities of size and contents.

The leukocytes are distinguished into several categories. The most populous are the neutrophils, which have a segmented nucleus and pinkish-brown granules in the cytoplasm. Their close relatives, eosinophils, have large red refractile granules, and basophils have many dark blue granules. Monocytes have blue-gray cytoplasm and an indented (kidney-shaped) nucleus. Lymphocytes have a generally round nucleus and cytoplasm in a variable amount that is blue and usually agranular.

The numbers of each of these cellular types are very carefully controlled under normal circumstances. These values are given in Table 46–1.

THE BONE MARROW

In the normal adult, the cells of the blood originate in the bone marrow, but the active marrow is confined to selected areas of bones: the ends of the long bones, the flat bones of the head and pelvis, the ribs, and the vertebral bodies. In children, active marrow also occurs in the shaft of the long bones, and in the fetus, in the spleen and liver.

Morphology

The marrow is examined after removal by aspiration or by biopsy, usually from the posterior superior iliac spine.

In the aspirated sample, the cells are spread and stained with polychrome stains that allow detailed examination and classification. The biopsy (a core of bone marrow removed intact by a large needle) permits evaluation of the structure of the marrow.

The normal marrow consists of hematopoietic precursors of granulocytes (usually the predominant cells), erythrocytes (1/3 to 1/5 the number of granulocyte precursors), some lymphocytes and plasma cells, and a few scattered precursors of platelets (megakaryocytes). All these cells constitute about 60% of the "space"; the rest of the marrow is taken up by fat cells and small amounts of supportive cells (blood vessels and fibroblasts).

Granulocytes

The most immature granulocytic precursor that is morphologically defined is the myeloblast. Since it is highly replicative, the chromatin of its nucleus is not condensed but is dispersed and contains nucleoli. The cytoplasm is rich in RNA and is hence a deep blue in the usual polychrome stains; no organelles are seen. As the cell matures, the chromatin of the nucleus becomes more condensed, the nucleoli disappear, and cytoplasmic organelles appear. In the earliest differentiated form, the progranulocyte, "primary" granules, which are deeply basophilic, appear; these contain microbicidal components (defensins, permeability-increasing protein, lysozyme, myeloperoxidase) and hydrolytic enzymes (neutral and acid proteases).

At the next step in maturation, a prominent Golgi apparatus appears, which is essential in "packaging" the definitive secondary granules. The Golgi apparatus itself does not stain but can be detected early when it contains the developing granules as a globule near the nucleus. It displaces the nucleus and eventually fits into the concavity of the nucleus as it matures. As soon as the specific granules (neutrophilic, eosinophilic, or basophilic) appear, the cell is classified as a myelocyte. As the nucleus undergoes further condensation and change in shape, it is called a metamyelocyte, a stab, and finally, as it forms into segments separated by thin strands, a segmented neutrophil. The granulocyte and basophil usually form three or four segments, the eosinophil, two.

The maturation of the erythrocytic precursors follows a similar scheme. The earliest precursor, the rubriblast, is much like the myeloblast except that the concentration of

RNA in the cytoplasm is higher and it is therefore more blue. As the cell matures, the chromatin of the nucleus becomes very condensed and does not segment but simply becomes smaller. The cytoplasm does not acquire organelles but rather hemoglobin; thus, it becomes progressively pinker until, when fully mature, it is virtually the same color as the red cell. The last step, the ejection of the nucleus, leaves only a remnant of RNA and other residual material. This material stains the cell a faint blue in the usual staining technique (which fixes the cells before applying the stain) or as blue-staining material in the reticulocyte staining technique (in which the stain reacts with the cell before fixation). These cells, which lack a nucleus but contain cytoplasmic remnants, are called reticulocytes and remain in the marrow for about 2 days; they spend about 1 day maturing in the spleen and then circulate in the peripheral blood for 1 day, where they constitute about 1% of the cells.

Platelets

The precursors of platelets, megakaryocytes, also originate as an immature blast cell. As they mature, they make copious amounts of cytoplasm, which gradually differentiates into platelet-like domains. The nucleus undergoes endoreduplication in which it replicates but does not divide. Thus, the fully mature megakaryocytes may contain the amount of DNA contained in 32 to 64 cells.

Monocytes

Monocytes constitute a minor population in the marrow and, under normal conditions, their presence is scarcely noted. Lymphocytes originate in the marrow but develop and mature elsewhere, for the most part.

Cellular Ontogeny in the Marrow

The homeostasis of the marrow is maintained by a delicate balance between proliferation and differentiation. All the cells of the marrow are derived from the stem cell, which is defined better by its characteristics than by its morphology (Fig. 46–1). This cell is capable of reproducing itself but is also capable of differentiating into any of the marrow elements; this proliferation and differentiation are under the control of a variety of polypeptides called cytokines (e.g., stem cell factor [SCF], granulocyte-macrophage colony stimulating factor [GM-CSF], granulocyte-colony stimulating factor [G-CSF], interleukin [IL]-3), which react with specific membrane surface receptors of the cell. These cytokines may be stimulatory or inhibitory, and their interplay results in the normal functioning of the marrow.

The lymphocyte lineage differentiates very early under the influence of a variety of cytokines, particularly IL-7. These cells then migrate to the thymus, spleen, and lymph nodes where, under specific controls, they differentiate into the full panoply of the immune system; this process is described in Chapter 48.

The stem cell that will differentiate into the other marrow elements is detected in culture by its ability to form mixed colonies, the so-called GEMM (granulocyte, erythrocyte, megakaryocyte, monocyte) colonies. Under the influence of the cytokine GM-CSF, the granulocyte-macrophage lineage splits from the erythrocyte-mega-

TABLE 46–1	Normal Values for Blood Cells		
Cell Type	**Sex**	**Mean**	**Range**
Hemoglobin	Women	14.0 g/dl	12–16 g/dl
	Men	15.5 g/dl	13.5–17.5 g/dl
Hematocrit	Women	41%	36–46%
	Men	47%	41–53%
Reticulocyte count		1%	0.5–1.5%
		60,000/μl	35,000–85,000/μl
Mean corpuscular volume (MCV)		89 fl	82–98 fl
Platelet count		250,000/μl	150,000–400,000/μl
Total white count		7400/μl	4500–11,000/μl
Neutrophils		59%	
		4400/μl	1800–7700/μl
Lymphocytes		34%	
		2500/μl	1000–4800/μl
Monocytes		4%	
		300/μl	
Eosinophils		3%	
		200/μl	
Basophils		1%	
		65/μl	

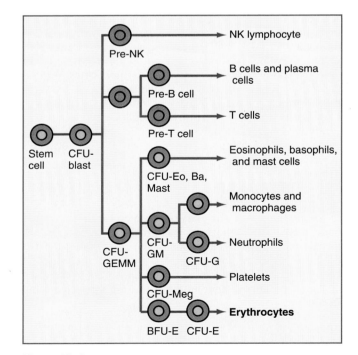

Figure 46–1

Schema of the development of the cells of the bone marrow.

karyocyte lineage; this lineage is further split between granulocytes (stimulated by the cytokine G-CSF) and monocytes-macrophages, each proceeding along a specific differentiation pathway. The granulocyte lineage further splits into neutrophils, eosinophils, and basophils before they reach final differentiation and maturation. The maturation of the macrophage-monocyte lineage proceeds separately; differentiation to macrophages does not occur for the most part until the cells migrate to peripheral sites.

The split into erythrocyte and megakaryocyte lineages occurs early and is under the influence of two cytokines, erythropoietin (EPO) and (presumably) thrombopoietin (TPO). The rate of secretion of EPO by the kidney is determined by the supply of oxygen available at the sensing cell. This cytokine, which is a glycoprotein of 35 kD molecular weight, then circulates to the marrow where it engages specific receptors on cells undergoing differentiation to the erythrocytic series. This interaction causes the cells to differentiate and to proliferate more rapidly, thus increasing the production of red cells.

A similar series of events presumably controls the production of platelets. Two cytokines, IL-11 and TPO, have recently been found, and the control of their secretion is not clear; presumably, some measure of the need for platelets increases its output. The result is an increase in the number of megakaryocytes and hence of platelets.

REFERENCES

Moore MAC: Clinical implications of positive and negative hematopoietic stem cell regulators. Blood 1991; 78:1.
Williams DA: In search of the self-renewing hematopoietic stem cell. Blood Cells 1991; 17:296.

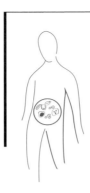

47

Disorders of the Hematopoietic Stem Cell

Abnormalities in the proliferation or differentiation and maturation of the stem cell have widespread implications for diseases of the hematopoietic system, and these abnormalities are likely to affect all the lineages of blood cells. Such disorders originating in the stem cell can be classified into three categories (Table 47–1):

1. Myeloaplastic disorders—characterized by a deficiency of production of the cells of the marrow but, for the most part, the cells that are produced are normal.
2. Myelodysplastic disorders—characterized by disordered and ineffective production of marrow cells, often with peripheral cytopenias, and the cells that are produced can usually be demonstrated to be abnormal in morphology and biochemistry.
3. Myeloproliferative disorders—characterized by overproduction of one or more of the cell lineages; the cells that are produced may also have dysplastic characteristics but these are usually less apparent than in the myelodysplastic disorders.

Because all three categories of disorders involve primarily the stem cell, they often merge into one another, and the boundaries are not always distinct. Thus, a patient with aplastic anemia (a myeloaplastic disorder) may exhibit changes characteristic of the myelodysplastic disorders. Furthermore, in all these disorders, there is a chance of their evolving into acute leukemia.

THE MYELOAPLASTIC DISORDERS

The myeloaplastic disorders are characterized by diminished production of cells in the marrow, resulting in peripheral cytopenia. When the stem cell is affected, the proliferation of all cell lineages is diminished and pancytopenia results; this is generically called "aplastic anemia" even though it is clear that the major difficulties are not related to anemia. In other cases, only a single line may be afflicted by problems with proliferation, as in the case of amegakaryocytic thrombocytopenia.

Myeloaplastic disorders may result from a wide variety of causes. In some instances, there is a congenital abnormality of the stem cell. In others, the stem cell may acquire a mutation that results in diminished production. The stem cell may be normal, but its proliferation and/or differentiation may be suppressed (e.g., by immune or by toxic influences) or may not be stimulated (e.g., by a lack of a cytokine). The clinical result is the same—deficiency of hematopoietic cells.

Congenital Myeloaplastic Disorders

Rarely, congenital defects in the stem cell result in aplastic anemia. The best known syndrome is Fanconi's anemia, which may not become apparent until adulthood. It is often associated with other abnormalities of the skin, genitourinary system, or musculoskeletal system and is characterized by specific chromosomal abnormalities that may become more apparent after exposure to oxidant and other drugs. There appear to be multiple forms, but all result in bone marrow failure, which is likely to be fatal.

Other syndromes, such as Shwachman-Diamond syndrome, dyskeratosis congenital, and reticular dysgenesis are also associated with aplastic pancytopenia but are even more rare.

Acquired Aplastic Anemia

Primary failure of proliferation of cells of the marrow results in pancytopenia of variable degree. This can occur secondary to drugs that interrupt cellular proliferation (chemotherapeutic agents) or to irradiation of the sites of production, or as an idiopathic acquired condition, which may or may not have followed some toxic exposure.

Basis of the Disease

Acquired aplastic anemia may be related to an external toxic or suppressive influence (drugs, viruses) or to poorly defined (probably autoimmune) causes. In both cases, all the cell lines of the marrow are affected.

Chemical substances have their effect in a number of ways, depending upon their structure. The cytotoxic drugs designed to treat malignancy usually interrupt the cell cycle or alter intracellular processes so that cell death supervenes; these seldom cause long-lasting aplastic anemia unless all the stem cells are victims. In some instances, the toxicity of the compound appears to reside in faulty detoxification, resulting in toxic intermediates in

TABLE 47–1	**Classification of the Disorders of the Stem Cell**

I. Myeloaplastic disorders
   A. Congenital
      1. Fanconi's
      2. Others more rare
   B. Acquired
      1. Suppression of hematopoiesis by toxin
      2. Idiopathic acquired
II. Myelodysplastic disorders
   A. Refractory anemia
      1. With ringed sideroblasts
      2. With excess blasts
      3. In transition to leukemia
   B. Chronic myelomonocytic leukemia
   C. Myelofibrosis (myeloid metaplasia)
   D. Paroxysmal nocturnal hemoglobinuria
III. Myeloproliferative diseases
   A. Polycythemia vera
   B. Chronic myelogenous leukemia
   C. Essential thrombocythemia
IV. Acute leukemia
   A. Acute lymphocytic leukemia
   B. Acute myelocytic leukemia
      1. Acute promyelocytic leukemia
      2. Other variations

some patients. Stem cell function can also be markedly reduced by certain viruses, particularly non-A, non-B, non-C viral hepatitis; in this case, the suppression of hematopoiesis may be long lasting.

Idiopathic acquired aplastic anemia is thought to be due primarily to autoimmune suppression of the stem cells. The evidence is somewhat indirect (recovery after therapy directed against immune reactions and indications of increased cytotoxic T cell activity) but is sufficient to merit consideration when planning therapeutic intervention.

Clinical and Laboratory Findings

Aplastic anemia is a disease of young adults, with a peak incidence at age 20 to 25, and of the elderly, with a less evident peak about age 60 to 65. Its incidence in the population ranges from 1.5 to 15 per million; higher incidences are found in countries in Eastern Asia. Men and women are nearly equally affected, and there is little familial predisposition.

The degree of severity may vary greatly, and the prognosis varies with the severity. Usually all three cell lines in the peripheral blood are deficient in number but normal in morphology, although the red cells may be large and have an elevated mean corpuscular volume (MCV). The reticulocyte count is reduced, frequently to very low numbers (< 5000/mm^3). The marrow is hypoplastic and may contain primarily lymphocytes. There are generally no other abnormalities of blood chemistries unless the course is complicated by infection.

If the diagnosis is made, immediate and aggressive therapy is needed if the condition is felt to be consistent

with severe aplastic anemia (SAA), as the prognosis of these patients is very poor if the condition is not successfully treated.

Therapy

The treatment of aplastic anemia is of three kinds: supportive, immunosuppressive, and marrow replacement. Supportive treatment consists of transfusions of red blood cells or platelets as needed and the appropriate use of antibiotics for infections. Transfusions should be limited in patients who are candidates for bone marrow transplantation, as they may induce alloimmunization and increase the risk of failure of the transplant; most importantly, no transfusions of blood from potential marrow donors should be given. Adrenocortical and androgenic steroids have been given in the past but are of minimal benefit.

The most definitive treatment of SAA is bone marrow transplantation, preferably from an human leukocyte antigen (HLA)-identical sibling; haploidentical and unrelated HLA-identical donors have also been used with much less success. Transplantation is age-limited (patients older than 50 years generally cannot tolerate the procedure) and is complicated by infections, graft-versus-host disease, and graft rejection. The overall success rate in aplastic anemia is 70%.

Immunosuppression using antithymocyte (or antilymphocyte) globulin (ATG) (derived from the serum of horses immunized with human lymphocytic cells) and cyclosporin (a T cell suppressing agent) is about equally successful in treating aplastic anemia and is used most frequently when bone marrow transplantation is not an option. The treatment may result in serum sickness. Relapse may occur and re-treatment may be necessary. The overall survival is about 60% following this treatment. Fifteen to 30% of patients who recover after ATG treatment have paroxysmal nocturnal hemoglobinuria (PNH; see later) or some other form of myelodysplasia.

THE MYELODYSPLASTIC DISORDERS

The myelodysplastic disorders are characterized by altered proliferation, usually resulting in cytopenia and abnormal cells. These appear to be due to abnormalities affecting the stem cell, since all three lines are usually affected, sometimes one more than the another. All may result in acute myeloblastic leukemia in some patients.

Myelodysplastic Syndromes (MDSs)

Myelodysplastic syndromes usually present in a slow and insidious development of bone marrow failure characterized by anemia and thrombocytopenia or a combination of both. MDSs usually have been found in the elderly but, in recent years, have been diagnosed at almost every age and appear to be increasing in younger age groups, especially those who have been treated with combination chemotherapy and irradiation therapy or a combination of the two. MDSs especially appear to occur after treatment for Hodgkin's disease or ovarian carcinoma but may occur after any chemotherapy with alkylating agents, including that given to patients treated with cyclophosphamide as an immunosuppressive agent for diseases such as systemic lupus, autoimmune hemolytic anemia, and thrombocytopenia. Typically, MDSs present with progressive symptoms and clinical signs of cytopenias (anemia and thrombocytopenia) along with increased fatigability and decreased exercise tolerance. Physical examination may reveal pallor, purpura, or petechiae, and laboratory examination reveals anemia and/or thrombocytopenia. The anemia in MDSs is typically macrocytic, with a mean corpuscular volume of 100 to 110 μL. The peripheral smear may show a dimorphic population of red blood cells, with one normochromic and normocytic and the other abnormal. The bone marrow is typically hypercellular with increased iron stores and morphologically abnormal erythroid precursors, which appear megaloblastoid with dyserythropoiesis. Hypocellular bone marrow in MDSs tends to impart a poor prognosis. Increased immature myeloid forms (blasts) may herald a more aggressive course and progression to acute leukemia.

The MDSs have been classified on morphologic grounds; Table 47–2 outlines the major clinical features and relative incidence of the five types of MDS. Refractory anemia (RA) is the most common type and may be present with or without ringed sideroblasts (RA or RAS). Median survival is approximately 3 to 4 years. RA is often associated with a specific chromosome abnormality, deletion of the long arm of chromosome 5, designated the 5q- syndrome. This group rarely proceeds to acute leukemia.

The other three categories, refractory anemia with excess blasts (RAEB), chronic myelomonocytic leukemia (CMML), and refractory anemia in transition (RAEBIT) carry a poorer prognosis with survival ranging from 1 to 2 years. Death in MDSs is usually due either to marrow failure or evolution to acute myeloid leukemia. The acute leukemia arising from MDSs is difficult to treat, and complete remissions are rarely obtained.

Treatment of MDSs is primarily directed toward improving the cytopenias and their clinical manifestations. Transfusions of red blood cells and, less often, platelets are the mainstay of treatment. Some patients with refractory anemia with ringed sideroblasts (RAS) respond to large doses of pyridoxine (vitamin B$_6$). Growth factors, especially recombinant human erythropoietin (rhu-EPO) may improve the anemia in some patients, and myeloid growth factors or granulocyte-colony stimulating factor (G-CSF or GM-CSF) may improve marrow function and the granulocytopenia in some patients. Other maturation agents have not been successful. Chemotherapy, usually low-dose cytosine arabinoside (AraC), has been used when increased numbers of blasts appear in the bone marrow, but the role of this drug is controversial; more recently, 5-azacytidine has been used with success. Bone marrow transplantation in younger patients should be strongly considered when an appropriate donor is available.

Paroxysmal Nocturnal Hemoglobinuria

Paroxysmal nocturnal hemoglobinuria (PNH) is an acquired stem cell disorder that is characterized by intravascular hemolysis, unusual venous thromboses, and evidence of diminished hematopoiesis. It may occur at any age but particularly in young adulthood and affects men and women equally. It is uncommon but not rare; estimates of 1/100,000 population have been made.

Basis of the Disease

Paroxysmal nocturnal hemoglobinuria is the result of the somatic mutation of a gene (the pig-A gene) on the X chromosome of a stem cell. The gene product that is missing is necessary for the biosynthesis of the glycosylphosphatidyl inositol (GPI) anchor, which is added to proteins post-translationally to anchor them into the external plasma membrane of the cell. Since this anchor cannot be synthesized in the defective cells, the proteins dependent upon it for their expression do not appear on the outer membrane of the cell. To date, at least 20 such proteins have been identified, and it is the lack of these proteins that are thought to underlie the pathogenesis of the disease.

Although the mutation occurs in a single cell (in most cases), the progeny of that cell may become predominant in the marrow and, in many patients, nearly

TABLE 47–2	Classification of the Myelodysplastic Syndromes		
Diagnosis (Relative Incidence)	**Patient Characteristics**	**Peripheral Blood**	**Bone Marrow**
Refractory anemia (56%)	Elderly patient; anemia	May have abnormal red cell morphology	<5% blasts
Refractory anemia with ringed sideroblasts (21%)	Elderly; anemia	May have dimorphic picture (microcytic/hypochromic and macrocytic)	Hypercellular; iron stain shows iron in a ring around red cell nuclei
Refractory anemia with excess blasts (10%)	May have pancytopenia	<5% blasts	5–20% blasts
Chronic myelomonocytic leukemia (11%)	Similar to above	Absolute monocytosis <5% blasts	5–20% blasts
Refractory anemia in transformation (1%)	Any age; symptoms of brief duration	>5% blasts	20–30% blasts

completely replace the normal cells. It is not clear how this happens, as the defective stem cell does not appear to have any proliferative advantage in cell culture studies.

Clinical Findings

Hemoglobinuria results from the intravascular hemolysis of the abnormal red cells. These cells lack the proteins that down-regulate the activation of complement at the cell surface (CD55 and CD59); thus, minimal activation of complement results in rupture of the membrane. The hemoglobinuria is nocturnal because complement is activated at night and is paroxysmal because complement is activated by such things as infections and physical stress. It results in a marked loss of iron in the urine, and many patients become iron deficient. It can result in acute renal failure if it is severe and in chronic renal damage if it is prolonged over years. Many patients, particularly those with small abnormal populations of red cells (less than 20 to 30%), rarely or never have overt hemoglobinuria but nearly always have hemosiderinuria.

Venous thromboses occur in about 40% of patients. These are frequently in hepatic, portal, splenic, or splanchnic veins and may occur in the cerebral veins as well. They are probably caused by defective platelets, which aggregate and lead to clot formation.

All patients have evidence of diminished hematopoiesis if carefully assessed. Sometimes this is manifest as leukopenia or thrombocytopenia alone. The diminution may be so severe as to resemble that seen in aplastic anemia, and it may precede the evolution of the abnormal cells of PNH or may occur at any time during the course of the disease.

Laboratory Findings

The laboratory findings are those of intravascular hemolysis (see previous) often coupled with neutropenia and/or thrombocytopenia. The diagnostic tests used for PNH classically rest on the hemolysis of the abnormal red cells by the activation of complement (Ham [acidified serum lysis] test or sugar water test). The diagnosis can be made more definitively by the demonstration of blood cells lacking the glucosephosphate isomerase (GPI)-linked proteins (e.g., CD59) using flow cytometry; cells completely lacking the proteins (PNH III cells) and cells partially deficient (PNH II cells) can be identified in this way.

Treatment

The only definitive treatment for PNH now available is bone marrow transplantation from an HLA-identical sibling. This is generally recommended for young patients who have complicated disease. If diminished hematopoiesis is the major problem, antithymocyte globulin may be used as in aplastic anemia; however, the abnormal clone may increase in size as a result. Glucocorticoids may diminish the activation of complement when given in moderately high doses (15 to 30 mg/day in adults); this

treatment should be given every other day to avoid toxicity. Anabolic steroids (danacrine or fluoxymesterone) may also improve the anemia. All patients (except those receiving transfusions) should take iron and folic acid supplements.

Outcome

Paroxysmal nocturnal hemoglobinuria is a chronic disease, and the survival is highly variable. Abdominal venous thrombosis, particularly of the hepatic veins, is a serious adverse prognostic indicator, as is continuing diminished hematopoiesis. Retrospective studies suggest that the mean survival is 8 to 12 years, but many patients survive for many years. In over half of these long-term survivors, the abnormal cells may virtually or completely disappear. Rarely (in 2 to 3% of patients), PNH evolves into acute leukemia.

Myelofibrosis

Myelofibrosis (also called agnogenic myeloid metaplasia) is characterized by abnormal hematopoiesis and replacement of the bone marrow by fibrous tissue. This replacement has the effect of disrupting the structure of the marrow, which permits the circulation of immature cells (leukoerythroblastic blood film) and which causes hematopoiesis to be diverted to the spleen, liver, and other organs. The cause of the disorder is not entirely clear, but it has been suggested that the primary problem is dysplasia of megakaryocytes (often very evident in examination of the bone marrow), which results in the local elaboration of cytokines that promote the growth of fibrous tissue. The fibrous tissue in the marrow is not clonal in origin, whereas the abnormal blood cells are.

Clinical Features

Myelofibrosis is usually a chronic disease of the middle aged and elderly; it can occur and progress with great rapidity in some cases. The patient become anemic and frequently has splenomegaly and hepatomegaly. As the disease progresses, the anemia worsens and other cytopenias may become evident. The spleen enlarges and may become massive in size; it is often symptomatic due to small infarcts (resulting in left upper quadrant or left shoulder pain or splenic rub) or due to its size (causing early satiety and left abdominal discomfort). Anemia is usually present, and marked leukocytosis and thrombocytosis may be seen, but if the spleen is trapping the cells, both leukopenia and granulocytopenia may result. Immature granulocytes and erythrocytes may circulate, and the platelets may be large and bizarre. The bone marrow cannot be aspirated, but the biopsy shows strands of fibrous tissue with nests of hematopoietic cells. Megakaryocytes are frequently plentiful and are often bizarre in morphology, with hyposegmentation of the nucleus. Megaloblastic features are sometimes seen in erythroid and granulocytic precursors.

Prognosis and Treatment

Myelofibrosis tends to be a chronic, debilitating disease; the mean survival from diagnosis is 5 to 10 years. Progression is noted by increased size of the liver and spleen and by the greater number and immaturity of cells circulating in the peripheral blood. In a few cases, this process terminates as acute leukemia.

As in other stem cell disorders, the most definitive treatment is bone marrow transplantation; this is not often an option because of the age of the patient. Mild chemotherapy, such as 6-mercaptopurine (100 mg/day) may be used if the process progresses to a proliferative phase. Splenectomy may become necessary if the spleen is symptomatic because of its size, because of infarctions, or because of hypersplenism.

MYELOPROLIFERATIVE DISORDERS

The third category of stem cell disorders are those characterized by excessive proliferation of one or more of the cell lines derived from the stem cell; Dameshek coined the term *myeloproliferative disorders*. In all, the cells are normally differentiated (except for the acute leukemias) but appear to have escaped the usual controls on growth. As in the case of the other stem cell disorders, the ultimate result of the defect may be acute myeloblastic leukemia.

Polycythemia Rubra Vera

The red cell mass is normally maintained within quite narrow limits though the control of the production of erythropoietin (EPO). This homeostatic control is lost when, for reasons not well understood, a clone of stem cells produces erythroid precursors autonomously. In cell culture of the marrow, these precursors grow in the absence of added erythropoietin, whereas normal precursors do not. The overproliferation of red cell precursors results in an increase in the red cell mass and in the hematocrit, and the production of erythropoietin is suppressed.

Clinical and Laboratory Findings

Polycythemia vera is a disease of older individuals. It may be manifest clinically by plethora of the face and superficial blood vessels and by splenomegaly (present in $> 60\%$ of patients). Patients may occasionally have erythromyalgia of the feet and may complain of generalized pruritus, especially after a bath. The hematocrit is usually $> 53\%$, but it is sometimes necessary to determine the red cell mass (> 36 ml/kg in men and 32 ml/kg in women), as alterations in the plasma volume may falsely raise (spurious or stress erythrocytosis) or lower the hematocrit. The red cells are normal in appearance but may be hypochromic if iron deficiency is present, which is relatively common. The white count is often elevated above 12,000/mm³, and the platelet count is usually above 450,000/mm³. Arterial hypoxia, a frequent cause of physiologic elevation of the red cell mass, is not present, distinguishing polycythemia vera from a number of causes of physiologic erythrocytosis due to hypoxia (lung disease, living at high altitude, or in heart anomalies with shunting of blood) (Fig. 47–1). The plasma erythropoietin level is usually undetectable. In addition, the leukocyte alkaline phosphatase is often elevated in the absence of infection, and the serum vitamin B_{12} level and B_{12} binding capacity are elevated. Other causes of increased red cell mass include nonphysiologic secretion of erythropoietin by tumors of the kidney or cerebellum, hemoglobinopathy due to hemoglobin that binds O_2 too tightly, and increased carboxyhemoglobin due to smoking; the level of EPO is elevated in these instances.

Course of the Disorder and Treatment

Polycythemia vera is a chronic disorder that is complicated by thromboses (frequently arterial) that terminates in either leukemia or myelofibrosis ("spent" polycythemia). Surgery in the patient whose disease is not under control may be dangerous. Treatment has consisted of phlebotomy to reduce the hematocrit, P^{32}, and chemotherapeutic agents. In well-studied cases, deaths from thrombosis were higher in patients undergoing phlebotomy and from leukemia and other neoplasms in patients receiving alkylating agents (chlorambucil) or P^{32}. More recently, the use of hydroxyurea, which does not seem to have the same oncogenic effect as the alkylating agents, has been used with great success, even though it is somewhat more difficult to adjust the dosage than with other forms of therapy. Thus, patients with nonaggressive and mild disease may be treated with phlebotomy, whereas those with increased platelet counts or any tendency to thrombosis should be treated with hydroxyurea if possible.

Chronic Myelogenous Leukemia (CML)

Chronic myelogenous leukemia is a malignant stem cell disorder often classified as a myeloproliferative disease because it shares a major feature of myeloproliferative diseases: uncontrolled growth or expansion of stem cells leading to increased numbers of all marrow elements, especially myeloid cells and megakaryocytes. CML was the first hematologic disorder defined by a specific chromosome abnormality. The Philadelphia (Ph[1]) chromosome is a translocation of the long arm of chromosome 22 to chromosome 9, a translocation that uncovers the c-abl oncogene and the breakpoint cluster region (bcr). The product of this translocation is a tyrosine kinase (P210), which promotes granulocyte proliferation. The Ph[1] chromosome is usually documented by standard cytogenetic analysis but, more recently, has also been demonstrated by two very sensitive techniques, polymerase chain reaction (PCR) and fluorescent *in situ* hybridization (FISH).

Chronic myelogenous leukemia usually occurs in adults but can occur at any age. The cause is usually not known, although exposure to radiation, as after the atomic

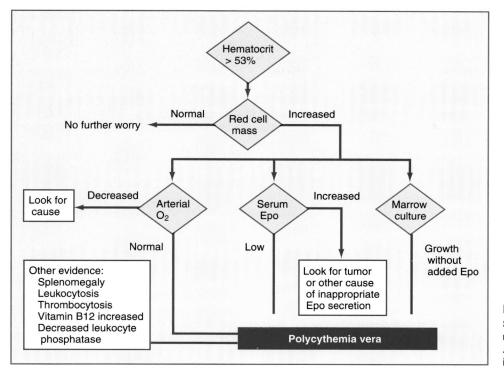

Figure 47–1

Scheme for the differential diagnosis of an increased hematocrit. *Arrows* point to subsequent studies that are needed.

bomb explosions in Japan in 1945, have been associated with increased incidence of CML.

This leukemia is often found incidentally when an elevated white blood cell count, predominantly of granulocytes and granulocyte precursors, is found. Initially, CML must be distinguished from a leukemoid reaction or from "other" myeloproliferative disorders; this is accomplished by peripheral blood evaluation, a low-leukocyte alkaline phosphatase (LAP), and chromosome analysis as described previously. Thrombocytosis is often present and may be marked. When platelets are significantly elevated, presenting features may include purpura or mucous membrane bleeding. The spleen is usually enlarged and may be noticed by the patient or found on routine examination.

Bone marrow examination usually reveals myeloid hyperplasia with a shift toward myeloid immaturity but without a significant increase in blast forms. Megakaryo-

cytes may be increased, as may reticulin fibers or fibrosis, and the absence of iron on bone marrow biopsy may be spurious, with iron demonstrated on bone marrow evaluation after initial treatment. Table 47–3 describes the differential diagnosis between CML, myeloid metaplasia, and a leukemoid reaction.

Treatment is initially aimed at decreasing the peripheral white blood cell count and splenomegaly. In the past, the alkylating agent busulfan was given, but more recently, the antimetabolite hydroxyurea (a ribonucleotide reductase inhibitor) is used as initial "debulking" treatment.

Alpha-interferon has assumed an important role in treatment of CML. Alpha-interferon, alone or combined with cytosine arabinoside given subcutaneously or intravenously, may decrease the number of Ph[1]-positive cells in the bone marrow and enrich the normal clone of cells that is usually present at diagnosis. Long-term treatment

TABLE 47–3	**Differential Diagnosis of an Elevated White Blood Count**		
	Myelofibrosis with Myeloid Metaplasia	**Chronic Myelogenous Leukemia**	**Leukemoid Reaction**
WBC	Usually >100,000/μl with early myeloid forms	May be >100,000/μl with early myeloid forms	Rarely >100,000/μl; promyelocytes or blasts are rare
RBC morphology	Nucleated RBC and teardrop cells	Occasional nucleated RBC	Usually normal
Leukocyte alkaline phosphatase (LAP score)	Normal or high	Low (<20)	High
Bone marrow	Usually "dry tap" with fibrosis	Panhypercellular	Myeloid hyperplasia
Philadelphia chromosome	Absent	Present (about 90% of cases)	Absent

RBC = Red blood cell; WBC = white blood cell.

with alpha-interferon may be necessary to achieve adequate response. Side effects of alpha-interferon include fever, malaise, anorexia, weight loss, and other flu-like symptoms and may limit its usefulness in some patients.

Bone marrow transplantation represents the only potentially curative means of treating CML. Allogeneic transplant is most common but requires an HLA-matched sibling donor. Recently, matched unrelated donor (MUD) transplants have been employed but with increased toxicity due to graft-versus-host disease.

Most patients with CML present in the "chronic" phase of disease, which usually lasts from 3 to 5 years but may be considerably shorter or longer. Adverse prognostic features include advanced age, basophilia, severe thrombocytosis, or more than one chromosome abnormality, including multiple Ph[1] chromosomes or other chromosome breaks and translocations. These same chromosome abnormalities may herald the appearance of the "accelerated" phase, during which the white blood cell count and splenomegaly become more difficult to control and the patient may require red blood cell transfusion or other blood product support. Either thrombocytopenia or marked thrombocytosis may herald the accelerated phase, and often fever, increased weakness, increased spleen size, and discomfort occur. The "blast crisis" phase of the disease represents a genuine acute leukemia and usually is of myeloid phenotype, while approximately 20% may bear lymphoid markers by terminal deoxynucleotidyl transferase (Tdt) and immunophenotype and may respond to traditional lymphoid treatment with vincristine and prednisone. The treatment of blast crisis is difficult and unsatisfactory even with aggressive treatment with drugs and schedules similar to those for acute myeloid leukemia. Usually, blast crisis ends in death between 3 and 6 months after its appearance.

Essential Thrombocythemia

The least common of the myeloproliferative diseases is that characterized by an increased platelet count. It is, like polycythemia vera, a disease of the middle aged and elderly and is due to a clonal growth of stem cells that produce excess numbers of megakaryocytes. The clinical manifestations are primarily those of thrombosis in small or large vessels. Thrombosis in small vessels may lead to gangrene of the tips of the fingers and toes and, more seriously, to neurologic symptoms. Thrombosis of large vessels leads to stroke, myocardial infarction, and venous thromboembolism. In addition, hemorrhage, primarily from the gastrointestinal tract, may be seen.

The diagnosis is made primarily from an increased platelet count ($>600,000/mm^3$) in the absence of other causes (infection, iron deficiency, inflammation, nonhematologic malignancy, other myeloproliferative disease) that persists over at least 2 months. The platelets may appear abnormal as well and, when carefully examined, may be qualitatively abnormal in function. The bone marrow is usually cellular and contains large number of megakaryocytes, which may be abnormal in appearance. Splenomegaly may be present.

The rate of complication from thrombosis is suffi-

ciently high as to mandate treatment in most patients. The platelet count may be rapidly lowered in patients with cerebral symptoms by plateletapheresis. The most commonly used chemotherapeutic agent is hydroxyurea, although trials of analgeride, a megakaryocyte inhibiting agent, have been reported to be successful. P^{32} may also be used with success at some risk for leukemia. Patients with this disorder rarely progress to leukemia but may have agnogenic myeloid metaplasia (myelofibrosis) as a late complication.

ACUTE LEUKEMIA

The acute leukemias are characterized by their cells of origin and are divided into two broad categories: acute lymphoblastic leukemia (ALL) and acute myeloblastic leukemia (AML). Either can occur at any age, but ALL is primarily a disease of children and represents $>90\%$ of the acute leukemias in this age group. AML is the predominant type of acute leukemia in adults, representing at least 80% of acute leukemias in the age group over 20 years. It is important to differentiate ALL from AML. Both require aggressive and often long-term treatment with chemotherapy, but the drugs themselves and schedules of treatment differ markedly.

Traditionally, diagnosis is initially suspected by morphologic evaluation of the peripheral blood and bone marrow aspiration and biopsy (Table 47–4) and may then be confirmed by using histochemical stains and immunophenotyping of surface and cytoplasmic markers. More recently, chromosome studies have assumed a more important place in distinguishing the acute leukemias and may be important in prognosis and treatment planning. For example, ALL with a positive Ph[1] chromosome follows a more virulent course than other ALL and may be treated more aggressively, up to and including early bone marrow transplantation. On the other hand, favorable myeloid leukemias (AMC) may be demonstrated in those groups showing chromosome abnormalities including a t(8–21) and translocation; t(15,17) and inversion-16 chromosomes.

Because of the heterogeneity within the broad categories of leukemia (AML and ALL), a French, American, and British (FAB) group subdivided these leukemias based primarily on morphologic grounds (Table 47–5). Among the myeloblastic leukemias, morphologic subtypes may be relatively distinctive and may correlate clinically with course and prognosis. These may also be characterized by the chromosome abnormalities described previously. For example, acute promyelocytic leukemia (M3) may be associated with bleeding phenomena due to disseminated intravascular coagulation (DIC) and also characterized by the presence of the t(15,17) translocation described. Other morphologic subtypes associated with specific chromosome abnormalities include M2 with t(8–21), and the inversion 16 (inv 16) with an M4 subtype also characterized by abnormal eosinophils. Acute monocytic leukemia (M5) may be associated clinically with gingival hypertrophy, skin infiltration with leukemic cells, and occasionally with lymph node enlargement. Among the lymphoblastic leukemias, the L1 subtype is found

	AML	ALL
TABLE 47–4	**Laboratory Aids to Distinguish Between Acute Myeloblastic Leukemia (AML) and Acute Lymphoblastic Leukemia (ALL)**	
1. Morphology of leukemic blasts	Granules in cytoplasm; Auer rods* may be present	Agranular, basophilic cytoplasm
	Multiple nucleoli	Regular, folded nucleus with one prominent nucleolus
	FAB (see Table 47–5) subclassification M_1–M_7	FAB subclassification, L_1–L_3
2. Histochemistry	Myeloperoxidase-positive	Myeloperoxidase-negative; PAS-positive
3. Cytoplasmic markers	—	Terminal deoxynucleotidyl transferase (Tdt)–positive
4. Surface markers (% of cases)	—	B cell markers (5%)
		T cell markers (15–20%): CD 2, 3, or 5
		CALLA (50–65%): CD 10
5. Cytogenetic and oncogenetic abnormalities	M_3: t (15,17) Abnormal retinoic acid receptor gene	L3: t (8,14) abnormal c-*myc*
	M_5: t (9,11)	Some ALL: Ph¹ bcr:*abl* fusion gene

* Auer rods are a linear coalescence of cytoplasmic granules that stain pink with Wright's stain.
CALLA = Common acute lymphoblastic leukemia antigen; FAB = French-American-British classification system; PAS = periodic acid–Schiff.

predominantly in children, and L2, in adults. The L3 subtype (analogous with Burkitt's lymphoma) may carry a poor prognosis unless treated very aggressively.

Diagnosis of acute leukemia is rarely difficult, although separation of ALL and AML may require the sophisticated techniques described previously. Presenting symptoms may be subtle and related to cytopenias (anemia and thrombocytopenia), causing fatigue, malaise, bleeding phenomena, and infection. These symptoms specifically relate to deficiencies of red blood cells, platelets, or white blood cells, respectively. Most often, these deficiencies are related to infiltration of the bone marrow with malignant cells, which prevents normal marrow function. Bone marrow aspiration and biopsy, along with complete characterization of the leukemic cells by morphology, histochemical stains, immunophenotyping, and chromosome analysis, should be performed to plan treatment properly. Supportive care in the form of transfusions of red blood cells or platelets, hydration, aggressive antibiotic therapy for infection, and the initiation of allopurinol to prevent hyperuricemia and renal damage should be initiated immediately.

Diagnosis of acute leukemia (either ALL or AML) should be considered a medical emergency. If the white blood cell count is > 100,000 μl, the patient is at high risk for leukostasis (described as obstruction of small blood vessels by the rigid blast cells). Therapeutic leukopheresis should be initiated, and specific chemotherapy initiated immediately.

Specific therapy of acute leukemia consists primarily of aggressive chemotherapy. The goal of treatment is to destroy the leukemic cells and produce a complete remission during which leukemia cells cannot be found in the peripheral blood or bone marrow by any technique available. To accomplish this goal, multiple courses of chemotherapy (in AML) and often very prolonged chemotherapy lasting 2 to 3 years are necessary in ALL.

Initial chemotherapy is usually termed "induction" and is aimed at producing complete remission. In AML, appropriate drugs include cytosine arabinoside, usually given as a 7-day infusion or in much higher doses every 12 hours for 6 days along with a second drug, usually an anthracycline such as daunorubicin, idarubicin, or mitoxantrone, with the latter given for 3 days during the initial course. Induction chemotherapy for AML produces complete remission in approximately 75% of patients under 60 years of age and in about 50% of patients over 60. Prolonged complete remission may ensue in younger patients but is less usual in the older age group, even with comparable chemotherapy.

Chemotherapy given soon after the induction of complete remission is termed "consolidation" chemotherapy and may employ the same drugs that placed the patient into remission, often either as the single drug cytosine arabinoside or with combination chemotherapy. In AML, it is clear that consolidation chemotherapy is necessary, though an exact schema is not universally agreed upon. Maintenance chemotherapy and central nervous system prophylaxis usually are not necessary in AML, although they are of critical importance in ALL. Long-term disease-free survival in younger patients with AML has been described in up to 30% of patients treated by conventional means and in a similar proportion of patients who go on to either allogeneic or autologous bone marrow transplantation. While potentially curable,

TABLE 47–5	**French-American-British (FAB) Classification of Acute Leukemia**

Acute Myelocytic Leukemia

M_1—Acute myelocytic leukemia without differentiation
M_2—Acute myelocytic leukemia with differentiation (predominantly myeloblasts and promyelocytes)
M_3—Acute promyelocytic leukemia
M_4—Acute myelomonocytic leukemia
M_5—Acute monocytic leukemia
M_6—Erythroleukemia
M_7—Megakaryotic leukemia

Acute Lymphocytic Leukemia

L_1—Predominantly "small" cells (twice the size of normal lymphocyte), homogeneous population; childhood variant
L_2—Larger than L_1, more heterogenous population; adult variant
L_3—"Burkitt-like" large cells, vacuolated abundant cytoplasm

allogeneic transplantation requires a suitable family donor, which limits the population available for it.

Treatment of ALL also requires prolonged chemotherapy. Initial induction usually involves multiple agents, including vincristine, prednisone, daunorubicin, cyclophosphamide, and L-asparaginase. In children, up to 90% of patients achieve complete remission, and an increasing proportion of patients are alive and in complete remission >5 years after initial induction. This achievement requires persistence and aggressive long-term maintenance chemotherapy lasting up to 2 to 3 years and early prophylaxis of the central nervous system with intrathecal chemotherapy with or without whole brain radiation.

Treatment of acute promyelocytic leukemia is unique. Treatment with all trans retinoic acid (ATRA), a vitamin A derivative, binds to the retinoic acid preceptor (RAR), a part of the t(15,17) translocation. In most patients, this stops the process of DIC and may lead to maturation of the leukemic clone into "normal" granulocytes. Treatment with all trans retinoic acid may be complicated by the so-called "ATRA syndrome" characterized by leukocytosis, serositis, and pulmonary leukostasis. This syndrome requires aggressive therapy with corticosteroids, hydroxyurea, leukopheresis, or the initiation of chemotherapy. Consolidation with conventional chemotherapy is necessary following initial remission with ATRA.

REFERENCES

Boultwood J, Lewis S, Wainscoat JS: The 5 q- syndrome. Blood 1994; 84:3253.

Franzman C, Bennett JM: Classification of acute leukemias. Contemp Oncol 1992; June:46.

Linker CA: Treatment of acute leukemia in adults. Curr Opin Oncol 1992; 4:53.

Rosse WF, Ware RJ: The molecular biology of paroxysmal nocturnal hemoglobinuria. Blood 1995; 86:3277–3286.

Schiffer CA, Lee EJ: Approaches to the therapy of relapsed acute myeloid leukemia. Oncology 1989; 3:23.

Warrell RP Jr, Dethe H, Wang ZY, Degos L: Acute promyelocytic leukemia. N Engl J Med 1993; 329:177.

Warrell RP Jr, Frankel SR, Miller WH, et al: Differentiation therapy of acute promyelocytic leukemia with trerinoin (all-trans retinoic acid). N Engl J Med 1991; 324:1385.

48

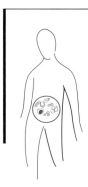

Disorders of Lymphocytes

ONTOLOGY OF LYMPHOCYTES

Lymphocytes are derived from hematopoietic stem cells; a precursor differentiates from the precursor that will differentiate into myeloid cells (see Chapter 46). From this precursor are derived three cell lines: B cells, T cells, and natural killer (NK) cells. These differentiation steps are directed by cytokines and cellular interactions in a very complex pattern.

B Cells

B lymphocytes are the cells that ultimately differentiate into antibody-producing plasma cells through a series of steps proceeding from pre–B cells through B cells to plasma cells. The cells at each step are identified by two characteristics:

1. The immunoglobulin genes undergo rearrangements that will permit the expression and secretion of immunoglobulins
2. Cell surface markers appear that can be detected by monoclonal antibodies (these markers are obviously functional molecules but their function often is not known)

These steps are replicated in the cells of the various lymphocytic neoplasms (Fig. 48–1).

The final step consists of differentiation into plasma cells, again under external influence of T cells. Plasma cells lose most of the surface markers and are characterized by the massive production of the immunoglobulin antibody dictated by the Ig gene rearrangements. This production is shown by an enlarged Golgi apparatus, which displaces the nucleus, and by deep blue cytoplasm because of the mRNA being generated.

T Cells

T lymphocytes (so called because they are associated with the thymus in their development) perform a large number of regulatory as well as effector reactions of the immune system. Their ontogenesis is complicated and different from that of the B cells.

Cells destined to be T cells acquire an antigen, CD7, which they maintain throughout their development. These cells migrate from the bone marrow to the cortex of the thymus, where they undergo a series of changes orchestrated by the thymic cells and by various cytokines (Fig. 48–2).

As cells migrate toward the medulla of the thymus, they acquire both the CD4 and the CD8 surface markers and begin to synthesize the T cell receptor. This receptor, crucial to many T cell functions, is composed of a heterodimer, $\alpha\beta$ being the most common combination. The components of these complexes each belong to the immunoglobulin superfamily and, like the immunoglobulin genes, must undergo a series of rearrangement of DNA, which gives them a range of diversity like the immunoglobulin molecules. These cells acquire the CD3 complex as well as the CD4 and CD8 molecules. As they proceed through the thymus, most are destroyed by apoptosis or programmed cell death initiated by self-antigens presented to T cells by the epithelial cells of the thymus; thus, clonal selection occurs that allows only the T cells bearing non–self-recognizing receptors to survive.

As cells mature, they lose either the CD4 or the CD8 surface molecule; which molecule is retained has a great influence on the interactions of the cell and its functions. CD4+ cells generally serve as helper cells in the immune system, whereas CD8+ cells generally have suppressor functions.

NK Cells

A third category of lymphocytes develops in the cells that do not bear the defining surface molecules of B cells or T cells and whose immunoglobulin and TcR genes do not undergo rearrangement. These cells are able to destroy cells without using immunoglobulin-like molecules; hence the name *natural killer* cells. They are characterized morphologically by their large size with abundant cytoplasm, which contains large azurophilic granules; they are sometimes called large granular lymphocytes (LGL). What is unique about NK cells (even among LGL cells) is the presence of the CD56 antigen (an isoform of the neural adhesion molecule N-CAM) and CD16, the third type of Fc receptor (FcRIII), which is also present on granulocytes and macrophages.

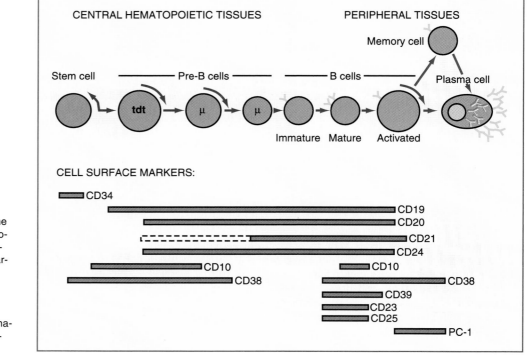

Figure 48-1

The maturation of B lympho-cytes. In the upper schema, the changes in immunoglobulin pro-duction and maturation are de-picted. In the lower, the appear-ance and disappearance of surface markers are shown. (Adapted from Handin RI, Lux SE, Stossel TP (eds.): Blood: Principles and Practice of Hema-tology. Philadelphia, JB Lippin-cott, 1995.)

LOCALIZATION OF LYMPHOCYTES

Lymphocytes are normally present in several types of tissue, including lymph nodes, aggregations associated with the gastrointestinal tract, spleen, and blood. Different varieties of lymphocytes are found in different locations.

Lymph Nodes

The structure of the normal lymph node is shown in Figure 48-3. The major components are the follicles, which consist of a germinal center and a mantle zone; these are arranged in the cortical area of the organ. The follicles contain mainly B cells that are polyclonal in origin; they contain cells that bear either $\kappa\lambda$ light chains. The cells of the mantle zone are somewhat less developed and bear surface-bound $\delta\mu$ chains.

T cells are found throughout the remainder of the lymph node. In the paracortical areas, the proportion of CD4 to CD8 cells is about 3:1 to 4:1, the same as in the peripheral blood. Few T cells occur in the germinal centers; those that are there are mainly CD8 in pheno-type.

Lymphoid organs associated with mucosal surfaces (pharyngeal tonsils and Peyer's patches) are organized much like the discrete lymph nodes, except that there are no afferent lymph channels to bring antigens to the reac-tive cells. Rather, antigen penetrates across the mucosa and is brought into immediate contact with the reactive areas. The constitution of the follicles and intrafollicular areas is not different from that seen in lymph nodes.

Spleen

The distribution of lymphocytes in the spleen is much like that in the lymph node. The follicles contain mostly

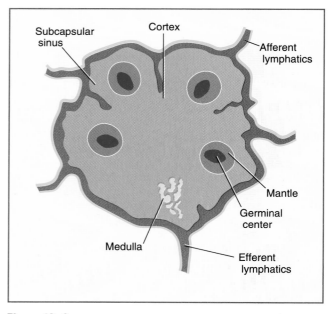

Figure 48-2

The structure of the normal lymph node. The cortical area contains the follicles, which consist of a germinal center and a mantle zone. The medulla contains a complex of channels that lead to the efferent lymphatics.

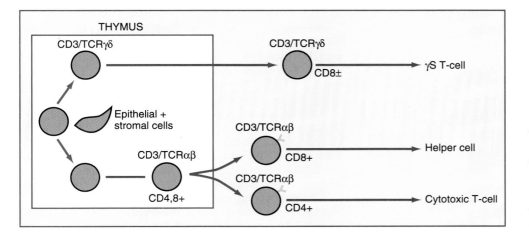

Figure 48-3

T lymphocyte maturation takes place in the thymus and involves changes in surface markers. (Adapted from Handin RI, Lux SE, Stossel TP (eds.): Blood: Principles and Practice of Hematology. Philadelphia, JB Lippincott, 1995.)

B cells. The cells in the periarteriolar sheaths are mainly CD4 T cells.

Peripheral Blood

Lymphocytes compose 20 to 40% of the circulating peripheral blood cells; this proportion is higher in young children. The majority are morphologically small, resting cells. About 80 to 85% are T cells; 75 to 80% of these are CD4, and the remainder, CD8 cells. These cells are polyclonal as assessed by the rearrangement of the T cell receptor. The B cells represent 15% of circulating lymphocytes and are also polyclonal as assessed by the expression of both $\kappa\lambda$ light chains on the surface immunoglobulins and by the diversity of the immunoglobulin chain rearrangements.

DISORDERS OF THE LYMPHATIC SYSTEM

Congenital Disorders

There are a number of congenital defects in lymphocytes that result in immunodeficiency disorders. These are described in Chapter 109.

Infectious Disorders

Lymphocytes play a major role in the response to any infection. This is sometimes seen in an increase in lymphocytes in the peripheral blood in viral diseases (mumps, hepatitis, varicella, and infectious mononucleosis) or in certain bacterial diseases (pertussis, brucellosis, and some forms of syphilis). This response is always polyclonal.

Enlargement of the lymph nodes, either locally or generally, may also accompany infection as part of the response to the invasion. This may result in striking enlargement of lymph nodes in local infections; such nodes show an active but normal architecture. The organism may invade the lymph node directly, as in the case of

tuberculosis and the other fungal diseases; biopsy of the node is of particular diagnostic value in such cases.

Neoplastic Disorders

Chronic Lymphocytic Leukemia

Chronic lymphocytic leukemia (CLL) is a malignant lymphoproliferative disorder characterized by accumulation of small lymphocytes. CLL is the most common form of leukemia worldwide and, while it can occur at any age, more than 90% occur in patients over 50 years of age. Men develop CLL twice as often as do women, and it is more common in white than in black populations.

The diagnosis of CLL is often suspected or found incidentally when a routine complete blood count reveals leukocytosis composed primarily of small lymphocytes. Often, review of previous blood counts confirms that lymphocytosis may have been present for many years. Diagnosis of CLL is based on the presence of at least 15,000 lymphocytes/μl in peripheral blood, with at least 40% of the cells in the bone marrow being lymphocytes. Usually, these lymphocytes are small and "well differentiated" and are the same cells present in enlarged or involved lymph nodes or in the spleen. Lymphadenopathy and/or splenomegaly are commonly present at the discovery of disease or may develop with progression of CLL over time.

Chronic lymphocytic leukemia cells may exhibit poor immunologic competence, manifested as hypogammaglobulinemia, an increase in infection, or the presence of autoimmune phenomena such as Coombs positive autoimmune hemolytic anemia (AIHA), immune thrombocytopenic purpura (ITP), or, more rarely, immune granulocytopenia. The presence of pure red cell aplasia as a presenting feature of CLL has also been reported but is unusual. Table 48-1 outlines some of the immune disorders associated with CLL.

Chronic lymphocytic leukemia represents a clonal proliferation, usually of B lymphocytes, and this clonality is demonstrated by immunoglobulin gene rearrangement, the presence of a single light chain ($\kappa\lambda$) as well as the

TABLE 48–1 Immune Disorders in CLL

Autoantibody production
Autoimmune hemolytic anemia
  Coombs' test positive in 20 to 30% of patients with CLL
  Hemolysis rare
  Usually responds to corticosteroids
Autoimmune thrombocytopenic purpura
  Thrombocytopenia also possibly due to bone marrow replacement
    by CLL or to splenic sequestration
  Usually responds to corticosteroids
Disorders of immunoglobulin synthesis
Monoclonal gammopathy
  Monoclonal spike present in 10% of patients with CLL—IgG or IgM
Hypogammaglobulinemia
  Present in majority of cases, particularly stages III and IV
  Results in increased susceptibility to bacterial infection

CLL = Chronic lymphatic leukemia.

presence of characteristic B-cell immunologic markers, including CD19, CD20, and the presence of CD5. CLL lymphocytes may express other antigens including Ia, the C3 receptor, and the receptor for the Fc portion of immunoglobulin. B cells demonstrate impaired responsiveness to mitogens.

Occasionally, "typical" appearing CLL may be derived from T lymphocytes. The T-lymphocyte clonality is confirmed by immunophenotyping. T-cell CLL has a poorer prognosis compared with its B-cell counterpart, and skin involvement is often seen in these patients.

A more virulent form of T-cell CLL is associated human T-cell leukemia virus (HTLV)-I infection. HTLV-I may be acquired through blood transfusion in the United States, although it was first demonstrated in a rural population in Kyushu, Japan. This disease may present with hypercalcemia, lytic bone lesions, and severe debility. It may be rapidly progressive. Conventional therapy with alkylating agents or with other more aggressive forms of treatment is rarely effective.

The cause of CLL is not known, and, despite occasional familial clustering, no firm genetic basis for the disease has been discovered. Likewise, causes of other leukemias, including exposure to radiation, alkylating agents, and other mutagens, do not appear to cause CLL. Chromosome abnormalities may also occur, and trisomy has been associated with a poorer prognosis.

TABLE 48–2 Clinical Staging for CLL

Level of Risk	Stage	Descriptions
Low	0	Lymphocytosis only in blood and bone marrow
	I	Lymphocytosis plus enlarged lymph nodes
Intermediate	II	Lymphocytosis plus enlarged liver or spleen (±enlarged nodes)
	III	Lymphocytosis plus anemia (not autoimmune) (±enlarged nodes, spleen, or liver)
High	IV	Lymphocytosis plus thrombocytopenia (not autoimmune) (±anemia, enlarged nodes, liver, or spleen)

Table 48–2 lists the clinical staging system for CLL. Stages range from very low "level" disease with stage 0, which represents lymphocytosis alone, through stages I and II, which reflect the development of increasing tumor mass with lymph node enlargement and hepatosplenomegaly. Stages III and IV denote bone marrow replacement and the presence of anemia and thrombocytopenia; anemia or thrombocytopenia due to autoimmune processes, not uncommon in CLL, is not considered reason to promote the severity of the disease to stage III or IV. The disease may present at any stage, but at diagnosis, most patients are categorized as stage 0, I, or II.

Patients at stages 0, I, or II may be observed without treatment until he or she develops bulky lymph node enlargement; disease symptoms such as fevers, night sweats, malaise, or fatigue; or the presence of cytopenia as related to either bone marrow infiltration or to immune phenomena as described previously (AIHA and ITP).

Initial treatment of the disease most often involves the use of a single alkylating agent such as chlorambucil or cyclophosphamide with the addition of prednisone if symptoms are present or if autoimmune phenomena occur. A variety of schedules employing chlorambucil on a daily, biweekly, or 5-days-a-month schedule may be effective. Multiagent chemotherapy with the addition of vincristine or an anthracycline may be beneficial, and "low-dose" CHOP (cyclophosphamide, hydroxydaunorubicin, vincristine, and prednisone) has been reported to have additional benefit.

More recently, fludarabine has made a significant impact on the treatment of advanced disease and may be employed as initial treatment. Fludarabine appears to produce significant tumor debulking and may produce complete remission in CLL, whereas "partial" remission usually is obtained with alkylating agents. Cell destruction appears to be through the mechanism of programmed cell death, termed "apoptosis."

Bulky tumor mass, lymph node enlargement, and bulky splenomegaly may be treated with radiation therapy, and splenectomy may be a viable option with autoimmune phenomena or splenic pain or enlargement not responsive to other treatment.

Chronic lymphocytic leukemia occasionally may transform into a clinically more malignant neoplasm, with features of high-grade lymphoma. This most often is defined histologically as a diffuse large-cell lymphoma and is termed "Richter's syndrome." Prolymphocytic leukemia, "a larger, less-mature" lymphoid cell, characterized by bulky splenomegaly and usually the absence of lymph node enlargement, may occur either as an evolution of typical CLL or *de novo*.

Increased infections during the evolution of CLL should be treated with antibiotics, and the frequency of these infections may be decreased by the use of intravenous gammaglobulin (IV-IgG).

Hairy Cell Leukemia

Hairy cell leukemia (HCL), also called leukemic reticuloendotheliosis, is a neoplastic disorder characterized by "hairy cells" in the peripheral smear and bone marrow.

Hairy cells look like lymphocytes with fine cytoplasmic projections. Unlike typical B cells, they are capable of phagocytosis. The cells stain positive for tartrate-resistant acid phosphatase (TRAP) and are positive for the low-affinity interleukin-2 receptor (CD2S+). The bone marrow is often inaspirable, but the appearance on biopsy is characteristic.

Hairy cell leukemia is a rare form of leukemia, constituting 1 to 2% of all leukemias. It is more common in men than in women and usually presents as a slowly developing pancytopenia with splenomegaly. Splenectomy may be useful if the spleen enlarges painfully or severe cytopenia develops. Chemotherapy with standard alkylating agents has not helped most patients with HCL. Most patients with HCL, however, respond to alpha-interferon, 2′-deoxycoformycin (Pentostatin), or 2-chlorodeoxyadenosine with a complete hematologic remission. Granulocyte colony-stimulating factor (G-CSF) administration may also correct the leukopenia. The median survival for patients with HCL is 3 to 5 years; some patients live many years after diagnosis with little treatment.

Lymphomas

The lymphomas are a group of malignant lymphoid neoplasms arising in lymph nodes or in any extranodal lymphoid tissue. The lymphomas are heterogenous malignancies from the pathologic, clinical, and treatment viewpoints. The two major groups of lymphomas include Hodgkin's disease and the non-Hodgkin's lymphomas. In both groups, the most common clinical presentation is an asymptomatic enlarged lymph node in the cervical, axillary, or inguinal region, usually first noticed by the patient. Usually the duration of lymph node enlargement is uncertain.

Lymphomas emphasize the importance of a careful and thorough physical examination prior to the initiation of lymph node biopsy or other diagnostic procedures. Cervical lymphadenopathy is most often associated with infections such as streptococcal pharyngitis or other bacterial infections, infectious mononucleosis or other viral illnesses, toxoplasmosis, and, rarely, cat scratch fever. Axillary lymphadenopathy, when unilateral, should direct a physician to a careful breast examination and examination of the skin of the chest, axillary area, and lower back. Inguinal lymphadenopathy may reflect skin infections in the lower extremities, genitalia, or perianal area. Sexually transmitted diseases, including human immunodeficiency virus (HIV), should be considered with any lymph node enlargement and should be excluded as a cause. Scrofula, or tuberculous lymphadenitis, may present as asymptomatic isolated lymph node enlargement and, while unusual, may be becoming more prevalent. Table 48–3 outlines various common causes of lymph node enlargement. If the cause of lymph node enlargement is not obvious after careful consideration of these conditions, excisional lymph node biopsy should be considered. Histologic examination including immunophenotyping studies, cultures, and, possibly, molecular studies for chromosome abnormalities and gene rearrangements should be done.

TABLE 48–3	Common Causes of Lymphadenopathy

Infection
  Bacterial: Localized infection with regional adenopathy (e.g., streptococcal pharyngitis, foot ulcer with inguinal adenopathy)
  Viral: Infectious mononucleosis, cytomegalovirus, cat scratch fever
  Retroviral: HIV, HTLV-1
  Parasitic: Toxoplasmosis
  Spirochetal: Syphilis
  Mycobacterial: Tuberculosis, *Mycobacterium avium* (in immunosuppressed patients)
  Fungal: Actinomycosis, cryptococcosis (in immunosuppressed patients)
Drug reaction
  Serum sickness
  Phenytoin (may cause "pseudolymphoma")
Malignancy
  Solid tumors—metastatic patterns
    Cervical adenopathy: head and neck cancer
    Supraclavicular adenopathy: gastrointestinal tumors
    Axillary adenopathy: breast cancer
    Inguinal adenopathy: carcinoma of the anus
  Lymphoma
Miscellaneous
  Sarcoidosis

HIV = Human immunodeficiency virus; HTLV-1 = human T-cell lymphoma virus-1.

NON-HODGKIN'S LYMPHOMA. Non-Hodgkin's lymphomas are a heterogeneous group of malignant neoplasms characterized by monoclonal proliferation of a malignant cell of lymphoid origin, usually either a T cell or a B cell. As in Hodgkin's disease, the cause of most non-Hodgkin's lymphomas is not known. Viruses have been implicated in African Burkitt's lymphoma (the Epstein-Barr virus), in acquired immunodeficiency syndrome (AIDS)–related lymphomas (HIV), and in lymphomas arising from immunosuppressive therapy after organ transplantation (Epstein-Barr virus). In contrast to African Burkitt's lymphoma, a disease with the same appearance arising in the United States carries no viral association but is characterized by translocations from chromosomes 8 and 14, which carry the genes for immunoglobulin heavy chains and light chains. These translocations also contain the oncogene c-*myc*, which may enhance sensitivity to chemotherapy.

Non-Hodgkin's lymphomas are classified by pathologic subtype, immunophenotype, and clinical stage. Pathology depends on the overall pattern of lymph node or tissue architecture and on the morphology of the cell that predominates in the neoplastic tissue. Neoplastic cells may replace the entire node in a diffuse pattern, which obliterates the normal pattern of germinal centers, or may appear as follicles that mimic but distort the normal architecture. This pattern of follicles defines the tumor as "follicular center cell" in origin and suggests B cell origin.

The predominant cell further classifies lymphoma. The major lymphoma cell types are small, well-differentiated lymphocytes, small lymphocytes with cleaved nuclei (follicular center cells), or a large lymphoid cell that appears less mature and may often appear plasmacytoid. Lymph nodes or any tissue from which a diagnosis of non-Hodgkin's lymphoma is suspected should be meticulously examined pathologically for morphology and by careful attention to immunologic surface markers to define the cell of origin (B cell, T cell, NK cell, or other lymphoid cell) and the exact subset of each of these categories represented by the lymphoma.

Clinical staging of non-Hodgkin's lymphoma is very similar to that described for Hodgkin's disease (Table 48–4). In contrast, non-Hodgkin's lymphomas are much more likely to present with advanced-stage disease (80% of the follicular center-cell lymphomas are stage IV at presentation). Additionally, the non-Hodgkin's lymphomas are more likely than Hodgkin's to occur in extranodal sites (gastrointestinal tract, central nervous system, or bone marrow), and non-Hodgkin's lymphomas do not typically follow the orderly, meticulous anatomic progression described for Hodgkin's disease.

True stage I or II non-Hodgkin's lymphomas are unusual but if present may be treated with local radiation therapy. Often, chemotherapy is given prior to local treatment. Patients with stage III and IV disease are usually treated with chemotherapy. Paradoxically, the high-grade or intermediate-grade lymphomas tend to be treatable and potentially curable with aggressive chemotherapy, as compared with the low-grade lymphomas, which generally are considered to be treatable but not curable.

Chemotherapy for low-grade lymphomas is similar to that described for chronic lymphocytic leukemia. A single alkylating agent, chlorambucil or cyclophosphamide, may often control the disease and may be employed on multiple occasions throughout the duration of the disease. Corticosteroids (prednisone, methylprednisolone, or dexamethasone) are often added to multiagent programs.

Following the use of an alkylating agent and steroid, cyclophosphamide, vincristine, and prednisone (COP) or an anthracycline antibiotic such as doxirubicin can be used.

Multiple chemotherapy programs have been developed in an attempt to take advantage of cell cycling and to avoid progression between treatments. These more aggressive programs have been employed mostly for intermediate- and high-grade lymphomas and include CHOP, Pro-MACE-CytaBOM, M-BACOD, and MACOP-B. The more complex regimens appear to give a higher degree of complete response and in many intermediate- and high-grade lymphomas may impart a better long-term prognosis or cure rate than does CHOP. The proper course of treatment for each disease and stage is controversial.

Non-Hodgkin's lymphomas occuring in extranodal sites such as the central nervous system and gastrointestinal tract are common in HIV-infected patients. These are typically high-grade B-cell lymphomas and often respond very poorly to therapy. Chemotherapy programs and the use of recombinant growth factors such as erythropoietin (Epo), granulocyte stimulating factor (G-CSF), and antiretroviral drugs may prove to alter this course.

The classification systems for non-Hodgkin's lymphomas are being revised. The one commonly used has been the so-called International Working Formulation, which in Table 48–5 is juxtaposed with the now outdated Rappaport system. A newer system of staging based on immunophenotype divides the non-Hodgkin's lymphomas into broad categories based on origin, such as "B cell neoplasms" or "T cell and putative NK cell neoplasms," with a third category for "Hodgkin's disease." This staging system is complex. It does recognize a number of unique types of lymphoma such as mucosal associated lymphoid tumor (MALT) involving the gastrointestinal tract and other unique types based on immunophenotype and clinical behavior.

TABLE 48–4	Staging Criteria for Hodgkin's Disease	
Stage	**Ann Arbor Criteria**	**Cotswold's Criteria**
I	Single lymph node region (LNR) (I) or a single extralymphatic site (ELS) (I_E)	Single LNR or lymphoid structure
II	Two or more LNRs on the same side of the diaphragm (II) or a solitary ELS and one or more LNRs on the same side of the diaphragm (II_E)	Two or more LNRs on the same side of the diaphragm*†
III	LNR on both sides of the diaphragm (III); with spleen involvement (III_S) or solitary involvement of an ELS (III_E) or both (III_{ES}); III_1 = upper abdomen; III_2 = lower abdomen	LNS or ELS on both sides of the diaphragm: III_1 = with or without involvement of spleen, splenic, hilar, celiac, or portal nodes; III_2 = involvement of para-aortic, iliac, and mesenteric nodes
IV	Diffuse involvement of ELSs with or without lymph node enlargement	Involvement of one or more ELSs in addition to a site given the designation E
	Presence of constitutional symptoms (fever, night sweats, loss of 10% of body weight) = B; absence = A	A and B mean the same as Ann Arbor; X = bulky disease (nodes > 10 cm, chest mass > 1/3 chest diameter)

* The mediastinum is considered a single site, whereas hilar lymph nodes are considered separately for each side.
† The number of anatomic sites should be indicated by a subscript Arabic number.

TABLE 48–5	Classification of the Non-Hodgkin's Lymphomas
International Working Formulation	**Rappaport Classification**
I. Low-grade lymphoma	
a. Small lymphocytic cell	Diffuse lymphocytic, well-differentiated
b. Follicular, mixed cleaved cell	Nodular lymphocytic, poorly differentiated
c. Follicular, mixed small cleaved and large cell	Nodular mixed lymphocytic-histiocytic
II. Intermediate-grade lymphoma	
d. Follicular, large cell	Nodular histiocytic
e. Diffuse, small cleaved cell	Diffuse lymphocytic, poorly differentiated
f. Diffuse, mixed small cleaved cell	Diffuse mixed lymphocytic-histiocytic
g. Diffuse large cell	Diffuse histiocytic
III. High-grade lymphoma	
h. Large cell immunoblastic	Diffuse histiocytic
i. Lymphoblastic cell	Diffuse undifferentiated
j. Small noncleaved cell (Burkitt and non-Burkitt)	

TABLE 48-6	Subtypes of Hodgkin's Disease (Rye Classification Modified)		
Subtype	**Relative Frequency (%)**	**Description**	**Prognosis**
Lymphocyte predominance	5–15	Few RS cells; mostly lymphocytes, histiocytes	Most favorable
Nodular sclerosis	40–75	Often in young, often mediastinal; fibrous tissue, lacunar cells	Usually responds well to radiation
Mixed cellularity	20–40	Often in more elderly; many nonimmunologic cells, many RS cells	Responds less well to radiation
Lymphocyte depletion	5–15	Abundant RS cells, some "malignant appearing"; may have abdominal only	Least favorable even with chemotherapy

RS = Reed-Sternberg.

As in Hodgkin's disease, bone marrow transplantation and peripheral stem cells offer the possibility of curing non-Hodgkin's lymphomas. Patients with high-grade lymphomas who have failed initial treatment or relapsed after initial treatment should be considered for bone marrow transplantation if a suitable donor or autologous stem cells are available for marrow reconstitution.

HODGKIN'S DISEASE. Hodgkin's disease is primarily a disease of young adults but is "bimodal" in its distribution, with another peak around 60 years of age. Younger patients have a better prognosis than do older ones.

Hodgkin's disease usually presents with asymptomatic lymph node enlargement and is often found on routine examination or by routine chest radiograph, which reveals a mediastinal mass. Some patients with Hodgkin's disease may present with "B" symptoms, including fever, night sweats, or weight loss and, more rarely, may present with dyspnea, shortness of breath, and the superior vena cava (SVC) syndrome.

Hodgkin's disease is classified by pathologic subtype, clinical stage, and the presence or absence of "B" symptoms. The four pathologic subtypes include lymphocyte predominance, nodular sclerosis, mixed cellularity, and lymphocyte depletion (Table 48-6). In all four subtypes, the finding of Reed-Sternberg cells confirms the diagnosis of Hodgkin's disease. Typical Reed-Sternberg cells are large and binucleate, with each nucleus revealing a prominent nucleolus, giving it the appearance of "owl's eyes." The origin of the Reed-Sternberg cell remains unknown.

Nodular-sclerosis Hodgkin's disease is the most common type. Pathologically, broad bands of fibrosis are prominent, and "lacunar" cells and scattered Reed-Sternberg cells are characteristic. This subtype of Hodgkin's disease typically presents as asymptomatic cervical lymph node enlargement or an asymptomatic mediastinal mass, often in young women. Hodgkin's disease of mixed cellularity subtype demonstrates a histologic background, which is more heterogeneous and more cellular, with infiltration of lymphocytes, eosinophils, plasma cells, and Reed-Sternberg cells. This type is more common in young to middle-aged men rather than in women. Lymphocyte-predominant Hodgkin's disease may carry a better prognosis. It presents in asymptomatic young men or women. Lymphocyte-depleted Hodgkin's disease is uncommon and occurs more often in older patients who present with "B" symptoms.

Hodgkin's disease is frequently curable with appropriate chemotherapy, radiation therapy, or combined modality treatment. Treatment planning is based on meticulous staging to define stage I, II, III, and IV, as outlined in Table 48-4. The presence or absence of symptoms is also part of staging and designates the patient as either "A" (asymptomatic) or "B" with the symptoms just described. The staging process is rigorous and should include all of the basic tests outlined in Table 48-7, up to but not necessarily including staging laparotomy.

Hodgkin's disease tends to follow a logical anatomic progression or "next-door" pattern of lymph node involvement. For example, a patient with cervical lymph node enlargement may have supraclavicular, mediastinal, or axillary adenopathy but is unlikely to have abdominal involvement. One exception is involvement of cervical lymph nodes and splenic involvement with no intervening axillary or mediastinal node involvement; splenic involvement may indicate hematogenous rather than contiguous spread.

The principle of contiguous anatomic progression is important in considering which tests to employ in the staging evaluation. This is most difficult to define within the abdomen. Computerized axial tomography that shows enlarged lymph nodes suggests the presence of intra-abdominal disease. Lymphangiogram may confirm a "foamy" pattern with abdominal lymph nodes and suggest the presence of Hodgkin's disease. Staging laparotomy is the most definitive pathologic staging technique and should include multiple lymph node sampling, splenec-

TABLE 48-7	Staging Evaluation for a Patient with Lymphoma

1. Complete history and physical examination
2. Complete blood count, differential, platelet count, urinalysis
3. Screening blood chemistries
4. Chest x-ray, CT scan of chest, abdomen, and pelvis
5. Bone marrow aspirate and biopsy
6. Consider lymphangiogram, gallium scan
7. Staging laparotomy if therapy will be changed by documentation of subdiaphragmatic disease

CT = Computed tomography.

tomy, and liver biopsy. Staging laparotomy should be considered in two situations: (1) if the findings of laparotomy will unequivocally alter the course of treatment and (2) if abdominal and pelvic radiation is considered in young women of childbearing age, when the laparotomy would transpose the ovaries out of the radiation field. Open laparotomy is traditional, but newer techniques of laparoscopy, even with splenectomy, may decrease the morbidity of this procedure. This procedure is important to establish whether a patient has disease below the diaphragm. If that patient has stage II-A or III-A disease, staging can be important in planning for radiation therapy and in determining the extent to which the abdomen will be treated.

The treatment of Hodgkin's disease depends on stage, bulk of disease, and the presence or absence of symptoms. Radiation therapy alone is the recommended treatment for patients with stage I and II-A disease. Some patients with stage II or III-A disease may have massive lymph node enlargement, especially in the mediastinum, and chemotherapy should be employed as a debulking treatment, to be followed by radiation therapy to areas involved with disease. Treatment of patients with stage II-B disease is controversial, and chemotherapy followed by radiation rather than radiation therapy alone, because of a high relapse rate after the latter, should be considered. Patients with stage III-B and IV disease are considered to have widespread disease and should be treated with chemotherapy.

Radiation therapy is delivered in tumoricidal doses to areas of known disease and to adjacent areas, including the next most proximal node-bearing area considered to be free of disease. For example, a patient with stage I Hodgkin's disease and a cervical node may receive a mantle port designed to treat cervical, supraclavicular, axillary, mediastinal, and hilar lymph nodes. A patient with inguinal lymph node involvement only would receive an "inverted Y" port to encompass inguinal, iliac, and para-aortic nodes.

Side effects of radiation depend on the field irradiated and the dose. Most frequently, sore throat, dysphagia, nausea, vomiting, and diarrhea may be present. These may be treated symptomatically or with delays in treatment. Delayed effects of radiation include pneumonitis, hypothyroidism (if the thyroid has been included in the field), radiation pericarditis, and accelerated coronary artery disease. Ovarian function will be suppressed or destroyed unless the ovaries have been moved out of the field of radiation at the time of laparotomy.

Combination chemotherapy for Hodgkin's disease may be curative in a large number of patients. The original multiagent chemotherapy program MOPP (nitrogen-mustard, vincristine, procarbazine, and prednisone) first provided cures in patients with stages III-B and IV disease. MOPP remains a useful program for advanced-stage Hodgkin's disease. The immediate side effects of chemotherapy, including nausea and vomiting and bone marrow suppression, have been substantially decreased by the use of newer antiemetic agents and myeloid growth factors (G-CSF). Delayed effects of chemotherapy include sterility in both men and women and the potential for the late development of acute myeloid leukemia in a small but

definite proportion of patients. The risk of leukemia and other secondary neoplasms appears to be directly related to the alkylating agents used in these chemotherapy programs. Alternative treatment regimens including ABVD (adriamycin, bleomycin, vincristine, and dacarbazine) or BCVPP (bischlorethylnitrosourea, cyclophosphamide, vinblastine, prednisone, and procarabine) appear to have the same efficacy as MOPP with less long-term toxicity.

Long-term prognosis for patients with Hodgkin's disease is related to staging, diagnosis, and response to treatment. Patients with stage I-A and II-A disease have a 5-year survival of over 90%, while most patients with stage III-A disease have a 5-year survival of >80%. "B" symptoms decrease the survival figures at each stage, with stage III-B and IV patients having a 5-year survival of >50%. Five-year disease-free survival rates can translate to cure rates in most instances.

Relapsed Hodgkin's disease may be treated either with combination chemotherapy or, more recently, with allogeneic or autologous bone marrow transplantation as salvage therapy. This should be considered in an initial relapse when the first remission was obtained by chemotherapy or combined modality treatment.

Increased risk of infection is a major concern in Hodgkin's disease due to immunologic abnormalities reflecting abnormal or suppressed T cell function. These include greater incidence of herpes zoster, fungal infections such as cryptococcus, and other "opportunistic" infections such as pneumocystis (Pneumocystis carinii). Patients who have undergone splenectomy are at increased risk for bacterial infections with pneumococci and meningococci and should all receive pneumococcal vaccine.

PLASMA CELL DISORDERS

The plasma cell disorders or "dyscrasias" include a group of B-cell neoplasms that arise from a differentiated clone of immunoglobulin-secreting cells and produce a monoclonal immunoglobulin (or part of an immunoglobulin). If the monoclonal immunoglobulin is of the IgM class, the disease is Waldenstrom's macroglobulinemia and the malignant cells are plasmacytoid lymphocytes. If the monoclonal immunoglobulin is of the IgG, IgA, IgD, or, rarely, the IgE class, the disease is termed "multiple myeloma" and the malignant cells are plasma cells. Normal plasma cells represent the most specialized cells in the B cell lineage. Figure 48–1 illustrates one scheme of maturation proceeding from a pluripotent stem cell to an early B cell to a well-differentiated plasma cell, indicating the malignant diseases that can arise from neoplastic proliferation at each stage of B-cell maturation.

Plasma cells normally secrete immunoglobulins and are responsible for maintaining humoral immunity, especially to bacterial and other infectious agents. The basic structure of all immunoglobulins is the same and includes two heavy ("H") polypeptide chains and two light ("L") polypeptide chains, bound together by disulfide bonds. Both H chains and L chains have "constant" regions of amino acid sequence and "variable" regions that allow for antibody specificity. The five subclasses of immunoglobulin: immunoglobulin γ (IgG), μ (IgM), α (IgA), δ (IgD), and ϵ (IgE) are determined by the constant region of their H chains. Light chains are of two types: kappa and lambda. Each antibody molecule has two identical H chains and two identical L chains; hybrid molecules are not synthesized. Protein electrophoresis provides the first step in detecting a monoclonal immunoglobulin in serum. Analysis of the protein "M spike" by agar gel immunoelectrophoresis or immunofixation using specific antibodies (e.g., anti-human IgG, anti-kappa) further defines the exact type of monoclonal immunoglobulin.

Monoclonal immunoglobulin elevations can be found in conditions other than multiple myeloma or Waldenstrom's macroglobulinemia. Approximately 10% of patients with CLL have monoclonal IgG or IgM peaks (M proteins) in their serum. In addition, an M protein on serum electrophoresis may be found in patients with no detectable associated disease. The peak is usually < 2 gm/dl and is accompanied by no other clinical or laboratory evidence of multiple myeloma or Waldenstrom's macroglobulinemia. This finding, formerly called "benign monoclonal gammopathy" and now designated monoclonal gammopathy of unknown significance (MGUS), increases in frequency with age above 60 years. Approximately 10% of these patients later develop a true immunoproliferative disorder.

Multiple Myeloma

Multiple myeloma is a malignant disease of plasma cells that is characterized by the presence of monoclonal immunoglobulin or light chains in the serum and urine and bone destruction caused by focal plasma cell tumors (plasmacytomas). The typical patient is older than 50 and presents with bone pain, mild anemia, and an elevated sedimentation rate. Initial bone radiography may be normal or may demonstrate only osteoporosis, although widespread lytic lesions are typical. Less frequently, the patient has hypercalcemia and renal disease ("light chain nephropathy") at the time of diagnosis. Serum immunoelectrophoresis generally shows a monoclonal elevation of one immunoglobulin (e.g., IgG$_\kappa$), with reciprocal depression of the other classes of immunoglobulins (e.g., IgA and IgM). Free κ or λ light chains (Bence Jones protein) may be excreted in excess in the urine and are usually detected by urine immunoelectrophoresis. About 20% of patients with multiple myeloma do not have a serum M protein but have free light chains detectable in urine and serum ("light chain disease"); about 1% of patients with multiple myeloma have neither monoclonal nor free light chains detectable. These patients with "nonsecretory" myeloma can be shown to have a malignant clonal proliferation of plasma cells by immunofluorescent staining of the bone marrow. The plasma cells reveal light chain restriction and stain with either the anti-kappa or anti-lambda antiserum but not with both reagents.

Bone marrow aspiration is important for the diagnosis of myeloma, although the nonhomogeneous distribution of tumor in the marrow means that myeloma cannot be ruled out by normal findings. If clinical suspicion is strong and the initial marrow is not diagnostic, it should be repeated, perhaps at a different site. Plasma cells usu-

TABLE 48–8	Clinical Syndromes of Multiple Myeloma

I. Due to marrow involvement with plasma cells
  A. Anemia
  B. Hypercalcemia
  C. Osteoporosis and osteolytic lesions
  D. Osteosclerosis (POEMS syndrome)
  E. Extraosseous plasmacytomas
II. Due to abnormal protein
  A. Hyperviscosity
  B. Amyloidosis
  C. Effective hypogammaglobulinemia (from hypercatabolism)
III. Due to excretion of Bence Jones protein
  A. Renal failure (hypercalcemia and amyloid may play role)

POEMS = Polyneuropathy, organomegaly, endocrinopathy, monoclonal gammopathy, and skin changes.

ally make up fewer than 5% of bone marrow cells; more than 10 to 20% plasma cells are required to make a bone marrow diagnosis of multiple myeloma. Some of the plasma cells may have bizarre morphology, with binucleated and multinucleated plasma cells, or they may be normal in appearance.

The clinical manifestations of multiple myeloma center on the systemic effects of the monoclonal protein (the paraprotein) and the concomitant humoral immunodeficiency state, as well as the effects of the bone and bone marrow invasion by malignant cells. Table 48–8 outlines the common clinical syndromes associated with multiple myeloma. Despite high levels of paraprotein, syndromes of hyperviscosity are rare in myeloma.

The prognosis of multiple myeloma is a reflection of the tumor cell burden. A poor prognosis is associated with a high tumor cell burden, as reflected by anemia, decreased renal function, hypercalcemia, extensive bony involvement, and large monoclonal protein peaks. A patient without any of these poor prognostic criteria may have a median survival of 5 years; a patient in the poor prognosis category is likely to have a median survival of < 2 years. The development of a staging system that correlates clinical criteria with the "measured" myeloma cell mass has been useful for predicting prognosis and selecting therapy.

The treatment of a patient with multiple myeloma requires meticulous attention to supportive care as well as expertise in the administration of chemotherapy. Cautious exercise and ambulation are important to retard bone resorption. Bone lesions may require local radiation therapy to prevent a pathologic fracture. Adequate hydration and avoidance of intravenous dye injection (e.g., for intravenous pyelography) help to prevent renal failure. Administration of pneumococcal vaccine and early detection and treatment of infections are important. Administration of intravenous gamma globulin to correct the profound hypogammaglobulinemia may help decrease the incidence of severe infections, but this therapy is costly.

The current chemotherapy of multiple myeloma centers on the use of cell cycle–nonspecific cytotoxic drugs (alkylating agents, nitrosoureas, and anthracycline antibiotics) and corticosteroids. Alkeran and prednisone or bischlorethylnitrosourea, cyclophosphamide, and prednisone are most often used first. VAD (vincristine, adriamycin, and dexamethasone) is often employed in advancing or refractory disease. Improvement in symptoms ensues in the majority of patients. Clinical remission is associated with a decrease of <1 log of tumor cells (e.g., 10^{12} to 10^{11}). Eradication of all tumor cells and cure of multiple myeloma are not attainable with available therapy, but bone marrow transplantation combined with intensive chemotherapy has been successful in a small number of cases, especially in young patients with myeloma.

Waldenstrom's Macroglobulinemia

Waldenstrom's macroglobulinemia is a clonal disease of IgM-secreting plasmacytoid lymphocytes. It is a chronic disorder that usually affects older people. The patient commonly presents with anemia and symptoms due to the physical properties of the elevated monoclonal IgM. IgM is a large molecule and remains primarily in the intravascular space. If the IgM level is elevated, plasma viscosity may be high. Nosebleeds, retinal hemorrhages, mental confusion, and congestive heart failure are typical presentations of the hyperviscosity syndrome. Some IgM molecules precipitate in the cold. The patient with this type of IgM may manifest the clinical picture of cryoglobulinemia. Blue (cyanotic) fingers, toes, nose, and earlobes on exposure to cold are typical. Foot and leg ulcers may develop, and vascular occlusion with gangrene may ensue. Leukocytoclastic vasculitis is seen on biopsy of these skin lesions. Some monoclonal IgM molecules may have activity directed against red cells, particularly the "I" antigen (see Hemolytic Anemias in Chapter 50). This type of IgM, a cold agglutinin, agglutinates red cells at temperatures below 37°C (e.g., in the extremities). These patients present with Raynaud's phenomenon and a hemolytic anemia. Keeping patients with cryoglobulinemia or the cold agglutinin syndrome warm is a primary part of their treatment. Peripheral neuropathy is a rare presentation of Waldenstrom's macroglobulinemia. A few patients have been described in whom the IgM monoclonal protein had antimyelin activity. Splenomegaly and lymphadenopathy may develop during the course of Waldenstrom's macroglobulinemia but are rarely a major cause of disability. Bone pain and hypercalcemia rarely occur.

The treatment of Waldenstrom's macroglobulinemia is directed at relief of symptoms. If the symptoms are primarily due to the elevated IgM (hyperviscosity syndrome), plasmapheresis is a useful tool and may be combined with chemotherapy. If the IgM is a cold agglutinin or a cryoglobulin, the plasmapheresis must be done in a warm environment. Chemotherapy (with alkylating agents such as chlorambucil or cyclophosphamide) may be useful to decrease the lymphadenopathy and splenomegaly but does not alter the natural history of the disease. Recently, 2-CDA (2-chlorodesoxyadenosine) has been used with beneficial effect. The median survival is about 3 years, although some patients may live 10 or more years with indolent disease.

Rarer Plasma Cell Dyscrasias

Rarely, a patient may present with heavy chain disease, a disorder that has some characteristics of myeloma or Waldenstrom's macroglobulinemia but behaves clinically more like lymphoma. Analysis of the serum reveals only the heavy chain of IgG, IgA, or IgM. Gamma chain disease is associated with lymphadenopathy and edema of the soft palate. Alpha chain disease ("Mediterranean lymphoma") is characterized by intestinal infiltration by lymphoma; chain disease is associated with chronic lymphocytic leukemia.

Plasma cell leukemia may either be primary or appear secondary to multiple myeloma. It responds poorly to therapy. *Osteosclerotic myeloma,* or POEMS syndrome, is characterized by polyneuropathy, organomegaly, endocrinopathy, an M protein, and skin changes and primarily produces a chronic demyelinating myelopathy with osteosclerosis. *Primary amyloidosis* represents pathologic tissue deposition of monoclonal light chains (variable portions), resulting in abnormal cardiac, hepatic, gastrointestinal, neurologic, or renal function, depending on the sites of deposition of the light chains as insoluble, Congo red-birefringent fibrils. Congestive heart failure, hemorrhage, nephrotic syndrome, and peripheral neuropathy are common complications. Treatment is supportive.

REFERENCES

Foon KA, Rai KR, Gale RP: Chronic lymphocytic leukemia: New insights into biology and therapy. Ann Intern Med 1990; 113:525.

Longo DL, Glatstein E, Duffey PL, et al: Radiation therapy versus combination chemotherapy in the treatment of early-stage Hodgkin's disease: Seven year results of a prospective randomized trial. J Clin Oncol 1991; 9:906.

Williams SF, Golomb HM (eds.): Non-Hodgkin's lymphoma. Semin Oncol 1990; 17:1.

49

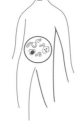

Disorders of Granulocytes and Monocytes

The main function of leukocytes is to maintain host defenses against infection, particularly bacterial infections. Mononuclear phagocytes (monocytes and tissue macrophages) and granulocytes accomplish this by ingestion and killing of microorganisms, digestion of tissue debris, and release of inflammatory cytokines and mediators. Lymphocytes participate in the activation and effector functions of the immune system, and macrophage/monocytes play essential roles in the responses of lymphocytes.

NEUTROPHIL STRUCTURE AND FUNCTION

Polymorphonuclear leukocytes make up the largest percentage of circulating leukocytes (50 to 70%). Originating in the bone marrow from pluripotential stem cells induced to differentiate by colony-stimulating factors (CSFs), they are nondividing, terminally differentiated cells that are motile, phagocytize a variety of microorganisms and inert particles, and release enzymes from cytoplasmic granules, both into phagocytic vacuoles and into the extracellular milieu. The three phases of microbial attack by neutrophils are *chemotaxis*, the directed movement along a concentration gradient of attractant substance toward a target organism; *phagocytosis*, the engulfment of the microbe in a membrane-lined phagocytic vacuole; and *microbial killing*, a chemical attack on the ingested microorganisms via the release of granule contents into the phagocytic vacuoles (bactericidal proteins, myeloperoxidase, cathepsins) plus the formation of oxygen-free radicals such as superoxide and hydroxyl ion.

Chemotaxis (the directed movement toward a chemical stimulus) involves the margination of circulating neutrophils along the endothelial lining of postcapillary venules, their penetration through the vascular wall via intercellular junctions, and their directed migration toward the extravascular source of the infection. The initial adhesion of neutrophils to the vascular endothelium is mediated by surface glycoproteins on the neutrophils (CDll/CD18 family), which bind to adhesion molecules expressed on activated endothelium (ICAM1, ELAM-1). The migration of the neutrophils takes place along a chemical gradient of an attracting substance, which may be N-methylated bacterial peptides, complement fragments (C5a), or leukotriene B. Leukocyte proteases are responsible for the production of complement-derived chemotaxins, whereas lipoxygenases mediate production of arachidonic acid–derived leukotrienes and hydroxyacids. These latter substances also have chemotactic and leukocyte-activating functions. Chemotactic substances binding to tissue sites may also serve to localize neutrophil accumulation.

Recognition of microorganisms or other particulate substances is required for subsequent ingestion by phagocytes. Opsonins, or proteins that coat microorganisms and promote their avid uptake by neutrophils, include the complement fragment C3b, the large plasma protein fibronectin, and immunoglobulins, particularly IgG. These substances adhere to the surface of microorganisms and promote binding to C3b and Fc receptors on the neutrophil plasma membrane. Phagocytosis, the localized invagination of the leukocyte surface membrane to form a vacuole or vesicle, follows, with internalization and then fusion of the phagocytic vacuoles with intracellular enzyme-containing granules.

Microbicidal activity of neutrophils combines two interacting functions: degranulation and activation of the respiratory burst. Neutrophils possess a double set of cytoplasmic granules. The primary or azurophilic granules contain lysozyme, acid hydrolases, neutral proteases including cathepsin G and elastase, myeloperoxidase, and basic proteins. Specific granules contain lysozyme, transcobalamin III, apolactoferrin, collagenase, and the C5-cleaving protease. These enzymes aid in the digestion of the bacterial cell wall, dissolve connective tissue, degrade cellular debris, or bind specific substances useful to bacterial metabolism such as iron.

The same stimuli that activate phagocytosis and granule release also initiate the respiratory burst by activating a plasma membrane-bound oxidase that catalyzes one-electron reduction of oxygen to superoxide (O_2^-) in the presence of the electron acceptor nicotinamide-adenine dinucleotide phosphate (NADPH). Interaction of O_2^- with H_2O yields hydroxyl radical OH^-, which is directly bactericidal. In addition, H_2O_2 and Cl^- in the presence of myeloperoxidase form the microbicidal hypochlorite ion OCl^-. These reactions are essential for the killing of catalase-positive microorganisms.

Granulocytes have a short lifespan in the circulation (half-life about 6 hours) and after release from the bone marrow go through the blood into the tissues, where they may live for a few days. In the blood, about 50% of granulocytes normally are marginated along vascular endothelium, remaining in dynamic equilibrium with the circulating neutrophil pool. Epinephrine, stress, or corticosteroids shift more granulocytes to the circulating pool.

Neutrophil dysfunctions include congenital or acquired defects in adhesion, chemotaxis, or microbial killing capacity. An example of the latter is chronic granulomatous disease, a group of disorders in which superoxide is not properly synthesized. In adults, such defects are usually acquired either transiently (as after hemodialysis or cardiopulmonary bypass, owing to interactions of circulating neutrophils with foreign surfaces) or in association with disease. In myelodysplasias and leukemias, neutrophil function may be abnormal. Drugs like corticosteroids and alcohol can also depress normal neutrophil function.

MONOCYTE STRUCTURE AND FUNCTION

Monocytes represent a second type of circulating and fixed (tissue macrophage) phagocyte of even greater functional versatility than neutrophils. They constitute a much smaller fraction of the circulating leukocytes, about 4 to 8%, and are longer lived. The circulating monocytes display slower chemotaxis than do neutrophils, appear later at sites of inflammation, and participate in the killing of intracellular microorganisms, both bacterial and parasitic. When monocytes are exposed to lipopolysaccharide or γ-interferon, they become "activated" and display increased motility, metabolic activity, size, and microbicidal potency. Like neutrophils, monocytes express increased surface CDll/CD18 glycoproteins upon activation. The three basic functions of mononuclear phagocytes are secretion, ingestion, and interaction with lymphocytes. Monocytes synthesize more than 50 different protein mediators and enzymes, release interleukins that affect lymphocyte function and cause fever, present antigen to T cells for immune responses, and have very active arachidonic acid metabolism resulting in production of prostaglandins (PGE_2, which regulate bone marrow and immunologic cell proliferation), leukotrienes, and thromboxane. Activated monocytes, by producing tissue factor, also potentiate blood coagulation; they also bear the urokinase-plasminogen activator receptor (UPAR) and by this propagate clot lysis. The process of pinocytosis permits macrophages to ingest and process large volumes of fluid, including plasma. Activated monocytes are also tumoricidal, producing both active oxygen and active nitrogen metabolites.

A series of reciprocal interactions between monocytes and lymphocytes is necessary for normal immune function. Monocytes and macrophages activate T cells by presenting antigen; special subpopulations of monocytes subserve this function, especially the Langerhans (skin) cells. Dendritic cells are a recently identified minor population of monocytic cells with long surface processes that appear to be the antigen-presenting cells of the blood, whereas Langerhans cells have a similar function in the skin. Lymphokines secreted by activated T cells cause accumulation and activation of monocytes. One such lymphokine, interleukin-2, is the T cell growth factor that permits expansion of T cell populations in immune responses. In addition, macrophages stimulate proliferation and differentiation of B lymphocytes via secretion of interleukin-1. PGE_1 secreted by monocytes and macrophages, in contrast, downregulates lymphocytic responses.

NEUTROPENIA

The normal white blood cell count varies between 5000 and 10,000/μl, with 50 to 70% neutrophils. The normal lower limit for neutrophil concentration is approximately 2000/μl for whites and 1500/μl for blacks, the difference resulting from different sizes of marginated pools. Normal bone marrow contains a postmitotic compartment of mature neutrophils sufficient for 7 to 10 days, although under stress, neutrophil transit time in the marrow from early differentiation to the appearance of mature forms in the blood can be as short as 5 days (Fig. 49–1).

Neutropenia can result from depressed production of leukocytes, increased peripheral destruction, increased marginal pooling, or an increased rate of loss into tissues (Table 49–1). Decreased production may be part of a generalized reduction in marrow function (congenital stem cell disorders, aplastic anemia, leukemia, myelodysplasia or vitamin deficiency [B_{12} or folate], or suppression by a toxic drug or by irradiation) or may be specifically targeting granulocytes (congenital disorders of granulocyte differentiation, idiosyncratic drug reactions [e.g., chlorpromazine], or immune suppression). The state of marrow production can often be determined by examination of the bone marrow.

Increased destruction of neutrophils may result from overutilization in the course of a severe infection; this is usually due to some diminished ability of the marrow to compensate for the loss. More chronic forms of increased destruction often involve immune mechanisms, even though the direct evidence of this (i.e., the equivalent of the Coombs' test for red cells) is not generally available. Immune destruction may be idiopathic when no other cause can be found. It may be related to drugs, as in the case of the other blood elements. It is frequent in collagen vascular diseases, particularly in Felty's syndrome accompanying rheumatoid arthritis; splenomegaly seen in this setting may play a role in the increased destruction. It is frequent in the disorder characterized by excess large granular lymphocytes; the reason for the neutropenia is not known. In newborns, transplacental transfer of isoimmune antibodies can cause profound neutropenia; infants 3 to 6 months old also often get a form of autoimmune neutropenia.

Increased pooling of the neutrophils may occur in an enlarged spleen; some destruction presumably takes place there as well. Activation of the complement components, particularly C5, as by a dialysis membrane, will result in massive margination of neutrophils, particularly in the lungs. Some are also destroyed in this process. Chronic, benign excessive margination has also been described.

Evaluation of neutropenia involves a search for underlying disease, examination of the bone marrow, testing

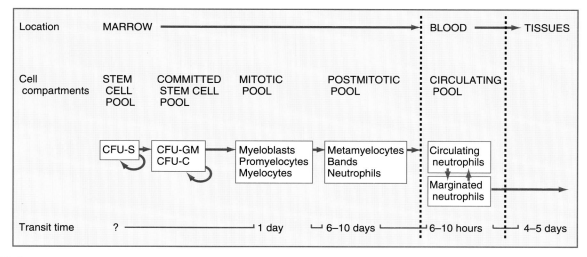

Figure 49-1
Compartments and kinetics of neutrophils. CFU = colony-forming unit.

for antibodies directed against leukocytes, and elimination of drugs. An absolute neutrophil count of less than 1000/ μL is worrisome, and one below 500/μL is considered life threatening. Meticulous oral and anal hygiene, stool softener therapy, and immediate evaluation of fever or any sign of infection are required throughout the duration of neutropenia. Rapid initiation of broad-spectrum antibiotics for fever or infection is needed, with attention to the danger of superinfection. Transfusion of neutrophil concentrates has not proved to be of benefit in recent controlled trials, probably because of a combination of dysfunction of neutrophils that occurs during preparation of the cells for transfusion and the brief half-life of neutro-

phils in the circulation (approximately 6 hours) following their infusion. Instead, current therapy favors administration of G-CSF or GM-CSF (see Chapter 48) to stimulate endogenous production of neutrophils in the bone marrow. Such treatment can shorten periods of neutropenia and enhance granulocyte function in many clinical settings, ranging from cyclic neutropenia to chemotherapy-induced neutropenia and immune neutropenia.

NEUTROPHIL LEUKOCYTOSIS

Neutrophil leukocytosis, or a persistent increase in circulating neutrophil levels above 7500/μL, is frequently observed in bacterial infection, inflammatory diseases, and hemorrhage and in association with malignancy or myeloproliferative disease (Table 49-2). There are also familial leukocytoses, which are benign. Transient leukocytosis can be induced by stress or severe exercise. A leukemoid reaction can usually be distinguished from the high white cell count of myeloproliferative disease or leukemia by

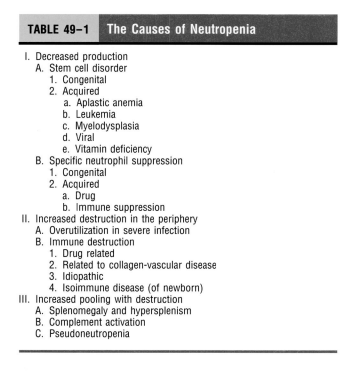

TABLE 49-1	The Causes of Neutropenia

I. Decreased production
  A. Stem cell disorder
    1. Congenital
    2. Acquired
      a. Aplastic anemia
      b. Leukemia
      c. Myelodysplasia
      d. Viral
      e. Vitamin deficiency
  B. Specific neutrophil suppression
    1. Congenital
    2. Acquired
      a. Drug
      b. Immune suppression
II. Increased destruction in the periphery
  A. Overutilization in severe infection
  B. Immune destruction
    1. Drug related
    2. Related to collagen-vascular disease
    3. Idiopathic
    4. Isoimmune disease (of newborn)
III. Increased pooling with destruction
  A. Splenomegaly and hypersplenism
  B. Complement activation
  C. Pseudoneutropenia

TABLE 49-2	Causes of Neutrophil Leukocytosis

  I. Familial
 II. Infections
  A. Acute bacterial infections
  B. Chronic bacterial infections
III. Inflammation
IV. Tumor necrosis
 V. Drugs
  A. Cytokine injection (G- or GM-CSF)
  B. Corticosteroids
  C. Lithium
VI. Malignancy
  A. Myeloproliferative disease
  B. Metastatic cancer
  C. Tumor necrosis

CSF = Colony-stimulating factor; G = granulocyte; GM = granulocyte/macrophage.

the maturity of the leukocytes, an orderly "left shift" or appearance of band forms and a few metamyelocytes, and an elevated leukocyte alkaline phosphatase.

EOSINOPHILIA

An increased eosinophil count in the peripheral blood usually reflects parasitic infection (especially with helminths), allergic reactions, or other underlying disorders such as collagen vascular disease. Tissue eosinophilia may exist without high blood eosinophil counts. Eosinophils participate in many immune processes by secreting lipid mediators, eliciting release of mediators from mast cells, and interacting with lymphocytes.

REFERENCES

Antman KS, Griffin JD, Elias A, Socinski MA, Ryan L, Cannistra SA, Oette D, Whitley M, Frei E 3d, Schnipper LE: Effect of recombinant human granulocytemacrophage colony stimulating factor on chemotherapy-induced myelosuppression. N Engl J Med 1988; 319:593.

Metcalf D: The molecular control of cell division, differentiation, committment and maturation in hematopoietic cells. Nature 1989; 339:27.

50

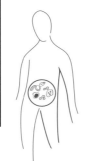

Disorders of Red Cells

SHAPE AND STRUCTURE OF RED CELLS

The human red cell is a biconcave disc about 7 μm in diameter that is filled with hemoglobin. The membrane consists of two structures: a lipid bilayer, which provides a water-impermeable barrier, and the cytoskeleton, which gives form and consistency to the membrane. The lipid bilayer consists of equimolar amounts of phospholipid and cholesterol molecules arranged so that the hydrophobic "tails" face one another and the head groups face toward the cytoplasm and the external world. Any molecules integrally attached to or penetrating this bilayer must have a hydrophobic portion that can be inserted into the lipid.

The cytoskeleton consists of heterodimers of $\alpha\beta$-spectrin, elongated molecules that form a meshwork under the lipid bilayer. Other proteins that afford attachment to the lipid bilayer are attached at the junctions of the mesh. Further attachment of the lipid bilayer to the underlying skeleton is provided by ankyrin, a molecule that affixes to the anion transporter, band 3 protein. The cytoskeleton is largely responsible for the shape of the cell. Cell shape is also influenced by changes caused by abnormal amounts of contents (hemoglobin) or volume. The red cell is elastic (able to deform and reassume the previous shape). If it is held in an abnormal shape sufficiently long to allow for altered patterns of protein interactions, the cell may assume the abnormal shape (e.g., the irreversibly sickled cell in sickle cell disease). The cytoskeleton may bear the scar of resealing the membrane after traumatic rupture (see later). Abnormalities in any of the components of the cytoskeleton are likely to result in characteristic shape changes.

BIRTH AND DEATH OF RED CELLS

In the adult, erythropoiesis can be assessed by bone marrow aspirate and through biopsy. More formal estimates can be made from studies of iron incorporation into hemoglobin, but this is seldom done. Most frequently, the rate of hematopoiesis is estimated roughly from the reticulocyte count, which represents the production of 1 to 2 days from the marrow (0.5 to 1.5%, 30,000 to 80,000/μL).

The normal red cell circulates about 120 days and then is destroyed by age-dependent mechanisms. When knowledge of the survival of red cells in the circulation is needed, the red cells may be removed, labeled with chromium 51 (^{51}Cr), and reinjected; the level of the isotope is then followed for 1 to 2 weeks. A relative measure ($T_{1/2}$) is obtained (normally 25 to 27 days). The site of accumulation of isotope (e.g., the spleen) may indicate where the cells are being destroyed.

ANEMIA

When the concentration of hemoglobin in the peripheral blood is less than normal, anemia is present; considered in this sense, anemia is a symptom rather than a diagnosis. However, some disorders are characterized and denominated by the anemia that they engender (e.g., autoimmune hemolytic anemia).

In its simplest consideration, anemia is caused by either a decrease in production or an increase in destruction. There are formal ways of measuring each of these, as outlined previously, but in a practical sense, this is seldom necessary. If the deficient production of red cells is the reason for the anemia, this will be evident in the fact that marrow production, reflected in the reticulocyte count, is less than that expected for the degree of anemia. If increased destruction or loss of red cells (hemolysis) is the reason for the anemia, the marrow production of red cells and hence the reticulocyte count will be elevated commensurate with the degree of anemia.

Hemolytic Anemias

If the patient is anemic, the reticulocyte count is elevated, and there is no sign or history of recent blood loss or recovery from erythropoietic suppression, then the anemia may be presumed to be caused by hemolysis. Other evidence of hemolysis includes

1. Elevated level of unconjugated bilirubin in serum from the breakdown of the heme of hemoglobin
2. Decreased serum level of haptoglobin, a protein that binds hemoglobin; this finding may be somewhat difficult to interpret, as haptoglobin is an acute phase reactant

3. Signs of intravascular hemolysis, including
   A. Elevation of the plasma hemoglobin
   B. Presence of hemoglobin in the urine (care must be taken to distinguish hemoglobinuria from hematuria [red cells present] and from myoglobinuria [detected by specific test]); all three will be detected as blood by the "dipstick" tests of urine commonly employed
   C. Presence of hemosiderin (iron confined to shed tubular cells) if intravascular hemolysis has occurred for several days
   D. Elevation of the plasma lactic acid dehydrogenase and, to a lesser degree, aspartate aminotransferase (AST) (serum glutamic-oxaloacetic transaminase [SGOT]); however, the plasma ALT will not be elevated, as red cells do not contain much of this enzyme

The *causes* of hemolytic anemia may be classified into two major categories (Table 50–1):

1. The congenital causes (usually resulting in defective red cells that do not survive normally)
2. The acquired causes (usually due to destructive factors acting on normally formed red cells)

No simple test distinguishes these categories, but an accurate history, particularly one that documents previous results of the examination of the blood, is very useful in making this distinction (Fig. 50–1).

The Congenital Hemolytic Anemias

Most patients with a congenital hemolytic anemia have a personal and family history of anemia, jaundice at birth, or previously abnormal blood examination results; some forms of congenital hemolytic anemia may be so mild as to have escaped notice or to have become apparent only when other events intervene, such as pregnancy, severe illness, or exposure to environmental factors.

Congenital hemolytic anemias are due to abnormalities of one of the three components of the red cell: (1) the membrane, (2) hemoglobin, or (3) the enzymes of the cells.

MEMBRANE ABNORMALITIES
Basis of the Disorders. Congenital hemolytic anemias due to membrane abnormalities generally are characterized by abnormalities in shape. The two most common of these are hereditary spherocytosis (HS), in which some of the cells are spherical on the peripheral blood (appearing as small cells without central pallor) (Fig. 50–2), and hereditary elliptocytosis (HE), in which the cells appear to be elliptical in shape or, in more severe abnormalities, acquire a fragmented appearance. In both instances, the defect is in the cytoskeleton rather than the lipid bilayer.

Hereditary spherocytosis results when the lipid bilayer is insufficiently well attached to the underlying cytoskeleton. Many abnormalities have been described that lead to this result, including a relative deficiency of spectrin, a lack of ankyrin and other proteins that traverse the

TABLE 50–1	The Causes of Anemia Due to Increased Destruction of the Red Cells

I. Congenital defects
  A. Membrane abnormalities
    1. Hereditary spherocytosis
    2. Hereditary elliptocytosis
      a. Hereditary pyropoikilocytosis
      b. Abnormalities of hemoglobin
    3. Abnormalities of structure
      a. Abnormalities resulting in defective molecular interaction
        (1) Sickle cell diseases
        (2) Hemoglobin C disease
      b. Unstable hemoglobins
    4. Defects in production
      a. α Thalassemia
      b. β Thalassemia
  B. Enzyme abnormalities
    1. Embden Meyerhof pathway
      a. Pyruvate kinase
      b. Others, including hexokinase and triose phosphate isomerase
    2. Hexose monophosphate shunt
      a. Glucose-6-dehydrogenase deficiency
      b. Others
    3. Nucleotide catabolism pathway
      a. 5-Nucleotidase deficiency
II. Acquired causes
  A. Dysplastic hematopoiesis
    1. Paroxysmal nocturnal hemoglobinuria
  B. Immune destruction
    1. Warm antibody
    2. Cold antibody
      a. Cold agglutinin disease
      b. Paroxysmal cold hemoglobinuria
    3. Drug-dependent immune hemolysis
      a. Drug alters cell
      b. Drug part of antigen
  C. Traumatic hemolysis (see Table 50–7)
  D. Toxic causes of hemolysis (See Table 50–8)
  E. Hemolysis caused by entrapment
    1. Splenomegaly
    2. Hemophagocytic syndromes

lipid bilayer and are attached to the cytoskeleton, and a lack of cytoskeletal proteins to which the anchoring proteins are attached. As the cell circulates, the lipid membrane is lost, and the spherocytosis is the result of the necessity of covering the same (or slightly less) cell contents with less membrane.

Hereditary elliptocytosis results when the cytoskeleton is unstable, usually because of abnormalities in spectrin and other essential structural proteins. When the disorder is in its mildest form, the cell is unable to revert to the biconcave shape and is deformed during its traversal of the capillaries, which have a diameter less than 7 μm; in most cases, the cells do not hemolyze. If the abnormality causes greater instability of the cytoskeleton, the cell fragments during the circulation but without some of the characteristics seen in traumatic hemolytic anemia (see later); the more severe variant is called "pyropoikilocytosis" because the cells are further unstabilized and hemolyzed *in vitro* when the temperature is raised to 50°C.

Clinical Findings. Both HS and HE can vary greatly in severity. When the defect causes severe abnormalities, it

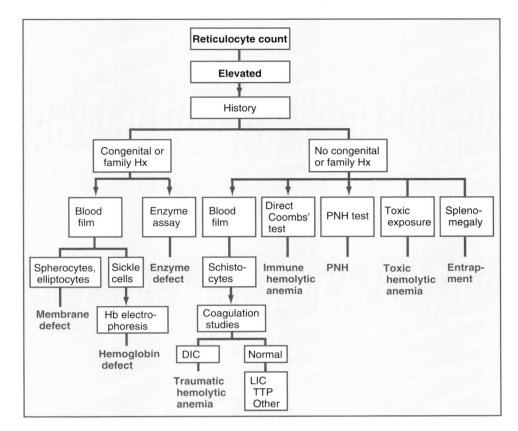

Figure 50-1
Diagnostic algorithm for anemia with an elevated reticulocyte count. DIC = Disseminated intravascular coagulation ; Hx = history; LIC = localized intravascular coagulation; PNH = paroxysmal nocturnal hemoglobinuria; TTP = thrombotic thrombocytopenic purpura.

is usually detected by hyperbilirubinemia and anemia at birth or shortly thereafter. On the other hand, milder forms may not be detected until very much later in life, often during routine examination or during family studies. The degree of anemia is frequently increased by infections or inflammation, when the rate of hematopoiesis is temporarily diminished. The spleen is frequently enlarged, although seldom massively so. Gallstones are usually present. In very severe cases, ulcers in the malleolar regions of the legs may be seen.

Laboratory Findings. The characteristic cells are found on blood film; in the case of HS, the spherocytosis may be confirmed by an abnormality in the osmotic lysis test and the autohemolysis test.

Treatment. The treatment of HS is splenectomy; this removes the major site in the body where the anatomy of the fine circulation prevents the undeformable spherocytes from passage. In milder forms of the disorder, this may not be necessary but is usually recommended if the patient is anemic at any time. Because of the possibility of sepsis, splenectomy in childhood is often delayed as long as possible. The gallbladder may also need to be removed if it contains stones and becomes inflamed; it should not be removed without removing the spleen, as intrahepatic bilirubin stones may result. Splenectomy may also be indicated in HE if sufficiently severe anemia is present; it is not as effective a treatment as it is in HS.

Hemoglobin Abnormalities

Since hemoglobin is the main intracellular molecule of the red cell, abnormalities in its structure or production can lead to hemolysis. The normal adult hemoglobin (HbA) consists of two α chains and two β chains; variations in either of these chains may result in abnormalities. Two other hemoglobins are present in small amounts in the adult: hemoglobin F and hemoglobin A_2. Hemoglobin F, which consists of two α and two β chains, is the main hemoglobin prior to birth but is replaced within 6 months so that it represents less than 1% of the hemoglobin in normal adults. Hemoglobin A_2, which consists of two α and two δ chains, is a minor component, representing between 2.5 and 4.0% of the total hemoglobin in adults. Abnormalities in these hemoglobins do not cause symptoms, but alterations in their concentration may be very helpful in diagnosis.

STRUCTURAL ABNORMALITIES. The structure of hemoglobin is highly conserved in evolution, and the four types of chains (α, β, γ, and δ) are very similar to one another. The assembled molecule consists of two pairs of α-non α dimers that exist in a globular form with an outer surface that does not interact with other molecules of hemoglobin. Each chain is folded in such a way that it can contain the very hydrophobic heme molecule in a "heme pocket" and can interact with the other chains in forming the tetrameric molecule. Within the heme pocket, specific

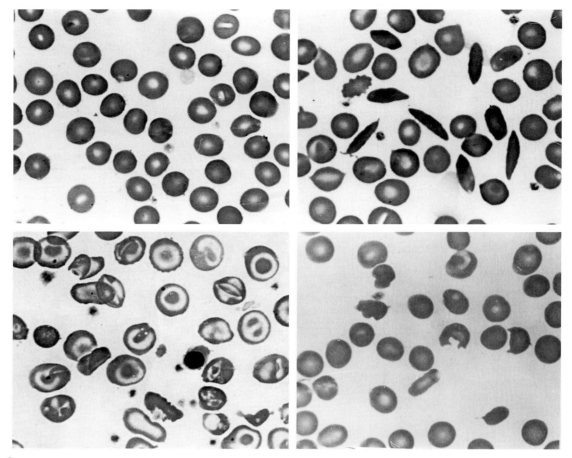

Figure 50–2
Photomicrographs of peripheral blood smears. *Upper left*, Spherocytes, round dense cells lacking a central pallor in a patient with hereditary spherocytes. *Upper right*, Sickle cells, typical of sickle cell anemia. *Lower left*, Target cells, typical of thalassemia. *Lower right*, Schistocytes, Typical of microangiopahthic hemolytic anemia.

amino acid residues are needed to react with heme and maintain the iron of heme in the reduced state.

Structural abnormalities in hemoglobin usually result from mutations of one of the genes encoding the hemoglobin chains. These mutations are usually single base substitutions, resulting in the substitution of amino acids into the molecule that alter function or molecular interactions. These abnormalities are usually one of the following:

1. Alterations in the interaction with other hemoglobin molecules
2. Alterations in the stability of the hemoglobin molecule
3. Alterations in the uptake or delivery of oxygen
4. Alterations in the ability to reduce oxidized iron in heme
5. Alterations that do not change the function or interactions of hemoglobin

ALTERATIONS IN INTERACTION WITH OTHER HEMOGLOBIN MOLECULES (SICKLE CELL AND RELATED DISEASES)

Basis of the Disorder. Since hemoglobin is packed into red cells at nearly maximal concentration, any alteration in the interaction of neighboring molecules is likely to result in precipitation of the molecule. By far the most common and serious of these alterations is the substitution of valine for glutamate at the $\beta6$ position (HbS). This permits the deoxygenated form of the molecule to form a dimer because this residue fits into a complementary hydrophobic area of the β chain of a nearby molecule. This dimer is able to add similar dimers to form a long chain, and several (~14) of these chains form bundles (paracrystals) within the cell. This distorts the cell to the shape of a sickle and markedly increases the intracellular viscosity and decreases the deformability of the cell; these three effects work together to result in the clinical symptoms.

These reactions occur most readily when only HbS is present, as in the homozygous condition (HbSS) or in the double heterozygote for β thalassemia in which the thalassemia gene is totally silent (HbS-$\beta°$ thalassemia) (Table 50–2); the latter condition is slightly milder than the former because of the decreased intracellular concentration of hemoglobin. Paracrystal formation occurs much less readily when HbA is present in the cell, either in the usual heterozygote carrier (sickle cell trait, HbAS) or in the double heterozygote for HbS and the form of thalassemia that makes a small quantity of A (β^+ thalassemia). HbF is even more effective in interfering with the reac-

TABLE 50–2	Sickle Cell Syndromes								
		Hemoglobin (%)					Average		
Phenotype	Genotype	S	A	A$_2$	F	Other	Hb	Severity
Sickle cell disease	SS	80–97	0	< 3.5	1–15		7.5–8.5	Marked
S-β^0 Thalassemia	S-β^0	80–95	0	> 3.5	1–15		8.0–9.0	Marked
S-β^+ Thalassemia	S-β^+	70–90	10–25	> 3.5	1–15		8.5–10.0	Moderate
Sickle cell trait	AS	25–40	60–75	< 3.5	< 1		Normal	Virtually asyptomatic
Sickle cell-HPFH	S-HPFH	65–85	0	< 2.5	10–30		8.0–13.0	Asymptomatic to moderately severe
SC disease	S, C	50	0	< 3.5	1–3	C = 50%	8.5–12.0	Mild to moderate

tion, and small amounts in the cell diminish the sickling effect. Hemoglobin C (which has a lysine at the 6 position) is able to take part in the reaction, and persons doubly heterozygous for S and C often have clinical symptoms; two other abnormal hemoglobins (D$_{Los\ Angeles}$ and O$_{Arab}$), while much less common than HbC, likewise increase the formation of the sickle paracrystals in the double heterozygous state; such patients may be very symptomatic.

The cellular abnormalities induced by the formation of paracrystals result in hemolysis of the cells, either directly or through alterations of the membrane. However, the effects on the circulation of the cells are more important. Obstruction of arterioles results in hypoxia, which, if repeated or sufficiently extensive, results in necrosis and organ damage. The increased cellular viscosity results in increased blood viscosity, particularly if the hematocrit is > 30%, and this results in abnormal perfusion with consequent hypoxia and tissue injury.

Clinical Findings. The clinical effects of sickle cell disease vary greatly from patient to patient and from age to age. In children, the spleen is impaired by the accumulation of sickled cells, which results in an inefficient clearance of gram-positive organisms, particularly *Streptococcus pneumoniae*, and children younger than 5 years old are very prone to sepsis for that reason. The patient may begin to have painful episodes, brought about by vaso-occlusion in the vessels of the long bones and other sites. These episodes are sudden in onset, last 5 to 10 days, and usually resolve without residua; they tend to increase in frequency when the person is in his or her mid-20s but decrease after the age of 30.

Patients with sickle cell disease are prone to "pneumonia" or "acute chest syndrome." This probably represents impaired circulation in the lungs due to small occlusions or increased viscosity of the blood; the hypoxic area that results is likely to become infected, and the patient probably will become febrile. This process can be very rapidly progressive with greater and greater hypoxia; this may cause sickling on the arterial side of the circulation, with disastrous results including multiple organ damage (brain, kidneys, pancreas, liver, bone marrow) because of the problems with perfusion. When the brain is affected, the patient may become comatose without localizing neurologic signs but may recover almost completely on appropriate treatment (full-exchange transfusion).

Other organs may be damaged more gradually by the difficulties with perfusion. Ulcers that are very difficult to heal may occur on the lower legs. Bones, particularly the heads of the femur and humerus, may undergo aseptic necrosis. The kidneys and heart may fail. Neovascularizing retinopathy may occur, and blindness may result from hemorrhage into the vitreous humor. Strokes may also occur.

The patient with SC disease is likely to have a more benign course than the patient with SS disease. The painful episodes are less well defined and often very infrequent. Some of the complications primarily attributable to increased blood viscosity (acute chest syndrome, aseptic necrosis of the hips and shoulders, retinopathy) occur with some frequency in SC disease; this is in part the result of the increased viscosity, because the hematocrit is often nearly normal.

Some of the effects of the disease are discernible on physical examination of the patient. Scleral icterus is usually present, and the conjunctival vessels may be seen to end in abrupt terminations. Ischemic retinopathy, including hypoxic "spots" and neovascularization (so-called "sea fans") may be seen, particularly in the periphery of the fundus. The heart is often enlarged, and flow murmurs are nearly always present. The spleen is usually not palpable in adult patients with HbSS but is often enlarged in patients with HbSC or other "milder" variants. If aseptic necrosis is present, the motion of the affected joint may be decreased; in the hip, this is demonstrated by elicitation of pain on flexion and internal rotation. Ulcers or the scars of ulcers may be found over the lower leg, and signs of previous neurologic damage may be found. Hypertension is almost never seen, except in patients with renal damage.

Laboratory Findings. All patients with HbSS are anemic, and it is useful to know what the usual degree of anemia is for each patient since changes may signify other clinical problems. The reticulocyte count should be markedly elevated; if it is not, then the cause should be sought. The white blood cell count and platelet count are frequently somewhat above normal, perhaps as a result of the asplenia. Sickled cells are nearly always found on the peripheral blood film (see Fig. 50–2). The serum unconjugated (indirect) bilirubin is elevated. The serum creatinine is lower than normal (unless renal failure has supervened) because of the increased glomerular filtration rate of kidneys that cannot concentrate urine. The urine may contain protein.

The diagnosis of the hemoglobinopathies is made primarily from electrophoresis. Although there are tests that measure the insolubility of HbS, they are inadequate to detect variations and should not be used. Careful evaluation of HbA_2 will help in the detection of the β-thalassemia trait except when HbC is also present.

Other laboratory and radiologic findings are specific to complications of the disease. Aseptic necrosis of bone can often be detected by radiograph, but computed tomography (CT) or magnetic resonance imaging (MRI) scan may be needed.

Treatment. Until recently, the treatment of sickle cell disease was the treatment of its complications. The painful episode is treated with hydration, and analgesia given is sufficient doses to obtain relief. The chest complications are treated with antibiotics (if pneumonia is thought to be present), oxygen supplementation, and, if arterial hypoxia supervenes, complete-exchange blood transfusion. Proliferative retinopathy may be treated with laser therapy. The ulcers of the legs are treated with local therapy. The effects of chronic organ damage (renal and heart failure) are treated with the usual measures; transfusion also may be needed.

Transfusion is reserved for specific clinical complications, including (1) increasing anemia (hemoglobin <20% below the usual or reticulocyte count markedly reduced); (2) incipient and established stroke, particularly in children; (3) progressive acute chest syndrome or acute multiorgan damage syndrome (rapid and immediate complete exchange is suggested [see later]); and (4) extensive and prolonged surgery. The role of transfusion in the pregnant patient is currently under debate; the preponderance of data suggests that chronic transfusion is not necessary.

Recently, the use of hydroxyurea has been shown to benefit patients with HbSS by increasing the level of fetal hemoglobin. The dose must be carefully adjusted, as marrow suppression is the principal toxicity.

Outcome. Mortality from sickle cell disease (HbSS) occurs either in infancy or in adulthood. In infancy, there is increased mortality from overwhelming infection and pneumonia unless prophylaxis with penicillin is instituted. Young adults begin to die of the complications, and the mean age at death is 46 years for women and 43 years for men. In HbSC disease, the mean age at death is about 63 for women and 60 for men.

ALTERATION IN THE STABILITY OF THE HEMOGLOBIN MOLECULE

Basis of the Disorders. The hemoglobin molecule has evolved to have a stable structure; disruption of this organization results in denaturing of the hemoglobin molecule and its precipitation within the cell as a Heinz body (best seen in supravital staining). The presence of an insoluble body within the cell causes changes in the membrane and causes the cell to be retained by the spleen, resulting in hemolysis. The catabolism of heme from denatured hemoglobin is different from that of heme removed in a more orderly fashion; it ends up as a brown-colored dipyrrole (mesobilifuchsin) rather than a tetrapyrrole (bilirubin and its metabolites); the dipyrrole is excreted in the urine as a dark pigment.

Clinical and Laboratory Findings. Most of these abnormal hemoglobins can be detected on electrophoresis. If the spleen has been removed, it is easy to demonstrate the Heinz bodies. The instability of the hemoglobin may be demonstrated by heating a solution to 52°C with a small amount of propanol and observing a precipitate.

OTHER SIGNIFICANT HEMOGLOBINOPATHIES. As oxygen is taken up by the tetrameric molecule of hemoglobin, the subunits move against one another so that subsequent oxygen molecules are more readily taken on than the first. This process may be hindered by changes in amino acids in any of the interfaces so that oxygen is either more tightly held than normal or is more easily given up. In the former case, relative tissue hypoxia will result and the patient will become polycythemic; in the latter case, the patient will become anemic. These abnormalities are rare in the population and are best detected by hemoglobin electrophoresis and by obtaining an oxygen dissociation curve.

The iron molecule in heme must be in the ferrous form to pick up oxygen. In this form, it is able to react with neighboring histidine molecules on either side of the heme pocket. If any of these histidines are changed (usually to tyrosine), the iron cannot be reduced and the patient has methemoglobin.

BIOSYNTHETIC ABNORMALITIES. A large number of different abnormalities of the globin genes may interrupt their biosynthesis; when this occurs, the general term *thalassemia* is applied. The abnormality can be in any of the globin genes—α, β, γ, δ, ϵ, or ζ; however, only those affecting the α and the β globin gene are of clinical importance (Table 50–3).

The β Thalassemia Syndromes. Abnormalities of the β globin gene were the first described. When only one of the two β globin genes is affected (the heterozygous state), the result is very mild anemia (hemoglobin 11 gm/dL ± 1 gm/dL), microcytosis and decreased mean corpuscular volume (MCV) (77 ± 5 fl), and a slightly hyperactive bone marrow. The blood picture looks much like iron deficiency, with which it is sometimes confused. The level of hemoglobin A_2 is increased (>4%), and the amount of hemoglobin F may be elevated. This condition is relatively asymptomatic.

When both β globin genes are abnormal, the results are much more serious. If the abnormality results in a gene that produces no hemoglobin, the patient will have β thalassemia major. This is characterized by extreme anemia requiring transfusion at an early age; markedly hypochromic and targeted red cells (see Fig. 50–2), often showing dense inclusions that are precipitated (excess) α globin chains; limited reticulocytosis (somewhat lower than expected for the degree of anemia); and marked erythroid hypercellularity. Although a large part of the anemia is due to ineffective erythropoiesis, the red cells

TABLE 50-3	Classification of the Thalassemias			
	α Globin genes (n)	Abnormal hemoglobin	Usual hemoglobin	Clinical severity
Alpha Thalassemias				
α_2 Heterozygote	3	Bart's (γ_4) (?)	Normal	Asymptomatic
α_2 Homozygote	2	Bart's (γ_4)	Slight anemia	Asymptomatic
α_1 Heterozygote	2	Bart's (γ_4)	Slight anemia	Asymptomatic
α_1/α_2 Double heterozygote	1	Hemoglobin H, Bart's (γ_4)	Moderate anemia, Heinz-like bodies	Mild
α_1 Homozygote	0	All Bart's	Death in infancy (hydrops fetalis)	Severe
Beta Thalassemias				
β^0 or β^+ Heterozygote	4	High A_2	Slight anemia	Mild
β^0/β^+, β^+/β^+ Double heterozygotes	4	High F, High A_2	Moderate to marked hypochromic anemia	Moderate
β^0 Homozygote	4	High % F	Very severe hypochromic anemia	Severe

are also hemolyzed prematurely, probably because of abnormalities generated by the precipitated α globin chains. Erythroid overgrowth of the marrow may distort the bones of the head, face, rib cage, and pelvis, and masses of extraosseous erythroid tissue may accumulate. These patients must be transfused from an early age and tend to accumulate iron from transfusions as well as from excessive absorption.

In other patients, the defect may not affect synthesis as greatly (β^+ thalassemia gene); these patients will have more moderate anemia, requiring transfusion at very much less frequent intervals. The other manifestations of the disease are also less notable.

At the present time, the best therapy available for patients with β thalassemia major is transfusion. Hypertransfusion to nearly normal levels of hemoglobin prevents many of the late complications of the disorder (particularly bony deformities and excessive splenomegaly and hypersplenism) at the cost of slightly higher amounts of blood than are needed. Bone marrow transplantation at an early age has been shown to be effective in those patients with an appropriate sibling donor.

The Thalassemia Syndromes. Each chromosome 16 normally contains 2 α globin genes that are identical (indicating that the reduplication has occurred recently); thus, the genome contains a total of four α globin genes. The most common cause of α thalassemia is the elimination of one of the globin genes on a chromosome due to unequal crossing over; the resulting "gene" is called the a_2 thalassemia gene and it has a frequency of about 0.30 in African populations. In the heterozygous state, it results in minimal diminution of the hemoglobin and hematocrit; in the homozygous state, the patient may be slightly anemic but is otherwise unaffected. Confusion with iron deficiency is frequent.

In non-African populations, both α globin genes on the same chromosome may be missing or inoperative; this "gene" is called the α_1 thalassemia gene. The heterozygous state is like the homozygous state of α_2 thalassemia; in both cases, two α globin genes are still functioning. The homozygous state of α_1 thalassemia is fatal before or

at birth, as no non-β globin chains are being made; these infants are extremely anemic and hydropic. The double heterozygous state, $\alpha\alpha_2$ thalassemia, results in a single active α globin gene; as a result, β globin molecules are made in great excess, and these combine in tetramers containing four β globin molecules (β_4), which is called hemoglobin H. These β_4 tetramers are visible as precipitates in supravital preparation of blood; they are unstable and cause hemolytic anemia with pigmenturia, like other unstable hemoglobins (see previous).

The diagnosis of the α thalassemia minor syndromes in the adult is difficult without resorting to analysis of the DNA to detect the missing genes. In the newborn, the presence of the tetramer of γ chains, called hemoglobin Bart's, may be seen. Hemoglobin H is also detected as a fast-running hemoglobin variant and is unstable in the tests for unstable hemoglobins.

Enzyme Abnormalities

The red cell has a limited repertoire of metabolic pathways consisting of (1) the glycolytic pathway, (2) the hexose monophosphate (HMP) shunt, and (3) the nucleotide catabolism pathways. Congenital deficiencies in any of these can cause hemolytic anemia.

THE GLYCOLYTIC PATHWAY
The Basis of the Disorders. The red cell contains the enzymes of the glycolytic pathway but does not contain the elements necessary for the further oxidation through the citric acid cycle. Therefore, all the energy it needs must be generated by the less efficient system. Deficiencies of almost all the enzymes of glycolysis have been described, but all are of rare occurrence except deficiency of pyruvate kinase, the last enzyme of the pathway.

The major effect of defects in the glycolytic pathway is the deprivation of the cell of energy. In the overall balance, two molecules of ATP are used in phosphorylation reactions, and four molecules of ATP are generated; hence, any interruption of the sequence is likely to tip over an already precarious energy balance. Although it is not clear how depletion of energy results in hemolysis, it occurs without discernible morphologic change.

The Clinical Findings. The degree of anemia is highly variable, even for a single-enzyme defect. When the defect results in severe hemolysis, the clinical signs are usually present at birth; when they are less severe, they may become apparent only upon stress to erythropoiesis such as infection. Pyruvate kinase deficiency is usually evident only in the red cells; some of the other enzyme deficiencies (e.g., triose isomerase) also manifest as neurologic disease and may result in early death.

The Laboratory Findings. The diagnosis is established by demonstration of the deficiency of the enzyme. For pyruvate kinase, this must be carefully done, as the abnormality may be small and easily missed; screening tests are available that will detect the moderate and severe abnormalities. More recently, the exact defect in the DNA has been identified for a number of the enzyme deficiencies, and molecular genetic techniques looking for these defects have been used to diagnose their presence.

Treatment and Outcome. Splenectomy is useful in the treatment of severe pyruvate kinase deficiency; this removes a sequestered site where young red cells (containing residual mitochondria and hence residual capacity to produce ATP) normally remain for 1 to 3 days. Often, transfusion can be avoided by this procedure.

THE HMP SHUNT. One of the important functions of the red cell is that of maintaining the iron of hemoglobin in the reduced state while the cell circulates in an oxidative environment. This is mainly accomplished by the generation of protons through the metabolism of glucose-6-phosphate. The failure of this system permits oxidative radicals to oxidize hemoglobin and membrane proteins, resulting in the hemolysis of the cell.

Glucose-6-Phosphate Dehydrogenase Deficiency. The initial step of the HMP shunt is the dehydrogenation of glucose-6-phosphate by the enzyme glucose-6-phosphate dehydrogenase. This enzyme, whose gene is on the X chromosome, is often deficient in populations exposed to malaria. Male hemizygotes are more affected than female heterozygotes; homozygotes are rare. Over 400 different defects have been identified, many at the DNA level, and the resultant deficiency ranges from none at all to a very severe lack. The wild-type enzyme is called B; about 30% of Africans have a normally active variant, A$^+$, and a further 10% have a defective variant A$^-$; these individuals have hemolytic anemia when confronted with an oxidative stress (e.g., a drug or infection) but are usually normal. Persons of Mediterranean ancestry often have a more defective variant and may have hemolytic anemia most of the time. Some of these individuals are prone to severe hemolysis after ingesting the fava bean (favism). Many drugs have been implicated in causing hemolysis, but in the moderately deficient cells, only a few truly do so (Table 50–4).

TABLE 50–4	Drugs Implicated in Causing Hemolysis in Patients with G-6-PD Deficiency

I. Antimalarials
  1. Primiquine
  2. Pamaquine
II. Sulfonamides and sulfones
  1. Sulfanilamide, sulfapyridine, sulfadimidine
  2. Dapsone, sulfoxone
  3. Septrin
III. Various
  1. Nitrofurans
  2. Vitamin K analogues
  3. Probenecid
  4. Methylene blue

G-6-PD = glucose 6-phosphate dehydrogenase.

The Acquired Hemolytic Anemias

With one exception (paroxysmal nocturnal hemoglobinuria [PNH]), the acquired hemolytic anemias are characterized by the fact that the red cells are normal when formed and are destroyed as they circulate because they are changed by an outside influence, such as reaction with antibody or reaction with a toxin (see Table 50–1).

DYSPLASTIC CAUSES. In the myelodysplastic syndromes, the red cells are often abnormal and do not survive normally. However, the only instance in which the problem is frequently thought of as primarily a hemolytic anemia is in the case of PNH.

IMMUNE CAUSES. Probably the most common causes of acquired hemolytic anemia are immune, in which an antibody is the proximate cause of the destruction of the cell (Table 50–5). The direct antiglobulin (Coombs') test, which measures IgG antibody and remnants of complement components on the membrane of the patient's red cells, shows positive results in more than 98% of cases and affords an excellent screening test. The clinical syndrome depends upon the isotype and reaction characteristics of the antibody, particularly whether it is able to react with the cell at body temperature.

Warm-Reacting Antibody
Basis of the Disorder. Most autoimmune antibodies able to react with their antigen (which is usually a membrane protein) at 37°C are IgG. They attach to the red cell and can react with receptors on phagocytes (particularly those of the spleen), causing the cells to be engulfed. When this process is incomplete, spherocytes result, which then may be trapped in the spleen. Complement may or may not be fixed; when it is, hemolysis by these processes is often more severe. Rarely, complement may lyse the cells directly.

    Warm-reacting IgG antibodies may arise in the absence of other illness as a circumscribed error of the immune system (idiopathic). They may be seen in other abnormalities of the immune system, such as malignancy of the immune system (chronic lymphocytic leukemia or

TABLE 50-5	Characteristics of Antibodies in Immune Hemolytic Anemia				
	Warm-Antibody Disease	**Cold Agglutinin Disease**	**Paroxysmal Cold Hemoglobinuria**	**Drug-Related Immune, Type I**	**Drug-Related Immune, Type II**
Antibody isotype	IgG (rarely IgA)	IgM	IgG	IgG	IgM, IgG
Optimum temperature of reaction	37°C	0°C	0°C	37°C	37°C
Direct Coombs' test	IgG ± C3	C3 only	C3 only	IgG only	C3 only
Agglutination in saline	None (rarely +)	++++	+	0–+	0–++(with drug)
Lysis by complement *in vitro*	Rare	Poor	Well	None	Sometimes well
Clinical severity	Mild to very severe	Mild to moderate	Moderate to severe	Mild to moderate	Mild to severe
Response to prednisone	Often	None	Often	If needed	Not needed
Response to splenectomy	Often	Rare	None	Not needed	Not needed

lymphoma); viral diseases affecting the immune system (HIV infection or Epstein-Barr virus infection); more general abnormalities of the immune self-recognition system (e.g., systemic lupus erythematosus, rheumatoid arthritis); and congenital abnormalities of the immune system. In childhood, IgG antibodies may occur in the course of response to a viral infection, but this is rare in adults.

Clinical and Laboratory Manifestations. The degree of anemia is highly variable but is frequently severe; the disorder may be fatal if not properly treated. There are few physical findings except for pallor and perhaps splenomegaly that is seldom massive. The blood counts other than those related to the red cells are usually normal, although simultaneous immune thrombocytopenia is not rare. Spherocytes are usually seen in the peripheral blood (similar to those in Fig. 50–2A), and the direct Coombs' test may have a positive result, usually showing IgG alone or IgG and complement (C3).

Treatment. Treatment is aimed at reducing the production of antibody or reducing the hemolysis of cells affected by antibody. Prednisone is given, initially at doses of about 1 mg/kg (60 mg in the adult). If it is effective, the dose is reduced rapidly to 20 mg/day; it is further reduced slowly by changing doses at monthly intervals until the minimum effective dose is achieved. If possible, prednisone should be given on alternate days. If prednisone is ineffective or the dose required for continued remission is too high, (more than 20 mg every other day), splenectomy should be considered; this procedures improves hemolysis in ∼80% of patients, particularly if complement is not fixed by the antibody. If both prednisone and splenectomy fail, chemotherapy with cyclophosphamide (100 mg/day in adults) or azathioprine may be given; the response to chemotherapy may take several weeks.

Cold-Reacting Antibody

Basis of the Disorder. Antibodies reacting with polysaccharide antigens usually bind more avidly at reduced temperatures. These antibodies are usually IgM (cold agglutinins) but may be IgG (Donath Landsteiner antibodies).

Because they do not react at body temperature, they do not cause hemolysis by reacting with phagocytes, as they are not on the membrane when the red cell is in proximity of those cells. They fix complement, and most of the hemolysis that they engender is caused by this reaction.

Cold agglutinins arise either as paraproteins from monoclonal proliferation of lymphocytes (chronic cold agglutinin disease) or in response to viral infections (*Mycoplasma Pneumoniae* or the Epstein Barr virus of infectious mononucleosis). Donath-Landsteiner antibodies arise as a complication of syphilis in response to viral diseases of childhood, or as an autoimmune disease.

Clinical and Laboratory Characteristics of Cold Agglutinin Disease. Cold agglutinins may cause agglutination of red cells peripherally in the venules, resulting in acrocyanosis, a purplish discoloration of terminal parts of limbs. Sometimes this agglutination makes the eating of cold foods or drinks painful. Other symptoms are generally lacking. The spleen may be enlarged.

The diagnosis is made by the demonstration of cold-agglutinating antibodies in the serum of the patient; although small amounts of cold agglutinins occur in normal serum, the amount occurring in the serum of symptomatic patients is usually far greater. In addition to titer (the highest dilution of the serum that will cause agglutination), the specificity of the antibody is important (Table 50–6). Anti-I antibodies react more strongly (to a higher

TABLE 50-6	Specificity of Cold Agglutinins Related to Clinical Associations		
Specificity	**Reaction with Red Cells**	**Neoplastic Causes**	**Infectious Causes**
Anti-I	Adult > fetal	Benign monoclonal, CLL	Mycoplasma
Anti-i	Fetal > adults	Aggressive lymphoma	Infectious mononucleosis
Anti-Pr	Adult = fetal	Benign (usually)	

CLL = Chronic lymphatic leukemia.

titer) with adult cells than fetal (cord) red cells and are seen in the more benign lymphoproliferative disorders (benign monoclonal gammopathy, chronic lymphatic leukemia) or in *M. Pneumoniae* infections. Anti-i antibodies react more strongly with fetal cells than adult cells and are seen in more aggressive lymphomas and in infectious mononucleosis. In nearly all patients with cold agglutinin disease, the direct Coombs' test results are positive with anti-C3 antiserum and negative with anti-IgG.

The degree of anemia is highly variable but usually is not severe; the hematocrit is usually lower in winter than in summer in seasonally cold climates. Agglutination (distinct from rouleaux) may be seen on the peripheral blood film, and the MCV may be falsely elevated because of the agglutination; this can be corrected by warming the blood before analysis.

Paroxysmal cold hemoglobinuria (PCH), which is caused by IgG cold-reacting antibody, is uncommon, but the clinical syndrome may be very severe, particularly the postviral childhood form. It often presents with hemoglobinuria following exposure to cold but may be manifest only as hemolytic anemia. Some patients have Raynaud's phenomenon but do not have acrocyanosis as do patients with cold agglutinins. The direct Coombs' test results may be positive with anti-C3 but not with anti-IgG; in many patients, the direct Coombs' test results are negative with the usual reagents. Normal red blood cells may lyse when reacted with the patient's serum and a source of complement at 0°C followed by incubation at 37°C (the Donath-Landsteiner test); this test is not very sensitive.

Treatment. Avoidance of the cold is of paramount importance, as this will usually reduce the hemolysis and other clinical signs. In cold agglutinin disease, the amount of antibody in the serum can be rapidly and temporarily reduced by whole body volume plasmapheresis (done carefully so as not to allow the blood to become cooled). *This is necessary for patients undergoing surgery requiring general anesthesia.* Chemotherapy with alkylating agents may be of benefit in some patients with chronic cold agglutinin syndrome. Chemotherapy appropriate to the underlying disease is clearly indicated in those patients with CLL or lymphoma; since the antibody is a product of the tumor, it may be used as a marker to assess the burden of tumor.

Paroxysmal cold hemoglobinuria may be treated with prednisone, as are other IgG-mediated hemolytic anemias, but splenectomy or intravenous gamma globulin is not useful. Chronic PCH may require chemotherapy with an alkylating or antimetabolic agent. The transient childhood variant can usually be managed with transfusion if needed.

DRUG-DEPENDENT IMMUNE HEMOLYTIC ANEMIA (DDIHA)
Basis of the Disorder. Drugs may invoke an immune response that will result in immune hemolytic anemia by two mechanisms: type 1, in which the drug (e.g., α-methyldopa) may alter a protein of the cell surface so that it is antigenic (the antibody that results cross-reacts with the normal protein to induce hemolysis even when the drug is not present), and type 2, in which the drug may

serve as a hapten by combination with a surface protein, and the resulting antibody may cause hemolysis when the drug is present. In either case, hemolysis results from the same reactions as immune hemolytic anemia without drugs—IgG antibodies (the more common) react with phagocytes, resulting in spherocytes, and IgM antibodies fix complement, resulting in lysis from those reactions.

Clinical and Laboratory Findings. In type 1 DDIHA, hemolysis occurs 3 to 6 weeks after the initiation of the drug and continues for 3 to 4 months after its discontinuation; spherocytosis is evident, and the direct Coombs' test results are positive with anti-IgG. Antibody against normal red cells can be detected in the serum without the addition of the drug. In type 2 DDIHA, hemolysis occurs 1 to 2 weeks after initiation of the drug (unless the patient is previously sensitized, in which case it occurs in 1 to 5 days); spherocytosis may be present, and the direct Coombs' test results are commonly positive with anti-C3 only. The exception is that due to penicillin, in which the direct Coombs' test results are positive with anti-IgG only. Antibody cannot be detected in the serum unless the drug is added to the reaction mixture.

Treatment. Stopping the drug is usually all that is needed to resolve the problem.

TRAUMATIC CAUSES OF HEMOLYTIC ANEMIA (TRAUMATIC HEMOLYTIC ANEMIA [THA])
Basis of the Disorder. The normal red cell is constructed so as to be able to circulate through the endothelially lined vascular system without damage. When incomplete obstructions in the microvasculature or unendothelialized surfaces are present (usually prostheses such as heart valves and vascular replacements), the cells may be broken by trauma imposed by the impulsion of the blood. The result is intravascular hemolysis characterized by schistocytes (see Fig. 50–2).

The most common impediments to flow in the microcirculation are fibrin strands associated with intravascular coagulation, either localized intravascular coagulation (LIC) or disseminated intravascular coagulation (DIC). This impediment must be on the arteriolar side, as only there are forces generated by the impulsion of the blood sufficient to fracture the cells. The red cells drape themselves over these strands and are cut in two by the force of blood flow. The membranes of the resulting fragments reseal, and they continue to circulate; however, their shape is altered by the seam, and they appear as schistocytes. True schistocytes, with sharp points at the seam, are indicative of traumatic hemolysis.

Clinical and Laboratory Findings. The clinical and laboratory findings vary greatly according to the cause of the intravascular impediment to flow (Table 50–7). In all cases, schistocytes on the peripheral blood film and evidence of intravascular hemolysis (increased plasma hemoglobin, increased lactate dehydrogenase (LDH), hemosiderinuria, and possibly hemoglobinuria) should be present. Thrombocytopenia is often present as well, particularly in DIC and thrombotic thrombocytopenic purpura–hemolytic uremic syndrome (TTP-HUS) (see later); DIC can be readily

TABLE 50–7	Characteristics of Various Types of Traumatic Hemolytic Anemia			
	Schistocytes	Thrombocytopenia	Prolonged PT and PTT	Increased Fibrin Split Products
Macrovascular (Prostheses)	Yes	No	No	Small
Microvascular				
Thrombotic thrombocytopenic purpura	Yes	Marked	No	Small
Disseminated intravascular coagulation	Yes	Moderate	Yes	Marked
Other	Yes	Not severe	No	Small

PT = Prothrombin time; PTT = partial thromboplastin time.

diagnosed by the prolonged prothrombin time and partial thromboplastin time, decreased fibrinogen, and increased fibrin split products. Thrombocytopenia and signs of consumption of procoagulants are not usually present in macrovascular causes of trauma.

Defective prosthetic heart valves are the most common cause of macrovascular traumatic hemolytic anemia. Earlier versions of valves often had plastic that would not endothelialize, but more recently, the presence of THA is more likely to be evidence of faulty placement or seating of the valve. THA occurs only when there is blood flow with a large difference in pressure, usually across a perivalvular leak. Rarely, the aperture of an aortic valve may be too small to allow adequate ventricular ejection, resulting in turbulence and trauma.

Thrombotic thrombocytopenic purpura and the closely related syndrome, HUS, are relatively frequent causes of traumatic hemolytic anemia. They are characterized by arteriolar fibrinous clots, probably caused by loss of endothelium in small arterioles; in TTP, these lesions occur widely. In HUS, they occur primarily in the kidney. These clots contain platelets and fibrin, and the platelet count is reduced, often markedly. The clinical symptoms depend upon the location and number of these lesions but classically include neurologic symptoms (bizarre behavior, nonfocal neurologic signs, coma) and renal failure (particularly in HUS). A strain of *Escherichia coli*, 0157:H7, has increasingly been implicated in the genesis of the syndrome, but the exact relationship has not been established; other organisms that, like *E. coli* 0157:H7, produce a "shiga toxin" have also been implicated in the pathogenesis of TTP and HUS.

Disseminated intravascular coagulation, in which the coagulation system is primarily activated in the circulating plasma, results in the formation of fibrin clots. When these are located at sites of sufficient flow pressure to rupture the red cells, hemolysis results. Platelets and the plasma procoagulants are consumed in the process, but the platelet count is rarely as low as is seen in TTP unless there is also some other reason (immune complexes). Because the formation of plasma clots is so widespread, the amount of fibrin split products that result is very large; these are detected as fibrin monomer, D-dimer, and others (see chapter 53, page 415).

There are a number of other conditions that result in traumatic rupture of the red cell during its circulation; in almost all, there is localized intravascular coagulation and the laboratory findings are like those of mild TTP. Malig-

nant hypertension may erode the arterioles of the kidney and result in the syndrome. Some cancers, particularly widely spread adenocarcinomas, may have localized intravascular clotting. Congenital arteriovenous malformations (hemangiomas) may do the same.

Treatment. Except for in TTP, the main focus of therapy is the treatment of the underlying disease, if possible. This may require replacement of the defective heart valve or other intravascular prosthesis; the severity of the hemolysis will determine in large part the necessity for this. Treatment of sepsis or other causes of DIC is important, as other measures (platelet transfusion, transfusion of procoagulants) will be of limited efficacy if the underlying cause cannot be corrected.

Mild TTP may on occasion respond to plasma infusion, but *most cases require plasmapheresis that is frequent and intense. This must be initiated as soon as the diagnosis is made.* Plasmapheresis may need to be continued for several weeks. Prednisone (1 gm/kg) is usually given, and in some cases, vincristine I mg/M²/week may be given. The hematocrit, platelet count, and plasma LDH are useful indicators of response. If the initial therapeutic measures are not successful in 7 to 10 days, splenectomy is often done.

TOXIC CAUSES OF HEMOLYSIS. The membrane of the red cell may be altered by toxins that are ingested from the outside or are produced by processes within the body (Table 50–8). These changes may not have morphologic correlates and are best suspected by knowledge of the history of the patient.

Internal Toxins
Liver Failure. When mild liver failure supervenes, the red cells acquire superfluous membrane; this is reflected as target cells. This defect is acquired by normal transfused cells within a few days and does not result in a shortened life span. With severe liver failure, further modifications of the membrane take place, characterized biochemically by excessive phospholipids (the phospholipid-to-cholesterol ratio exceeds 1) and morphologically by bizarre crenated forms. These are fundamentally echinocytes with a rigid membrane; as the cells circulate, they lose the spines characteristic of echinocytes and become acanthocytes. These cells are destroyed in the spleen. Their presence is a bad prognostic sign.

TABLE 50-8	Causes of "Toxic" Hemolytic Anemia

I. Internal toxins
   A. Liver disease
      1. Target cells (nonhemolytic)
      2. Acanthocytosis (spur cell anemia)
      3. "Zieve's syndrome" (with hyperlipidemia)
   B. Renal disease
   C. Hypophosphatemia
   D. Hypercupremia of Wilson's disease
II. External toxins
   A. Microorganisms invading red cell
      1. Malaria
      2. Borrelia
      3. Babesiosis
   B. Toxic animal or plant product
      1. Snake envenomation
      2. Spider bite (especially brown recluse)
      3. Clostridial infection (phospholipase mediated)
   C. Toxic chemicals
      1. Solvents (e.g., chloroform)
      2. Oxidants (e.g., Dapsone)
      3. Metals (e.g., copper)

Renal Failure. Occasionally, patients with renal failure have hemolytic anemia. The red cells have no morphologic abnormality but may have altered ion exchange. *Hypophosphatemia* with serum levels of phosphate < 1 mg/dL may result in diminished red cell adenosine triphosphate (ATP) and consequent stiffening of the membrane. This results in hemolysis.

External Toxins. A variety of chemicals, drugs, and natural products may affect the red cell and cause hemolysis. In some instances, deficiency of the enzyme glucose-6-phosphate may predispose this hemolysis (see previous); in others, drugs produce sufficient oxidative stress in the presence of normal amounts of the enzyme. This often results in precipitation of hemoglobin as Heinz bodies (seen particularly if the spleen has been removed) or as "bite cells" as the denatured hemoglobin is removed during passage through the spleen. The oxidative stress may also cause methemoglobinemia.

Copper may precipitate hemoglobin and cause membrane damage; this occurs in Wilson's disease and in copper ingestion or injection through a renal dialysis apparatus. Solvents may alter the membrane; chloroform poisoning is an example. Animal products such as snake and spider venoms may also result in hemolysis; the history of such contact is important. Clostridial infections may release phospholipases that can digest the phospholipids and cause hemolysis.

Whenever the cause of acquired hemolysis is obscure, a search for possible toxic causes by a very careful history will sometimes reveal the reason.

ENTRAPMENT CAUSES. Throughout the circulation, red blood cells are able to flow easily from the arterial side to the venous side except in one organ—the spleen. As noted previously, the spleen is structured so that blood must pass through a "pool" of blood in the cords of Billroth and through a narrow opening into the venous sinus before regaining the circulation. If the spleen is enlarged for any reason, the pool of blood becomes larger and the cells may be destroyed in the spleen. This is anatomic hypersplenism and is usually accompanied by thrombocytopenia and neutropenia, as these cells are entrapped in the same way. Splenomegaly of this magnitude can occur with circulatory changes in the portal system resulting in portal hypertension, with a variety of hematologic diseases such as myelodysplasia and lymphoma, from storage diseases such as Gaucher's disease and from a number of other causes. Whatever the cause, the cytopenias associated with anatomic hypersplenism can be corrected by splenectomy.

Blood cells can be destroyed by elements of the phagocytic system if these elements become deranged (hemophagocytic syndrome), as by virus (the viral hemophagocytic syndrome) or in a fulminant reaction (histiocytic medullary reticulosis). In either case, macrophages that have ingested red cells, platelets, or granulocytes will be found on bone marrow biopsy.

The Anemias of Reduced Production

The other primary cause of anemia is an inadequate production of red cells. Since the life span of the red cell in the circulation is about 120 days, 1% must be renewed each day to maintain the normal level of hemoglobin and hematocrit. This results in the production of 30,000 to 80,000 reticulocytes per mm^3, or about 0.5 to 2% of the red cells. As previously noted, if the need for red cells is increased, this total number should also be increased; if it is not, a relative hypoproduction is present.

The causes of hypoproduction are multiple (Table 50–9, Fig. 50–3). The MCV of the red cells, which is obtained with the usual flow cytometric blood count, can be of immense help in determining the cause. The MCV is indirectly an indicator of the relative rates of cytoplasmic and nuclear productive capacity. If the cytoplasmic productive capacity is greater than the nuclear, then the MCV is increased as more cytoplasm is made per cell. If cytoplasmic production is diminished but nuclear production is relatively normal, the MCV is diminished. If the problem is primarily one of cellular proliferation rather than specific deficient production of either cytoplasm or nucleus, then the MCV is normal.

Normal MCV

A primary lack of sufficient proliferation of red cell precursors is manifest by normal-appearing red cells (normochromic and normocytic) and an inadequate reticulocyte count. Although the bone marrow may be abnormal for other reasons, the red cell precursors are normal in morphology but deficient in number.

STEM CELL DISORDERS. In any syndrome involving abnormalities of the stem cell, anemia is likely to result (with the exception of some of the myeloproliferative diseases). If the stem cells are diminished in number (as in the myeloaplastic syndromes), are defective (as in the myelodysplastic syndromes), or are replaced (as in the acute

TABLE 50-9	The Causes of Anemia Due to Decreased Production

I. Normal MCV (82-96 fl)
  A. Stem cell disorders
    1. Myeloaplastic (see above)
    2. Myelodysplastic (see above)
    3. Acute leukemia
    4. Drug effect or toxicity
  B. Lack of erythropoietin (Epo)
    1. Renal failure
    2. Antibodies to Epo
    3. Abnormal hemoglobin with reduced oxygen affinity
  C. Erythropoietic suppression
    1. Anemia secondary to chronic disease
    2. Anemia due to virus, particularly parvovirus
    3. Specific immune inhibition (pure red cell aplasia)
II. Increased MCV (> 98 fl)
  A. Vitamin deficiency
    1. Folic acid
    2. Cobalamine (Vitamin B_{12})
  B. Myelodysplasia
III. Decreased MCV (< 82 fl)
  A. Iron-deficient hematopoiesis
    1. Iron deficiency
    2. Poor iron reutilization
  B. Deficient heme synthesis
    1. Congenital lack of ALA synthase (X-linked anemia of Rundles and Falls)
    2. Secondary to toxin exposure
    3. Myelodysplastic (refractory anemia with ringed sideroblasts)
  C. Defective globin synthesis
    1. Thalassemias (see above)

ALA = δ-Aminolevulinic acid; MCV = mean corpuscular volume.

myeloproliferative syndromes), normocytic anemia with reduced reticulocyte count will result. In all cases, the abnormality of the stem cells results in abnormalities in number, morphology, or both of the other cells of the blood; these abnormalities are often paramount in delineating the nature of the stem cell defect.

The stem cell may be suppressed by drugs, either idiosyncratically or as part of the action of the drug. The result is a hypoproliferative anemia with normal red cells.

LACK OF ERYTHROPOIETIN. The main stimulus for the production of red cells is the hormone erythropoietin (Epo). If Epo is not available to stimulate the bone marrow, reduced production of red cells will result. Since only the red cells are affected by the lack of erythropoietic, the other blood cells will be normal in number and morphology.

Lack of erythropoietin nearly always arises from disease of the kidney, which eliminates the primary site of production of the cytokine. Although there is nearly always evidence of renal malfunction, the degree of abnormality in Epo production may not correspond to the degree of renal disease; i.e., severe anemia may occur with only moderate decrease in renal function. The serum erythropoietin level is less than one would expect for the degree of anemia. In general, the anemia responds to the administration of erythropoietin.

Other causes of erythropoietin deficiency (abnormal hemoglobin that delivers oxygen too readily or antibodies to erythropoietin) are very rare.

ERYTHROPOIETIC SUPPRESSION. Erythropoiesis may be specifically suppressed without affecting the other marrow elements.

Anemia Secondary to Chronic Disease. Specific suppression of erythropoiesis most commonly occurs because of some inflammatory condition (infection or autoimmune disease), and the syndrome is designated "the anemia secondary to chronic disease." The cause of the suppression is obscure, and no direct tests defining this state are available; the diagnosis is usually made by the identification of the underlying disease and the elimination of other causes of normochromic, normocytic anemia. The serum erythropoietin is usually appropriately elevated, and the administration of exogenous erythropoietin is not usually helpful. The anemia resolves when the inflammatory origin resolves.

Anemia Due to Parvovirus Infection. A strain of parvovirus, B19, specifically invades red cell precursors and suppresses their proliferation for a period of 1 to 3 weeks. This usually occurs in patients with hyperactive erythropoiesis due to hemolytic anemia and may be the cause of sudden onset of severe anemia.

Pure Red Cell Aplasia. Erythropoiesis may be suppressed specifically by immune processes; this results in pure red cell aplasia, in which the bone marrow is normal except that it almost completely lacks red cell precursors. The treatment is that of any other autoimmune disease—prednisone and, if necessary, cytotoxic therapy (e.g., cyclophosphamide) or cyclosporine.

Increased MCV

The MCV is usually determined and reported by the hematologic analytic devices currently in use; these estimate the volume displacement of individual particles as they pass through the machine. The MCV may be falsely elevated if the cells adhere to one another, as in cold agglutinin (and, rarely, warm agglutinin) hemolytic anemia. Since reticulocytes contain more water than mature cells, their MCV is greater, and if they are plentiful, the measured MCV may be increased. When the MCV is truly elevated, it indicates that cellular proliferation is impaired because of disturbances in nuclear replication, whereas cytoplasmic maturation is normal. Although the red cells are the most strikingly abnormal, such processes affect the other hematopoietic cell lines as well.

VITAMIN DEFICIENCIES. This process occurs when either cyanocobalamine or folic acid is available in insufficient amounts. This results in characteristic abnormalities of nuclear metabolism, which are manifest as megaloblastic hematopoiesis.

The Basis of the Disorder. Both folic acid and cobalamine (vitamin B_{12}) are necessary for the production of DNA,

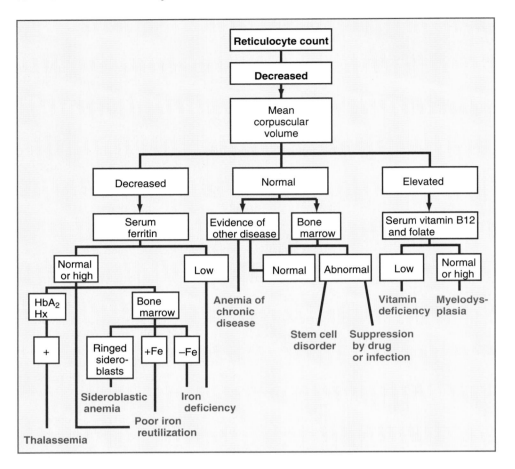

Figure 50−3

Diagnostic algorithm for anemia with a decreased reticulocyte count. The same designations used as in Figure 50−1. Hx = history.

and in their absence, the nucleus of the cell cannot undergo mitosis normally. Folic acid is derived from vegetable food sources, where it is present in the poly- (usually hepta-) glutamyl form. The main cause of folic acid deficiency is dietary insufficiency when the diet lacks fresh fruits and vegetables, as the absorption of the vitamin is rarely impaired. The compound is markedly heat sensitive and is largely destroyed in cooking. Deficiency can also arise as the result of overutilization, as in patients with hemolytic anemia.

Cobalamine is a tetrapyrrole molecule containing cobalt bonded to a 5′deoxyadenosyl and a benzimidazole moiety. It is also involved in one carbon unit metabolism as a cofactor in two enzymatic reactions:

1. It transfers the methyl group from N^5-methyltetrahydrofolate to homocysteine to form methionine
2. It is involved in the isomerization of L-methylmalonyl CoA to succinyl CoA (a reaction that does not involve folic acid)

Cobalamine is absorbed from animal food sources by a complex series of reactions. The released compound is bound in the stomach by a protein, the R binder. This is digested in the upper intestine and is replaced by intrinsic factor (IF), a protein made in the parietal cells of the stomach. The cobalamine-IF complex is absorbed in the distal ileum through specific receptors. The cobalamine is then transported by a specific protein, transcobalamine II, to the cells, where it is taken in through specific receptors.

The most common cause of deficiency of cobalamine is malabsorption, as any diet containing animal products will usually contain enough of the compound for normal needs. Pernicious anemia is due to a lack of IF, usually due to an autoimmune reaction manifest by anti−parietal cell and anti-IF antibodies, and is the most common cause of this malabsorption. Resection or disease of the terminal ileum will remove the site of absorption. The fish tapeworm, *Diphyllobothrium latum*, utilizes the compound during its passage through the gut. Bacteria in isolated pockets (such as diverticuli or postoperative sacs) may multiply and alter the absorption of the compound.

The pathophysiology of degeneration of myelinated nerves in B_{12} deficiency is not clear. It may be due to the fact that in this state, methylmalonic-CoA concentration increases and is incorporated into lipids. This results in lipid molecules with an uneven number of carbons and with side-chains of methyl groups, effects that might lead to unstable myelin and then demyelination.

The Clinical Syndrome. The major manifestation of uncomplicated deficiency of either folate or cobalamine is megaloblastic anemia that may be very slow in onset. The history may be useful in documenting malnutrition or alcohol ingestion (both suggestive of folate deficiency) or surgery that may have removed the stomach or terminal ileum. In cobalamine but not in folate deficiency, there are neurologic symptoms, which include loss of proprioception in the lower extremities, loss of perception of vibration in the same distribution, loss of sense of smell, unusual cerebral symptoms, and even dementia. Both deficiencies may be manifest by loss of glossal papillae and a sore tongue.

The degree of anemia may be profound because of the slow onset. Frequently, white cells, platelets, or both will be diminished in number as well. Many of the red cells appear large and ovoid (macrovalocytes), although in severe cases there may be considerable variability in size and shape of the other cells; the MCV will be greater than normal. A few of the neutrophils may have more than the usual number of lobes. The reticulocyte count is usually low.

The most striking and diagnostic finding is megaloblastosis of the marrow. The dissociation of maturation of the nucleus and cytoplasm is best seen in the red cell series, where the usual clumping and pyknosis of the nucleus is impaired, even though the cytoplasm matures normally. Thus, cells have a large nucleus with open (uncondensed) chromatin and cytoplasm that is nearly fully hemoglobinized. The granulocyte precursors are larger than normal and often have an enlarged nucleus, best seen in the "giant band" form.

Signs of ineffective erythropoiesis are present. The marrow has erythroid hypercellularity even though the reticulocyte count is low. The serum LDH may be elevated because the precursors are being destroyed in the marrow. The serum haptoglobin may be diminished as well.

The diagnosis is best made by determination of the serum levels of the vitamins; if the folate-deficient patient has been given folate, the determination of the red cell folate will be helpful, as this will reflect folate stores at the time the cell was made. Slightly subnormal B$_{12}$ levels are sometimes difficult to interpret. The diagnosis of pernicious anemia can be affirmed by demonstrating the presence of anti-IF and anti–parietal cell antibodies. The absorption of B$_{12}$ can be assessed by the Schilling test, in which radiolabeled B$_{12}$ is given orally and the amount excreted in the urine after a parenteral flushing dose of the vitamin is determined; this test depends upon reliable urine collection and reasonably normal renal function. If this test is abnormal, the second stage (giving the B$_{12}$ along with exogenous IF) may be performed; this will determine if the malabsorption is due to IF deficiency. If this is also abnormal, the gut may be "sterilized" with antibiotics to rid it of bacteria, and stage 1 may then be repeated; if removal of the bacteria is helpful, then the cause for their presence should be sought. *The Schilling test is expensive and should be used only when it is not clear why the patient is B$_{12}$ deficient.*

Therapy. The treatment of a vitamin deficiency is replacement. Folate can be given as 1 mg/day or with an improved diet. Cobalamine usually is given parenterally, often with a loading during first treatment. The usually chronic dose is 1 mg/month. After treatment, there should be a prompt and striking rise in the reticulocyte count about 5 to 10 days after its initiation.

Dysplasia. When the proliferation of the marrow elements is dysplastic, alterations in nuclear maturation may often be part of the problem, and megaloblastic-like proliferation and macrocytosis may result; the various forms of myelodysplasia are discussed previously. It is important to note, however, that macrocytosis may be the first sign of the alteration of marrow function. Macrocytosis with a normal serum folate and serum B$_{12}$ level should lead to the suspicion of myelodysplasia, particularly in an older patient.

Anemia with Decreased Production and Decreased MCV

When the MCV is below normal, the production of cytoplasm is less than the cellular production. In almost all cases, this results in decreased effective production of cells, although the ineffective production of cells may be increased. The reduced production of cytoplasm is due to the reduced production or availability of one of the three components of hemoglobin—iron, globin, or heme.

ANEMIA DUE TO IRON-DEFICIENT HEMATOPOIESIS
Basis of the Disorder. The source of iron is dietary and is found in both vegetables (e.g., beans) and meat; the iron present in meat is more readily available. For iron other than that complexed in heme to be absorbed, it must be freed from its binding; this is clearly incomplete, and less than a third of the iron ingested is available for absorption. Iron is absorbed in the upper intestine, and this absorption is improved by acidification provided by the stomach and reduction provided by, for instance, vitamin C.

The iron in the circulation is attached to the iron-binding protein, transferrin. It is transferred to erythroid precursors and other iron-requiring cells (such as those of the liver) directly through receptors or into iron-storing cells. The proportion going to each destination depends upon the amount of erythropoiesis that is going on.

Iron enters the erythropoietic cell by endocytosis while attached to its plasma carrier, transferrin. It is stored in ferruginous micelles within the cytoplasm. As heme is made, iron is transferred to the mitochondria where it is inserted into the protoporphyrin molecule by the enzyme ferrochelatase.

Once the iron has been incorporated into heme and has circulated with the cell, it is removed when the cell is destroyed and is shunted to cells that store it in ferritin. The synthesis of ferritin is carefully controlled; in general, the amount of ferritin present in the body is proportional to the amount of iron that must be stored and is reflected in the serum level of apoferritin, which can be determined clinically.

From the storage pool, iron can be mobilized to enter the plasma attached to transferrin. In general, the iron that was last put into storage is the first that is mobilized for utilization. This process is controlled by factors that are poorly understood but can be interrupted by reactions occurring during inflammation.

IRON DEFICIENCY

Clinical and Laboratory Findings. Iron deficiency has been divided into four stages:

1. Stage 1—depletion of body iron stores with normal laboratory values
2. Stage 2—laboratory evidence of depletion of iron stores but normal hemoglobin
3. Stage 3—diagnostic evidence of iron depletion, slight anemia, and normal MCV
4. Stage 4—severe iron deficiency with obvious hypochromia of the red cells and reduction in MCV and moderate to marked anemia

In the early stages of iron deficiency, few symptoms are encountered. As the severity progresses, the symptoms become obvious. Patients with moderate or severe iron deficiency often have fatigue out of proportion to the decrease in hemoglobin; this has been attributed to the absence of iron from some of the important energy-producing reactions. Some patients may relate that they ingest ice or other substances (starch or clay) as a pica. In severe iron deficiency, the nails may be reversed in their curvature ("spoon nails," or koilonychia); this may also be hereditary and not related to iron deficiency. The incidence of cheilosis (cracking at the corners of the mouth) is said to be higher in patients who are iron deficient. The spleen is rarely enlarged.

In established iron deficiency, the hematocrit is diminished; the longer and more severe the deficiency, the lower the hematocrit. The MCV is also diminished and may be below 55 fL in severe iron deficiency. The other blood elements are usually normal, but the platelet count may be elevated (as high as 1.5 million/mm^3). The serum iron is usually low, and the saturation of the iron binding capacity (effectively transferrin) is less than 15%. The serum transferrin is usually below 12 ng/ml but may be artificially elevated as part of an acute phase reaction. No iron will be found on bone marrow biopsy, the diagnostic gold standard of true iron deficiency.

Once the diagnosis of iron deficiency is established, it is necessary to find the cause. This is most often excessive loss due to the loss of blood (or, more rarely, of hemoglobin in the urine); the gastrointestinal tract is the most common site of this loss. Dietary deficiency due to malnutrition, excessive use of iron-binding medications (phosphates, phytates), and loss of gastric tissue, which provides a more suitable pH in the upper intestine for absorption, should be considered as a cause.

Therapy. Iron replenishment and correction of the cause are important in the treatment of iron deficiency. If possible, iron should be given orally, although this is sometimes not tolerated because of gastrointestinal systems. Several forms are available, and all are equally efficacious (if they are not packaged in delayed-release tablets). The hemoglobin should correct to normal within a month to 6 weeks of therapy. Once the hemoglobin has been corrected, treatment should continue for 4 to 6 months to allow the body to build up stores of iron.

Oral medication may fail or may not be tolerated. Failure may be due to incorrect diagnosis (e.g., thalassemia, nonreutilization of iron [see later], lead poisoning, concomitant folate or vitamin B$_{12}$ deficiency), to iron loss at a greater rate than can be compensated for, or to noncompliance with medication. If it is determined that iron cannot be adequately given orally, parenteral forms are available for intramuscular or intravenous use. The most common of these is iron-dextran. The total dose of iron needed, allowing for 1 gm of iron stores, is calculated, and the appropriate amount of drug is given, either as intramuscular injections (2 ml to each buttock three times a week) or as an infusion over 4 to 6 hours.

POOR IRON UTILIZATION AND REUTILIZATION. In certain states, iron may be present in the body but is not available to be used. Most commonly, this occurs in states of inflammation. For reasons not well understood, inflammation (and sometimes the presence of malignancy) prevents the mobilization of iron from storage sites; thus, the serum transferrin is desaturated, and suboptimal amounts of iron are available for hematopoiesis. This leads to the paradoxical state of iron-deficient hematopoiesis in the presence of plentiful stores of iron. The result is microcytic anemia with a low reticulocyte count and a low serum iron and reduced saturation of transferrin but normal or elevated levels of serum ferritin and storage iron on bone marrow biopsy. If the underlying cause can be treated, then iron-sufficient hematopoiesis may supervene. It is important to note that only a small proportion of patients with anemia secondary to chronic disease have this block in iron metabolism.

ANEMIA DUE TO ABNORMALITIES OF HEME SYNTHESIS

The Basis of the Disorders. The biosynthesis of heme begins with the condensation of glycine and succinyl CoA by the enzyme δ-aminolevulinic acid synthase to form δ-aminolevulinic acid (δ-ALA); pyridoxyl-5-phosphate is a cofactor in this reaction. Two molecules of δ-ALA are combined to form a molecule of porphobilinogen by the enzyme δ-aminolevulinic acid dehydrase. Four molecules of porphobilinogen combine to form first a linear tetrapyrrole, which is then circularized into urobilinogen. The side-chains of this molecule are modified, and one species, protoporphyrin IX, is able to form the heme molecule when iron is inserted into the midst of the four tetrapyrroles.

The first step, the combination of glycine and succinyl CoA, is the most important of this series; defects at this step result in the deficiency of heme synthesis that is seen clinically. When heme is not synthesized, the iron that is imported into the cell resides either in the mitochondria (where it is usually inserted into the heme moiety) or just outside. In either case, iron is seen in the cytoplasm of the late orthochromatic normoblasts, a stage when it should have all been incorporated into heme. This iron is often in granules that surround the nucleus; hence the name "ringed sideroblast."

Congenital Defects in Heme Synthesis. Rarely, δ-aminolevulinic acid synthase, the crucial enzyme at the initiation of heme synthesis, is hereditarily defective; since it is located on the X-chromosome, this results in a more severe syndrome in male hemizygotes than in female heterozygotes. Since relatively little heme is synthesized, the red cells are markedly hypochromic, and the patient is very anemic. The marrow has erythroid hyperplasia, and all of the cells are ringed sideroblasts. In the much less severe heterozygous state, only a portion of the red cells are hypochromic, and only a portion of the erythroid precursors are ringed sideroblasts. In some families, the condition can be ameliorated by high doses of pyridoxine, since the enzyme defect appears to involve interaction with that cofactor. This syndrome has been called "the X-linked hypochromic anemia of Rundles and Falls."

Sideroblastic Anemia Secondary to Toxin Exposure. δ-Aminolevulinic acid synthase can be inhibited by toxic substances. The most common is ethyl alcohol, which may inhibit some step in pyridoxine metabolism. Many patients may show ringed sideroblasts while they are drinking alcohol heavily; these rapidly disappear when the drinking is stopped. Ringed sideroblasts have also been reported in patients receiving antituberculous therapy that includes isoniazide, a drug known to antagonize pyridoxine.

Lead salts inhibit the dehydratase that combines two molecules of δ-ALA (the second step in heme synthesis) and the transfer of iron into the mitochondrion. The defect in the dehydratase has little effect on heme synthesis, as the enzyme is present in 80-fold excess. The second defect results in cytoplasmic iron accumulation, which may appear as ringed sideroblasts. Lead also inhibits the 5′-nucleotidase that is responsible for catabolism of the mRNA and DNA of the cell; this results in the artifactual presence of large basophilic stipples in the erythrocytes on the standard Wright stain.

Acquired Sideroblastic Anemia. Ringed sideroblasts may also occur as the result of somatic mutations of genes responsible for the proteins of the heme biosynthetic pathway. In some patients, this appears to be a distinct defect in the erythropoietic line, as this appears to be the only cell affected and there is no further progression. This probably occurs because of somatic mutation of the gene for δ-aminolevulinic acid synthase; since this gene is located on the X-chromosome, a single somatic "hit" is enough to result in manifestations of disordered heme synthesis.

In other patients, the defect appears to be part of a stem cell–generated myelodysplastic disorder, as the other cell lines are abnormal as well (resulting particularly in thrombocytopenia), and the disease progresses, often ending in acute leukemia. This, like the other myelodysplastic syndromes, is a disease of older patients.

REFERENCES

Brittenham GM: Disorders of iron metabolism: Iron deficiency and overload. *In* Hematology: Basic Principles and Practice. 2nd ed. New York, Churchill-Livingstone, 1995.

Dacie JV: The Haemolytic Anaemias. Parts 1–5. New York, Churchill-Livingstone.

Embury SH, Hebbel RP, Mohandas N, Steinberg MH: Sickle Cell Disease: Basic Principles and Clinical Practice. New York, Raven Press, 1994.

Herbert V: Biology of disease. Megaloblastic anemias. Lab Invest 1985; 52:3.

Rosse WF: Clinical Immunohematology: Basic Concepts and Clinical Applications. Boston, Blackwell Scientific Publications, 1990.

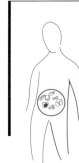

51

Transfusion and Bone Marrow Transplantation

In many hematologic diseases and hematologic complications of other diseases, it is advantageous or necessary to supplement or replace the components of the blood or bone marrow by transfusion or transplantation of the tissue from homologous donors. This process is limited greatly by differences in tissue antigens between donor and recipient; nevertheless, the process can be successfully accomplished if certain requirements are observed.

TRANSFUSION

Blood transfusion originally involved the infusion of whole blood from the donor to the recipient. Although this is still possible and sometimes indicated, in current practice specific components of the blood (red cells, platelets, plasma, or plasma components) are usually given for particular indications.

Transfusion of Red Cells

Indications

Red cells are transfused for the following indications:

1. Replacement of shed blood. The patient who is actively bleeding needs both the oxygen-carrying capacity of the red cells and the volume-producing capacity of the red cells and the plasma. For that reason, either whole blood or packed red cells and plasma (reconstituted blood) are given.
2. Anemia not due to blood loss. Oxygen-carrying capacity but not volume is needed, and packed red cells usually suffice. The level of anemia requiring transfusion varies greatly from patient to patient. If the anemia is acute, then oxygen hunger may occur at hemoglobin levels around 8 gm/dl, whereas patients more chronically anemic may be able to tolerate much lower levels of oxygen. The age of the patient is also important in determining when blood should be given; older patients tolerate hypoxia less well than younger ones. At any rate, blood should be transfused when the signs of oxygen hunger are present (increased heart or respiratory rate, extreme fatigue, onset of neurologic symptoms). If it is delayed until the blood pressure falls, it may be too late.

3. Replacement of abnormal cells. In some instances, particularly in the sickling disorders, the patient's red cells may be pathogenetic and need to be replaced; this is particularly true in sickle cell disease when obstructive manifestations such as acute chest syndrome, acute stroke, acute sequestration syndromes, and acute multiple organ damage syndromes occur. This replacement may be accomplished by partial exchange (removal of part of the patient's blood with replacement by transfusion) or by complete exchange (exchange of the patient's blood using a plasmapheresis apparatus).

Compatibility Testing

Early experiments with transfusion of blood often resulted in massive hemolysis of the transfused red cells due to the immunologic incompatibility of the donor and the recipient. Later it became possible to reduce the incidence of this complication by seeking donors the compatibility of whose cells could be assured by *in vitro* testing.

ANTIGEN MATCHING. If the antigens of the donor match the antigens of the recipient, the cells of the donor are compatible with those of the recipient and no immunologic reaction is possible. About 600 different antigens have been identified on human red cells; most of these are of little consequence. Only two antigen groups are sufficiently polymorphic in the population and sufficiently antigenic to make antigen matching routinely useful:

1. ABO blood groups are the antigens involved in the reactions that initially limited transfusion, as incompatible transfusion (the blood of the donor bears antigens not present on the cells of the recipient) almost invariably results in hemolysis.
2. $Rh_0(D)$ is a strong immunogen; alloimmunization of child-bearing women may cause hemolytic disease of the newborn.

Antigen matching may be used in special circumstances:

1. If the recipient has several antibodies, it may be easier to begin testing for compatibility by selecting donors that have the same major antigens, since none of the antibodies can be against shared antigens.

2. Patients with sickle cell disease are readily alloimmunized because of racially determined discrepancies of antigenic constitution; therefore, it is sometimes useful to do limited antigen matching in selecting donors.

ANTIBODY DETECTION. The other method of determining compatibility is the detection of antibodies in the serum of the recipient that are incompatible with the cells of the donors. This is usually done in two ways:

1. Screening of the serum: the serum of the recipient is reacted with red cells of known and maximally diverse antigenic constitution; if any reaction is detected, the specificity of the antibody is determined.
2. Cross-match: the cells of the donor are reacted with the serum of the recipient and any reaction determined by several sensitive tests.

If the ABO and $Rh_0(D)$ antigens match and no antibodies are found in the serum of the recipient, the blood of the donor is deemed compatible with respect to red cells.

Consequences of Incompatibility

If, for clerical or immunologic reasons, the red cells of the donor *are* immunologically incompatible with antibodies in the serum of the recipient, one of three types of hemolytic transfusion reactions may ensue:

1. Major hemolytic transfusion reaction: this occurs primarily with incompatibility within the ABO blood groups. The antibody, present in large amounts, activates complement, causing the intravascular hemolysis of the donor red cells; this results in hemoglobinemia and hemoglobinuria, which, if sufficiently great, results in renal failure. This, combined with other complications, including shock and disseminated intravascular coagulation, may result in death.
2. Minor hemolytic transfusion reaction: in most other hemolytic reactions, insufficient complement is activated to result in massive hemolysis, but the donor cells are destroyed over a period ranging from hours to days. This results in signs of hemolysis (increased bilirubin, increased lactate hydrogenase [LDH]), a positive direct antiglobulin test (the donor cells bind antibody), and a loss of the gain in hemoglobin and hematocrit expected. This reaction is rarely serious but complicates medical care.
3. Delayed hemolytic transfusion reaction: in some cases, antibodies caused by previous transfusion or pregnancy may be so low in titer as to be undetectable at the time of compatibility testing. When red cells bearing the antigen are infused, an anamnestic response may result in generation of sufficient antibody to lyse the transfused cells. This usually is seen 5 to 7 days after the transfusion and may manifest as hemoglobinuria. If the reaction is severe, some of the complications of the major hemolytic transfusion reaction may occur, but rarely is the reaction fatal.

Nonhemolytic Complications

The nonhemolytic complications of blood transfusion may be divided into four categories:

1. Acute allergic and febrile reactions: components of transfused blood (including platelets and plasma) may trigger allergic reactions, which range from urticaria to hypotension to bronchospasm and, in the most serious form, anaphylactic shock. These reactions can be avoided by removing the offending protein from the transfusate; the patients may be treated by antihistaminics or, if needed, epinephrine. Febrile reactions occur when leukocytes are present in the transfused preparation and may be due to the release of cytokines or pyrogens from these cells. The febrile reaction is treated with antipyretics.
2. Graft-versus-host reactions: when immunocompromised patients are transfused with preparations containing viable lymphocytes, the latter cells may establish themselves and mount a reaction against the tissues of the recipient. For that reason, such patients should receive only blood preparations that have been irradiated with x-rays to inactivate any lymphocytes.
3. Transfusions may transmit a number of infectious diseases. Occasionally, due to contamination, bacterial infections may be transmitted; this is most common with platelet transfusions, as they are kept at room temperature for several days. Hepatitis (B, C, and others), cytomegalovirus, human immunodeficiency virus (HIV), human T-cell leukemia/lymphoma virus-1 (HTLV-1), and other viral diseases may be transmitted, although rigid testing regimens have done much to eradicate this problem.
4. Iron overload: each unit of red cells that is transfused adds about 250 mg to the body burden of iron. Since the means of excreting this iron are limited, it tends to accumulate, especially in patients who have a chronic need for transfusion. When the total burden is greater than about 20 to 30 gm, the adverse effects of hemochromatosis may be seen.

Transfusion of Platelets

One of the advances that has made the modern treatment of many hematologic and oncologic diseases possible is the development of methods for acquiring and transfusing platelets. Platelets may be obtained from donated whole blood that is separated into components (red cells, platelets, and plasma) by differential centrifugation; however, it requires the platelets from about six donations to make an effective dose for transfusion to an adult. For that reason, platelets are increasingly obtained by platelet apheresis, using a mechanical device that centrifuges the blood in line, so that a therapeutic dose of platelets can be obtained from a single donor.

The problems and methodology for assessing compatibility are considerably different from those used for transfusing red cells. This is because

1. The tests of compatibility for platelets are much more difficult and less reliable than those developed for red cells
2. The range of important antigens (antigens polymorphic in the population and immunogenic) is much greater for platelets, making the selection of donors more difficult

Indications for Platelet Transfusion

Platelet transfusion is particularly useful when the platelet count is reduced due to diminished production (e.g., chemotherapy or in aplastic anemia). Platelet transfusions are of much less value in situations where the platelets are being rapidly destroyed.

Several guidelines have been developed for giving platelets prophylactically:

1. For otherwise uncomplicated patients with a platelet count < 5000 to 20,000/mm³; the exact level at which such prophylactic transfusions are useful is a matter of debate. The figures quoted are probably too low and too high, respectively
2. For patients with active bleeding and a platelet count < 30,000 to 50,000/mm³
3. For patients requiring surgery with a platelet count < 70,000/mm³

Platelet transfusions may also be required in patients with normal numbers of defective platelets, such as those of Glanzmann's disease or Bernard-Soulier defect; in these cases, necessity is often determined by active bleeding, except where surgery is necessary.

Compatibility Testing in Platelet Transfusion

The refined techniques of compatibility testing used in the transfusion of red cells have not been fully developed for platelets, but the principles are the same.

Antigen Matching

The antigens of importance on the platelet are of three categories:

1. Antigens shared with red cells: these are primarily the ABO antigens. Their role in incompatible platelet transfusions is not clear, but the best results have been obtained when the plasma of the recipient does not contain antibodies to A or B antigens on the donor platelets.
2. Histocompatibility antigens that are also present on lymphocytes (as well as most other body tissues): platelets bear class I human leukocyte antigen (HLA) antigens (particularly HLA-A and HLA-B), although the quantity may vary greatly. These antigens are usually assessed by lymphocytotoxicity. Because of the pleomorphism of the HLA antigens, matching for very specific so-called "private" antigens (of which there

are over 120) may be difficult; frequently, matches must be made with related so-called "cross-reacting" or public antigens (of which there are less than 20).
3. Antigens specific to platelets: several glycoproteins of the platelet are allomorphic and antigenic; these antigens must be assessed directly by testing platelets or derivatives from the platelet membrane. It is not entirely clear how often antibodies to these antigens play a role in incompatible platelet transfusion, and they are seldom matched in selecting platelet donors.

Antibody Detection

The techniques of detecting antibodies on the surface of platelets that have been used in the past are somewhat cumbersome and difficult to interpret; for these reasons, they are not used routinely. Instead, the antibodies of most importance in transfusion therapy, those against the histocompatibility antigens, are detected using lymphocytes in the lymphocytotoxicity assays. The assumption is that significant antibodies to lymphocytes will be significant for platelets, a case that may not always be true. In these assays, antibodies to specific HLA antigens can be detected in some patients, and this information may be of value in selecting donors of platelets. More commonly, such specificity is difficult to identify, limiting the usefulness of antibody detection in selecting compatible donors.

The Usual Practice in Platelet Transfusion

Because of the difficulties in selecting compatible donors and the relative innocuousness of incompatible transfusions, an algorithm that is commonly used has been adopted for platelet transfusion:

1. Platelets derived from random donors of blood are transfused until they become ineffective (i.e., there is no significant elevation of the platelet count 1 hour after the transfusion is completed).
2. Single-donor platelets may be given; if the response is suboptimal, then donors with the same or similar HLA phenotypes may be sought (HLA-matched platelets). The serum of the patient may be examined for antibodies to antigens on platelets (primarily by lymphocytotoxicity assays), and platelets bearing antigens reacting with identified specific antibodies may be avoided.
3. If the patient becomes refractory to HLA-matched platelet transfusions, then cross-match procedures may be instituted, in which the donor platelets are mixed with the recipient's serum, and evidence of antibody on the platelets is sought. Often, however, the patient is refractory to all platelet transfusions.

This procedure is convenient but unsatisfactory in that the patient may become universally refractory owing to alloimmunization, and platelet transfusions will not be useful. Attempts are being made to find ways to reduce alloimmunization by platelet transfusions:

1. The HLA antigens on leukocytes are much more immunogenic than the same antigens on platelets; studies have suggested that careful removal of all leukocytes, as by filtering the blood or platelet product, may reduce the incidence of alloimmunization.
2. As indicated previously, the complexity of the public HLA antigens is very much less than that of the private HLA antigens (the ones usually discussed); some studies have shown that antigen matching for these public antigens, which is not difficult if the panel of donors is sufficiently large, may reduce the rate of alloimmunization by transfusion.

When the patient becomes totally refractory to even the best-matched platelets, attempts to give platelets by continuous transfusion, the administration of intravenous gamma globulin, and other steps are usually not helpful. This markedly restricts the options and the prognosis of the patient if he or she remains thrombocytopenic.

Transfusion of Granulocytes

Although it would certainly be useful to be able to give the neutropenic patient granulocytes, this has not proved to be practical in adults. The survival of granulocytes in the circulation is so short ($T_{1/2}$ of about 6 hours), granulocytes are in such low numbers in the peripheral blood, and the preservation of granulocytes in a useful form is so difficult that transfusions of granulocytes are not generally available.

ALLOGENEIC BONE MARROW TRANSPLANTATION (BMT)

In a number of hematologic disorders, the ideal treatment consists of replacement of the diseased bone marrow with normal bone marrow. While simple in concept, BMT is complex for two reasons:

1. Except in the case of monozygotic twins, the histocompatibility antigens of the donor are different than those of the recipient (this difference may be minimized by careful testing and selection of appropriate donors but is probably always present to a greater or lesser extent). This means that the immune system of the recipient must be suppressed so that it will not recognize the incompatibilities and will allow the donor marrow to survive.
2. If immune competent cells are infused into the immunocompromised recipient, they may react against the antigens of the recipient (host) that are different from those of the donor (graft). This results in graft-versus-host disease, which may destroy enough of the host's tissues to be fatal.
3. Because of the necessary immunosuppression, the patient is subject to infections and other complications that may prove fatal.

These complications are magnified in the elderly, and BMT is seldom considered for patients over 45 to 55 years of age. For all these reasons, allogeneic BMT is undertaken with considerable caution.

Selection of Donors

The major impediment to successful BMT is the immunologic incompatibility between donor and recipient. These immunologic differences are mainly carried on proteins bearing histocompatibility antigens. The major antigens are part of a complex of proteins involved in self and nonself recognition that are coded for by genes of the major histocompatibility complex (MHC) on chromosome 6. These antigens are of two classes:

1. Class I—these antigens are of three types: HLA-A, HLA-B, and HLA-C. HLA-A and HLA-B proteins are very polymorphic, comprising some 90 antigens; these antigens are not randomly distributed, as some are very much more common than others. These antigens are readily detected on lymphocytes by specific antibodies. Subtle differences can also be identified by analysis of the gene, using the technology of polymerase chain reaction (PCR).
2. Class II—a group of related proteins that are less readily detected by alloantibodies are termed HLA-DR and HLA-DQ. In the past, incompatibilities among these proteins have been detected by the mixed lymphocyte reaction, in which unlike antigens stimulate the proliferation of lymphocytes. They may also be detected serologically on B lymphocytes, but they are best defined by analysis of their genes using PCR.

Since the genes for these molecules are located in a single stretch of chromosome, they are usually inherited as a package; the HLA-A, -B, and -DR genes on one chromosome of a parent will be transmitted intact to the offspring unless there is "crossing over" between the genes of the group. Thus, the best allogeneic donors are siblings, as they are most likely to share the largest degree of histocompatibility. Since each parent has two MHC loci, which are passed on randomly to the offspring, there is a one in four chance that two siblings will share the antigen complexes.

Although the recipient may have eight molecules or more from this complex (three class I, five class II), compatibility is usually determined for the HLA-A, HLA-B, and HLA-DR antigens, as these appear to be the most important in the immunologic acceptance of the bone marrow. When random antigen-matched, unrelated donors are selected, great care is taken to be certain that these (and perhaps some of the other antigens) are as well matched as possible to avoid the complications of BMT.

Complications of Allogeneic BMT

Graft Rejection

The immune system of the recipient may react against the infused bone marrow cells, resulting in their not replacing the endogenous marrow. Very strong immunosuppression with antimetabolites, radiography, and other specific immunosuppressive drugs may be used to diminish this effect.

Graft-Versus-Host Disease

The lymphocytes administered with the bone marrow may engraft and set up an immune reaction against the tissues of the recipient. This is frequently transient and not severe but may become chronic and debilitating. The organs most frequently affected are the skin, the gastrointestinal tract, and the liver.

Infections

Because of the marked immunosuppression that is needed, recipients of BMT are very susceptible to infections. During the early phases when the marrow is regenerating, bacterial infections are common. After the return of granulocytes, viral (particularly cytomegalovirus) and fungal infections are also seen.

Because of these complications, the mortality rate due to the transplantation process remains between 10 and 60%. It is lower for children and very much higher for matched but unrelated donors.

Indications for Allogeneic BMT

Allogenic BMT should be attempted in the following situations:

1. Severe aplastic anemia—since the survival of severe aplastic anemia is so poor, BMT is clearly indicated if an appropriate donor is available. The same is true of patients with PNH complicated by serious thrombosis or hematopoietic deficiency.
2. Acute leukemia—BMT is usually given to patients with acute myelogenous or acute lymphocytic leukemia during the first remission; younger patients do better than older ones.
3. Chronic myelogenous leukemia—in eligible patients, transplantation early in the disease has proved useful; the leukemic clone is eradicated in the process. Unfortunately, many patients are too old to benefit from this procedure.
4. Lymphomas and multiple myeloma—BMT is being used in those cases in which other manifestations of the disease cannot be eradicated by therapy; this indication is not as clear as with the primary bone marrow neoplasms.
5. Genetic diseases—BMT is used in genetic diseases, both hematologic (thalassemia, sickle cell disease) and nonhematologic (Fabry's disease, Hunter's, osteopetrosis).

52

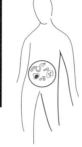

Platelets and Primary Hemostasis

Normal hemostasis depends on the complex interplay of multiple components to rapidly produce a hemostatic plug at a site of vascular injury. As with many biologic processes, however, this reaction is tightly regulated to prevent formation of an occlusive plug on normal endothelium. Consequently, disorders in the hemostatic process may result in either hemorrhagic or thromboembolic manifestations, depending on the specific defect. Furthermore, the defect may be either inherited or acquired, and multiple defects can be present concomitantly, complicating diagnosis and management. Evaluation of the patient with a disorder of hemostasis, therefore, requires a complete personal history, with special consideration for medications and systemic illnesses, family history, and careful physical examination. This information is used with the results of selected screening assays (Table 52–1), guiding therapeutic management of these patients as well as further diagnostic evaluation as indicated.

PRIMARY HEMOSTASIS

Platelets are small, anucleate cells that form the initial hemostatic plug following vascular injury. They are formed from megakaryocytes, which are large, multinucleate cells found in the bone marrow. Megakaryopoiesis is a complex process that is dependent on both early- and late-acting hematopoietic growth factors. Once formed, committed megakaryocyte progenitor cells undergo final maturation in response to the lineage-specific cytokine thrombopoietin. Formation of platelets involves the demarcation membrane system, which divides the megakaryocyte cytoplasm into smaller regions, although the precise mechanism whereby this process occurs remains unknown. Once formed, platelets circulate for an average of 7 to 10 days before being removed by the reticuloendothelial system in the spleen. The normal platelet count is maintained between 150,000/μl and 450,000/μl.

The platelet surface contains specific *receptors* that mediate adhesion to damaged endothelium, activation and secretion of intracellular contents, and aggregation of the platelets at the site of injury (Table 52–2). These receptors are derived from several different receptor families, including the integrins (glycoproteins IIb–IIIa, Ia–IIa, and Ic–IIa), leucine-rich glycoproteins (glycoprotein Ib–IX), selectins (P-selectin), and seven transmembrane

domain proteins (thrombin receptor). The glycoprotein IIb–IIIa complex, an integrin restricted to platelets and megakaryocytes, is the predominant platelet surface receptor, with 40,000 to 80,000 receptors present on the surface of a resting platelet. In contrast, the glycoprotein P-selectin is not found on the platelet surface until the platelet has been activated, making it a useful marker of platelet activation. The thrombin receptor mediates platelet activation by a tethered ligand mechanism, with receptor cleavage by thrombin exposing a new amino terminus that inserts into the membrane and mediates platelet activation.

Several types of *granules* that contain a variety of biologically active substances are present within the platelet cytoplasm. The dense bodies contain adenosine diphosphate (ADP), adenosine triphosphate (ATP), calcium, and serotonin, important components for enhancing platelet aggregation at a site of injury. The α-granules are the most abundant, containing von Willebrand factor (vWF), platelet factor 4, fibrinogen, multimerin, factor V, and platelet-derived growth factor. P-selectin is also found within the α-granules, becoming exposed on the surface following fusion of the granule membrane with the surface membrane.

The process whereby circulating platelets interact with a damaged vascular surface is referred to as *primary hemostasis*. Contraction of the vessel is a mechanical response that occurs immediately after vascular injury. In addition, injury exposes the vascular subendothelium, which contains multiple adhesive proteins (including collagen, laminin, fibronectin, vitronectin, and vWF) that provide binding sites for platelet surface receptors (see Table 52–2). At high shear rates, vWF is essential for platelet adhesion to the subendothelium, which is mediated by the platelet surface glycoprotein Ib–IX complex.

Bound platelets rapidly undergo a change in shape, losing their discoid shape and becoming more spherical with extended pseudopods. Activation results in secretion of the contents of the platelet granules, referred to as the release reaction. Released ADP and thromboxane A$_2$ result in platelet recruitment, leading to further stimulation, aggregation, and augmentation of the nascent hemostatic plug. ADP also results in structural rearrangement of surface glycoprotein IIb–IIIa, forming the fibrinogen receptor on the platelet surface. Bound fibrinogen can act as a bridge between receptors on adjacent platelets in the pres-

TABLE 52–1 Screening Coagulation Tests Used in the Assessment of a Patient with a Disorder of Hemostasis

Screening Test	Mechanism Investigated	Commonly Abnormal With
Complete blood count and peripheral smear	Platelets, primary hemostasis	Quantitative platelet defects
Bleeding time (BT)	Primary hemostasis	Quantitative and qualitative platelet defects, vWD
Prothrombin time (PT)	Secondary hemostasis, extrinsic pathway	Defects in vitamin K–dependent factors, liver disease, DIC, oral anticoagulants
Activated partial thromboplastin time (aPTT)	Secondary hemostasis, intrinsic pathway	Defect in factors VIII (hemophilia A), IX (hemophilia B), XI, or XII; severe vWD; heparin; lupus anticogulants
Thrombin clot time (TCT)	Conversion of fibrinogen to fibrin	Hypofibrinogenemia, DIC, heparin, factor II inhibitors

DIC = Disseminated intravascular coagulation.

ence of calcium ions. Lastly, activated platelets undergo a rearrangement of surface phospholipids, resulting in the generation of a procoagulant surface that is essential for several of the reactions of secondary hemostasis.

Clinical manifestations of a disorder of primary hemostasis include mucosal and cutaneous bleeding, petechiae, purpura, and prolonged oozing of blood after trauma or surgery. Laboratory assessment includes a complete blood count and review of the blood smear, to evaluate platelet number and gross morphology as well as erythrocyte morphology (e.g., the presence of schistocytes in patients with thrombotic thrombocytopenic purpura). Bone marrow aspiration and biopsy is helpful in many patients with a quantitative platelet disorder. Additional studies that may prove useful in the evaluation of a patient with thrombocytopenia include an antiplatelet antibody analysis, drug-induced antiplatelet antibody analysis, or investigation for the presence of anti-PL^{A1} antibodies.

An initial screening tool for qualitative defects of primary hemostasis is the bleeding time. This test requires making a small incision on the volar surface of the forearm while maintaining a constant pressure on the upper arm with a blood pressure cuff. A prolonged bleeding time (greater than 9 minutes) may occur with (1) thrombocytopenia (platelet counts < 100,000/μl); (2) qualitative platelet defects; (3) von Willebrand disease (vWD); and (4) various vascular defects. Qualitative platelet defects

can be more completely characterized by platelet aggregation studies, and vWF is characterized by ristocetin cofactor activity, immunologic assays, and multimer analysis.

QUANTITATIVE PLATELET DISORDERS

Thrombocytopenia

Thrombocytopenia is defined as an absolute decrease in the platelet count below 150,000/μl. In general, the development of hemorrhagic complications is inversely proportional to the platelet count. Platelet counts in the 40,000/μl to 60,000/μl range may be associated with an increased risk of post-traumatic bleeding, and platelet counts below 20,000/μl are associated with an increased frequency of spontaneous bleeding. The mechanisms for thrombocytopenia include: (1) decreased or ineffective platelet production; (2) shortened platelet survival due to increased destruction; (3) splenic sequestration; and (4) intravascular dilution of circulating platelets (Table 52–3).

Disorders Resulting in Decreased Platelet Production

Decreased platelet production can occur with systemic infections, nutritional defects (e.g., folate or vitamin B$_{12}$ deficiency), radiation, systemic chemotherapy, or marrow replacement by tumor or fibrosis. Numerous drugs can inhibit megakaryopoiesis, including ethanol, anticonvulsants, and thiazide diuretics. Less commonly, inherited disorders may result in thrombocytopenia, including congenital megakaryocyte hypoplasia, the sex-linked *Wiskott-Aldrich syndrome*, and the autosomal dominant disorders *May-Hegglin* anomaly and *Alport's syndrome*.

Disorders Resulting in Increased Platelet Destruction

Drug-Induced Thrombocytopenia

Many commonly used drugs can result in thrombocytopenia due to increased peripheral destruction (Table 52–4).

TABLE 52–2 Platelet Surface Glycoproteins

Receptor	Ligands	Function
Glycoprotein Ib-IX	vWF	Initial platelet adhesion, especially in high-shear stress
Glycoprotein IIb-IIIa	vWF, fibrinogen, collagen, fibronectin, and vitronectin	Platelet aggregation
Glycoprotein Ia-IIa	Collagen	Platelet adhesion
Glycoprotein Ic-IIa	Fibronectin, laminin	Platelet adhesion
Vitronectin receptor	Vitronectin	Platelet adhesion
P-selectin (GMP 140)	Leukocyte L-selectin	Platelet-leukocyte adhesion
Thrombin receptor	Thrombin	Platelet activation
Thromboxane A$_2$ receptor	Thromboxane A$_2$	Platelet activation

TABLE 52–3	Causes of Thrombocytopenia
Mechanism	**Examples**
Decreased or ineffective platelet production	Drugs (ethanol, anticonvulsants)
	Infections
	Nutritional defects (vitamin B$_{12}$ deficiency)
	Myelophthisic processes
	Radiation or systemic chemotherapy
Increased platelet destruction	Drug-induced thrombocytopenia
	Alloimmune thrombocytopenia (PTP, NAIT, platelet refractoriness)
	Autoimmune thrombocytopenia (ITP, HIV)
	Consumptive thrombocytopenia (TTP, HUS, DIC)
Abnormal distribution	Splenic sequestration
Intravascular dilution	Massive transfusion

DIC = Disseminated intravascular coagulation; HIV = human immunodeficiency virus; HUS = hemolytic uremic syndrome; ITP = immune thrombocytopenic purpura; NAIT = neonatal alloimmune thrombocytopenia, PTP = post-transfusion purpura; TTP = thrombotic thrombocytopenic purpura.

In general, drug-induced thrombocytopenias are associated with an increase in platelet-associated IgG, resulting in increased platelet clearance in the reticuloendothelial system. Quinidine, for example, can act as a hapten with a platelet surface glycoprotein (glycoproteins Ib–IX or IIb–IIIa) to elicit an immune response. The thrombocytopenia can be severe (less than 20,000/μl) and complicated by hemorrhage. Heparin can also result in an immune-mediated thrombocytopenia by forming an immunogenic complex with platelet factor 4. In contrast to the other drug-induced thrombocytopenias, however, heparin-induced thrombocytopenia can paradoxically result in life-threatening thromboembolic events. In most cases of drug-induced thrombocytopenia, the mainstay of treatment consists of withdrawing the offending agent. If the platelet count is markedly low or the patient is bleeding, however, platelet transfusions and/or steroids may be necessary.

TABLE 52–4	Drugs Implicated in Immune-Mediated Thrombocytopenias

Quinidine/quinine
Gold salts
Methyldopa
Valproic acid
Chlorothiazides
Imipramine
Heparin
Penicillin/ampicillin/cephalosporins
Carbamazepine
Rifampin
Digotoxin/digoxin
Procainamide

Alloimmune Thrombocytopenias

Alloantigens are genetically determined molecular variations of proteins or carbohydrates that can be recognized by the host immune system as foreign compounds, leading to the generation of IgG alloantibodies that result in the premature destruction of the cells carrying the alloantigens. Clinical situations in which this can be observed include during pregnancy or with transfusion therapy. *Post-transfusion purpura* (PTP) is a rare syndrome characterized by the abrupt onset of severe thrombocytopenia 5 to 10 days following transfusion of one or more units of blood. Alloantibodies to at least six different platelet antigens have been reported, although most bind to the PL^{A1} antigen located on surface glycoprotein IIIa. Characteristically, PTP occurs in PL^{A1} negative individuals who were previously exposed during pregnancy or prior transfusion. The mechanism whereby autologous platelets, which lack the alloantigen, are destroyed remains unknown, and the thrombocytopenia may persist for up to a month or longer in duration. Bleeding complications are not uncommon, especially early in the course, and can be fatal. Treatment consists of plasmapheresis or intravenous immunoglobulin therapy.

Neonatal alloimmune thrombocytopenia (NAIT) is caused by the maternal production of IgG alloantibodies that are capable of crossing the placenta and destroying fetal platelets that bear paternally derived alloantigens. The syndrome occurs with a frequency of 1 in 1000 to 2000 newborn infants in western populations, and the PL^{A1} antigen is implicated in most cases. Hemorrhagic complications are not uncommon, and delivery by caesarian section is recommended if the diagnosis is confirmed prenatally. Response to transfusion with washed, irradiated maternal platelets can be both therapeutic and diagnostic. *Platelet refractoriness*, defined by the failure to achieve adequate platelet increments in multiply transfused thrombocytopenic patients, is a common alloimmunization syndrome. This is most frequently due to incompatibilities in the HLA system but may also include platelet-specific epitopes.

Autoimmune Thrombocytopenias

Autoantibodies to platelets may develop in a variety of disorders, including lymphoproliferative malignancies, autoimmune disorders, and infection with human immunodeficiency virus (HIV) or other viral illnesses. As many as 15% of patients with systemic lupus erythematosus may develop a significant immune-mediated thrombocytopenia during the course of their disease. Thrombocytopenia is also a common manifestation in patients with the primary antiphospholipid antibody syndrome. The antiplatelet antibodies appear to be distinct from the antiphospholipid antibodies in these patients, however, since they respond differently to therapy. Treatment of immune thrombocytopenia in these autoimmune disorders is similar to the treatment of idiopathic thrombocytopenic purpura and is described further later. Treatment of immune thrombocytopenia in patients with acquired immunodeficiency syndrome (AIDS) includes the antiviral agent zidovudine, although patients with severe thrombocytopenia will also need additional treatment, as for patients with severe idiopathic thrombocytopenic purpura.

Idiopathic (autoimmune) thrombocytopenic purpura (ITP) is an immune-mediated destruction of platelets that occurs in the absence of any toxin or drug exposure. Most of these patients have abnormally high levels of IgG on the platelet surface, and autoantibodies directed against epitopes on platelet glycoproteins Ib or IIb–IIIa have been identified. In the circulation, platelet survival is markedly decreased, with the IgG-coated platelets being cleared in the spleen and, less frequently, the liver.

Idiopathic thrombocytopenic purpura can occur at any age and is clinically associated with the development of petechiae (most commonly in the lower extremities), ecchymoses, mucosal bleeding, and epistaxis. Severe complications include gastrointestinal or intracranial hemorrhage, which occurs more commonly with platelet counts below $10,000/\mu l$ or with a rapidly falling platelet count. A preceding viral infection may have occurred 1 to 2 weeks prior to presentation, most commonly among pediatric patients. On physical examination, the spleen is usually not enlarged, in contrast to patients with splenic sequestration syndromes, and findings may be limited to evidence of hemorrhage.

Laboratory assessment confirms thrombocytopenia, often severe, with normal coagulation studies. Giant platelets may be seen on the peripheral blood smear, suggestive of increased marrow production, and the other cell lines are normal. Bone marrow examination usually reveals an increased or normal number of megakaryocytes, consistent with peripheral destruction. Confirmatory tests include evaluation for the presence of antiplatelet antibodies and demonstration of shortened platelet survival. Platelet survival studies can be performed by infusing [111]Indium-labeled platelets (preferably autologous) and measuring residual radioactivity at defined intervals following the injection. In addition, scintillation counting can be used to localize the accumulation of the label in specific organs of the body, which can be useful if splenectomy is a therapeutic consideration.

The clinical course of ITP depends on the age of onset. ITP in childhood is most frequently acute in onset, and the syndrome usually resolves within several weeks, with or without specific treatment. In contrast, the disorder in adults (and in as many as 10 to 20% of children) is more commonly insidious in onset and tends to follow a more chronic course. Characteristically, the thrombocytopenia will not resolve without some form of treatment, and prolonged courses of therapy may be needed before a response is obtained. Relapses are not uncommon and may occur in the setting of an infection. ITP developing or exacerbating during pregnancy can result in significant fetal thrombocytopenia, since the antibody is usually IgG and can cross the placenta. Hemorrhagic complications that can occur at the time of delivery include intracerebral hemorrhage, subdural and subgaleal hematomas, and increased bruising.

The initial therapy in most patients with ITP is prednisone (1 mg/kg/day), which results in an elevation in the platelet count in ~60 to 80% of adult patients. The response generally occurs within 2 weeks of initiation of therapy, and if a response has not occurred within 4 weeks, an alternative therapy should be considered. In addition, about half of the adult patients who achieve a remission with prednisone will relapse following discontinuation of the drug. Splenectomy is the treatment of choice in patients who fail to respond to steroids or relapse after steroids are withdrawn. Remission is achieved in up to 80% of patients following splenectomy and is maintained in over half without any additional therapy. A search for accessory spleens should be done in those patients who relapse following a successful initial response to splenectomy. Intravenous immunoglobulin (1 gm/kg) can produce a transient, relatively rapid elevation in the platelet count and can be given while waiting for an increase in the platelet count with prednisone. Platelet transfusions are generally not useful, although they should be used in those patients presenting with severe hemorrhagic complications. In patients with chronic ITP, alternative therapeutic modalities include vincristine, azathioprine, cyclophosphamide, danazol, and colchicine.

Consumptive (Nonimmune) Disorders Resulting in Thrombocytopenia

A wide variety of nonimmunologic mechanisms may result in the development of thrombocytopenia by increased platelet destruction (Table 52–5).

Thrombotic thrombocytopenic purpura (TTP) is a rare disorder characterized by diffuse microvascular occlusion of arterioles and capillaries, resulting in ischemic dysfunction of multiple organs. The underlying pathophysiologic process is incompletely understood, although several platelet-aggregating factors as well as ultra-large vWF multimers have been observed in the plasma of these patients. Organ dysfunction most frequently involves the central nervous system, resulting in altered mental status, focal deficits, and seizures, and the kidneys, resulting in oliguric renal failure. Classical laboratory findings of TTP include thrombocytopenia, often se-

TABLE 52–5	Disorders Resulting in Thrombocytopenia due to Increased Platelet Destruction by Nonimmunologic Mechanisms

Thrombotic thrombocytopenic purpura (TTP)
HELLP syndrome (hemolysis, elevated liver enzymes, and low platelets)
Pregnancy
Infections
Extracorporeal circulation (coronary artery bypass grafting; hemodialysis)
Burns
Hemolytic uremic syndrome (HUS)
Pre-eclampsia/eclampsia
Disseminated intravascular coagulation
Congenital or acquired cardiac disease
Kasabach-Merritt syndrome (hemangioma-thrombocytopenia syndrome)

vere, and evidence of microangiopathic hemolytic anemia (anemia, schistocytes, reticulocytosis, elevated lactate dehydrogenase, elevated bilirubin, and absent haptoglobin). Many of these patients also have fever.

If untreated, the mortality rate of TTP exceeds 90%. Rapid initiation of appropriate therapy reduces mortality to 10 to 20%, and TTP should therefore be considered a true medical emergency. The mainstay of therapy for TTP consists of plasma exchange, which should be initiated as soon as the diagnosis is made. Prednisone (up to 200 mg/day) is also used in most cases, and some mild cases (e.g., no neurologic manifestations, mild anemia, and thrombocytopenia) may respond to steroid therapy alone. Laboratory monitoring to assess response to therapy should include daily blood counts, reticulocyte count, LDH, and review of the blood smear. Refractory TTP may respond to therapy with vincristine, splenectomy, or intravenous immunoglobulin. As many as 64% of patients in one study relapsed, with most relapses occurring within the first month after discontinuation of therapy.

The *hemolytic uremic syndrome* (HUS) is a nephrotropic variant of TTP that predominantly affects young children. The typical presentation is oliguric renal failure in a young child following a prodromal illness consisting of a gastroenteritis with bloody diarrhea. The enteritis results from infection with an organism producing a shigatoxin or shiga-like toxin, most commonly *Escherichia coli* serotype O157:H7 in western countries. Severe cases should be treated with plasma exchange therapy, but mildly affected patients may need little treatment other than careful management of fluid and electrolyte balance.

Both TTP and HUS have been reported in association with certain chemotherapeutic agents, particularly mitomycin C, as well as following high-dose chemotherapy and bone marrow transplantation. The *HELLP syndrome* (hemolysis, elevated liver enzymes, and low platelets) occurs during pregnancy and appears to represent a severe form of pre-eclampsia. Thrombocytopenia also occurs in ~15 to 20% and ~50% of patients who develop pre-eclampsia and eclampsia, respectively. Characteristically, the thrombocytopenia and other manifestations of the HELLP syndrome resolve following delivery. Other causes of nonimmune platelet destruction include disseminated intravascular coagulation, sepsis, and cardiopulmonary disorders (see Table 52–5).

Platelet Sequestration

Hypersplenism is a syndrome characterized by the association of splenomegaly with one or more cytopenias. Thrombocytopenia results from increased splenic platelet pooling, with a massively enlarged spleen able to hold up to 90% of the total platelet mass. Total platelet mass and platelet lifespan are usually near normal. The thrombocytopenia is rarely severe (50,000 to 100,000/μl), and most patients have no hemorrhagic manifestations. Treatment should be aimed at the underlying cause of the splenomegaly, and only rarely is splenectomy indicated for management of the thrombocytopenia.

Thrombocytopenia Secondary to Intravascular Dilution

Dilutional thrombocytopenia can develop following massive transfusions of crystalloid, colloid, or packed cells and can last for several days. In certain settings, especially aggressive resuscitation efforts for trauma patients, concomitant causes of thromboctyopenia (e.g., disseminated intravascular coagulation) may develop, which can complicate management. In patients with a normal bone marrow, the condition is generally transient, and platelet transfusions should be reserved for patients with hemorrhagic complications or severe progressive thrombocytopenia (<50,000/μl).

THROMBOCYTOSIS

Thrombocytosis is defined as an increase in platelet count above 450,000/μl and occurs in three forms: (1) physiologic or transitory; (2) reactive or secondary; and (3) primary or "essential" thrombocytosis.

Transitory or Physiologic Thrombocytosis

A physiologic thrombocytosis may occur following stress or exercise and represents mobilization of preformed platelets from the spleen or lung under the influence of epinephrine. Since this process also occurs in splenectomized individuals, this may represent platelet release from the lungs.

Secondary Thrombocytosis

A reactive, or secondary, thrombocytosis results from an increased platelet production in response to hemorrhage, hemolysis, certain infections (e.g., tuberculosis), iron deficiency, inflammatory diseases, or malignancy. Reactive thrombocytosis following splenectomy may result in platelet counts in excess of 1,000,000/μl and may last for several weeks. In general, a secondary thrombocytosis does not result in hemorrhagic or thrombotic complications, and therapy to directly lower the platelet count is not necessary. Successful treatment of the underlying disease usually results in a return of the platelet count to normal levels.

Primary (Essential) Thrombocytosis

Essential thrombocytosis is a myeloproliferative disorder arising from neoplastic transformation of a pluripotent stem cell. It is characterized by an elevated platelet count, splenomegaly, platelet dysfunction, and, in contrast to physiologic or secondary thrombocytosis, an increased risk of hemorrhagic as well as thromboembolic events. Giant platelets may be seen in the circulation, and platelet aggregation studies are frequently abnormal. Vaso-occlusive manifestations include erythromelalgia, transient ischemic attacks, and amaurosis fugax, with occlusion of larger vessels being distinctly less common. Hemorrhagic complications are predominantly mucosal and can be exacerbated by the use of aspirin. The diagnosis and treatment of essential thrombocytosis are discussed in more detail in Chapter 47.

QUALITATIVE PLATELET DISORDERS

Qualitative platelet defects can result in a prolonged bleeding time in the presence of a normal platelet count. These disorders may produce abnormalities in platelet adhesion, aggregation, or the release reaction.

Disorders of Platelet Function

Inherited Disorders of Platelet Function

The *Bernard-Soulier syndrome* is a rare autosomal recessive disorder characterized by a deficiency of the platelet surface glycoprotein Ib–IX complex, which mediates initial adhesion of the platelet to vWF. Giant platelets are observed on the blood smear, and the bleeding time is markedly prolonged because of failure of the platelets to adhere to the subendothelium. In contrast to the Bernard-Soulier syndrome, *Glanzmann's thrombasthenia* is an autosomal recessive disorder characterized by deficiency of the glycoprotein IIb–IIIa complex. This receptor complex binds to fibrinogen and mediates platelet aggregation. Laboratory evaluation includes a normal platelet count and morphology but a prolonged bleeding time. Platelet aggregation studies reveal absent aggregation to all agonists but normal agglutination to ristocetin. Clinical manifestations for these two disorders include menorrhagia, easy bruising, epistaxis, and gingival bleeding, and therapy consists of platelet transfusions for hemorrhagic complications. Since alloantibodies to the absent surface glycoproteins can develop in these patients, platelet transfusions should be utilized only in urgent clinical situations.

Inherited disorders of platelet granules may also result in a hemorrhagic diathesis. Patients whose platelets lack dense bodies have d-storage pool disease, manifested by variable mucocutaneous hemorrhage and bleeding after delivery, tooth extractions, and surgery. The *grey platelet syndrome* is a rare disorder characterized by the absence of α-granules and a mild bleeding disorder. Inherited disorders with a qualitative platelet defect in association with other manifestations include the *Hermansky-Pudlak syndrome* (oculocutaneous albinism, ceroidlike inclusions in reticuloendothelial cells, and a hemorrhagic diathesis due to δ-storage pool disease), the *Chediak-Higashi syndrome* (partial oculocutaneous albinism, giant lysosomal granules, and recurrent pyogenic infections), and the *Wiskott-Aldrich syndrome* (eczema, thrombocytopenia, and immunodeficiency). Therapy for all of these disorders includes avoidance of aspirin and other antiplatelet agents, hormonal control of menses, and platelet transfusions for hemorrhagic complications.

Acquired Disorders of Platelet Function

In contrast to the inherited qualitative platelet defects, acquired disorders are quite common and frequently associated with drug ingestion, predominantly aspirin, or an underlying systemic disorder, such as uremia. Many drugs can result in platelet dysfunction by a variety of mechanisms. Aspirin and nonsteroidal anti-inflammatory medications inhibit cyclo-oxygenase and thereby prevent platelet synthesis of prostaglandin endoperoxides and thromboxane A_2. In contrast to aspirin, which has an irreversible effect on the enzyme, the cyclo-oxygenase inhibitory effect of the nonsteroidals is reversible. Certain antibiotics, especially penicillins in large dose, interfere with platelet function, although clinically significant hemorrhagic events are seldom due to antibiotic-induced platelet dysfunction as a single mechanism. Other medications that have been implicated in acquired platelet functional defects include heparin, plasma expanders such as dextran, and certain psychotropic medications.

Prior to the development of dialysis, hemorrhage was a common cause of morbidity and mortality in patients with renal failure. Hemorrhagic manifestations include subdural hematomas, gastrointestinal tract bleeding, epistaxis, and mucosal bleeding. Hemorrhage following surgery or biopsy is a common clinical problem. The most consistently abnormal test of hemostasis in patients with renal failure is the bleeding time, although a prolonged bleeding time is not an accurate predictor of increased hemorrhagic risk. Factors that contribute to the hemorrhagic manifestations of uremia include dysfunctional platelets, anemia, vWF dysfunction, concomitant medications, and thrombocytopenia. Therapeutic management includes dialysis, correcting the anemia to a hematocrit of ~25 to 30%, and the use of conjugated estrogens in patients with hemorrhagic manifestations. Desmopressin (DDAVP) stimulates release of endogenous vWF from endothelial cells, which frequently results in a shortening of the bleeding time and decreased hemorrhagic manifestations. Infusion of cryoprecipitate, which contains vWF, has a similar effect and can be used if DDAVP has no effect. In general, platelet transfusions are of little benefit since the infused platelets rapidly acquire the functional defect and should be reserved for emergency situations, such as uncontrolled hemorrhage.

VASCULAR PURPURAS

Abnormalities of the blood vessels that can lead to hemorrhagic manifestations include vasculitides, vascular malformations, collagen disorders, and the purpuras (Table 52–6). *Hereditary hemorrhagic telangiectasia* (Osler-Weber-Rendu disease) is an autosomal-dominant disorder with an estimated frequency of 1 in 50,000, although it may be significantly more common in certain populations. Clinical manifestations include mucosal telangiectasias, epistaxis, gastrointestinal hemorrhage, and larger arteriovenous malformations that can occur in the lung or brain. Hereditary hemorrhagic telangiectasia has been genetically linked to chromosome 9q33–34 in some families and

TABLE 52–6	Vascular Abnormalities Resulting in a Hemorrhagic Diathesis

Purpura simplex (easy bruising)
Henoch-Schonlein purpura
Kasabach-Merritt syndrome
Metabolic purpuras (scurvy, hypercortisolism)
Dysproteinemias
Senile purpura ("age spots")
Hereditary hemorrhagic telangiectasia
Inherited connective tissue disorders
Drug-induced purpuras
Psychogenic purpura

chromosome 12q in others. The gene on chromosome 9 encodes the transforming growth factor β receptor endoglobulin, which is an abundant integral membrane protein on endothelial cells. Recurrent gastrointestinal hemorrhage presents a significant problem for these patients, resulting in chronic iron deficiency anemia. Therapy consists of efforts to maintain local hemostasis and vigorous iron replacement therapy to correct for recurrent blood loss.

The *Kasabach-Merritt syndrome* is a consumptive coagulopathy that develops within giant hemangiomas, occurring most frequently in the pediatric population. Certain inherited disorders of connective tissue can result in hemorrhagic manifestations, especially type IV Ehlers-Danlos syndrome and pseudoxanthoma elasticum. *Henoch-Schonlein purpura* is an immune complex–mediated vasculitis that results in arthritic symptoms, abdominal pain, nephritis, and palpable purpura. Acquired causes of nonthrombocytopenic purpura include *scurvy* from a lack of vitamin C and the easy bruising noted in patients with hypercortisolism.

PLASMA PROTEIN DISORDERS AFFECTING PRIMARY HEMOSTASIS

Inherited Disorders

von Willebrand factor is a large adhesive glycoprotein found in the plasma, in platelet α-granules, in Weibel-Palade bodies in endothelial cells, and in the basement membrane of blood vessels. The protein circulates as disulfide-linked multimers that range in size from 500 kDa to more than 20,000 kDa, with the larger multimers having a high affinity for binding collagen as well as platelets. In the circulation, vWF binds to and stabilizes coagulation factor VIII but does not bind to platelets. Following endothelial disruption, however, vWF binds to exposed subendothelial collagen. This binding results in a change in protein conformation that enables vWF to interact with the platelet surface glycoprotein Ib–IX, mediating initial platelet adhesion. Following platelet activation, vWF will also bind to glycoprotein IIb–IIIa, but this interaction is not involved in the initial binding to the subendothelium.

von Willebrand disease results from qualitative as well as quantitative defects in the vWF molecule (Table 52–7). The prevalence of vWD in the general population is almost 1%, although the more severe forms are considerably less common. The most common form, type 1, is inherited as an autosomal-dominant trait. This form is defined as a partial *quantitative* decrease in a qualitatively normal-appearing molecule. In contrast, type 2 refers to a *qualitative* deficiency, which may be inherited as an autosomal dominant or recessive trait, depending on the subtype. Depending on the appearance of the multimers and the functional defect observed, Type 2 vWD is further subdivided into types 2A, 2B, 2M, and 2N (see Table 52–7). Type 3 vWD is an autosomal-recessive disorder characterized by virtually complete absence of vWF. The prevalence of type 3 vWD is approximately 1 in 1 million.

Clinical manifestations of vWD include epistaxis, easy bruising, mucosal bleeding, gastrointestinal hemorrhage, and menorrhagia. Bleeding is also common following surgical procedures and dental extractions. The bleeding tendency is variable in any individual patient over time, however, and also varies between afflicted members of the same family. Patients with type 3 vWD manifest the most severe hemorrhagic tendency, and, because of the associated decrease in factor VIII, these patients may also develop hemarthroses and deep hematomas. Interestingly, patients with type 2N vWD phenotypically appear to have hemophilia A rather than vWD, due to a mutation in the factor VIII binding site of the vWF molecule. The inheritance pattern is autosomal dominant, however, indicating that this is not a primary defect of coagulation factor VIII (see Chapter 52 for discussion of factor VIII deficiency).

The laboratory diagnosis of vWD can be difficult due to heterogeneity within a particular individual over time, frequently necessitating repeat testing in patients in whom the disorder is clinically suspected. In addition, von Willebrand factor is an acute phase reactant, and circulating levels increase with stress, pregnancy, and age. The bleeding time is variable and frequently normal in mildly affected patients. Complete assessment includes a vWF antigen determination, ristocetin cofactor assay, factor VIII activity, and a multimer analysis, which will allow appropriate disease classification (see Table 52–7). Additional screening tests that should be performed in these patients include a platelet count (decreased in patients with type 2B) and an aPTT (prolonged in patients with severe vWD due to a decrease in coagulation factor VIII). Lastly, ristocetin-induced platelet aggregation will be increased in patients with type 2B vWD, which can help with identification of this subtype.

The choice of therapy in any single patient depends on the type and severity of vWD as well as the specific clinical setting. Desmopressin (DDAVP) elevates the vWF activity to adequate levels in most patients with type 1 vWD by stimulating release of endogenous endothelial stores. DDAVP has essentially no effect in patients with severe vWD, however, and is contraindicated in patients with type 2B due to the potential for exacerbating the thrombocytopenia. Patients who do not respond to DDAVP can be treated with intermediate purity factor

TABLE 52-7 Quantitative and Qualitative Defects of the von Willebrand Factor (vWF) Resulting in von Willebrand Disease (vWD)

Subtype	Pathophysiologic Defect	Clinical Features	Laboratory Features	Therapeutic Options
1	Partial quantitative deficiency	Mild to moderate bleeding	Proportionate decrease in vWF:Ag and ristocetin cofactor activity; normal multimer pattern	DDAVP Intermediate purity factor VIII preparations
2A	Qualitative defect with decreased platelet-dependent function and absent HMW multimers	Generally mild to moderate bleeding	Variable decrease in vWF:Ag and ristocetin cofactor; factor VIII may also be low; absent HMW multimers	DDAVP usually ineffective Intermediate purity factor VIII preparations
2B	Qualitative defect characterized by increased affinity for platelet glycoprotein Ib	Generally mild to moderate bleeding	Variable decrease in vWF: Ag, ristocetin cofactor and factor VIII; absent HMW multimers; thrombocytopenia; increased platelet sensitivity to ristocetin	DDAVP contraindicated Intermediate purity factor VIII preparations
2M	Qualitative defect with decreased platelet-dependent function but normal HMW multimers	Variable bleeding disorder	Variable decrease in vWF:Ag, ristocetin cofactor; distribution and/or satellite binding pattern may be abnormal	Intermediate purity factor VIII preparations DDAVP may be useful in certain cases
2N	Markedly decreased affinity for factor VIII	Variable bleeding disorder	Disproportionately low factor VIII activity	
3	Severe quantitative deficiency state	Severe bleeding disorder	Generally undetectable vWF: Ag, ristocetin cofactor activity, and factor VIII	DDAVP ineffective Intermediate purity factor VIII preparations

DDAVP = Desmopressin; HMW = high molecular weight.

VIII concentrates, which contain significant amounts of vWF (in contrast, monoclonal antibody purified or recombinant factor VIII concentrates contain essentially no vWF). Since cryoprecipitate is not treated to inactivate viruses, it should not be used in these patients when specific replacement therapy is desired. Estrogen therapy has been used to control menorrhagia, and antifibrinolytic therapy can be useful, particularly during dental procedures.

Acquired Disorders

Acquired inhibitors to vWF have been described in patients with benign monoclonal gammopathy, multiple myeloma, lymphoproliferative disorders, and several autoimmune disorders such as systemic lupus erythematosus. Bleeding episodes in these patients can be acutely managed with DDAVP in patients with low-titer inhibitors or an intermediate purity factor VIII preparation (containing significant amounts of vWF) in patients with higher-titer antibodies. Immunosuppressive therapy, intravenous immunoglobulin, and plasmapheresis have all been used in the management of these patients. Acquired von Willebrand disease that is not immune mediated has been reported in patients with myeloproliferative syndromes, uremia, cardiac defects, and in the presence of certain drugs.

REFERENCES

Coller BS: Inherited disorders of platelet function. *In* Bloom AL, Forbes CD, Thomas DP, Tuddenham EGD (eds.): Haemostasis and Thrombosis. 2nd ed. New York, Churchill Livingstone, 1994, pp 721–766.

Ware HA, Coller BS: Platelet morphology, biochemistry, and function. *In* Beutler E, Lichtman MA, Coller BS, Kipps TJ (eds.): Williams Hematology. 5th ed. New York, McGraw-Hill, 1995, pp 1161–1201.

Warkentin TE, Kelton JG: Acquired platelet disorders. *In* Bloom AL, Forbes CD, Thomas DP, Tuddenham EGD (eds.): Haemostasis and Thrombosis. 2nd ed. New York, Churchill Livingstone, 1994, pp 767–815.

White III GC, Montgomery RR: Clinical Aspects of and Therapy for von Wildebrand disease. *In* Hoffman R, Benz Jr EJ, Shattil SJ, Furie B, Cohen HJ, Silberstein LE (eds.): Hematology. Basic Principles and Practice. 2nd ed. New York, Churchill Livingstone, 1995, pp 1725–1736.

53

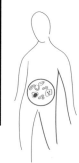

Blood Coagulation and Its Disorders

SECONDARY HEMOSTASIS AND CLOT STABILIZATION

Following formation of the initial platelet plug, secondary hemostasis consolidates this relatively loose structure into a stable clot held together by a meshwork of tightly cross-linked fibrin strands. The plasma proteins involved in blood coagulation circulate in the plasma as inactive zymogens or procofactors in concentrations far in excess of the amounts required for normal hemostasis. Following vascular injury and exposure of the subendothelium, the blood is exposed to tissue factor, which initiates the *extrinsic pathway* of secondary hemostasis (also referred to as the initiation phase; Fig. 53–1). Exposed tissue factor binds to factor VIIa, which then activates factor IX to factor IXa and factor X to factor Xa in the presence of Ca^{2+} ions. This process is rapidly downregulated by tissue pathway factor inhibitor (TPFI), which binds to the tissue factor–factor VIIa–factor X complex to form an inactive quaternary structure.

A sustained procoagulant response requires incorporation of the components of the *intrinsic pathway*, resulting in the amplification phase of secondary hemostasis (see Fig. 53–1). This critical amplification step is promoted by the generation of a small amount of thrombin during the initiation phase of the procoagulant response. Thrombin feedback activates factor XI, factor V, and factor VIII. Factor XIa activates factor IX to factor IXa, which then interacts with factor VIIIa in the presence of Ca^{2+} and a phospholipid membrane surface to form the "intrinsic factor X-ase complex." Factor Xa then interacts with the cofactor factor Va in the presence of Ca^{2+} ions and a phospholipid membrane surface to form the prothrombinase complex. These two procoagulant enzyme complexes rapidly convert their zymogen substrates to active enzymes to rapidly produce thrombin at the site of injury.

Thrombin proteolytically cleaves fibrinogen, a large asymmetric protein (MW $\sim$ 340,000 daltons) consisting of three pairs of polypeptide chains (referred to as $A\alpha\beta\gamma$). The resulting fibrin monomers polymerize to form an insoluble meshwork that is subsequently cross-linked by the transglutaminase factor XIIIa, resulting in a clot that is resistant to lysis. In addition to converting fibrinogen to fibrin, thrombin has a number of additional functions that are essential for a normal procoagulant response. As just mentioned, thrombin feedback activates factor V, factor VIII, and factor XI, resulting in amplification of the procoagulant response (see Fig. 53–1). Thrombin also activates platelets, thereby exposing procoagulant phospholipids (providing a surface membrane for the factor X-ase and prothrombinase complexes) and inducing the release of a number of platelet-activating substances, including thromboxane, Ca^{2+} ions, adenosine disphosphate (ADP), von Willebrand factor, fibronectin, and thrombospondin. Thrombin also activates factor XIII, which then cross-links the fibrin polymers. Lastly, thrombin also has a role in the activation of protein C, one of the natural anticoagulants, as described further later.

The liver is the site of synthesis for most of the coagulation proteins. Factors II, VII, IX, and X, and the anticoagulant proteins C and S require vitamin K for γ-carboxylation of specific glutamic acid residues in the phospholipid binding domain. In the absence of vitamin K (or in the presence of warfarin), abnormal proteins are formed that lack the γ-carboxyglutamic acid residues and therefore do not function in blood clotting. Factors V, XI, XII, fibrinogen, and antithrombin III are also synthesized in the liver but do not require vitamin K for their synthesis. Factor VIII is also synthesized in the liver (liver transplantation increases factor VIII levels to normal in patients with hemophilia A), but the concentration of factor VIII does not fall in end-stage liver disease. In fact, factor VIII levels may actually rise in patients with liver disease, in parallel with von Willebrand factor, which is synthesized in the vascular endothelium. This suggests that factor VIII is synthesized in the vascular endothelium as well as in the liver.

The clinical manifestations of a patient with a disorder of one of the procoagulant proteins involved in secondary hemostasis differ from the manifestations of a patient with a disorder of primary hemostasis and include joint and muscle hemorrhage, easy bruising, and bleeding following trauma or surgery. Screening laboratory studies to investigate abnormalities in the procoagulant proteins include the prothrombin time (PT), the activated partial thromboplastin time (aPTT), and the thrombin clot time (TCT) (Table 53–1), but diagnosis of a specific deficiency requires determination of factor levels. Because of recent advances in available therapeutics, it is essential that the specific deficiency state be clearly defined for optimal management.

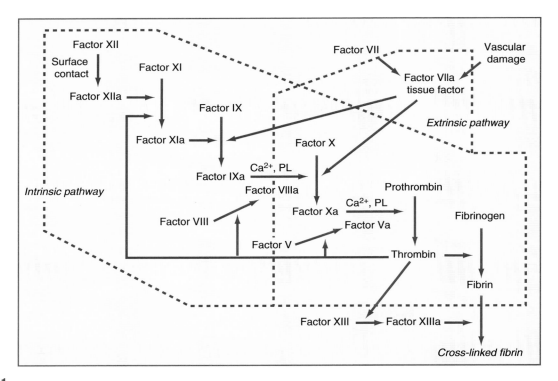

Figure 53-1

Secondary hemostasis. The extrinsic pathway begins with the exposure of tissue factor and initiates secondary hemostasis. The intrinsic pathway is essential for the continued generation of thrombin, which activates several factors in this component of secondary hemostasis by feedback. The prothrombin time (PT) measures the extrinsic pathway, and the activated partial thromboplastin time (aPTT) measures the intrinsic pathway of coagulation. PL = Phospholipid.

Inherited Disorders of Secondary Hemostasis

Hemophilia A

Classic hemophilia, or hemophilia A, is an X-linked hemorrhagic disorder with a frequency of 1 in 5000 male births, making it the most common inherited disorder of

TABLE 53-1	Screening Coagulation Test Abnormalities in Inherited Disorders of Secondary Hemostasis and von Willebrand Factor (vWF)			
	Results in a Prolongation of			
Deficiency of	**PT**	**aPTT**	**TCT**	**Bleeding Time**
Factor VII	+	−	−	−
Factor X	+	+	−	−
Factor V	+	+	−	−
Factor II	+	+	−	−
Fibrinogen	+	+	+	+
Factor XII	−	+	−	−
Factor XI	−	+	−	+/−
Factor IX	−	+	−	−
Factor VIII	−	+	−	−
Factor XIII	−	−	−	−
vWF	−	+/−	−	+

aPTT = Activated partial thromboplastin time; PT = prothrombin; TCT = thrombin clotting time.

secondary hemostasis. Hemophilia A results from a functional deficiency of factor VIII, which slows the rate of activation of factor X by the "intrinsic factor X-ase complex" and thereby results in loss of the amplification phase of secondary hemostasis (see Fig. 53-1). The gene for factor VIII has been cloned, sequenced, and localized to the long arm of the X chromosome (Xq28). It is an unusually large gene, occupying ~0.1% of the entire X chromosome. Deletions, insertions, inversions, and missense mutations have been identified throughout the factor VIII genes of patients with hemophilia A. Although many different mutations have been identified, as many as 50% of patients with severe hemophilia A will have an inversion involving intron 21, an unusually long intron spanning 32 kb. Lastly, there is a significant rate of spontaneous mutation in this large gene, since as many as 30% of patients have no family history.

The clinical manifestations of hemophilia A are directly related to the circulating level of factor VIII in the affected individual. Severe hemophilics have less than 1% of the normal level of factor VIII and manifest severe recurrent bleeding episodes, including spontaneous hemarthroses, intramuscular hematomas, pseudotumors, hematuria, intracranial bleeding, epistaxis, and gingival bleeding. Mild hemophilics, on the other hand, have >5% of the normal level of factor VIII. These patients seldom develop spontaneous bleeding complications but do have an increased hemorrhagic tendency following trauma or surgical procedures. Moderate hemophilics have between 1%

and 5% of the normal level of factor VIII and display hemorrhagic tendencies between the two extremes.

The laboratory diagnosis of hemophilia A includes a normal PT, TCT, and bleeding time but a prolonged aPTT that corrects when patient plasma is mixed with normal pooled plasma. Confirmation requires determination of a decreased factor VIII level, which also helps to predict the clinical manifestations of the disease. Carrier detection and prenatal diagnosis can be performed by restriction fragment length polymorphism analysis of the affected family.

Elevation of circulating plasma factor VIII to hemostatic levels is critical for the appropriate management of these patients when bleeding complications develop or for preoperative therapy. Desmopressin (DDAVP) may be useful in some patients with mild hemophilia because it stimulates the vascular endothelium to release endogenous factor VIII. In most patients, however, replacement therapy with high-purity plasma factor VIII concentrates or recombinant factor VIII represents the mainstay of treatment. Factor VIII concentrates derived from human plasma are solvent-detergent treated or heat treated to inactivate hepatitis viruses and human immunodeficiency virus (HIV), which previously represented a major scourge for the hemophilic population. Dosing and duration of therapy are determined by the location and severity of a specific bleeding episode or by the type of surgery to be performed. One unit of factor VIII per kilogram of body weight should increase the factor VIII level by 2%, and the infused protein has a plasma half-life of about 8 to 12 hours.

Special considerations for the patient with hemophilia include the avoidance of aspirin and other anti-platelet drugs; no intramuscular injections; no invasive procedures without appropriate factor VIII replacement therapy; and the rapid initiation of replacement therapy for all bleeding or potential bleeding episodes. In severe hemophilics with recurrent bleeding, programs of home therapy and/or factor VIII prophylaxis can be useful. The potential long-term complications for these patients include progressive arthropathy due to recurrent intra-articular hemorrhage; hepatitis; and the development of a factor VIII inhibitor, which may occur in as many as 15 to 20% of patients (discussed further later).

Hemophilia B

Hemophilia B is also a sex-linked hemorrhagic disorder, caused by a deficiency of factor IX, with an estimated incidence of 1 in 30,000 births. Factor IX is also located on the long arm of chromosome X (Xq27.1), and, as with deficiency of factor VIII, deficiency of factor IX slows the amplification pathway of secondary hemostasis (see Fig. 53–1). Clinically, hemophilia B and hemophilia A are identical, and screening coagulation studies reveal a prolonged aPTT that corrects with mixing studies (see Table 53–1). Documentation of a decreased factor IX activity level is essential for the diagnosis of hemophilia B. Treatment of hemorrhagic episodes consists of replacement therapy with monoclonal antibody-purified plasma factor IX preparations. Recombinant factor IX prepara-

tions are currently under investigation. The half-life of factor IX *in vivo* is ~ 18 to 24 hours, and so maintenance therapy may be needed only once daily. Fresh frozen plasma (FFP) or factor IX concentrates (also known as prothrombin complex concentrates [PCCs]) used to be administered to patients with hemophilia B. These concentrates should no longer be used in this clinical setting, since they also contain factor VII, factor X, and prothrombin, and infusion of factor IX concentrates has been associated with the development of consumptive thrombohemorrhagic disorders. As with hemophilia A, factor IX inhibitors may develop in as many as 5 to 10% of patients with hemophilia B treated with factor IX preparations.

Other Clotting Factor Deficiencies

Factor VII deficiency is a rare autosomal recessive trait with an estimated incidence of 1 in 500,000. Clinical manifestations include easy bruising, epistaxis, gastrointestinal hemorrhage, soft tissue hemorrhage, and menometrorrhagia in women. Characteristically, factor VII deficiency presents with a prolonged PT and normal aPTT, TCT, and bleeding time (see Table 53–1). Therapy for hemorrhagic episodes consists of FFP or PCCs, but this can be complicated by the short biologic half-life of factor VII (2 to 6 hours). However, only 10 to 20% of factor VII activity may be necessary for adequate hemostasis.

Factor X deficiency is also an autosomal recessive trait with an estimated incidence of less than 1 in 500,000. Clinical manifestations are similar to those for factor VII deficiency, but laboratory analysis reveals a prolonged PT and aPTT (see Table 53–1). Management of hemorrhagic episodes consists of FFP or PCCs. *Factor V deficiency*, or parahemophilia, is a rare autosomal recessive disorder that also affects the "prothrombinase complex." As with factor X deficiency, laboratory analysis reveals a prolonged PT and aPTT. In contrast to factor X, however, approximately 20% of the factor V in the blood is contained within the platelet α-granules. Interestingly, hemorrhagic complications are variable in severity between different kindreds and occasionally correlate better with the platelet level of factor V rather than the plasma level. Treatment for factor V deficiency consists of FFP for bleeding episodes and for surgical prophylaxis.

Prothrombin deficiency is an extremely rare disorder, with fewer than 30 well-characterized kindred. Clinical manifestations include easy bruising, bleeding with surgery, and menorrhagia; hemarthroses are uncommon. Laboratory analysis reveals a prolonged PT and aPTT, and diagnosis requires a specific factor II level. FFP is used for the treatment of hemorrhagic episodes and for preoperative management; acute hemorrhagic episodes can be treated with PCCs.

Fibrinogen deficiency may be due to the lack of production of the normal molecule (afibrinogenemia or hypofibrinogenemia) or to the production of a structurally abnormal protein (dysfibrinogenemia). Congenital afibrinogenemia is a rare autosomal recessive disorder that results in hemorrhagic problems from birth. Laboratory analysis reveals all of the screening tests to be prolonged in these patients (see Table 53–1). In contrast, dysfibrinogenemias may be associated with a hemorrhagic tendency in some patients, although most are not associated with any clinical manifestations, and several actually result in a prothrombotic tendency. Treatment of patients with afibrinogenemia and hemorrhagic dysfibrinogenemias consists of cryoprecipitate for bleeding episodes and for preoperative therapy. The half-life of fibrinogen is 4 days, so adequate replacement therapy can be readily achieved and maintained in most cases.

Factor XI deficiency is inherited as an autosomal recessive trait, but heterozygotes for the deficiency state may manifest minor hemorrhagic symptoms. Factor XI deficiency is most common in individuals of Ashkenazi Jewish descent, although it is also seen in multiple other ethnic groups. Spontaneous hemorrhages are relatively uncommon, with most bleeding events being associated with surgical and/or dental procedures. The aPTT is prolonged, and diagnosis requires determination of the factor XI level. The bleeding tendency does not correlate well with the extent of the deficiency, however, and some patients with very low levels have essentially no hemorrhagic problems. Therapy consists of FFP for bleeding episodes and preoperative prophylaxis.

Factor XII deficiency results in a marked prolongation of the aPTT that corrects with mixing studies, but there is no hemorrhagic tendency associated with this deficiency state. Similarly, deficiency of high–molecular weight kininogen or prekallikrein will also prolong the aPTT with no increased hemorrhagic risk. It is important to correctly identify these deficiency states because these patients should not receive prophylactic plasma therapy. In contrast, *factor XIII deficiency* is a rare autosomal recessive disorder characterized by a hemorrhagic diathesis but normal screening hemostasis assays. The bleeding diathesis commonly presents at birth with umbilical stump hemorrhage and continues throughout life. Laboratory diagnosis requires demonstration that the fibrin clot dissolves in 8 M urea, indicating that the fibrin polymers have not been cross-linked by factor XIII. Therapy consists of FFP for hemorrhagic episodes as well as prophylactically. The half-life is long (~9 days), and as little as 3 to 5% of the normal level of factor XIII may provide normal hemostasis.

Acquired Disorders of Secondary Hemostasis

Vitamin K Deficiency

Vitamin K is required for the post-translational γ-carboxylation of specific glutamyl residues in factors VII, IX, X, and II and in the anticoagulant proteins C and S. Very little vitamin K is actually stored in the body, and the fat-soluble vitamin is usually obtained in dark green, leafy vegetables (vitamin K_1) and through synthesis by the normal gastrointestinal bacterial flora. Consequently, deficiency states are not uncommon. Common clinical situations producing vitamin K deficiency include (1) vitamin K deficiency of the newborn, secondary to lack of vitamin K synthesis by intestinal bacteria until the gut is colonized; (2) malabsorption syndromes, such as regional enteritis and adult celiac disease; (3) prolonged parenteral feeding, especially in combination with antibiotic therapy resulting in sterilization of the bowel; and (4) ingestion of oral anticoagulants. The hallmark of early vitamin K deficiency is an isolated prolongation of the PT, due to the short half-life of factor VII. With sustained vitamin K deficiency, the aPTT also becomes prolonged due to decreases in factors IX, X, and II (Table 53–2). Hemorrhagic manifestations include ecchymoses, gingival bleeding, hematomas, hematuria, and gastrointestinal bleeding. Therapy consists of vitamin K replacement, which can be administered orally, subcutaneously, or intravenously. Intravenous infusions have been associated with adverse reactions and so should be infused slowly. In general, intramuscular injections should be avoided, as these can result in large hematomas. In patients with significant hemorrhagic symptoms in whom rapid (albeit temporary) correction of the deficiency state is essential, FFP and/or PCCs can be used.

Liver Disease

Patients with advanced liver disease commonly suffer hemorrhagic tendencies. Impaired liver function can result in multiple abnormalities of blood clotting, including (1) decreased synthesis of coagulation factors by the hepatocytes; (2) propagation of disseminated intravascular coagulopathy due to failure to clear activated clotting factors and reduced levels of regulatory proteins (antithrombin III and protein C); (3) thrombocytopenia, generally due to sequestration in a spleen enlarged by portal hypertension; (4) platelet dysfunction due to interference from elevated levels of fibrin degradation products or other inhibitors of platelet function not adequately cleared by the liver; and (5) enhanced fibrinolysis from an increased release of tissue plasminogen activator from vascular endothelial cells and decreased hepatic synthesis of α_2-plasmin inhibitor. Clinical laboratory findings include a prolonged PT and aPTT, elevated fibrin degradation products, and thrombocytopenia. In contrast to vitamin K deficiency, all factors, procoagulant and anticoagulant, synthesized in the liver will be decreased, with the exception of factor VIII, which is characteristically elevated (see Table 53–2). In fact, a low factor VIII level should raise the suspicion for a superimposed consumptive process. Therapy includes vitamin K supplementation and blood products for hemorrhagic episodes.

Disseminated Intravascular Coagulation

Disseminated intravascular coagulation (DIC) occurs when the normal hemostatic regulatory systems break down or are overwhelmed. The procoagulant response is activated intravascularly, leading to the generation of thrombin in a diffuse, nonlocalized fashion. Tissue ischemia and organ damage may result from the widespread deposition of fibrin thrombi in the microvasculature. In addition to the procoagulant response, the fibrinolytic

TABLE 53–2		**Clinical Laboratory Abnormalities That Can Be Used to Help Distinguish Among Vitamin K Deficiency, Liver Disease, and DIC**				
Disorder	PT	aPTT	Factor II	Factor V	Factor VIII	Platelets
Vitamin K deficiency	↑	NL or ↑	↓	NL	NL	NL
Liver disease	↑	↑	↓	↓	NL	NL or ↓
"Acute" DIC	↑	↑	↓	↓	↓	↓

aPTT = Activated partial thromboplastin time; DIC = disseminated intravascular coagulation; NL = normal; PT = prothrombin.

pathway is also activated, leading to the generation of the fibrin-degrading enzyme plasmin (Fig. 53–2). The concomitant activation of these two competing mechanisms can lead to the consumption of clotting factors and platelets, resulting in clinically significant hemorrhage. The variable clinical picture observed with this syndrome is determined by the extent to which these two processes are activated.

It should always be remembered that DIC is a secondary process that is initiated by an underlying primary pathophysiologic process. The causes of DIC are extensive and include infections, malignancy, acquired and congenital vascular abnormalities, obstetric complications, transfusion reactions, trauma, envenomation, and a wide variety of other mechanisms (Table 53–3). In some cases, DIC may represent the most florid manifestation of an illness, such as the hemorrhagic complications that accompany meningococcal sepsis. In others, such as malignancy, laboratory abnormalities indicative of ongoing DIC may be present, although the extent of the abnormalities will not be as severe and there may be no associated clinical manifestations. However, "low-grade" DIC may rapidly evolve into an acute process with an associated change in clinical status. Establishing the severity of the consumptive process is essential if therapeutic interventions of the hemostatic process itself are being considered.

Laboratory diagnosis of DIC depends on a pattern of laboratory test results, no single one of which is diagnostic, in a certain clinical setting. In acute uncompensated DIC, the PT and aPTT are prolonged, the levels of fibrinogen, factor V, and factor VIII are low, and thrombocytopenia is present (see Table 53–2). Evidence of fibrinolytic activity is manifested by elevated levels of fibrin split products and D-dimers. The latter result from plasmin digestion of fibrin strands that have been cross-linked by factor XIIIa and are diagnostic of a fibrinolytic (as opposed to fibrinogenolytic) process. Schistocytes can be seen on the peripheral blood smear, resulting from shear damage sustained by erythrocytes passing through intravascular fibrin strands. In contrast to acute DIC, chronic (or compensated) DIC may actually manifest normal or minimally abnormal screening tests. However, fibrin split products or D-dimers are usually elevated, indicating the presence of a lytic state.

Appropriate interpretation of the laboratory data requires integration with the specific clinical scenario. For example, microangiopathic hemolytic anemia may be seen with DIC as well as thrombotic thrombocytopenic purpura (TTP), but the clinical management of these two

Figure 53–2

The mechanism of action of the antithrombin III and protein C natural anticoagulant pathways. In the presence of thrombomodulin, thrombin is converted from a procoagulant enzyme to an anticoagulant enzyme, converting protein C to activated protein C. Deficiency of either protein C or protein S results in a hypercoagulable state in certain pedigrees. Factor V_{Leiden} results from a single amino acid mutation at Arg_{506} in the factor Va heavy chain that renders the activated molecule *resistant* to activated protein C. In contrast to the protein C pathway, which inactivates the procoagulant cofactors, antithrombin III binds to and neutralizes the procoagulant enzymes. Heparin produces an anticoagulant effect by accelerating the inactivation of these serine proteinases by antithrombin III. PL = Phospholipid.

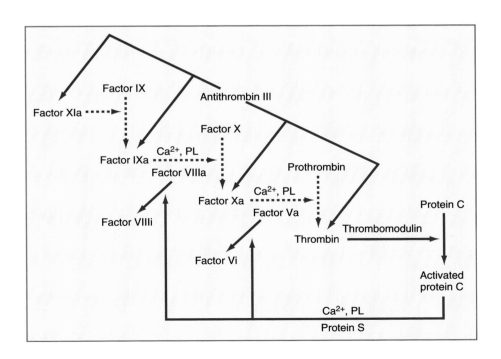

TABLE 53–3	Clinical Settings Associated with the Development of Disseminated Intravascular Coagulation (DIC)

Predominantly Acute Setting

Sepsis
Abruptio placentae
Amniotic fluid embolism
Snake bite
Massive hemolytic reactions
Trauma, hyperthermia
Acute promyelocytic leukemia

Predominantly Chronic Setting

Malignancy
Arteriovenous malformations
Arterial aneurysm
Pre-eclampsia
Dead fetus syndrome
Malignant hypertension
Severe hepatic cirrhosis

disorders is extremely different. Similarly, the coagulopathy of liver disease manifests many of the same laboratory abnormalities seen in DIC. The presence of an elevated factor VIII in liver disease can help distinguish the two processes, although this is by no means diagnostic, and both ongoing DIC and liver disease can be present in the same patient. Lastly, some patients with laboratory abnormalities consistent with DIC may actually have a localized consumptive process, secondary to an arterial aneurysm or cavernous hemangioma (Kasabach-Merritt syndrome). Treatment of the vascular abnormality may result in correction of the coagulopathy.

The therapeutic management of DIC, therefore, must emphasize treatment of the underlying disease, such as the use of antibiotics in the septic patient or by delivery of the fetus in the case of abruptio placentae. Correction or removal of the inciting process is essential to provide resolution of the consumptive process. Specific treatment of the hemostatic defects is unnecessary in compensated cases or when hemorrhagic complications are mild. If significant depletion of clotting factors (e.g., fibrinogen < 100 mg/dl or prolongation of the PT) and/or platelets (e.g., platelet count $< 20,000/mm^3$) occur, prophylactic replacement therapy may help reduce the hemorrhagic risk. Laboratory testing must be used to determine the response to therapy as well as to guide subsequent management. The use of heparin in DIC is controversial, although it may be of benefit in the treatment of DIC associated with acute promyelocytic leukemia. Antifibrinolytic agents such as ϵ-aminocaproic acid have also been used in the treatment of DIC, but isolated interruption of the fibrinolytic mechanism may result in an increased risk of prothrombotic events. Lastly, antithrombin III concentrates have been used in DIC associated with certain syndromes, although their clinical efficacy as a therapeutic modality in this situation remains to be defined.

FACTOR INHIBITORS

Antibodies to procoagulant proteins are encountered most commonly as alloantibodies that develop following replacement therapy in patients with hemophilia or other inherited deficiency states. Factor inhibitors may arise in ~ 15 to 20% of patients with hemophilia A and about 5% of patients with hemophilia B, most commonly occuring in patients with a severe clinical phenotype. The existence of an alloantibody in a patient with hemophilia is suspected when bleeding manifestations become more severe, when response to replacement therapy is less than expected, or when mixing studies no longer correct. Therapeutic options that can be used to achieve hemostasis during acute bleeding episodes include high-dose replacement therapy for lower titer inhibitors, porcine factor VIII for non–cross-reacting factor VIII inhibitors, or bypassing agents such as PCCs or recombinant factor VIIa. High-titer inhibitors have been treated with plasmapheresis, extracorporeal adsorption therapy, and intravenous immunoglobulin. Long-term management of these patients includes attempts to eliminate the inhibitor by immunosuppressive or cytotoxic therapy or by induction of immune tolerance.

Spontaneously occurring autoantibodies are most commonly directed against factor VIII. Clinical conditions associated with the development of these autoantibodies include the postpartum state, immunologic or lymphoproliferative disorders, and old age. Clinical manifestations range from no symptoms in individuals in whom the inhibitor spontaneously resolves to life-threatening hemorrhagic episodes. The therapeutic approach to these patients is similar to treatment of patients with hemophilia and an acquired antibody.

Although spontaneously occurring antibodies to factor V are relatively rare, factor V inhibitors may develop as alloantibodies following exposure to bovine thrombin products. Bovine thrombin is frequently used as a topical hemostatic agent or as a component of fibrin glue. However, many of these "thrombin" products contain a significant amount of bovine factor V as well as other bovine proteins. Antibodies to the bovine proteins may cross-react with human factor V or human factor II, resulting in prolongations of the PT and aPTT that do not correct with mixing studies. Clinical manifestations are variable, but severe hemorrhage is encountered in some cases. Platelet transfusions may be useful in these patients, since they include factor V in the α-granules, which may sequester the protein from the antibody. Treatment of factor II inhibitors includes FFP and PCCs.

NATURAL ANTICOAGULANTS AND THE FIBRINOLYTIC PATHWAY

The generation of an explosive procoagulant response is essential to prevent excessive hemorrhage from a damaged blood vessel. Conversely, it is also critical that this process be contained and prevented from disseminating widely throughout the vasculature. Several natural antico-

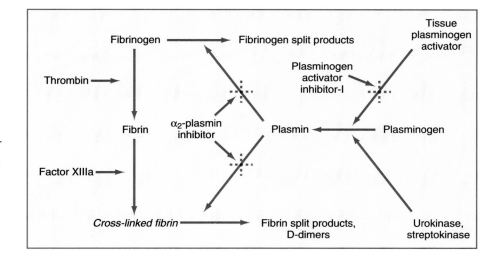

Figure 53-3
The fibrinolytic pathway. Tissue plasminogen activator, urokinase, and streptokinase all convert plasminogen to plasmin. Plasmin degrades cross-linked fibrin to fibrin split products and D-dimers. The fibrinolytic pathway is downregulated by plasminogen activator inhibitor-I, which inactivates tissue plasminogen activator, and α_2-plasmin inhibitor, which inactivates plasmin.

agulant mechanisms exist to downregulate essentially every step of the procoagulant response and maintain it only at the site of vascular injury. TFPI downregulates the initiation steps of the procoagulant response, antithrombin III neutralizes the serine proteinases (factors IIa, Xa, IXa, XIa, and XIIa), and the activated protein C system inactivates the essential cofactors factor Va and factor VIIIa (Fig. 53-3).

In addition to the natural anticoagulant mechanisms, the fibrinolytic pathway provides the mechanism whereby an already-formed fibrin clot can be actively remodeled and eventually removed during the course of vascular repair (see Fig. 53-2). Plasminogen is activated by plasminogen activators (tissue plasminogen activator, urokinase) to plasmin, a serine proteinase that degrades the

fibrin clot as well as proteolytically cleaves fibrinogen, factor V, and factor VIII to prevent additional fibrin formation. As with the procoagulant response, the fibrinolytic system is also tightly regulated by specific inhibitors that limit the generation (plasminogen activator inhibitor 1) and activity (α_2-plasmin inhibitor) of plasmin.

Inherited abnormalities of the natural anticoagulant or fibrinolytic mechanisms, as well as a number of acquired disorders, can result in an increased risk of thromboembolic disease (Table 53-4). Venous thromboembolism has an estimated annual incidence of 1 in 1000, resulting in significant morbidity as well as mortality. Evaluation of the patient with a venous thromboembolic event includes a thorough history, especially family history, and a complete physical examination. Laboratory analysis for a primary hypercoagulable state should be guided by the clinical assessment as well as any screening laboratory results, although these are generally not abnormal in the majority of patients with a primary hypercoagulable state.

PRIMARY HYPERCOAGULABLE STATES

Antithrombin III Deficiency

Antithrombin III (ATIII) is a serine proteinase inhibitor that functionally neutralizes thrombin and factors Xa, IXa, XIa, and XIIa. Inhibition occurs by formation of an equimolar complex between ATIII and the individual proteinase, a process accelerated by the anticoagulant heparin. *In vivo*, endothelial surface heparans and other glycosaminoglycans may serve to enhance the inactivation of the procoagulant serine proteinases by ATIII. Deficiency of ATIII is an autosomal dominant disorder characterized by an increased risk for venous thromboembolism, particularly in young adults. The prevalence of ATIII deficiency in the general population has been estimated to vary from 1 in 2000 to 1 in 5000. The incidence of venous thrombosis in an ATIII-deficient individual increases with age, and recurrent thrombosis may occur in as many as 60%

TABLE 53-4	Hypercoagulable States

Primary (Inherited) Hypercoagulable States

Antithrombin III deficiency
Protein C deficiency
Protein S deficiency
Activated protein C resistance
Dysfibrinogenemia
Homocystinemia
Abnormalities of fibrinolysis
    Hypoplasminogenemia
    Dysplasminogenemia
    Abnormal tissue plasminogen activator release
Elevated plasminogen activator inhibitor
    Elevated lipoprotein (a)

Secondary (Acquired) Hypercoagulable States

Antiphospholipid antibodies
Malignancy
Myeloproliferative syndromes
Paroxysmal nocturnal hemoglobinuria
Pregnancy
Therapy-related states
Nephrotic syndrome
Inflammatory bowel disease
Behçet's syndrome
Sepsis

of patients following an initial event. Conversely, ATIII deficiency accounts for only about 2% to 6% of all patients presenting with a new deep venous thrombosis.

Acquired ATIII deficiency states may be seen with liver disease, nephrotic syndrome, consumptive thrombohemorrhagic states, or in association with certain medications, including heparin and L-asparaginase. Laboratory diagnosis of ATIII deficiency includes both functional and antigenic assays. Therapy consists of anticoagulation for thromboembolic events, although higher doses of heparin may be required to achieve a therapeutic effect. ATIII concentrates are available, although their role as a therapeutic agent remains undefined.

Protein C, Protein S, and Activated Protein C Resistance

Thrombomodulin is a constitutively expressed endothelial cell surface protein that is a receptor for thrombin. When thrombin binds to thrombomodulin, it no longer functions as a procoagulant protein and instead becomes a potent activator of protein C, a vitamin K–dependent zymogen. In the presence of protein S, calcium ions, and a phospholipid membrane surface, activated protein C proteolytically inactivates factor Va and factor VIIIa (see Fig. 53–2). Hypercoagulable states have been described involving thrombomodulin, protein C, protein S, and, most recently, a specific mutation in factor V that renders it resistant to inactivation by protein C.

The clinical phenotype of *protein C deficiency* is heterogenous. In some kindreds, protein C deficiency is clearly inherited as an autosomal dominant trait, with as many as 75% of the affected individuals experiencing a venous thromboembolic event. In contrast, other kindreds have been described in which individuals with heterozygous protein C deficiency are totally asymptomatic. Homozygous deficiency of protein C is generally associated with very low levels of the protein ($<1\%$) and presents clinically as neonatal purpura fulminans. Heterozygous members of these pedigrees are generally asymptomatic, suggesting an autosomal recessive mode of inheritance. Interestingly, mutation analysis in these different families reveals that similar mutations have been identified in kindreds with an increased prothrombotic risk as in those that are asymptomatic, suggesting that additional factors may be involved in determining the clinical phenotype.

Laboratory diagnosis of protein C deficiency requires demonstration of a decreased level of protein C in a patient not receiving warfarin therapy and who is not vitamin K deficient. Treatment consists of long-term anticoagulant therapy for patients with venous thromboembolic events. A potential therapeutic complication in patients with protein C deficiency is the development of warfarin-induced skin necrosis. Because of the short half-life of protein C (~ 6 hrs), it can be rapidly depleted when initiating warfarin therapy, potentially enhancing the hypercoagulable state and leading to the transient development of an increased hypercoagulable state. For this reason, patients with protein C deficiency should always

receive overlapping doses of therapeutic heparin when starting warfarin therapy. Lastly, protein C concentrates have been used in the management of purpura fulminans due to homozygous deficiency.

Protein S is also a vitamin K–dependent protein, but, in contrast to the other vitamin K–dependent clotting factors, protein S is a cofactor for activated protein C rather than a zymogen. Approximately 60% of the total protein S in the circulation is in a complex with the complement component C4b-binding protein, an acute phase reactant. Only the free (nonbound) form of protein S can function as a cofactor for activated protein C. Consequently, in acute inflammatory states, the increase in the level of C4b-binding protein results in a decrease in the level of free protein S with a normal total protein S (free + bound). Documentation of protein S deficiency, therefore, requires confirmation of a low level at a time when the patient is clinically stable and not on oral anticoagulant therapy.

Protein S deficiency is inherited as an autosomal dominant trait, and the heterozygous state is associated with an increased risk of thromboembolic events. Predominant venous thrombotic events include deep venous thrombosis, superficial thrombophlebitis, and pulmonary embolism, but thromboses of axillary, mesenteric, and cerebral veins have also been described. Protein S deficiency has also been associated with an increased frequency of arterial thromboembolic events, particularly in young adults. These patients are at an increased risk of recurrent thromboembolic events and generally require lifelong anticoagulant therapy following a first event. Warfarin-induced skin necrosis has been reported with protein S deficiency, but it is less common than with protein C deficiency. Lastly, acquired deficiency states occur during pregnancy and with the use of oral contraceptives, but it is unclear if an acquired deficiency state results in an increased prothrombotic risk.

Activated protein C (APC) exerts its anticoagulant effect by proteolytically neutralizing factor Va and factor VIIIa. Some patients with recurrent venous thromboembolic events have a *resistance to APC* using a modified aPTT-based assay. The majority of these patients have a single point mutation in the factor V gene, replacing Arg_{506} with a glutamine residue (referred to as Factor V_{Leiden}). This renders the APC cleavage site at this position resistant to proteolysis, making Factor Va_{Leiden} resistant to neutralization by APC.

Activated protein C resistance has subsequently become recognized as the most common inherited disorder resulting in a hypercoagulable state. Depending on patient selection criteria, as many as 19 to 60% of patients with venous thromboembolic disease were resistant to APC. Furthermore, in certain populations, as many as 2.0 to 8.5% of normal individuals may also have this mutation. Racial differences do exist, since APC resistance has been reported to be relatively uncommon among certain ethnic populations. The estimated increase in the risk of venous thrombosis with APC resistance is ~ 5- to 10-fold for heterozygotes and 50- to 100-fold for homozygotes. In general, APC resistance is not associated with an increased frequency of arterial thromboembolic events, although several kindreds have been described with an increased frequency of stroke involving affected members.

Clinical laboratory diagnosis of APC resistance consists of an aPTT-based assay to which APC is added. Addition of APC to plasma from a normal individual prolongs the aPTT. In contrast, addition of APC to plasma from a patient with APC resistance does not prolong the aPTT to the same extent. Several alternative approaches exist for characterization of plasma samples in the presence of heparin and lupus anticoagulants. An abnormal plasma-based APC resistance assay should be further evaluated by genotype analysis to determine heterozygosity versus homozygosity. Genotypic determination is essential for therapeutic recommendations as well as for pedigree analysis.

Abnormalities of Fibrinolysis

Congenital defects in several of the components of the fibrinolytic system have been associated with thrombosis (see Table 53–4). At least 30 families have been described with inherited abnormalities of plasminogen, and both qualitative and quantitative abnormalities have been described. Clinical manifestations are variable, and diagnosis requires determination of a plasminogen level. No patients with tissue plasminogen activator (tPA) deficiency have been clearly documented, but several kindreds with an inherited defect in tPA release have been described. Documentation of tPA release defects is difficult and requires a provocative test to stimulate release of tPA from the vascular endothelium. In the normal individual, tPA levels increase two to three times above a baseline level after stimulation, but this response is blunted in certain individuals. Lastly, several individuals with elevated levels of plasminogen activator inhibitor I (PAI I) and thrombosis have been reported. However, PAI-I levels are also frequently elevated as an acute phase reactant, and documentation of a true inherited disorder requires testing on several occasions. Treatment of thrombotic episodes secondary to inherited disorders consists of anticoagulant therapy.

Defects in the fibrinolytic system can also result in a hemorrhagic state that is not detected by routine screening assays. Deficiency of α_2-plasmin inhibitor as well as PAI-1 has been reported to result in a hemorrhagic diathesis. Both of these disorders require specific coagulation testing for confirmation of diagnosis.

SECONDARY HYPERCOAGULABLE STATES

Antiphospholipid Antibodies

Antiphospholipid antibodies include lupus anticoagulants, identified by interference with phospholipid-dependent coagulation tests, and anticardiolipin antibodies, identified by the ability to bind to immobilized cardiolipin in an enzyme-linked immunosorbent assay. Many of these patients will also manifest a false-positive Venereal Disease Research Laboratory (VDRL) because of interaction of the antibodies with the cardiolipin in the assay. Antiphospholipid antibodies have been most frequently described in patients with systemic lupus erythematosus (SLE), although about half of the patients with a serologic diagnosis of an antiphospholipid antibody do not have SLE. These patients include individuals with other autoimmune disorders or malignancy, individuals taking certain medications (e.g., chlorpromazine, quinidine, procainamide, or hydralazine), or otherwise healthy people.

Thromboembolic events, including both arterial and venous events, occur in ~40% of patients with antiphospholipid antibodies who have SLE. The frequency of thromboembolic events in patients with antiphospholipid antibodies who do not have SLE varies, with some patients having a high frequency of thromboembolic complications (e.g., those patients with a primary antiphospholipid antibody syndrome), whereas other patients have infrequent complications (e.g., those with infection-associated antibodies). Other clinical manifestations associated with the presence of antiphospholipid antibodies include neurologic symptoms, especially amaurosis fugax, transient ischemic attacks, and headaches; recurrent fetal loss; livedo reticularis; cardiac valvular abnormalities; and thrombocytopenia.

Clinical laboratory determination of an antiphospholipid antibody can be difficult due to antibody heterogeneity and requires demonstration of a lipid-dependent inhibitor of coagulation or an anticardiolipin antibody. In many cases, the antibody is identified during the evaluation of an isolated elevated aPTT in an otherwise normal individual. Thromboembolic events are treated with anticoagulant therapy, and at least a subset of these patients appears to require a high therapeutic international normalized ratio (INR) to prevent recurrent events. However, because many of these patients will never sustain a thromboembolic event, anticoagulant therapy for an individual with an antiphospholipid antibody but with no prior thrombosis is not recommended.

Malignancy

Armand Trousseau first described the association between thrombophlebitis and malignancy over 120 years ago. It has subsequently been demonstrated that certain neoplasms, especially adenocarcinomas of the pancreas, stomach, and the biliary tree, are associated with an increased frequency of thromboembolic events. Conversely, as many as 10% of patients with a deep venous thrombosis and no identifiable risk factor may subsequently develop a malignancy. Evaluation for a malignancy in a patient presenting with a new thromboembolic event should be pursued based on clinical assesment.

THERAPY OF THROMBOEMBOLIC DISEASE

Therapeutic modalities used in the treatment of thromboembolic disease include antiplatelet, anticoagulant, and fibrinolytic therapy (Table 53–5).

TABLE 53–5	Therapeutic Agents Used in the Treatment and Prevention of Thrombotic Disorders		
Agent	**Mechanism of Action**	**Useful Laboratory Tests**	**Antidote**
I. Antiplatelet Agents			
Aspirin	Inhibits platelet cyclo-oxygenase	Platelet aggregation studies; bleeding time	Platelet transfusion
Ticlopidine	Inhibits ADP-mediated platelet aggregation	Platelet aggregation studies	Platelet transfusion
Dipyridamole	Inhibits cyclic AMP phosphodiesterase	—	Platelet transfusion
Antibody 7E3	Antibody to glycoprotein IIb-IIIa	Platelet aggregation studies	Platelet transfusion
Disintegrins	Interfere with fibrinogen binding to glycoprotein IIb-IIIa	Platelet aggregation studies	Platelet transfusion
II. Anticoagulants			
Heparin	Accelerates antithrombin III inhibition of thrombin and thrombin generation	aPTT; heparin levels	Protamine sulfate
LMWH, heparinoid	Accelerates antithrombin III inhibition of factor Xa	Anti–factor Xa levels	Protamine sulfate partially reverses effect
Warfarin	Interferes with γ-carboxylation of vitamin K–dependent clotting factors	PT	(1) Vitamin K; (2) FFP; (3) PCCs
Hirudin	Specific leech antithrombin	aPTT	FFP, PCCs
Argatroban, PPACK	Synthetic antithrombins	—	FFP, PCCs
III. Thrombolytic Agents			
Streptokinase	Activation of plasminogen to plasmin	TCT; fibrinogen; FSP	Cryoprecipitate
Urokinase	Activation of plasminogen to plasmin	TCT; fibrinogen; FSP	Cryoprecipitate
t-PA	Activation of plasminogen to plasmin	TCT; fibrinogen; FSP	Cryoprecipitate

PT = prothrombin time; aPTT = activated partial thromboplastin; LMWH = low–molecular weight heparin; TCT = thrombin clotting time; FFP = fresh frozen plasma; PCCs = prothrombin complex concentrates; FSP = fibrin(ogen) split products; t-PA = tissue plasminogen activator.

Antiplatelet Therapy

Antiplatelet therapy has been shown to be of the most value in the treatment of arterial thromboembolic disease by blocking platelet deposition on the surface of a disrupted atherosclerotic plaque. The most commonly used antiplatelet agent is *aspirin*, which irreversibly inhibits platelet cyclo-oxygenase, resulting in inhibition of arachidonic acid-mediated platelet aggregation. Clinical situations in which aspirin has been proven to be useful include (1) the treatment of patients with unstable angina and (2) the secondary prevention of stroke. *Ticlopidine* is an antiplatelet agent that interferes with ADP-mediated aggregation. In general, it is used as a secondary agent if aspirin is not tolerated or does not result in clinical improvement. *Dipyridamole* is an inhibitor of cyclic adenosine monophosphate phosphodiesterase and may be of use in combination with warfarin to decrease the rate of systemic embolization in patients with prosthetic heart valves. Several new therapeutic agents have been shown to be of benefit in certain clinical situations, including the chimeric antiglycoprotein IIb/IIIa monoclonal antibody 7E3 (abciximab) and the disintegrins.

Anticoagulant Therapy

Anticoagulant therapy interferes with secondary hemostasis to delay formation of a fibrin clot. *Heparin* is a parenteral anticoagulant that markedly enhances the rate of inhibition of factor II, and, to a lesser extent, factor X and factor IX, by antithrombin III. Standard heparin is a complex mixture of polysulfated glycosaminoglycans purified from porcine intestinal mucosa or bovine lung. Ad-

ministered intravenously or subcutaneously, standard heparin is an excellent anticoagulant that has been shown to be efficacious in a number of clinical situations. It can be used in the management of venous thromboembolic disease and unstable angina and other unstable coronary syndromes, and for thromboembolic prophylaxis. It is the anticoagulant of choice during pregnancy. Monitoring is performed with the aPTT, with the therapeutic range corresponding to *ex vivo* heparin levels of 0.2 to 0.4 U/ml, determined by protamine titration. Complications of heparin therapy include hemorrhage, osteopenia, and heparin-induced thrombocytopenia.

Low–molecular weight heparins (LMWHs) are prepared from standard heparin by enzymatic cleavage or chemical hydrolysis. The ability of heparin to catalyze the inhibition of thrombin by antithrombin III is critically dependent on molecular size, with a minimum oligosaccharide chain length of 18 being necessary for thrombin inhibition. In contrast, inhibition of factor Xa can occur with significantly shorter oligosaccharide chains. Consequently, the LMWHs have a more pronounced anti–factor Xa effect rather than an anti-thrombin effect. A significant therapeutic advantage of the LMWHs is that they tend to have fewer hemorrhagic complications while providing antithrombotic effects comparable to those of standard heparin.

Warfarin is an oral anticoagulant that blocks the regeneration of vitamin K from its epoxide, thereby interfering with the post-translational carboxylation of specific glutamic acid residues located in clotting factors II, VII, IX, and X and the anticoagulant proteins C and S. Inhibition of this process leads to the synthesis of functionally inactive blood clotting factors, resulting in an anticoagulated state. Although warfarin is rapidly absorbed from the gastrointestinal tract, there is a 24- to 36-hour delay before any observable anticoagulant effect is noted, representing the time required for the descarboxylated vitamin K–dependent clotting factors to replace the normal proteins as they are cleared from the circulation. Anticoagulant therapy with warfarin must be monitored to obtain a desired antithrombotic effect without exposing the patient to an excessive hemorrhagic risk, and the PT is the optimal test for this purpose. Because of variable responsiveness of individual thromboplastins to the anticoagulant effects of warfarin, the international normalized ratio (INR) was developed as a mechanism to standardize monitoring. An INR of 2.0 to 3.0 is recommended for most clinical situations requiring warfarin therapy, with the exception of mechanical prosthetic heart valves, which should be anticoagulated to an INR of 2.5 to 3.5. Reversal of an overanticoagulated patient can be achieved with vitamin K supplementation or, in more acute situations, with FFP.

Fibrinolytic Therapy

Thrombolytic agents function by activating plasminogen to plasmin, which thereby promotes clot lysis. The most commonly used fibrinolytic agents include streptokinase, urokinase, and tissue plasminogen activator, which differ in their mechanism of plasminogen activation, survival time in the circulation, and specificity for fibrin (as opposed to fibrinogen). Thrombolytic therapy is most efficacious in the treatment of patients with acute myocardial infarction, although there are also data to support its use in certain patients with thromboembolic strokes, peripheral arterial thrombosis, and venous thromboembolic disease. Hemorrhagic complications are not uncommon, and intracranial hemorrhage may occur in as many as 0.5 to 1.0% of patients treated with fibrinolytic agents. Laboratory tests that can be used to monitor fibrinolytic therapy include the thrombin clotting time (TCT), the euglobulin clot lysis time, and the fibrinogen level, although short-term infusions of fibrinolytic agents may not require specific monitoring to acheive a desired therapeutic effect. Reversal can be achieved with the use of cryoprecipitate as a source of fibrinogen, and antifibrinolytic agents can be used in situations with life-threatening hemorrhage.

REFERENCES

Dahlbäck B: Inherited thrombophilia: Resistance to activated protein C as a pathogenic factor of venous thromboembolism. Blood 1995; 85: 607–614.
Dalen JE, Hirsh J (eds.): Fourth ACCP Consensus Conference on Antithrombotic Therapy. Chest 1995; 108(Supplement): 225S–522S.
Hoffman M, Roberts HR: Hemophilia and related conditions—inherited deficiencies of prothrombin (factor II), factor V, and factors VII to XII. *In* Beutler E, Lichtman MA, Coller VS, Kipps TJ (eds.): Williams Hematology. 5th ed. New York, McGraw-Hill, 1995, pp 1413–1439.
Ratnoff OD: Hemostatic defects in liver and biliary tract disease and disorders of vitamin K metabolism. *In* Ratnoff OD, Forbes CD (eds.): Disorders of Hemostasis. 2nd ed. Philadelphia, WB Saunders, 1991, pp 459–479.
Seligsohn U: Disseminated intravascular coagulation. *In* Beutler E, Lichtman MA, Coller BS, Kipps TJ (eds.): Williams Hematology. 5th ed. New York, McGraw-Hill, 1995, pp 1497–1516.

Oncologic Disease

Section VIII

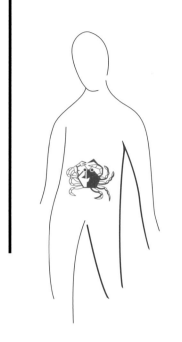

54

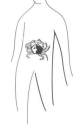

General Considerations in Oncology

In the United States, cancer accounts for more than 550,000 deaths annually, a toll second only to that from cardiovascular diseases. Current statistics suggest that approximately 30% of Americans develop cancer in their lifetimes, of whom two thirds will die as a result of their disease. The leading sites of cancer are the prostate gland and lung in males, the breast and lung in females, and the colorectal region in both sexes (Fig. 54–1). During the past 25 years, cancers of the skin, breast, pancreas, bladder, and testes have increased in incidence, while gastric and invasive cervical cancers have declined. Recently, lung cancer in men has declined in association with a decrease in smoking, but the drop is more than compensated for by an increased incidence in women. Striking geographic differences exist in specific cancer rates. In Japan, for example, gastric and hepatocellular carcinomas are common, while breast and colon carcinomas are relatively rare. Presumably, the differences reflect environmental factors, as Japanese immigrants to the United States display American cancer rates within just one or two generations of residence.

ETIOLOGY

Oncogenes

The last decade has focused attention on the genes that control cell proliferation as being the targets for mutations leading to the disruption in normal cell growth that results in cancer. Some of these gene mutations may be inherited through the germ line and explain the high incidence of cancer in some families. Others may be acquired through exposure to environmental carcinogens, viruses, or other agents. The occurrence of cancer in an individual is the end result of more than one mutation in normal cellular DNA, and a number of distinct changes in the cellular genome are necessary for full expression of a cancer cell.

Two elements of the human genome have received the most attention in research involving human DNA and cancer: the oncogenes and the tumor suppressor genes. Proto-oncogenes (or cellular oncogenes) are normal constituents of all cells and are critically important in regulating normal cell growth and differentiation. Proto-oncogenes are highly conserved in vertebrate evolution and are prime candidates for a substrate upon which the multitude of carcinogenic stimuli may play. Oncogenes are tumor-promoting segments of DNA that are activated or potentiated by a perturbation of the proto-oncogenes. The tumor suppressor genes are recessive genes that also act to control normal cell proliferation. An imbalance between the activation of oncogenes and the inactivation of tumor suppressor genes is important in carcinogenesis.

More than 20 proto-oncogenes have been identified. Their products are proteins located in the nucleus, cytoplasm, and plasma membrane of cells. Some of the functions of these proteins are known (Table 54–1). Many are tyrosine kinases and some are growth factors (e.g., platelet-derived growth factor and epidermal growth factor). One example of activation of a proto-oncogene is the Philadelphia chromosome (Ph^1), consisting of reciprocal translocation between chromosomes 9 and 22 in chronic myelogenous leukemia (CML). Ph^1 (Fig. 54–2) exists in the hematopoietic cells of nearly all patients with CML. The c-abl proto-oncogene is localized to chromosome 9 near the breakpoint and is invariably translocated to chromosome 22, with the breakpoint on 22 occurring in a tightly restricted region called the "breakpoint cluster region (bcr)." The resulting bcr : c-abl fusion gene encodes a chimeric fusion protein, p210 (i.e., molecular weight of 210 kd). Unlike the native c-abl gene product, p145, the fusion protein, p210, undergoes autophosphorylation of its tyrosine residues and possesses potent tyrosine kinase activity that may be fundamental to the pathogenesis of CML. The recent demonstration that a disease resembling CML develops in mice in which the blood stem cells had been transfected with a bcr : c-abl fusion gene confirms the importance of the chromosomal translocation in the pathogenesis of this disease.

Although cellular oncogenes promote cell growth, normal cells also possess recessive tumor suppressor genes that constrain cell growth. Tumor suppressor genes were first described for the rare childhood tumor, retinoblastoma. This tumor is associated with the inactivation of both functional copies of the RB gene on chromosome 13. Another syndrome associated with loss of the tumor suppressor genes is familial polyposis, a disorder predisposing to colon cancer. The gene adenomatous polyposis coli (APC gene) is located on the long arm of chromosome 5.

Proto-oncogenes and tumor suppressor gene sites in

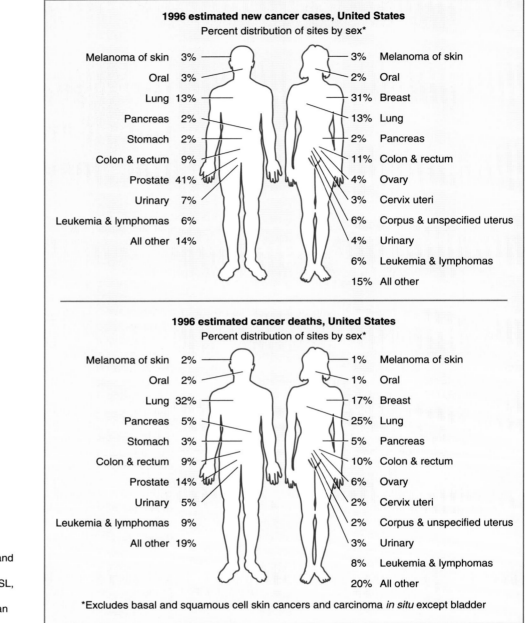

Figure 54–1
Estimated new cancer cases and cancer deaths in the United States in 1996. (From Parker SL, Tong T, Bolden S, Wingo PA: Cancer statistics, 1996. CA Can J Clin 1996; 46:5–27.)

cellular DNA are prime targets for various carcinogens. It is unlikely that any one carcinogen acts on a single site to produce cancer; most cancers result from a sequence of events that disturb the cellular balance between promotion and inhibition of growth.

The cells of several human malignancies, including bladder cancer and acute myelogenous leukemia, contain *ras* oncogenes that result from point mutations in normal *ras* genes. *Ras* genes normally encode guanosine triphosphate (GTP)-binding proteins (see Table 54–1); the mutated *ras* proteins contain single amino acid substitutions and are capable of neoplastic transformation.

Amplification of proto-oncogene sequences has been detected in some tumors, such as N-*myc* in neuroblastoma and *neu* in breast cancer. In these cancers, proto-onco-

gene amplification is associated with a poor prognosis, suggesting that its enhanced expression may be critically related to disease progression.

Environmental Carcinogens

Tobacco is the major environmental carcinogen, contributing to 25% of all cancer deaths. Tobacco exposure strongly potentiates the carcinogenic effect of other agents, most notably asbestos and alcohol; it leads not only to cancer of the lung but also of the head, neck, esophagus, and bladder, among others. This synergistic effect exemplifies how environmental carcinogens cause cancer. Lung cancer, for example, is thought to result

TABLE 54–1	Proto-Oncogene Families	
Family	**Cardinal Properties**	**Examples**
Tyrosine-specific protein kinase	Protein phosphorylation with specificity for tyrosine. Most kinases localize to the cell surface, and some members are bona-fide receptors.	c-*erb*B (EGF-receptor; erythroleukemia) c-*fms* (CSF-1 receptor; sarcoma) c-*abl* (CML) c-*src* (sarcoma)
Serine-threonine	Protein phosphorylation with specificity for serine or threonine. Proteins are homologous to tyrosine kinase. Proteins localize to the cytosol.	c-*mos* sarcoma) c-*raf*
Receptor for thyroid hormone	Homology to steroid receptors	c-*erb*A
GTP-binding proteins	Bind guanine nucleotides and hydrolyze GTP. Are analogous to G proteins that modulate receptor signals, including transducin, Gi, Gs, and Go.	c-Ha-*ras* (sarcoma) ci-Ki-*ras*
Growth factor	Beta chain of platelet-derived growth factor	ci-*sis* (sarcoma)
Nuclear proteins	Generally short half-life and rapid inducibility, DNA binding or transcription factors	c-*myc* (carcinomas; leukemia; sarcoma) c-*fos* (osteosarcoma) p53 (colon cancer)
Other	Blocks apoptosis ?G-protein	bcl-2 (follicular B cell lymphoma)

CML = Chronic myelogenous leukemia; CSF = colony-stimulating factor; EGF = epidermal growth factor; GTP = guanosine triphosphate.
Adapted from Nienhuis AW, Sherr CJ: Oncogenes in hematopoietic neoplasms. *In* HEMATOLOGY—1987. The Educational Program of the American Society of Hematology.

from a multistage process characterized by several exposures, some acting as initiators (true carcinogens) and others as promoters (cocarcinogens). The actual induction of carcinogenesis by a chemical carcinogen may involve covalent modification of host DNA, dose dependence, and the existence of a lag period between exposure and malignant transformation.

Occupational exposure to chemical carcinogens (e.g., asbestos, vinyl chloride) accounts for about 5% of all cancers. In certain occupations, as in furniture makers with a high exposure to wood dusts, nasal sinus cancers are an occupational hazard. Other important known carcinogens include smokeless tobacco, which is increasingly popular among young adults in the southwestern United States and is associated with oropharyngeal carcinoma.

Medications form another major category of chemical carcinogens. For example, alkylating agents used to treat lymphoma, multiple myeloma, and ovarian cancer may induce acute myelogenous leukemia. Maternal ingestion of prenatal diethylstilbestrol leads to the later development of adenocarcinomas of the vagina and cervix in some daughters exposed *in utero*.

Immunosuppression either by medication, as in patients with renal transplants, or by the acquired immunodeficiency syndrome (AIDS)–causing HTLV-III (human T cell lymphotropic virus III) virus predisposes to certain cancers, particularly high-grade lymphomas. Other viruses have been linked to human cancer. The HTLV-I retrovirus is commonly found in patients with adult T cell leukemia/lymphoma. Also well established are the association of the papilloma virus (type 16) with cervical cancer and the hepatitis B virus with hepatoma.

Evidence derived from animal and epidemiologic studies as well as from limited clinical trials suggests that diet plays an important causative and protective role in carcinogenesis. However, data regarding the carcinogenicity of specific dietary factors are largely inconclusive. Possible associations include high dietary fat intake with colon and breast cancer and aflatoxin with liver cancer.

Protective roles have been postulated for micronutrients and trace metals such as selenium, carotene, vitamins E and C, and calcium, although controlled trials have failed to demonstrate a protective effect of β carotene.

Hormones are important in the development of certain cancers. Breast and uterine cancers are associated with high levels of estrogen, both endogenous and exogenous. Prostate cancer is sensitive to male hormones. Androgen ablation, either by orchiectomy or by medication, is the treatment of choice.

Radiation-induced carcinogenesis has been observed in atomic bomb survivors, patients receiving therapeutic

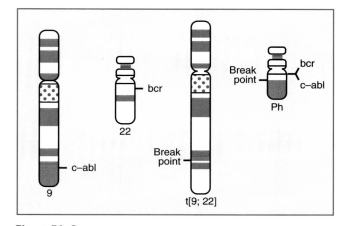

Figure 54–2

Reciprocal translocation resulting in the formation of the Philadelphia (Ph¹) chromosome pathognomonic of chronic myelogenous leukemia (CML). The c-*abl* proto-oncogene on chromosome 9 is translocated to the breakpoint cluster region (bcr) on chromosome 22. A new bcr:*abl* fusion gene is created on the Ph¹ chromosome, which encodes a fusion protein, p210, likely to be important in the pathogenesis of CML. (Adapted from Champlin RE, Golde DW: Chronic myelogenous leukemia: Recent advances. Blood 1985; 65:1039; with permission.)

TABLE 54–2	Some Hereditary Neoplasms and Preneoplastic Syndromes	
	Inheritance	**Clinical Features**
Hereditary Neoplasms		
Retinoblastoma	AD	Susceptibility to other cancers, particularly osteosarcoma; deletion in long arm of chromosome 13 in some cases
Multiple endocrine neoplasia I	AD	Adrenal, pancreatic, pituitary, parathyroid tumors; carcinoid tumors
Multiple endocrine neoplasia II	AD	Medullary thyroid carcinoma, pheochromocytoma; parathyroid tumors and neurofibromas in some
Polyposis coli	AD	Multiple adenomatous polyps; adenocarcinoma of large bowel
Dysplastic nevus syndrome	AD	Hereditary melanomas derived from nevi
Li-Fraumeni syndrome	AD	Susceptibility to cancer in childhood, particularly osteosarcoma, sarcoma, brain tumors, leukemia, and breast cancer when older
Hereditary Preneoplastic Syndromes		
Neurofibromatosis	AD	Multiple neurofibromas; café au lait spots; some develop neurofibrosarcomas, gliomas, acoustic neuromas, leukemias
Xeroderma pigmentosum	AR	Skin cancers; defective repair of DNA damaged by ultraviolet light
Bloom's syndrome; Fanconi's anemia	AR	Acute leukemia; other malignancies; associated with chromosomal instability
X-linked lymphoproliferative syndrome	XR	Immunoblastic sarcoma; B cell lymphoma; associated with abnormal immune response to EBV

AD = Autosomal dominant; AR = autosomal recessive; EBV = Epstein-Barr virus; XR = X-linked recessive.
Adapted from Fraumeni JF Jr: Epidemiology of cancer. *In* Wyngaarden JB, Smith LH Jr (eds): Cecil Textbook of Medicine. 18th ed. Philadelphia. WB Saunders, 1988, pp 1095–1096.

irradiation for Hodgkin's disease and phosphorus-32 for polycythemia vera, children exposed to x-rays prenatally, and patients irradiated in the distant past for nonmalignant conditions such as thymus enlargement. Radiation exerts its carcinogenic effects in a dose-dependent manner and spares no organ, although bone marrow, breast, and thyroid are the most radiation sensitive. The time lag varies: radiation-induced leukemia first appears at 2 to 5 years and peaks at 6 to 8 years, whereas solid tumors develop after a latency period of at least 5 to 10 years. Experts estimate that natural background irradiation (i.e., cosmic rays, radium, and other radionucleotides in the earth's crust) causes fewer than 2% of all cancers. Exposure to ultraviolet irradiation, however, is the major risk factor for the development of melanoma and nonmelanoma skin cancers.

Genetic Susceptibility

More than 200 single gene disorders have been linked to the development of neoplasms. Certain genes create a >90% risk of developing cancer (hereditary retinoblastoma, familial polyposis coli, Li-Fraumeni syndrome). Table 54–2 lists some hereditary neoplasms and preneoplastic syndromes. Most cancers demonstrate a minor familial component (twofold to threefold excess risk). Exceptions include early and multifocal breast and colon cancers, in both of which familial risks increase to 20 to 30 times that of the general population. Appropriate management of hereditary cancers includes avoidance of environmental carcinogens (e.g., ultraviolet light in the dysplastic nevus syndrome), prophylactic treatment (e.g., colectomy in polyposis coli), early detection (e.g., thyrocalcitonin determinations in multiple endocrine neoplasia), and genetic counseling (e.g., retinoblastoma).

SCREENING FOR EARLY CANCER DETECTION

Periodic, thorough physical examinations as well as analyses of simple blood tests (i.e., a complete blood count and routine chemistries) and urine are critical for the early detection of malignancy. Rectal, breast, and testicular examinations are the most effective means of diagnosing early cancers of the prostate and rectum, breast, and testes, respectively. A microcytic anemia in a nonmenstruating patient should alert one to the possibility of an occult gastrointestinal malignancy. Similarly, microscopic hematuria in an asymptomatic patient should prompt a search for a bladder or kidney cancer.

More complex screening procedures must take into account cost-benefit ratios. Costs include not only the dollar cost to society, but the risk of the procedure to the individual. Costs can be reduced by using epidemiologically derived data to restrict screening to (1) individuals at highest risk of developing cancer and (2) cancers whose early detection and treatment lead to significantly increased survival.

The American Cancer Society recommends screening as detailed in Table 54–3. Only one of the recommendations results from controlled, randomized, prospective clinical trials: mammography in women over the age of 40 years. The basis for the remaining recommendations is less firm. The recommendations do not include chest radiographs and sputum cytologies even in populations at high risk for developing lung cancer, as several studies demonstrate that this approach fails to detect lung cancers at an effectively treatable stage.

Tumor Markers

Routine radiographs rarely detect tumor masses <1 cm^3, a size that reflects approximately 1 billion tumor cells. This has prompted a search for tumor-specific products—tumor markers—in body fluids. A number of available tumor markers are useful as indices of response to treatment and early disease recurrence (Table 54–4). How-

TABLE 54–3	American Cancer Society Recommendations for Screening of Asymptomatic Individuals		
Test	**Sex**	**Age**	**Frequency**
Sigmoidoscopy	M & F	Over 50 yr	Every 3–5 yr after 2 negative examinations 1 yr apart
Stool guaiac test	M & F	Over 50 yr	Every year
Digital rectal examination	M & F	Over 40 yr	Every year
Papanicolaou (PAP) test	F	All women who have reached age 18 yr or have been sexually active	Every year*
Pelvic examination			
Endometrial biopsy	F	High-risk† or menopausal on estrogen therapy	Every year
Breast self-examination	F	Over 20 yr	Every month
Breast physical examination	F	20–40 yr	Every 3 yr
		Over 40 yr	Every year
Mammography	F	35–39 yr	One baseline study
		40–49 yr	Every 1–2 yr
		Over 50 yr	Every year
Health counseling	M & F	Over 20 yr	Every 3 yr
Cancer check-up‡	M & F	Over 40 yr	Every year

* After three or more consecutive satisfactory normal annual examinations, PAP test may be done less frequently at the discretion of the physician.
† History of infertility, obesity, failure of ovulation, abnormal uterine bleeding, or estrogen therapy.
‡ To include examination for cancers of the thyroid, testicles, prostate, ovaries, lymph nodes, oral region, and skin.

ever, lack of sensitivity and specificity precludes their use as screening tests for asymptomatic populations.

SYSTEMIC EFFECTS OF CANCER

Most symptoms caused by cancer are due to the physical presence of the tumor. Common examples are headache caused by brain metastases from lung cancer, backache from prostatic metastases to the spine, and jaundice caused by biliary tract obstruction from a pancreatic cancer. Cancer also can cause indirect effects on the host. Some of these effects are common, generalized, and poorly understood (e.g., anorexia). Some less common effects such as cerebellar degeneration are known as paraneoplastic syndromes and are due to tumor-related mediators, some of which are now well defined.

Anorexia and Cachexia

Complex factors act to produce tumor cachexia. They include anorexia due to aberrations in taste and smell, depression, and malaise; gastrointestinal dysfunction due to obstruction and the deleterious effects of chemotherapy, radiation, and surgery; and increased catabolism due to fever, tumor-induced alterations in protein and energy metabolism, and loss of protein into third spaces (e.g., ascites).

TABLE 54–4	Tumor Markers Useful in Following Known Malignancies	
Tumor Marker*	**Positive in Some**	**False Positives in**
Carcinoembryonic antigen (CEA)	Gastrointestinal (GI), lung, breast cancers	Smokers, cirrhotics Inflammatory bowel disease Rectal polyps Pancreatitis
Alpha-fetoprotein (αFP)	Hepatocellular, gastric, pancreatic, colon, and lung cancers Nonseminomatous germ cell cancers	Pregnancy Alcoholic and viral hepatitis Cirrhosis
Human chorionic gonadotrophin (beta subunit of hCG)	Trophoblastic tumors Germ cell neoplasms Adenocarcinomas of ovary Pancreatic, gastric, and hepatocellular cancers	Pregnancy (the alpha subunit crossreacts with luteinizing hormone)
Prostate-specific antigen	Prostatic cancer (especially if bony metastases are present), myeloma, bony metastases from nonprostatic cancers	Benign prostatic hypertrophy, osteoporosis, hyperthyroidism, hyperparathyroidism
CA 125 (ovarian tumor marker)	80% of ovarian cancer 20% of nongynecologic cancers	1% healthy control, 5% benign diseases
Beta$_2$-microglobulin	Multiple myeloma	

* Note that none of these tumor markers is specific enough to be useful in screening programs, except possibly prostate-specific antigen.

TABLE 54–5	Hematologic Manifestations of Malignancy	
Manifestation	**Associated Tumors**	**Contributing Factors**
Anemia	About 50% of all advanced malignancies	Chronic disease; extrinsic blood loss; bone marrow invasion by tumor or suppression by therapy; autoimmune hemolytic anemia; disseminated intravascular coagulation (DIC); microangiopathic hemolytic anemia; erosion of the tumor into a blood vessel; splenic sequestration
Thrombocytopenia	Lymphoma, chronic lymphocytic leukemia (CLL), carcinoma	Immune thrombocytopenia
Erythrocytosis	Hepatoma, hypernephroma, cerebellar hemangioblastoma	Inappropriate production of erythropoietin
Leukemoid reaction	Carcinomas of lung, pancreas, stomach; hepatoma; lymphomas	Tumor necrosis; tumor elaboration of colony stimulating factors; marrow invasion by metastases
Eosinophilia	Lymphomas, especially Hodgkin's disease; melanoma; brain tumors	Tumor elaboration of eosinophilopoietin
Thrombocytosis	Carcinoma; lymphoma	
Bleeding diatheses	Myeloma; Waldenström's macroglobulinemia	Platelet dysfunction; abnormal fibrin polymerization
	Myeloproliferative diseases	Platelet dysfunction

Hypercoagulability
    Migratory thrombophlebitis (Trousseau's syndrome)
    Disseminated intravascular coagulation
    Nonbacterial thrombotic endocarditis
	Mucin-secreting adenocarcinoma of gastrointestinal tract; carcinomas of lung, breast, ovary, prostate	Tumor cell expression of tissue factor; mucin activation of Factor X; prothrombinase-promoting tumor cell activity

Hematologic Manifestations

Malignancy can cause prominent abnormalities in coagulation and all hematopoietic cell lines (Table 54–5). Most can be reversed only by successfully treating the underlying malignancy.

Endocrine Manifestations

Some tumors develop a remarkable capacity to express one or another of the body's natural hormones (Table 54–6). Such hormone production is usually independent of normal regulatory mechanisms.

Neurologic Manifestations

Metastases to the brain, epidural space, and meninges constitute the major cause of neurologic dysfunction in cancer patients. Neurologic symptoms may also result from metabolic abnormalities, opportunistic infections of the central nervous system, and vascular disease due to hemorrhage (intraparenchymal, subdural, and subarachnoid) and infarction (thrombotic and embolic).

Tables 119–2 and 119–3 list some of the remote effects of cancer on the central nervous system; these can be presenting signs of occult malignancy.

Cutaneous Manifestations

The skin is a common site of metastatic cancer. In addition, paraneoplastic skin lesions include a variety of erythemas (e.g., necrolytic migratory erythema), pigmented lesions (e.g., acanthosis nigricans), and miscellaneous lesions (e.g., dermatomyositis). They can occur before, concomitant with, or after the diagnosis of malignancy. Their association with malignancy may be specific (e.g., necro-

TABLE 54–6	Ectopic Hormones Produced by Malignancy	
Hormone	**Manifestations**	**Associated Tumors**
ACTH	Cushing syndrome (psychosis, hyperglycemia, generalized weakness)	Lung (especially oat cell); thymus; pancreas, medullary thyroid, pheochromocytoma
HHM factor	Hypercalcemia	Carcinomas of lung (especially epidermoid and large cell), kidney, head and neck, and ovary
Somatomedins (also called NSILA)	Hypoglycemia	Mesenchymal tumors (especially mesothelioma), hepatoma, adrenal carcinomas, gastrointestinal tumors
ADH	Hyponatremia, hyperosmolar urine, high urinary sodium concentration	Small cell carcinoma of lung
hCG	Gynecomastia in men; oligomenorrhea in premenopausal women	Germ cell tumors, lung cancer

ACTH = Corticotropin; ADH = antidiuretic hormone; hCG = human chorionic gonadotropin; HHM = humoral hypercalcemia of malignancy (a parathyroid hormone–like peptide); NSILA = nonsuppressible insulin-like activity.

lytic migratory erythema and glucagonoma) or generalized (e.g., dermatomyositis).

Renal Manifestations

Etiologies of renal dysfunction in malignancy include direct tumor or amyloid infiltration, urinary tract obstruction, electrolyte imbalances (e.g., hypercalcemia, hyperuricemia) and the toxicities of chemotherapy. Glomerular lesions associated with the nephrotic syndrome constitute the primary paraneoplastic manifestation. In Hodgkin's disease, the malignancy most commonly associated with the nephrotic syndrome, the prominent renal lesion is lipoid nephrosis. In contrast, membranous glomerulonephritis is the most frequent glomerular lesion observed in patients with carcinoma.

REFERENCES

Blot WJ: The epidemiology of cancer. *In* Bennett JC, Plum F (eds.): Cecil Textbook of Medicine. 20th ed. Philadelphia, WB Saunders, 1996, pp 1013–1017.

Devita VT, Hellman S, Rosenberg SA (eds.): Cancer: Principles and Practice of Oncology. 4th ed. Philadelphia, JB Lippincott, 1993.

Ponder BAJ (ed.): Genetics of malignant disease. Brit Med Bull 1994; 50:517–745.

55

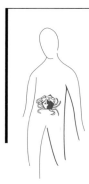

Principles of Cancer Therapy

Advances in the fields of surgery, radiation therapy, and medical oncology have made many cancers curable or amenable to palliation. This chapter outlines the basic principles governing the use of these modalities. Therapy of specific tumors is discussed in chapters related to diseases of the affected organ.

FORMING A TREATMENT PLAN

The first step in the evaluation of a patient diagnosed as having cancer is a thorough review of the diagnostic biopsy material with an experienced pathologist. Accurate classification of tumors and valuable prognostic information may be obtained by careful analysis of morphology, histochemical stains, cell surface immune markers, hormone receptors, karyotype, oncogene expression, and electron microscopic appearance. Certain malignancies such as lymphomas, leukemias, and lung cancers require accurate subclassification, because prognosis and treatment are different and distinct for the various subtypes.

Determination of the stage of the cancer at diagnosis is essential. Most cancers are staged according to the TNM system, which incorporates information about the size of the primary tumor (T), involvement of regional lymph nodes (N), and the presence or absence of metastases (M). Staging of lymphomas and hematologic malignancies is discussed in Chapter 50. This requires knowledge of the usual pattern of metastasis for the neoplasm in question. Staging procedures, particularly if invasive or costly, should be carried out only if the derived information will alter the therapeutic approach or significantly change the prognosis. Low-yield procedures, such as bone scans in asymptomatic patients with localized breast cancer, should be avoided.

The biologic aggressiveness and curability of the tumor must be assessed. Patients with indolent malignancies such as early-stage chronic lymphocytic leukemia and systemic low-grade lymphomas are not curable with available chemotherapy and often can be safely followed without therapy for several years. In contrast, those with biologically aggressive high-grade lymphomas are eminently curable with combination chemotherapy and should generally be treated even in the absence of symptoms.

Patients with curable malignancies (e.g., Hodgkin's disease) should receive an optimal therapeutic regimen that is not compromised in any way, as the potential toxicities of treatment are generally justified. Even when curative therapy is available, however, patients with serious underlying medical conditions may not be suitable candidates.

In patients with incurable cancers, one often can achieve a significant prolongation of survival. In these instances, the physician must consider the probability of extending meaningful survival as well as the impact of the therapeutic program on the quality of the patient's remaining life. Ultimately, effective palliation of symptoms and improvement of the functional status and quality of life of the incurable cancer patient represent the physician's twin objectives. Effective palliation requires close observation for the development and treatment of the complications of malignancy, such as bony metastases, metabolic disturbances, visceral obstruction, persistent pain, and emotional distress.

PRINCIPLES OF ONCOLOGIC SURGERY

Definitive surgical resection with attainment of tumor-free margins is the treatment of choice for the majority of localized solid tumors. However, because many malignant tumors have already micrometastasized at the time of diagnosis, surgery is increasingly being integrated with other modalities to achieve local as well as distant disease control and to minimize the magnitude and morbidity of operative procedures. For example, conservative surgery, local radiation therapy, and adjuvant chemotherapy are widely applied to the treatment of localized breast cancer as well as to childhood rhabdomyosarcoma. In rare circumstances, such as with solitary lung metastases in sarcoma patients and solitary hepatic metastases in colorectal cancer patients, resection of isolated metastases may be curative. Although not itself curative, cytoreductive or debulking surgery plays a role in the treatment of some cancers (e.g., ovarian), presumably by increasing the growth fraction of the remaining cells, thereby rendering them more susceptible to the effects of chemotherapy.

Regional lymph node dissection, as in axillary lymph node sampling for breast cancer, provides prognostic information about the likelihood of distant tumor recurrence and serves as a guide to the administration of adjuvant therapy.

Surgical intervention also can offer palliation of symptoms resulting from complications of cancer such as intestinal or biliary obstruction, hemorrhage (e.g., from gastric carcinoma), perforation (e.g., in the setting of chemotherapy for gastrointestinal lymphoma), and compression of vital structures (e.g., spinal cord compression). Reconstructive and plastic surgery also figures prominently in the rehabilitation of treated cancer patients. Examples include breast reconstruction after mastectomy and lysis of radiation-induced contractures.

PRINCIPLES OF RADIATION THERAPY

Radiation exerts its biologic effect by ejecting electrons from target molecules, a process called ionization. Ionizing radiation may interact with DNA directly or indirectly, the latter by generating free radicals. The biologic end point is loss of cellular reproductive capacity.

Radiation therapy is delivered in the form of electromagnetic waves such as x-rays or gamma rays or as streams of particles such as electrons. High-energy (megavoltage) beams in the form of gamma rays generated by radioactive isotopes (e.g., cobalt-60) or x-rays generated by linear accelerators are ideal for the treatment of visceral tumors, as they penetrate to great depths before reaching full intensity and thereby spare toxicity to skin. Electron beam irradiation is most useful in the treatment of superficial tumors, as energy is deposited at the skin and quickly dissipates, sparing toxicity to deeper tissues.

Fractionation

Radiation therapy is generally administered in fractions of 1.8 to 2.5 Gy (180 to 250 rads)/day, 5 days a week. Fractionation improves the therapeutic index (the margin of safety between therapeutic and toxic doses), presumably because sublethal radiation injury is repaired more effectively in normal tissues than in tumors. Weekend treatment breaks allow the patient to recover from acute toxicities and the tumor to regress and reoxygenate. Such improved oxygenation renders the tumor more susceptible to subsequent radiation therapy because hypoxic cells at the center of poorly vascularized neoplasms are two to three times more resistant to radiation than their well-oxygenated counterparts.

Clinical Considerations

The goal of radiation therapy is to deliver a tumoricidal dose while sparing normal tissues. The probability of both achieving tumor control and producing toxicity in normal tissue increases with dose in a sigmoid-curve relationship (Fig. 55–1). Greater separation of these curves results in an improved therapeutic index. The tumoricidal dose depends on the inherent radiation sensitivity of the neoplasm as well as its volume. The tumoricidal dose for

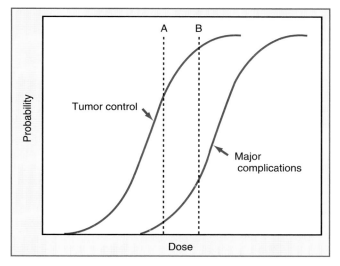

Figure 55–1

Sigmoid curves of tumor control and complications. *A,* Dose for tumor control with minimal complications. *B,* Maximum tumor dose with significant complications. (From Hellman S: Principles of radiation therapy. *In* Devita VT, Hellman S, Rosenberg SA [eds.]: Cancer: Principles and Practice of Oncology. 3rd ed. Philadelphia, JB Lippincott, 1989, p 1021; with permission.)

lymphomas, for example, is 40 to 50 Gy (4000 to 5000 rads), whereas that for most solid tumors ranges from 50 Gy for microscopic disease to 70 Gy for 4-cm tumors. The normal tissue tolerance to radiation also varies considerably (Table 55–1). Cell renewal tissues requiring rapid, continued proliferation for their function—skin, bone marrow, and gastrointestinal mucosa—are most vulnerable to acute toxicities (e.g., stomatitis, diarrhea, cytopenias). Late toxicities such as fibrosis, necrosis, and nonhealing ulcerations are determined by the total radiation dose and fraction size rather than by the proliferative potential of the affected tissue.

Radiation therapy is preferable to surgery in the management of localized tumors such as laryngeal carcinomas or certain deep-lying malignant brain tumors whose resection would be associated with significant

TABLE 55–1	Normal Tissue Tolerance to Radiation Therapy*	
Organ	**Toxicities**	**Dose Limit (Gy)†**
Bone marrow	Aplasia, pancytopenia	2.5
Liver	Acute and chronic hepatitis	25.0
Stomach, intestine	Ulceration, diarrhea, hemorrhage	45.0
Brain	Infarction, necrosis	60.0
Spinal cord	Infarction, necrosis	45.0
Heart	Pericarditis, pancarditis, coronary artery disease	45.0
Lung	Pneumonitis, fibrosis	15.0
Kidney	Nephrosclerosis	20.0
Skin	Dermatitis, sclerosis	55.0

* Assuming 2 Gy/fraction, 5 fractions/wk.
† Dose for 5% injury in 5 yr; 1 Gy = 100 rads.

functional impairment or mutilation. Tumors curable by radiation include Hodgkin's and non-Hodgkin's lymphomas, seminomas, and localized carcinomas of the larynx, cervix, and prostate.

Radiation therapy is frequently administered in an "adjuvant" setting with surgery, chemotherapy, or both. Postoperative adjuvant radiation therapy may eradicate residual foci of microscopic tumor and decrease the likelihood of local recurrence. It may also permit a more conservative surgical approach, such as is attained by employing lumpectomy and radiation therapy rather than mastectomy for localized breast cancers. The addition of adjuvant chemotherapy in such a setting may further increase the likelihood of cure by eradicating occult distant micrometastases. Examples of this principle include the administration of adjuvant radiation therapy and chemotherapy after resection of localized breast and rectal carcinomas. Adjuvant radiation therapy to sanctuary sites, such as the central nervous system and testes, which are not accessible to systemic chemotherapy, increases the likelihood of cure in malignancies such as acute lymphocytic leukemia and small cell lung cancer.

Chemotherapy and radiation therapy are combined in the primary treatment of a number of malignancies, including bulky Hodgkin's lymphomas, limited-stage small cell lung cancer, and anal carcinoma. In another dimension, chemoradiation therapy is administered in supralethal doses as a preparative regimen for bone marrow transplantation (discussed later).

Radiation therapy can be a potent palliative modality, as is illustrated in the treatment of painful bony metastases. It is also employed as the primary therapy for many oncologic emergencies, including the superior vena cava syndrome, spinal cord compression, and brain metastases.

PRINCIPLES OF CHEMOTHERAPY

Many cancers have established metastatic clones by the time they become clinically detectable. Systemic chemotherapy and hormonal therapy play a major role in the management of the 60% of cancer patients who are not curable by regional modalities. The advent of effective combination chemotherapy has produced cures in a number of advanced malignancies (Table 55–2) and meaningful remissions in many others (Table 55–3).

Tumor Kinetics

Exponentially growing tumors double approximately 30 times before becoming clinically detectable (10^9 cells give a 1-cm mass). Each tumor has a characteristic doubling time ranging from 2 to 5 days for Burkitt's lymphoma to over 100 days for adenocarcinomas of the lung and breast. Tumor kinetics are best described by the Gompertz growth curve (Fig. 55–2)—over a short time, tumor growth appears exponential; with time, a progressively greater percentage of the cell population enters a nonproliferative pool by virtue of cell death, differentiation, and entry into the G_0 or resting phase of the cell

TABLE 55–2	Adult Tumors Curable with Chemotherapy

Tumor	Long-Term Disease-Free Survival (%)
Choriocarcinoma	90
Burkitt's lymphoma (stage I)	90
Testicular carcinoma	90
Diffuse large cell non-Hodgkin's lymphoma	50–60
Hodgkin's disease	60
Acute lymphocytic leukemia	35–45
Acute myelogenous leukemia	20
Ovarian carcinoma	10–20
Small cell lung carcinoma	10

cycle. Eventually, a plateau is reached, where the rate of new cell production equals that of cell death. The exponential increase in the proportion of nonproliferating cells decreases the susceptibility of large tumors to antineoplastic agents, which are most active against rapidly dividing cells. This principle provides the rationale for "debulking" tumors (by surgery or irradiation) so as to recruit residual G_0 cells into an active proliferative state with an enhanced susceptibility to chemotherapy.

Most chemotherapeutic agents exploit kinetic differences between normal and malignant cells by acting preferentially on dividing cells. Such "cell cycle–specific" agents (e.g., cyclophosphamide, methotrexate, cytosine arabinoside) achieve a kill rate of certain lymphoproliferative tumor cells that is several thousandfold greater than that of bone marrow stem cells that are partially in a resting phase. This results in rapidly reversible cytopenias but permanent tumor eradication.

Mechanisms of Action of Antineoplastic Drugs

All chemotherapeutic agents act by interfering with cell division. Antimetabolites, acting as fraudulent analogues of vital physiologic substrates, inhibit the synthesis of

TABLE 55–3	Adult Tumors Responsive to Chemotherapy

Tumor	Partial or Complete Response (%)
Chronic lymphocytic leukemia	75
Chronic myeloproliferative disorders	80
Hairy cell leukemia	75
Multiple myeloma	75
Low- and intermediate-grade non-Hodgkin's lymphoma	80
Mycosis fungoides	75
Breast carcinoma	65
Bladder carcinoma	40–50
Gastric carcinoma	35
Head and neck carcinoma	65
Ovarian carcinoma	75
Prostate carcinoma	75
Islet cell tumors	50

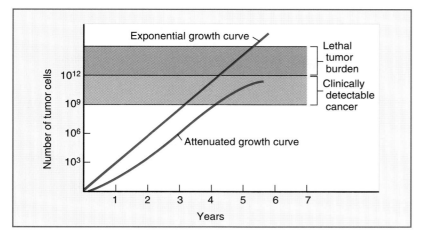

Figure 55–2

A schematic plot to describe models of exponential and gompertzian growth curves. (From Chabner BA: Introduction to oncology. *In* Wyngaarden JB, Smith LH Jr, Bennett JC [eds.]: Cecil Textbook of Medicine. 19th ed. Philadelphia, WB Saunders, 1992, p 1021.)

DNA or their nucleotide building blocks. Examples include methotrexate, a folic acid analogue; cytosine arabinoside, a pyrimidine analogue; and 6-mercaptopurine, a purine analogue. Alkylating agents such as cyclophosphamide chemically interact with DNA. They contain highly reactive alkyl groups that cause DNA breaks and cross-link complementary DNA strands that prevent replication. Cisplatin, a heavy metal compound, achieves its cytotoxicity by a similar mechanism. Many of the antitumor antibiotics, such as the anthracyclines, daunomycin and doxorubicin, intercalate themselves between strands of the DNA double helix and thereby inhibit DNA, RNA, and ultimately protein synthesis. The vinca alkaloids, vincristine and vinblastine, are plant products that arrest cells in the metaphase of mitosis by binding to tubulin and thereby inhibit microtubular function. The enzyme L-asparaginase depletes cells of the nonessential amino acid asparagine. Most human tissues have the capacity to synthesize asparagine by the action of L-asparagine synthetase. Some tumor cells, particularly those of T cell line-

age, lack this enzyme. As a result, depletion of circulating pools of asparagine by L-asparaginase results in inhibition of protein synthesis and ultimately cytotoxicity.

Toxicity

Safe administration of antineoplastic drugs, with their narrow therapeutic indices, requires knowledge of their routes of metabolism and elimination. Dose modification in the setting of renal or hepatic dysfunction minimizes toxicity. Major dose modifications of the anthracyclines and vinca alkaloids are required when hepatic dysfunction exists and of cisplatin, methotrexate, streptozotocin, bleomycin, and hydroxyurea when azotemia is present. The toxic manifestations of chemotherapy are legion and spare no organ. The patterns of toxicity of some commonly used drugs are outlined in Table 55–4.

Dose Intensity

Most antineoplastic agents produce a steep dose-response curve. Dose intensity and dose rate (drug delivered per unit time) are powerful determinants of response to therapy and overall survival. The strong correlation between the dose and cure rates of chemosensitive malignancies such as Hodgkin's disease justifies the enhanced toxicity of aggressive treatment in these settings.

Resistance to Chemotherapy

The major cause of treatment failure is drug resistance. Although most neoplasms arise from a single clone, random mutations lead to marked cellular heterogeneity with regard to radiation sensitivity and susceptibility to cytotoxic drugs. The probability of drug resistance within a tumor is proportional to the size of the neoplasm and the rate at which the drug-resistant gene mutates (Goldie-Coldman hypothesis). This principle explains the greater curability of small cancers with a low likelihood of drug resistance and the relative refractoriness of widely meta-

TABLE 55–4	Major Toxicities of Commonly Used Cancer Chemotherapeutic Agents
Effect	**Examples**
Short-Term	
Nausea, vomiting	Cisplatin, doxorubicin
Alopecia	Doxorubicin
Myelosuppression	Alkylating agents
	Cyclophosphamide
	Methotrexate
	Etoposide
Hypersensitivity	Bleomycin, L-asparaginase
Tissue necrosis	Doxorubicin, vincristine
Stomatitis	Methotrexate
Renal failure	Cisplatin
Hemorrhagic cystitis	Cyclophosphamide
Ileus	Vincristine
Long-Term	
Leukemia	Alkylating agents
Cardiomyopathy	Doxorubicin
Pulmonary fibrosis	Bleomycin
Hemolytic-uremic syndrome	Mitomycin
Peripheral neuropathy	Vincristine, cisplatin, paclitaxel
Premature menopause, sterility	Alkylating agents

static cancers that are likely to contain cells resistant to several drugs. Many solid tumors have long doubling times because of a high rate of cell loss; by the time they become clinically detectable (approximately 30 doublings), they have undergone numerous divisions and mutational events. This biologic characteristic may account for their relative resistance to chemotherapy compared with rapidly dividing lymphoproliferative malignancies such as high-grade lymphomas. The practice of giving adjuvant chemotherapy shortly after tumor resection when the systemic tumor burden is low derives from this principle. Such an approach may bring a cure to patients with malignancies that have a propensity to recur, such as breast and rectal carcinomas and osteogenic and soft-tissue sarcomas.

Chemotherapy selectively eradicates sensitive tumor clones and permits the overgrowth of resistant cell populations. Mechanisms of drug resistance include impaired drug uptake or activation, enhanced drug inactivation, increased expression of the target enzyme by gene amplification, and altered target proteins. Some tumor cells develop pleiotropic (multidrug) resistance to several classes of drugs that are structurally and functionally distinct (vinca alkaloids, anthracyclines, dacarbazine). Such multidrug-resistant cells contain amplified gene sequences that encode a 170-kd protein, P-glycoprotein, involved in drug efflux. Overexpression of this protein results in decreased intracellular drug accumulation and clinical resistance.

Combination Chemotherapy

The cure of advanced malignancies, when possible, has been achieved primarily with combination chemotherapy. The rationale for combination regimens stems from the fact that antineoplastic agents have diverse mechanisms of action. Hence, tumor cells resistant to one drug may still be sensitive to another. The most effective regimens consist of drugs that are individually effective against the neoplasm and have nonoverlapping toxicities, thereby permitting administration of full dosage of all drugs (e.g., mustard, Oncovin [vincristine], procarbazine, prednisone [MOPP] for Hodgkin's disease). Proper scheduling of combination regimens is integral to their efficacy. The administration of nonmyelosuppressive drugs, such as bleomycin or methotrexate, with leucovorin rescue between cycles of myelotoxic drugs, such as the alkylating agents or anthracyclines, allows the bone marrow to recover despite continued treatment. Treatment breaks of 2 to 3 weeks between cycles also permit recovery of sensitive normal tissues, such as gastrointestinal mucosa and bone marrow. Newer approaches include instituting alternating cycles of equally effective non–cross-resistant combinations and the early introduction of all effective drugs in an effort to prevent the emergence of resistance.

As mentioned previously, combination chemotherapy has been successfully integrated with radiation therapy in the treatment of certain cancers such as bulky Hodgkin's disease. A regimen of high-dose chemotherapy and total body irradiation followed by reconstitution with allogeneic or autologous bone marrow or peripheral blood stem cells has been administered with varying degrees of success to patients with acute and chronic leukemias, refractory lymphomas, and a number of chemoradiation-sensitive solid tumors, including small cell lung, breast, ovarian, and testicular cancers. Allogeneic human leukocyte antigen (HLA)–matched bone marrow transplantation has become the treatment of choice for younger patients with chronic myelogenous leukemia in chronic phase, acute lymphocytic leukemia in second remission, and acute myelogenous leukemia in relapse. Bone marrow transplantation as a treatment of refractory lymphomas and solid tumors is promising but remains experimental in view of its extreme toxicities, which include interstitial pneumonitis, graft-versus-host disease, opportunistic infections, and hepatic veno-occlusive disease.

HORMONAL THERAPY

A number of cancers, most notably breast and prostate, respond to manipulations of their hormonal milieu. Manipulation involves alteration in steroid hormone levels or their activity. Steroid hormones enter the cell and bind to cytoplasmic receptors. The hormone-receptor complex is translocated to the nucleus, where it influences the transcription of messenger RNA for growth-inhibitory or -stimulatory proteins.

Steroid antagonists, such as the antiestrogen tamoxifen used in the treatment of breast cancer, compete with endogenous hormones for binding to receptor sites. Hormone antagonist-receptor complexes fail to initiate transcription changes induced by the native hormone. Estrogen and progesterone receptor levels in breast cancer tissue correlate well with hormonal dependence and predict responsiveness to hormonal therapy.

Aminoglutethimide inhibits adrenal steroidogenesis by blocking the enzymatic conversion of cholesterol to pregnenolone as well as the aromatization in peripheral tissues of androgens to estrone, a major source of estrogen in postmenopausal women. This agent has almost entirely replaced surgical adrenalectomy in the treatment of breast cancer.

Estrogens such as diethylstilbestrol and analogues of luteinizing hormone–releasing hormone, which are potent inhibitors of testosterone production, help to palliate prostate cancer.

Glucocorticoids are used extensively in the treatment of lymphomas, lymphocytic leukemias, multiple myeloma, and breast cancer.

BIOLOGIC RESPONSE MODIFIERS

Human beings possess cellular and humoral antitumor capacity. Three classes of cytotoxic lymphocytes exist—lymphokine-activated killer (LAK) cells, natural killer cells, and natural cytotoxic cells. Biologic substances such as interferons and interleukins potentiate the antitumor effects of lymphocytes. The reinfusion of LAK cells that are derived from patients with renal cell carcinoma and malignant melanoma and then expanded *in vitro* with exogenous interleukin-2 (IL-2) has produced significant regressions of these chemoresistant tumors. Broad application of this technique has been limited by its serious toxicities, which include a capillary leak syndrome, hypotension, and marked fluid retention.

Naturally occurring products of lymphocytes (lymphokines), such as interferons, are antiproliferative and immunomodulatory and are endowed with direct antitumor activity. Alpha-interferon has been successfully used to treat hairy cell leukemia, chronic myelogenous leukemia, and low-grade non-Hodgkin's lymphomas. More modest responses have been observed with solid tumors such as renal cell carcinoma and Kaposi's sarcoma.

Monoclonal antibodies against specific tumor antigens have been utilized in purging autologous bone marrow from patients with B cell lymphoma and acute lymphocytic leukemia. Similarly, T cell antibodies have been used to purge allogeneic marrow of T lymphocytes in order to prevent graft-versus-host disease. The use of monoclonal antibodies against the idiotype of the immunoglobulin on the surface of B cell lymphomas and leukemias has also been attempted but has met with limited success owing to the emergence of mutations within the idiotype.

REFERENCES

Chabner BA, Longo DL (eds.): Cancer Chemotherapy and Biotherapy: Principles and Practice. 2nd ed. Philadelphia, Lippincott-Raven, 1996.

Drugs of choice for cancer chemotherapy. Med Lett 1995; 37:25–32.

Salmon SE, Bertino JR: Principles of cancer therapy. *In* Bennett JC, Plum F (eds.): Cecil Textbook of Medicine. 20th ed. Philadelphia, WB Saunders, 1996, pp 1036–1049.

56

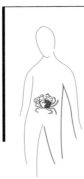

Oncologic Emergencies

The natural history of malignancies leads to several types of medical emergencies. Many gastrointestinal and genitourinary tumors present with acute obstruction or hemorrhage. Bone marrow infiltrated by tumor or suppressed by chemotherapy can lead to life-threatening infection. Tumor erosion into a blood vessel and tumor- or treatment-induced thrombocytopenia can precipitate life-threatening hemorrhage. Other types of oncologic emergencies include those summarized in Table 56–1, a few of which are discussed in detail here.

HYPERCALCEMIA

Hypercalcemia occurs in 10 to 20% of cancer patients. It is seen in association with solid tumors in the presence (e.g., breast cancer) or absence (e.g., renal cell and squamous cell lung cancers) of bone metastases as well as with hematologic malignancies (e.g., myeloma and adult T cell lymphoma). Tumor cells in bone can directly stimulate bone resorption or induce bone resorption by secreting cytokines (interleukin-1, tumor necrosis factors) or prostaglandin E_2. Tumor-derived parathyroid hormone–like peptides and growth factors appear to be important humoral mediators of cancer-associated hypercalcemia.

Common presenting symptoms include an altered mental status (ranging from apathy to coma), generalized muscle weakness, nausea and vomiting, abdominal pain, polyuria (resulting from a reversible renal tubular defect in urine concentrating ability), and polydipsia. Clinical findings associated with hypercalcemia include an altered mental status, dehydration, renal insufficiency, hyporeflexia, pancreatitis, peptic ulcer, hypertension, cardiac arrhythmias, prolonged PR interval, shortened QT interval, and widening of the T wave on electrocardiogram (ECG).

Although definitive treatment of hypercalcemia requires tumor control, interim therapy should be aimed at enhancing calcium excretion and diminishing calcium resorption from bone.

Repleting intravascular volume is of primary importance in the management of hypercalcemia. This enhances the glomerular filtration rate and increases the clearance rates of sodium and calcium. Once the patient is euvolemic, a diuretic such as furosemide, which diminishes renal tubular reabsorption of sodium and calcium and promotes calciuresis, may be administered. During this time, fluid and electrolyte balance must be carefully monitored and congestive heart failure vigorously treated. Such therapy usually lowers serum calcium by 2 to 4 mg/dl within 24 hours.

Glucocorticoids are most useful in the treatment of hypercalcemia associated with hematologic malignancies and breast cancer, as they are effective antineoplastic agents in these diseases. Steroids also act by decreasing intestinal absorption and increasing renal excretion of calcium, as well as by blocking activation of osteoclasts by osteoclast-activating factors and reducing prostaglandin synthesis. Calcium levels decline only after several days of steroid therapy.

Refractory hypercalcemia may be treated with the antitumor antibiotic mithramycin, which directly inhibits bone resorption. Its effects are usually detectable within 24 to 48 hours and can last for a week or more. The adverse effects of mithramycin (including bone marrow suppression, postural hypotension, and hepatocellular and renal damage) limit its usefulness as a first-line agent.

Calcitonin, a polypeptide hormone secreted by thyroid parafollicular cells, is moderately effective in treating malignancy-associated hypercalcemia. Its hypocalcemic effect is due to inhibition of bone resorption and is manifest within hours of administration. Concomitant administration of steroids may prolong its hypocalcemic effect.

Diphosphonates, synthetic analogues of pyrophosphate, inhibit osteoclastic bone resorption and are effective in treating malignancy-associated hypercalcemia.

Oral phosphates can be used for chronic maintenance of normocalcemia, but their use should be limited to patients with normal renal function who are not hyperphosphatemic.

SPINAL CORD COMPRESSION

Extradural spinal cord compression (SCC) is found at autopsy in as many as 5% of patients with cancer. Vertebral or occasionally paravertebral metastases derived from carcinomas of the lung, breast, and prostate, as well as lymphoma and myeloma, account for most cases.

Back pain, with or without a radicular component, is the presenting symptom in nearly all patients with SCC; the pain is frequently worse when the patient is supine.

TABLE 56–1 Some Oncologic Emergencies

Type of Emergency	Most Common Manifestations	Most Common Etiologies
Hemodynamic		
Superior vena cava syndrome	Superficial thoracic vein collaterals Neck vein distention Facial edema Tachypnea	Bronchogenic carcinoma Lymphoma
Pericardial tamponade	Congestive heart failure (CHF)–like symptoms Kussmaul's sign Pulsus paradoxus Distant heart sounds	Lung carcinoma Breast carcinoma Lymphoma
Hyperviscosity syndrome	Confusion, coma Stroke Hypervolemia Retinopathy	Waldenström's macroglobulinemia Myeloma
Thrombosis	Trousseau's syndrome (migratory thrombophlebitis) Nonbacterial thrombotic endocarditis (NBTE) Disseminated intravascular coagulation (DIC)	Mucinous adenocarcinomas Myeloproliferative disorders Prostatic carcinoma Acute promyelocytic leukemia
Neurologic		
Increased intracranial pressure	Mental status changes Seizures Signs of herniation	Brain metastases Primary brain tumors Carcinomatous or lymphomatous meningitis
Spinal cord compression	Pain (usually radicular) Weakness Autonomic dysfunction Sensory abnormalities	Carcinoma of lung, breast, prostate Lymphoma Myeloma
Metabolic		
Hypercalcemia	Anorexia, nausea, and vomiting Abdominal pain Apathy, coma Muscle weakness Polyuria, azotemia Cardiac conduction abnormalities	Carcinoma of breast, lung, kidney, head, and neck Myeloma
"Tumor lysis syndrome"	Acute renal failure	Undifferentiated lymphomas (particularly Burkitt's and lymphoblastic lymphomas) Acute lymphoblastic leukemia Anaplastic small cell carcinoma
Hypoglycemia	Confusion, loss of consciousness	Insulinoma Mesenchymal tumors Hepatoma
Hyponatremia	Confusion, coma Seizures Anorexia	SIADH (usually small cell carcinoma)

SIADH = Syndrome of inappropriate antidiuretic hormone.

Later signs and symptoms include weakness, sensory loss, autonomic dysfunction, and ataxia.

Unless diagnosed and treated early, SCC leads to irreversible neurologic deficits, making prompt diagnosis and initiation of appropriate treatment a crucial matter. A high index of suspicion must be employed in any older patient presenting with back pain of recent onset, especially if there is a history of malignancy. Once SCC enters into the differential diagnosis of neurologic symptoms, diagnostic and therapeutic measures must be undertaken immediately. Interim medical management includes the use of high-dose steroid therapy in an attempt to decrease pressure on the cord.

Although plain films are likely to demonstrate extensive vertebral involvement or destruction by tumor, magnetic resonance imaging (MRI) or myelography is re-quired to diagnose SCC, to demonstrate the number of lesions, and to define the upper and lower margins of the blockage to free flow of spinal fluid. If myelography is performed, spinal fluid should be obtained for cell count and chemical and cytologic analysis. In the rare case that myelography is contraindicated and MRI is unavailable, computed tomography (CT) scanning with contrast enhancement can be helpful.

Available treatment approaches are listed in Table 115–10. They include radiation therapy and surgical decompression with or without postoperative radiation. Surgery causes more morbidity and mortality and is usually reserved for: (1) cases in which there has not been a previous diagnosis of malignancy and there is no more accessible site for biopsy, (2) lesions known to be radiation resistant, and (3) tumors involving areas already

TABLE 56–2	Management of Increased Intracranial Pressure from Brain Tumors

Stable Patient

1. Dexamethasone (or equivalent corticosteroid), 4 mg qid po; double q48h as necessary to control symptoms

Unstable Patient (Cerebral Herniation)

1. Dexamethasone, 100 mg IV stat; continue at 24 mg qid
2. Mannitol, 0.5–1 gm/kg IV stat; repeat as necessary
3. Intubate; control ventilation to keep Pa_{CO_2} at 25–30 mm Hg

IV = Intravenous.

treated with radiation. In certain instances, chemotherapy can be used as adjunct therapy but is not recommended as the primary mode of treatment.

In general, neurologic prognosis (sphincter control and independence of ambulation) depends on the degree of impairment when treatment is initiated and on the radiation sensitivity of the primary tumor.

INCREASED INTRACRANIAL PRESSURE

Patients with mass lesions or diffuse infiltrative processes such as lymphomatous or carcinomatous meningitis may present with signs and symptoms of increased intracranial pressure (ICP).

Early signs of increased ICP include headache, seizures, lethargy, confusion, and papilledema. Additional signs and symptoms of neurologic dysfunction reflect the anatomic site of metastasis. An MRI scan with contrast enhancement is the safest and most reliable diagnostic test and should be promptly obtained in all patients with suspected mass lesions in the brain. Prompt recognition of the cause of increased ICP and rapid institution of medical therapy (prior to definitive diagnosis and treatment of the precipitating cancer) are essential for preservation of cerebral function.

While definitive diagnostic and therapeutic measures are being planned and executed, medical therapy including pharmacologic doses of intravenous steroids, diuretics, and fluid restriction can temporarily decrease ICP (Table 56–2). Anticonvulsant therapy is not routinely administered except to patients presenting with seizures. Patients with elevated ICP, carcinomatous meningitis, and melanoma have seizures more frequently and should be considered for prophylactic anticonvulsant therapy.

Care must be taken to exclude nonmalignant intracranial masses, particularly in patients without a previous diagnosis of malignancy or widely disseminated cancer. For example, there is an increased incidence of benign meningioma in women with breast cancer. Similarly, brain abscesses occur more commonly in the immunocompromised cancer patient. Radiation-induced brain necrosis may be difficult to differentiate from recurrent tumor. Surgical intervention is indicated in these instances of uncertain diagnosis.

Once a diagnosis of brain metastasis is established, radiation therapy should be instituted promptly. Fifty to 75% of patients so treated demonstrate neurologic improvement, although in many, tumors eventually recur.

SUPERIOR VENA CAVA SYNDROME

The onset of a superior vena cava (SVC) syndrome creates a subacute or acute medical emergency whose diagnosis and treatment usually require the multidisciplinary efforts of the medical oncologist, surgeon, and radiation therapist. The SVC is the major venous channel for blood return from the head, neck and upper extremities, and thorax. A thin-walled vessel enclosed in a relatively unyielding compartment, its low intravascular pressures make it particularly vulnerable to extrinsic compression by an adjacent mass.

Common presenting symptoms include distended thoracic and neck veins, facial edema, tachypnea, cyanosis, upper extremity edema, Horner's syndrome, and vocal cord paralysis. Chest radiography almost invariably shows a mass—usually in the right superior mediastinum. Lung carcinoma and lymphoma cause most cases of the SVC syndrome; fewer than 5% result from benign causes such as thyroid goiter, pericardial constriction, idiopathic sclerosing mediastinitis, and thrombosis of the SVC.

Sputum cytology, bronchoscopy, mediastinoscopy, or lymph node biopsy usually yields a tissue diagnosis, although a diagnostic thoracotomy may be required.

Radiation therapy is generally the therapeutic modality of choice, although chemotherapy may be equally efficacious in patients with small cell lung carcinoma. The vast majority of patients have prompt palliation of symptoms. Failure to respond usually signifies thrombotic obstruction of the SVC. Supportive medical therapy with steroids, diuretics, anticoagulation, and (in the case of SVC thrombosis) fibrinolytic therapy may help to ameliorate symptoms.

REFERENCES

Morris JC, Holland JF: Oncologic emergencies. *In* Holland JF, Frei E, Bast RC, Kufe DW, Morton DL, Weichselbaum RR (eds.): Cancer Medicine. 4th ed. Philadelphia, Lea & Febiger, 1996.

Posner JB: Neurologic Complications of Cancer. Philadelphia, FA Davis, 1995.

Metabolic Disease

Section IX

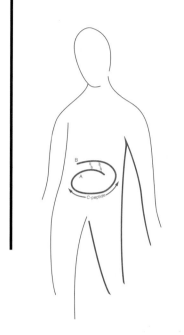

57

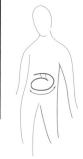

Introduction To Metabolic Disease

A disorder is classified as a disease of metabolism when the fundamental pathogenic mechanism includes one of numerous chemical transformations that occur within living organisms. Such chemical reactions are divided into two large categories. Anabolic reactions are usually energy requiring and generally result in the synthesis of molecules larger than those of the initial reactants. Catabolic reactions are energy-yielding processes that cause degradation of larger molecules into smaller products. Many diseases of metabolism involve specific enzyme defects that alter anabolic or catabolic processes. Defects that can be attributed to an underlying genetic abnormal-

ity are termed inborn errors of metabolism. Other metabolic diseases are acquired rather than hereditary.

The diseases discussed in this section are chiefly those whose manifestations are multisystemic or in which biochemical and genetic factors dominate the clinical presentation. A complete discussion of all known inborn errors of metabolism falls beyond the scope of this text. Many inborn errors are life limiting, leading to death in infancy or early childhood. This section focuses upon the more common hereditary or acquired metabolic diseases encountered in adults.

58

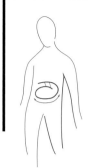

Eating Disorders

OBESITY

United States government task forces have defined *overweight* as the 85th percentile of the United States population aged 20 to 29 years. Application of sex-specific cutpoints shows that up to 50 million Americans are overweight, and 12 million are severely overweight.

Clinicians most frequently use body weight or preferably the body mass index (BMI) (weight [kg]/height [m]^2) to judge if a patient is "overweight." Very muscular individuals may be moderately overweight and not obese. Others with small frames and low muscle mass may be obese without fulfilling criteria for overweight. Nevertheless, most seriously overweight patients are also obese. An obesity classification scheme based on BMI is presented in Table 58–1.

Obesity and overweight are largely genetically determined and are strongly conditioned by available palatable food and sedentariness. A child of two obese parents has about an 80% chance of becoming obese, whereas the risk is only 15% for the offspring of two parents of normal weight. Moreover, a correlation between parental and child BMI is found across a broad spectrum of values, suggesting both polygenic inheritance of obesity and several contributing metabolic mechanisms. The precise causative mechanisms remain unknown.

Pathogenesis

How does obesity occur? Fat accounts for 21 to 37% of the weight of middle-aged men and women (Table 58–2). At some time in life, the obese individual consumed more calories than he or she expended *and* appetite was not subsequently reduced to compensate for the increase in stored energy. The usual tight regulation of the size of the adipose organ indicates that neural or humoral signals from the adipose organ are transmitted to the brain, which in turn regulates food seeking and consumption (Fig. 58–1). Failure of fat cells to send adequate signals or failure of the brain to respond to appropriate signals causes obesity (Table 58–3).

Mechanisms controlling fat cell size and numbers are still poorly understood. Several facts are clear. The enzyme lipoprotein lipase, produced by the adipocyte and residing on its capillary endothelium, permits fat cells to take up fatty acids from circulating chylomicrons (dietary fat) and very low density lipoproteins. Fat cells with enhanced lipoprotein lipase activity may have a competitive advantage in assimilating lipoprotein triglyceride. Adipocytes can also take up fatty acids circulating bound to albumin. Breakdown and release of adipocyte triglyceride are regulated by a second enzyme, hormone-sensitive lipase, which responds to signals increasing intracellular cyclic adenosine monophosphate (AMP) (i.e., circulating or neuronally derived catecholamines, glucagon, gonadotropins) and is inhibited by insulin (see Fig. 59–1). The adipocytes of obese individuals may resist lipolytic stimuli from nerves or circulating catecholamines. Gluteal fat in both men and women, for example, has a lower lipolytic response to alpha-adrenergic stimulation than does abdominal fat. Abdominal fat in men appears to have more alpha$_2$-adrenergic receptor function (antilipolytic) than abdominal fat in women, leading to the "beer belly" in men more often than in women.

Well-fed fat cells can grow to a maximum of 1 μg. Storage of more fat requires an increase in adipocyte number by differentiation of preadipocytes (see Fig. 59–1). The signal for this hyperplasia is unknown and is a critical link if excess caloric consumption can drive an increase in adipocyte number. The converse—that increased adipocyte number drives increased food intake—is also possible.

Well-fed fat cells elaborate a hormone, leptin, which circulates to the brain, binds to receptors, and in turn causes release of glucagon-like peptide-1 (GLP-1) or another neurotransmitter, that directly or indirectly suppresses appetite (see Fig. 59–1). GLP-1 is capable of inhibiting neuropeptide Y, the most powerful known stimulant of feeding. Some genetically obese mice do not produce leptin, but obese humans, perhaps because their adipocytes are so well fed, actually have high circulating leptin levels. It remains to be shown if obese humans have defective leptin receptors or defective synthesis of GLP-1 or another neurohormone in response to leptin stimulation.

Whatever the cause of obesity, the condition itself is intractable once it occurs. Increased fat cell numbers are maintained, and, when deprived of calories, fat cells seem to communicate their underfed status to the brain, thus stimulating appetite. Moreover, caloric restriction to

TABLE 58–1	Obesity Classification Based on Body Mass Index (BMI)*	
	Classification	**BMI**
	Underweight	<20
	Normal	20–25
	Overweight	25–30
	Obese	30–40
	Severely obese	>40

* In kilograms per square meter.

achieve weight loss is associated with reductions in energy expenditure in the obese to levels far below those in naturally lean individuals.

Anatomy

It has been puzzling that obesity is associated with risk factors for vascular disease, but that in prospective studies obesity is poorly predictive of vascular disease. Regional patterns of body fat distribution may partially explain this inconsistency. It appears that the form of obesity that characteristically occurs in men, called android or abdominal obesity, is closely associated with metabolic complications such as hypertension, insulin resistance, hyperuricemia, and dyslipoproteinemia. The typical female or gynecoid obesity, with fat deposited in hips and gluteal and femoral regions, has much less metabolic significance. The waist-to-hip circumference ratio has been used to distinguish these forms of obesity. In men, a ratio above 1.0 and in women above 0.6 suggests the undesirable male obesity pattern. Thus, it is better to be shaped like a pear than like an apple. The BMI range associated with the lowest mortality is 20 to 25 kg/m².

Medical Consequences

Clinically Severe Obesity

Subjects weighing 45 kg or 100 lb (~60%) more than desirable are designated severely obese. This corresponds to a weight of 240 lb in a woman 63 inches tall or 260 lb in a man of 68 inches. Cardiorespiratory problems present the greatest risk (Table 58–4). Chronic hypoventilation is

TABLE 58–2	Variation of Fat and Lean Body Mass (LBM) with Age			
	Men		**Women**	
Age	**LBM (% Body Weight)**	**Fat (% Body Weight)**	**LBM (% Body Weight)**	**Fat (% Body Weight)**
25	81	19	68	32
45	74	26	58	42
65	65	35	51	49

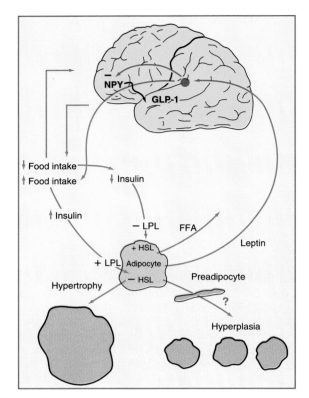

Figure 58–1
Pathogenesis of obesity. Increased food intake stimulates insulin secretion. Insulin, in turn, stimulates lipoprotein lipase (+LPL), permitting uptake of circulating triglyceride by the adipocyte, and insulin simultaneously inhibits hormone-sensitive lipase (−HSL) and the release of adipocyte free fatty acids (FFA). The overfed adipocyte may hypertrophy, or a stimulus, currently unknown, may trigger differentiation of preadipocytes. The well-fed adipocyte secretes leptin, which circulates and binds to receptors in the hypothalamus, causing glucagon-like peptide-1 (GLP-1) release and inhibiting neuropeptide-Y (NPY), a powerful stimulator of appetite and feeding. Reduced food intake, in contrast, lowers insulin, leading to LPL suppression, activation of HSL, and FFA release.

common and leads to hypercapnia, pulmonary hypertension, and right heart failure. Left ventricular dysfunction also occurs and may be related to both hypertension and hypervolemia. Severe episodic hypoxia can cause arrhyth-

TABLE 58–3	Possible Causes of Obesity
Neurologic	Reduced sympathetic activity
	Increased parasympathetic activity
	Insensitivity to satiety signals
	Increased neuropeptide Y
	Decreased leptin receptors
	Decreased glucagon-like peptide-1
Adipocyte	Increased stimulus/response to preadipocyte differentiation
	Increased lipoprotein lipase activity
	Diminished hormone-sensitive lipase
	Reduced leptin secretion
Other	Insulin resistance/hyperinsulinemia

TABLE 58–4	Medical Complications of Severe Obesity

Sudden death
Obstructive sleep apnea
Pickwickian syndrome: daytime hypoventilation, somnolence, polycythemia, and cor pulmonale
Congestive heart failure
Nephrotic syndrome/renal vein thrombosis
Immobility limiting daily activities

mias, and sudden death is 10 times more common in the severely obese. Most devastating, however, are the psychosocial consequences of the disorder. Self-esteem and body image are impaired, immobility greatly limits work and recreational activities, and humiliation is a daily experience when body size is too large for conventional scales, furniture, vehicles, and clothes.

Moderate Obesity

A weight more than 20% above ideal poses increased risk of early mortality. Subjects more than 30% overweight have about a 50% greater mortality rate than those of average weight. Such naked statistics, however, can be deceiving. Overweight young adults (<45 years), for example, appear at risk from complications of moderate obesity, whereas obesity is less of a risk factor in older people. Restated, obesity does not appear to be a major risk factor in the age range where mortality is greatest. Moreover, there has been a slight increase in obesity prevalence in the United States in the past two decades, whereas total mortality rates have fallen by 20 to 30%.

Some disorders are clearly related to obesity. Hypertension is more frequent in obese people than in those of normal weight. This may be due to sympathetic hyperactivity or to hyperinsulinemia, but neither mechanism is clearly established. Type II diabetes mellitus can be unmasked and aggravated by excess weight, and this may be the most important medical complication of moderate obesity. The cause appears to be insulin resistance, but many obese individuals never develop hyperglycemia. Obesity is often associated with high triglyceride and low high-density lipoprotein (HDL) concentrations, particularly when mild glucose intolerance is also present. Finally, obesity clearly increases the risk of cholelithiasis and endometrial carcinoma.

Treatment

Clinically Severe Obesity

Severe caloric restriction (200 to 800 kcal/day), with or without anorectic drugs, should be tried first. A 90% failure rate is the rule. Subjects more than 100 lb overweight who have failed medical treatment may be candidates for surgery (gastroplasty or gastric bypass) to reduce stomach size. Patients in general lose 40 to 50% of

excess weight within a year of gastric surgery, but some consume calorically dense liquids and regain weight. The long-term safety and efficacy of this surgery are not certain. The once common intestinal bypass surgery for morbid obesity has been abandoned because of unacceptable long-term complications.

Moderate Obesity

Americans spend over \$30 billion annually on weight loss programs and diet products. Low-calorie diets remain the most widely advocated treatment for obesity. The recommendation to count calories and eat less of everything has intuitive appeal but little success. Behavior modification techniques focusing on stimulus control, the obese eating style, group and spouse support, reinforcement procedures, and exercise are far more effective. Nevertheless, 95% of graduates of such programs return to their initial weight within 5 years. More popular but even less successful are innumerable eating plans based on marked diet imbalance (e.g., rice diet, ice cream diet, Fit-for-Life diet). These are only transiently helpful because a diet very low in either fat or carbohydrate rapidly becomes monotonous and unpalatable. Diets very low in carbohydrate are also ketogenic and inhibit appetite. Most dramatic in effect, but potentially hazardous, are the very low calorie diets that approximate a supplemented fast, rely on withdrawal of most conventional foods, and entail purchase and consumption of an expensive diet supplement. No diet calling for 800 or fewer calories should be undertaken without medical supervision. More than 50 deaths, some from documented ventricular tachycardia and fibrillation, occurred with the early "liquid protein," very low calorie diets.

No program consisting of caloric restriction alone has been generally successful beyond 12 to 18 months despite the enormous commercial success of diet books and systems.

Anorectic drugs are potentially addicting, often unsafe, and only marginally effective. Patients with any history of drug abuse should avoid any of the amphetamines. These agents may be useful in the short term when incorporated in a program that includes diet counseling, behavior modification, and close medical supervision.

When the pathophysiology of obesity is better defined, then more specific and effective measures should emerge.

ANOREXIA NERVOSA AND BULIMIA NERVOSA

These two psychiatric disorders are characterized by a distorted body image and abnormal eating patterns. Neither has a distinctive pathognomonic feature; the two disorders share some common features, and they may overlap (Table 58–5). Bulimia nervosa is not associated with cachexia, whereas this is the most prominent aspect of anorexia nervosa. The primary treatment of both disorders is psychiatric, although they may manifest important medical complications.

TABLE 58–5	Diagnostic Criteria for Anorexia Nervosa and Bulimia Nervosa

Anorexia Nervosa

A. Refusal to maintain body weight at or above a minimally normal weight for age and height (e.g., weight loss leading to maintenance of body weight less than 85% of that expected or failure to make expected weight gain during period of growth, leading to body weight less than 85% of that expected).

B. Intense fear of gaining weight or becoming fat, even though underweight.

C. Disturbance in the way in which own body weight or shape is experienced, undue influence of body weight or shape on self-evaluation, or denial of the seriousness of the current low body weight.

D. In postmenarchal females, amenorrhea, i.e., the absence of at least three consecutive menstrual cycles (a woman is considered to have amenorrhea if her periods occur only following hormone administration, e.g., estrogen).

Bulimia Nervosa

A. Recurrent episodes of binge eating. An episode of binge eating is characterized by both of the following:
   1. Eating, in a discrete period of time (e.g., within any 2-hour period), an amount of food that is definitely larger than most people would eat during a similar period of time and under similar circumstances
   2. A sense of lack of control over eating during the episode (e.g., a feeling that one cannot stop eating or control what or how much one is eating)

B. Recurrent inappropriate compensatory behavior in order to prevent weight gain, such as self-induced vomiting; misuse of laxatives, diuretics, enemas, or other medications; fasting; or excessive exercise.

C. The binge eating and inappropriate compensatory behaviors both occur, on average, at least twice a week for 3 months.

D. Self-evaluation is unduly influenced by body shape and weight.

E. The disturbance does not occur exclusively during episodes of anorexia nervosa.

From American Psychiatric Association (1994). *Diagnostic and Statistical Manual of Mental Disorders* (4th ed., pp 549–550). Washington, DC: American Psychiatric Association. Copyright 1994 by the American Psychiatric Association. Reprinted by permission.

Anorexia Nervosa

Prevalence

The overall prevalence of anorexia nervosa is estimated to be 0.3 to 0.6% in the general population. In amenorrhea clinics, between 5 and 15% of patients may be affected, and in a London study the prevalence among girls 16 to 18 years old was about 1%. The disorder affects girls at least 10 times as often as boys, with typical onset in adolescence but occurrence as late as the menopause.

Pathogenesis and Clinical Features

Some individuals can recall life situations or events that triggered their preoccupation with thinness. The usual pubertal weight increase may be critical in most girls. The restriction of food intake is initially voluntary, and a compulsion to lose weight may lead to self-induced vomiting, abuse of purgatives and diuretics, and exhausting exercise. Patients view their own body dimensions as excessive, but their view of other people is not abnormal.

In typical cases, the diagnosis of anorexia nervosa presents little difficulty. In atypical cases, occurring for example in men and older women, careful evaluation for malignancy, acquired immunodeficiency syndrome (AIDS), malabsorption, and hyperthyroidism may be necessary. Weight loss in anorexia nervosa usually begins within a few years of menarche, although onset may occur at ages 11 to 40 years. Amenorrhea is the rule, secondary to weight loss and low gonadotropin levels. Men will complain of poor libido and impotence. Stunted growth and fractures of vertebrae and long bones may be seen when the disease begins in early adolescence.

Physical examination reveals little subcutaneous fat, with gaunt facies, atrophic breasts and buttocks, and often extensive growth of fine lanugo hair on neck and extremities. Bradycardia and hypothermia may occur, presumably because of low tri-iodothyronine (T_3) levels. Hypovolemia from starvation and mild diabetes insipidus may cause hypotension.

Laboratory findings are not diagnostic but usually include low gonadotropins and gonadal hormones, hypercorticolism, and low T_3 and increased reverse T_3 as in *sick euthyroidism*. Occasionally there is pancytopenia, rarely with increased infections; hypoglycemia, occasionally with coma; and occasionally hypoalbuminemia and hypercholesterolemia. Hypokalemia is rare in patients who are not purging. Abdominal radiographs may show gastric distention and megaduodenum, and echocardiography may demonstrate mitral valve motion abnormalities and reduced left ventricular mass.

Treatment and Prognosis

All patients should be evaluated by a psychiatrist or psychologist experienced in treating anorexia nervosa. Patients weighing 65% or more of ideal body weight may be successfully managed as outpatients. Those under 65% of ideal body weight are candidates for inpatient psychiatric and nutritional care. If the patient is unable or unwilling to consume 500 kcal more than needed for daily energy requirements, use of peripheral parenteral nutritional supplementation (see Chapter 59) or tube feeding should be considered.

Hypothalamic and endocrine problems generally resolve when 85% of normal body weight is restored. Amenorrhea may persist for several more months, but menses usually return without specific intervention.

The mortality rate for patients with anorexia nervosa is about 6% per decade. At least 50 to 60% regain normal weight and eating habits and have return of menses. In 20%, the condition remains chronic despite therapy. Prognosis is poorer in those with bulimic features or long duration of illness.

Bulimia Nervosa

Prevalance

The lifetime prevalence of bulimia, in a large Canadian study, was 1.1% for women and 0.1% for men. Less-comprehensive studies have suggested that up to 20% of college students report bulimic symptoms. Within families of patients with bulimia, serious depression and substance abuse, particularly alcoholism, occur six times more frequently than expected by chance. The increase in weight and adiposity at puberty is probably the stimulus for bulimia, just as for anorexia nervosa. The hallmark of bulimia is not induced vomiting but binge eating; bulimia is synonymous with paroxysmal hyperphagia. Binges leave the patient embarrassed, guilty, and focused again on maintaining weight below an arbitrary level. This end is achieved by prolonged fasting, self-induced vomiting, nonprescription anorectics, and use of substances like diuretics and laxatives. In marked contrast to patients with anorexia nervosa, bulimics generally feel out of control and often welcome help.

Because bulimics are not wasted, physical findings may be subtle or absent. Calluses or scratches on the dorsum of the hand may result from abrasion by teeth during induced gagging. Puffy cheeks from parotid or other salivary gland enlargement are present in up to 50% of patients, and serum salivary amylase levels may be elevated. Erosions occur on the lingual, palatal, and posterior occlusal surfaces of the teeth from acid-induced enamel dissolution and decalcification.

Frequent binge eating and vomiting may cause gastric or esophageal perforation or bleeding, pneumomediastinum, or subcutaneous emphysema. Heavy use of ipecac to induce vomiting may cause myopathic weakness and electrocardiographic abnormalities from emetine toxicity.

Loss of gastric fluids can result in metabolic alkalosis with elevated carbon dioxide and hypochloremia. Diuretic abuse can produce both hypokalemia and hyponatremia. Menstrual irregularities are common, but amenorrhea is rare.

Treatment and Prognosis

Bulimics, in general, do not need hospitalization, but outpatient psychiatric treatment is beneficial. Cognitive behavioral therapy, examining the way the patient thinks followed by deliberate modification of the thought process, is probably superior to therapy directed at managing anxiety or treatment with antidepressant drugs. At least a third of patients relapse within a 2-year follow-up period, most within the first 6 months, and require additional treatment. Successfully treated bulimics still remain at high risk for alcohol and other drug dependence.

REFERENCES

Brownell KD, Fairburn CG (eds.): Eating Disorders and Obesity. A Comprehensive Handbook. New York, The Guilford Press, 1995.

Herzog DB, Copeland PM: Eating disorders. N Engl J Med 1985; 313: 295–303.

Pi-Sunyer FX: Obesity. *In* Wyngaarden JB, Smith LH Jr, Bennett JC (eds.): Cecil Textbook of Medicine. 20th ed. Philadelphia, WB Saunders, 1996.

59

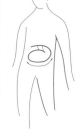

Principles of Nutritional Support in Adult Patients

NUTRITIONAL ASSESSMENT

Every hospitalized patient deserves objective consideration of nutritional status. Severely malnourished patients have poorer outcomes, irrespective of disease entity or reason for hospitalization. Types of patients benefiting from nutritional support have been identified (Table 59–1). In general, patients who have recently lost $\geq 10\%$ of their body weight and those $\geq 30\%$ below ideal body weight are considered candidates for nutritional support. Patients who will be without adequate nutrition for ≥ 7 days should be supported from admission. Finally, patients with a variety of specific disease entities (see Table 59–1) will have quicker recoveries and shorter hospital stays if nutritional needs are met.

A number of aspects of nutritional assessment and support are controversial. Laboratory markers of malnutrition are capricious. Hypoalbuminemia may be due to protein-calorie malnutrition but is equally likely to be due to fluid shifts in recumbent and overhydrated patients, to losses in the urine, gastrointestinal (GI) tract, or third space, and to cytokine effects reducing hepatic albumin production. Lymphopenia, similarly, has causes other than malnutrition, particularly the corticotropin (ACTH) and corticosteroid response to acute biologic stress. Parenteral nutrition was previously provided to a wide variety of surgical patients in the belief it supported rapid recovery and wound healing. It is now clear that surgical patients with severe malnutrition benefit from total parenteral nutrition (TPN), whereas those with borderline or mild degrees of malnutrition do not have survival improved by TPN, and they suffer more infectious complications than patients not given TPN.

ROUTE OF NUTRITIONAL SUPPORT

Support should be by the enteral route unless contraindications (Fig. 59–1) are present. Most critically ill patients will tolerate enteral feeding. Use of the gut avoids gut starvation and atrophy and undesirable increases in mucosal permeability to bacteria. Absorption through the small intestine presents most nutrients to the enterohepatic circulation, reduces tides of glycemia and lipemia, permits first-pass hepatic extraction of nutrients, and stimulates physiologic endocrine responses to feeding. Conversely,

parenteral nutrition is plagued by mechanical complications of catheter insertion in 4 to 6% of cases. These include pneumothorax and hemothorax and injury to vessels, brachial plexes, and thoracic duct. Infectious complications occur in about 5% of patients receiving parenteral nutrition and include tunnel and line sepsis, metastatic abscess, and right heart endocarditis. Severe hyperglycemia, fluid, acid-base, and electrolyte disturbances, as well as nutritional deficiencies are more common with parenteral nutrition unless great attention is paid to detail.

Peripheral parenteral nutrition (PPN) may be used to provide partial or total nutrition for up to 2 weeks. Thereafter, venous access becomes difficult. PPN solutions cannot contain more than 10% dextrose, and 5% is typically used (Table 59–2). Solutions of high osmolality cause painful thrombophlebitis. Thus, PPN requires relatively high volumes to deliver a modest number of calories, and patients must be able to tolerate these volumes.

WATER

Adults daily require about 30 ml of water per kilogram of body weight or roughly 1 ml/kcal of energy. Elderly patients and others incapable of expressing their thirst require careful attention to serum osmolality. This should be routinely calculated and adjusted, if indicated, by increasing or decreasing total fluid volume (see Chapter 26). Patients with ascites, edema, heart failure, or intrinsic kidney disease may have low urine output and require less water. Those with fistulas, GI drainage, or impaired renal water conservation may require large volumes of water and electrolytes.

CALORIES AND PROTEIN

Protein and carbohydrates provide about 4 kcal of energy per gram, and fat, 9 kcal/gm. In a typical American diet, about 16% of calories are protein, 37% fat, and 47% carbohydrate. Nonstressed patients should be provided total energy at 30 kcal/kg ideal body weight, and protein should constitute at least 4 kcal/kg or 1 gm/kg/day. Stressed patients, such as those with major trauma, burns,

TABLE 59–1	Indications for Adult Enteral Nutritional Support (ENS) and Parenteral Nutritional Support (PNS)	
Strongly Supported By Outcome Studies	**Moderately Supported By Research Studies**	**Recommended By Expert Panels**
Acute renal failure (ENS or PNS) Prolonged (>7d) acute pancreatitis (ENS or PNS) Acute respiratory failure with mechanical ventilatory support (ENS or PNS) Acute exacerbation of Crohn's disease (PNS) Short bowel syndrome (PNS or ENS) Severely malnourished patients preoperatively (PNS or ENS) Enterocutaneous fistulas (PNS)	Acute alcoholic liver disease (ENS or PNS) Severe but stable chronic obstructive pulmonary disease and cystic fibrosis (ENS) Chronic Crohn's disease (ENS) Acute ulcerative colitis (ENS or PNS)	Severely malnourished cancer patients suffering time-limited radiation or chemotherapy enteritis (ENS or PNS) Support of acquired imunodeficiency syndrome patients (ENS or PNS) Chronic renal failure (ENS or PNS) Intensive care/critically ill patients (>7d) (ENS or PNS) Neurologic impairment of oral intake (ENS) Anorexia nervosa with 30% recent weight loss or ≤65% of ideal body weight (ENS or PNS) Any patient with predicted severe inadequate nutrition >7 days (ENS or PNS)

inflammatory bowel disease, or infections, may require increasing protein up to 1.5 gm/kg/day to avoid catabolism of muscle protein.

Peripheral and central parenteral nutrition solutions (see Table 59–2) are formulated with amino acids rather than proteins. Two liters of a 5% amino acid solution is equivalent to about 80 gm of protein. Disease-specific amino acid mixtures are commercially available for parenteral nutrition, but their superiority over balanced mixtures of essential and nonessential amino acids is uncertain. Preparations for patients with renal disease contain only essential amino acids to limit the nitrogen load, whereas those for patients with liver failure are enriched in branched-chain amino acids (valine, leucine, and iso-

leucine). Chronic liver disease is associated with low plasma levels of these amino acids.

Most of the calories in parenteral nutrition formulations are derived from dextrose and fat (see Table 59–2). Dextrose concentrations as high as 25 to 30% can be infused through centrally placed catheters, whereas 10% is the practical maximum through peripheral lines. Lipid emulsions, unless contraindicated by pancreatitis or severe hypertriglyceridemia, can be used to advantage to provide 20 to 40% of total calories. Lipid emulsions are isotonic rather than hypertonic and provide essential fatty acids. In certain patients, lipid also limits the risk of severe hyperglycemia, hepatic steatosis, and hypercapnea from excessive dextrose administration.

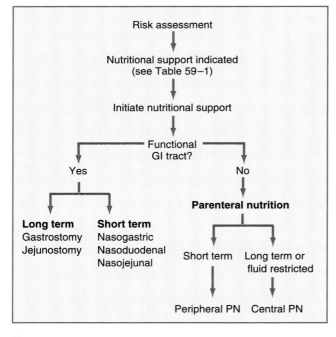

Figure 59–1

Algorithm for selecting type of nutritional support. GI = Gastrointestinal; PN = parenteral nutrition.

TABLE 59–2	Typical Nutrient Contents of Peripheral Parenteral Nutrition (PPN) or Central (CPN) Solutions	
	CPN	**PPN**
Nonprotein calories	1 kcal/ml	0.5 kcal/ml
Dextrose	20% (680 kcal/L)	5.0% (170 kcal/L)
Fat	3% (272 kcal/L)	3.8% (340 kcal/L)
Amino acids	5% (200 kcal/L)	4.25% (170 kcal/L)
Electrolytes (per liter)		
Cations	Sodium	45.0 mEq
	Potassium	31.0 mEq
	Calcium	4.5 mEq
	Magnesium	5.0 mEq
Anions	Chloride	35.0 mEq
	Phosphate	12.5 mM
	Acetate	29.5 mEq
Trace elements (per day)	Zinc	2.5 mg
	Copper	1.0 mg
	Manganese	0.25 mg
	Chromium	0.01 mg
Multivitamins (per day) (A, D, E, B_1, B_2, niacin, B_6, C, K, biotin, pantothenic acid)	One vial	

Most commercially available enteral feeding formulas also contain about 1 kcal/ml energy, although products as calorically dense as 1.5 kcal/ml are available. Calories are generally supplied by soy protein, corn starch or syrup, and vegetable oil. Since much of their carbohydrate is complex, these formulas have relatively low osmolality (300 to 500 mosm), and moderate volumes will not cause diarrhea. Most are also lactose and gluten free and have little residue.

VITAMINS AND MINERALS

Commercial enteral solutions contain sufficient vitamins, electrolytes, and trace minerals to guarantee adequate nutrition when provided in 2- to 3-L volumes each day. The majority contain <2 gm of sodium and are acceptable when salt intake must be limited.

Parenteral solutions routinely have water soluble and miscible vitamins as well as standard additions of trace minerals. Notable exceptions are vitamin B_{12}, which should be administered intramuscularly every month during long-term parenteral nutrition, and selenium and molybdenum, which may become deficient after several months.

Hospitals often recommend a standard electrolyte mix such as that in Table 59–2, but physicians should monitor these carefully and stipulate different concentrations when indicated. Potassium uptake by cells may be large during the first 10 days of central parenteral nutrition, requiring relatively high initial potassium infusion rates.

HOME NUTRITIONAL SUPPORT

More than 300,000 Americans receive home enteral tube feeding (HETF). The major indications cited are malignancy ($\sim 40\%$) and neurologically impaired swallowing ($\sim 30\%$). The ease of endoscopic placement of gastrostomy tubes has dramatically increased demand for HETF.

At least 50,000 Americans receive home parenteral nutrition (HPN), a number exceeding the annual prevalence in the rest of the world. Usually accepted indications are Crohn's disease, ischemic bowel disease, fistulas, and gastrointestinal motility disorders. In the United States, about 40% of patients receiving HPN have cancer, and 5% have acquired immunodeficiency syndrome.

Home nutritional support in Crohn's disease has been provided for up to 20 years and generally leads to long-term survival. HETF or HPN is also justified in a few other conditions. The use of home nutritional support to prolong life by weeks or months in the terminally ill, however, is widely debated. Cost aside, physicians must ask whether nutritional support in such patients actually prolongs life or merely prolongs the dying process.

REFERENCES

American Society for Parenteral and Enteral Nutrition: Guidelines for the use of parenteral and enteral nutrition in adult and pediatric patients. J Parenteral Enteral Nutr 1993; 17:15A–525A.

Sax, HC, Soriba WM: Enteral and parenteral feedings: Guidelines and recommendations. Med Clin North Am 1993; 77:863–880.

The Veterans Affairs Total Parenteral Nutrition Cooperative Study Group: Perioperative total parenteral nutrition in surgical patients. N Engl J Med 1991; 325:525–532.

60

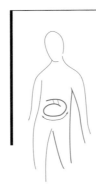

Hyperuricemia and Gout

Gout is characterized by hyperuricemia, an acute inflammatory arthritis, deposits of sodium urate crystals called tophi, and uric acid kidney stones.

PREVALENCE

About 0.7% of men and 0.1% of women develop gout. As many as 2 million Americans may have the disorder. Annual incidence rates in men correlate with the uric acid level and range from 0.1% at levels <7 mg/dl to 5% in those >9 mg/dl.

MECHANISMS OF HYPERURICEMIA

Gout is due to overproduction or undersecretion of uric acid or to both factors (Table 60–1). Probably only 10% of cases are due to overproduction. Uric acid is the catabolic endproduct of adenine and guanine, the purine bases essential for nucleic acids and metabolically active purine nucleotides. Uric acid is also derived from dietary purines. Of the 600 to 700 mg of uric acid excreted daily, roughly a third derives from the diet and two thirds from endogenous sources. Striking pathologic overproduction of uric acid may occur in states of greatly enhanced nucleic acid turnover, as in lymphomas, hematologic malignancies and treatment of these disorders (tumor lysis syndrome), hemolysis, and psoriasis (Table 60–2). Rare genetic diseases such as hypoxanthine-guanine phosphoribosyltransferase (HPRT) deficiency and overproduction or overactivity of the enzyme phosphoribosylpyrophosphate synthetase may also cause severe hyperuricemia.

Roughly 90% of gout is due to underexcretion of uric acid. The site or nature of the responsible renal defect has not been defined. Virtually 100% of uric acid filters through the glomerulus, and the proximal tubule reabsorbs almost all of it. The proximal tubule then engages in energy dependent secretion and reabsorption processes, with a net 6 to 12% of the filtered uric acid passing through the remaining nephron and out in the urine.

Uric acid reabsorption is linked to sodium reabsorption. When the plasma volume is contracted by diuretics, starvation, dehydration, or diabetes insipidus, the sodium-avid kidney also holds on to uric acid. Certain organic

acids interact with mechanisms for urate reabsorption and secretion. Large quantities of salicylates and probenecid inhibit uric acid reabsorption. In contrast, acetoacetate, β-hydroxy butyrate, lactate, and low-dose salicylates inhibit uric acid secretion. This latter mechanism may cause hyperuricemia in starvation and in both diabetic and alcoholic ketoacidosis (see Table 60–2).

PATHOGENESIS OF GOUT ARTHRITIS

Irrespective of mechanism, hyperuricemia per se would not be a problem if uric acid were highly soluble. However, it is not. Monosodium urate solubility is reduced by low pH, low temperature, and high ionic strength. Solubility in plasma is 10.6 mg/dl and is less at the 29 to 32°C temperatures of peripheral joints. Crystallization from biologic fluids, however, is difficult to predict and requires factors other than supersaturation. Crystals themselves are not irritating, and urate crystals can be found in asymptomatic joints of patients with gout. When phagocytized by polymorphonuclear (PMN) leukocytes, however, urate crystals induce release of leukotrienes, cytokines, and chemotactins, which can elicit an intense inflammatory reaction. Lysosomal and other enzymes released can lead to joint destruction.

PATHOGENESIS OF RENAL DISEASE

At a pH of 5.5 and below, uric acid rather than monosodium urate is found in urine. Solubility in urine is determined primarily by pH and ionic strength and ranges from 10 to 40 mg/dl, averaging about 23 mg/dl. Subjects excreting 600 mg/day need urine volumes of at least 2.6 L to avoid supersaturation. When uric acid excretion exceeds 1000 mg daily, the incidence of stones approaches 50%. Over 80% of stones are uric acid, but uric acid crystals may seed stones containing predominantly calcium oxalate or phosphate. The presence of uric acid in any stone should raise the possibility of hyperuricosuria.

With acute urate overproduction, as in the tumor lysis syndrome, serum urate levels can reach 12 to 36 mg/dl, and urate crystals can cause tubular obstruction and acute renal failure, usually without nephrolithiasis.

TABLE 60–1 Classification of Hyperuricemia and Gout

Primary (Presumably Genetic)

I. Metabolic (overproduction)
   A. Idiopathic (10% of primary gout)
   B. Associated with specific enzyme defects (<1% of primary gout)
      1. Phosphoribosylpyrophosphate synthetase overproduction
      2. Partial deficiency of hypoxanthine-guanine phosphoribosyl transferase
      3. "Complete" deficiency of hypoxanthine-guanine phosphoribosyl transferase
II. Renal (idiopathic underexcretion—90% of primary gout)

Secondary (Acquired)

I. Metabolic
   A. Increased nucleic acid turnover (e.g., chronic hemolysis, lymphoproliferative or myeloproliferative disorders)
   B. Glucose-6-phosphatase deficiency (i.e., type I glycogen storage disease)
II. Renal
   A. Acute or chronic renal failure
   B. Volume depletion
   C. Altered tubular handling by drugs or endogenous metabolic products

The syndrome can occur in untreated as well as treated malignancies. Finally, a disorder termed urate nephropathy, caused by sodium urate crystals in renal interstitial tissue, may rarely be a cause of mild proteinuria, defects in concentrating the urine, and a fall in glomerular filtration rate (GFR).

PATHOGENESIS OF TOPHI

Tophi are deposits of solid urate crystals that elicit a foreign body reaction of mononuclear cells with granu-

TABLE 60–2 Some Drugs and Conditions Increasing Serum Uric Acid Concentrations

Drugs

Diuretics
Low-dose salicylates
Ethanol
Cyclosporine
Ethambutol
Levodopa
Nicotinic acid
Pyrazinamide
Methoxyflurane
Cytolytic agents
Vitamin B_{12} (pernicious anemia)

Conditions

Leukemias
Lymphomas
Psoriasis
Renal failure
Lactic acidosis
Starvation
Obesity
Lead poisoning
Trisomy 21
Glycogen storage disease

loma formation. Occurring after long-standing severe hyperuricemia, tophi may involve the joint and cause a destructive arthropathy. Tophi have been described in virtually every organ outside the central nervous system. They may cause overlying skin to ulcerate and extrude urate crystals.

CLINICAL FEATURES

Acute Gouty Arthritis

Clinical gout is uncommon before the 40s; its peak age of onset in men is about 45 years, usually after 20 to 30 years of sustained hyperuricemia. The primary manifestation is a painful arthritis, usually involving the lower extremities. Ninety percent of initial attacks are monoarticular, and at least half involve the first metatarsophalangeal joint (podagra). Other initial sites of involvement, in order of frequency, include the ankles, heels, knees, wrists, fingers, and elbows. Acute gouty arthritis may be precipitated by events such as trauma, surgery, alcohol ingestion, or systemic infection. Although the course of an untreated attack varies, initial episodes are usually self-limited. However, more than 50% of patients experience recurrent arthritis within 1 year of the first attack. Later attacks tend to be more prolonged and severe and more commonly involve multiple joints.

A presumptive diagnosis of gout can be made if the patient is hyperuricemic and has the classic clinical features described previously. Unfortunately, a substantial minority of patients with acute gout exhibit *normal* uric acid levels. A dramatic response to colchicine is highly suggestive but not pathognomonic of acute gout. When the diagnosis is in doubt, acute gouty arthritis can be confirmed by demonstration of negatively birefringent, needle-shaped urate crystals within the white blood cells of synovial fluid examined under a polarizing lens. Synovial fluid analysis otherwise exhibits nonspecific signs of acute inflammation. The synovial fluid leukocyte count ranges from 1000 to more than 70,000/μl, with a predominance of polymorphonuclear cells. Concentrations of glucose and uric acid in synovial fluid are usually similar to those in serum.

Chronic Tophaceous Gout

Tophi detectable on physical examination develop in 10 to 20% of gouty patients. They appear 10 to 15 years after the initial arthritic attack and are found in cartilage, tendons, bursae, soft tissues, and synovial membranes at a rate that parallels the degree and duration of hyperuricemia. Common sites include the external ear and pressure points such as the Achilles tendons and olecranon bursae. Gouty tophi may spontaneously ulcerate and extrude a pasty material consisting of pure urate. Although tophi themselves are painless, their presence in and around joints ultimately can limit joint mobility or cause a destructive arthropathy.

Nephrolithiasis

Uric acid stones occur in 10 to 20% of patients with gout, and this relatively low percentage reflects the modest contribution of uric acid overproduction to the syndrome. Uric acid stones, lacking calcium, are radiolucent. Gouty patients also have an increased incidence of calcium oxalate stones, and a quarter of calcium oxalate stone formers have either hyperuricemia or hyperuricosuria. Patients with normal serum uric acid levels may also have uric acid stones, as would be predicted from the low solubility of this organic acid.

Uric acid gravel appears as red-orange sand, and uric acid stones are also pigmented because the pigment uricine is adsorbed. Stones can be passed painlessly, but when they exceed 0.5 cm they usually cause flank pain radiating to the groin and gross or microscopic hematuria. Occasionally stones may obstruct, causing gross hematuria or hydronephrosis, but most stones pass spontaneously, albeit while providing the patient with a very memorable and painful experience.

Hyperuricemic Acute Renal Failure

Acute urate nephropathy in the tumor lysis syndrome may be heralded by oliguria or anuria and nonspecific constitutional symptoms like nausea, vomiting, and lethargy. Its occurrence is readily suspected in untreated patients with a large tumor burden from leukemia or lymphoma or after chemotherapy for these disorders. Suspicion is further enhanced by hyperuricemia, hyperkalemia, lactic acidosis, hyperphosphatemia, and hypocalcemia. Nephrolithiasis is uncommon in this syndrome.

TREATMENT

Arthritis

Acute gouty arthritis responds to nonsteroidal antiinflammatory drugs. Seventy-five mg of indomethacin may be administered initially, followed by 50 mg every 6 to 8 hours for 2 days. Colchicine, 0.6 to 1.2 mg daily, may be administered as prophylaxis against recurrent attacks. Prednisone, 40 to 60 mg daily for 2 to 3 days, may be used in patients with gastrointestinal bleeding or peptic ulcer disease in whom nonsteroidals are relatively contraindicated.

Colchicine historically had been used as a diagnostic therapeutic agent and as the mainstay of acute therapy. However, gastrointestinal toxicity occurs so frequently at therapeutic doses that it is now rarely considered a first-line agent to abate arthritic attacks.

Hypouricemic drugs are not used during acute gouty arthritis because they may aggravate the attack. They are initiated in less than full doses 1 to 2 weeks after an acute attack has subsided and while the patient is on prophylactic colchicine.

Hyperuricemia

Allopurinol and its major metabolite, oxypurinol, are inhibitors of the enzyme xanithine oxidase. Allopurinol is the drug of choice in recurrent uric acid nephrolithiasis. Allopurinol is also widely used to treat hyperuricemia and gout despite the fact that most patients are low excretors rather than overproducers. The preference for allopurinol is based largely on concern that uricosurics might increase risk of urolithiasis, a concern generally valid only during initial treatment when uric acid excretion is transiently increased. The daily single dose of allopurinol needed to normalize the uric acid level ranges from 100 to 600 mg, with a mean of 300 mg. Lower doses should be used in renal insufficiency. In patients at risk for tumor lysis syndrome, allopurinol in doses of 600 to 900 mg daily should be started a couple days before chemotherapy and thereafter tapered to maintain uric acids < 7 mg/dl.

Allopurinol has been used for more than 20 years and is well tolerated. However, gastric upset, diarrhea, or rash occurs in about 3% of patients; and 0.4% experience severe hypersensitivity with renal insufficiency, hepatitis, and skin injury (exfoliative dermatitis, Stevens-Johnson syndrome, and others). Renal failure patients are at particularly high risk if appropriately low doses are not used.

Uricosuric drugs offer an alternative to allopurinol in patients with hyperuricemia and low urinary excretion rates. Probenecid is started at 250 mg twice daily and increased to 500 mg twice daily after 1 to 2 weeks to maintain serum urate below 7 mg/dl. Sulfinpyrazone is begun at 50 mg twice daily and increased to 300 to 400 mg/day. Urine output to 3 L daily should be promoted, particularly in the early weeks of uricosuria. These drugs should not be used when the glomerular filtration rate is below 30 ml/min.

Acute Urate Nephropathy

Acute renal failure from hyperuricemia rarely responds to vigorous hydration, diuretics, and urine alkalinization. After initial support with hemodialysis to correct both hyperuricemia and acute electrolyte imbalance, prognosis is good for return to near normal renal function.

Asymptomatic Hyperuricemia

In men with uric acid levels > 13 mg/dl and women > 10 mg/dl, treatment of asymptomatic hyperuricemia is probably justified to avoid possible nephrotoxicity. Moreover, the majority of patients excreting more than 1 gm of uric acid daily will get nephrolithiasis and should be treated with allopurinol, if feasible. Most modest hyperuricemics, however, never develop gout or tophi and should not be treated until arthritis appears. There is no evidence that mild hyperuricemia is nephrotoxic. Despite the association of hyperuricemia with insulin resistance, diabetes mellitus, hypertension, and hypertriglyceridemia (one of the syndrome Xs), there is no direct connection between uric acid and atherogenesis.

REFERENCES

Becker MA, Roessler BJ: Hyperuricemia and gout. *In* Scriver CR, Beaudet AL, Sly WS, Valle D (eds.): The Metabolic and Molecular Bases of Inherited Disease. 7th ed. New York, McGraw-Hill, 1995.
Hirshfield MS: Gout and uric acid metabolism. *In* Bennett JC, Plum F (eds.): Cecil Textbook of Medicine. 20th ed, Philadelphia, WB Saunders, 1996.

61

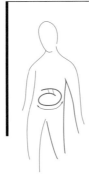

Disorders of Lipid Metabolism

PLASMA LIPOPROTEIN PHYSIOLOGY

The major properties of the plasma lipoproteins are summarized in Table 61–1. Normal men and women daily consume 80 to 120 gm of fat (triglyceride [TG]). Dietary fat is hydrolyzed by pancreatic lipase, absorbed by the intestinal mucosal cells, and secreted into the mesenteric lymphatics as chylomicrons (Fig. 61–1). One hundred grams of dietary fat mixed in an adult plasma volume of 25 dl can theoretically increase plasma TG by 4000 mg/dl! The liver also transforms plasma free fatty acids, unneeded when there is a surfeit of calories from the diet, into TG and daily secretes an additional 10 to 30 gm of very low density lipoprotein (VLDL) TG into the plasma. This potentially further increases TG by 1000 mg/dl. Both chylomicrons and VLDL acquire a 9000 molecular weight peptide called apolipoprotein C-II (apo C-II) from plasma high-density lipoproteins (HDL). Apo C-II is a critical cofactor for lipoprotein lipase, which is located on the capillary endothelium of muscle and adipose tissue. After hydrolysis of chylomicron and VLDL TG, excess phospholipid, cholesterol, and apoproteins transfer to HDL and increase HDL mass. The remnants remaining after hydrolysis of chylomicron TG are cleared very rapidly by the liver and do not normally accumulate in plasma. This process is mediated by apolipoprotein E (apo E) on the chylomicron surface, which binds to hepatic heparan sulfate proteoglycans and accounts for the rapid clearance of chylomicron remnants from the blood stream. Apo E on the chylomicron surface is then specifically bound to the low-density lipoprotein (LDL)-receptor–related protein (LRP) in the hepatocyte cell membrane and internalized (see Fig. 61–1).

Some VLDL remnants (10 to 30%) are also cleared directly by the liver, but the majority are converted to intermediate-density lipoproteins (IDL). IDL are normally short-lived and by the action of lipases are converted to the final VLDL catabolic product, LDL (see Fig. 61–1). In contrast to VLDL, which survive about 20 minutes in plasma, LDL circulate for 3 to 5 days. Although LDL normally account for 70% of the total plasma cholesterol, they are basically metabolic garbage. Most LDL clearance from plasma takes place when apo B on the LDL surface binds to the B,E receptor (LDL receptor) on membranes of many tissues, particularly the liver.

Lp(a) lipoproteins are secreted by the liver, consti-

tute ≤ 10% of the total plasma lipoprotein mass, possess regions homologous to plasminogen, and are associated with vascular disease risk. Genetic heterogeneity produces 100-fold concentration differences among individuals, and levels are little affected by diet, habits, and most lipid-lowering drugs.

High-density lipoproteins are secreted into plasma by both intestine and liver. It is thought that HDL readily accept cholesterol from cells and other lipoproteins. This cholesterol initially is absorbed onto the HDL surface, where it is substrate for the plasma enzyme lecithin: cholesterol acyltransferase (LCAT). LCAT transfers a fatty acid from phosphatidyl choline to the 3-hydroxyl group of cholesterol. This produces cholesteryl esters that move from the hydrophilic HDL surface into the hydrophobic HDL core. The HDL surface is then free to accept more cholesterol from cells or other lipoproteins. The cholesteryl esters in the HDL core can be removed and transferred by a plasma protein and are the major source of cholesteryl esters contained in chylomicrons, VLDL, and LDL.

At least 10 well-characterized apolipoproteins are located on lipoprotein surfaces. These stabilize the lipoprotein micelle, are recognized by cell membrane receptors, and serve as enzyme cofactors. Their major lipoprotein associations are listed in Table 61–1. The usefulness of quantifying these apolipoproteins in clinical practice is uncertain.

EVALUATION OF SERUM LIPOPROTEIN CONCENTRATIONS

Cholesterol levels should be measured in children who have a parent with hyperlipidemia or coronary heart disease before age 55 years. Routine screening of other children is not recommended. Every adult should have a total serum cholesterol and HDL-cholesterol determined during his or her 20s. A total cholesterol value < 200 mg/dl at any time of day does not require retesting for 5 years. A level > 200 mg/dl should lead to measurement of total cholesterol, TG, and HDL-cholesterol after a 14-hour fast. Similar testing is indicated in adults who have first-degree relatives with vascular disease or lipid disorders. An HDL-cholesterol level below 35 mg/dl in men and below 45 mg/dl in women signifies clearly increased

TABLE 61–1	Properties of Lipoproteins		
Liproprotein Class	**Origin**	**Major Apoprotein Groups**	**Major Core Lipid**
Chylomicrons	Intestine	B-48, C, E	Dietary tri-glycerides
VLDL	Liver	B-100, C, E	Hepatic tri-glycerides
LDL	VLDL catabo-lism	B-100	Cholesteryl esters
Lp(a)	Liver	B-100, (a)	Cholesteryl esters
HDL	Liver, intestine	A, C	Cholesteryl esters

HDL = High-density lipoprotein; LDL = low-density liprotein; VLDL = very low density lipoprotein.

TABLE 61–2	Approach to Elevated LDL-Cholesterol (LDL-C) Levels in Adults Without Coronary Heart Disease (CHD)*
LDL-C Level	**Approach**
<130 mg/dl	Desirable; repeat in 5 yr
130–159 mg/dl	Diet
160–189 mg/dl	Diet; consider drugs if two CHD risk factors present
190–220 mg/dl	Intensive diet in men <35 years and premenopausal women; diet and drugs in all others

* Recommendations of the Adult Treatment Panel, National Cholesterol Education Program. CHD risk factors include male ≥45 yr, female ≥55 yr or menopause without estrogen replacement, family history of CHD before age 55 yr, smoking, hypertension, diabetes mellitus, and HDL-cholesterol <35 mg/dl. Subtract a risk factor if HDL-cholesterol ≥60 mg/dl.

risk. If TG levels are over 500 mg/dl, then specific treatment of hypertriglyceridemia should be undertaken. The highest total cholesterols commonly encountered (600 to 2000 mg/dl) are usually due to increases in chylomicrons and VLDL. Elevated cholesterols, therefore, cannot be interpreted without knowledge of TG levels.

If TG levels are <400 mg/dl, then the LDL-cholesterol (LDL-C) is calculated as follows:

$$LDL\text{-}C = Total\ C - (HDL\text{-}C + VLDL\text{-}C)$$
$$= Total\ C - (HDL\text{-}C + TG/5)$$

A therapeutic strategy based on LDL is indicated in Table 61–2.

Elevated HDL levels are thought to confer protection against coronary heart disease (CHD) and do not require treatment. Low HDL levels justify aggressive modification of other factors, including even mild LDL elevations (>130 mg/dl).

ELEVATED CHYLOMICRONS, VLDL, AND IDL

Disorders Manifest in Childhood

The occurrence of eruptive xanthomas, lipemia retinalis, hepatosplenomegaly, and abdominal pain in an infant or small child suggests a primary defect in clearance of chylomicrons and VLDL. This may be due to a defi-

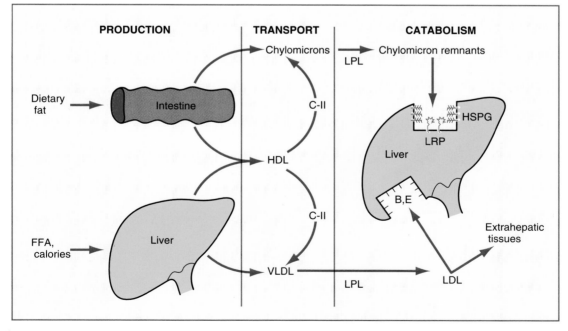

Figure 61–1

Normal metabolism of plasma lipoproteins. See text for details. B,E = Membrane receptor for lipoproteins containing apo B and apo E (synonomous with the LDL receptor); FFA = free fatty acids; HDL = high density lipoproteins; HSPG = heparan sulfate proteoglycan; LDL = low-density lipoproteins; LRP = LDL-receptor–related protein; VLDL = very low density lipoproteins.

ciency of lipoprotein lipase (assayed in plasma after heparin injection) or of apo C-II, the cofactor for lipoprotein lipase. These abnormalities have a prevalence less than one or two in a million.

Disorders Manifest in Adulthood

Chylomicrons and VLDL are both catabolized by lipoprotein lipase, and the enzyme is saturable. The enzyme prefers chylomicrons, so VLDL usually accumulate first until TG levels exceed 500 mg/dl. At higher levels, both VLDL and chylomicrons contribute to the hypertriglyceridemia. Testing to resolve the independent contribution of these two lipoproteins is rarely indicated, and tests for lipoprotein lipase and apo C-II should be reserved for cases arising in childhood. Most hypertriglyceridemia in adults appears to be due to VLDL overproduction, although defective catabolism is responsible in a subset of patients.

Moderate to severe hypertriglyceridemia is relatively common in men and women older than 30 years. The disorder is usually genetic and is commonly associated with hypertension, hyperuricemia, and abnormal glucose tolerance (syndrome X). Hypertriglyceridemia may be aggravated by obesity, even moderate alcohol consumption, exogenous estrogens, and drugs such as diuretics and beta-adrenoreceptor blockers. Common secondary causes of hypertriglyceridemia are renal disease with proteinuria, both hyper- and hypothyroidism, exogenous and endogenous glucocorticoids, and type II diabetes mellitus. A very severe form of hypertriglyceridemia (2000 to 6000 mg/dl) can occur in patients with chronic insulin deficiency and very mild acidosis. This abnormality is completely corrected by insulin administration. The hypertriglyceridemia occurring in acute diabetic ketoacidosis is usually milder (250 to 800 mg/dl) and also responds to insulin.

The importance of hypertriglyceridemia in vascular disease risk is controversial. A National Institutes of Health (NIH) consensus conference concluded that TG levels under 250 mg/dl were normal, those 250 to 500 mg/dl were borderline, and only higher values were considered abnormal. Nevertheless, TG levels in the upper normal range (120 to 250 mg/dl) are very prevalent in CHD populations, and within this range the inverse relationship between TG and HDL-cholesterol is strongest. The association of hypertriglyceridemia and diabetes mellitus, obesity, and hypertension has further confounded efforts to define its independent role in vascular disease.

Dysbetalipoproteinemia

This disease is characterized by the accumulation of chylomicron remnants and IDL in plasma. It is caused by homozygosity for a species of apo E (E_2), which does not bind normally to the B,E receptor and probably not to the LRP (see Fig. 61–1). This leads to defective hepatic clearance of chylomicron remnants and ineffective catabolism of IDL to LDL. Less commonly, heterozygosity for

a variant apo E results in an autosomal dominant form of dysbetalipoproteinemia.

Apo E_2 differs from normal apo E_3 and apo E_4 because of a point mutation causing a cysteine-for-arginine substitution. Homozygosity for apo E_2 occurs in 1 to 2% of the population, but fewer than 1 in 1000 develops hyperlipidemia. Dysbetalipoproteinemia occurs only if the E_2 homozygote also has an additional disorder such as hypothyroidism or familial hypertriglyceridemia. This abnormality is suspected in individuals who have elevated levels of both cholesterol and TG. Diagnosis requires demonstration of the apo E_2 homozygosity (not generally available) or unusual cholesterol enrichment of the VLDL. If the ratio of cholesterol to TG in VLDL, isolated by ultracentrifugation, is higher than 0.40, then dysbetalipoproteinemia is likely. This form of hyperlipoproteinemia causes palmar and tuboeruptive xanthomas as well as coronary and peripheral vascular disease. The condition is worth identifying because it is exquisitely sensitive to weight reduction, cholesterol-lowering diets, and drugs such as clofibrate, gemfibrozil, lovastatin, and fenofibrate.

Familial Combined Hyperlipoproteinemia

Familial combined hyperlipoproteinemia has been used to describe families with a mixture of lipoprotein abnormalities that appear to segregate as an autosomal dominant trait. Affected members may have high VLDL levels, high LDL levels, or elevations of both VLDL and LDL. The basic abnormality is probably VLDL overproduction. Subjects who do not effectively catabolize VLDL show only hypertriglyceridemia. Those who are very efficient in VLDL catabolism manifest only increased cholesterol and LDL levels. Others show combined elevations of TG (VLDL) and cholesterol (LDL). Family screening is required for a confident diagnosis, but the label is often loosely used to describe anyone with both VLDL and LDL elevations. The abnormality occurs frequently in patients with CHD, and affected patients often require diet and several lipid-lowering drugs to achieve normal lipid concentrations. This is one of the most difficult treatment problems.

TREATMENT OF HYPERTRIGLYCERIDEMIA
General Principles

The treatment of the hyperlipoproteinemias requires a systematic approach (Table 61–3). In general, the abnormality should be documented twice before treatment is undertaken. About half of affected individuals are sensitive to diet (>10% reduction in lipids), and the extent of sensitivity should be defined by administering a very strict diet for 2 to 3 weeks (Table 61–4). Patients are retested once or preferably twice on this diet, and the results provide a point of reference for all future diet and drug interventions. If diet reduces cholesterol and LDL to target values—as in Table 61–2—or triglycerides <120 mg/dl, then it may be liberalized to give greater menu

TABLE 61-3   Treatment of Hyperlipoproteinemia

1. Document abnormality twice after a 14-hr fast while on typical American diet. Provisionally classify as cholesterol or triglyceride problem. Test total cholesterol, TG, HDL-C.
2. Evaluate potential for control with diet modification—fish-vegetarian diet for 3 wk; retest after 2 and 3 wk.
3. Return to conventional lipid-lowering diet (30% fat with equal proportions of polyunsaturated, monounsaturated, and saturated fats) for 4 wk; retest.
4. If target values are not achieved, add lipid-lowering medicine or food supplements. Retest 4 wk after each change in regimen.

Maintenance

5. Patient keeps lipid record on flow sheet and has rapid access to test results.
6. Minimum follow-up test frequency is every 4 mo.

HDL-C = High-density lipoprotein cholesterol; TG = triglyceride.

variety. Skinned, defatted fowl may substitute for some fish entrees, and lean red meat may be consumed once or twice each week. If target values are not achieved, then drug treatment is considered (Table 61–5). Compliance is best when patients chart their lipid levels, have ready access to test results, and have follow-up testing every 3 to 4 months. Assessment of drug effects takes no more than 1 to 2 months, and in general the efficacy of individual agents should be established before combinations are prescribed.

TABLE 61-4   Fish-Vegetarian Diet

Permissible Foods/Beverages

Fish (including clams, oysters, lobster, shrimp, and scallops)
Bread
Pasta (with vegetable oil, tomato, or clam sauce if desired)
Potato
Rice
Vegetables (all)
Fruits (except avocado) and fruit juices
Vegetable oils, margarine, and mayonnaise
Peanut butter
Nuts (except for coconut and macadamia)
Cereal (except granola-type "natural" cereals)
Low-fat crackers (matzo, Ry Krisp, Stoned Wheat Thins)
Angel food cake (plain)
Skim (not 1%) milk
Coffee, tea, soda
Alcohol
Nondairy creamers
    Coffee-Rich
    Poly-Rich
    Poly-Perx

Foods to Be Omitted

Meat (including fowl)
Baked goods (including desserts and "chips")
Dairy products (including eggs, butter, and cheese)

Restaurants

None

Fast Foods

None

TABLE 61-5   Drugs for Hyperlipoproteinemia

Cholesterol Problems

Resins (cholestyramine, colestipol)
Niacin (regular or timed release)
Lovastatin, pravastatin
Simvastatin, fluvastatin
Combinations
Others (probucol, fibrates)

Triglyceride Problems

Fibrates (clofibrate, gemfibrozil, fenofibrate, etc.)
Niacin
Fish oils
Combinations

Diet

Reduced fat consumption is the only treatment for patients with deficiencies of lipoprotein lipase or apo C-II. The daily fat intake is limited to 25 gm by restricting all fat-enriched foods, including those made from vegetable oils. Adults with more common forms of severe hypertriglyceridemia and levels over 1000 mg/dl should also follow a low-fat diet to reduce TG levels to <500 mg/dl. Subjects with milder TG elevations benefit from a diet that is close to a fish-vegetarian diet (see Table 61–4). This very strict diet typically lowers cholesterol levels by 15 to 20% and TG levels by 30 to 40% in hypertriglyceridemics. A second major objective of diet is to reduce body fat content. Most hypertriglyceridemics show marked improvement while actively losing weight, and a significant proportion are cured after weight reduction. Finally, alcohol should be restricted to one or two servings a week, and this alone may correct the problem. If TG levels of 300 mg/dl or less are not sustained by diet, then exercise programs or drugs are appropriate in many patients.

Exercise

Triglyceride levels are reduced after even a single exercise session, and exercise has been shown to augment lipoprotein lipase activity. The efficacy of regular aerobic exercise in mild to moderate hypertriglyceridemia has been repeatedly demonstrated, and exercise has great potential in promoting weight loss. The program goal should be 45 minutes of submaximal exercise on 5 days each week. The type of aerobics, duration, and intensity should be explicitly defined by the physician to promote compliance.

Drugs

The fibrate class of drugs (see Table 61–5) enhances lipoprotein lipase activity and may have dramatic effects in severe hypertriglyceridemics requiring drug treatment. Fibrates are most effective in patients with dysbetalipoproteinemia and in others with high VLDL levels reflected by high total cholesterol levels (500 to 1000 mg/dl) as well as high triglyceride levels (1000 to 10,000 mg/dl). When hypertriglyceridemia is due primarily to chylomicronemia and the cholesterol is only modestly elevated (250 to 500 mg/dl), the fibrates are less effective than dietary fat restriction. Use of niacin in moderate hypertriglyceridemia (500 to 1000 mg/dl) can be gratifying but requires considerable patience by both physician and patient. The starting dose is 100 mg three times daily after meals, with very slow dose escalation to 1.5 to 4.5 gm/day. The user should be thoroughly familiar with niacin's side effects and their significance and control. Fish oils reduce hepatic VLDL production and are a popular but still experimental treatment for hypertriglyceridemia. The minimum effective dose is 12 to 16 gm/day (e.g., 4 gm with each meal and at bedtime), and TG levels are usually reduced by 40% in moderately severe hypertriglyceridemia (500 to 1500 mg/dl).

Fibrates and fish oils can increase LDL levels while lowering VLDL and chylomicrons. Occasionally, LDL levels are raised above 160 mg/dl (see Table 61–2), and this undesirable effect must be weighed against the potential gain.

ELEVATED LDL

Polygenic Hypercholesterolemia

An individual's total cholesterol level is, on average, intermediate between that of his or her parents. About 60 to 70% of a patient's cholesterol or LDL level is, therefore, genetically determined, with the remaining contribution from age, sex, diet, and other factors. The nature of these genetic effects is not defined. Subjects in the upper range of the normal distribution have an increased CHD risk, and the upper 50% contribute about 80% of CHD cases. Those in the highest 25% are generally considered targets for diet or even drug intervention.

Familial Monogenic Hypercholesterolemia

About 1 in 500 North Americans has a monogenic disorder producing an abnormality of the B,E receptor (see Fig. 61–1). Affected individuals exhibit roughly half the normal number of receptors when their fibroblasts are grown in tissue culture. As a consequence, they generally have total cholesterol levels around 370 mg/dl and more than twice the average concentration of LDL. Increased LDL is manifest in the first year of life and is associated with early corneal arcus, xanthomas of the Achilles tendon and extensor tendons of the hands, and a risk of CHD that is about 25 times that in unaffected relatives. Heterozygous men have a 50% chance of myocardial infarction by 50 years of age, and the comparable risk in women is 10 to 20%. Homozygotes or those heterozygotic for two abnormal alleles (compound heterozygotes) have cholesterol levels of 650 to 1000 mg/dl severe xan-

thomatosis, and they typically die of cardiovascular disease before age 30.

TREATMENT OF HYPERCHOLESTEROLEMIA

General Principles

The general principles in the treatment of hypercholesterolemia are the same as defined for hypertriglyceridemia and as outlined in Table 61–3.

Diet

Limitation of dietary saturated fat is central to both cholesterol- and TG-lowering diets. Carbohydrates are often substituted for the saturated fats, but high-carbohydrate diets may increase TG and reduce HDL. Monounsaturated fats may prove better substitutes for saturated fat. Reduction of dietary cholesterol has a small additional LDL-lowering effect. In practice, the optimal diet approaches the fish-vegetarian diet used to establish diet sensitivity (see Table 61–4). The average hypercholesterolemic lowers total cholesterol by 12% (range, 0 to 40%) on this diet. When diet responders show secondary failure, the usual cause is noncompliance. This can be identified by asking patients to complete a 7-day diet diary and reviewing the record with them. Subjects who travel extensively and eat frequently in restaurants have greatest trouble with diet prescriptions. When large populations have been studied, most cholesterol-lowering diets have been disappointing, with mean total cholesterol reductions in the range of 5%.

Exercise

Although trained endurance athletes have LDL levels about 10% lower than those of controls, endurance training is generally not effective in reducing LDL concentrations. As noted previously, exercise effects in hypertriglyceridemics are much more substantial.

Drugs

Several considerations govern choice of drugs for hypercholesterolemics not controlled by diet. The drugs are usually prescribed for years to decades, and most are moderately expensive. The risk-benefit profile must be carefully assessed because any significant morbid or mortal effects can offset the modest potential gains. Annoying side effects limit compliance with some agents. Only a few drugs have been shown to prolong life, and this outcome has been shown only in middle-aged men.

The resins (see Table 61–5) are safe and effective and are the only agents appropriate for children. The starting dose is 2 scoops or unit dose packets before supper; this dose is enough in many mild hypercholesterolemics, and more than 6 unit doses a day is rarely worth the cost and inconvenience. A large bowl of wheat or corn bran cereal can prevent constipation during resin use, but some patients still feel bloated. Resins are contraindicated in the hypertriglyceridemias, and TG levels should be reduced to under 300 mg/dl before resins are used in mixed or combined hyperlipidemics.

Niacin is useful in patients with LDL elevations, and the same precautions apply that were noted for niacin use in hypertriglyceridemia. The drug can cause fatty liver and cirrhosis, and the long-term safety is not established. Lovastatin, pravastatin, simvastatin, and fluvastatin are a series of drugs that competitively inhibit hydroxymethyl glutaryl coenzyme A (HMG-CoA) reductase, the rate-limiting enzyme in cholesterol biosynthesis. This inhibition induces an increase in hepatic B,E receptors, and LDL typically are lowered by 30%. Reductase inhibitors are appropriate for hypercholesterolemics of any age who have established CHD and for other adults with moderately severe hypercholesterolemia (LDL > 190 mg/dl). These drugs are expensive but well tolerated, and compliance is excellent. Use in combination with niacin, fibrates, or cyclosporine may cause myositis and even rhabdomyolysis. The reductase inhibitors occupy a unique position in primary and secondary CHD intervention. They have been shown to both prevent cardiac endpoints (myocardial infarction and CABG surgery) and prolong life.

The fibrates are not approved for simple hypercholesterolemia. They typically lower LDL levels by only 8 to 10% but may produce dramatic results in some patients. Many patients, particularly those who have heterozygotic familial hypercholesterolemia, require two or three drugs to achieve adequate control. Resins plus niacin plus lovastatin or resins plus fibrates have been widely used. Resins or reductase inhibitors plus fish oils are also effective in mixed hyperlipidemics. Familial monogenic hypercholesterolemia homozygotes are poorly responsive to diet and drugs and are considered candidates for liver transplantation. Finally, estrogen replacement therapy after the menopause can significantly lower LDL levels while increasing HDL.

LIPIDS AND VASCULAR DISEASE

Intervention studies in the last decade have shown that cholesterol reduction using diet, drugs, or surgery reduces the risk of development or progression of CHD. In general, a 1% fall in LDL-cholesterol has been associated with roughly a 2% reduction in disease end points. Arteriographic studies have shown small but convincing regressions of arterial lesions. With use of the more powerful reductase inhibitors, LDL-cholesterols have been reduced by up to 35%, and death rates in men with coronary heart disease have been reduced by 30%. Thus, few experts doubt the wisdom of treating lipid disorders in young men and women known to have coronary or peripheral vascular disease or in older patients with moderately severe LDL elevations.

There is still considerable debate about the cost-effectiveness of screening the general population for lipid disorders and treating individuals found to have cholesterol elevations. The reference ranges established by the National Cholesterol Education Program would lead to 27% of adult Americans being classified as having "high cholesterol" and another 30% as having "borderline high" values. Indeed, almost half of all postmenopausal women have total and LDL-C levels over 240 mg/dl and 160 mg/dl, respectively. It has been estimated that about 100,000 people must be treated annually to prevent 70 heart disease deaths.

Nevertheless, general agreement exists that eating less saturated fat and cholesterol and adopting diet and exercise habits to reduce obesity will benefit the health of most people. Preliminary data suggest a significant fall in American cholesterol levels in the past decade, and vascular disease rates have been falling for almost three decades. These public health effects will probably have a much greater impact than medical intervention approaches.

REFERENCES

Brown MS, Goldstein JL: Drugs used in the treatment of hyperlipoproteinemias. *In* Gilman AG, Rall TW, Nies AS, Taylor P (eds.): The Pharmacological Basis of Therapeutics. 8th ed. New York, Pergamon Press, 1991.

Scriver CR, Beaudet AL, Sly WS, Valle D (eds.). The Metabolic and Molecular Bases of Inherited Disease. 7th ed. New York, McGraw-Hill, 1995.

Summary of the Second Report of the National Cholesterol Education Program (NCEP) Expert Panel on Detection, Evaluation and Treatment of High Blood Cholesterol in Adults (Adult Treatment Panel II). JAMA 1993; 264: 3015–23.

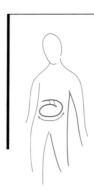

62

Disorders of Metals and Metalloproteins

WILSON'S DISEASE

Wilson's disease, or hepatolenticular degeneration, is an autosomal recessive disorder affecting 1 to 3 per 100,000 population. It is caused by defective hepatic excretion of copper. The consequence is copper-induced injury to many organs, particularly the liver and brain.

Normal Copper Metabolism

Copper is an essential trace element. Organ meats (particularly liver), nuts, seafood, and seeds are rich dietary sources. Humans ingest about 1 to 3 mg/day. Unlike iron, absorption does not appear to be tightly regulated. Copper absorption can be reduced by zinc. Zinc induces production of the cysteine-rich protein metallothionein, which retains copper in intestinal mucosal cells. Copper so bound is poorly absorbed and lost when the cells slough. Albumin and other proteins transport copper from the mucosal cell to the liver, which takes up most absorbed copper. Copper may be stored in the liver, bound in part to metallothionein; may be secreted into plasma bound to ceruloplasmin, which transports 80% of plasma copper; or may be excreted in bile, perhaps bound to ceruloplasmin fragments. Copper is essential for several enzyme systems, including superoxide dismutase, which detoxifies free radicals.

Large doses of copper consumed accidentally or intentionally can cause severe hemolysis and acute liver and kidney failure.

Pathogenesis

The genetic defect accounting for defective copper excretion in Wilson's disease has been localized to chromosome 13, and the gene product is thought to be a transmembrane copper transporter. Biliary copper excretion is low, and copper slowly accumulates in the liver. Signs and symptoms of organ dysfunction do not appear before age 6 years, but two thirds of patients have hepatic and/or brain dysfunction between ages 8 and 20 years. Delay of symptoms to age 60 has been described.

Organ dysfunction appears to result from copper-induced hepatic inflammation and destruction or from ab-

normal release of hepatic copper into the circulation, with toxic effects in many extrahepatic organs. Copper-induced liver disease may present like acute viral hepatitis, chronic active hepatitis, or postnecrotic cirrhosis. When copper release from the liver is abrupt and massive, a transient Coomb's negative hemolytic anemia is produced. Prolonged increased release of copper not bound to ceruloplasmin causes basal ganglion and, in some cases, cerebral cortex destruction. Prominent symptoms include tremor, muscular rigidity, and dystonic postures. Kidney damage may present as nephrolithiasis when renal tubular dysfunction causes hypercalcuria, and some patients develop the Fanconi syndrome, with aminoaciduria, glucosuria, and rickets. Copper deposits at the periphery of the cornea produce the almost diagnostic yellow-brown to green deposits called Kayser-Fleischer rings.

Diagnosis

No laboratory test is diagnostic, but complementary results on two or more tests (Table 62–1) are very helpful. Liver biopsies should be assayed for copper content, which is higher in early disease and less elevated in late disease. High hepatic levels do occur in some other liver diseases such as primary biliary cirrhosis. Ceruloplasmin levels are low in 95% of cases, but low levels are not the *cause* of Wilson's disease. Confusion may arise because ceruloplasmin is an acute phase reactant that is also increased in pregnancy and by estrogens; under such circumstances, apparently normal ceruloplasmin levels may be seen in Wilson's disease. Total serum copper levels may be low but may overlap the normal range. Urinary copper excretion is almost always high, reflecting use of an ancillary route of excretion. Ultimately, the combination of laboratory tests with a consistent clinical presentation yields a secure diagnosis.

Treatment

D-Penicillamine in typical doses of 500 mg twice daily can increase urinary copper to 1500 to 3000 μg/day. About 5 to 10% of patients develop severe penicillamine side effects such as rash, fever, lymphadenopathy, cytopenias, lupus erythematosus, Goodpasture's syndrome,

TABLE 62-1	Diagnostic Copper Testing in Wilson's Disease	
Test	**Levels in Normal People**	**Levels in Wilson's Disease**
Liver copper content (μgCu/g dry weight)	10–50	100–2000
Serum ceruloplasmin (mg/dl)	20–45	0–20
Serum copper (μg/dl)	70–160	25–70
Urinary copper (μg/day)	3–35	100–1000

and nephrotic syndrome. Recently zinc, which stimulates metallothionein synthesis and reduces copper absorption, has shown clinical efficacy at doses of 50 mg three times daily. Triethylene tetramine (trientine) has been used as a safe alternative chelator but has not been consistently available. Fulminant or progressive liver failure has been successfully treated with liver transplantation. Treatment by any modality can prolong life and interrupt hepatic and brain deterioration.

HEMOCHROMATOSIS

Hemochromatosis is a disorder characterized by excessive body iron storage causing multiorgan dysfunction. The condition may result from ingestion of excessive iron or multiple transfusions. This section, however, deals with hereditary hemochromatosis. This autosomal recessive disorder is carried by 5 to 10% of whites, and 1 in every 200 to 400 individuals is homozygotic. Hemochromatosis is only a tenth as common in blacks and is rare in Asians.

Normal Iron Metabolism

The body of a normal adult man contains about 4 gm of iron. More than half is contained in hemoglobin, and about 15% is in myoglobin, heme enzymes, and nonheme enzymes. Reserve iron is normally about 1 gm. Most

TABLE 62-2	Iron Indices in Normal Subjects and in Patients with Symptomatic Hemochromatosis	
Index	**Normal Subjects**	**Patients with Hemochromatosis**
Plasma iron (μg/dl)	50–150	180–300
Total iron binding capacity (μg/dl)	250–375	200–300
Percent transferrin saturation	20–40	80–100
Serum ferritin (ng/ml)	10–200	900–6000
Urinary iron after 0.5 gm desferrioxamine	0–2	9–23
Liver iron (μg/100 mg dry weight)	30–140	600–1800

(70%) is stored in ferritin, a readily available storage form, and the remainder in hemosiderin, a product of lysosomal enzyme degradation of ferritin.

Men lose about 1 mg of iron daily, mostly from the gastrointestinal tract. Women lose more, about 1.4 mg daily, because of menstruation. An additional 1000 mg of iron is needed for each pregnancy. Western diets contain about 6 mg iron per 1000 kcal, and absorption takes place in the duodenum and upper jejunum. We normally absorb the 1.0 to 1.4 mg/day that is lost and can increase absorption when needed to about 3 to 4 mg/day with an unsupplemented diet. It is not known how the intestinal mucosal cell determines whether to transport iron into the mesenteric circulation or store it as ferritin, ultimately to be excreted when the cell turns over. It is possible that the mucosal cell responds to the availability of circulating iron bound to transferrin.

Iron transport in the circulation is on transferrin, a large liver protein whose synthesis is stimulated by iron deficiency. Transferrin synthesis is reduced by cytokines released under conditions of cell death, inflammation, or malignancy. When iron stores are normal, the plasma iron concentration is at least 50 μg/dL and transferrin is 20 to 40% saturated (Table 62–2). Transferrin releases its iron only after binding to specific receptors on proliferating, differentiating, or heme-synthesizing cells. There are nearly one million such receptors on the normoblast, whereas the mature red blood cell has none.

Pathogenesis of Hereditary Hemochromatosis

The gene for hemochromatosis is on chromosome 6, tightly linked to the human leukocyte antigen (HLA) locus. The abnormal gene product has not been identified but is neither a mutant ferritin nor a mutant transferrin. It could be a cellular membrane or cytosolic iron-binding protein. Affected homozygotes absorb about 3 mg or two to three times the normal amount of iron each day, and this can increase body stores by about 7 gm each decade. Most patients are 40 to 60 years old before symptoms occur after accumulating 20 to 40 gm of surplus iron. Homozygotes are of course equally represented in men and women, but men are 10 times more likely to develop organ dysfunction, perhaps because of the absence of menses and greater alcohol consumption.

Alcohol can mobilize iron stored in tissue ferritin, and this iron is capable of generating free (hydroxyl and ferryl) radicals that can cause lipid peroxidation and cell injury. Moreover, even without parenchymal cell damage, tissue iron, like alcohol, directly stimulates collagen production and fibrosis. A liver fibrotic from virtually any cause can give rise to hepatocellular carcinoma.

Clinical Features and Pathology

Children may be affected, but most symptomatic patients are over 40 years. Lethargy and weakness, common nonspecific constitutional complaints, are present in more than 80%. The skin has a fivefold increase in iron content and may be bronzed to slate-gray from excessive melanin and hemosiderin pigmentation. The liver can be enlarged and firm, and elevated transaminases are characteristic in the early clinical stages. In the absence of alcoholism, fibrosis does not occur until iron content exceeds 2.2% of the liver's dry weight. Biopsy shows considerable hemosiderin in hepatocytes and bile duct epithelium and a diagnostic absence of iron loading in Kupffer cells. Signs of cirrhosis may appear with advanced disease, but severe portal hypertension and ascites are less common than in alcoholic cirrhosis.

Hemosiderin deposits can be seen in the pancreatic islets with iron localized to the insulin-producing beta cells. Alpha cells and exocrine cells are spared. Insulinopenia usually causes diabetes mellitus in advanced hereditary hemochromatosis, but there may also be insulin resistance secondary to hepatic cirrhosis. Gonadal atrophy is common in men and women due to pituitary hypogonadotropism. Symptoms include low libido, amenorrhea, impotence, and scant axillary and pubic hair. In contrast to alcoholic cirrhosis, excessive estrogen production and gynecomastia are rare.

Cardiac abnormalities may cause the first overt symptoms. Hemosiderin accumulates in both myocardial fibers and interstitial cells, with less involvement of conducting tissue and the sinoatrial node. Necrosis of myocardial cells and fibrosis can occur. The predominant clinical presentation is dilated cardiomyopathy, often with ventricular ectopy. Finally, arthralgias and signs of degenerative joint disease are found in 45% of patients. Chondrocalcinosis and, occasionally, pseudogout can occur. The mechanism is unknown, although it has been speculated that iron inhibits pyrophosphatase, thereby increasing pyrophosphate crystals.

Diagnosis

In view of the high prevalence of homozygotic hereditary hemochromatosis and the expense of treating organ failure, it has been shown that screening the general population for the disorder is cost effective. Initial testing should consist of serum iron and iron-binding capacity with calculation of percent transferrin saturation (see Table 62–2). Saturations of 50% in women and 60% in men should lead to testing of ferritin concentrations. If the ferritin is twice the upper normal limit, a liver biopsy should be performed to quantify liver iron and assess the extent of fibrosis or cirrhosis. Even if the ferritin is normal, the homozygotic state cannot be excluded, and repeat testing every 2 years is recommended. Alternatively, in patients with high transferrin saturations and normal ferritins, the physician may choose to recommend phlebotomy at 3-month intervals.

Treatment and Prognosis

Initial iron depletion is accomplished by removing 500 ml blood once or twice a week until a microcytic anemia develops or until the transferrin saturation and serum ferritin fall below the lower normal limits. Each unit of blood removes only 200 to 250 mg of iron, so at least 2 to 3 years of weekly phlebotomies are required. Lifelong maintenance phlebotomy, every 2 to 6 months, is then initiated using the serum ferritin to guide therapy.

Early detection and treatment prevents the morbid consequences of hemochromatosis. Untreated symptomatic patients have a 5-year survival of 20%. Even with cirrhosis, phlebotomy can increase 10-year survival to 75%. Cardiac failure often improves but can worsen despite iron depletion. Hypogonadism is not corrected by phlebotomy, and diabetes may improve but rarely disappears.

THE PORPHYRIAS

Porphyrias are disorders caused by partial deficiencies of one of the eight enzymes involved in heme production (Fig. 62–1). A different form of porphyria is associated with six of the eight enzymes. Symptoms of the porphyrias include neurovisceral disturbance and/or photosensitivity and are caused by abnormal accumulation of heme synthesis intermediates. Inheritance may be autosomal recessive or dominant, and factors extrinsic to the patient usually determine if the enzyme deficiency becomes clinically manifest. This section deals with the three most common varieties of porphyria, which illustrate the cardinal biochemical and clinical features (Table 62–3).

Acute Intermittent Porphyria (AIP)

Acute intermittent porphyria is an autosomal dominant disorder, and the activity of the involved enzyme, porphobilinogen (PBG) deaminase (see Fig. 62–1), is almost always ≤50% of normal. The majority of subjects (~90%) with the heritable disorder never develop symptoms of porphyria. Attacks are precipitated in the minority by external stimuli to hepatic heme synthesis, particularly drugs inducing the mitochondrial cytochrome P-450.

The flux of intermediates through the heme synthetic pathway is usually at a level where enzyme substrates are efficiently processed despite reduced enzyme activity. The rate-limiting step, controlling the stream of intermediates in hepatic heme biosynthesis, is the inducible enzyme δ-aminolevulinic acid (ALA) synthase (see Fig. 62–1). In all the forms of porphyria, including AIP, this enzyme functions normally. When defects occur beyond ALA production, it is possible for ALA synthase to be induced and for ALA to be overproduced, driving the subsequent series of reactions. In AIP, the defect is at the third enzymatic step (see Fig. 62–1), so both ALA and PBG accumulate (see Table 62–3).

It is believed that symptoms in AIP are largely, if not exclusively, the result of central or peripheral nervous system dysfunction. There are two unproven theories of causation. One holds that ALA itself is neurotoxic. A second theory suggests that restricted hepatic heme production affects metabolism of a critical neurotransmitter or its precursor.

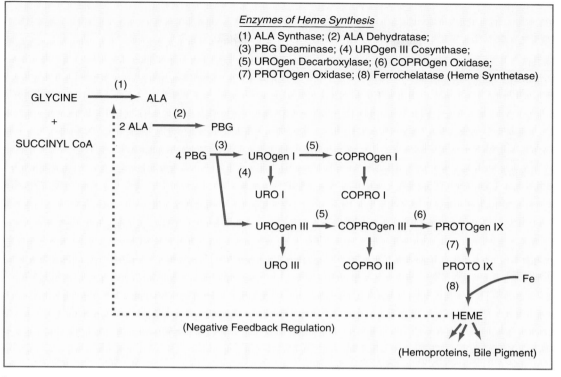

Figure 62–1

Pathway of heme biosynthesis. ALA = δ-Aminolevulinic acid; COPRO = coproporphyrin; PBG = porphobilinogen; PROTO = protoporphyrin; URO = uroporphyrin. (Adapted from Bissell DM; Porphyria. *In* Wyngaarden JB, Smith LH Jr [eds.]: Cecil Textbook of Medicine. 18th ed. Philadelphia, WB Saunders, 1988, p 1183.)

Symptoms in AIP are listed in Table 62–3. Abdominal pain, sometimes mistakenly prompting surgical exploration, is found in more than 90% of acute attacks. With accompanying nausea, vomiting, and altered bowel function, primary gastrointestinal pathology is usually suspected. Sympathetic nervous system symptoms of tachycardia and hypertension may be pronounced. Hypertension can become sustained. Neuropathy, occurring in more than 60% of cases, may present as muscle weakness, even involving the cranial nerves, with respiratory paralysis and death. Prominent mental symptoms such as anxiety, paranoia, and depression may mistakenly be taken as evidence of a primary affective disorder. Seizures, particularly with syndrome of inappropriate antidiuretic hormone (SIADH) and hyponatremia, are not uncommon.

Acute intermittent porphyria is rare before puberty, and sex hormones may precipitate attacks. A host of drugs can do likewise, and Table 62–4 contains a partial list. Fasting and calorically restricted diets have precipitated attacks. In some cases, stress, infectious and other illnesses, and even surgery under local anesthesia have caused attacks.

Treatment of AIP is largely preventive. Patients must avoid alcohol, offending drugs, hypocaloric diets, and other precipitating factors. Narcotic analgesics are safe and effective during attacks, and at least 300 gm/day of dietary carbohydrate have traditionally been provided. Intravenous infusions of hemin, a heme derivative processed from red blood cells, inhibit ALA-synthase and reduce ALA and PBG production. This treatment, used for almost two decades, probably has modest efficacy. β-Adrenoreceptor blockers effectively treat hypertension and tachycardia.

Porphyria Cutanea Tarda (PCT)

Several thousand cases of PCT have been identified, but accurate prevalence figures are not available. The affected enzyme is uroporphyrinogen (UROgen) decarboxylase, which is at step 5 in heme biosynthesis (see Fig. 62–1). The major porphyrins accumulating in plasma are uroporphyrin, which is behind the partial enzymatic block, and 7-carboxylate porphyrin, the first product of the enzyme's sequential action on uroporphyrin. UROgen and 7-carboxylate porphyria cause the photosensitivity in PCT.

Photosensitivity of the skin is seen in all porphyrias except those with blocks before porphyrin production, i.e., AIP and ALA-dehydratase deficiency (see Fig. 62–1). Most porphyrins absorb light at 400 nm wavelength and then release energy-generating oxygen free radicals that are particularly damaging to lipid membranes.

Porphyria cutanea tarda usually begins in adulthood with symptoms and signs as noted in Table 62–3. In those with familial disease, the factors inducing heme

TABLE 62-3	Three Most Common Porphyrias			
Disorder	Prevalence	Affected Enzyme (see Fig. 62-1)	Symptoms and Signs	Screening Test
Acute intermittent porphyria (AIP)	5-10/100,000	(3) PBG deaminase	Abdominal pain Vomiting Constipation Muscle weakness Hypertension Tachycardia Mental changes	Urine: ALA, PBG; PBD deaminase in red blood cells
Porphyria cutanea tarda (PCT)	Uncertain, but most common porphyria	(5) UROgen decarboxylase	Symptoms in light-exposed skin Fragility Vesicles Bullae Hyperpigmentation Hypertrichosis	Urine: URO, 7-carboxylate porphyrin, COPRO
Erythropoietic protoporphyria (EPP)	Several hundred known worldwide	(8) Ferrochelatase	Symptoms in light-exposed skin Burning Edema Itching Erythema Anemia	Plasma and red blood cell PROTO (not urine)

ALA = δ-Aminolevulinic acid; COPRO = coproporphyrin, PBG = porphobilinogen PROTO = protoporphyrin; URO = uroporphyrin; UROgen = uroporphyrinogen.

synthesis are those discussed for AIP. There is also substantial evidence that UROgen decarboxylase deficiency and PCT may be acquired and that acquired disease is far more common than the inherited forms. Moderate to severe alcoholism, estrogen in oral contraceptives, and hormone supplements are implicated in most cases currently recognized. Two other associations are particularly noteworthy. Most patients have evidence of iron overload and at least mild hemochromatosis. In addition, a number of patients with acquired immunodeficiency syndrome have manifested PCT.

As with AIP, prevention of attacks is the focal point of management. Environmental toxins such as chlorinated hydrocarbons, alcohol, estrogen, and other drugs (see Table 62-4) should be identified. Phlebotomy for hemochromatosis is effective treatment for PCT and is widely employed (see previous). Chloroquine has been used in refractory cases.

Erythropoietic Protoporphyria (EPP)

Erythropoietic protoporphyria has been described in more than 300 patients worldwide. Unlike PCT, it typically is manifest in childhood. The deficient enzyme, ferrochelatase, is at the eighth and final step in heme biosynthesis and incorporates ferrous ion in protoporphyrin to produce heme. Since the enzyme block in EPP is so late, massive amounts of protoporphyrin accumulate in erythrocytes, plasma, and feces. Protoporphyrin is not found in urine since it is not water soluble.

Cutaneous damage in EPP occurs as described for PCT, and signs and symptoms (see Table 62-3) are similar to those of PCT, except that vesicles and bullae are less common. Sun avoidance and highly protective sun screens (SPF 26 or higher) are the primary approach to management. β-Carotene may also offer some photoprotection. Anemia, which would occur if heme production were severely limited, is not common.

TABLE 62-4	Some Drugs Precipitating Attacks of Acute Intermittent Porphyria

Barbiturates
Chlorpropamide
Danazol
Dapsone
Diphenylhydantoin
Ergot preparations
Ethanol
Glutethimide
Griseofulvin
Meprobamate
Progestins
Sulfonamide antibiotics
Tolbutamide
Valproic acid

REFERENCES

Bothwell TH, Charlton RW, Motulsky AG: Hemochromatosis. In Scriver CR, Beaudet AL, Sly WS, Valle D (eds.). The Metabolic and Molecular Bases of Inherited Disease. 7th ed. New York, McGraw-Hill, 1995.

Danks DM: Disorders of copper transport. *In* Scriver CR, Beaudet AL, Sly WS, Valle D (eds.). The Metabolic and Molecular Bases of Inherited Disease. 7th ed. New York, McGraw-Hill, 1995.

Deiss A: Wilson's disease. *In* Bennett JC, Plum F (eds.): Cecil Textbook of Medicine. 20th ed, Philadelphia, WB Saunders, 1996.

Edwards CQ, Kushner JP: Screening for hemochromatosis. N Engl J Med 1993; 328:1616–20.

Kappas A, Sassa S, Galbraith RA, Nordmann Y: The porphyrias. *In* Scriver CR, Beaudet AL, Sly WS, Valle D (eds.). The Metabolic and Molecular Bases of Inherited Disease. 7th ed. New York, McGraw-Hill, 1995.

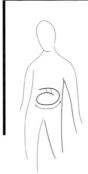

63

Disorders of Amino Acid Metabolism

There are more than 80 recognized abnormalities of amino acid metabolism. Most have been identified through detection of abnormal quantities of one or several amino acids in the urine. The kidney normally reabsorbs more than 95% of filtered amino acids, but saturation of reabsorptive mechanisms by high plasma levels or modification of the transporter can cause aminoaciduria.

Individual disorders of amino acid metabolism are rare. Many are benign, while others are associated with seizures, mental retardation, growth retardation, nephropathy, hepatic cirrhosis, and other organ dysfunction (Table 63–1). The best known, for which all newborns are screened, is phenylketonuria, which affects only 1 in 10,000 births. Physicians of adult patients are more likely to encounter secondary aminoacidurias. In these cases, a drug, toxin, or disease process damages the proximal renal tubules, producing a generalized aminoaciduria and other defects of the Fanconi syndrome.

This chapter focuses on two disorders of amino acid metabolism that are very relevant to adult medicine: homocysteinemia and cystinuria.

HOMOCYSTEINEMIA

Homocysteine is not normally incorporated into human proteins but is an intermediate in methionine metabolism. It is produced, for example, when methionine donates a methyl group in a reaction producing cysteine. Homocysteine so generated is metabolized in one of three reactions (Fig. 63–1). The enzyme methionine synthase, which requires methylcobalamin (vitamin B_{12}) and folate, catalyzes conversion to methionine (see Fig. 63–1). Another enzyme, cystathionine β-synthase, which has tightly bound pyridoxal-phosphate (vitamin B_6), catalyzes the condensation of serine with homocysteine to produce cystathionine. In a third reaction, catalyzed by betaine-homocysteine methyl transferase, betaine produced from choline donates a methyl group to again convert homocysteine to methionine.

The prototypic form of homocysteinemia (and homocysteinuria) is the rare genetic disease cystathionine β-synthase deficiency. Homozygotes for this autosomal recessive disorder may have ectopic lenses, severe osteoporosis, and mental retardation. Most striking, however, is their predisposition to both venous and arterial thrombo-

embolic events and arteriosclerosis. The latter is characterized by marked fibrous thickening of the intima with a notable absence of lipid deposits. It is believed that elevated plasma homocysteine may alter platelet function, injure endothelium, activate clotting factors, or reduce activity of natural anticoagulants. It is not known if one mechanism predominates. The homocysteinemia in many cases is responsive to pyridoxine (see Fig. 63–1).

There is considerable current interest in the possibility that mild forms of homocysteinemia may occur commonly and contribute to coronary and peripheral arterial disease in the general population. A large number of case-control and cross-sectional studies have shown higher homocysteine levels in patients with stroke, carotid stenosis, and myocardial infarction. Since folate deficiency is probably the most common vitamin deficiency in developed countries and since folate, vitamin B_{12}, and vitamin B_6 can lower homocysteine levels (see Fig. 63–1), the prospects for intervention using vitamins are intriguing. However, research is needed to prove efficacy and validate the homocysteinemia-atherosclerosis connection.

CYSTINURIA

The overall prevalence of homozygous cystinuria is about 1 in 7000, making this one of the most common genetic disorders. The affected gene encodes a transporter protein of 633 amino acids, which is strongly expressed in the kidney and intestine. This transporter, a membrane glycoprotein, mediates the absorption of cystine, arginine, ornithine, lysine, and some neutral amino acids.

The dibasic amino acids are very soluble, but cystine is the most insoluble of all amino acids. When urinary cystine concentrations exceed 300 mg/L, distinctive hexagonal crystals appear and can usually be found in the first urine specimen after waking. The cyanide-nitroprusside test is widely used to confirm cystinuria. Quantitative urine collections, unnecessary when typical crystals are demonstrated, show excretion of more than 250 mg of cystine per gram of creatinine. Normal excretion is less than 20 mg.

Cystine stones readily form in acid urine. They are yellow-brown in color, in contrast to the black color of the more common calcium oxalate stones. They are radio-

TABLE 63–1	**Examples of Disorders of Amino Acid Metabolism**		
Disorder	**Amino Acid**	**Process Affected**	**Clinical Features**
Phenylketonuria	Phenylalanine	Phenylalanine oxygenase	Mental retardation if untreated
Hypertyrosinemia	Tyrosine	Fumarylacetoacetate hydrolase	Hepatic cirrhosis and renal tubular failure
Hyperhistidinemia	Histidine	Histidine ammonia-lyase	Benign
Maple syrup urine disease	Leucine, isoleucine, valine	Branched-chain–α-ketoacid lipoate oxidoreductase	May be mild or cause mental retardation and even neonatal collapse
Cystinosis	Cystine	Lysosomal membrane transporter	Renal tubular Fanconi syndrome by age 1 yr; renal failure by 10 yr; cystine deposits throughout body compromise organ function
Alcaptonuria	Homogentisic acid from phenylalanine and tyrosine	Homogentisic acid oxidase	Gray-blue pigmentation of ear cartilage (ochronosis), degenerative arthritis

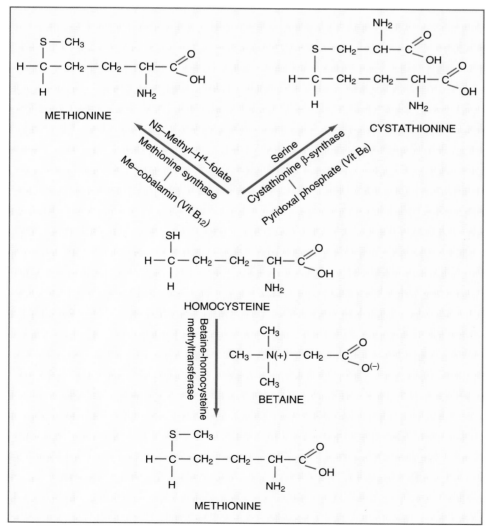

Figure 63–1

Metabolism of homocysteine, producing methionine, cystathionine, and methionine.

paque and can form staghorn calculi. All kidney stones should be chemically analyzed because stones initiated by cystine crystallization often have a mixed composition, and cystine may not predominate.

Renal colic, hematuria, obstructive uropathy, or secondary infection typically afflict cystinuric patients in their 20s or 30s. Episodes of urolithiasis and urinary tract infection then tend to be recurrent until adequate therapy is initiated. The most important aspect of treatment is ingestion of sufficient fluids to yield 3 to 4 L/day of urine. Alkalinization of the urine is useful since cystine solubility sharply increases above pH 7.5. Preparations of citric acid and sodium or potassium citrate are used for alkalinization. Finally, chemicals with free sulfhydryl groups, capable of forming much more soluble mixed disulfides on reaction with cystine, can dramatically lower urinary cystine. D-Penicillamine has traditionally been used for this purpose when hydration and urinary alkalinization are inadequate. However, the drug is quite toxic.

Tiopronin (α-mercaptopropionylglycine, Thiola®, Mission Pharmacal Co., San Antonio, TX) at doses of 200 to 300 mg tid is also effective and appears less toxic than D-penicillamine. Recently, captopril at a dose of 50 mg tid has been used with some success.

REFERENCES

Mudd SH, Levy HL, Skovby F: Disorders of transsulfuration. *In* Scriver CR, Beaudet AL, Sly WS, Valle D (eds.). The Metabolic and Molecular Bases of Inherited Disease. New York, McGraw-Hill, 1995, pp 1279–1327.

Robinson K, Mayer E, Jacobsen DW: Homocysteine and coronary artery disease. Cleve Clin J Med 1994; 61:438–450.

Scriver CR: Hyperaminoaciduria (with a classification of the inborn and developmental errors of amino acid metabolism). *In* Bennett JC, Plum F (eds.): Cecil Textbook of Medicine. 20th ed, Philadelphia, WB Saunders, 1996.

64

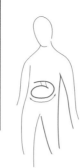

Inherited Disorders of Connective Tissue

The genetically transmitted disorders reviewed in this chapter are characterized by structural changes in skin, muscle, bone, and the nervous system. Each involves defective synthesis, secretion, or catabolism of the fibrillar or nonfibrillar components of connective tissue.

Collagen and elastic fibers are the major connective tissue fibrillar components. The nonfibrillar or amorphous ground substance consists of proteoglycans including fibronectin, which binds cells to the fibrils, and the high–molecular weight carbohydrate polymers dermatan sulfate, hyaluronic acid, heparan sulfate, chondroitin sulfate, and keratan sulfate. The effects of abnormalities of the fibrillar or nonfibrillar components of connective tissue may be widespread or relatively localized, depending on the tissue distribution of the affected protein or carbohydrate.

The connective tissue diseases are generally grouped according to the similarities of the clinical states rather than according to the type of fibrillar or nonfibrillar component affected (Table 64–1). Thus, Ehlers-Danlos syndrome consists of at least 10 separate disorders, most involving collagen production. However, at least one form of Ehlers-Danlos syndrome is due to a functional defect in a nonfibrillar component, fibronectin.

OSTEOGENESIS IMPERFECTA

Collagen defects cause this heterogeneous group of disorders characterized by abnormalities of bones, teeth, hearing, and soft tissues (see Table 64–1). Blue sclerae and bone deformities or fractures usually lead to diagnosis in childhood. The clinical course varies from perinatal death due to poor calvarial mineralization to normal life expectancy with slightly reduced bone mass. There is no specific therapy.

EHLERS-DANLOS SYNDROME

A number of variants of this syndrome are recognized. They differ in mode of inheritance, genetic defect, and clinical features (see Table 64–1). Loose joints and blue sclerae are found in some variants, but the skin changes of Ehlers-Danlos syndrome are not found in Marfan's syndrome or osteogenesis imperfecta. The skin is unusually soft, velvety, and hyperextensible, having a rubber-like quality that allows it to be stretched away from the underlying structures, promptly returning to its original position upon release. With aging, the skin may sag and become redundant, particularly over the elbows. The skin is very fragile, and minor trauma may produce gaping wounds. Minor injuries may also produce large hematomas that may organize into tumorlike calcified masses. Hyperextensibility of the joints allows affected patients to perform unusual contortions. Chronic or recurrent joint dislocations are common, particularly affecting the hips, knees, shoulders, and temporomandibular joints. Many patients suffer inguinal, hiatal, and umbilical hernias as well as gastrointestinal or genitourinary diverticulae.

Life expectancy may be shortened by rupture of arteries and viscera (most marked in the type IV variant), or the clinical consequences may be remarkably benign. Therapy is directed at symptoms since correction of the connective tissue defects is not currently possible.

MARFAN'S SYNDROME

Marfan's syndrome, due to abnormalities of the ubiquitous extracellular protein fibrillin I, is characterized by tall stature, lens dislocation, pectus deformities, and cardiovascular abnormalities. More than 20 mutations in the fibrillin gene are recognized, and there is considerable clinical heterogeneity. Moreover, fibrillin mutations account for a variety of other syndromes sharing features of Marfan's syndrome (dominant ectopia lentis, mitral valve prolapse with skeletal feature, and dominant aortic aneurysm without typical ocular and skeletal features).

Tall stature does not distinguish Marfan's syndrome, but arm span greater than height (dolichostenomelia) is more specific. Pectus excavatum occurs more commonly than pectus carinatum, and elements of both may be present. Upward dislocation of the lens is probably present at birth in 50 to 80% of cases and generally is not progressive. Joint laxity and arachnodactyly (spider fingers) have little diagnostic specificity.

Progressive dilation of the ascending aorta usually begins in the 20s, leading to aortic valve incompetence and aortic valve dissection. This complication used to limit life expectancy to 40 to 50 years. Prophylactic β-adrenergic blockade slows the process. Prophylactic repair

TABLE 64–1	Heritable Disorders of Connective Tissue		
	Incidence Per 100,000 Births	Genetic Abnormality	Major Clinical Manifestations
Abnormalities of Fibrous Proteins			
Osteogenesis imperfecta	~5	Mutations alter ability of $\alpha1(I)$ or $\alpha2(I)$ chains of type I collagen to be secreted, to form fibrils or to be mineralized	Blue sclerae; thin, easily fractured bones; short stature
Ehlers-Danlos syndrome (EDS) types I–IX	~20	Highly heterogeneous; includes defects in synthesis of both types I and III collagen, and defects in post-translational modification of collagen	Marked joint laxity; soft, velvety, hyperextensible skin; easy bruising and "cigarette-paper" scars; vascular or bowel rupture in EDS type IV
Marfan's syndrome	~10	Abnormal synthesis, secretion, or accumulation of fibrillin I, a major microfibril component of elastic tissue and the zonular fibrils of the lens	Tall stature, long fingers and toes (arachnodactyly), long arms and legs (dolichostenomelia); inward displacement of sternum (pectus excavatum); dislocation of lens (ectopia lentis); lax joints; aortic dilatation, dissection, and rupture
Pseudoxanthoma elasticum	~0.6	Unknown, presumed to affect elastin	Redundant, lax inelastic skin on face, neck, axilla, abdomen and thighs; hypertension; coronary and cerebral artery occlusion; gastrointestinal and urinary tract bleeding
Abnormalities of Ground Substance			
EDS, type X	—	Mutation alters functional properties of fibronectin	See above
Mucopolysaccharidoses (Hurler, Scheie, Hunter, Sanfilippo, Marquis, Maroteaux-Lamy)	~10	Deficient activity of lysosomal enzymes degrading proteoglycans (dermatan, chondroitin, heparan, and keratan sulfate)	Manifest generally before 4 years, with corneal clouding, organomegaly, skeletal malformations, and mental retardation

or replacement of the aortic root when its diameter reaches 55 mm can generally prevent cardiovascular catastrophe. Median life expectancy in Marfan's syndrome may now exceed 70 years.

MUCOPOLYSACCHARIDOSES

The mucopolysaccharidoses (MPSs), like other lysosomal storage diseases, are generally progressive and involve many organs (see Table 64–1). The stored materials are glycosaminoglycans (GAGs) derived from the degradation of proteoglycans in the nonfibrillar connective tissue. Some MPS genetic defects involve complete deficiencies of a lysosomal enzyme, whereas others yield enzymes with reduced activity. GAG accumulation in neurons leads to mental retardation and neurologic deficits. Accumulation in smooth muscle cells and macrophages can cause arteriosclerosis and myocardial and cerebral infarcts. Reticuloendothelial cell accumulation produces hepatosplenomegaly.

Most patients with MPSs appear normal at birth but show signs of GAG organ involvement in childhood.

Since urinary GAG excretion is increased, a positive urinary toluidine-blue test leads the clinician to characterize the excreted GAGs and then demonstrate the enzyme defect in cultured fibrobasts, leukocytes, or other tissues. Some varieties have been successfully managed with bone marrow transplantation; gene infusion therapy may prove curative in the future. Currently, children with the most serious MPS, Hurler's syndrome, typically die by 10 years. In contrast, patients with Scheie syndrome and a mild form of Hunter's can live to their 60s.

REFERENCES

Byers PH: Disorders of collagen biosynthesis and structure. *In* Scriver CR, Beaudet AL, Sly WS, Valle D (eds.): The Metabolic and Molecular Bases of Inherited Disease. 7th ed. New York, McGraw-Hill, 1995.

Neufeld, EF, Muenzer J: The mucopolysaccharidoses. *In* Scriver CR, Beaudet AL, Sly WS, Valle D (eds.): The Metabolic and Molecular Bases of Inherited Disease. 7th ed. New York, McGraw-Hill, 1995.

Pyeritz RE, McKusick VA: The Marfan syndrome: Diagnosis and management. N Engl J Med 1979; 300:772–777.

Endocrine Disease

Section X

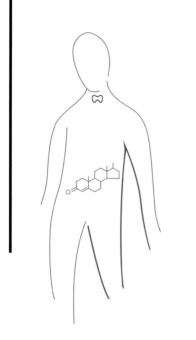

65

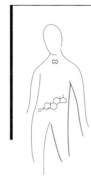

Hypothalamic-Pituitary Axis

ANATOMY

The pituitary gland, weighing 500 to 900 mg, lies at the base of the skull in the sella turcica, within the sphenoid bone. The cavernous sinus containing the carotid arteries and cranial nerves III, IV, and VI borders laterally on the pituitary gland. The optic chiasm courses over the superior aspect, separated from the gland by the diaphragma sella of the dura, while the roof of the sphenoid sinus forms the floor of the sella turcica. Two thirds of the pituitary gland is composed of an anterior lobe, and one third, of a posterior lobe.

The anterior pituitary gland receives a rich vascular supply, largely from the median eminence of the hypothalamus via a hypothalamic-pituitary portal circulation. Hypothalamic stimulatory and inhibitory hormones are transported via the hypothalamic-pituitary portal circulation directly to specific cells of the anterior pituitary gland, where they regulate synthesis and secretion of the pituitary trophic hormones (Fig. 65–1).

Each of the anterior pituitary hormones, adrenocorticotropic hormone (ACTH), growth hormone (GH), prolactin (PRL), and thyroid-stimulating hormone (TSH) are secreted by a specific pituitary cell type. Luteinizing hormone (LH) and follicle-stimulating hormone (FSH) are secreted by the same cell. GH, PRL, and ACTH are polypeptide hormones, whereas FSH, LH, and TSH are glycoproteins that share the same α-subunit, but each has a distinctive β-subunit. Arginine vasopressin (AVP) is also known as antidiuretic hormone (ADH); it is synthesized in the supraoptic and paraventricular nuclei of the hypothalamus and transported through long axons into the posterior pituitary (Table 65–1).

ANTERIOR PITUITARY HORMONE PHYSIOLOGY AND TESTING

Growth Hormone

Growth hormone is a 191–amino acid peptide with a molecular weight of 22,000 daltons. Secretion is stimulated by the 40– and 44–amino acid hypothalamic growth hormone–releasing hormones (GHRH) and inhibited by the hypothalamic tetradecapeptide somatostatin. These hypothalamic factors bind to pituitary somatotroph cells and regulate GH secretion. GH binds to receptors in the liver and induces insulin-like growth factor I (IGF-I), which circulates in the blood bound to binding proteins (BPs), the most important of which is IGF-BP3. IGF-I mediates most of the growth-promoting effects of growth hormone. GH also affects carbohydrate metabolism.

Evaluation of GH Reserve

Provocative tests that indirectly stimulate the somatotroph are required in the assessment of children with short stature who may be GH deficient, as basal GH levels are frequently very low even in normal individuals. GH levels may also be important in the work-up of adults with suspected hypopituitarism.

Insulin-induced hypoglycemia is the most reliable stimulus of GH hypersecretion. Insulin (0.05 to 0.1 units/kg) is administered intravenously to reduce the patient's blood glucose levels to 50% of initial blood glucose or to 40 mg/dl with serial sampling of serum GH and glucose. A normal response is when peak GH levels occur at 60 minutes in excess of 7 ng/ml. Arginine infusion over 30 minutes has a peak GH stimulatory effect 1 hour after administration. L-dopa, a precursor of dopamine and norepinephrine, crosses the blood-brain barrier and stimulates GH secretion from the pituitary somatotroph. Clonidine and propranolol are alternate orally administered agents, used to assess GH reserve. Arginine, L-dopa, clonidine, and propranolol are safer in older individuals or patients with central nervous system disorders than is insulin-induced hypoglycemia. Multiple tests are performed to diagnose GH deficiency in a single patient, as only 90% of normal individuals respond adequately to any single test. IGF-BP3 levels can be used as a screening test for GH deficiency, as IGF-BP3 levels are regulated by GH; GH deficiency is indicated by low IGF-BP3 levels.

A single dose of GHRH stimulates GH secretion to normal levels ($>7~\mu g/ml$) in those GH deficiency patients in whom the GH deficiency results from hypothalamic dysfunction. Patients with GH deficiency due to hypopituitarism do not respond to GHRH. Pretreatment with multiple GHRH injections can result in a subsequently adequate GH response in some patients with hypothalamic GHRH deficiency who had minimal response to a single dose of GHRH. However, GHRH offers no substantial improvement over standard stimulation tests.

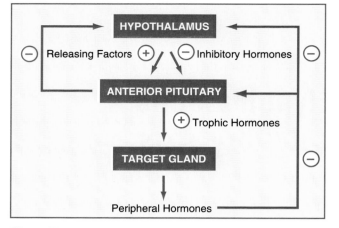

Figure 65-1
Feedback control of the hypothalamic-pituitary-target gland axis.

Tests for GH Hypersecretion

Growth hormone is secreted in a pulsatile fashion, and the measurement of random GH levels is of no value. Moreover, cirrhosis, starvation, anxiety, type 1 diabetes mellitus, and acute illness can be associated with GH hypersecretion. However, measurement of IGF-I levels is a useful indicator of GH hypersection, as this level does not fluctuate throughout the day. IGF-I levels are elevated in almost all patients with GH hypersecretion. A simple and specific dynamic test for GH hypersecretion is the administration of oral glucose. Seventy-five to 100 gm glucose administered orally suppresses GH levels to less than 2 ng/ml after 120 minutes in healthy volunteers. In acromegaly, GH levels may increase, remain unchanged, or decrease (however, not below 2 ng/ml) after an oral glucose load. IGF-I and oral glucose suppression tests are the cornerstones in the laboratory confirmation of GH hypersecretion in patients with acromegaly (see later).

Twenty to 50% of acromegalic patients exhibit a paradoxical increase in GH secretion after administration of thyrotropin-releasing hormone (TRH).

Prolactin

Prolactin, a 198–amino acid 22,000 dalton polypeptide, is synthesized and secreted by pituitary lactotrophs. The human PRL molecule is 16% homologous with GH and 13% homologous with human placental lactogen. PRL secretion is under predominantly inhibitory control by hypothalamic dopamine. TRH and vasoactive intestinal polypeptide (VIP) are prolactin-releasing factors. PRL secretion is episodic. Estrogens increase basal and stimulated PRL secretion; glucocorticoids and thyroid hormone blunt TRH-induced PRL secretion. PRL levels increase during pregnancy, enhancing breast development. Postpartum PRL stimulate milk production. However, elevated PRL levels are not required to maintain lactation, and basal PRL secretion falls as the suckling reflex maintains lactation.

Evaluation of PRL Reserve

Basal PRL levels increase three- to fivefold above baseline 15 to 30 minutes after TRH administration (200 mcg intravenous bolus). Age and sex affect PRL response to TRH.

Evaluation of PRL Hypersecretion

Basal PRL levels are used in the assessment of hyperprolactinemia. Basal PRL levels greater than 200 ng/ml are highly suggestive of PRL-secreting adenomas (see Prolactinoma).

TABLE 65-1	Hypothalamic-Pituitary-Target Organ Hormone Axis			
Hypothalamic Hormone	**Pituitary Target Cell**	**Pituitary Hormone Affected**	**Peripheral Target Gland**	**Peripheral Hormone Affected**
Stimulatory				
1) Anterior pituitary				
Thyrotropin-releasing hormone (TRH)	Thyrotroph	Thyroid-stimulating hormone (TSH)	Thyroid gland	Thyroxine (T_4) Triodothyroxine (T_3)
Growth hormone–releasing hormone (GHRH)	Somatotroph	Growth hormone (GH)	Liver	Insulin-like growth factor-I (IGF-I)
Gonadotropin-releasing hormone (GnRH)	Gonadotroph	Luteinizing hormone (LH)	Ovary	Progesterone
		Follicle-stimulating hormone (FSH)	Testis	Testosterone
			Ovary	Estradiol
			Testis	Inhibin
Corticotropin-releasing hormone	Corticotroph	Adrenocorticotrophic hormone (ACTH)	Adrenal gland	Cortisol
2) Posterior pituitary				
Vasopressin			Kidney	
Oxytocin			Uterus, breast	
Inhibitory				
Somatostatin	Somatotroph	GH		

Thyroid-Stimulating Hormone

Thyroid-stimulating hormone, a 28,000 dalton glycoprotein hormone is synthesized and secreted by the pituitary thyrotroph cells. It is composed of an α-subunit, structurally identical to the α-subunit of the other glycoprotein hormones, FSH, LH, and human chorionic gonadotropin (hCG). The β-subunit differs in the glycoprotein hormones and confers biologic specificity. TSH secretion is stimulated by the hypothalamic tripeptide TRH. The inhibitory effect of hypothalamic somatostatin augments the negative feedback inhibition of TSH secretion by peripheral thyroid hormones. TSH attaches to receptors on the thyroid gland and activates adenylyl cyclase, stimulating iodine uptake and the synthesis and release of the thyroid hormones, thyroxine (T_4) and tri-iodothyronine (T_3). T_4 and T_3 in turn exert negative feedback inhibition on pituitary TSH secretion.

Evaluation of TSH Secretion

Basal measurements of peripheral thyroid gland function are initially evaluated via thyroid function tests (free thyroxine [FT_4], free tri-iodothyronine [FT_3], or free thyroxine index [FT_1]). Normal thyroid function studies in a euthyroid patient imply adequate TSH secretion with no need for TSH measurement. However, low thyroid function tests mandate measurement of TSH to differentiate primary thyroid gland failure (elevated TSH) from hypothyroidism secondary to hypothalamic/pituitary gland failure (low or inappropriately normal TSH). In hyperthyroid states, thyroid function tests are elevated and TSH is suppressed if the hyperthyroidism is due to a thyroid gland disorder and TSH is elevated if due to the rare TSH-secreting pituitary adenoma.

Thyroid-stimulating hormone is measured by ultrasensitive assays (immunoradiometric assays), which can accurately distinguish low, normal, and high TSH levels. The ultrasensitive TSH assay has largely replaced the need for further dynamic testing, particularly the TRH test.

Adrenocorticotropic Hormone

Adrenocorticotropic hormone, a 39–amino acid peptide, is synthesized as part of a larger 241–amino acid precursor molecule, pro-opiomelanocortin (POMC), which is subsequently enzymatically cleaved into β-lipotropin (β-LPH), ACTH, joining peptide, and an NH2 terminal peptide in the anterior pituitary. ACTH is then cleaved into α-melanocyte-stimulating hormone (N-acetyl ACTH [1–13] NH_2 [α-MSH]) and corticotropin-like peptide (ACTH [18–39]), while β-LPH is split into γ LPH and β-endorphin.

Hypothalamic corticotropin-releasing hormone (CRH) stimulates ACTH secretion by pituitary corticotroph cells. ACTH in turn stimulates cortisol production by the adrenal gland, which exerts a negative feedback effect on ACTH and CRH. ACTH is secreted in bursts and is under circadian control, reaching maximal levels in the last hours before awakening followed by a steady decline to a nadir in the evening. Both psychological and physical stress increase ACTH and cortisol secretion, whereas glucocorticoids inhibit ACTH secretion as well as CRH and AVP synthesis and release. ACTH binds to adrenal receptors and stimulates steroidogenesis, resulting in cortisol synthesis and secretion. ACTH also promotes maintenance of adrenal size by increasing protein synthesis.

Evaluation of ACTH Secretion

Excess ACTH secretion results in Cushing syndrome, which may be due to a pituitary adenoma (Cushing disease) or to ectopic ACTH secretion (see Chapter 67). ACTH deficiency results in adrenocortical insufficiency, with decreased secretion of cortisol and adrenal androgens. Aldosterone secretion is largely regulated by the renin-angiotensin axis; therefore, aldosterone secretion remains intact.

BASAL ACTH LEVELS. Random basal ACTH measurements are unreliable because of the short plasma half-life and pulsatile secretion of the hormone. Interpretation of plasma ACTH levels requires concomitant assessment of plasma cortisol levels. As ACTH regulates cortisol secretion, plasma cortisol levels better reflect hypothalamic-pituitary-adrenal function. An 8 a.m. cortisol level > 10 μ/dl effectively excludes adrenal insufficiency but cannot be used to assess adrenal reserve. Simultaneously measured ACTH levels can be used to differentiate primary from secondary adrenal insufficiency. Plasma ACTH levels will be normal to high in adrenal insufficiency due to a primary adrenal disorder and will be low to absent in adrenal insufficiency secondary to hypothalamic-pituitary hypofunction. ACTH levels are also useful in establishing the etiology of Cushing syndrome (see Chapter 67).

EVALUATION OF ACTH RESERVE. To assess adequacy of ACTH reserve under conditions of stress, provocative testing is performed. If compromised adrenal function is suspected, these tests are potentially hazardous and patients should be closely monitored by a physician. Prolonged ACTH deficiency results in adrenal atrophy. Thus, adrenal cortisol reserve can be measured as an indirect test of pituitary ACTH status. Two hundred and fifty μg of cortrosyn (synthetic ACTH 1-24) administered intravenously or intramuscularly results in an increment ≥ 7 mcg/dl in serum cortisol or peak levels > 20 mcg/dl, within 60 minutes, in normal individuals. An inadequate response implies either impaired pituitary ACTH secretion or primary adrenal failure.

A subnormal cortrosyn-stimulating test requires subsequent direct evaluation of pituitary ACTH secretion via insulin-induced hypoglycemia or corticotropin-releasing factor (CRF) test.

The insulin-induced hypoglycemia test is performed by administering 0.05 to 0.1 units/kg regular insulin intravenously, which usually decreases blood sugar to 50% of baseline within 30 minutes. Neuroglycopenia associated with hypoglycemia (blood glucose < 40 mg/dl) stimulates the hypothalamic-pituitary-adrenal axis due to stress. A peak cortisol level of at least 20 mcg/dl, or doubling of the baseline cortisol at 30 to 45 minutes after onset of hypoglycemia, confirms normal ACTH reserve. Insulin-induced hypoglycemia is the most reliable test of the ACTH secretory response to stress. The test is contraindicated in elderly patients and patients with cerebrovascular and seizure disorders and cardiovascular disease. A physician should always be in attendance during testing. Ovine CRF (1 μg/kg, intravenous) directly stimulates pituitary corticotrophs to secrete ACTH, with a peak response within 15 minutes and subsequent peak cortisol response at 30 to 60 minutes. Patients with adrenal insufficiency secondary to hypopituitarism demonstrate an absent ACTH response to CRF; hypothalamic dysfunction results in a delayed peak. Patients with pituitary corticotroph cell adenomas often show exaggerated ACTH response to CRF, whereas ectopic ACTH-secreting tumors do not exhibit a further increase in ACTH levels.

EVALUATION OF ACTH HYPERSECRETION. Pituitary corticotroph adenomas in Cushing disease or ectopic ACTH-secreting tumors result in ACTH hypersecretion and hypercortisolism. Diagnosis is discussed in Chapter 67.

Gonadotropins (LH and FSH)

Hypothalamic GnRH, a 10–amino acid peptide secreted in a pulsatile fashion every 60 to 120 minutes, regulates LH and FSH secretion from the pituitary gonadotrophs. LH and FSH, glycoprotein hormones composed of α- and β-subunits, are secreted by the same cell. The LH β-subunit, conferring biologic specificity, closely resembles the hCG β-subunit.

Gonadotroph secretion is regulated by hypothalamic GnRH, and feedback inhibition, by gonadal steroids (estrogen and testosterone) and peptides (inhibin and activin). Basal LH and FSH are secreted in a pulsatile fashion, concordant with the pulsatile release of GnRH. GnRH release determines the onset of puberty and generates the mid-cycle gonadotropin surges necessary for ovulation. Feedback regulation of gonadotropin secretion is complex. Gonadal steroids exert both positive and negative feedback effects on gonadotroph secretion. In addition, the gonadal polypeptide inhibin, produced by ovarian granulosa cells and testicular sertoli cells, negatively inhibits FSH secretion, while activins stimulate FSH secretion. LH and FSH bind to receptors in the ovary and testis and stimulate sex steroid secretion (mainly LH) as well as gametogenesis (mainly FSH). LH stimulates gonadal steroid secretion by testicular Leydig cells and by the ovarian follicles. In females, the ovulatory LH surge results in rupture of the follicle and then luteinization. In males, FSH stimulates Sertoli cell spermatogenesis, and in females, follicular development.

Evaluation of Hypothalamic-Pituitary-Gonadal Axis

Luteinizing hormone and FSH levels vary with age and with the menstrual cycle in women. Prepubertal gonadotropin levels are low, and postmenopausal women have elevated levels. Male FSH and LH levels are pulsatile but fluctuate less than those in females. During the follicular phase of the menstrual cycle, LH levels rise steadily, with a mid-cycle spike that stimulates ovulation. FSH rises during the early follicular phase, falls in the late follicular phase, and peaks mid-cycle concurrently with the LH surge. Both LH and FSH levels fall after ovulation. LH and FSH levels in males are measured by three pooled samples drawn 20 minutes apart, which compensates for the normal pulsatile secretion. The normal values for FSH are 4 to 20 mlU/ml. Concurrently, testosterone levels are measured, with normal values in males being above 280 ng/dl.

Gonadotropin and sex steroid estimations in females are more complex. However, women with regular menstrual cycles and a documented normal luteal phase serum progesterone concentration are unlikely to have significant gonadotropin dysfunction. In amenorrheic women, measurement of serum LH, FSH, estradiol, prolactin, and hCG can differentiate between primary ovarian failure with elevated FSH and LH and normal prolactin levels; hyperprolactinemia with elevated prolactin and normal follicular phase LH, FSH, and estradiol levels; and pregnancy with a positive hCG, normal to high prolactin, normal to high LH, and high estradiol.

Gonadotropin deficiency is best diagnosed by concurrent measurement of serum gonadotropins and gonadal steroid concentrations. Low or normal FSH/LH levels in the face of low testosterone (in males) and estradiol (in females) confirms the diagnosis. Low gonadal steroids in the face of elevated gonadotropins suggest primary gonadal failure.

Gonadotropin-releasing hormone, 100 μg intravenously, directly stimulates the pituitary gonadotrophs to secrete gonadotropins. LH levels usually increase three-fold and peak within 30 minutes, while FSH levels plateau after 1 hour. Pituitary hypogonadism may be present despite a normal GnRH test. Thus, pituitary and hypothalamic hypogonadism cannot be reliably distinguished by this test.

NEURORADIOLOGIC EVALUATION OF THE PITUITARY

Clinical features of pituitary hormone excess or deficiency or headache or visual field abnormalities, suggesting hypothalamic-pituitary dysfunction, require neuroradiologic assessment of the hypothalamus and pituitary to confirm the existence and extent of lesions. Endocrine evaluation should precede imaging studies, as 10 to 25% of the normal population are found to harbor nonfunctional asymptomatic pituitary microadenomas at autopsy. Furthermore, patients with pituitary microadenomas may have false-negative neuroradiologic studies.

Magnetic resonance imaging (MRI) is the imaging procedure of choice for hypothalamic-pituitary lesions. Rarely, arteriography may be required to confirm the presence of intrasellar/parasellar aneurysms. Lesions as small as 3 to 5 mm can be visualized by MRI performed in both sagittal and coronal planes at 1.5- to 2-mm intervals. The contrast agent gadolinium is used to help differentiate small pituitary lesions from normal anterior pituitary tissue.

Microadenomas are defined as pituitary lesions < 10 mm in diameter. Lesions <5 mm in diameter may not be visualized by MRI and do not alter the normal pituitary contour, whereas lesions >5 mm in diameter may cause deviation of the pituitary stalk and convexity of the superior pituitary margin.

Macroadenomas are pituitary lesions >10 mm in diameter. They are easily differentiated from normal surrounding pituitary tissue by MRI. They cause marked deviation of the pituitary stalk to the opposite side. Adenomas exceeding 1.5 cm frequently demonstrate suprasellar extension with compression and displacement of the optic chiasm. MRI may also demonstrate lateral extension of large adenomas into the cavernous sinus.

PITUITARY AND HYPOTHALAMIC DISORDERS

These disorders present with a variety of clinical manifestations, including headache, visual loss, several distinctive syndromes of pituitary hormone hypersecretion and hyposecretion, and incidentally discovered sellar enlargement.

Pituitary adenomas associated with hormonal hypersecretion are the most frequently occurring lesions. The earliest clinical manifestations are usually the characteristic signs and symptoms caused by the hormone hypersecretion (see later). Subsequently, local manifestations of tumor enlargement develop, including headache, visual abnormalities (including visual field defects and diplopia), sellar enlargement, and hypopituitarism. Visual loss can occur with hypothalamic or pituitary lesions and manifests typically as a bitemporal hemianopia. Neuro-ophthalmologic evaluation, including visual field assessment and MRI, should be performed. Visual field defects may be the presenting feature of nonsecretory pituitary tumors. Extension of large tumors laterally into the cavernous sinus can compress the third, fourth, or sixth cranial nerves and lead to diplopia or abnormalities of extraocular eye muscle movements. Hypopituitarism should be excluded in these patients, and serum PRL should be measured.

HYPOTHALAMIC DYSFUNCTION

In children and young adults, craniopharyngioma is the most frequent cause of hypothalamic dysfunction. Primary central nervous system tumors, pinealomas, and dermoid and epidermoid tumors also cause hypothalamic dysfunction in adulthood. The major clinical manifestations of tumors that could cause hypothalamic dysfunction include visual loss, symptoms of raised intracranial pressure

(headache and vomiting), hypopituitarism including growth failure, and diabetes insipidus (DI). Hypothalamic disturbances include disorders of thirst (leading to dehydration or polydipsia and polyuria), appetite (with resultant hyperphagia and obesity), temperature regulation, behavior, and consciousness (with resultant somnolence and emotional lability). DI is a common manifestation of hypothalamic lesions but rarely occurs with primary pituitary lesions. Diagnosis is confirmed by MRI. As hypopituitarism occurs frequently with hypothalamic lesions, complete assessment of anterior pituitary function should be performed.

Craniopharyngioma is treated primarily with surgical resection and then radiotherapy. Biopsy of other types of hypothalamic tumors is usually required for histologic diagnosis prior to surgical resection, since some such as germinoma may be very radiosensitive.

HYPOPITUITARISM

Hypopituitarism results from diminished secretion of one or more pituitary hormones. The syndrome is due either to anterior pituitary gland destruction or to pituitary gland dysfunction secondary to deficient hypothalamic stimulatory/inhibitory factors that normally regulate pituitary function. Hypopituitarism can be caused by congenital or acquired lesions (Table 65–2). Pituitary insufficiency is usually a slow, insidious disorder. Pituitary lesions may result in single or multiple hormone losses.

GH Deficiency

Growth hormone deficiency during infancy and childhood manifests as growth retardation, short stature, and fasting hypoglycemia. A syndrome of adult GH deficiency may present as increased abdominal adiposity, reduced strength and exercise capacity, cold intolerance, and impaired psychosocial well-being. Adult GH deficiency is usually accompanied by other symptoms of panhypopituitarism.

TSH Deficiency

Thyroid-stimulating hormone deficiency causes thyroid gland involution and hypofunction. Clinical features of hypothyroidism include lethargy, constipation, cold intolerance, bradycardia, weight gain, poor appetite, dry skin, and delayed reflex relaxation time. Secondary hypothyroidism can be differentiated from primary hypothyroidism by the presence of a low circulating TSH in the presence of low thyroid hormone levels.

Gonadotropin Deficiency

Central hypogonadism during childhood results in failure to enter normal puberty. Females have delayed breast development, scant pubic and axillary hair, and primary

TABLE 65–2	Etiology of Hypopituitarism

Type of Disorder	Cause
Congenital	Septo-optic dysplasia
	Prader-Willi syndrome
	Lawrence-Moon-Biedle syndrome
	Isolated anterior pituitary hormone or releasing factor deficiency
Tumors	Pituitary
	Secretory adenomas
	Nonsecretory adenomas
	Hypothalamic
	Craniopharyngioma
	Hamartoma
	Pinealoma
	Dermoid
	Epidermoid
	Glioma
	Lymphoma
	Meningioma
Immunological	Autoimmune lymphocytic hypophysitis
Infiltrative	Hemachromatosis
	Langerhans cell histiocytosis
	Sarcoidosis
	Metastatic carcinoma (breast and bronchus)
	Amyloidosis
Infectious	Tuberculosis
	Mycoses
	Syphilis
Physical trauma	Cranial trauma and hemorrhage
	Ionizing radiation
	Stalk section
	Surgery
Vascular	Postpartum pituitary necrosis (Sheehan's syndrome)
	Pituitary apoplexy
	Carotid aneurysm

amenorrhea. In boys, the phallus and testes remain small, and body hair is sparse. Sex steroids are required for closure of the epiphyses of the long bones. Thus, in isolated gonadotropin deficiency, growth continues (as GH is intact) as there is failure of epiphyseal fusion, resulting in tall adolescents with eunuchoid proportions (upper-to-lower segment ratio < 1). In adult women, hypogonadism presents as breast atrophy, loss of pubic and axillary hair, and secondary amenorrhea. Hypogonadal adult males develop testicular atrophy, decreased libido, impotence, and loss of body hair.

ACTH Deficiency

Adrenocorticotropic hormone deficiency results in adrenal failure, causing lethargy, weakness, nausea, vomiting, dehydration, orthostatic hypotension, and, if untreated, coma. If adrenal insufficiency is not recognized and treated, it can lead to death.

ADH (Vasopressin) Deficiency

Vasopressin deficiency occurs with posterior pituitary dysfunction and leads to DI with polyuria, polydipsia, and nocturia.

Diagnosis

The diagnosis of pituitary hormone deficiency has been discussed previously in relation to the individual hormones. Quadruple bolus testing (Table 65–3) can be performed to assess anterior pituitary reserve. The hypothalamic-releasing hormones TRH, CRF, GHRH, and GnRH are administered intravenously sequentially over 1 minute, followed by venous sampling for anterior pituitary hormones. This test is rarely needed.

Treatment

Patients with panhypopituitarism must have adequate replacement of thyroxine, glucocorticoids, and appropriate sex steroids. Children with short stature due to GH deficiency should receive GH replacement therapy. GH replacement therapy for adults who develop GH deficiency is of uncertain value. Testosterone therapy in males restores libido and potency, beard growth, and muscle strength. Estrogen replacement therapy in females maintains secondary sex characteristics and prevents hot flashes. Human menopausal gonadotropins and human chorionic gonadotropin (hCG) given intramuscularly or GnRH administered by infusion pumps may be given to induce ovulation. In patients with combined TSH and ACTH deficiency, glucocorticoids should be replaced prior to thyroxine, as thyroxine may aggravate adrenal insufficiency and may precipitate acute adrenal failure.

EMPTY SELLA SYNDROME

The empty sella syndrome occurs when the arachnoid membranes herniate through an incompetent diaphragma sella and extend into the sella turcica, partially filling it with cerebrospinal fluid and compressing the pituitary gland. Primary empty sella syndrome is the most common cause of an enlarged sella turcica. This results from a congenital weakness in the diaphragma sella, most often occurring in obese women, hypertensive patients, or patients with raised intracranial pressure. Secondary empty sella syndrome can occur following pituitary surgery or

TABLE 65–3	Hypothalamic Peptides Administered in the Quadruple Bolus Test for Anterior Pituitary Reserve

Hypothalamic Releasing Hormone	Pituitary Hormone Assayed
TRH 200 μg	TSH, PRL
CRF 1 μg/kg	ACTH
GHRH 1 μg/kg	GH
GnRH 100 μg	FSH, LH

ACTH = Adrenocorticotropic hormone; CRF = corticotropin-releasing factor; FSH = follicle-stimulating hormone; GH = growth hormone; GHRH = growth hormone–releasing hormone; GnRH = gonadotropin-releasing hormone; LH = luteinizing hormone; PRL = prolactin; TRH = thyrotropin-releasing hormone; TSH = thyroid-stimulating hormone.

radiation therapy and can also occur following postpartum pituitary infarction (Sheehan's syndrome). Empty sella syndrome is usually asymptomatic and detected incidentally on routine imaging of the head. Some patients have a history of chronic headache. Visual field abnormalities are very rare. Endocrine function is usually normal, although partial hypopituitarism has been reported; therefore, tests of anterior pituitary function should be performed to exclude isolated or multiple pituitary trophic hormone deficiencies. The diagnosis of empty sella syndrome is confirmed by MRI, which demonstrates fluid in the sella turcica.

PITUITARY TUMORS

The pituitary comprises five different cell types, each of which, either singly or in combination, can give rise to pituitary adenomas, which secrete hormones, characteristic to the particular cell type. Pituitary tumors may also be "nonfunctioning." These tumors do not secrete biologically active hormones but may secrete the α-subunit common to the glycoprotein hormones. Prolactinomas are the most common secretory pituitary tumors. Pituitary tumors are usually benign neoplasms. Isolated reports of pituitary carcinomas with distant metastases have been described.

Secretory pituitary tumors are usually diagnosed by the constellation of signs and symptoms due to hypersecretion of the particular pituitary trophic hormone. GH adenomas cause acromegaly, prolactinomas cause amenorrhea and galactorrhea in females or sexual dysfunction in males, and ACTH-secreting adenomas result in Cushing disease. Large pituitary adenomas (secretory or nonsecretory) can result in signs and symptoms due to pressure on surrounding structures. Headache is a frequent symptom, possibly due to pressure on the diaphragma sella. If the tumor extends into the suprasellar space, the optic chiasm may be compressed, resulting in bitemporal hemianopia or a superior bitemporal defect. Lateral extension into the cavernous sinus can result in ophthalmoplegia, diplopia, or ptosis due to dysfunction of the third, fourth, fifth, and sixth cranial nerves. Compression of surrounding normal pituitary tissue due to an enlarging tumor mass can cause hyposecretion of one or several pituitary trophic hormones, resulting in signs and symptoms of hypopituitarism. Destructive pituitary lesions result in hormone loss, which follows a particular pattern: initially, GH, followed by LH/FSH, then TSH, ACTH, and, lastly, PRL.

Prolactinomas

Women present commonly with microprolactinomas, whereas macroadenomas are seen more frequently in males. Hyperprolactinemia in women can cause hypogonadotropic hypogonadism, resulting in estrogen deficiency. Gonadotropin levels are normal, and sex steroids are decreased. PRL inhibits pulsatility in gonadotropin secretion and suppresses the mid-cycle LH surge with consequent anovulation. In hyperprolactinemic males, testosterone levels are usually suppressed.

Clinical Features

Irrespective of the cause of hyperprolactinemia, the clinical features are the same. Prolactinomas are often recognized earlier in females who present with menstrual irregularities, as opposed to males, who manifest decreased libido and impotence.

Ninety percent of hyperprolactinemic women complain of amenorrhea, galactorrhea, or infertility. If the prolactinoma occurs before the onset of menarche, adolescents can present with primary amenorrhea. Prolactinomas account for 15 to 20% of secondary amenorrhea. Anovulation is associated with infertility. Galactorrhea may accompany, precede, or follow the menstrual irregularities, may not be clinically obvious, and may only be discovered during breast examination.

Estrogen deficiency may cause osteopenia, vaginal dryness, hot flashes, and irritability. Prolactin stimulates adrenal androgen production, and androgen excess can result in weight gain and hirsutism. Hyperprolactinemia may be associated with anxiety and depression.

Males usually present with loss of libido and impotence due to hypogonadism. These symptoms are not often attributed to a prolactinoma, resulting in frequent delay in diagnosis in males until visual impairment, headache, and hypopituitarism develop.

Diagnosis

Several physiologic conditions (pregnancy, stress, nipple stimulation), as well as certain medications (phenothiazines, methyldopa, cimetidine, metoclopramide) and pathologic states (hypothyroidism, chronic renal failure, chest wall lesions), affect PRL secretion. These conditions can be associated with mildly elevated prolactin levels; however, basal PRL levels in excess of 200 ng/ml usually imply prolactinoma. The diagnosis should be confirmed by MRI.

Treatment

Medical management with bromocriptine, a dopamine agonist, at a dosage of 2.5 to 15 mg/d orally in divided doses restores gonadal function and fertility in the majority of patients. Bromocriptine causes tumor shrinkage in a significant number of patients with macroadenomas. Surgery is indicated in patients with visual field abnormalities or neurologic symptoms. Trans-sphenoidal microsurgery is the procedure of choice. Patients who are intolerant to bromocriptine or have residual tumor postoperatively may benefit from radiation therapy, although the incidence of hypopituitarism after radiation is high.

Acromegaly and Gigantism

In childhood, hypersecretion of GH leads to gigantism, while in adults whose long bone epiphyses are fused, GH excess causes acromegaly with local overgrowth of bone in the acral areas. GH hypersecretion is almost always due to a GH-secreting pituitary adenoma. Ectopic GH secretion has been described with pancreatic, breast, and lung tumors. Ectopic GHRH secretion can occur with pancreatic islet cell tumors and bronchial or intestinal carcinoids. Both ectopic GH and GHRH present clinically with acromegaly but are extremely rare.

Clinical Features

The clinical features of acromegaly are insidious, and it may take several years for the disfiguring features to be diagnosed. Untreated acromegaly causes increased morbidity and mortality late in the course of the disorder. The most classical clinical feature is the acral enlargement, manifested as widening of the hands and feet and coarsening of the facial features; frontal sinuses enlarge leading to prominent supraorbital ridges, and the mandible grows downward and forward, resulting in prognathism and widely spaced teeth. Ring, glove, and shoe size increase due to soft tissue enlargement of hands and feet. The bony and soft tissue changes are accompanied by endocrine, metabolic, and systemic manifestations (Table 65–4).

Diagnosis

Insulin-like growth factor-1 mediates the classical acral changes that occur with acromegaly. IGF-1 levels are elevated in virtually all acromegalic patients. Biochemical confirmation of the diagnosis is obtained by measuring GH levels 2 hours after an oral glucose load. MRI or computed tomography scan of the pituitary will help lo-

calize the tumor and assess tumor size. Ninety percent of acromegalic patients have tumors larger than 1 cm. If no pituitary mass is detected, an extrapituitary source of ectopic GH or GHRH should be sought, utilizing imaging studies of the chest and abdomen.

Treatment

Trans-sphenoidal microsurgery is the initial therapy of choice, resulting in rapid reduction of GH levels with a low surgical morbidity. Cure rates are proportional to preoperative tumor size, with a 90% success rate in small or moderate-sized tumors (<2 cm). Radiotherapy is an effective method of reducing GH hypersecretion; however, the time until onset of its effect is longer, and the incidence of hypopituitarism is high. Medical management utilizes bromocriptine and octreotide. Bromocriptine is effective in suppressing GH in only a minority of acromegalic patients. However, octreotide acetate, a long-acting somatostatin analog, is very effective in reducing GH and IGF-1 levels to normal in the majority of acromegalic patients treated; it has been reported to shrink tumors in some cases. Octreotide is administered as a subcutaneous injection, three times daily, and requires chronic therapy. Side effects include diarrhea, abdominal cramps, flatulence, and, possibly, asymptomatic gallstone formation.

ACTH-Secreting Pituitary Tumors

(See Chapter 67.)

Gonadotropin-Secreting Pituitary Tumors

Gonadotropin-secreting pituitary tumors are rare and have been reported mainly in males. The majority of tumors are large at the time of presentation and hypersecrete only FSH. Patients usually present with signs and symptoms of local pressure, such as visual impairment. Patients may also present with hypogonadism with low or normal testosterone levels or low or normal sperm counts due to down-regulation of the pituitary gonadal axis by the high levels of circulating gonadotrophs. Rarely, excess LH may stimulate increased testosterone levels.

Surgical removal of gonadotropin-secreting adenomas is the usual primary treatment. However, patients frequently require subsequent radiotherapy to adequately control LH/FSH hypersecretion.

Thyrotropin-Secreting Pituitary Tumor

These tumors are extremely rare, presenting with hyperthyroidism, goiter, and inappropriately elevated TSH in the presence of elevated thyroid hormone levels. TSH-secreting tumors are usually plurihormonal, secreting GH, PRL, and the glycoprotein hormone α-subunit, as well as TSH. Initially, tumor bulk is reduced with either surgery

TABLE 65–4	Clinical Features of Acromegaly	
Type of Change	**Change**	**Manifestations**
Somatic	Acral changes	Enlarged hands and feet
	Musculoskeletal changes	Arthralgias
		Prognathism of jaw
		Malocclusion of teeth
		Carpal tunnel syndrome
		Proximal myopathy
	Skin changes	Sweating
	Colon changes	Polyps
		Carcinoma
	Cardiovascular symptoms	Cardiomegaly
		Hypertension
	Visceromegaly	Tongue
		Thyroid
		Liver
Endocrine-metabolic	Reproduction problems	Menstrual abnormalities
		Galactorrhea
		Decreased libido
	Carbohydrate metabolism changes	Impaired glucose tolerance
		Diabetes mellitus
	Lipid changes	Hypertriglyceridemia

or radiotherapy. These tumors are often resistant to removal, requiring several surgical procedures or multiple doses of radiotherapy. Octreotide acetate has been found to be useful in decreasing TSH secretion in patients with these tumors and has been shown to shrink the tumor in some cases. Iodine-131 (^{131}I) ablation or thyroid surgery may be required to control thyrotoxicosis.

THE POSTERIOR PITUITARY GLAND

The posterior pituitary gland secretes ADH, or AVP, and oxytocin. These hormones are synthesized in the supraoptic and paraventricular nuclei in the hypothalamus in cell bodies of neurons that extend from the hypothalamus to the posterior pituitary. ADH, a 1084-dalton nonapeptide with a ring structure and disulfide linkage, helps to regulate water balance and is a potent vasoconstrictor. ADH binds to receptors on the renal tubule, increasing the water permeability of the luminal membrane of the collecting duct epithelium, thus facilitating reabsorption of water. Maximal ADH effect results in a small volume of concentrated urine with a high osmolarity (as high as 1200 mOsm/kg). Deficiency of ADH results in a large volume of very dilute urine (as low as 100 mOsm/kg). In addition to the renal tubular effects, ADH also binds to peripheral arteriolar receptors, causing vasoconstriction and resultant increase in blood pressure. However, there is a countereffect to the hypertensive effect of ADH in that ADH also causes bradycardia and inhibition of sympathetic nerve activity.

Deficiency of ADH or insensitivity of the kidney to ADH results in DI, which is manifested as polyuria and polydipsia. Inappropriate secretion of ADH in excess amounts results in the syndrome of inappropriate antidiuretic hormone secretion (SIADH) and causes a hyponatremic state.

Oxytocin, a 1007-dalton nonapeptide that also has a ring structure and disulfide linkage, causes uterine smooth muscle contraction. It is released by nipple stimulation and facilitates milk ejection by causing mammary duct myoepithelial cell contraction in response to nipple stimulation.

DI

Diabetes insipidus results from lack of ADH secretion. DI can be of a central (neurogenic) origin when there is failure of the posterior pituitary to secrete adequate amounts of ADH, or it can be of nephrogenic origin resulting from failure of the kidney to respond to adequate amounts of circulating ADH. Irrespective of the cause, patients are polyuric, secreting large volumes of dilute urine. This causes cellular and extracellular dehydration, stimulating thirst, resulting in polydipsia. The causes of central DI are entirely different from those of nephrogenic DI (Table 65–5). Several of the causes of hypopituitarism, especially those that involve the hypothalamus, can also cause DI.

TABLE 65–5	Causes of Diabetes Insipidus (DI)

Causes of Central DI

Idiopathic
Familial
Hypophysectomy
Infiltration of hypothalamus and posterior pituitary
   Langerhans cell histiocytosis
   Granulomas
Infection
Tumors (intrasellar and suprasellar)
Autoimmune

Causes of Nephrogenic DI

Idiopathic
Familial
Chronic renal disease, e.g., chronic pyelonephritis, polycystic kidney disease, or medullary cystic disease
Hypokalemia
Hypercalcemia
Sickle cell anemia
Drugs
   Lithium
   Fluoride
   Demeclocycline
   Colchicine

Differential Diagnosis

Diabetes insipidus (central or nephrogenic) must be distinguished from primary polydipsia. Primary polydipsia is a compulsive psychoneurotic disorder manifested as a disorder of thirst, in which patients drink in excess of 5 L of water a day. This results in decreased ADH secretion and subsequent water diuresis. One possible distinguishing clinical feature is that patients with DI prefer cold beverages. Several tests can be performed to confirm the diagnosis of DI and differentiate the syndrome from primary polydipsia. Initially, random simultaneous samples of plasma and urine for sodium and osmolarity are obtained. In DI (central or nephrogenic), inappropriate water diuresis will result in a urine osmolarity that is less than that of plasma osmolarity. Plasma osmolarity may be elevated, depending on the patient's state of hydration. However, in primary polydipsia, both plasma and urine are dilute.

The primary test used to differentiate among the causes of polyuria is the water deprivation test. The patient is denied fluids for 12 to 18 hours, and body weight, blood pressure, urine volume, urine specific gravity, and plasma and urine osmolarity are measured every 2 hours. Careful supervision is required, as patients with DI may become rapidly dehydrated and hypotensive if denied access to water. If the body weight falls more than 3%, the study should be terminated. A normal response is a decrease in urine output to 0.5 ml/min, as well as an increase in urine concentration to greater than that of plasma. Patients with DI (either central or nephrogenic) maintain a high urine output, which continues to be dilute (specific gravity less than 1.005 [200 mOsm/kg of water]) despite water deprivation. Patients with primary polydipsia increase their urine osmolarity to values greater than plasma osmolarity. Water deprivation is continued until the urine osmolarity plateaus (an hourly increase of < 30 mOsm/kg for three successive hours). At that point, 5 μg of AVP is administered subcutaneously, and the urine osmolarity is measured after 1 hour. Patients with complete central DI increase urine osmolarity above plasma osmolarity, whereas in nephrogenic DI, the urine osmolarity increases less than 50% in response to AVP. Partial central DI also shows an increase in urine osmolarity, but it is less than 50%, whereas patients with primary polydipsia have increases of < 10%. ADH levels should be measured during the water deprivation test. Patients with nephrogenic DI have normal or increased levels of ADH during water deprivation, unlike those with complete central DI, who have suppressed levels. Patients with partial central DI show a smaller than normal increase in plasma ADH during water deprivation.

Treatment

Central DI

Desmopressin acetate (DDAVP), a synthetic analog of ADH, is usually administered intranasally or orally in the treatment of DI. Frequency of administration is determined by the severity of the DI. Adequacy of replacement is monitored by regular measurement of serum osmolarity and sodium.

Nephrogenic DI

As far as possible, the underlying disease process should be reversed. Specific treatment of nephrogenic DI aims to maintain a state of mild sodium depletion with reduction in the solute load on the kidney and subsequent increased proximal tubular reabsorption. Diuretics with dietary salt restriction can be used to achieve this goal.

SIADH

Syndrome of inappropriate secretion of antidiuretic hormone is characterized by plasma ADH concentrations that are inappropriately high for plasma osmolarity, resulting in water retention leading to hyponatremia and decreased plasma osmolarity (< 280 mOsm/kg). Urine osmolarity is inappropriately concentrated relative to the low plasma osmolarity and is higher than the plasma osmolarity. The diagnosis can only be made in the absence of hypervolemia (nephrotic syndrome, cardiac failure, cirrhosis) and with normal renal, adrenal, and thyroid function. The clinical signs and symptoms depend upon the degree of the hyponatremia and the rate of fall of the plasma osmo-

TABLE 65–6	Disorders Associated with Syndrome of Inappropriate Antidiuretic Hormone Secretion (SIADH)
Type of Disorder	**Disorder**
Pulmonary disorders	Malignant
	Oat cell carcinoma
	Benign
	Tuberculosis
	Pneumonia (viral, bacterial)
	Abscess
CNS disorders	Meningitis (viral, bacterial, TB, fungal)
	Brain abscess
	Head trauma
Adverse drug effects	Clofibrate
	Chlorpropamide
	Cyclophosphamide
	Phenothiazine
	Carbamazepine
Tumors (ectopic production of ADH)	Lymphoma
	Sarcoma
	Carcinoma of duodenum or pancreas

larity. Headache, anorexia, vomiting, and confusion may be found with serum sodiums between 115 and 120 mEq/l, while disorientation, stupor, coma, seizures, paralysis, and focal neurologic findings may be present with serum sodiums < 110 mEq/l.

Causes

Several benign and malignant conditions are associated with SIADH (Table 65–6).

Treatment

The underlying condition associated with SIADH should be treated. Further management aims to normalize the plasma osmolarity while avoiding further expansion of the extracellular fluid. Fluid restriction is thus the cornerstone of treatment.

REFERENCES

Cunnah D, Besser M: Management of prolactinomas. Clin Endocrinol 1991; 34:231.

Klinbanski A, Zervas NT: Diagnosis and management of hormone-secreting pituitary adenomas. N Engl J Med 1991; 324:822.

Molitch ME: Gonadotroph cell pituitary adenomas. N Engl J Med 1991; 324:626.

Thorner MO, Vance ML, Horvath E, Kovacs K: The anterior pituitary. *In* Wilson J, Foster DW (eds.): Williams Textbook of Endocrinology. 8th ed. Philadelphia, WB Saunders, 1992.

Vance ML: Hypopituitarism. N Engl J Med 1994; 330:1651.

66

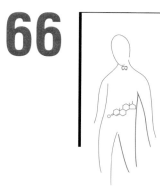

The Thyroid Gland

The thyroid gland secretes thyroxine (T_4) as well as smaller amounts of tri-iodothyronine (T_3), both of which modulate energy utilization and heat production and facilitate growth. The gland consists of two lateral lobes joined by an isthmus. The weight of the adult gland is approximately 10 to 20 gm. Microscopically, the thyroid is composed of several follicles containing colloid and surrounded by a single layer of thyroid epithelium. The follicle cells synthesize thyroglobulin, which is then stored as colloid. Biosynthesis of T_4 and T_3 occurs by iodination of tyrosine molecules in thyroglobulin.

THYROID HORMONE PHYSIOLOGY

Thyroid Hormone Synthesis

Dietary iodine is essential for synthesis of thyroid hormones. The recommended daily iodine intake is 150 μg/day. Average diets in the United States contain 250 to 750 μg/day of iodine due to enrichment of foods with iodine. Iodine is converted to iodide in the stomach; after rapid absorption from the gastrointestinal tract, iodide is distributed in the extracellular fluids. The thyroid follicular cells actively transport iodide from the blood stream across the follicular cell basement membrane. The trapped iodide is enzymatically oxidized by thyroid peroxidase; thyroid peroxidase also mediates the iodination of the tyrosine residues in thyroglobulin to form monoiodotyrosine (MIT) and di-iodotyrosine (DIT). The iodotyrosine molecules couple to form thyroxine (3,5,3'5'–tetraiodothyronine) or triiodothyronine (3,5,3'–triiodothyronine). Once iodinated, thyroglobulin containing newly formed T_4 and T_3 is stored in the follicles. Secretion of free T_4 and T_3 into the circulation occurs after proteolytic digestion of thyroglobulin. Thyroid hormone secretion is stimulated by thyroid-stimulating hormone (TSH). MIT and DIT are also released from thyroglobulin during proteolytic digestion; iodotyrosine deiodinase deiodinates MIT and DIT within the thyroid gland, and the released iodine then re-enters the thyroid iodine pool.

Thyroid Hormone Transport

Thyroxine and T_3 are tightly bound to carrier proteins in the serum. The unbound or free fractions are the biologically active fractions and represent only 0.04% of the total T_4 and 0.4% of total T_3. The three major proteins that transport thyroid hormones are thyroxine-binding globulin (TBG), thyroxine-binding prealbumin (TBPA), and albumin.

Peripheral Metabolism of Thyroid Hormones

The normal thyroid gland secretes daily approximately 100 nmol of T_4, 5 nmol of T_3, and < 5 nmol of reverse T_3, a biologically inactive form of T_3. Most of the circulating T_3 is derived from 5'-deiodination of circulating T_4 in the peripheral tissues. Approximately 35 nmol of T_3 is derived from T_4 daily. Deiodination of T_4 can occur at the outer ring (5'-deiodination), producing T_3(3,5,3'-triiodothyronine), or at the inner ring, producing reverse T_3(3,3'5'-triiodothyronine). T_3 is three to eight times more potent than T_4. Different iodothyronine deiodinases catalyze the monodeiodination of T_4 to T_4 or reverse T_3(rT_3).

Control of Thyroid Function (Fig. 66–1)

The hypothalamic thyrotropin-releasing hormone (TRH) is transported via the hypothalamic-hypophysial portal system to the anterior pituitary gland where it binds to thyrotroph receptors and stimulates the synthesis and release of TSH. TSH, in turn, increases thyroidal iodide uptake and iodination of thyroglobulin; it also releases T_3 and T_4 from the thyroid gland by increasing hydrolysis of thyroglobulin. TSH also stimulates thyroid cell growth; excess secretion of TSH over time results in thyroid enlargement (goiter). TRH and TSH release are under negative feedback inhibition by circulating levels of T_4 as well as T_3.

Physiologic Effects of Thyroid Hormones

Thyroid hormones exert metabolic effects in several body tissues by increasing oxygen consumption and heat production, thereby increasing basal metabolic rate. Thyroid hormones also have specific effects on several organ systems (Table 66–1). These effects are exaggerated in hyperthyroidism and lacking in hypothyroidism, accounting

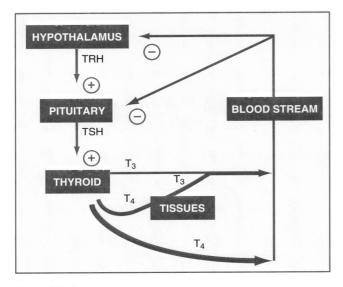

Figure 66–1
Hypothalamic-pituitary-thyroid axis. T_3 = Tri-iodothyronine; T_4 = thyroxine; TRH = thyrotropin-releasing hormone; TSH = thyroid-stimulating hormone.

for the well-recognized signs and symptoms of these two disorders.

THYROID EVALUATION

The thyroid can be evaluated for functional status (euthyroid, hyperthyroid, or hypothyroid), the etiology of thyroid dysfunction, and structural abnormalities of the thyroid gland, which may be responsible for dysfunction.

Thyroid gland function and structures can be evaluated in several different ways: (1) serum thyroid hormone levels, (2) evaluation of thyroid gland size and architec-

TABLE 66–1	Physiologic Effects of Thyroid Hormone
Cardiovascular effects	Increased heart rate and cardiac output
Gastrointestinal effects	Increased gut motility
Skeletal effects	Increased bone turnover and resorption
Pulmonary effects	Maintenance of normal hypoxic and hypercapnic drive in the respiratory center
Neuromuscular effects	Increased muscle protein turnover and increased speed of muscle contraction and relaxation
Lipids and carbohydrate metabolism effects	Increased hepatic gluconeogenesis and glycogenolysis as well as intestinal glucose absorption; increased cholesterol synthesis and degradation; increased lipolysis
Sympathetic nervous system effects	Increased numbers of beta-adrenergic receptors in the heart, skeletal muscle, lymphocytes, and adipose cells; decreased cardiac alpha-adrenergic receptors; increased catecholamine sensitivity
Hemopoietic effects	Increased red blood cell 2,3-diphosphoglycerate facilitating oxygen dissociation from hemoglobin with increased oxygen available to tissues

ture, (3) measurement of thyroid autoantibodies, and (4) thyroid gland biopsy (by fine-needle aspiration [FNA]).

Tests of Serum Thyroid Hormone Levels

Total serum T_4 and T_3 measures the total amount of hormone bound to thyroid-binding proteins and in the free state by radioimmunoassay. Total T_4 and total T_3 levels are elevated in hyperthyroidism and low in hypothyroidism. Changes in serum concentration of thyroid-binding proteins modify the total T_4 or T_3, but not the free serum T_4 or T_3. Increase in TBG (as with pregnancy or estrogen therapy) increases the total T_4 and T_3 in the absence of hyperthyroidism. Similarly, T_4 and T_3 are low despite euthyroidism in conditions in which thyroid-binding proteins are low (e.g., cirrhosis or nephrotic syndrome). Thus, further tests must be performed to assess the free hormone level that reflects biologic activity. Free T_4 level can be estimated by calculating the free T_4 index or can be measured directly by dialysis.

Free thyroxine index (FTI) is an indirect method of assessing free T_4. It is derived by multiplying the total T_4 by the T_3 resin uptake, which is inversely proportional to the binding sites on TBG.

Free T_4 can be measured directly by dialysis. This method separates the free from the bound hormone without disturbing the equilibrium between them, by direct equilibrium dialysis or by ultrafiltration of undiluted serum and subsequent quantitative assay of free T_4. Direct measurement of free T_4 is most accurate and is preferred to the FTI.

Serum TSH is measured by a third-generation immunometric assay, which employs at least two different monoclonal antibodies against different regions of the TSH molecule, resulting in highly accurate detection of TSH levels to below the normal range. Thus, the TSH assay can establish the diagnoses of primary hyperthyroidism and subclinical hyperthyroidism, in which the TSH level is suppressed. In primary (thyroidal) hypothyroidism, serum TSH is supranormal. In secondary (pituitary) or tertiary (hypothalamic) hypothyroidism, the TSH is usually low but may be normal.

Serum thyroglobulin measurements are useful in the follow-up of patients with papillary or follicular carcinoma. Following thyroidectomy and iodine 131 (^{131}I) ablation therapy, thyroglobulin levels should be < 10 μg/L. Levels in excess of this value indicate the presence of metastatic disease.

Calcitonin measurements are invaluable in the assessment of medullary carcinoma of the thyroid and for following the effects of therapy of this entity.

Thyroid Imaging

Iodine 123 (^{123}I) or technetium 99m (^{99m}Tc) pertechnetate is useful in assessing the functional activity of the thyroid gland (thyroid uptake and scan). These radionuclides are concentrated in the gland, and after subsequent scanning of the gland with a gamma camera, information about the size and shape of the gland and the location of the functional activity in the gland is obtained (thyroid scan). Functioning thyroid nodules are called "warm" or "hot" nodules; "cold" nodules are nonfunctioning. Malignancy is usually associated with a cold nodule; 16% of surgically removed cold nodules are malignant.

Thyroid ultrasound is useful in the differentiation of solid from cystic nodules. It can also guide the operator during FNA of a nodule that is difficult to palpate.

Thyroid Antibodies

Autoantibodies to several different antigenic components in the thyroid gland, including thyroglobulin (TgAb), thyroid peroxidase (TPO Ab, formerly called antimicrosomal antibodies), and the TSH receptor, can be measured in the serum. A strongly positive test for TgAb or TPO Ab indicates autoimmune thyroid disease. Elevated thyroid receptor–stimulating antibody occurs in Graves' disease (see later).

Thyroid Biopsy

Fine-needle aspiration of a nodule to obtain cells for cytology is the best way to differentiate benign from malignant disease. FNA requires adequate tissue samples and interpretation by an experienced cytologist.

HYPERTHYROIDISM

Thyrotoxicosis is the clinical syndrome that results from elevated circulating thyroid hormones. Clinical manifestations of thyrotoxicosis are due to the direct physiologic effects of the thyroid hormones, as well as to the increased sensitivity to catecholamines. Tachycardia, tremor, stare, sweating, and lid lag are due to catecholamine hypersensitivity.

Signs and Symptoms of Hyperthyroidism

Table 66–2 lists the signs and symptoms of hyperthyroidism with their frequency of occurrence. Thyrotoxic crisis or "thyroid storm" is a life-threatening complication of hyperthyroidism, which can be precipitated by surgery, radioactive iodine therapy, or severe stress (e.g., uncontrolled diabetes mellitus, myocardial infarction, acute infection). The syndrome presents as an acute exacerbation of the hypermetabolism and the excessive adrenergic symptoms of thyrotoxicosis. Patients develop fever, flushing, sweating, marked tachycardia, atrial fibrillation, and cardiac failure. Marked agitation, restlessness, delirium, and coma occur frequently. Gastrointestinal manifestations may include nausea, vomiting, and diarrhea. Hyperpyrexia out of proportion to other clinical findings is the hallmark of thyroid storm.

TABLE 66–2	Prevalence of Symptoms and Signs in Patients with Thyrotoxicosis
Symptom	**Prevalence (%)**
Nervousness	99
Increased sweating	91
Hypersensitivity to heat	89
Palpitation	89
Fatigue	88
Weight loss	85
Tachycardia	82
Dyspnea	75
Weakness	70
Increased appetite	65
Eye complaints	54
Swelling of legs	35
Diarrhea	23
Anorexia	9
Sign	**Prevalence (%)**
Tachycardia	100
Goiter	100
Skin changes	97
Tremor	97
Thyroid	77
Eye signs	71
Atrial fibrillation	10
Splenomegaly	10
Gynecomastia	10
Liver palms	8

From Williams RH: Thiouracil treatment of thyrotoxicosis. J Clin Endocrinol Metab 1946; 6:1–22.

Differential Diagnosis

Thyrotoxicosis usually reflects hyperactivity of the thyroid gland due to Graves' disease, toxic adenoma, multinodular goiter, or thyroiditis. However, it may be due to excessive ingestion of thyroid hormone or, rarely, thyroid hormone production from an ectopic site—struma ovarii (Table 66–3 and Fig. 66–2). Clinically, Graves' disease

TABLE 66–3	Causes of Thyrotoxicosis

Common Causes

Graves' disease
Toxic adenoma (solitary)
Toxic multinodular goiter

Less Common Causes

Subacute thyroiditis (de Quervain's or granulomatous)
Hashimoto's thyroiditis with transient hyperthyroid phase
Thyrotoxicosis factitia
Postpartum (probably variant of silent thyroiditis)

Rare Causes

Struma ovarii
Metastatic thyroid carcinoma
Hydatidiform mole
TSH-secreting pituitary tumor
Pituitary resistance to T_3 and T_4

T_3 = Tri-iodothyronine; T_4 = thyroxine; TSH = thyroid-stimulating hormone.

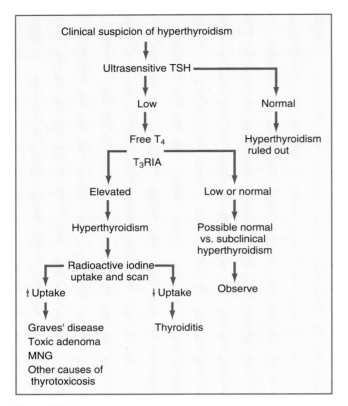

Figure 66–2
Algorithm for differential diagnosis of hyperthyroidism. MNG = multinodular goiter; T_3 = tri-iodothyronine; T_3RIA = tri-iodothyronine radioimmunoassay; T_4 = thyroxine; TSH = thyroid-stimulating hormone.

presents insidiously with a nontender smooth symmetric thyroid enlargement, often with a bruit, whereas thyroiditis presents acutely with tenderness of the thyroid gland to palpation.

GRAVES' DISEASE

Graves' disease, the most common cause of thyrotoxicosis, is an autoimmune disease, more common in women, with a peak age incidence of 20 to 40 years. One or more of the following features are present: (1) goiter; (2) thyrotoxicosis; (3) eye disease ranging from tearing to proptosis, extraocular muscle paralysis, and loss of sight due to optic nerve involvement; and (4) thyroid dermopathy, usually presenting as marked skin thickening without pitting in a pretibial distribution (pretibial myxedema).

Pathogenesis

Thyrotoxicosis in Graves' disease is due to overproduction of an antibody that binds to the TSH receptor. These thyroid-stimulating immunoglobulins (TSIs) increase thyroid cell growth and thyroid hormone secretion. Ophthalmopathy is due to infiltration of the extraocular eye muscles by an acute inflammatory reaction consisting of lymphocytes and mucopolysaccharides. The inflammatory reaction that contributes to the eye signs in Graves' disease may be caused by lymphocytes sensitized to antigens common to the orbital muscles and thyroid.

Clinical Features

The common manifestations of thyrotoxicosis (see Table 66–1) are characteristic features of younger patients with Graves' disease. In addition, patients may present with a goiter or the eye signs characteristic of Graves' disease. Older patients often do not manifest the florid clinical features of thyrotoxicosis, and the condition is termed "apathetic hyperthyroidism"; such patients may have flat affect, emotional lability, weight loss, muscle weakness, or congestive heart failure and atrial fibrillation resistant to standard therapy.

Eye signs of Graves' disease may be due to thyrotoxicosis (spasm of the upper lids) or to inflammatory infiltrate of the orbital tissues, periorbital edema, conjunctival congestion and swelling, proptosis, extraocular muscle weakness, and/or optic nerve damage with visual impairment.

Pretibial myxedema (thyroid dermopathy) occurs in 2 to 3% of patients with Graves' disease and presents as thickening of the skin over the lower tibia without pitting. Onycholysis, characterized by separation of the fingernails from their beds, often occurs in Graves' disease.

Laboratory Findings

Elevated free T_4 and a suppressed TSH confirm the clinical diagnosis of thyrotoxicosis. TSI is usually elevated and is especially useful in patients with eye signs who do not have other characteristic clinical features. Increased uptake of ^{123}I differentiates Graves' disease from early subacute or Hashimoto's thyroiditis, in which uptake is low in the presence of hyperthyroidism. Magnetic resonance imaging (MRI) or ultrasonography of the orbit usually reveals orbital muscle enlargement, whether or not there are clinical signs of ophthalmopathy.

Treatment

Three treatment modalities are employed to control the hyperthyroidism of Graves' disease:

1. Antithyroid drugs: The thiocarbamide drugs, propylthiouracil, methimazole, and carbimazole, block thyroid hormone synthesis by inhibiting thyroid peroxidase. Propylthiouracil also partially inhibits peripheral conversion of T_4 to T_3. Medical therapy must be administered for a prolonged period (12 to 18 months), until the disease undergoes spontaneous remission. Upon cessation of medication, only a small percentage of patients (20 to 30%) remain in remission, and the patients who relapse must then undergo definitive surgery or radioactive iodine treatment. Side effects of the thiocarbamides include pruritis and rash (about 5%

of patients), cholestatic jaundice, acute arthralgias, or, rarely, agranulocytosis (0.5% of patients). Patients must be instructed to discontinue the medication and consult a physician if they develop fever or sore throat, as these may indicate agranulocytosis. At the onset of treatment, during the acute phase of thyrotoxicosis, beta-adrenergic blocking drugs help alleviate tachycardia, hypertension, and atrial fibrillation. As the thyroid hormone levels return to normal, treatment with beta blockers is tapered.

2. Radioactive iodine: In terms of cost, efficacy, ease, and short-term side effects, radioactive iodine has benefits that exceed both surgery and antithyroid drugs. ^{131}I is probably the treatment of choice in adults with Graves' disease. Patients with severe thyrotoxicosis, very large glands, or underlying heart disease should be rendered euthyroid with antithyroid medication prior to receiving radioactive iodine, since ^{131}I treatment can cause release into the circulation of preformed thyroid hormone from the thyroid gland; this can precipitate cardiac arrhythmias and exacerbate symptoms of thyrotoxicosis. Following administration of radioactive iodine, the thyroid gland shrinks, and patients become euthyroid over a period of 6 weeks to 3 months. Approximately 10 to 20% of patients become hypothyroid within the first year of treatment, and thereafter, at a rate of 3 to 5% per year. Fifty to 80% of patients who have received radioactive iodine ultimately become hypothyroid. Serum TSH levels should be monitored and replacement with levothyroxine instituted if the TSH rises. Hypothyroidism may also develop after surgery or antithyroid medication, mandating lifelong follow-up in all patients with Graves' disease.

3. Surgery: Subtotal thyroidectomy is the treatment of choice for patients with very large glands and obstructive symptoms or multinodular glands or for patients desiring to become pregnant within the next year. An experienced thyroid surgeon is essential. Preoperatively, patients should receive antithyroid drugs for approximately 6 weeks so that they will be euthyroid at the time of surgery. Two weeks prior to surgery, patients should receive oral saturated solution of potassium iodide (SSKI) daily to decrease the vascularity of the gland. With adequate preoperative preparation prior to thyroidectomy, immediate operative mortality is very low. Permanent hypoparathyroidism and recurrent laryngeal nerve palsy occurs in less than 2% of patients. Ten percent of patients develop recurrent thyrotoxicosis; they should generally then be treated with radioactive iodine.

TOXIC ADENOMA

Solitary toxic nodules occur more frequently in older patients. Toxic adenomas are usually benign. Clinical manifestations are those of thyrotoxicosis. Physical examination demonstrates a distinct solitary nodule. Laboratory investigation reveals suppressed TSH and markedly elevated T_3 levels, often with only moderately elevated T_4. Thyroid scan shows a "hot nodule" of the affected lobe with complete suppression of the unaffected lobe. Solitary toxic nodules are usually managed with radioactive iodine. However, unilateral lobectomy, after the administration of antithyroid drugs to render the patient euthyroid, may be required for large nodules.

TOXIC MULTINODULAR GOITER

Toxic multinodular goiter occurs in older patients with long-standing multinodular goiter. Thus, the presenting clinical features are frequently tachycardia, heart failure, and arrhythmias.

Physical examination reveals a multinodular goiter. Diagnosis is confirmed by laboratory features of suppressed TSH, markedly elevated T_3, moderately elevated T_4, and a thyroid scan with multiple functioning nodules. The treatment of choice is subtotal thyroidectomy. However, as these patients are frequently elderly with underlying heart disease, surgery is sometimes contraindicated. The toxic nodules are then treated with ^{131}I, but the multinodular goiter remains, with the possibility that other nodules will become toxic and require future ^{131}I treatment.

THYROIDITIS

Thyroiditis may be classified as acute, subacute, or chronic. Although thyroiditis may eventually result in clinical hypothyroidism, the initial presentation is often that of hyperthyroidism due to acute release of T_4 and T_3. Hyperthyroidism due to thyroiditis can be readily differentiated from other causes of hyperthyroidism by the radioactive iodine uptake, which is markedly suppressed.

Acute suppurative thyroiditis, a rare complication of septicemia, presents with high fever, redness of the overlying skin, and thyroid gland tenderness; it may be confused with subacute thyroiditis. If blood cultures are negative, needle aspiration should identify the organism. Intensive antibiotic treatment and, occasionally, incision and drainage are required.

Subacute Thyroiditis

Subacute thyroiditis (de Quervain's thyroiditis or granulomatous thyroiditis) is an acute inflammatory disorder of the thyroid gland, probably secondary to viral infection, which undergoes complete resolution within months in 90% of cases. Subacute thyroiditis is characterized by fever and anterior neck pain. The patient may have symptoms and signs of hyperthyroidism such as sweating, palpitations, anxiety, tachycardia, tremor, and hyperreflexia. The classical feature on physical examination is an exquisitely tender thyroid gland. Laboratory findings vary with the course of the disease. Initially, serum T_4 is elevated, the serum TSH is depressed, and the radioactive iodine uptake is very low, while the patient may be symptomatically thyrotoxic. Subsequently, the thyroid status will fluctuate through euthyroid and hypothyroid phases and may return to euthyroidism. Increase in radioactive iodine uptake on scan reflects recovery of the gland. Treatment usually includes nonsteroidal anti-inflammatory drugs, but a short course of prednisone may be required if pain and fever are severe. During the hypothyroid phase, replacement therapy with levothyroxine may be indicated by clinical symptoms.

Chronic Thyroiditis

Chronic thyroiditis (Hashimoto's thyroiditis, lymphocytic thyroiditis) results from destruction of normal thyroidal architecture by lymphocytic infiltration, resulting in hypothyroidism and goiter. Riedel's struma is probably a variant of Hashimoto's thyroiditis, characterized by extensive thyroid fibrosis resulting in a rock-hard thyroid mass. Hashimoto's thyroiditis is more common in women and is probably the most common cause of goiter and hypothyroidism in the United States. Occasionally, patients with Hashimoto's thyroiditis may have transient hyperthyroidism with low radioactive iodine uptake. This is due to release of T_4 and T_3 into the circulation and can be differentiated from subacute thyroiditis, in that the gland is nontender to palpation and antithyroid antibodies are present in high titer. Early in the disease, TgAb is markedly elevated; it may disappear later. TPO Ab also is present early and generally remains present for years. Radioactive iodine uptake may be high, normal, or low. Serum T_3 and T_4 are either normal or low; when low, the TSH is elevated. FNA of the thyroid reveals lymphocytes and Hurthle cells (enlarged basophilic follicular cells). Hypothyroidism and marked glandular enlargement (goiter) are indications for levothyroxine therapy. Adequate doses of levothyroxine are administered to suppress TSH levels and shrink the goiter.

THYROTOXICOSIS FACTITIA

Thyrotoxicosis factitia presents with typical features of thyrotoxicosis due to ingestion of excessive amounts of thyroxine, often in an attempt to lose weight. Serum T_3 and T_4 levels are elevated, and TSH is suppressed, as is the serum thyroglobulin concentration. Radioactive iodine uptake is absent. Patients may require psychotherapy.

RARE CAUSES OF THYROTOXICOSIS

Struma ovarii occurs when an ovarian teratoma contains thyroid tissue, which secretes thyroid hormone. Diagnosis is confirmed by demonstrating uptake of radioiodine in the pelvis on body scan.

Hydatidiform mole is due to proliferation and swelling of the trophoblast during pregnancy, with excess production of chorionic gonadotrophin, which has intrinsic TSH-like activity because it shares a common α-subunit with TSH. The hyperthyroidism remits with surgical and medical treatment of the molar pregnancy.

HYPOTHYROIDISM

Hypothyroidism is a clinical syndrome due to deficiency of thyroid hormones. In infants and children, hypothyroidism causes retardation of growth and development and may result in permanent motor and mental retardation. Congenital causes of hypothyroidism include agenesis (complete absence of thyroid tissue), dysgenesis (ectopic or lingual thyroid gland), hypoplastic thyroid, thyroid dyshormogenesis, and central hypothyroidism. Adult-onset hypothyroidism results in a slowing of metabolic processes and is reversible with treatment. Hypothyroidism (Table 66–4) is usually primary (thyroid failure), but may be secondary (hypothalamic or pituitary deficiency) or due to resistance at the thyroid hormone receptor. The biosynthetic abnormalities causing hypothyroidism and goiter include (1) impaired iodine transport; (2) defective peroxidase activity; (3) defective iodotyrosyl coupling; (4) defective iodotyrosine deiodinase; and (5) defective thyroglobulin synthesis. In adults, autoimmune thyroiditis (Hashimoto's thyroiditis) is the most common cause of hypothyroidism. This may be isolated or part of the polyglandular failure syndrome, type II (Schmidt's syndrome). Other associated diseases of Schmidt's syndrome include insulin-dependent diabetes mellitus, pernicious anemia, vitiligo, gonadal failure, hypophysitis, celiac disease, myasthenia gravis, and primary biliary

TABLE 66–4	Causes of Hypothyroidism

Primary Hypothyroidism

Autoimmune
  Hashimoto's thyroiditis
  Part of polyglandular failure syndrome, type II
Iatrogenic
  ^{131}I therapy
  Thyroidectomy
Drug-induced
  Iodine deficiency
  Iodine excess
  Lithium
  Amiodarone
  Antithyroid drugs
Congenital
  Thyroid agenesis
  Thyroid dysgenesis
  Hypoplastic thyroid
  Biosynthetic defect

Secondary Hypothyroidism

Hypothalamic dysfunction
  Neoplasms
  Tuberculosis
  Sarcoidosis
  Langerhans cell histiocytosis
  Hemochromatosis
  Radiation treatment
Pituitary dysfunction
  Neoplasms
  Pituitary surgery
  Postpartum pituitary necrosis
  Idiopathic hypopituitarism
  Glucocorticoid excess (Cushing syndrome)
  Radiation treatment

cirrhosis. The possibility that a patient with Hashimoto's thyroiditis has these associated diseases should be carefully considered. Iatrogenic causes of hypothyroidism include ^{131}I therapy, thyroidectomy, and treatment with lithium or amiodarome. Iodine deficiency or excess can also cause hypothyroidism.

Clinical Manifestations

The clinical presentation of hypothyroidism (Table 66–5) depends on age of onset and severity of thyroid deficiency. Infants with congenital hypothyroidism (also called cretinism) may present with feeding problems, hypotonia, inactivity, open posterior fontanelle, and/or edematous face and hands. Mental retardation, short stature, and delayed puberty occur, if treatment is delayed. Hypothyroidism in adults usually develops insidiously. Patients often have fatigue, lethargy, and gradual weight gain for years before the diagnosis is established. Characteristic symptoms include fatigue, lethargy, weakness, cold intolerance, dry skin, coarse hair or hair loss, weight gain, constipation, myalgias, arthralgias, and menstrual abnormalities. Signs include cool dry skin, coarse thin hair, hoarse voice, brittle nails, and hypertension. A delayed relaxation phase of deep tendon reflexes ("hung-up" reflexes) is a valuable clinical sign characteristic of severe hypothyroidism. Increased blood levels of carotene may give the skin (especially the palm) an orange hue. Subcutaneous infiltration by mucopolysaccharides, which bind water, causes the edema (termed myxedema), which is responsible for the thickened features and puffy appearance of patients with severe hypothyroidism. Cardiovascular complications include bradycardia and myocardial dilatation. Congestive heart failure, pericardial effusions, pleural effusions, and ascites may occur with advanced disease.

Severe untreated hypothyroidism can result in myxedema coma. This disorder, the ultimate stage of long-standing hypothyroidism, is characterized by hypothermia, extreme weakness, stupor, hypoventilation, hypoglycemia, and hyponatremia. Decompensation is often precipitated by cold exposure, infection, or psychoactive drugs.

Laboratory Tests

Laboratory abnormalities in patients with primary hypothyroidism include an elevated serum TSH and low free and total T_4. The pituitary is quite sensitive to decreased circulating levels of thyroid hormones (primarily T_3) and responds by increasing TSH output. Thus, in mild hypothyroidism, a patient will have an elevated serum TSH level with a low normal serum T_4 level. In the setting of primary hypothyroidism, a patient with a serum TSH >8 μU/mL (the upper limit of normal is 4 to 5 μU/mL) should be treated with L-thyroxine, even with normal T_4 levels.

Secondary hypothyroidism is characterized by a low or low normal morning serum TSH in the setting of hypothalamic or pituitary dysfunction. Often, the serum total and free T_4 levels are at the lower limit of normal. Secondary hypothyroidism may be due to a lack of the nocturnal surge of serum TSH or due to biologically inactive but immunologically active TSH, so that morning serum TSH level may be only mildly subnormal. A diurnal TSH test can be performed, if needed, to confirm the diagnosis of central hypothyroidism. In this test, a midnight serum TSH value <1.5 times the afternoon value is consistent with central hypothyroidism.

Hypothyroidism is often associated with other abnormal laboratory values, including hypercholesterolemia and elevated creatine phosphokinase with an increase in MB (the fraction characteristic of cardiac muscle) bands. Anemia in patients with hypothyroidism is usually normocytic, normochromic but may be macrocytic (vitamin B_{12} deficiency due to associated pernicious anemia) or microcytic (due to nutritional deficiencies or menstrual blood loss in women).

Differential Diagnosis

Since the initial manifestations of hypothyroidism are subtle, the early diagnosis of hypothyroidism demands a high index of suspicion in patients presenting with one or more of the signs or symptoms listed in Table 66–5. Early symptoms that are often overlooked include menstrual irregularities (usually menorrhagia), arthralgias, and myalgias.

Laboratory diagnosis may be complicated by the finding of a low total T_4 in euthyroid states associated with low TBG, such as nephrotic syndrome, cirrhosis, or TBG deficiency; in these situations TSH and free T_4 levels are normal. A low total T_4 may also be found in the "euthyroid sick syndrome," a condition occurring in acutely ill patients. In such patients, total and, occasionally, free T_4 levels are low and serum TSH is usually normal but may be mildly elevated. These patients, who should not be treated with L-thyroxine replacement, may be distinguished from patients with primary hypothyroidism by absence of a goiter, absence of antithyroid anti-

TABLE 66–5	Clinical Features of Hypothyroidism
Symptoms	Signs
Childen	
Learning disabilities	Mental retardation
Short stature	Delayed bone age
	Delayed puberty
Adults	
Fatigue	Dry, coarse, cold skin
Cold intolerance	Coarse, thin hair
Weakness	Hoarse voice
Lethargy	Brittle nails
Weight gain	Periorbital, peripheral edema
Constipation	Delayed reflexes
Myalgias	Slow reaction time
Arthralgias	Orange skin hue
Menstrual irregularities	Bradycardia
Hair loss	Pleural, pericardial effusions

bodies, and elevated serum rT_3 levels, as well as clinical presentation.

Treatment

Hypothyroidism should be treated with synthetic L-thyroxine. Although T_3 is the more bioactive thyroid hormone, peripheral tissues convert T_4 to T_3 to maintain physiologic levels of the latter. Thus, administration of L-thyroxine results in bioavailable T_3 and T_4. Tri-iodothyronine (liothyronine; T_3) should be avoided because of its rapid absorption and disappearance form the blood stream, resulting in uneven blood levels. L-thyroxine has a half-life of 8 days, so it needs to be given only once a day. The average replacement dose for adults is 100 to 150 μg/day. In healthy adults, 100 μg/day is an appropriate starting dose. In elderly patients or those with cardiac disease, L-thyroxine should be increased gradually, with a beginning dose of 25 μg daily, increasing this dose by 25 μg every 2 weeks. The therapeutic response to L-thyroxine therapy should be monitored clinically and with serum TSH levels. As overtreatment may cause osteopenia, normal serum TSH levels should be sought. Patients with secondary hypothyroidism should be treated with L-thyroxine until their free T_4 is in the mid-normal range. Appropriate treatment of these patients will result in suppressed serum TSH levels.

In patients with myxedema coma, a suggested treatment regimen is 100 μg of intravenous L-thyroxine daily. Hydrocortisone (100 mg intravenous three times a day) and intravenous fluids should also be given. The underlying precipitating event should be corrected. Respiratory assistance and treatment of hypothermia with warming blankets may be required. Although myxedema coma carries a high mortality despite appropriate treatment, many patients improve in 1 to 3 days, and full recovery is the norm.

GOITER

Enlargement of the thyroid gland is called goiter. Patients with goiter may be euthyroid (simple goiter), hyperthyroid (toxic nodular goiter or Graves' disease), or hypothyroid (nontoxic goiter or Hashimoto's thyroiditis). Thyroid enlargement (often focal) also may be due to a thyroid adenoma or carcinoma. In nontoxic goiter, inadequate thyroid hormone synthesis leads to TSH stimulation with resultant enlargement of the thyroid gland. Iodine deficiency (endemic goiter) was once the most common cause of nontoxic goiter; with the use of iodized salt, it is now almost nonexistent in North America. Low iodine leads to impaired thyroid hormone production, increased TSH secretion, and hyperplasia of thyroid cells. Thyroid hormone replacement rapidly shrinks the goiter, although iodine must also be given to correct the underlying deficiency.

Dietary goitrogens can cause goiter, and iodine is the most common goitrogen. Large doses of iodine can cause goiter in a susceptible individual. Mild iodine excess is unlikely to be harmful. Other possible goitrogens include lithium and vegetable products such as thioglucosides found in cabbage. Thyroid hormone biosynthetic defects can cause goiter associated with hypothyroidism or, with adequate compensation, euthyroidism.

A careful thyroid examination coupled with thyroid hormone tests can delineate the cause of the goiter. A smooth symmetric gland, often with a bruit, along with thyroid tests indicating hyperthyroidism, is suggestive of Graves' disease. A nodular thyroid with laboratory evidence of hypothyroidism and positive antithyroid antibodies is consistent with Hashimoto's thyroiditis. A diffuse, smooth goiter with laboratory tests of hypothyroidism but without antithyroid antibodies may be indicative of iodine deficiency or a biosynthetic defect. As the thyroid enlargement seen with goiters represents compensated hypothyroidism, laboratory studies often reveal only mild hypothyroidism. Goiters may become very large, extend substernally, and cause dysphagia, respiratory distress, or hoarseness. An ultrasound or radioiodine scan delineates the thyroid gland, and a thyroid uptake and scan can determine the functional activity of the goiter.

Goiters, with the exception of those due to neoplasms or autonomous nodules, are treated with thyroid hormone at a dose that suppresses TSH (100 to 200 μg/day). This treatment, which will correct the hypothyroidism and result in slow regression of the goiter, should be continued indefinitely. Long-standing goiters may not regress but usually will not grow on L-thyroxine therapy. Surgery is indicated for nontoxic goiter only if obstructive symptoms develop or substantial substernal extension is present.

SOLITARY THYROID NODULES

Thyroid nodules are common. They can be detected clinically in about 4% of the population and are found in about 50% of the population at autopsy. Benign thyroid nodules are usually follicular adenomas, colloid nodules, benign cysts, or nodular thyroiditis. Patients with Hashimoto's thyroiditis may have one prominent nodule on clinical examination, but thyroid ultrasound may reveal multiple nodules. Although the majority of nodules are benign, a small percentage of them are malignant, so a practical approach must be pursued to detect these lesions. Additionally, most thyroid cancers are of low-grade malignancy. A careful history and physical examination and laboratory tests can be helpful in differentiating benign from malignant lesions (Table 66–6). For example, lymph node involvement or hoarseness is strongly suggestive of a malignant tumor.

The major etiologic factor for thyroid cancer is childhood or adolescent exposure to head and neck radiation. Previously, radiation was used to treat an enlarged thymus, tonsilar disease, hemangioma, or acne. Recently, exposure to radiation from nuclear plants (e.g., Chernobyl, Ukraine) has contributed to an increased incidence of thyroid cancer. The incidence of thyroid cancer is linearly related to the radiation dose up to 1500 rads. TSH is possibly a cocarcinogen; thus, patients exposed to high-risk radiation may benefit from TSH suppression by thyroid hormone. Patients with a history of irradiation should

TABLE 66–6	High-Risk Factors for Malignancy in a Thyroid Nodule

Technique for Detection or Evaluation	Factor
History	Head/neck irradiation
	Exposure to nuclear radiation
	Rapid growth
	Recent onset
	Young age
	Male sex
	Familial incidence (medullary)
Physical	Hard consistency of nodule
	Fixation of nodule
	Lymphadenopathy
	Vocal cord paralysis
	Distant metastasis
Laboratory/imaging	Elevated serum calcitonin
	"Cold" nodule on ^{123}I scan
	Solid lesion on ultrasound
L-thyroxine therapy	No regression

^{123}I = Iodine 123.

have their thyroid carefully palpated every 2 years. In the absence of palpable disease, imaging procedures are not warranted.

The thyroid status of a patient with a thyroid nodule may dictate further evaluation. A hyperthyroid patient is most likely to have a toxic nodule or thyroiditis, while a hypothyroid patient probably has a prominent nodule in a gland with Hashimoto's thyroiditis. These patients are unlikely to have malignant lesions. Euthyroid patients with a solitary nodule should undergo an FNA biopsy. This is a safe procedure that has reduced the need for diagnostic thyroid surgery. An expert cytologist can identify most benign lesions (75% of all biopsies). Additionally, malignant lesions (5% of biopsies), such as papillary, anaplastic, and medullary carcinoma, can be specifically identified. Follicular neoplasms, however, cannot be diagnosed as benign or malignant by FNA; this cytology report, along with "suspicious" cytology, requires surgical excision.

Previously, thyroid scans have been used to evaluate single thyroid nodules. "Hot" thyroid nodules are almost always benign. Most cancers are "cold," but since most benign lesions are also "cold," these patients still require FNA. Thus, thyroid scans have largely been supplanted by aspiration for evaluation of thyroid nodules.

Benign thyroid nodules should be treated with L-thyroxine suppression therapy with a follow-up thyroid examination in 6 months. A significant decrease in the size of the nodule occurs in 10 to 20% of the cases and may be monitored by ultrasound. Most benign lesions and some cancers remain unchanged in size. An increase in size of the nodule while on suppression therapy warrants a re-evaluation.

THYROID CARCINOMA

The most common type of thyroid carcinoma is papillary carcinoma (60%). Follicular carcinoma (20%), anaplastic

carcinoma (14%), medullary carcinoma (5%), and lymphoma (1%) occur less frequently. Papillary carcinoma is associated with local invasion and lymph node spread. Poor prognosis is associated with thyroid capsule invasion, size >2.5 cm, age of onset >45 years, tall-cell variant, and lymph node involvement. Follicular carcinoma is slightly more aggressive than papillary carcinoma and can spread by local invasion of lymph nodes or hematogenously to bone, brain, or lung. Patients may present with metastases before diagnosis of the primary thyroid lesion. Anaplastic carcinoma tends to occur in older individuals (>50 years), is very aggressive, and rapidly causes pain, dysphagia, and hoarseness. Death usually occurs in the first year.

Medullary carcinoma of the thyroid is derived from calcitonin-producing parafollicular cells and is more malignant than papillary or follicular carcinoma. This type of cancer is multifocal and spreads both locally and distally. It may be either sporadic or familial. When familial, it is inherited in an autosomal dominant pattern and is part of multiple endocrine neoplasia (MEN) type 2A (medullary carcinoma of the thyroid, pheochromocytoma, and hyperparathyroidism) or MEN type 2B (medullary carcinoma of the thyroid, mucosal neuromas, intestinal ganglioneuromas, marfanoid habitus, and pheochromocytoma). Measurement of basal serum calcitonin levels can usually confirm the etiology of this type of thyroid carcinoma. Measurement of serum calcitonin after pentagastrin stimulation should be performed in all first-degree relatives of patients with medullary carcinoma of the thyroid. Measurements of the RET protooncogene mutations in family members of affected individuals have allowed preclinical diagnosis of this genetic disorder.

Treatment

Lobectomy can be performed for papillary and follicular carcinoma <1.5 cm in size. These patients require lifelong L-thyroxine suppressive therapy and yearly thyroid examinations. Larger papillary or follicular tumors require near-total thyroidectomy, with modified neck dissection if there is evidence of lymph node metastases. Postoperatively, the patient should receive triiodothyronine (T$_3$) for about 3 months. The medication is stopped for 2 weeks, and the patient is scanned with 3 mCi of ^{131}I. If uptake occurs, the patient is treated with ^{131}I until no further uptake is observed. The patient is then treated with a sufficient dose of L-thyroxine to suppress serum TSH to undetectable levels. Frequent neck examinations for masses should be accompanied by measurement of serum thyroglobulin levels. A rise in serum thyroglobulin levels suggests recurrence of thyroid cancer. Solitary metastatic lesions that take up ^{131}I can be treated with radioactive iodine, while those that do not take up ^{131}I can be treated with local x-ray therapy. Medullary carcinoma of the thyroid should be tested by total thyroidectomy with removal of the central lymph nodes in the neck. Completeness of the procedure and monitoring for recurrence is determined by measurement of serum calcitonin.

The treatment for patients with anaplastic carcinoma is different. Treatment consists of isthmusectomy to confirm the diagnosis and to prevent tracheal compression, followed by palliative x-ray treatment. Thyroid lymphomas are also treated with x-ray therapy.

The prognosis for well-differentiated thyroid carcinomas is good. Age at the time of diagnosis and sex are the most important prognostic factors. Men over 40 and women over 50 have a higher recurrence and death rate than younger patients. The 5-year survival rate for invasive medullary carcinoma is 50%, while the mean survival for anaplastic carcinoma is 6 months.

REFERENCES

Bayer MF: Effective laboratory evaluation of thyroid status. Med Clin North Am 1991; 75:1.

Dayan CM, Daniels GH: Chronic autoimmune thyroiditis. N Engl J Med 1996; 335:99.

Helfand M, Crapo LM: Screening for thyroid disease. Ann Intern Med 1990; 112:840.

Larsen PR: The thyroid. *In* Bennett JC, Plum F (eds.): Cecil Textbook of Medicine. 20th ed. Philadelphia, WB Saunders, 1996.

Singer PA: Thyroiditis, acute, subacute and chronic. Med Clin North Am 1991; 75:61.

Weetman AP, McGregor AM: Autoimmune thyroid disease: Further developments in our understanding. Endocrine Rev 1994; 15:788.

67

Adrenal Gland

PHYSIOLOGY

The adrenal glands lie at the superior pole of each kidney and are composed of two distinct regions, the cortex and the medulla. The adrenal cortex consists of three anatomic zones: the outer zona glomerulosa, which secretes the mineralocorticoid aldosterone; the intermediate zona fasciculata, which secretes cortisol; and the inner zona reticularis, which secretes adrenal androgens. The adrenal medulla, lying in the center of the adrenal gland, is functionally related to the sympathetic nervous system and secretes the catecholamines epinephrine and norepinephrine in response to stress.

The synthesis of all steroid hormones begins with cholesterol and is catalyzed by a series of regulated, enzyme-mediated reactions (Fig. 67–1). Glucocorticoids are pleotropic hormones that affect metabolism, cardiovascular function, behavior, and the inflammatory/immune response (Table 67–1). Cortisol, the natural human glucocorticoid, is secreted by the adrenal glands in response to ultradian, circadian, and stress-induced hormonal stimulation by adrenocorticotropic hormone (ACTH; corticotropin). Plasma cortisol has a marked circadian rhythm, with highest levels in the morning. ACTH, a 39–amino acid neuropeptide, is part of the proopiomelanocortin (POMC) precursor molecule, which also contains β-endorphin, β-lipotropin, corticotropin-like intermediate-lobe peptide (CLIP), and various melanocyte-stimulating hormones (MSH). The secretion of ACTH by the pituitary is primarily regulated by the 41–amino acid polypeptide corticotropin-releasing hormone (CRH) and the decapeptide vasopressin; both are delivered from the parvocellular division of the paraventricular nucleus of the hypothalamus to the pituitary via the hypophysial portal system. Glucocorticoids exert negative feedback upon CRH and ACTH secretion. The hypothalamic-pituitary-adrenal (HPA) axis (Fig. 67–2) interacts with and influences the function of the reproductive, growth, and thyroid axes at multiple levels, with major participation of glucocorticoids at all levels.

The renin-angiotensin system (Fig. 67–3) is the major factor controlling aldosterone secretion. The juxtaglomerular cells of the kidney secrete renin in response to a decrease in circulating volume and/or a reduction in renal perfusion pressure. Renin is the rate-limiting enzyme that cleaves the 60 kDa angiotensinogen, synthesized by the liver, to the decapeptide angiotensin I. Angiotensin I is rapidly converted to the octapeptide angiotensin II by angiotensin-converting enzyme (ACE) in the lungs and other tissues. Although angiotensin I has no biologic activity, angiotensin II is a potent vasopressor and also acts to stimulate aldosterone production. Angiotensin II does not stimulate cortisol production. Angiotensin II is the predominant regulator of aldosterone secretion, but plasma potassium, sodium status, and ACTH also influence aldosterone secretion. ACTH probably mediates the circadian rhythm of aldosterone, resulting in the highest plasma concentration of this hormone in the morning. Aldosterone binds to the type I mineralocorticoid receptor, while cortisol binds to the type II glucocorticoid receptor. Binding of aldosterone to the renal cytosol mineralocorticoid receptor provides energy for the transepithelial movement of sodium from the cell via the sodium-potassium pump. Thus, aldosterone leads to Na^+ movement into the extracellular fluid and K^+ and H^+ secretion into the urine. The resultant increase in plasma Na^+ and decrease in plasma K^+ provide a feedback mechanism to suppress renin and, subsequently, aldosterone secretion.

Both cortisol and aldosterone circulate in either the free form or bound to corticosteroid-binding globulin (CBG) and albumin. Approximately 5% of cortisol and 40% of aldosterone exist in the unbound form.

Adrenal androgens include dehydroepiandosterone (DHEA) and its sulfate, DHEAS, and androstenedione. They are synthesized in the zona reticularis under the influence of ACTH and other ill-defined adrenal androgen–stimulating factors. While the adrenal androgens have minimal intrinsic androgenic activity, they contribute to androgenicity by their peripheral conversion to testosterone and dihydrotestosterone. In adult males, excessive adrenal androgen has no clinical consequences; however, in females, peripheral conversion of excess adrenal androgen secretion results in acne, hirsutism, and virilization. Because of gonadal production of androgens and estrogens and the secretion of norepinephrine by sympathetic ganglia, deficiencies of adrenal androgens and catecholamines are not clinically recognized.

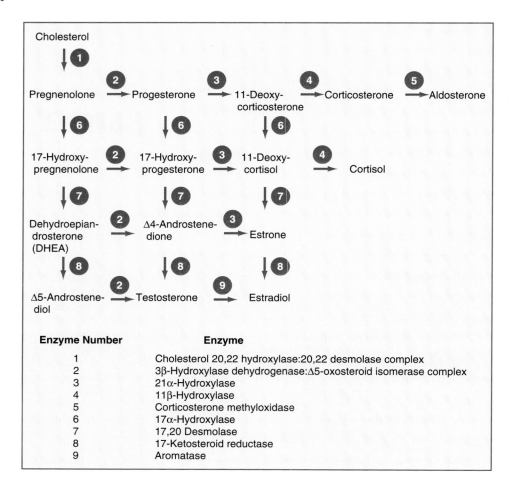

Figure 67-1
Pathways of steroid biosynthesis.

Enzyme Number	Enzyme
1	Cholesterol 20,22 hydroxylase:20,22 desmolase complex
2	3β-Hydroxylase dehydrogenase:Δ5-oxosteroid isomerase complex
3	21α-Hydroxylase
4	11β-Hydroxylase
5	Corticosterone methyloxidase
6	17α-Hydroxylase
7	17,20 Desmolase
8	17-Ketosteroid reductase
9	Aromatase

ADRENAL INSUFFICIENCY

Glucocorticoid insufficiency can either be primary, resulting from the destruction or dysfunction of the adrenal cortex, or secondary, caused by ACTH hyposecretion (Table 67–2). Autoimmune destruction of the adrenal glands (Addison's disease) is the most common cause of primary adrenal insufficiency in the industrialized world, accounting for about 65% of cases. Both glucocorticoid and mineralocorticoid secretion are diminished in this condition, which, if untreated, is usually fatal. Adrenal medulla function is usually spared. Approximately 70% of the patients with Addison's disease have antiadrenal antibodies.

Tuberculosis was formerly the most common cause of adrenal insufficiency; however, it now accounts for less than 20% of cases of adrenal insufficiency in the industrialized world. Calcified adrenal glands can be seen in 50% of cases of tuberculous adrenal insufficiency. Fungal and cytomegalovirus infections, metastatic infiltration of the adrenals, sarcoidosis, amyloidosis, hemochromatosis, traumatic injury to both adrenals, bilateral adrenal hemorrhage, and sepsis (usually meningococcemia) are less frequent causes of adrenal insufficiency. Patients with human immunodeficiency virus (HIV) infection often have decreased adrenal reserve without overt adrenal insufficiency. Congenital causes of adrenal dysfunction include congenital adrenal hyperplasia (discussed later), ad-

TABLE 67-1	Actions of Glucocorticoid

1. Maintains metabolic homeostasis
   A. Regulates blood glucose level/permissive effects on gluconeogenesis/increases glycogen synthesis
   B. Raises insulin levels/permissive effects on lipolytic hormones
   C. Increases catabolism/decreases anabolism (except fat)/inhibits growth hormone axis
   D. Inhibits reproductive axis
   E. Mineralocorticoid activity of cortisol
2. Affects connective tissues
   A. Causes loss of collagen and connective tissue
3. Affects calcium homeostasis
   A. Stimulates osteoclasts/inhibits osteoblasts
   B. Reduces intestinal calcium absorption/stimulates PTH release/increases urinary calcium excretion/decreases reabsorption of phosphate
4. Maintains cardiovascular function
   A. Increases cardiac output
   B. Increases vascular tone
   C. Permissive effects on pressor hormones/increases sodium retention
5. Affects behavior and cognitive function
6. Affects immune system
   A. Increases intravascular leukocyte concentration
   B. Decreases migration of inflammatory cells to sites of injury
   C. Suppresses immune system (thymolysis, suppression of cytokines, prostanoids, kinins, serotonin, histamine, collagenase, and plasminogen activator)

PTH = Parathyroid hormone.

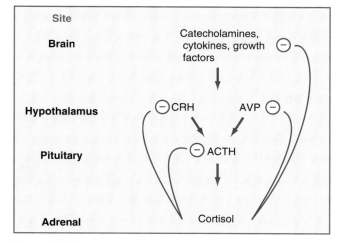

Figure 67–2
The brain-hypothalamic-pituitary-adrenal axis.

renal unresponsiveness to ACTH, congenital adrenal hypoplasia, and two demyelinating lipid metabolism disorders, adrenoleukodystrophy and adrenomyeloneuropathy. The latter two disorders are caused by abnormal fatty acid metabolism leading to accumulation of very long chain saturated fatty acids in the brain, adrenal cortex, and other organs. Iatrogenic causes of adrenal insufficiency include bilateral adrenalectomy, agents that inhibit cortisol biosynthesis (metyrapone, aminoglutethimide, trilostane, ketoconazole), adrenolytic drugs (o,p'-DDD), and the glucocorticoid antagonist mifepristone (RU 486).

Addison's disease may be part of two distinct autoimmune polyglandular syndromes. Type I autoimmune polyglandular syndrome, also termed autoimmune polyendocrine-candidiasis-ectodermal dystrophy (APECED) or autoimmune polyglandular failure syndrome, is marked by the triad of hypoparathyroidism, adrenal insufficiency, and mucocutaneous candidiasis. Other less common manifestations include hypothyroidism, gonadal failure, gastrointestinal malabsorption, insulin-dependent diabetes melli-

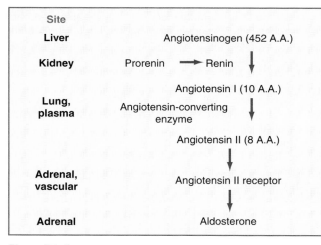

Figure 67–3
The renin-angiotensin-aldosterone axis. AA = Amino acids.

TABLE 67–2	Syndromes of Adrenocortical Hypofunction

I. Primary adrenal disorders
  A. Combined glucocorticoid and mineralocorticoid deficiency
    1. Autoimmune
      a. Isolated autoimmune disease (Addison's disease)
      b. Polyglandular failure syndrome, type I
      c. Polyglandular failure syndrome, type II
    2. Infectious
      a. Tuberculosis
      b. Fungus
      c. Cytomegalovirus
    3. Vascular
      a. Bilateral adrenal hemorrhage
      b. Sepsis
      c. Coagulopathy
      d. Thrombosis/embolism
      e. Infarction
    4. Infiltration
      a. Metastatic carcinoma/lymphoma
      b. Sarcoidosis
      c. Amyloidosis
      d. Hemochromatosis
    5. Congenital
      a. Congenital adrenal hyperplasia
        1. 21α-hydroxylase deficiency
        2. 3β-hydroxylase dehydrogenase: Δ⁵-oxysteroid isomerase complex deficiency
        3. 20,22-Desmolase deficiency
      b. Adrenal unresponsiveness to ACTH
      c. Congenital adrenal hypoplasia
      d. Adrenoleukodystrophy
      e. Adrenomyeloneuropathy
    6. Iatrogenic
      a. Bilateral adrenalectomy
      b. Drugs—metyrapone, aminoglutethimide, trilostane, ketoconazole, o,p'-DDD, RU 486
  B. Mineralocorticoid deficiency without glucocorticoid deficiency
    1. Corticosterone methyloxidase deficiency
    2. Isolated zona glomerulosa defect
    3. Heparin therapy
    4. Critically ill patients
    5. Converting enzyme inhibitors
II. Secondary adrenal disorders
  A. Secondary adrenal insufficiency
    1. Hypothalamic/pituitary dysfunction
    2. Exogenous glucocorticoids
    3. Following removal of an ACTH-secreting tumor
  B. Hyporeninemic hypoaldosteronism
    1. Diabetic nephropathy
    2. Tubulointerstitial diseases
    3. Obstructive uropathy
    4. Autonomic neuropathy
    5. Nonsteroidal anti-inflammatory drugs
    6. Beta-adrenergic drugs

ACTH = Adrenocorticotropic hormone (corticotropin).

tus, alopecia areata and totalis, pernicious anemia, vitiligo, chronic active hepatitis, keratopathy, hypoplasia of dental enamel and nails, hypophysitis, asplenism, and cholelithasis. This syndrome presents in childhood. Type II autoimmune polyglandular syndrome, also called Schmidt's syndrome, is marked by Addison's disease, autoimmune thyroid disease (Graves' disease or Hashimoto's thyroiditis), and insulin-dependent diabetes mellitus. Other less frequently associated diseases include pernicious anemia, vitiligo, gonadal failure, hypophysitis, celiac disease, myasthenia gravis, primary biliary cirrhosis, Sjögren's syndrome, lupus erythematosus, and Parkinson's disease. This syndrome usually presents in adults and is associated with HLA haplotypes B8 and DR3.

Adrenal insufficiency commonly presents as weight loss, increasing fatigue, vomiting, diarrhea or anorexia, and salt craving. Muscle and joint pain, abdominal pain, and postural dizziness may also occur. Signs of increased pigmentation (on the extensor surfaces, creases of the palm, and buccal mucosa) often occur as the result of the increased production of ACTH or other POMC-related peptides by the pituitary. Laboratory abnormalities may include hyponatremia and hyperkalemia, metabolic acidosis, azotemia, hypercalcemia, anemia, lymphocytosis, and eosinophilia. Hypoglycemia may also occur, especially in children.

The diagnosis of acute adrenal insufficiency is a medical emergency, and treatment should not be delayed pending laboratory results. In a critically ill patient with postural hypotension and hypovolemia, a plasma sample for cortisol, ACTH, and renin should be obtained, and then treatment should be immediately initiated with an intravenous bolus of 100 mg of hydrocortisone and parenteral isotonic saline administration. A plasma cortisol level >18 μgm/dl rules out the diagnosis of adrenal crisis, while a value <18 μgm/dl in the setting of shock may be consistent with adrenal insufficiency. In a patient with chronic symptoms (e.g., fatigue, anorexia, postural dizziness), a 1-hour cosyntropin test should be performed. In this test, 0.25 mg ACTH[1-24] (cosyntropin) is given intravenously, and plasma cortisol is drawn at 0, 30, and 60 minutes. A normal response is a plasma cortisol level >20 μgm/dl at any time during the test. A patient with a basal morning plasma cortisol level <12 μgm/dl *and* a stimulated cortisol level <18 μgm/dl probably has frank adrenal insufficiency and should receive treatment. A person with a basal morning plasma cortisol level between 12 and 18 μgm/dl probably has impaired adrenal reserve and should receive cortisol replacement under stress conditions (see later).

Once the diagnosis of adrenal insufficiency is made, the distinction between primary and secondary adrenal insufficiency needs to be ascertained. Secondary adrenal insufficiency results from inadequate stimulation of the adrenal cortex by ACTH. This can occur due to lesions anywhere along the hypothalamic-pituitary axis or as a sequela of prolonged suppression of the HPA axis by exogenous glucocorticoids. Secondary adrenal insufficiency presents with manifestations similar to those of primary adrenal insufficiency but with a few important differences. Since ACTH and other POMC-related peptides are reduced in secondary adrenal insufficiency, hyperpigmentation does not occur. Additionally, since mineralocorticoid levels are normal in secondary adrenal insufficiency, symptoms of salt craving as well as the laboratory abnormalities of hyperkalemia and metabolic acidosis are not present. However, hyponatremia is often present due to the inappropriate ADH secretion that accompanies glucocorticoid insufficiency. Since corticotropin secretion is the most preserved of the pituitary hormones, a patient with secondary adrenal insufficiency due to a pituitary lesion usually has concomitant symptoms and/or laboratory abnormalities consistent with hypothyroidism, hypogonadism, or growth hormone deficiency.

Laboratory studies that distinguish primary from secondary adrenal insufficiency in the presence of cortisol deficiency include basal morning plasma ACTH sample and a standing (after 2 hours) plasma renin level. A plasma ACTH level of >50 pg/ml (normal is 5 to 30 pg/ml) is consistent with primary adrenal insufficiency, while a value <20 pg/ml probably represents secondary adrenal insufficiency. An upright plasma renin level of >3 ng/ml/hr is consistent with primary adrenal insufficiency, while a value of <3 ng/ml/hr probably represents secondary adrenal insufficiency. The 1-hour cosyntropin test is suppressed in secondary as well as primary adrenal insufficiency.

Secondary adrenal insufficiency occurs commonly after discontinuation of long-term glucocorticoid administration. When prolonged glucocorticoid therapy is necessary, alternate-day glucocorticoid treatment results in less suppression of the HPA axis than daily therapy. The natural history of recovery from iatrogenic adrenal suppression includes, sequentially, a gradual increase in ACTH levels, followed by the normalization of plasma cortisol levels, followed then by a normalization of the cortisol response to ACTH. Complete recovery of the HPA axis can take up to 1 year; the rate-limiting step appears to be recovery of the CRH neurons.

Treatment

After stabilization of acute adrenal insufficiency, patients with Addison's disease require lifelong replacement of both glucocorticoids and mineralocorticoids. Most physicians tend to overtreat patients with glucocorticoids and undertreat them with mineralocorticoids. As overtreatment with glucocorticoids results in insidious weight gain and osteoporosis, the minimal cortisol dose tolerated without symptoms of glucocorticoid insufficiency (usually joint pain) is recommended. An initial regimen of 15 to 20 mg of hydrocortisone first thing in the morning and 5 mg of hydrocortisone at around 4:00 p.m. mimics the physiologic dose and is recommended. Although glucocorticoid replacement is fairly uniform in most patients, mineralocorticoid replacement varies greatly. The initial dose of the synthetic mineralocorticoid fludrocortisone (Florinef), should be 100 μg/day and should be adjusted to keep the standing plasma renin between 1 and 3 ng/ml/hr. A standing plasma renin level above 3 ng/ml/hr while the patient is on the correct glucocorticoid dose suggests undertreatment with fludrocortisone.

Under the stress of a minor illness (nausea, vomiting, or fever $>100.5°$F), the hydrocortisone dose should be doubled for as short a period of time as possible. The inability to ingest hydrocortisone pills may require parenteral hydrocortisone administration. Patients undergoing a major stress (i.e., surgery requiring generalized anesthesia or major trauma) should receive 150 to 300 mg of parenteral hydrocortisone daily (in three divided doses) with a rapid taper to normal replacement during recovery. All patients should wear a Medic Alert bracelet and should be instructed in the use of intramuscular emergency hydrocortisone injections.

HYPORENINEMIC HYPOALDOSTERONISM

Mineralocorticoid deficiency may also occur due to decreased renin secretion by the kidney. Resultant hypoangiotensinemia leads to hypoaldosteronism. Hyperkalemia and hyperchloremic metabolic acidosis occur. Plasma sodium concentration is usually normal, but sodium conservation is often deficient. Plasma renin and aldosterone levels are low and unresponsive to stimuli. Diabetes mellitus and chronic tubulointerstitial diseases of the kidney are the most common underlying conditions leading to impaired renin secretion by the renal juxtaglomerular apparatus. A subset of hyporeninemic hypoaldosteronism is due to autonomic insufficiency. Stimuli mediated by baroreceptors, such as upright posture or volume depletion, do not elucidate a normal renin response. Administration of pharmacologic agents such as nonsteroidal anti-inflammatory agents, angiotensin-converting enzyme inhibitors, and beta-adrenergic antagonists can also produce conditions of hypoaldosteronism. Potassium restriction and fludrocortisone, or furosemide, either singly or in combination, are usually effective in correcting the hyperkalemia and acidosis due to hypoaldosteronism.

Rarely, mineralocorticoid deficiency occurs in association with hyperreninism. The causes include a deficiency of corticosterone methyloxidase, the enzyme complex responsible for the final step of aldosterone biosynthesis, or an autoimmune-mediated destruction of the aldosterone-producing cells in the zona glomerulosa. Chronic administration of heparin and related compounds may also produce a state of hyperreninemic hypoaldosteronism.

CONGENITAL ADRENAL HYPERPLASIA

Congenital adrenal hyperplasia (CAH) refers to a group of congenital disorders of adrenal steroid biosynthesis resulting in glucocorticoid and mineralocorticoid deficiency. Due to deficient cortisol biosynthesis, a compensatory increase in ACTH occurs, inducing adrenal hyperplasia and overproduction of the steroids preceding the blocked enzyme (see Fig. 67–1). There are five major types of CAH, and the clinical manifestations of each disorder depend on which steroids are in excess and which are deficient. All of these syndromes are transmitted in an autosomal recessive pattern. 21-α-hydroxylase deficiency is the most common disorder and accounts for about 95% of the cases of CAH. In this condition, there is a failure to convert 17-hydroxyprogesterone and progesterone to 11-deoxycortisol and 11-deoxycortisone, respectively, with deficient cortisol and aldosterone production. Cortisol deficiency leads to increased ACTH release, causing overproduction of 17-hydroxyprogesterone and progesterone. Increased ACTH production also leads to increased biosynthesis of androstenedione and DHEA, which can be converted to testosterone. Patients with 21-α-hydroxylase

deficiency can be divided into two clinical phenotypes, classic 21-α-hydroxylase deficiency, usually diagnosed at birth or during childhood, and late-onset 21-α-hydroxylase deficiency, which manifests during or after puberty. Two thirds of patients with classic 21-α-hydroxylase deficiency have various degrees of mineralocorticoid deficiency (salt-losing form), while the remaining one third are not salt losing (simple virilizing form). A more profound enzymatic block appears to occur in the salt-losing form. Both decreased aldosterone production and increased concentrations of precursors that are mineralocorticoid antagonists, progesterone and 17-hydroxyprogesterone, contribute to salt loss in the salt-losing form.

Neonatal girls with classic 21-α-hydroxylase deficiency have masculinization of the genitalia, and neonatal boys may exhibit phallic enlargement. Both sexes may exhibit salt loss resulting in hyponatremia, hyperkalemia, acidosis, dehydration, and hypotension. Adrenal crisis usually occurs in the second week of life. Prepubescent children usually present with precocious puberty (isosexual in males, heterosexual in females). Androgen excess leads to rapid bone maturation and eventual short stature. The most useful measurement for the diagnosis of classic 21-α-hydroxylase deficiency is plasma 17-hydroxyprogesterone. A value >200 ng/dl is consistent with the diagnosis. A cortisol deficiency is usually found, and all salt losers and many patients with the simple virilizing form have hyperreninemia and hypoaldosteronism. The aim of treatment for classic 21-α-hydroxylase deficiency is to replace glucocorticoids and mineralocorticoids, suppress ACTH and androgen overproduction, and allow for normal growth and sexual maturation. Physiologic doses of hydrocortisone reduce androgen production but not to normal levels. Supraphysiologic doses of hydrocortisone can normalize androgen levels, but this requires the patient to be exposed to the deleterious effects of hypercortisolism. The optimal approach to achieving adequate suppression of androgens without causing hypercortisolism has not yet been determined.

Late-onset 21-α-hydroxylase deficiency represents an allelic variant of classic 21-α-hydroxylase deficiency, characterized by a mild enzymatic defect. This is the most frequent autosomal recessive disorder in humans and is especially present in Ashkenazi Jews. The syndrome usually presents around puberty with signs of virilization (hirsutism and acne) and amenorrhea or oligomenorrhea. It should be considered in women with unexplained hirsutism and menstrual abnormalities. The diagnosis is made by finding an elevated plasma 17-hydroxyprogesterone level (>1500 ng/dl) 30 minutes after administration of 0.25 mg of synthetic ACTH[1-24]. Although the traditional treatment for late-onset 21-α-hydroxylase deficiency is dexamethasone (0.5 mg/day), the use of an antiandrogen such as spironolactone (100 to 200 mg/day) is probably more effective and has fewer side effects. Mineralocorticoid replacement is not needed in late-onset 21-α-hydroxylase deficiency.

11β-Hydroxylase deficiency accounts for about 5% of the cases of CAH. In this syndrome, the conversion of 11-deoxycortisol to cortisol and 11-deoxycorticosterone (DOC) to corticosterone (the precursor to aldosterone) is blocked. As DOC is a mineralocorticoid, the patients usually have hypertension and hypokalemia. Virilization occurs as with 21-α-hydroxylase deficiency, and a late-onset form presenting as androgen excess also occurs. The diagnosis is made by finding elevated plasma 11-deoxycortisol, either basally or after ACTH stimulation. 3β-Hydroxysteroid dehydrogenase Δ^5-/Δ^4 isomerase deficiency, 17α-hydroxylase deficiency, and 20,22-desmolase deficiency are all rare forms of congenital adrenal hyperplasia.

SYNDROMES OF ADRENOCORTICOID HYPERFUNCTION

Hypersecretion of the glucocorticoid hormone, cortisol, results in Cushing syndrome, a metabolic disorder affecting carbohydrate, protein, and lipid metabolism. Hypersecretion of mineralocorticoids such as aldosterone results in a syndrome of hypertension and electrolyte disturbances.

Cushing Syndrome

Pathophysiology

Increased production of cortisol is seen in both physiologic and pathologic states (Table 67–3). Physiologic hypercortisolism occurs in stress, during the last trimester of pregnancy, and in individuals chronically performing strenuous exercise. Pathologic conditions of elevated cortisol include exogenous or endogenous Cushing syndrome and several psychiatric states, including depression, alcoholism, anorexia nervosa, panic disorder, and alcohol or narcotic withdrawal.

Cushing syndrome may be due to exogenous ACTH or glucocorticoid administration or endogenous hyperproduction of these hormones. Endogenous Cushing syndrome is either ACTH dependent or ACTH independent. ACTH-dependent cases account for 85% of Cushing syndrome patients and include pituitary sources of ACTH (Cushing disease), ectopic sources of ACTH, and ectopic sources of CRH. Pituitary Cushing disease accounts for 80% of ACTH-dependent Cushing syndrome. Ectopic ACTH secretion occurs most commonly in patients with small cell lung carcinoma, in whom signs and symptoms of lung cancer are usually predominant, or in patients with intrathoracic (lung and thymic) carcinoid tumors. The remaining patients have pancreatic, adrenal, or thyroid tumors secreting ACTH.

Adrenocorticotropic hormone–independent cases account for 15% of Cushing syndrome and include adrenal adenomas, adrenal carcinomas, micronodular adrenal disease, and autonomous macronodular adrenal disease. The mean age of presentation for pituitary Cushing disease is in the 20s and 30s, while for ectopic Cushing syndrome and adrenal carcinoma, a bimodal age of onset is present, with increased incidence in children and young

TABLE 67–3	Syndromes of Adrenocortical Hyperfunction

I. States of glucocorticoid excess
  A. Physiologic states
    1. Stress
    2. Strenuous exercise
    3. Last trimester of pregnancy
  B. Pathologic states
    1. Psychiatric conditions (pseudo-Cushing disorders)
      a. Depression
      b. Alcoholism
      c. Anorexia nervosa
      d. Panic disorders
      e. Alcohol/drug withdrawal
    2. ACTH-dependent states
      a. Pituitary adenoma (Cushing disease)
      b. Ectopic ACTH syndrome
        1. Bronchial carcinoid
        2. Thymic carcinoid
        3. Islet cell tumor
        4. Small cell lung carcinoma
      c. Ectopic CRH secretion
    3. ACTH-independent states
      a. Adrenal adenoma
      b. Adrenal carcinoma
      c. Micronodular adrenal disease
  C. Exogenous sources
    1. Glucocorticoid intake
    2. ACTH intake
II. States of mineralocorticoid excess
  A. Primary aldosteronism
    1. Aldosterone-secreting adenoma
    2. Bilateral adrenal hyperplasia
    3. Aldosterone-secreting carcinoma
    4. Glucocorticoid-suppressible hyperaldosteronism
  B. Adrenal enzyme deficiencies
    1. 11β-Hydroxylase
    2. 17α-Hydroxylase
    3. 11β-Steroid dehydrogenase
  C. Exogenous mineralocorticoids
    1. Licorice
    2. Carbenoxolone
    3. Fludrocortisone
  D. Secondary hyperaldosteronism
    1. Associated with hypertension
      a. Accelerated hypertension
      b. Renovascular hypertension
      c. Estrogen administration
      d. Renin-secreting tumors
    2. Without hypertension
      a. Bartter's syndrome
      b. Sodium-wasting nephropathy
      c. Renal tubular acidosis
      d. Diuretic/laxative abuse
      e. Edematous states (cirrhosis, nephrosis, congestive heart failure)

ACTH = Adrenocorticotropic hormone (corticotropin); CRH = corticotropin-releasing hormone.

people 20 and under and in the 50s and 60s. The female-to-male ratio for non–cancer-related forms of Cushing syndrome is 4 : 1, while for adrenal carcinoma it is 1.5 : 1.0. Because of the usually insidious onset of Cushing syndrome, the median duration of symptoms before the diagnosis is made is 3 to 5 years.

TABLE 67–4	Common Symptoms and Laboratory Abnormalities of Hypocortisolism

Symptoms and Abnormalities	Occurrence (%)
Fat distribution (dorsocervical and supraclavicular fat pads, temporal wasting, centripetal obesity, weight gain)	95
Stunted growth (in children)	95
Arrested puberty (in children)	90
Menstrual irregularities (in women)	80
Central hypothyroidism	80
Thin skin/plethora	80
Moon facies	75
Increased appetite	75
Sleep disturbances	75
Hypertension	75
Hypercholesterolemia/hypertriglyceridemia	70
Altered mentation (poor concentration, decreased memory, euphoria)	70
Diabetes mellitus/glucose intolerance	65
Striae	65
Hirsutism	65
Proximal muscle weakness	60
Psychological disturbances (emotional lability, depression, mania, psychosis)	50
Leukocytosis	50
Decreased libido/impotence	50
Acne	45
Osteoporosis/pathologic fractures	40
Virilization (in women)	40
Easy bruisability	40
Poor wound healing	40

Clinical Manifestations

The more common clinical signs and symptoms and common laboratory findings of Cushing syndrome are listed in Table 67–4. Typically the obesity seen in Cushing syndrome is centripetal, with wasting of the arms and legs, making the syndrome quite distinct from the generalized weight gain seen in idiopathic obesity. The characteristic rounding of the face (moon facies) and a dorsocervical fat pad ("buffalo hump") may also occasionally occur in non–Cushing syndrome–related obesity, while facial plethora and supraclavicular and temporal filling are more specific for Cushing syndrome. Patients with Cushing syndrome may have proximal muscle weakness, often leading to inability to stand up from a squat. Menstrual irregularities often precede other cushingoid symptoms in females, while males frequently complain of poor libido and impotence. Adult-onset acne or hirsutism in females should also raise the suspicion of Cushing syndrome. Skin striae often occur; they are violacious (purple or dark red), with a width of at least 1 cm. Thinning of the skin on the top of the hands is a very specific sign in younger adults with Cushing syndrome that should always be sought during examination. Old pictures are extremely helpful to evaluate the physical stigmata of Cushing syndrome.

In pediatric patients with Cushing syndrome, growth arrest is the most common presentation. Pubertal arrest, virilization, and menstrual irregularities are also frequently seen.

Associated laboratory findings in Cushing syndrome include elevated plasma alkaline phosphatase, granulocytosis, thrombocytosis, hypercholesterolemia, hypertriglyceridemia, and glucose intolerance/diabetes mellitus. Central hypothyroidism occurs in about 70% of patients with Cushing syndrome and may occur in the absence of other signs of pituitary disease. Hypokalemic alkalosis is an infrequent finding in patients with Cushing syndrome and usually occurs in patients with severe hypercortisolism due to the ectopic ACTH syndrome.

Diagnosis

The diagnostic approach to patients with signs and symptoms of hypercortisolism consists of two steps (Fig. 67–4). First, patients with Cushing syndrome must be separated from those without the diagnosis. Once the diagnosis of Cushing syndrome is established, the etiology of the hypercortisolism must be ascertained. If the history and physical examination are suggestive of hypercortisolism, the diagnosis of Cushing syndrome can usually be established by collecting urine for 24 hours and measuring urinary free cortisol (UFC). UFC excretion reflects plasma unbound cortisol, which is filtered and excreted by the kidney. This test is extremely sensitive for the diagnosis of patients with Cushing syndrome, as 90% of affected patients have an initial UFC level of >90 μgm/24 hours. Patients with pseudo-Cushing states secondary to psychiatric disorders or alcoholism frequently have UFC levels between 90 and 300 μgm/24 hours. A UFC level of >300 μgm/24 hours is fairly specific for Cushing syndrome. Patients with Cushing disease usually have UFC levels between 300 and 1000 μgm/24 hours, while patients with the ectopic ACTH syndrome and cortisol-secreting adrenal adenomas or carcinomas frequently have UFC levels of >1000 μgm/24 hours.

Cortisol normally is secreted in a diurnal fashion, with the highest plasma concentration occurring in the early morning (between 6:00 and 8:00 a.m.) and the lowest concentration occurring around midnight. The normal 8:00 a.m. plasma cortisol level ranges between 5 and 25 μgm/dl and declines throughout the day. By 11:00 p.m., the values are usually <5μgm/dl. Most patients with Cushing syndrome lack this diurnal variation. Thus, while their morning cortisol levels may be similar to those of normals, their afternoon or evening concentrations are markedly higher. Late afternoon or night values >50% of the morning values are consistent with Cushing syndrome. Measurement of random morning cortisol levels is generally not helpful.

The overnight dexamethasone suppression test can also be used as a screening test to evaluate patients suspected of having hypercortisolism. One milligram of dexamethasone is given orally at 11:00 p.m., and plasma cortisol is determined the following morning at 8:00 a.m. A morning plasma cortisol level >5 μgm/dl suggests hypercortisolism. This test is easy and can be performed on an outpatient basis. The test is fairly sensitive, although

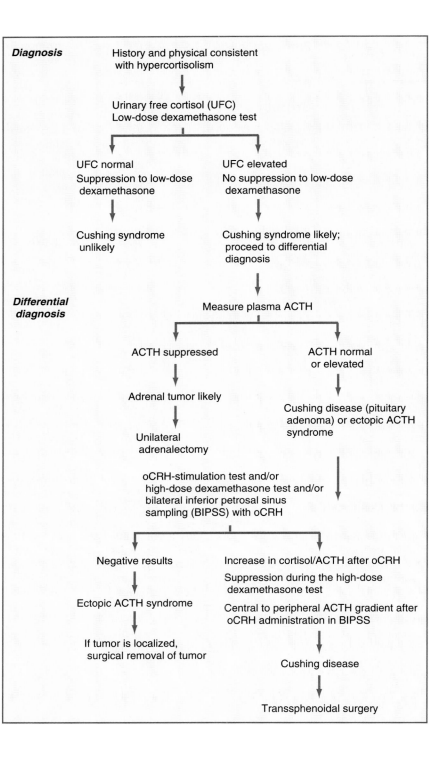

Figure 67–4

Flow chart to evaluate a patient with suspected Cushing syndrome. ACTH = Adrenocorticotropic hormone; oCRH = ovine corticotropin-releasing hormone.

some pituitary adenomas are very sensitive to dexamethasone and a false-negative result may be obtained in the presence of such tumors. However, the test also has a significant number of false-positive results, especially in obese and depressed patients, the two patient populations in whom the differentiation from mild Cushing syndrome may be most difficult. For these reasons, collection of urine for measurement of 24-hour UFC excretion is a better screening test for Cushing syndrome.

Differential Diagnosis

Once the diagnosis of Cushing syndrome is established, the etiology of the hypercortisolism needs to be ascertained. This is accomplished by biochemical studies, which evaluate the feedback regulation of the HPA axis by venous sampling techniques and by imaging procedures. Basal ACTH levels are normal or elevated in patients with pituitary Cushing disease and the ectopic

ACTH syndrome and are undetectable in primary adrenal Cushing syndrome.

In the dexamethasone suppression test (Liddle test), 0.5 mg of dexamethasone is given orally every 6 hours for 2 days, followed by 2 mg of dexamethasone every 6 hours for another 2 days. On the second day of the high dose of dexamethasone, UFC is suppressed to <90% of that of the baseline collection in patients with pituitary adenomas but not in patients with the ectopic ACTH syndrome or adrenal cortisol–secreting tumors. While the Liddle test is often helpful in establishing the etiology of Cushing syndrome, it has some disadvantages. The test requires 6 days of accurate urine collections, often necessitating inpatient hospitalization.

In approximately 50% of patients with bronchial carcinoids causing ectopic ACTH production, the carcinoids are suppressible by high-dose dexamethasone, giving a false-positive result. Additionally, since patients with Cushing syndrome are often episodic secretors of corticosteroids, considerable variation in daily UFC can occur, and false results can be found. Therefore, the Liddle test should be interpreted cautiously in patients who exhibit episodic secretion, and other confirmatory tests should be performed prior to sending a patient to surgery.

An overnight high-dose dexamethasone test is helpful in establishing the etiology of Cushing syndrome. In this test, a baseline 8:00 a.m. cortisol level is measured, and then 8 mg of dexamethasone are given orally at 11:00 p.m. At 8:00 a.m. the following morning, a plasma cortisol level is obtained. Suppression, which would occur in patients with pseudo-Cushing states and in patients with pituitary Cushing disease, is defined as a decrease in plasma cortisol to <50% of the baseline. Few patients with bronchial carcinoid have been examined, so the suppressibility of these tumors to high-dose overnight dexamethasone is not well established.

The ovine CRH (oCRH) test can also be helpful in determining the etiology of Cushing syndrome. Corticotrophs of normal individuals and of patients with pituitary Cushing disease respond to oCRH by increasing the synthesis and secretion of ACTH and, therefore, of cortisol. Thus, the oCRH test cannot be used to distinguish normal individuals from patients with pituitary Cushing disease. Patients with cortisol-secreting adrenal tumors have low or undetectable concentrations of ACTH that do not respond to oCRH. Patients with ectopic ACTH secretion have high basal ACTH levels that do not increase with oCRH. In patients with either primary adrenal hypercortisolism or the ectopic ACTH syndrome, cortisol levels do not change in response to oCRH. Discrepancies between the oCRH and dexamethasone test results require further work-up for ascertainment of the diagnosis.

Bilateral inferior petrosal sinus sampling (BIPSS) before and after intravenous administration of CRH is an extremely accurate and safe procedure to distinguish pituitary Cushing disease from both the ectopic ACTH syndrome and adrenal adenomas. However, the procedure requires a radiologist experienced in petrosal sinus sampling and is available in a limited number of tertiary care facilities.

Imaging techniques may be helpful in evaluating the etiology of hypercortisolism. These include magnetic resonance imaging (MRI) of the pituitary and computed tomography (CT) scan and MRI of the adrenal gland. CT scan and MRI of the chest and abdomen are useful when an ectopic ACTH-secreting tumor is suspected. Fewer than 10% of patients with Cushing disease develop pituitary tumors larger than 5 mm in diameter; it is only in these tumors that CT scan or plain radiographs are helpful. Imaging of the pituitary by MRI combined with intravenously administered gadolinium is therefore the procedure of choice. This test can detect many pituitary tumors as small as 3 mm in diameter and therefore identifies approximately 40 to 50% of pituitary ACTH-secreting tumors.

Treatment

The preferred treatment for all forms of Cushing syndrome (pituitary adenomas, ectopic ACTH syndrome, adrenal adenoma, or adrenal carcinoma) is appropriate surgery. Pituitary Cushing disease is best treated by transsphenoidal surgery (TSS). In the hands of an experienced neurosurgeon, approximately 90 to 95% of patients who undergo initial surgery become hypocortisolemic postoperatively, and over 90% remain permanently cured. The success rate is lower for reoperations (50 to 70%). Transsphenoidal surgery has a very low rate of morbidity and mortality.

Patients with the ectopic ACTH syndrome should have their tumor localized by appropriate scans, followed by surgical removal. A unilateral adrenalectomy is the treatment of choice in patients with a cortisol-secreting adrenal adenoma. Patients with cortisol-secreting adrenal carcinomas should also be treated surgically; however, they have a poor prognosis, with only 20% surviving more than 1 year.

Patients who have failed initial pituitary surgery or have recurrent Cushing disease may be treated with pituitary radiation. Radiation has more long-term complications than TSS and results in cure in about 60% of patients. Almost all patients will eventually develop panhypopituitarism, so that thyroid, gonadal, and even steroid replacement may be needed.

Patients with Cushing disease who remain hypercortisolemic after pituitary surgery and radiation or who decline radiation should undergo bilateral adrenalectomy. About 10% of patients with Cushing disease who undergo bilateral adrenalectomy develop Nelson's syndrome (hyperpigmentation and an ACTH-secreting pituitary macroadenoma often causing visual field defects). This incidence of Nelson's syndrome is significantly reduced if the patient has undergone pituitary irradiation.

Medical treatment for hypercortisolism may be needed to prepare patients for surgery, in patients who are undergoing or have undergone pituitary irradiation and are awaiting its effects, in patients with mild Cushing syndrome, or in patients who are not surgical candidates or who elect not to have surgery. Ketoconazole, mitotane (o,p'DDD), metyrapone, aminoglutethimide, RU 486, and trilostane are the most commonly used agents for adrenal blockade and can be used alone or in combination.

Primary Mineralocorticoid Excess

Pathophysiology

Increased mineralocorticoid activity is manifested by salt retention, hypertension, hypokalemia, and metabolic alkalosis. In primary aldosteronism (see Table 67–3), this can be due to an aldosterone-producing adenoma (75%), bilateral adrenal hyperplasia (22%), adrenal carcinoma (1%), or glucocorticoid-remediable hyperaldosteronism (<1%). The adrenal enzyme defects, 11β-steroid dehydrogenase, 11β-hydroxylase, and 17α-hydroxylase deficiencies, and exogenous mineralocorticoid ingestion (licorice or carbenozolone) are also rare causes of mineralocorticoid excess. Secondary aldosteronism (see Table 67–3) results from an overactivation of the renin-angiotensin system.

Primary aldosteronism is usually recognized during evaluation of hypertension or hypokalemia and represents a potentially curable form of hypertension. Less than 2% of patients with hypertension have primary aldosteronism. The patients are usually between 30 and 50 years of age, and the female-to-male ratio is 2:1.

Clinical Manifestations

Hypertension, hypokalemia, and metabolic alkalosis are the main clinical manifestations of hyperaldosteronism, with most of the presenting symptoms related to hypokalemia. Mildly hypokalemic patients have symptoms of fatigue, muscle weakness, nocturia, lassitude, and headaches. If more severe hypokalemia exists, polydipsia, polyuria, paresthesias, and even intermittent paralysis and tetany can occur. Blood pressure can range from borderline to severely hypertensive levels, rarely with malignant hypertension. A positive Trousseau or Chvostek sign may occur because of metabolic alkalosis.

Diagnosis and Treatment

The initial approach to diagnose hyperaldosteronism is to document hypokalemia in the presence of hypertension (Fig. 67–5). Care must be taken that the patient is taking an adequate amount of salt and is not taking diuretics prior to potassium measurement. A low-sodium diet can mask hypokalemia, so if a diet history suggests salt intake of <120 mEq/day, 100 mEq of sodium chloride should be given for 4 days prior to potassium measurement. Additionally, the patient needs to be off of diuretic treatment for 3 weeks before potassium is measured. If hypokalemia is found under these conditions, a 24-hour urinary aldosterone level should be measured while the patient is on a diet containing adequate sodium (120 to 180 mEq/day), and an upright (standing for at least 2

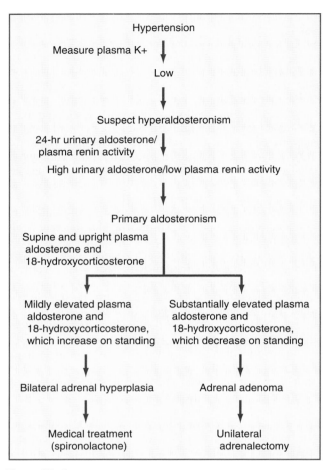

Figure 67–5
Flow chart to evaluate a patient with suspected primary hyperaldosteronism.

hours) plasma renin level should be obtained. An elevated urinary aldosterone level (>15 μgm/day) and a suppressed plasma renin level (<2 ng/ml/hr) suggest the diagnosis of hyperaldosteronism.

Once the diagnosis of primary aldosteronism has been demonstrated, it is important to distinguish between an aldosterone-producing adenoma and bilateral hyperplasia, as the former is treated with surgery and the latter is treated medically. The initial test, a postural challenge, involves testing a patient with adequate sodium intake (at least 4 days of more than 120 mEq/day) following an overnight bedrest. At 8:00 a.m., a supine blood sample is drawn for plasma aldosterone, 18-hydrocorticosterone, renin, and cortisol levels. The patient then stands for 2 hours, and at 10:00 a.m. an upright sample is drawn for the same hormones. A basal plasma aldosterone level of <8 ng/dl is usually found in normal individuals, a value between 8 and 20 ng/dl is usually found in patients with bilateral hyperplasia, and a value >20 ng/dl suggests the diagnosis of adrenal adenoma. After 2 hours in the upright posture, normal individuals will have a rise in renin and aldosterone but a decrease in cortisol because of the diminished influence of ACTH at 10:00 a.m., compared with at 8:00 a.m. Patients with bilateral hyperplasia are still sensitive to the same increases in renin that occur in the upright position and will have an increase in plasma aldosterone. Patients with an adenoma do not activate their renin system and usually have a fall in plasma aldosterone levels because of decreased stimulation by ACTH. An 8:00 a.m. plasma 18-hydroxycorticosterone level of >50 ng/dl, which falls with upright posture, occurs in most patients with an adenoma, while a level of <50 ng/dl, which rises with the upright posture, occurs in most patients with bilateral hyperplasia. These postural studies can usually confirm the diagnosis of primary aldosteronism and distinguish between an adrenal adenoma and bilateral hyperplasia. If these tests confirm the diagnosis of primary aldosteronism, a CT scan of the adrenal glands should be performed to localize the tumor. If a discrete adenoma is seen in one adrenal gland with a normal contralateral gland and biochemical tests consistent with an adenoma, the patient should undergo a unilateral adrenalectomy. However, patients with bilateral lesions on CT scan may in fact have only one functioning adenoma and would also benefit from surgery. Such patients who have biochemical studies consistent with an adenoma but CT results consistent with bilateral disease should undergo adrenal venous sampling for aldosterone and cortisol measurement. Patients with biochemical and localization studies consistent with bilateral hyperplasia should be treated medically, usually with spironolactone. Patients with biochemical studies consistent with bilateral hyperplasia should also be evaluated for dexamethasone-suppressible hyperaldosteronism by receiving a trial of dexamethasone, which will reverse the hyperaldosteronism in this rare autosomal dominant disorder.

Hyperaldosteronism secondary to activation of the renin-angiotensin system and hypertension can occur in patients with accelerated hypertension or renovascular hypertension, in those on estrogen therapy, and rarely, in patients with renin-secreting tumors. Hyperaldosteronism without hypertension occurs in patients with Bartter's syndrome, sodium-wasting nephropathy, or renal tubular acidosis and in patients abusing diuretic or laxatives.

ADRENAL MEDULLARY HYPERFUNCTION

The adrenal medulla synthesizes the catecholamines norepinephrine, epinephrine, and dopamine from the amino acid tyrosine. Norepinephrine, the major catecholamine produced by the adrenal medulla, has predominantly alpha-agonist actions, causing vasoconstriction. Epinephrine acts primarily on the beta receptors, having positive inotropic and chronotropic effects on the heart, causing peripheral vasodilation, and increasing plasma glucose concentrations in response to hypoglycemia. The action of circulating dopamine is currently unclear. Whereas norepinephrine is synthesized in the central nervous system and sympathetic postganglionic neurons, epinephrine is synthesized almost entirely in the adrenal medulla. The adrenal medullary contribution of norepinephrine secretion is relatively small. Bilateral adrenalectomy results in only minimal changes in circulating norepinephrine levels, although epinephrine levels are dramatically reduced. Thus, hypofunction of the adrenal medulla has little physiologic impact, whereas hypersecretion of catecholamines produces the clinical syndrome of pheochromocytoma.

Pheochromocytoma

Pathophysiology

Although pheochromocytomas can occur in any sympathetic ganglion in the body, more than 90% of pheochromocytomas arise from the adrenal medulla. The majority of extra-adrenal tumors occur in the mediastinum or abdomen. Bilateral adrenal pheochromocytomas occur in about 5% of the cases and may occur as part of familial syndromes. Pheochromocytoma occurs as part of multiple endocrine neoplasia (MEN) type 2A or 2B syndromes. The former (Sipple's syndrome) is marked by medullary carcinoma of the thyroid, hyperparathyroidism, and pheochromocytoma, while the latter is characterized by medullary carcinoma of the thyroid, mucosal neuromas, intestinal ganglioneuromas, marfanoid habitus, and pheochromocytoma. Pheochromocytomas are also associated with neurofibromatosis, cerebelloretinal hemangioblastosis (von Hippel-Lindau syndrome) and tuberous sclerosis.

Clinical Manifestations

Since the majority of pheochromocytomas secrete norepinephrine as the principal catecholamine, hypertension is the most common finding. Such hypertension is sometimes paroxysmal and may be associated with other symptoms, of which the most common is the triad of headache, palpitations, and sweating. Other symptoms may include flushing, anxiety, nausea, fatigue, weight loss, and abdominal and chest pain. These paroxysms may be precipitated by emotional stress, exercise, anesthesia, abdominal pressure, or intake of tyramine-containing foods. Some patients have orthostatic hypotension, which may be due to release of epinephrine and/or dopamine from the tumor. Wide fluctuations in blood pressure often occur, and the hypertension associated with pheochromocytoma usually does not respond to standard antihypertensive medicines.

Diagnosis and Treatment

The diagnosis of pheochromocytoma is made by demonstrating elevated urinary excretion of catecholamines or their metabolites, the metanephrines, and vanillylmandelic acid (VMA) during a period of hypertension. Measurement of urinary metanephrine levels is probably the single best test, but usually urinary total catecholamines, epinephrine, norepinephrine, and VMA are also measured. Measurement of plasma catecholamines may also be useful. The blood sample must be drawn when the patient is hypertensive and supine and must be obtained from an indwelling catheter to avoid the stress of venipuncture. A plasma norepinephrine level of >1500 pg/ml or an epinephrine level of >500 pg/ml is consistent with the diagnosis of a pheochromocytoma. If the values are borderline elevated, a clonidine suppression test should be performed. In this test, chlonidine (0.3 mg/kd) is given orally, and plasma catecholamines are measured before and 3 hours after administration. Normal individuals have a decrease in catecholamine levels into the normal range, while patients with a pheochromocytoma have unchanged or increased levels. Once the diagnosis of pheochromocytoma is made, a CT scan of the adrenals should be performed. Most intra-adrenal pheochromocytomas are readily visible on this scan. If the CT scan findings are negative, extra-adrenal pheochromocytomas can often be localized by ^{131}I-metaiodobenzylguanidine (MIBG) scan, radiolabelled octreotide scan, or abdominal MRI.

The treatment of pheochromocytoma is surgical if the lesion can be localized. Patients should undergo preoperative alpha blockade to improve surgical morbidity and mortality. Phenoxybenzamine and alpha-methyl-p-tyrosine (an inhibitor of tyrosine hydroxylase, the rate-limiting enzyme in catecholamine biosynthesis) should be given for 1 to 2 weeks prior to surgery. Beta-adrenergic antagonists should be used during the operation if the lesion secretes epinephrine. After surgery, large volumes of saline are often needed to maintain blood pressure. Approximately 5 to 10% of pheochromocytomas are malignant. Patients with malignant pheochromocytomas usually have a poor prognosis. ^{131}I-MIBG or chemotherapy may be useful. Alpha-methyl-p-tyrosine may be used to decrease catecholamine secretion from the tumor.

REFERENCES

Chrousos GP: The hypothalamic-pituitary-adrenal axis and immune-mediated inflammation. N Engl J Med 1995; 332:1351–1362.

Flack MR, Oldfield EH, Cutler GB Jr, Zweig MH, Malley JD, Chrousos GP, Loriaux DL, Nieman LK: Urine free cortisol in the high-dose dexamethasone suppression test for the differential diagnosis of the Cushing syndrome. Ann Intern Med 1992; 116:211–217.

Oldfield EH, Doppman JL, Nieman LK, Chrousos GP, Miller DL, Katz DA, Cutler GB Jr, Loriaux DL: Petrosal sinus sampling with and without corticotropin-releasing hormone for the differential diagnosis of Cushing's syndrome. N Engl J Med 1991; 325:897–905.

Tyrrell JB, Baxter JD: Disorders of the adrenal cortex. In Bennett JC, Plum F (eds.): Cecil Textbook of Medicine. 20th ed. Philadelphia, WB Saunders, 1996.

Young WF Jr, Hogan MJ, Klee GG, Grant CS, van Heerden JA: Primary aldosteronism: Diagnosis and treatment. Mayo Clin Proc 1990; 65:96–110.

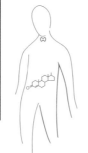

68

Female Reproductive Endocrinology

NORMAL SEXUAL DEVELOPMENT

In contrast to the testes, the ovary during fetal development does not actively participate in sexual differentiation. In the presence of an ovary or in the absence of a gonad, müllerian duct structures will develop, giving rise to the fallopian tubes, the uterus, and upper third of the vagina, and the external genitalia will remain open, resulting in the presence of labia, a vagina, and a urethral orifice in the perineum.

During childhood, the ovaries secrete small quantities of estradiol that are sufficient to suppress the release of the pituitary gonadotropins, follicle-stimulating hormone (FSH), and luteinizing hormone (LH). The normal time for onset of pubertal development is between ages 8 and 13 years. The initial event appears to be a decrease in the sensitivity of the hypothalamus to feedback inhibition by estrogens. As the hypothalamus becomes less sensitive, increasing quantities of gonadotropin-releasing hormone (GnRH) are secreted, which results in rising concentrations of the pituitary gonadotropins, FSH initially, and LH later. The increased circulating FSH concentrations stimulate the ovaries to secrete more estrogens. The estrogens are responsible for development of the secondary sexual structures including the breasts, labia minora and majora, vaginal mucosa, and uterine enlargement. Together with adrenal androgens, ovarian androgen production brings about development of axillary and pubic hair. The pubertal growth spurt is also a reflection of the action of sex steroid hormones on the epiphyseal plates of the long bones. Menarche, the onset of uterine bleeding, is a relatively late event in the pubertal process, occurring at an average age of 12.8 years in the United States. During the first year after menarche, the majority of menstrual cycles are anovulatory and reflect shedding of the uterine lining that has been built up under the stimulation of ovarian estrogen.

Normal, ovulatory menstrual cycles require the coordination of the hypothalamus, pituitary, and ovaries as well as the presence of an intact uterus and open vagina to allow egress of blood. The menstrual cycle is divided into two phases (Fig. 68–1). The follicular, or proliferative, phase begins with the first day of menstrual bleeding, which is termed day 1 of the cycle, and continues until ovulation occurs at approximately day 14 of a normal 28-day cycle. The period following ovulation until the onset of new menstrual bleeding represents the luteal, or secretory, phase and also averages 14 days in length. During the first half of the follicular phase, the pituitary gonadotrophs secrete increasing quantities of FSH, which in turn stimulates the ovarian follicles to secrete estradiol. During the second half of the follicular phase, the increasing concentrations of estradiol feed back in a negative fashion on the pituitary to decrease the secretion of FSH. The concentrations of LH rise gradually during the follicular phase. The follicular phase estrogen levels bring about proliferation of the lining of the endometrium and decrease the viscosity and increase the quantity of cervical mucus. FSH stimulates the development of several oocytes within primordial follicles. However, most of the follicles become atretic and disintegrate; generally only one follicle undergoes full development to become the preovulatory or graafian follicle. When the estradiol levels reach a certain concentration, there is a positive feedback effect at the level of the hypothalamus and pituitary, resulting in a surge in gonadotropins with an acute elevation of both FSH and LH. This brings about ovulation and the start of the luteal phase.

Following ovulation, the follicle is converted into the corpus luteum, which secretes both estradiol and progesterone. These hormones stimulate endometrial glandular secretion and prepare the endometrium for implantation of the blastocyst should conception occur. If fertilization does not take place, the corpus luteum regresses, the estrogen and progesterone levels decline, and the lining of the uterus sloughs, marking the beginning of a new menstrual cycle. Ovulatory menstrual cycles continue until the menopause, unless pregnancy, functional abnormalities, or a disease state intervenes.

PRECOCIOUS PUBERTY

Growth of the breasts and uterus, increased vaginal secretions, and increased growth velocity with or without the appearance of axillary or pubic hair before the age of 8 years constitute precocious puberty. This should be differentiated from premature thelarche, which refers to isolated breast enlargement, and premature adrenarche, which refers to the isolated development of axillary and

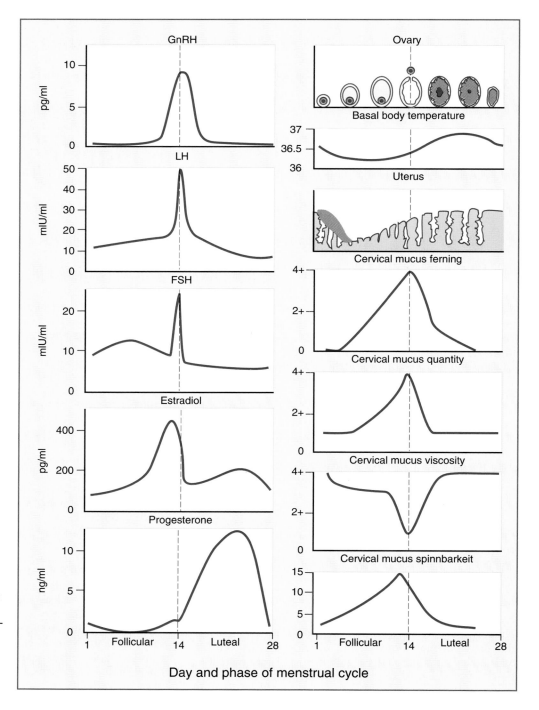

Figure 68-1
Schematic representation of the normal menstrual cycle. FSH = Follicle-stimulating hormone; GnRH = gonadotropin-releasing hormone; LH = luteinizing hormone. (From Braunstein GD: Female reproductive disorders. *In* Hershman JM (ed.): Endocrine Pathophysiology: A Patient-Oriented Approach. Philadelphia, Lea & Febiger, 1988, p 153.)

pubic hair without other signs of puberty due to a mild increase in the secretion of adrenal androgens. Complete or true precocious puberty in which all pubertal manifestations are present reflects premature activation of the hypothalamic-pituitary-ovarian axis. This may occur from structural central nervous system disorders such as a hypothalamic glioma or a GnRH-secreting hamartoma. In the majority of girls with precocious puberty, no structural lesions are identified and the condition is considered to be idiopathic. Primary hypothyroidism is a rare cause of precocious puberty and galactorrhea. Another etiology is the McCune-Albright syndrome, which also includes

fibrous dysplasia of the long bones and multiple café-au-lait spots. Incomplete isosexual precocious puberty refers to the appearance of an excessive estrogen effect from exogenous estrogen exposure, ovarian follicular cysts, or granulosa cell tumors of the ovary. Virilization reflecting excessive androgen effects is found in girls with congenital adrenal hyperplasia or androgen-secreting adrenal or ovarian neoplasms and is referred to as heterosexual precocity.

A careful history should be obtained to evaluate the possibility of environmental exposure to exogenous estrogens, and a detailed neurologic examination and search for the presence of café-au-lait spots or neurofibromas are necessary. The initial evaluation of isosexual precocious puberty should include measurements of LH and estradiol. If both are elevated for the patient's age, then precocious puberty is due to early activation of the hypothalamic-pituitary-ovarian axis. Magnetic resonance imaging of the hypothalamic-pituitary region is the procedure of choice to look for structural lesions. If the estradiol level is elevated but the LH is suppressed, a gonadotropin-independent cause of sexual precocity is present, and an evaluation of the ovaries through ultrasonography should be carried out, after the exogenous intake of estrogens has been eliminated from consideration. If there is evidence of virilization, then measurements of serum testosterone and dehydroepiandrosterone-sulfate (DHEAS) should be measured. DHEAS is a weak androgen, 95% of which comes from the adrenal gland. If testosterone is elevated and DHEAS is normal or low, then ultrasonography of the ovaries may reveal an androgen-secreting ovarian tumor. Elevations of both DHEAS and testosterone require further evaluation for congenital adrenal hyperplasia with ACTH stimulation testing. If the latter is normal, then suppression of adrenal gland androgen secretion with dexamethasone is indicated. If DHEAS does not fall, radiographic assessment of the adrenal glands for an adrenal neoplasm should be performed by computed tomographic scanning.

Central precocious puberty may be treated with a long-acting analogue of GnRH, which brings about down-regulation of the GnRH receptors on the gonadotrophs in the anterior pituitary, leading to a lowering of gonadotropin concentrations. Effective treatment of the cause of incomplete sexual precocity will cause regression of the pubertal changes.

AMENORRHEA

Primary amenorrhea is defined by an absence of menses in a phenotypic female by age 16 years, while secondary amenorrhea indicates an absence of menses for 3 or more months in a previously menstruating woman.

Primary Amenorrhea

A convenient way to categorize the causes of primary amenorrhea is by site of the lesion (Table 68–1). Lower tract abnormalities involving the vagina or uterus are associated with amenorrhea, but patients exhibit normal secondary sexual development of the breasts and axillary and pubic hair because the hypothalamic-pituitary-ovarian axis and estrogen secretion are normal. These patients also may have cyclical symptoms including premenstrual breast enlargement, weight gain, and bloating, as well as a mid-cycle ovulation pain (mittelschmerz). If the uterus is present but the vagina is obstructed, then often the patient will have a monthly lower abdominal mass with pain, caused by the collection of menstrual blood behind the obstruction. Surgical correction of an imperforate hymen or an atretic vagina is curative. Defective development of müllerian duct structures is associated with ab-

TABLE 68–1	Causes of Primary Amenorrhea

Lower Tract Defects
Vaginal aplasia or atresia
Imperforate hymen
Uterine Disorders
Congenital absence of the uterus
Destruction of the endometrium
Gonadal Disorders
Gonadal dysgenesis*
17α-Hydroxylase deficiency*
Resistant ovary syndrome*
Polycystic ovary disease
Testicular feminization
Adrenal Disorders
Congenital adrenal hyperplasia
Thyroid Disorders
Hypothyroidism*
Pituitary-Hypothalamic Disorders
Hypopituitarism*
Prolactin-secreting pituitary tumor*
Nutritional or exercise-induced delay*
Constitutional delay*

* Associated with lack of incomplete secondary sexual development.

sence of the fallopian tubes, uterus, and upper third of the vagina, as well as abnormalities of the urinary tract, vertebrae, and heart. These patients and those who have had their endometrium destroyed through infection will also have normal sexual development and cyclic symptoms of ovulation.

The most common gonadal disorder causing primary amenorrhea is 45X gonadal dysgenesis, or Turner's syndrome. This syndrome, which occurs in 1 in every 3000 to 5000 female infants, is characterized by short stature, and multiple somatic anomalies including epicanthal folds, low-set ears, webbed neck, multiple pigmented nevi, lymphedema of the hands and feet, renal malformations, and coarctation of the aorta. Short stature, streak ovaries, which lack germinal tissue, and multiple somatic anomalies as well as other forms of gonadal dysgenesis, including XX and XY gonadal dysgenesis, are also associated with streak ovaries but not with the somatic abnormalities. In fact, such individuals tend to be tall because their long bones continue to grow under the influence of growth hormone without undergoing epiphyseal fusion, which requires gonadal steroids. Patients with the 17α-hydroxylase enzyme deficiency affecting both the ovaries and adrenals are unable to synthesize cortisol and estrogen but do synthesize excessive adrenal mineralocorticoids, leading to the combination of primary amenorrhea, lack of secondary sexual characteristics, and hypertension. Patients who lack a normal FSH receptor in ovarian follicles may have primary amenorrhea with poor secondary sexual development. In contrast to patients with gonadal dysgenesis, girls with the resistant ovary syndrome will have primordial follicles present in the ovaries.

Although testicular feminization is not a disorder affecting genetic females, males with this syndrome lack normal androgen receptors and therefore appear as pheno-

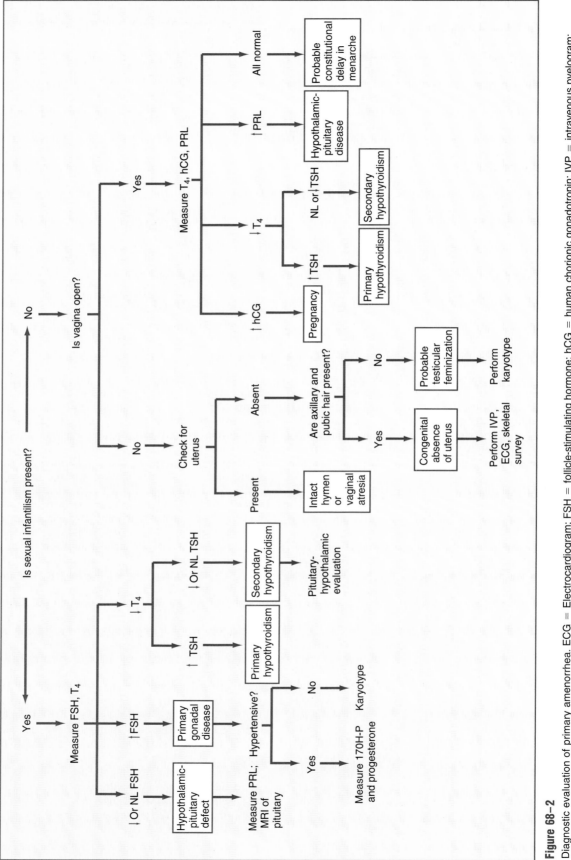

Figure 68-2

Diagnostic evaluation of primary amenorrhea. ECG = Electrocardiogram; FSH = follicle-stimulating hormone; hCG = human chorionic gonadotropin; IVP = intravenous pyelogram; MRI = magnetic resonance imaging; NL = normal; 17OH-P = 17α-hydroxyprogesterone; PRL = prolactin; T₄ = thyroxine; TSH = thyroid-stimulating hormone; ↓ = decreased, ↑ = increased.

typic females with primary amenorrhea and normal breast development; they lack pubic or axillary hair since the androgen receptors are absent in the hair follicles. Congenital adrenal hyperplasia, including deficiency of 21α-hydroxylase, 11β-hydroxylase, and 3β-hydroxysteroid dehydrogenase enzymes, may be associated with primary amenorrhea, hirsutism, and virilization. Severely affected girls with the 21α-hydroxylase and 11β-hydroxylase defects may present as female pseudohermaphrodites because of androgen-induced fusion of the labial-scrotal folds. Hypothyroidism during adolescence may result in sexual infantilism, as can hypopituitarism from structural abnormalities or lack of hypothalamic-releasing hormones. Prolactin-secreting pituitary tumors, although more commonly associated with secondary amenorrhea, may occur prepubertally and prevent normal gonadotropin release and function.

Primary amenorrhea may also occur in young women with anorexia nervosa or bulimia or who have had weight loss or malnourishment because of dieting. In each of these situations there is a functional hypothalamic defect that leads to an immaturity of the hypothalamus in regard to release of GnRH. Correction of the nutritional abnormality leads to the onset of pubertal development. Similarly, girls who exercise excessively and have little body fat may also have primary amenorrhea. This is commonly seen in ballerinas, gymnasts, and long-distance runners and remits when the amount of exercise is reduced and body fat increases. One of the most common causes of primary amenorrhea is constitutional delay in the onset of menses; this has a strong genetic component, with female relatives often giving a history of late onset of menstruation. These patients usually have some degree of pubertal development before age 16, but menses may be delayed for several years.

Once a history and physical examination rule out the presence of a systemic illness associated with weight loss that may lead to hypothalamic dysfunction, the algorithm presented in Figure 68–2 can be followed to derive the likely diagnosis in patients who do not have signs or symptoms of virilization. Therapy depends upon the underlying pathology. Because patients with long-standing estrogen deficiency develop osteopenia, estrogen replacement therapy should be given to those found to have primary hypogonadism and/or hypothalamic-pituitary disease. In the latter, ovulation induction through the use of gonadotropins can be achieved when pregnancy is desired. Primary amenorrhea associated with hypothyroidism responds to thyroid replacement.

Secondary Amenorrhea

Table 68–2 lists the various etiologies of secondary amenorrhea. Again, the problems can be classified according to the site of the lesion.

Pregnancy is the most common cause of secondary amenorrhea; it should be easily diagnosed by history and can be confirmed with one of the rapid, sensitive urine or serum pregnancy tests that measure human chorionic gonadotropin (hCG). A history of a uterine infection or prior surgical manipulation of the uterus may point to the

TABLE 68–2	Causes of Secondary Amenorrhea

Uterine Disorders

Pregnancy
Endometrial scarring
Endometrial atrophy

Ovarian Disorders

Premature menopause
   Chemotherapy or radiation
   Idiopathic or autoimmune
Ovarian tumors
Polycystic ovary disease

Adrenal Disorders

Late-onset congenital adrenal hyperplasia
Cushing syndrome
Virilizing adrenal tumors
Adrenocortical insufficiency

Thyroid Disorders

Hypothyroidism
Hyperthyroidism

Hypothalamic-Pituitary Disorders

Acquired hypopituitarism
Hyperprolactinemia
Drug suppression
Nutritional disorders

Extrahypothalamic Nervous System Disorders

presence of scarring involving the lining of the uterus, making it unresponsive to estrogen and progesterone. Atrophy of the lining of the uterus also may be found following prolonged administration of progestational agents such as the depot form of medroxyprogesterone acetate.

Chemotherapeutic drugs, especially alkylating agents used for treatment of malignancies, as well as pelvic irradiation, may lead to destruction of the ovarian follicles resulting in secondary amenorrhea. Premature ovarian failure with cessation of ovarian function in patients younger than 40 years may occur as an isolated phenomenon or as part of the polyglandular autoimmune failure syndrome associated with autoimmune thyroiditis, adrenal insufficiency, vitiligo, or diabetes mellitus. Premature ovarian failure is associated with menopausal symptoms including vasomotor instability and vaginal dryness. Ovarian tumors rarely cause amenorrhea unless they are androgen-secreting, which will lead to virilization in association with the amenorrhea. Estrogen-secreting ovarian tumors often will cause oligomenorrhea characterized by infrequent bleeding episodes with intramenstrual periods of greater than 35 days. The most common ovarian cause of secondary amenorrhea is the polycystic ovary syndrome. As originally described, this included the complex of obesity, oligo- or amenorrhea, hirsutism, and involuntary infertility associated with large ovaries containing multiple follicular cysts. It is now known that many individuals with polycystic ovaries may exhibit only menstrual dysfunction. These patients tend to have mild elevations of adrenal and ovarian androgens as well as an elevated LH : FSH ratio.

Overproduction of adrenal androgens may also be associated with secondary amenorrhea. Several forms of mild, attenuated or late-onset congenital adrenal hyperplasia have been noted. The most common lesion is a mild 21α-hydroxylase deficiency, which may present with primary or secondary amenorrhea with or without acne, hirsutism, or signs of virilization. Patients with Cushing syndrome and virilizing adrenal tumors may also develop secondary amenorrhea from adrenal androgen excess. Adrenal cortical insufficiency leads to a marked weight loss, which results in hypothalamic dysfunction and amenorrhea. Similarly, both hypothyroidism and hyperthyroidism, through changes in nutritional status as well as altered metabolism of sex steroid hormones, may be associated with menstrual disturbances; amenorrhea is most common in hyperthyroidism, and polymenorrhea (frequent periods with a cycle length of less than 21 days) is more common in hypothyroidism. With the exception of late-onset congenital adrenal hyperplasia, patients with underlying adrenal or thyroid disorders usually have sufficient manifestations of the underlying pathology to point toward the correct diagnosis.

A variety of pituitary and hypothalamic disorders may be associated with secondary amenorrhea. Pituitary destruction from infiltrative, infectious, vascular, immunologic, or neoplastic diseases may result in secondary amenorrhea, along with other signs and symptoms of trophic hormone deficiency. Hyperprolactinemia, whether drug-induced or due to a prolactin-secreting pituitary adenoma, is also associated with amenorrhea, with or without accompanying galactorrhea, as the elevated prolactin concentrations interfere with the normal cyclic release of gonadotropins. Primary eating disorders, as well as any systemic illness that leads to weight loss, are associated with hypothalamic dysfunction. Medications such as oral contraceptives or other drugs that elevate prolactin can suppress the hypothalamus and pituitary. Finally, there are situations in which hypothalamic dysfunction is a reflection of an underlying emotional stress or a psychiatric problem. Pseudocyesis, or false pregnancy, in which amenorrhea accompanies weight gain, breast enlargement and engorgement, and abdominal enlargement simulating pregnancy, is an example of how higher cortical areas can disrupt hypothalamic function.

The scheme presented in Figure 68–3 can be followed to elucidate the cause of secondary amenorrhea. In all patients, pregnancy must be ruled out; this can easily be accomplished through measurements of serum or urine hCG. A negative pregnancy test can be followed by administration of progesterone. Uterine bleeding occurring within the next 2 weeks indicates that there has been a sufficient amount of estrogen to build up the lining of the uterus, which was responsive to the estrogen. An absence of the bleeding may be due to severe estrogen deficiency or to a problem involving the endometrial lining. This can be differentiated by priming the lining of the uterus for 1 or 2 months with estrogen, followed by another progesterone withdrawal test. An absence of bleeding at that time indicates the presence of endometrial lining disorder; the patient should be referred to a gynecologist for direct examination of the endometrium. If bleeding does occur following the priming, then one can assume that the uterus is responsive and look for a disorder at another level. If the patient has had a marked weight loss, she should be evaluated for hyperthyroidism, adrenal insufficiency, nutritional disorder, or another systemic illness causing weight loss. In the absence of weight loss, the next question to address is whether the patient is hirsute or virilized. If she is not, then measurement of FSH and prolactin should be performed. An elevated FSH level indicates the presence of ovarian failure, while a normal or low FSH level, with or without an elevated prolactin level, indicates the presence of pituitary or hypothalamic disorder. If the patient is hirsute or virilized, then measurement of FSH, LH, testosterone, and DHEAS is appropriate to define whether the disorder lies within the ovaries or the adrenals.

The treatment of secondary amenorrhea depends upon the underlying condition. Patients with premature ovarian failure should be treated with estrogens for the vasomotor symptoms and vaginal dryness and to avoid osteopenia and coronary artery disease. Similarly, those with pituitary or hypothalamic dysfunction should receive estrogens unless a contraindication such as a prolactin-secreting pituitary tumor is present. Ovarian and adrenal neoplasms should be removed surgically; if malignant and persistent, they may be treated with inhibitors of androgen synthesis such as ketoconazole, or in the case of adrenal neoplasms, o-p'-DDD (mitotane). The treatment of polycystic ovary disease depends upon the manifestations. If amenorrhea is present, simple withdrawal with progesterone every 1 to 3 months is sufficient to bring about shedding of the lining of the uterus. Hirsutism and virilization may be treated with antiandrogens, glucocorticoids, or oral contraceptives. Fertility may be induced through the use of antiestrogens such as clomiphene citrate or direct stimulation of the ovaries with human menopausal gonadotropins.

HIRSUTISM

Hirsutism is inappropriate heavy hair growth in the androgen-sensitive areas of the body, such as the beard or mustache region. Virilization reflects hirsutism with progression to clitoral hypertrophy, deepening of the voice, temporal hair recession, and male pattern muscular development. The causes of hirsutism with and without virilization are listed in Table 68–3.

Approximately 10 to 15% of women have hirsutism, and the vast majority will have it on a familial basis or because of either polycystic ovary disease or idiopathic hirsutism. Patients with the familial variety generally have normal menses and no abnormalities in serum hormone concentrations. Patients with idiopathic hirsutism have either a mild increase in the production of testosterone from the ovaries or have increased sensitivity of the hair follicle to normal circulating levels of testosterone. Hirsutism is one of the common manifestations of polycystic ovary disease; a small percentage of such patients may also be virilized because of excessive production of an-

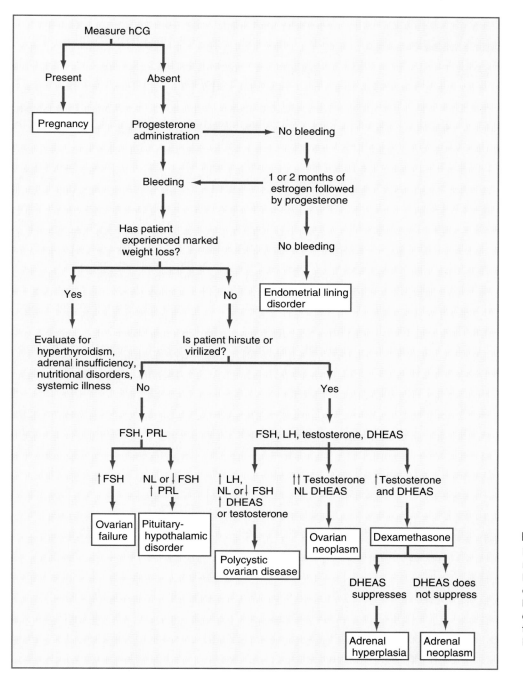

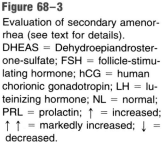

Figure 68–3

Evaluation of secondary amenorrhea (see text for details). DHEAS = Dehydroepiandrosterone-sulfate; FSH = follicle-stimulating hormone; hCG = human chorionic gonadotropin; LH = luteinizing hormone; NL = normal; PRL = prolactin; ↑ = increased; ↑ ↑ = markedly increased; ↓ = decreased.

drogens from both the ovary and adrenal glands. Hirsutism as the result of each of these three conditions has its onset in the perimenarchal age range, and the hirsutism is slowly progressive.

Late-onset congenital adrenal hyperplasia, especially mild 21α-hydroxylase deficiency, accounts for less than 5% of patients with hirsutism. The slight elevation of plasma ACTH in this syndrome leads to increased production of 17α-hydroxyprogesterone and adrenal androgens, which may be manifest by hirsutism, acne, and menstrual irregularities. The HAIR-AN syndrome refers to the clinical features of hyperandrogenism (HA), insulin resistance (IR), and acanthosis nigricans (AN). In this uncommon syndrome, the ovaries exhibit stromal hyperthecosis and follicular cysts, and the increased production of testosterone by the ovaries is a manifestation of the hyperinsulinism. Hirsutism may be a mild component of hypothyroidism and of growth hormone– or ACTH-secreting pituitary tumors. The underlying cause is generally apparent at the time that hirsutism is noted. Hirsutism with or without virilization is also seen in patients who use anabolic steroids and other medications with androgenic activity. Several drugs such as minoxidil and diazoxide may cause hypertrichosis, which is growth of a

TABLE 68–3	Causes of Hirsutism

Hirsutism Without Virilization

Normal individuals
  Familial
  Drug-induced
  Idiopathic
Pathologic conditions
  Ovarian disorders
    Polycystic ovary disease
    Hyperthecosis
    HAIR-AN syndrome
  Adrenal disorders
    Late-onset congenital adrenal hyperplasia
  Thyroid disorders
    Hypothyroidism
  Hypothalamic-pituitary disorders
    Acromegaly
    Cushing disease

Hirsutism With Virilization

Normal individuals
  Anabolic steroids
Pathologic conditions
  Ovarian disorders
    Polycystic ovary disease
    Virilizing ovarian tumors
  Adrenal disorders
    Congenital adrenal hyperplasia
    Adrenal carcinoma or adenoma

HAIR-AN = Hyperandrogenism, insulin resistance, and acanthosis nigricans.

downy type of hair that is more generalized than the hair growth seen in true hirsutism. Hypertrichosis also is found with starvation.

Hirsutism with virilization may occur in patients who are ingesting anabolic steroids and may also be present in individuals with polycystic ovary disease or congenital adrenal hyperplasia. A rapid onset of hirsutism and virilization raises the possibility of a virilizing ovarian or adrenal tumor.

The diagnostic evaluation should include a measurement of serum testosterone, DHEAS and 17α-hydroxyprogesterone (Fig. 68–4). Normal levels of all three hormones are compatible with idiopathic hirsutism or polycystic ovary disease. Further evaluation with measurements of LH and FSH will allow discrimination between the two. Normal or mildly elevated levels of testosterone, DHEAS, and 17α-hydroxyprogesterone are compatible with idiopathic hirsutism, polycystic ovary disease, or late onset congenital adrenal hyperplasia. A cortrosyn stimulation test with synthetic ACTH should be performed with measurements of 17α-hydroxyprogesterone, 17α-hydroxypregnenolone, DHEA, and 11-desoxycortisol to diagnose the different forms of congenital adrenal hyperplasia. Patients with marked elevations of serum testosterone but with normal levels of DHEAS or 17α-hydroxyprogesterone generally have an ovarian neoplasm or ovarian hyperthecosis, while those who have a slight increase in testosterone and marked elevations of DHEAS will have either an adrenal neoplasm or congenital adrenal hyperplasia. Differentiation of the latter two problems can be made through dexametha-

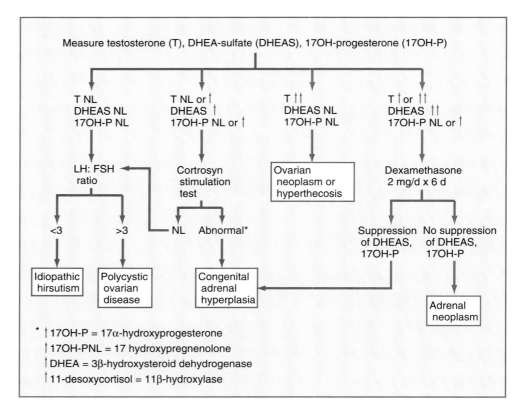

Figure 68–4

Laboratory evaluation of hirsutism (see text for details). DHEAS = dehydroepiandrosterone; NL = normal; 17OH-P = 17α-hydroxyprogesterone; ↑ = increased; ↑↑ = markedly increased.

sone suppression tests as well as cortrosyn stimulation testing.

Surgical removal of ovarian and adrenal neoplasms is the treatment of choice for those problems. Patients who are found to have late-onset congenital adrenal hyperplasia should be placed on glucocorticoids to suppress ACTH and thereby suppress adrenal androgen production. The treatment of the other causes of hirsutism consists of a combination of cosmetic and medical therapy. Cosmetic therapies include bleaching, which is good for sideburn hair, epilation through waxing, which is useful for body hair, depilation through shaving or topical creams, which are effective for excessive thigh and lower abdominal hair, and electrolysis, which is the only permanent form of hair removal.

Medical therapy consists of hormonal suppression with oral contraceptives, glucocorticoids, long-acting GnRH agonists, and ketoconazole, an antifungal agent that inhibits androgen production. Anti-androgens are also useful since they bind with the androgen receptor and displace the more potent androgens of ovarian and adrenal origin. In the United States, spironolactone and flutamide are the two most commonly used antiandrogens. 5α-reductase inhibitors, such as finasteride, are also useful for inhibiting hair growth, but the woman must use contraception because finasteride crosses the placenta and will inhibit labial-scrotal fold fusion in male fetuses should the woman conceive while taking the drug. Overall, the medical therapies are about 75% effective in reducing the rate of hair growth but generally do not cause all the pre-existing hairs to fall out. Since the hair turnover rate is relatively slow, patients should understand that a minimum of 3 to 6 months should elapse while on a medication to determine whether it is effective.

INFERTILITY

Of the 15% of couples who are infertile, approximately 40% are unable to conceive because of female factors, 40% because of male factors, and 20% from couple factors. Male factors include spermatogenic defects, obstruction of the tubal system transporting sperm from the testes to the urethra, retrograde ejaculation, medications, and immunologic abnormalities with antisperm antibodies. Common female factors include ovulatory problems with anovulation or oligo-ovulation, tubal disease, abnormalities affecting cervical mucus, and the presence of antisperm antibodies in the genital tract.

The initial evaluation of male factors consists of performance of a full semen analysis for sperm density, morphology, and motility. Ovulatory function is assessed through obtaining a history of the presumptive signs of ovulation such as premenstrual bloating, breast tenderness, menstrual cramps, and ovulatory pain (mittelschmerz) occurring 2 weeks before menses. Since progesterone slightly increases the core temperature, examining basal body temperature recordings for a sustained increase in temperature following ovulation may also provide good presumptive evidence of an ovulatory cycle. Finding an elevation of serum progesterone or endometrial biopsy results that show proliferative endometrium that is synchronous with the day of the menstrual cycle provides absolute evidence of ovulation. Cervical mucus is best assessed at mid-cycle around the time of ovulation when the quantity is the highest, viscosity lowest, and the spinnbarkeit (the ability of the cervical mucus to be stretched into a thin thread between two fingers or glass slides) is highest (see Fig. 68–1). A postcoital test in which the couple has intercourse within 2 hours before the examination of the cervical mucus also allows assessment of the number of spermatozoa present in the mucus and their motility. If the sperm are not motile, then the couple should be examined for the possibility of antisperm antibodies being present in either the male or female reproductive tracts. Fallopian tubal patency can be evaluated by hysterosalpingography, or at the time of laparoscopy, dye may be injected into the uterus and followed through the fallopian tubes. Laparoscopy is also useful in diagnosing endometriosis, which may cause infertility. If therapy directed at the underlying problem is unsuccessful, then one of the several types of assisted reproductive technologies such as *in vitro* fertilization, gamete intrafollicular transfer, or direct injection of sperm into ova may be tried.

DYSMENORRHEA

Colicky pelvic pain, nausea, vomiting, diarrhea, and headache just prior to and during menstruation characterize dysmenorrhea, which is due to prostaglandin-mediated uterine contractions. When severe, the woman may be totally disabled. Primary dysmenorrhea, in which no pathology is identified, generally responds to prostaglandin synthesis inhibitors such as indomethacin, ibuprofen, naproxen, or mefenamic acid. Secondary dysmenorrhea occurs in the presence of pelvic pathology, especially endometriosis. If prostaglandin synthesis inhibitors do not relieve the discomfort, then ovulation suppression through the use of oral contraceptives, GnRH agonists, or the androgenic progestogen danazol may be effective.

PREMENSTRUAL SYNDROME (PMS)

The premenstrual syndrome comprises physical symptoms such as weight gain, bloating, peripheral edema, headaches, and breast tenderness, as well as emotional symptoms including irritability, anxiety, depression, insomnia, fatigue, increased appetite, and inability to engage in social interactions. The syndrome is most commonly found during the late luteal phase just prior to menstruation, although it can begin at the time of ovulation and last throughout the luteal phase. The etiology is unknown and is probably multifactorial. Dysmenorrhea is also common with the syndrome. Therapy includes elimination of caffeine, alcohol, and salt as well as the use of the aldosterone-antagonist spironolactone for fluid retention or prostaglandin synthetase inhibitors for the dysmenorrhea and headaches. Inhibition of ovulation through the use of GnRH agonists with estrogen replacement therapy may also be helpful. Occasionally, antidepressant medication (e.g., fluoxetine) may provide symptomatic relief.

MENOPAUSE

The average age of menopause is 51 years, with 95% of American women having cessation of menses between the ages of 45 and 55 years. Although menses may abruptly cease, more commonly during the months to years prior to the menopause, episodes of irregular uterine bleeding occur as the result of a shortened follicular phase. Menopausal symptoms may actually begin prior to the cessation of menstruation. The most common vasomotor menopausal symptom is the hot flash or hot flush, which is a brief episode of cutaneous vasodilation with flushing and a sensation of warmth, with sweating involving the chest, neck, and face. The frequency of the episodes varies, but they may be severe and awaken the patient with drenching sweats so frequently that she develops chronic daytime somnolence and depression. Estrogen deficiency also leads to a decrease in vaginal secretions, resulting in vaginal dryness and dyspareunia, or painful intercourse. Long-term manifestations of estrogen deficiency include osteopenia and a rise in low-density lipoprotein, which may predispose the patient to heart disease. Estrogen administration ameliorates the vasomotor symptoms and vaginal dryness, decreases osteoclastic bone resorption (thereby decreasing the risk of osteoporotic bone fractures), and raises serum high-density lipoprotein levels, which decreases the risk of coronary artery disease. The risks of estrogen therapy include weight gain, increased incidence of gall stones and hypertension, bloating, and breast tenderness. If the patient has not undergone a hysterectomy, there is an increased risk of endometrial carcinoma; this risk may be mitigated by the co-administration or cyclic administration of a progesterone analogue. Because of the possibility of an increased risk for the occurrence of breast carcinoma in women taking estrogen replacement therapy, women on estrogens should have yearly breast examinations and mammograms.

REFERENCES

Franks S: Polycystic ovary syndrome. N Engl J Med 1995; 333:853.

Goldfien A, Monroe SE: Ovaries. *In* Greenspan FS, Baxter JD (eds.): Basic & Clinical Endocrinology. 4th ed. Norwalk, CT, Appleton & Lange, 1994, p 419.

Lobo RA: Treatment of the Postmenopausal Woman: Basic and Clinical Aspects. New York, Raven Press, 1994.

Redmond GP: Androgenic Disorders. New York, Raven Press, 1995.

Speroff L, Glass RH, Kase NG: Clinical Gynecologic Endocrinology and Infertility. 5th ed. Baltimore, Williams & Wilkins, 1994.

69

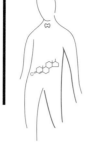

Cancer of the Breast, Cervix, Uterus, and Ovary

CANCER OF THE BREAST

Cancer of the breast is the most common malignancy in women in the United States. Approximately 182,000 women developed breast cancer in 1994, and more than 46,000 died of it. The lifetime risk of developing breast cancer is a staggering one in eight women. Although two thirds of cases occur after the menopause, 15% occur in women before the age of 40 years.

Etiology

The etiology of carcinoma of the breast is not known, but a number of risk factors are associated with it (Table 69–1).

Histologic Types

The most prevalent histologic types of breast cancer are infiltrating ductal carcinoma (80%), infiltrating lobular carcinoma (5 to 10%), and intraepithelial ductal carcinoma. The remainder represent various combinations of infiltrating ductal, mucinous, papillary, and lobular carcinomas. Ductal carcinoma is usually unilateral, while lobular carcinoma tends to be bilateral. Most breast cancers are adenocarcinomas, but occasionally medullary carcinoma (6%), mucinous, tubular, or squamous cell carcinoma, sarcomas, and Paget's disease occur.

Screening

Usually women detect their own breast cancers: all adult women should therefore be taught the importance and technique of self-examination of the breast. A breast examination by a physician should be performed on every woman over the age of 40. Mammography, an effective routine screening test, is recommended every 1 or 2 years for women aged 50 years or older, annually for women at any age with a personal history of breast cancer, and annually for women aged 40 and over who have a family history of breast cancer or other significant risk factors.

The smallest palpable mass is approximately 1 cm. Routine mammography can detect cancers less than 0.5

cm. The survival rate is significantly improved in women in whom cancer is detected by mammography, as opposed to palpation. The risk of frequent breast radiographs does not outweigh the potential benefits of screening, as the radiation dose is approximately one tenth of that used 20 years ago.

Clinical Presentation

The most common presentation of breast cancer is that of a painless, palpable breast mass in a postmenopausal woman. The more common signs and symptoms are listed in Table 69–2.

Diagnosis

It is often difficult to distinguish benign breast masses, such as fibroadenomas, lipomas, inflammatory masses, and cysts, from malignant ones, especially in premenopausal women. Definitive diagnosis requires histologic examination. A fine-needle aspiration (5% false-negative rate), a percutaneous needle biopsy, or an excisional or incisional biopsy is required for diagnosis. Mammography is helpful in examining the remainder of the breast, as well as the opposite breast, but is not universally diagnostic; 10% of cancers may not be detected with this technique. A biopsy should be done on a suspicious mass, even if the mammogram is negative. A mammogram may also be used to guide a biopsy when a mass is not palpable. An ultrasound study may detect and diagnose breast cysts and cancer.

Staging and Treatment

A chest radiograph is performed to assess the lungs, ribs, and spine for metastases. A bone scan is performed to rule out bone metastases; however, this is usually not necessary with small cancers. An abdominal computed tomography (CT) scan and liver function tests are also obtained to detect liver metastases. Occasionally, a serum carcinoembryonic antigen (CEA) level and/or a CA-15-3 level may be elevated. The presence or absence of estrogen and progesterone receptors in breast tumors should be

519

TABLE 69–1	Risk Factors for Cancer of the Breast

Increased Risk Factors

Increasing age
Familial history of breast carcinoma
First- and second-degree relatives with breast cancer (including relatives on the father's side), especially premenopausal cancer
Mutations in either BRCA1 or BRCA2 genes
Premalignant breast lesions (multiple papillomatosis, atypical hyperplasia)
Previous carcinoma in one breast, especially premenopausal
Early menstruation (<12 yr)
Late menopause (>52 yr)
Nulliparity
Radiation therapy to the chest
Family history of carcinoma of the ovary, uterus, or colon
Obesity (postmenopausal women)
Resident of North America or Europe
Possibly postmenopausal estrogen replacement therapy
Possibly high-fat diet or alcohol use

Lower Risk Factors

Term pregnancy under age 18 years
Early menopause
Castration before age 37 years
Asians residing in Asia

determined, as this may provide useful information concerning prognosis and subsequent hormone therapy.

The treatment of cancer of the breast is extremely complex and has changed rapidly over the years. Adverse prognostic factors include the presence of axillary node metastasis, high histologic grade, inflammatory carcinoma subtype, absence of estrogen receptors, and increased expression of oncogenes and epidermal growth factor receptors. Therapy is based on the histologic type, size, and location of the tumor, age of the woman, menopausal status, presence or absence of hormone receptors, preference of the patient, and experience of the physician (Table 69–3). Adjuvant combination chemotherapy and/or hormone therapy is usually recommended for women with positive axillary nodes. Postmenopausal women with metastatic disease who are hormone receptor positive are treated with various combinations or sequences of tamoxifen, progestin, and, occasionally, oophorectomy, adrenalectomy, and androgens. For those who are estrogen re-

TABLE 69–2	Symptoms and Signs of Breast Cancer

Early Disease

Palpable lump (75%)
Breast pain
Nipple discharge, retraction, or ulceration
Skin dimpling, edema, or erythema
Mass in the axilla
Scaling of the nipple

Advanced Disease

Fixation of the mass to the chest wall
Edema of the arm
Ulceration
Distant metastases to the lung, bone, liver, and brain
Weight loss (tumor cachexia)
Hypercalcemia

TABLE 69–3	Staging, Treatment, and Prognosis of Breast Cancer

Stage 0 (in situ carcinoma): 5-yr survival, over 95%
  a. Intraductal carcinoma in situ:
    Wide local excision, excisional biopsy with radiation therapy, or total mastectomy (with or without axillary node dissection)
  b. Lobular carcinoma in situ (commonly occurs bilaterally):
    No further treatment, unilateral or bilateral total mastectomy with or without low axillary lymph node dissection, or "lumpectomy" with radiation therapy

Stage I: Primary tumor <2 cm, negative axillary lymph nodes, and no distant metastases; 5-yr survival, 85%
    "Lumpectomy" or quadrantectomy, or modified radical or total mastectomy with axillary lymph node dissection

Stage IIA: Primary tumor <2 cm and positive axillary nodes, or primary lesion between 2 and 5 cm in diameter with negative nodes; 5-yr survival, 75%

Stage IIB: Tumor between 2 and 5 cm in diameter with positive nodes or a tumor >5 cm with negative nodes; 5-yr survival, 65%
    Modified radical mastectomy and axillary node dissection, or "lumpectomy" with axillary node dissection and postoperative radiation therapy

Stage IIIA: Primary tumor >5 cm with ipsilateral axillary node involvement or fixed lymph nodes; 5-yr survival, 50%
    Surgery, radiation, chemotherapy, hormone therapy in varying sequences

Stage IIIB: Internal mammary lymph nodes are involved; tumor extends to the chest wall and ulcerates the skin; 5-yr survival, 41%
    Surgery, radiation, chemotherapy, hormone therapy in varying sequences

Stage IV: Distant metastases; 5-yr survival, 10%
    Surgery, radiation, chemotherapy, hormone therapy in varying sequences

ceptor negative or who no longer respond to hormonal manipulation, combination chemotherapy is commonly given. Premenopausal women with positive axillary lymph nodes are also treated with adjuvant combination therapy. A number of different chemotherapeutic agents are used in varying dosages and combinations, including cyclophosphamide, doxorubicin, methotrexate, and 5-fluorouracil. Recently, taxol has been found to give a high response rate as initial therapy for metastatic breast cancer. Experimental high-dose chemotherapy with granulocyte colony-stimulating factor (G-CSF) or granulocyte-macrophage colony-stimulating factor (GM-CSF) or with autologous bone marrow transplantation is currently being studied.

CARCINOMA OF THE CERVIX

Carcinoma of the cervix accounts for 2.5% of all malignancies of women in the United States. Approximately 15,800 cases are diagnosed each year, and in 1995, 4800 women died from the disease. In addition, many more women have preinvasive cervical carcinoma, known as cervical intraepithelial neoplasia. Since the advent of cervical and vaginal cytology in the early 1940s, the incidence and mortality from invasive carcinoma of the cervix have been decreasing.

TABLE 69–4	Risk Factors for Carcinoma of the Cervix

Immunosuppression
History of genital warts
History of genital herpes
Multiple sexual partners
Partner with penile warts, dysplasia, or cancer
Low socioeconomic status
Intercourse before age 17 years
Early pregnancy
Cigarette smoking
Multiple pregnancies
In utero diethylstilbesterol exposure

Etiology and Risk Factors

Intraepithelial neoplasia and invasive carcinoma of the cervix are venereal in origin. A genital human papillomavirus (HPV) is either the cause of or a strong cofactor in the development of warts, intraepithelial neoplasia, or invasive carcinoma. Approximately 90 to 95% of squamous cell carcinomas of the cervix contain HPV DNA. Although more than 60 types of HPV infect humans, some are more commonly associated with lower genital tract neoplasia. Types 6 and 11 are believed to have a more benign behavior, while types 16, 18, 31, 33, and 35 result in higher-grade intraepithelial neoplasia and carcinomas. HPV is also thought to be responsible for adenocarcinoma of the cervix, as well as intraepithelial and invasive squamous cell carcinoma of the vagina and the vulva. Other risk factors are listed in Table 69–4.

Classification

Ninety per cent of all cervical carcinomas are squamous cell. Approximately 5 to 9% are adenocarcinomas, of which the majority are of endocervical cell type. Small cell carcinoma and sarcomas may occur but are rare.

Clinical Presentation

Almost all cases of intraepithelial neoplasia and many cases of early invasive cervical cancer are asymptomatic and are detected by a Papanicolaou (Pap) smear. Abnormal vaginal bleeding, vaginal discharge, bleeding after intercourse, and pelvic pain may result from an invasive malignancy. Advanced disease due to local extension or metastases is associated with severe chronic pelvic, low back, or leg pain; leg edema; a chronic cough; or weight loss.

Diagnosis

All women with an abnormal Pap smear or a suspicious cervical lesion should undergo a colposcopy-directed biopsy of the cervix. A cervical conization is required when colposcopy is unable to determine whether the lesion is intraepithelial. A careful pelvic and rectal examination to detect local extension is important for clinical staging. Liver function tests, a serum creatinine level, a serum squamous cell carcinoma antigen level, and a CEA level may also be useful. Squamous cell carcinoma antigen is elevated in 50% of women with invasive squamous cell carcinoma of the cervix, while CEA is elevated in approximately 10 to 20%. A chest radiograph and a magnetic resonance imaging (MRI) scan of the pelvis and abdomen are usually obtained. Cystoscopy and sigmoidoscopy are important in women with advanced disease.

Staging, Treatment, and Prognosis

These data are presented in Table 69–5.

Follow-up

A Pap smear and a careful physical examination should be done every 3 months for the first 2 years, and then every 6 months from years 3 to 5. Routine radiographic studies are not warranted in the absence of symptoms. Elevated levels of CEA or squamous cell carcinoma antigen can be followed serially in women with these laboratory abnormalities.

Symptoms of recurrent cervical cancer include vaginal bleeding or discharge; pelvic, back, or leg pain; leg edema; chronic cough; and weight loss. Central pelvic recurrences can be treated with radiation therapy if not given previously, or with pelvic exenteration if indicated. Distant metastases are treated with combination chemotherapy.

CANCER OF THE UTERUS

Endometrial carcinoma is the fourth most common cancer of women, accounting for 13% of all malignancies. Approximately 34,000 cases of endometrial carcinoma are diagnosed each year in the United States. The incidence of this tumor has decreased each year since 1975, however, and the death rate has declined since 1950. Since this cancer is usually diagnosed at an early stage, the cure rate is excellent, with an overall 5-year survival of 83%.

Risk Factors

Uterine cancer and its precursor, endometrial hyperplasia, occur most commonly in postmenopausal women. Women who undergo menopause after the age of 52 years are 2.5 times more likely to develop uterine cancer. Obesity greater than 50 pounds over ideal body weight increases the risk 10-fold, and previous pelvic radiation therapy (usually for cervical carcinoma) increases the risk 8-fold. Women who are on unopposed estrogen replacement therapy have a 3- to 7-fold increased risk of developing uterine cancer. On the other hand, oral contraception that includes progestins decreases the risk of developing endometrial cancer. Women who do not ovu-

TABLE 69–5	Staging, Therapy, and Prognosis for Carcinoma of the Cervix

Stage 0: Cervical intraepithelial neoplasia III
  a. Squamous cell carcinoma *in situ:* 5-yr survival, 100%
     Cryotherapy, laser vaporization, loop electrocautery, cone biopsy, or hysterectomy
  b. Adenocarcinoma *in situ:* 5-yr survival rate, 100%
     Conization for diagnosis (may be curative); hysterectomy

Stage IA1: Cancer involves the cervix with only minimal microscopic invasion; 5-yr survival, 100%
     Cone biopsy; hysterectomy

Stage IA2: Cervical stromal invasion <5 mm and <7 mm wide; 5-yr survival, 100%
     Depth of invasion <3 mm and no vascular space involvement—cone biopsy, abdominal hysterectomy; invasion >3 mm or vascular space involvement is treated like stage IB cancer

Stage IB: Cancer greater than stage IA2 confined to the cervix; 5-yr survival, 80–90%
     Radical abdominal hysterectomy with bilateral pelvic lymphadenectomy, or whole-pelvis external beam radiation therapy and intracavitary cesium

Stage IIA: Carcinoma extends into the vagina but not the lower third; 5-yr survival rate, 75–80%
     Radical abdominal hysterectomy or bilateral pelvic lymphadenectomy, or whole-pelvis external beam radiation therapy and intracavitary cesium

Stage IIB: Parametrial involvement but not to the pelvic side wall; 5-yr survival rate, 66–80%
     Whole-pelvis external beam radiation therapy followed by two intracavitary cesium insertions

Stage IIIA: Disease involving the lower third of the vagina; 5-yr survival rate, 50–60%
     Whole-pelvis external beam radiation therapy followed by two intracavitary cesium insertions

Stage IIIB: Extension to the pelvic side walls or obstruction of one or both ureters or a nonfunctioning kidney; 5-yr survival rate, 30–40%
     Whole-pelvis external beam radiation therapy followed by two intracavitary cesium insertions or interstitial iridium radiation

Stage IVA: Carcinoma involves the bladder or rectal mucosa; 5-yr survival rate, <20%
     Whole-pelvis external radiation therapy followed by two intracavitary cesium insertions or interstitial iridium radiation, or pelvic exenteration

Stage IVB: Distant metastases
     Palliation with radiation therapy to relieve symptoms and/or combination chemotherapy, including various doses and combinations of cisplatin, etoposide, bleomycin, mitomycin-C, 5-fluorouracil, carboplatin, and ifosfamide

late, secondary to polycystic ovaries, or who have not had children have a slightly increased risk, as do women with hypertension or diabetes.

Classification

Adenocarcinoma accounts for 60% of all endometrial carcinomas. Adenoacanthoma (adenocarcinomas associated with benign squamous metaplasia) accounts for approximately 20% of cases. Adenosquamous carcinoma, papillary adenocarcinoma, and uterine sarcoma also occur.

Clinical Presentation

More than 90% of women who have uterine cancer have a history of abnormal uterine bleeding. Postmenopausal bleeding, even if only staining or spotting, should be evaluated promptly. Advanced cases are associated with pelvic, back, and leg pain; increased frequency of urination; and weight loss. Advanced endometrial carcinoma can also manifest with symptoms similar to those of ovarian carcinoma, as it may spread within the abdominal cavity. Approximately 5% of women with cancer of the uterus are asymptomatic.

Diagnosis

A careful pelvic and abdominal evaluation, as well as an examination of groin and supraclavicular nodes, should be performed. All women with abnormal uterine bleeding should undergo an office endometrial biopsy or a dilation and curettage. A Pap smear is only occasionally diagnostic. A significant number of women with endometrial adenocarcinoma have an elevated serum CA-125.

Staging and Prognosis

Cancer of the uterus is surgically staged. Between 70 and 80% of all endometrial cancers are stage 1. The grade of the malignancy (well-differentiated, moderately differentiated, and poorly differentiated) is also part of the staging system (Table 69–6).

Treatment

Standard therapy for uterine cancer is an abdominal hysterectomy, bilateral salpingo-oophorectomy, cytologic ex-

TABLE 69–6	Staging of Uterine Cancer	
Stage	**Description**	**5-Yr Survival (%)**
IA	Cancer confined to the endometrium	95
IB	Tumor invades the myometrium, but <50%	80
IC	Tumor invades the uterine wall by more than half its thickness	70
IIA	Endocervical gland involvement	65
IIB	The cancer involves the cervical stroma	60
IIIA	Involvement of the surface of the uterus and/or fallopian tubes and/or positive peritoneal cytology	Up to 30
IIIB	Vaginal metastasis	30
IIIC	Metastasis to the pelvic and/or peri-aortic lymph nodes	30
IVA	The tumor involves the bladder or rectal mucosa	10
IVB	Distant metastases, intra-abdominal spread, or groin node metastases	5

amination of the peritoneal fluid and selective pelvic and aortic lymph node sampling. Most gynecologic oncologists measure estrogen and progesterone receptors from the tumor to guide subsequent hormone therapy if the tumor should recur. Postoperative pelvic radiation therapy is usually given to those with an increased risk of recurrent disease, such as a higher-grade lesion or a deeply invasive cancer. Progestational agents, such as megastrol acetate, or combination chemotherapy is given to women with advanced disease. Active drugs include cisplatin, carboplatin, doxorubicin, cyclophosphamide, mitoxantrone, and ifosfamide.

Follow-up and Recurrent Disease

A careful pelvic examination and Pap smear should be performed every 3 months for the first 2 years after treatment. Other diagnostic studies should be performed only in the presence of signs or symptoms. Recurrences confined to the central pelvis are managed with a pelvic exenteration, with reported 5-year survival rates of 40 to 50%. Recurrent cancer of the uterus outside the central pelvis is usually treated with hormone therapy or combination chemotherapy.

OVARIAN CARCINOMA

Carcinoma of the ovary is the eighth most common malignancy in women. Approximately 1 in every 70 women develops cancer of the ovary, and 1 in 100 dies of it. Approximately 24,000 cases of ovarian cancer are diagnosed in the United States each year, resulting in approximately 13,600 deaths.

Risk Factors

The incidence of epithelial carcinoma of the ovary is increased slightly in nulliparous women and in those who have a late menopause or a history of pelvic radiation therapy or a high-fat diet. Women who are of North American or northern European descent or have a personal history of endometrial, colon, or breast cancer are at higher risk, whereas the use of oral contraceptives, more than one full-term pregnancy, and breast feeding appear to decrease the risk of developing ovarian cancer. In some families, there is a hereditary predisposition.

Histologic Classification

Ninety per cent of malignant ovarian tumors are epithelial in origin; in decreasing frequency, these are serous, mucinous, endometrioid, clear cell, and undifferentiated carcinoma. Clear cell carcinoma and undifferentiated carcinoma have poorer prognoses than do the other epithelial cell types. Epithelial cancers are also graded—well-differentiated, intermediately differentiated, or poorly differentiated tumors. Approximately 40% are tumors of low

malignant potential or borderline tumors; these grow extremely slowly with an excellent prognosis. Approximately 5% of the cancers are germ cell tumors and occur in premenopausal women. Approximately 5% of cancers arise from the gonadal stroma (granulosa, theca, and Sertoli-Leydig cells).

Clinical Presentation

Unfortunately, three quarters of all women with epithelial ovarian carcinoma have advanced disease at the time of diagnosis. The diagnosis is frequently delayed because early symptoms tend to be nonspecific—vague pelvic or abdominal pain or fullness, indigestion, bloating, early satiety, or altered bowel habits. Advanced carcinoma often manifests with ascites or intestinal obstruction. Occasionally, women with early-stage disease are asymptomatic and are found to have an adnexal or pelvic mass on a routine physical examination. Gonadal stromal tumors can secrete estrogen or testosterone, which may result in abnormal uterine bleeding, precocious puberty, or virilization. Ovarian carcinoma may also be associated with a variety of paraneoplastic manifestations, including cerebellar degeneration, hypercalcemia, seborrheic keratosis, or disseminated intravascular coagulation.

Screening, Diagnosis, and Staging

The utility of an abdominal or vaginal ultrasound examination and measurement of the serum CA-125 level for routine screening is currently being studied, especially for those women at increased risk of developing ovarian carcinoma. A palpable ovary in a postmenopausal woman may suggest ovarian cancer, since normal ovaries often cannot be palpated. If enlarged ovaries or a pelvic mass is present, pelvic ultrasonography may help delineate the pathology. The pelvis, abdomen, chest, and peripheral lymph nodes should be carefully examined. Preoperative studies should include measurement of the serum CA-125, liver function tests, a chest radiograph, abdominal CT scan, and, if symptoms warrant, an upper gastrointestinal series, barium enema, or colonoscopy. Cancer of the ovary is surgically staged (Table 69–7).

Therapy

The mainstay of therapy is surgical resection, including a total abdominal hysterectomy, bilateral salpingo-oophorectomy, omentectomy, and selective pelvic and periaortic lymph node sampling. Unilateral salpingo-oophorectomy may suffice in premenopausal women with either a low-grade malignancy or a germ cell tumor. For women with advanced disease, aggressive surgical debulking is performed in an attempt to remove as much diseased tissue as possible. Combination multiagent chemotherapy is given postoperatively. Drugs active in ovarian carcinoma include cisplatin, carboplatin, cyclophosphamide, doxorubicin, etoposide, ifosfamide, hexamethylmelamine, mel-

TABLE 69-7	Staging and Survival Rates of Ovarian Cancer

Stage	Description
IA	Cancer is confined to the ovary; no ascites or tumor on the ovarian surface, and the capsule is unruptured; 5-yr survival rate for low-grade tumors, 91–98%; for high grade, 80%
IB	Cancer is confined to both ovaries; no ascites or tumor on the ovarian surface, and the capsule is unruptured; 5-yr survival rate for low-grade tumors, 91–98%; for high grade, 80%
IC	The cancer is either stage IA or IB, and there is tumor on the ovarian surface, the capsule has ruptured, ascites present, or the peritoneal cytology is positive; 5-yr survival rate, 60–100%
IIA	Cancer extends to the uterus and/or fallopian tubes
IIB	Cancer extends to the other pelvic organs
IIC	The cancer is either stage IIA or IIB, and there is tumor on the surface of one or both ovaries, the tumor has ruptured, ascites present, or the peritoneal cytology is positive; 5-yr survival rate, 40–60%
IIIA	The tumor is grossly limited to the pelvis with microscopic cancer on the abdominal tumor implants; the pelvic and periaortic nodes are histologically negative
IIIB	The tumor involves one or both ovaries, and there are tumor implants on the abdominal peritoneal surfaces <2 cm in diameter; the pelvic and periaortic lymph nodes are negative
IIIC	The tumor involves one or both ovaries, and there are tumor implants on the abdominal peritoneal surfaces >2 cm in diameter, or there are positive pelvic, periaortic or groin lymph nodes; 5-yr survival rate, 20–40%
IV	There are metastases to the liver or lung parenchyma, or there is a pleural effusion with cytologically positive fluid; 5-yr survival rate, 5%

phalan, and 5-fluorouracil (5-FU). Increasingly, taxol is being used in refractory disease. Open-field whole-abdomen radiation therapy or intra-abdominal radioactive phosphorus (^{32}P) may be used in early-stage disease or in women with minimal residual disease after surgery. Intraperitoneal chemotherapy is sometimes effective in carcinoma of the ovary. Good prognostic factors include young age, early stage, low histologic grade, low residual tumor volume, and rapid rate of tumor response.

REFERENCES

Cannistra SA: Cancer of the ovary. N Engl J Med 1993; 329:1550.

Cannistra SA, Niloff JM: Cancer of the uterine cervix. N Engl J Med 1996; 334:1030.

Harris JR, Lippman ME, Veronesi U, Willett W: Medical progress: Breast cancer. N Engl J Med 1992; 327:319, 390, 473.

Lewis BJ: Breast carcinoma. *In* Wyngaarden JB, Smith LH Jr, Bennett JC (eds.): Cecil Textbook of Medicine. 19th ed. Philadelphia, WB Saunders, 1992, pp 1381–1386.

Lippman ME, Lichter AS, Danforth DN Jr (eds.): Diagnosis and Management of Breast Cancer. Philadelphia, WB Saunders, 1988.

Merchant DJ (ed.): Contemporary management of breast disease II: Breast cancer. Obstet Gynecol Clin North Am 1994; 21:555.

NIH Consensus Conference: Ovarian cancer. Screening, treatment, and follow-up. JAMA 1995; 273:491.

Partridge EE: Endometrial cancer. Changing concepts in therapy. Surg Clin North Am 1991; 71:991.

70

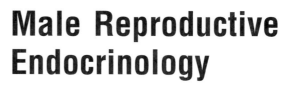

Male Reproductive Endocrinology

The testes are dual endocrine organs composed of Leydig or interstitial cells that secrete testosterone and estradiol and the sperm-producing seminiferous tubules, which occupy 80 to 90% of the testes. The testes are regulated by the gonadotropins, luteinizing hormone (LH) and follicle-stimulating hormone (FSH), secreted by the anterior pituitary under the influence of the hypothalamic decapeptide, gonadotropin-releasing hormone (GnRH) (Fig. 70–1). LH stimulates the Leydig cells to secrete testosterone, which feeds back in a negative fashion at the level of the pituitary and hypothalamus to inhibit further LH production. FSH stimulates sperm production through interaction with the Sertoli cells in the seminiferous tubules. Feedback inhibition of FSH is through gonadal steroids as well as through inhibin, a glycoprotein produced by Sertoli cells.

Biochemical evaluation of the hypothalamic-pituitary-Leydig axis is carried out by measurement of serum LH and testosterone concentrations, while a semen analysis and serum FSH determination will provide an assessment of the hypothalamic-pituitary-seminiferous tubular axis. Normal semen should have a volume of 2 to 5 ml and a sperm concentration $>20 \times 10^6$/ml. The ability of the pituitary to release gonadotropins can be dynamically tested through GnRH stimulation, and the ability of the testes to secrete testosterone can be evaluated through injections of human chorionic gonadotropin (hCG), a glycoprotein hormone that has biologic activity similar to that of LH.

HYPOGONADISM

Either testosterone deficiency or defective spermatogenesis leading to oligospermia or azoospermia constitutes hypogonadism. Often both coexist. The clinical manifestations of androgen deficiency depend upon the time of onset and degree of deficiency. Since testosterone is required for wolffian duct development into the epididymis, vas deferens, seminal vesicles, and ejaculatory ducts, as well as virilization of the external genitalia through the major intracellular testosterone metabolite, dihydrotestosterone, early prenatal androgen deficiency leads to ambiguous genitalia and male pseudohermaphroditism. Androgen deficiency occurring later during pregnancy may result in micropenis or cryptorchidism—the unilateral or bilateral absence of testes in the scrotum due to failure of normal descent. During puberty, androgens are responsible for male sexual differentiation, which includes growth of the scrotum, epididymis, vas deferens, seminal vesicles, prostate, penis, skeletal muscle, and larynx. Additionally, androgens stimulate axillary, pubic, and body hair growth, as well as increased sebaceous gland activity, and are responsible in part for the growth and fusion of the epiphyseal cartilaginous plates seen clinically as the pubertal growth spurt. Thus, prepubertal androgen deficiency leads to poor muscle development, decreased strength and endurance, a high-pitched voice, sparse axillary and pubic hair, and absence of facial and body hair. The long bones of the lower extremities and arms may continue to grow under the influence of growth hormone, leading to eunuchoidal proportions in which the arm span exceeds the total height by 5 cm or more, and there is a greater growth of the lower extremities relative to the total height. Postpubertal androgen deficiency may result in a decrease in libido, impotence, low energy, fine wrinkling around the corners of the eyes and mouth, and diminished facial and body hair.

Male hypogonadism may be classified into three categories according to the level of the defect (Table 70–1). Hypogonadism due to lesions in the hypothalamus or pituitary give rise to secondary or hypogonadotropic hypogonadism, since the low testosterone or ineffective spermatogenesis is a result of inadequate stimulation of the testes by insufficient or inadequate concentrations of the gonadotropins. In contrast, diseases directly affecting the testes will result in primary or hypergonadotropic hypogonadism, characterized by oligo- or azoospermia and low testosterone levels but with elevations of LH and FSH because of a decrease of the negative feedback regulation on the pituitary and hypothalamus by androgens and inhibin.

Hypothalamic-Pituitary Disorders

Panhypopituitarism occurs congenitally from structural defects or inadequate production or release of the hypothalamic-releasing factors. The condition may also be acquired through replacement by tumors, infarction from vascular insufficiency, infiltrative disorders, autoimmune diseases, trauma, and infections.

Isolated gonadotropin deficiency can involve either

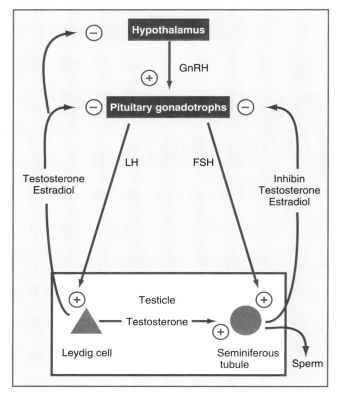

Figure 70–1

Regulation of the hypothalamic-pituitary-testicular axis. + = Positive feedback; − = negative feedback; FSH = follicle-stimulating hormone; GnRH = gonadotropin-releasing hormone; LH = luteinizing hormone.

LH or FSH but most commonly involves both hormones on a congenital basis. Kallmann's syndrome is a form of hypogonadotropic hypogonadism associated with problems in the ability to discriminate odors, either incompletely (hyposmia) or completely (anosmia). This syndrome results from a defect in the migration of the GnRH

TABLE 70–1	**Classification of Male Hypogonadism**

Hypothalamic-Pituitary Disorders (Secondary Hypogonadism)
Panhypopituitarism
Isolated gonadotropin deficiency
Complex congenital syndromes

Gonadal Disorders (Primary Hypogonadism)
Klinefelter's syndrome and associated chromosomal defects
Myotonic dystrophy
Cryptorchidism
Bilateral anorchia
Seminiferous tubular failure
Adult Leydig cell failure
Androgen biosynthesis enzyme deficiency

Defects in Androgen Action
Testicular feminization (complete androgen insensitivity)
Incomplete androgen insensitivity
5α-reductase deficiency

neurons from the olfactory placode into the hypothalamus. Thus, it represents a GnRH deficiency. The patients remain prepubertal, with small rubbery testes, and develop eunuchoidism. There are several other complex congenital syndromes, such as the Prader-Willi and Laurence-Moon-Biedl syndromes, that have hypogonadism as one of their manifestations.

Hyperprolactinemia, whether caused by a prolactin-secreting pituitary micro- or macroadenoma or drug induced, may result in hypogonadotropic hypogonadism because prolactin elevation inhibits normal GnRH release, decreases the effectiveness of LH at the Leydig cell level, and also inhibits some of the action of testosterone at the target organ level. Normalization of the prolactin through withdrawal of an offending drug, surgical removal of the pituitary adenoma, or the use of the dopamine agonist bromocriptine reverses this form of hypogonadism.

Another form of secondary hypogonadism in males is due to weight loss or systemic illness. This induces a defect in the hypothalamic release of GnRH, resulting in low gonadotropin and testosterone levels. This is commonly seen in patients with cancer, acquired immunodeficiency syndrome (AIDS), and chronic inflammatory processes.

Primary Gonadal Abnormalities

The most common congenital cause of primary testicular failure is Klinefelter's syndrome, which occurs in approximately 1 of every 1000 live male births and is usually due to maternal meiotic chromosomal nondisjunction that results in an XXY genotype. At puberty the clinical findings include varying degrees of hypogonadism, gynecomastia, small firm testes measuring < 2 cm in the longest axis (normal testes measure over 3.5 cm), azoospermia, eunuchoidal skeletal proportions, and elevations of FSH and LH. There are a number of chromosomal variants of Klinefelter's syndrome. Generally, as the number of X chromosomes increases there is a decrease in the IQ, whereas, as the number of Y chromosomes increases, macronodular acne and aggressive antisocial behavior are found. Primary gonadal failure is also found in patients with another congenital condition, myotonic dystrophy, which is characterized by progressive weakness; atrophy of the facial, neck, hand, and lower extremity muscles; frontal baldness; and myotonia.

Approximately 3% of full-term male infants have cryptorchidism, which spontaneously corrects during the first year of life in the majority, so that by 1 year of age the incidence is approximately 0.75%. When the testes are maintained in the intra-abdominal position, the increased temperature leads to defective spermatogenesis and oligospermia. Leydig cell function generally remains normal and therefore adult testosterone levels are normal. Cryptorchidism must be differentiated from retractile testes due to a hyperactive cremasteric reflex, which pulls the testes from the scrotum into the inguinal canal. A careful testicular examination in a warm room with gentle pressure applied over the lower abdomen will usually allow palpation of the testes in this situation. Another condition to be differentiated is bilateral anorchia, also known as the vanishing testicle syndrome. In this rare condition, the external genitalia are fully formed, indicating that ample quantities of testosterone and dihydrotestosterone were produced during early embryogenesis. However, the testicular tissue disappeared prior to or shortly after birth, resulting in an empty scrotum. Differentiation from cryptorchidism can be made through an hCG stimulation test. Patients with cryptorchidism will have an increase in serum testosterone following an injection of hCG, while patients with bilateral anorchia will not.

There are numerous causes of acquired gonadal failure. The adult seminiferous tubules are susceptible to a variety of injuries, and seminiferous tubular failure is found following infections such as mumps, gonococcal or lepromatous orchitis, irradiation, vascular injury, trauma, alcohol, and chemotherapeutic drugs, especially alkylating agents. The serum FSH concentrations may be normal or elevated, depending upon the degree of damage to the seminiferous tubules. The Leydig cell compartment may also be damaged by these same conditions. In addition, some men experience a gradual decline in testicular function as they age, possibly due to microvascular insufficiency. The decreased testosterone production may be clinically manifest by a lowered libido and potency, emotional lability, fatigue, and vasomotor symptoms such as hot flushes. The serum LH concentration is usually elevated in this situation.

Defects in Androgen Action

When testosterone enters target cells, it may be converted to the potent androgen dihydrotestosterone (DHT). When either testosterone or DHT binds to the androgen receptor, the receptor is activated and binds DNA, stimulating transcription, protein synthesis, and cell growth, which collectively constitutes androgen action. An absence of androgen receptors results in the syndrome of testicular feminization, a form of male pseudohermaphroditism. These genetic males have cryptorchid testes but appear to be phenotypical females. Because androgens are inactive during embryogenesis, there is failure of the labial-scrotal folds to fuse, resulting in the presence of a short vagina. The fallopian tubes, uterus, and upper portion of the vagina are absent because the testes secrete müllerian duct inhibitory factor during early fetal development. At the time of puberty, the patients have breast enlargement because the testes secrete a small amount of estradiol, and peripheral tissues convert testosterone as well as adrenal androgens to estrogens. Axillary and pubic hair do not grow, as these require androgen action for development. The serum testosterone concentrations are elevated due to continuous stimulation by LH, whose concentrations are raised because of the inability of the testosterone to act in a negative feedback fashion at the hypothalamic level. Patients may have incomplete forms of androgen insensitivity due to point mutations affecting the androgen receptor gene, and clinically they will demonstrate varying degrees of male pseudohermaphroditism.

Patients who lack the 5α-reductase enzyme required to convert testosterone to DHT will be born with a bifid scrotum, reflecting abnormal fusion of the labial-scrotal folds, and hypospadias, with the urethral opening in the perineal area or in the shaft of the penis. At puberty, there is a sufficient increase in androgen production to partially overcome the defect, the scrotum, phallus, and muscle mass enlarge, and the patients appear to develop into normal adult males.

These rare defects in androgen action must be differentiated from the even rarer congenital enzyme defects in the testicular androgen biosynthetic pathway, since both types of conditions will lead to ambiguous genitalia. These conditions can be differentiated biochemically, since patients with enzyme defects will have low serum testosterone concentrations, while patients whose defects are at the androgen action level will have raised testosterone concentrations.

Diagnosis

Figure 70–2 presents an algorithm for laboratory evaluation of hypogonadism. Serum concentrations of LH, FSH, and testosterone should be obtained, and a semen analysis should be performed. Since gonadotropins and testosterone are secreted in a pulsatile fashion every 60 to 90 minutes, equal aliquots of sera from three blood samples obtained at 20-minute intervals may be combined prior to measurement to derive average concentrations of these hormones. A low testosterone level with low gonadotropins indicates a hypothalamic-pituitary abnormality, which needs to be evaluated with serum prolactin determination and radiographic evaluation of the hypothalamic-pituitary region. Elevated concentrations of gonadotropins with a normal or low testosterone level reflect a primary testicular abnormality. If no testes are palpable in the scrotum and careful "milking" of the lower abdomen does not bring retractile testes into the scrotum, then an hCG stimulation test should be carried out. If serum testosterone concentrations rise, this indicates the presence of functional testicular tissue, and a diagnosis of cryptorchidism can be made. An absence of a rise in testosterone suggests bilateral anorchia. Small, firm testes that are present in the scrotum are highly suggestive of Klinefelter's syndrome; this needs to be confirmed with a chromosomal karyotype. Testes larger than 3.5 cm in the longest diameter that are of normal consistency or soft indicate postpubertal acquired primary hypogonadism. If the major abnormality is a deficient sperm count with or without an elevation of FSH, then one must differentiate between a ductal problem and an acquired primary hypogonadism. If sperm are present, then at least the ducts emanating from one testicle are patent; this indicates an acquired testicular defect. If there are no sperm in the ejaculate, this may be caused by a primary testicular problem or a ductal problem. The seminal vesicles secrete fructose into the seminal fluid. Therefore, the presence of fructose in the ejaculate should be followed by a testicular biopsy to see whether the defect results from spermatogenic failure or obstruction of the ducts leading from the testes to the

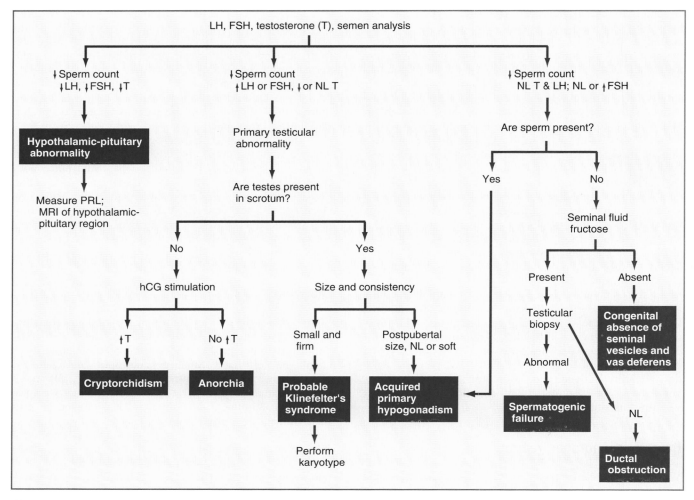

Figure 70–2

Laboratory evaluation of hypogonadism. FSH = follicle-stimulating hormone; hCG = human chorionic gonadotropin; LH = luteinizing hormone; MRI = magnetic resonance imaging; NL = normal; PRL = prolactin ↑ = elevated; ↓ = decreased or low.

seminal vesicles. Absence of seminal fluid fructose indicates a congenital absence of the seminal vesicles and vas deferens.

Male Infertility

Infertility affects approximately 15% of couples, and male factors appear to be responsible in approximately 40% of the cases. Female factors account for another 40%, while a couple factor is present in approximately 20% of the cases. In addition to the defects in spermatogenesis that occur in patients with hypothalamic, pituitary, testicular, or androgen action disorders, hyperthyroidism, hypothyroidism, adrenal abnormalities, and systemic illnesses may also result in defective spermatogenesis. Disorders of the vas deferens, seminal vesicles, and prostate may also lead to infertility, as can diseases affecting the bladder sphincter that may result in retrograde ejaculation, with the sperm passing into the bladder rather than through the penis. Anatomic defects of the penis, as seen

in patients with hypospadias, poor coital technique, and the presence of antisperm antibodies in either the male or in the female genital tract also are associated with infertility.

Therapy for Hypogonadism and Infertility

Treatment of androgen deficiency in patients who have hypothalamic-pituitary or primary testicular abnormalities is best accomplished with exogenous testosterone administration, both from patient acceptance and cost-effectiveness standpoints. Oral and sublingual preparations of testosterone are available, but these have potential hepatotoxicity and usually incompletely virilize the patient. Therefore, replacement therapy with the intramuscular injection of intermediate-acting testosterone esters or with a transdermal testosterone patch are the methods of choice. Testosterone therapy will increase libido, potency, muscle mass, strength, endurance, and hair growth on the face and body. Side effects include acne, fluid retention, erythrocytosis, and, rarely, sleep apnea. This therapy is contraindicated in patients with cancer of the prostate.

If fertility is desired, patients with hypothalamic abnormalities may develop virilization and spermatogenesis with the use of GnRH given in a pulsatile fashion subcutaneously with an external pump. Direct stimulation of the testes in patients with hypothalamic or pituitary abnormalities may be accomplished with the use of exogenous gonadotropins, which will increase testosterone and sperm production. If primary testicular failure is present and the patient has oligospermia, then an attempt can be made to concentrate the sperm for intrauterine insemination or *in vitro* fertilization. If the azoospermia is due to ductal obstruction, then repair of the obstruction may be undertaken, or aspiration of sperm from the epididymis may be accomplished for *in vitro* fertilization. However, if spermatogenic arrest has occurred and the patient has no sperm in the ejaculate, then fertility is not possible.

IMPOTENCE

Normal erection requires an intact central nervous system that allows psychogenic and sensory stimuli to be integrated and transmitted to the sympathetic nervous system that controls penile blood flow, patent arterial blood vessels capable of dilating and delivering blood to the penis, a normal corpora cavernosal sinus system that can become engorged with blood, an anatomically normal penis, and competence of the venous drainage system that does not leak blood from the penis during erection. The hypothalamic-pituitary-testicular axis must also be normal because testosterone is required for maintenance of normal libido and has a permissive effect in regard to erection. Thus, neurologic, vascular, urogenital, and endocrine abnormalities may result in erectile dysfunction, which can span the spectrum from total inability to obtain and maintain an erection to ability to obtain an erection but not maintain it sufficiently long to complete sexual activity. Diabetes mellitus is one of the most common endocrine abnormalities associated with impotence; at all ages the prevalence of impotence is higher in diabetics than in the population at large. Numerous drugs have also been associated with impotence, including antihypertensive agents, diuretics, tranquilizers, tricyclic antidepressants, H_2-receptor antagonists, and antiandrogens. Tobacco, alcohol, opiates, amphetamines, and cocaine are also associated with erectile dysfunction.

Approximately 80% of patients with impotence develop it because of a drug or underlying organic illness, while the other 20% have a primary psychogenic etiology. Organic impotence generally results in a gradual and total loss of potency, with maintenance of normal libido until a secondary psychogenic decrease occurs. Conversely, patients who have psychogenic impotence often will have erections under some circumstances but not in others and generally will experience an acute onset of sexual dysfunction temporarily related to a significant life event.

Since normal men will experience three to five erections per night during rapid eye movement sleep, nocturnal penile tumescence monitoring will allow assessment of the neurologic pathways and vascular integrity of the penis. Both the arterial blood supply and penile venous competence can be assessed through Doppler ultrasonography following the intracorporeal injection of prostaglandin E_1, which induces an erection.

Psychogenic impotence may be treated with behavioral therapy, which is successful in approximately half the individuals. Patients who develop impotence while on a prescription or recreational drug known to be associated with erectile dysfunction should have the drug discontinued or medication switched to one that is less likely to cause impotence. If impotence persists or if it is due to an organic illness or is psychogenic in origin but cannot be corrected through behavioral therapies, self-administered intracavernosal prostaglandin E_1 will effectively induce erections in up to 80% of men. The therapy may be associated with penile pain, hematoma, and, less commonly, penile fibrosis. Erections may also be induced with a vacuum device that brings about penile engorgement, which can be maintained through constrictive bands placed at the base of the penis. Close to 90% of patients will achieve an erection with this method. Finally, there are several types of penile prostheses that can be permanently implanted in the corpora cavernosa. Satisfactory results have been noted in 80 to 90% of couples.

GYNECOMASTIA

Gynecomastia refers to a benign enlargement of the male breast resulting from proliferation of the glandular component. This is a common condition found in as many as 70% of pubertal boys and approximately a third of adults 50 to 80 years old. Estrogens stimulate and androgens inhibit breast glandular development. Thus, gynecomastia is the result of an imbalance between estrogen and androgen action at the breast tissue level. This may be due to an absolute increase in free estrogens, a decrease in endogenous free androgens, androgen insensitivity of the tissues, or enhanced sensitivity of the breast tissue to estrogens. Table 70–2 lists the common conditions associated with gynecomastia.

Gynecomastia must be differentiated from fatty enlargement of the breasts without glandular proliferation and other disorders of the breasts, especially breast carcinoma. Male breast cancer usually presents as a unilateral, eccentric hard or firm mass that is fixed to the underlying tissues. It may be associated with skin dimpling or retraction as well as crusting of the nipple or nipple discharge. In contrast, gynecomastia occurs concentrically around the nipple and is not fixed to the underlying structures.

Painful and tender gynecomastia in a pubertal male should be followed with periodic examinations, because in the vast majority of patients, pubertal gynecomastia disappears within a year. Asymptomatic gynecomastia in an adult that is discovered on routine physical examination requires a careful history and physical examination

TABLE 70–2	Conditions Associated with Gynecomastia

Physiologic

Neonatal
Pubertal
Involutional

Pathologic

Neoplasms
    Testicular
    Adrenal
    Ectopic hCG production
Primary gonadal failure
Secondary hypogonadism
Enzyme defects in testosterone production
Androgen insensitivity syndromes
Liver disease
Malnutrition with refeeding
Dialysis
Hyperthyroidism
Excessive extraglandular aromatase activity
Drugs
    Estrogens and estrogen agonists
    Gonadotropins
    Antiandrogens or inhibitors of androgen synthesis
    Cytotoxic agents
    Alcohol
Idiopathic

HCG = Human chorionic gonadotropin.

for evaluation of alcohol, drug, or medication use; liver, lung, or kidney dysfunction; and signs and symptoms of hypogonadism or hyperthyroidism. If these are not present, then only follow-up is required. In contrast, if there is recent onset of progressive painful gynecomastia in an adult, then measurements of thyroid, liver, and renal function should be carried out. If these are normal, then serum concentrations of hCG, LH, testosterone, and estradiol should be measured. Further evaluation should be carried out according to the scheme outlined in Figure 70–3.

Removal of the offending drug or correction of the underlying condition causing the gynecomastia may result in regression of the breast glandular tissue. If the gynecomastia persists, a trial of antiestrogens such as tamoxifen may be given for 3 months to see whether there is regression. Gynecomastia that has been present for over a year usually contains a fibrotic component that does not respond to medications. Therefore, correction usually requires plastic surgical removal of the tissue.

TESTICULAR TUMORS

Testicular tumors represent 1 to 2% of malignancies in men and are the second most frequent cancer in men between the ages of 20 and 34 years. Germ cell neoplasms account for 95% of the tumors, while stromal or

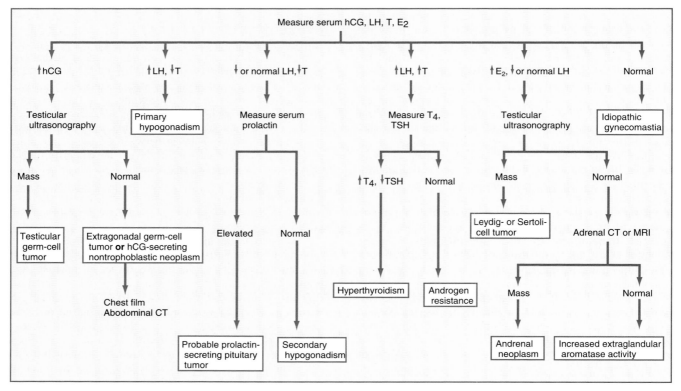

Figure 70–3

Diagnostic evaluation for causes of gynecomastia based on measurements of serum human chorionic gonadotropin (hCG), luteinizing hormone (LH), testosterone (T), and estradiol (E₂). CT = Computed tomography; MRI = magnetic resonance imaging; TSH = thyroid-stimulating hormone; ↑ = increased; ↓ = decreased. (From Braunstein GD: Gynecomastia. N Engl J Med 1993; 328:490–495. Reprinted by permission of *The New England Journal of Medicine,* Copyright 1993 Massachusetts Medical Society.)

Leydig cell neoplasms account for the other 5%. Approximately one third to one half of germ cell tumors are seminomas, while the rest are composed of α-fetoprotein–secreting embryonal cell neoplasms, teratomas, or the rare hCG-secreting choriocarcinoma. These tumors generally present as a testicular enlargement, which may be associated with pain and tenderness. A small number of patients will have gynecomastia, and less than 10% will have symptoms of distant metastases at the time of presentation. These tumors are staged through measurements of hCG and α-fetoprotein, imaging studies, and surgery. Seminomas are quite radiosensitive and may be cured through orchiectomy and local radiotherapy. Disseminated disease is treated with both radiotherapy and chemotherapy. Localized disease has a 5-year survival rate close to 100%, which drops to approximately 20% with widely disseminated disease. Nonseminomatous germ cell tumors are treated with surgery, radiation, and combination chemotherapy. Aggressive therapy is associated with 5-year survival rates of between 60 and 90%.

Leydig cell tumors also present as a testicular mass and, in some patients, gynecomastia. In children, the tumors are often associated with precocious sexual development. Most are benign and are cured by orchiectomy.

Testicular tumors must be differentiated from inguinal hernias, epididymitis, orchitis, hematomas, hydrocele, and infiltrative disorders. An ultrasound evaluation will discriminate between many of these conditions.

BENIGN PROSTATIC HYPERPLASIA

Adenomatous enlargement of the prostate is present in the majority of men older than 55 years, close to two thirds of whom will have symptoms of prostatism. These symptoms can be divided into those due to obstruction, such as decreased force of the urine stream, urinary retention, and renal insufficiency, and those due to irritative symptoms from abnormal bladder function. The latter include nocturia, frequency, a sensation of incomplete voiding, urgency, and urinary incontinence. An enlarged prostate is usually found on physical examination, although significant obstructive symptoms can be found with periurethral enlargement that may not be appreciated on digital examination of the prostate.

The mainstay of therapy for benign prostatic hyperplasia has been surgical resection of the prostate, either transurethrally or through an open prostatectomy. Significant complications of surgery include incontinence, impotence, retrograde ejaculation, and bladder neck contractures. The two most commonly used medical therapies are inhibition of dihydrotestosterone production in the prostate through the use of a 5α-reductase inhibitor, finasteride, which decreases prostate volume by an average of 20% over 3 to 6 months, and the α_1-adrenergic blocking drug terazosin, which relaxes the smooth muscle component of the prostate, decreasing bladder outlet obstruction.

CARCINOMA OF THE PROSTATE

Next to skin cancers, prostate cancers are the second most common tumors in men. Approximately 200,000 new cases are diagnosed each year and are more common among blacks and men with a strong family history of prostate cancer.

Early prostate cancer is asymptomatic and may be detected by routine digital examination or elevation of prostate-specific-antigen (PSA) or may be found in tissue obtained from surgery performed to relieve symptoms associated with benign prostatic hyperplasia. Locally invasive disease may cause urinary obstruction, producing symptoms similar to those of benign prostatic hyperplasia, or may obstruct the ureters, leading to hydronephrosis and uremia. Unfortunately, many patients present with symptoms of metastatic disease, such as bone pain or pathologic fractures. Staging of prostate cancer is carried out through combinations of radiographic assessment of local disease with transrectal ultrasonography or magnetic resonance imaging, tumor marker assessment with quantitative serum PSA and acid phosphatase measurements, and bone scans for detection of bone metastases. If the disease appears to be localized to the prostate area, then a staging pelvic lymphadenectomy may be performed to assess regional lymph node involvement.

Therapeutic approaches include radical prostatectomy, radiation therapy, hormonal therapy, and chemotherapy. For a clinically unapparent, incidentally found tumor in individuals whose life expectancy is less than 10 years because of age or concurrent illness, watchful waiting alone is reasonable. For those whose projected life expectancy is over 10 years, watchful waiting, radical prostatectomy, and radiation therapy are current options. Radical prostatectomy, radiation therapy, or hormonal therapy is appropriate for individuals whose tumors are confined to the prostate, with the choice being determined by the degree of histologic differentiation of the tumor. Radiation therapy is generally used for locally advanced disease that has extended outside of the prostate. Disseminated disease is usually treated with hormonal therapy. Since prostate cancer is androgen sensitive, hormonal therapy is directed at lowering serum testosterone. This can be done through surgical or medical castration. The latter can be accomplished by giving large doses of estrogen in the form of diethylstilbestrol or, more commonly, through a long-acting analogue of GnRH, which brings about down regulation of the GnRH receptors on the pituitary gonadotrophs, leading to a lowering of LH and FSH and a subsequent decrease of testosterone. Some physicians prefer to perform total androgen blockade by combining a GnRH agonist with an androgen receptor antagonist, such as flutamide. However, it is not clear that this combination is superior to GnRH agonist therapy alone. Chemotherapy has had limited success in patients with hormone-refractory metastatic disease. Serial prostate-specific antigen determinations are useful in monitoring the effects of therapy. A rising or persistently elevated level of prostate-specific antigen indicates residual cancer.

REFERENCES

Bardin CW, Swerdloff RS, Santen RJ: Androgens: Risks and benefits. J Clin Endocrinol Metab 1991; 73:4.

Braunstein GD: Gynecomastia. N Engl J Med 1993; 328:490.

Braunstein GD: Testes. *In* Greenspan FS, Baxter J (eds.): Basic and Clinical Endocrinology. Norwalk, CT, Appleton & Lange, 1994, pp 391–418.

Roth BJ, Nochols CR (eds.): Testicular cancer. Semin Oncol 1992; 19: 117.

Whitcomb RW, Crowley WF Jr: Male hypogonadotropic hypogonadism. Endocrinol Metab Clin North Am 1993; 22:125.

71

Diabetes Mellitus

Diabetes affects over 14 million people in the United States. Approximately 90% have type II diabetes (non–insulin dependent diabetes mellitus [NIDDM]), and the remainder have type I diabetes (insulin-dependent diabetes [IDDM]). Of those who have type II diabetes, approximately 50% are undiagnosed and are therefore untreated. Diabetes is an expensive disease; in 1994, patients diagnosed with diabetes accounted for 4.6% of the United States population yet were responsible for 14.6% of all direct health care expenditures. Diabetes is the major cause of adult blindness in people 20 to 74 years old, as well as the leading cause of nontraumatic lower extremity amputation and end-stage renal disease. Fortunately, the results of the Diabetes Control and Complications Trial (DCCT) proved that the development of the microvascular and neuropathic complications of diabetes can be delayed and the progression slowed by the lifelong maintenance of near-normal blood glucose levels. Now the major challenge in treating patients with diabetes is ensuring that all patients have adequate access to appropriate care that will provide them the opportunity to achieve and maintain near-euglycemia. As a first step in this process, at each visit diabetic patients should have all of their diabetes problems addressed and treated (if necessary). Table 71–1 lists the fundamental pieces of information that should be obtained for each diabetic patient seen.

BASIC CLASSIFICATION

The differences between type I and type II diabetes are listed in Table 71–2. Type I diabetes generally occurs in younger, lean patients and is characterized by the marked inability of the pancreas to secrete insulin. The distinguishing characteristic of a patient with type I diabetes is that if insulin is withdrawn, ketosis and, eventually, ketoacidosis develops. These patients are therefore insulin dependent (i.e., insulin is life sustaining), since they produce no endogenous insulin. It is important to identify patients with type I diabetes to provide appropriate care during periods of illness or surgery. For instance, patients with type I diabetes must have a continuous source of carbohydrate and insulin given when ill and unable to retain fluids or when not allowed to receive anything orally, as in the postoperative situation. Urine ketones

should be measured when patients with type I diabetes develop marked hyperglycemia, especially when associated with illness.

Patients with type II diabetes are often older (>40 years of age), have a family history of diabetes, and are obese, although 10% to 20% are lean. Type II diabetes is characterized by peripheral resistance to the action of insulin and decreased insulin secretion in spite of the presence of elevated serum glucose levels. These defects lead to decreased peripheral uptake of glucose, as well as increased hepatic glucose output, producing both postprandial and fasting hyperglycemia, respectively. Because patients with type II diabetes retain the ability to secrete some endogenous insulin, those who are taking insulin usually do not develop diabetic ketoacidosis (DKA) when they fail to take the insulin. Therefore, they are considered insulin requiring, not insulin dependent. Moreover, patients with type II diabetes often do not need treatment with oral antidiabetic medication or insulin if they lose weight or are hospitalized and do not eat.

Previously, differentiating between the two types of diabetes was relatively straightforward—if a patient developed diabetes in childhood, especially if accompanied by DKA, he or she was considered a type I diabetic patient. Now people are developing type II diabetes at younger ages (sometimes as young as 6 or 7 years of age), and to further complicate the issue, some present in DKA only to ultimately be controlled on diet or oral antidiabetic agents. Conversely, some elderly patients present with new-onset type I diabetes and DKA and are subsequently insulin dependent. Defining a patient as having type I versus type II diabetes can therefore be challenging, but a good clinical history often allows one to make the distinction. A strong family history of type II diabetes, obesity, and a Hispanic, black, or Native American heritage all make the diagnosis of type II diabetes more likely, regardless of age. A lean white patient without a family history of diabetes who developed diabetes in childhood is likely to have type I diabetes.

No definitive test exists for differentiating between the two types. Early in the course of diabetes, C-peptide (connecting peptide) levels are often measurable in patients with either type of diabetes; therefore, this does not distinguish between the two types of diabetes. If it is decided that an insulin-treated patient is likely to have type II diabetes and it is elected to discontinue the insu-

TABLE 71-1	Information to Obtain During Initial Diabetes Interview

- Type of diabetes: I or II (determine based on history, current therapy, and clinical judgment).
- Duration of diabetes.
- Diabetes treatment: Diet, oral antidiabetic agent(s), and/or insulin. Include dose and frequency of medications.
- Self-monitoring of blood glucose (SMBG): Does patient perform SMBG? If yes, note frequency and usual range of values at each time of day.
- Last HgbA$_{1c}$ level: Date and value (and normal range)
- Hypoglycemia: Does patient have episodes of unexplained hypoglycemia? If yes, note when, how often, and how patient treats these episodes. Also note whether patient has hypoglycemia unawareness.
- Microvascular complications
  Retinopathy—When was last dilated eye examination? What were the results?
  Nephropathy—Any known diabetic kidney disease? When was last measurement of urine protein and serum creatinine? Results? Is patient taking an angiotensin-converting enzyme inhibitor?
- Neuropathy: Does patient have a history of neuropathy? Symptoms of peripheral neuropathy? Autonomic neuropathy? (Be sure to ask about impotence if male.)
- Diabetic foot: Has patient had prior (or current) foot ulcers/amputations?
- Macrovascular complications
  Hypertension (HTN)—Does patient have HTN? If yes, what medications are taken?
  Coronary artery disease (CAD)—Does patient have known CAD? Family history of CAD?
  Peripheral vascular disease (PVD)—Symptoms of claudication, history of vascular bypass?
  Cerebrovascular—Has patient had cerebrovascular accident or transient ischemic attack?
  Lipids—Most recent lipid levels? Is patient taking lipid-lowering medication?
- Behavioral/general: Does patient smoke? Does patient receive annual flu shot? Does patient exercise? If yes, what type of exercise and frequency? Does patient adhere to a specific diet? For female patients: Is patient planning pregnancy? If not, is patient using adequate contraceptive techniques?

HgbA$_{1c}$ = Hemoglobin A$_{1c}$, or glycated hemoglobin.

lin, the insulin dose should be slowly tapered as an oral antidiabetic medication is added. The patient should perform self-monitoring of blood glucose (SMBG) and measure urine for ketones if hyperglycemia develops.

Other Types Of Diabetes

Maturity onset diabetes of the young (MODY) is a form of type II diabetes that affects many generations in the same family with an early onset of the disease. Several different genetic defects may cause this syndrome, most involving the glucokinase gene (an enzyme important for glucose-induced insulin secretion and glucose uptake by the liver).

Gestational diabetes is a form of impaired glucose tolerance that develops during pregnancy, when an inherited decrease in B cell reserve results in an inability of the pancreas to secrete adequate amounts of insulin to overcome the insulin resistance created by placental hormones. It occurs in 2 to 5% of all pregnancies (increasing with the increasing age of the mother) and results in fetal macrosomia, hypoglycemia, hypocalcemia, and/or hyperbilirubinemia if untreated. When gestational diabetes is suspected, patients should be screened at 25 weeks of gestation with a 50-gm glucose load. The diagnosis of gestational diabetes is suggested if the plasma glucose level 1 hour after the 50-gm screen is ≥ 140 mg/dl and should be followed by a full 3-hour glucose tolerance test (OGTT) (Table 71-3).

TABLE 71-2	Differentiating Between Type I and Type II Diabetes Mellitus (DM)

Characteristic	Type I Diabetes	Type II Diabetes
Synonyms	Insulin-dependent diabetes mellitus (IDDM)	Non–insulin dependent diabetes mellitus (NIDDM)
Age of onset	Usually <30 yr; sometimes in older adults	Usually >40 yr; sometimes in younger persons, even children
Genetic predisposition	Moderate (requires environmental factor[s] for expression)—only 50% of identical twins develop type I DM if one sibling affected	Strong—80–100% of identical twins develop type II DM if one sibling affected
Precipitating factors	Viral/toxic/other trigger precipitating autoimmune response	Obesity, age
Findings at diagnosis	80% Islet cell antibody (ICA) positive at diagnosis	Most patients had asymptomatic diabetes for 4–7 yr prior to "diagnosis"
Endogenous insulin levels	Very low to none	Present
Insulin resistance	Only present when blood glucose levels high	Almost always present
Response to prolonged fast	Hyperglycemia, ketoacidosis	Normal blood glucose levels
Response to stress, withdrawal of insulin	Ketoacidosis	Hyperglycemia without ketosis

TABLE 71–3	World Health Organization Criteria for the Diagnosis of Gestational Diabetes Mellitus*		
	Venous Plasma Glucose, mg % (mM)	**Venous Whole Blood Glucose, mg % (mM)**	**Capillary Blood Glucose, mg % (mM)**
Fasting	105 (5.8)	90 (5.0)	90 (5.0)
1 hr	190 (10.6)	170 (9.5)	190 (10.6)
2 hr	165 (9.2)	145 (8.1)	165 (9.2)
3 hr	145 (8.1)	125 (7.0)	145 (8.1)

* Two or more of these values after a 100-gm glucose tolerance test must be met or exceeded to make the diagnosis of gestational diabetes.

A condition known as malnutrition-related diabetes occurs in patients (usually in third world countries) who are suffering from malnutrition. These patients are usually 10 to 40 years of age, have markedly symptomatic diabetes and are ketosis resistant. Most require treatment with insulin.

A variety of types of diabetes may be caused by other illnesses or medications (formerly called "secondary diabetes"). Depending on the primary process involved (i.e., destruction of pancreatic B cells or development of peripheral insulin resistance), patients with these types of diabetes behave similarly to patients with type I or type II diabetes, respectively. Included in the differential diagnosis are (1) diseases of the pancreas that destroy the pancreatic B cell (e.g., hemochromatosis, pancreatitis, cystic fibrosis, pancreatic cancer); (2) hormonal syndromes that interfere with insulin secretion (e.g., pheochromocytoma) and/or cause peripheral insulin resistance (e.g., acromegaly, Cushing syndrome, pheochromocytoma); (3) drug-induced diabetes (e.g., by phenytoin, glucocorticoids, estrogens); (4) rare abnormalities of the insulin receptor; (5) several rare genetic syndromes in which diabetes mellitus occurs frequently; and (6) patients with an abnormal insulin molecule that is much less effective than normal.

DIAGNOSIS

Patients who present with symptoms of uncontrolled diabetes, such as polyuria, polydipsia, nocturia, and weight loss, with a confirmatory random blood glucose level of >200 mg/dl, are easy to diagnose as having diabetes. Young patients with new-onset type I diabetes who present with DKA are also easily identified. However, the asymptomatic patient with type II diabetes often goes undiagnosed for many years. The average patient with "new-onset" type II diabetes has actually had diabetes for 4 to 7 years before the diagnosis is made. Therefore, patients newly diagnosed with type II diabetes may have diabetic retinopathy, neuropathy, and/or nephropathy at the time of diagnosis.

In an asymptomatic patient with diabetes, a fasting plasma glucose (FPG) concentration of ≥140 mg/dl documented on two separate occasions is diagnostic. If an FPG is not diagnostic, an HgbA1c (hemoglobin A_{1C}) level (a measure of overall diabetic control for the prior 2 to 3 months) of >7.0% indicates the presence of diabetes that requires treatment. Oral glucose tolerance tests are time consuming and poorly reproducible and are therefore seldom indicated, except for the diagnosis of gestational diabetes.

Because insulin resistance increases with age, patients with risk factors for diabetes are more likely to develop the disease as they grow older; they should therefore be screened periodically. Risk factors for type II diabetes include obesity (>120% of desirable body weight), a family history of type II diabetes in a first-degree relative, Hispanic, black, or Native American race, age ≥65 years with any preceding risk factor, a history of prior impaired glucose tolerance (IGT), hypertension or significant hyperlipidemia (total cholesterol ≥240 mg/dl or triglyceride level ≥250 mg/dl), a history of gestational diabetes, or a history of the delivery of a baby ≥9 pounds in weight (suggesting gestational diabetes). An FPG concentration should be measured, and if it is ≤115 mg/dl in a patient with one or more risk factors, screening with a FPG concentration should be performed every 3 years for the development of overt diabetes. If the FPG concentration is between 115 and 140 mg/dl, a HgbA1c level should be measured. Patients with an FPG concentration between 115 and 140 mg/dl probably have an abnormality of glucose metabolism and should be followed carefully for the development of treatable diabetes. Risk factors such as obesity and inactivity should be treated, if possible. Even patients with a normal FPG concentration and one or more risk factors for diabetes often have an accompanying phenotype that favors the development of atherosclerotic macrovascular disease even before diabetes is manifest. Therefore, behavioral modification to promote weight loss and exercise, and aggressive treatment of lipid abnormalities and hypertension are warranted in all patients.

PATHOGENESIS

Type I Diabetes

Patients with type I diabetes appear to have a genetic susceptibility to develop diabetes; they are susceptible to a variety of triggers (viral, environmental, or toxin) that stimulate immunologically mediated destruction of the B cell. After 80 to 90% of the B cells are destroyed, hyperglycemia develops and diabetes is diagnosed. In studies on identical twin pairs in which one twin has type I diabetes, antibodies to the islet cell (ICA) and to insulin (IAA) may be positive for several years in the nondiabetic twin before overt diabetes develops. Autoantibodies to glutamate decarboxylase (GAD_{65}-AA) are also found and may be an extremely good marker for type I diabetes. As B cell mass declines, insulin secretion decreases until the available insulin is no longer adequate to maintain normal blood glucose levels. Although the specific genes related to type I diabetes have not been found, patients with type I diabetes are more likely to express DR3 and/or DR4 class II HLA molecules. (About 90 to 95% of patients with type I diabetes compared with 50 to 60% in the general population have these HLA haplotypes.)

Treatment with immunosuppressive agents in patients with new-onset type I diabetes has been attempted to prevent the ongoing immune-mediated destruction of B cells. This has been found to be effective, although diabetes returns immediately upon cessation of the immunosuppressive agent; the side effects and risks of long-term immunosuppression are felt to be greater than the risk of diabetes. Therefore, this therapy is not routinely employed. Another approach is to start children considered high risk for developing type I diabetes (i.e., those with positive antibodies, appropriate haplotype, decreased acute-phase insulin release but normal FPG) on low doses of insulin. This technique can delay the complete obliteration of the pancreas's ability to secrete insulin and allows the patient to have more years with less "brittle" diabetes (the presence of endogenous insulin makes treatment of diabetes much easier).

After the initial diagnosis, patients with type I diabetes often undergo a "honeymoon" period, in which the ability to secrete endogenous insulin returns transiently before it is lost forever. It is important to monitor patients clinically for the development of the honeymoon period, because insulin doses usually need to be decreased (and sometimes stopped) based on the patient's SMBG results. This period can last for up to 1 year, but once it ends, it is usually necessary to begin increasing the patient's insulin doses to maintain near-euglycemia.

Type II Diabetes

Type II diabetes has a powerful genetic predisposition (90 to 100% concordance in identical twin pairs), although the exact genetic basis is unknown. It is likely that more than one pathogenic mechanism will be found. Many patients with type II diabetes are asymptomatic, and their diabetes is either diagnosed during screening for diabetes or when the patient is seen for another, unrelated medical problem. Patients who develop type II diabetes exhibit peripheral insulin resistance along with insufficient pancreatic B cell secretion of insulin. As hyperglycemia develops, glucotoxicity occurs, which further decreases insulin secretion. The liver also is resistant to the inhibitory effects of insulin, and as a result, hepatic gluconeogenesis is not adequately suppressed, leading to fasting hyperglycemia. Most patients (90%) who develop type II diabetes are obese, and obesity itself is associated with insulin resistance, which further worsens the diabetic state.

Type II diabetes is becoming increasingly common because more people are living longer (diabetes increases with age). It is also occurring more frequently in younger people, as more individuals are exposed to high-calorie Western diets, leading to childhood obesity.

TREATMENT OF DIABETES

Treatment Goals

The treatment goals for patients with type I and type II diabetes are similar, although they are modified in certain circumstances (e.g., advanced age, hypoglycemia unawareness). Table 71–4 outlines recommended treatment guidelines. The Diabetes Control and Complications Trial (DCCT) demonstrated that maintaining blood glucose concentrations in a near-normal range prevents the development and/or progression of diabetic complications. Intensive treatment, with maintenance of an $HgbA_{1c}$ level of ~7.0% and an average blood glucose concentration of ~150 mg/dl, decreases the development of clinically significant diabetic retinopathy by 76%, proteinuria by 54%, and clinical neuropathy by 60%, as compared with incidence in the patients with less intensive ("standard") insulin therapy. However, intensive treatment is associated with a marked increase in episodes of hypoglycemia; this is one of the largest obstacles faced by patients striving to maintain near-normal blood glucose levels.

The findings of the DCCT are also thought to be applicable to patients with type II diabetes because there is no difference in the pathophysiology of development of the microvascular and neuropathic complications in either type of diabetes. However, controversy exists over the putative greater danger of hyperinsulinemia in type II diabetes as well as the greater risk of hypoglycemia in patients likely to have macrovascular disease. For young patients with type II diabetes, however, the risks of developing the microvascular and neuropathic complications of diabetes probably outweigh the risks associated with hyperinsulinemia and hypoglycemia.

When treating diabetes, glycated hemoglobin levels (such as $HgbA_{1c}$) are the best indicator of overall diabetic control, reflecting the average blood glucose levels over the past 8 to 12 weeks. Different assays are used to measure glycated hemoglobin levels, with differing normal ranges, so it is important to become familiar with the assay used locally. For clinical purposes, an acceptable $HgbA_{1c}$ level is <1.5% above the upper limit of normal of the assay used. Therefore, if the normal range (in nondiabetic controls) for the $HgbA_{1c}$ is 4.0 to 6.2%, an acceptable target for blood glucose control is ≤6.2% + 1.5% = 7.7%. An extremely motivated patient may wish to work to maintain an $HgbA_{1c}$ level of 7.0% (similar to the control in the DCCT trial); with proper management, this goal can often be achieved. Preprandial blood glucose levels should be 80 to 140 mg/dl (and can be 70 to 120 mg/dl in a patient trying hard to achieve near-euglycemia). The prebedtime snack blood glucose target level in patients taking insulin should be 100 to 140 mg/dl to avoid nocturnal hypoglycemia.

Some patients should not aim for near-normal blood glucose levels. In elderly patients who have a life expectancy of <5 years or in any patient with a terminal dis-

TABLE 71–4	Treatment Guidelines for Diabetes (Modified from the American Diabetes Association Recommendations)			
Intervention	Frequency—Patients on Insulin	Frequency—Patients Not on Insulin	Treatment Goal
HgbA$_{1c}$ level	Quarterly	p.r.n. to maintain near-euglycemia (usually quarterly)	Keep ≤8%, preferably ≤7%
FPG concentration	p.r.n.	p.r.n.—often 4–6 times/year	Keep ≤140 mg/dl
Fasting lipid profile (total, HDL, and LDL cholesterol, triglycerides)	Initially—subsequent frequency depends on results and treatment	Initially—subsequent frequency depends on results and treatment	LDL ≤130 mg/dl (no CAD) LDL ≤100 mg/dl (with CAD)
Urine dipstick protein measurement	Yearly	Yearly	Normal
Determination for microalbuminuria	Yearly (if urine protein dipstick negative)	Yearly (if urine protein dipstick negative)	Normal
Office visit for diabetes (to include weight, blood pressure, foot examination)	Quarterly	Quarterly to semiannually	Education, management of diabetes and lipid disorders, early detection and treatment of complications
Dilated retinal exam	Yearly	Yearly	Early detection and treatment of diabetic retinopathy
Self-monitoring of blood glucose	Daily—preprandially and before bedtime snack ideal (regimen based on patient's needs)	p.r.n.—based on clinical situation and patient preference	80–120 mg/dl preprandially, 100–140 mg/dl prebedtime snack (adjusted based on patient circumstances)
Telephone follow-up	p.r.n.	p.r.n.	Adjustment of insulin doses and encouragement to comply with regimen

CAD = Coronary artery disease; FPG = fasting plasma glucose; HDL = high-density lipoprotein; LDL = low-density lipoprotein; p.r.n. = as necessary.
Modified from American Diabetes Association Standards of Care for Patients with Diabetes Mellitus. Diabetes Care 1994; 17:616–623.

ease, tight control is unnecessary. Patients with known coronary artery disease or cerebrovascular disease should also have higher preprandial blood glucose targets (e.g., 100 to 180 mg/dl) to prevent excessive hypoglycemia. Some patients have advanced microvascular and neuropathic diabetic complications and may not benefit from maintenance of near-euglycemia. Finally, patients with hypoglycemia unawareness (the lack of adrenergic warning signs of hypoglycemia) or those with recurrent episodes of severe hypoglycemia (hypoglycemia requiring administration of treatment by another person) should also have higher target blood glucose levels.

Type I Diabetes

By definition, patients with type I diabetes require lifelong treatment with insulin. Short-, intermediate- and long-acting preparations of insulin exist. Recombinant human insulin is now most commonly used. Table 71–5 describes the properties of the various types of insulin. Commercially prepared mixtures of 70/30 and 50/50 insulin (70% neutral protamine Hagedorn [NPH] + 30% regular and 50% NPH + 50% regular insulin, respectively) are available but allow less flexibility than having a patient mix the components of the insulin dose individually.

When starting a patient on insulin, it is important to develop a regimen that best suits his or her lifestyle. Optimal diabetic control often requires SMBG four times per day (preprandially and before bedtime snack) or even more often. With frequent monitoring, it is possible to determine the activity of the various components of the insulin regimen; this allows for rational adjustments in insulin doses. Most patients with type I diabetes require at least a split/mixed insulin regimen (Table 71–6), which was the regimen used in the "standard" therapy group in the DCCT trial. Although some patients can achieve near-euglycemia on a split/mixed regimen, it provides little flexibility to the patient as to mealtimes and insulin injections. Often, a multiple injection regimen, in which regular insulin is adjusted before each meal with intermediate-acting insulin given at bedtime, is necessary to provide more flexibility and to achieve better glycemic control. With a multiple-injection regimen, patients can add insulin or subtract regular insulin (called compensatory doses) from their basic insulin dose in response to the immediate blood glucose level before the meal.

Type II Diabetes

For many patients with type II diabetes, especially those who are obese, diet and exercise should be the first treatment modalities attempted. Unfortunately, patients are often unsuccessful, and after a few months hyperglycemia persists and it is necessary to start an oral medication for the treatment of diabetes (Fig. 71–1). Three classes of oral antidiabetic agents are available—the sulfonylurea agents, the biguanides, and intestinal α-glucosidase inhibitors. Table 71–7 lists the available agents and their phar-

TABLE 71-5	Types and Properties of Insulin Preparations

Type of Insulin	Preparation	Onset of Action (hr)	Peak Effect (hr)	Usual duration of action (hr)
Short acting	Regular	0.5-1.0	2-4	4-6
Intermediate acting	NPH or Lente	3-4	8-14	16-24
Long acting	Ultralente			
	Beef	4-6	14-24	>32
	Human	4-6	10-20	24-28

NPH = Neutral protamine Hagedorn.

macologic properties. Tolazamide, chlorpropamide, glyburide, glipizide, and metformin are all equally effective as monotherapy for treating type II diabetes. Tolbutamide and acetohexamide are somewhat less effective. However, tolbutamide is useful in patients with renal insufficiency who might become hypoglycemic on a longer-acting agent. Acarbose, a α-glucosidase inhibitor that slows carbohydrate breakdown and glucose absorption, may be used as monotherapy, although it is somewhat less effective than the other two classes. Its effects are additive to those of the other two classes, and therefore, it may be used along with the sulfonylurea agents and/or metformin.

To choose between a sulfonylurea agent or metformin, it is important to recognize the pros and cons of each therapy. Sulfonylurea agents have few side effects and act rapidly, and many are available as generic preparations. However, they can cause hypoglycemia and weight gain. Metformin does not cause weight gain or hypoglycemia and has beneficial effects on the lipid profile. However, it has to be titrated gradually, causes frequent gastrointestinal side effects (although often temporary) and is more expensive. It also has the potential to cause lactic acidosis if given to patients with contraindications to its use; therefore, the prescribing instructions should be followed closely. Clinically, in an obese, dieting patient with type II diabetes, metformin is a good first agent to use because the patient can continue to diet without developing hypoglycemia and will not be discouraged by sulfonylurea agent-induced weight gain. On the other hand, in a moderately symptomatic lean patient

with type II diabetes, in whom achieving a rapid lowering of blood glucose levels is indicated, a sulfonylurea agent would be a good choice.

An FPG concentration should be measured 2 weeks after every dose change and the drug increased until the FPG is < 140 mg/dl. If treatment goals are not reached with monotherapy, then one or both of the other classes of medication can be added. For example, metformin can be added to a maximal-dose sulfonylurea agent therapy or vice versa, and if the control remains suboptimal, acarbose can be added, (see Fig. 71-1). If this also fails and the HgbA$_{1c}$ level remains ≥ 1.5% above the upper limit of normal, insulin should be started. When starting insulin, a variety of approaches are possible. Twice-daily insulin can be started without oral medications, or evening NPH insulin can be added to the combination of metformin plus a sulfonylurea agent, to metformin alone, or to a sulfonylurea agent alone. Because the latter two approaches tend to be easier for the patient to adjust to and generally produce similar diabetic control to twice-daily insulin regimens, bedtime insulin/daytime sulfonylurea agent therapy has become increasingly popular. If this fails, metformin can be added back to the regimen (if the patient was able to tolerate it). If all combinations of oral antidiabetic medications and insulin fail, then insulin alone can be attempted. Throughout the treatment of a patient with type II diabetes, adherence to diet and exercise should be stressed, since behavior modification can have a large impact on the degree of diabetic control reached.

TABLE 71-6	Possible Insulin Regimens

Regimen	Before Breakfast	Before Lunch	Before Supper	Before Bedtime
Split/mixed	NPH/regular*		NPH/regular	
Split/mixed variant†	NPH/regular		Regular	NPH
Multiple-injection regimen	Regular	Regular	Regular	NPH
Multiple injections using ultralente	Ultralente/regular (separate injections)‡	Regular	Ultralente/regular (separate injections)‡	
BIDS	Maximal dose of sulfonylurea agents (± metformin)			NPH
Insulin pump	Small amounts of regular insulin infused throughout 24-hr period (basal rate) with boluses of regular insulin given before each meal			

* Regular insulin should be injected 30 minutes before designated meal.
† Useful if a patient develops nocturnal/fasting hypoglycemia when NPH insulin given before supper.
‡ The zinc in ultralente and lente insulins binds regular insulin and delays its absorption. Therefore, giving two separate injections or using NPH instead of lente insulin is preferable.
BIDS = Bedtime insulin/daytime sulfonylurea agent therapy; NPH = neutral protamine Hagedorn.

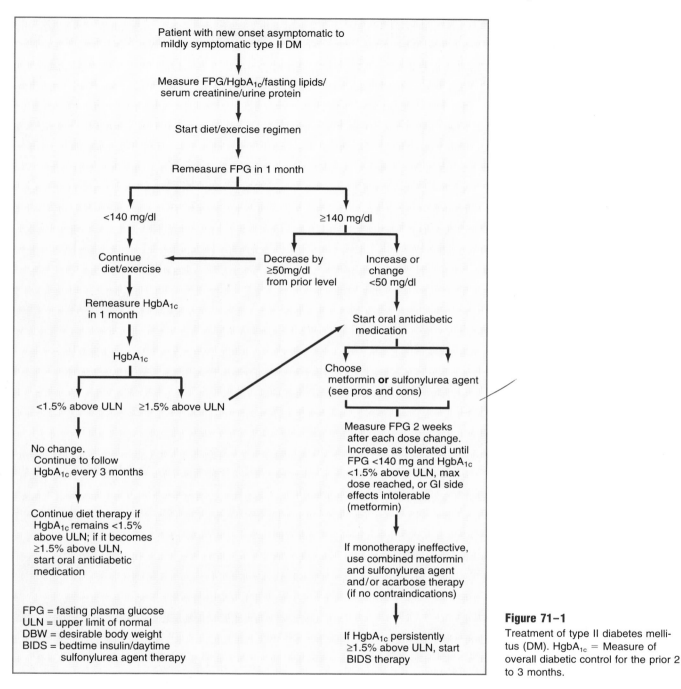

Figure 71-1
Treatment of type II diabetes mellitus (DM). HgbA$_{1c}$ = Measure of overall diabetic control for the prior 2 to 3 months.

COMPLICATIONS

Acute Complications

DKA

Diabetic ketoacidosis occurs when profound insulin deficiency is combined with elevated levels of the counterregulatory hormones (e.g., glucagon, cortisol, growth hormone, epinephrine, and norepinephrine) that render the available insulin ineffective. By definition, DKA occurs in patients with type I diabetes and, most commonly, when an intercurrent illness develops (e.g., infection), when a patient's insulin dose is inappropriately decreased or discontinued, or when the patient has new-onset type I diabetes. The primary features of DKA are dehydration, acidosis, and electrolyte depletion, which are explained by the effects of insulin deficiency on carbohydrate, protein, and lipid metabolism. Without effective circulating insulin levels, blood glucose concentrations rise, eventually producing an osmotic diuresis with loss of fluid and electrolytes. This results in dehydration (sometimes up to 4 to 6 L), depletion of total body potassium (up to ~10%), and lesser degrees of depletion of sodium, chloride, phosphate, and magnesium.

TABLE 71–7	Oral Antidiabetic Medications

Generic Name	Trade Name	Tablet Size(s) (mg)	Usual Daily Dose Range (mg)	Maximal Dose (mg)	Duration of Action (hr)	Comments
Tolbutamide	Orinase	250, 500	500–2000 (divided)	3000	6–12	Least effective
Chlorpropamide (use only in patients <65 yr of age)	Diabinese	100, 250	100–500 (single)	750	60	Can cause prolonged hypoglycemia, hyponatremia, Antabuse-like reaction
Acetohexamide	Dymelor	250, 500	250–1500 (single or divided)	1500	12–24	
Tolazamide	Tolinase	100, 250, 500	100–750 (single or divided)	1000	12–24	
Glyburide	Micronase, Diabeta	1.25, 2.5, 5.0	2.5–10.0 (single or divided)	20	12–24	Micronized glyburide
	Glynase	1.5, 3.0, 6.0	1.5–6.0 (single or divided)	12	12–24	
Glipizide	Glucotrol	5, 10	5–20 (single or divided)	40	10–24	Long acting
	Glucotrol XL	5, 10	5–10 (single)	20	24–48	
Metformin*	Glucophage	500, 850	1500–2000 (divided)	2500	~12	Do not use in patients with contraindications; gastrointestinal side effects common
Acarbose	Precose	50, 100	150–300 (divided)	300	~3	Gastrointestinal side effects common

* Use only in patients with a creatinine <1.5 mg/dl (males) or <1.4 mg/dl (females), normal hepatic function, no known conditions causing hypoxia and/or chronic acidosis; contraindicated in patients with alcoholism. Hold the drug if patient undergoes a surgical procedure, angiographic study, and/or becomes acutely ill.

Protein breakdown is accelerated, leading to an elevated flux of amino acids to the liver, enhancing gluconeogenesis (further worsening the hyperglycemia). Finally, in the absence of insulin, the activity of hormone-sensitive lipase, which breaks down stored triglycerides into free fatty acids, is increased. This increase in lipolysis leads to markedly increased levels of free fatty acids in the circulation. This increases the rate of hepatic ketone body formation; hepatic ketone bodies are weak acids, and once they deplete the available stores of buffer, ketoacidosis results.

Patients with DKA feel acutely ill and tend to seek medical attention within 2 days of the onset of the illness. Patients have polyuria, polydipsia, headache, nausea, vomiting, and abdominal pain. Patients may complain of dyspnea, which results from an increase in the depth of their respirations in an attempt to compensate for their metabolic acidosis (Kussmaul's respirations). Body temperature tends to be low or normal, even in the presence of infection. An elevated temperature almost always indicates infection. Patients can present with generalized neurologic abnormalities, usually in the form of depressed mental activity. The patient's level of consciousness is related to serum osmolality, not to the degree of acidosis.

Hyperosmolar Nonketotic Syndrome (HNKS)

Table 71–8 describes the differences between DKA and HNKS. Patients with HNKS have type II diabetes and tend to be older. The onset of symptoms is generally more gradual, usually over at least 7 to 10 days. Patients usually have a blood glucose level >800 mg/dl, a serum osmolality >350 mOsm/kg, marked dehydration, and the absence of ketoacidosis. (Serum osmolality = 2[Na + K] + [glucose]/18 + [BUN]/2.8.) The exact mechanism or mechanisms by which ketoacidosis is avoided are un-

TABLE 71–8	A Comparison of Diabetic Ketoacidosis (DKA) and Hyperosmolar Nonketotic Syndrome (HNKS)

Feature	DKA	HNKS
Age of patient	Usually <40 yr	Usually >60 yr
Duration of symptoms	Usually <2 days	Usually >5 days
Serum glucose concentration	Usually <800 mg/dl	Usually >800 mg/dl
Serum sodium concentration [Na+]	More likely to be normal or low	More likely to be normal or high
Serum bicarbonate concentration [HCO3−]	Low	Normal
Ketone bodies	At least 4+ in 1:1 dilution	<2+ in 1:1 dilution
pH	Low	Normal
Serum osmolality	Usually <350 mOsm/kg	Usually >350 mOsm/kg
Cerebral edema	Occasionally clinical symptoms	Rarely (never?) clinical
Prognosis	3–10% mortality	10–20% mortality
Subsequent course	Insulin therapy required in almost all cases	Insulin therapy not required in most cases

TABLE 71–9	Guidelines for Diagnosing and Treating Diabetic Ketoacidosis (DKA)

1. DKA suspected based on clinical history, signs, and symptoms
   a) Confirm quickly with fingerstick BG/urine ketone measurement/ABG (optional)
2. If urine ketones positive and ABG indicates acidosis, along with a normal to elevated BG level, DKA likely
   a) Measure Chem Panel (Na, K, HCO_3, Cl, BUN, Cr, Glu), serum ketones, CBC with differential STAT; also measure Ca and PO_4
   b) Obtain EKG, CXR (if indicated)
   c) If succusion splash or dilated stomach present on physical examination, nasogastric tube for emptying of stomach contents
   d) Work-up other precipitating factor(s)
3. Start
   a) IV fluids (usually NS) at 500–1000 ml/hr
   b) IV insulin drip at 5 units/hr
   c) Potassium replacement before laboratory results return if patient urinating and T waves nonpeaked (add 20 mEq KCl/L); if T waves flat or U waves present, add 40 mEq KCl/L; if T waves peaked and/or patient anuric, wait for measured potassium level to return before deciding on potassium replacement
4. Follow-up
   a) Fingerstick BG every 2 hr initially—the BG level should decrease by 100 mg/dl/hr; if BG levels do not fall by at least 10% after first 2–3 hr and patient is receiving adequate hydration, double the insulin infusion rate (this usually does not occur); double the rate every 2 hr until BG levels begin to decrease by at least 10%
   b) Measure urine output; measure urine ketones every 4 hr
   c) Obtain Chem Panel every 2 hr × 3; decrease frequency once patient improving; use Chem Panel to assess need for potassium replacement; bicarbonate level and anion gap useful to indicate improvement of acidosis and resolution of DKA (usually not necessary to measure repeat ABG)
   d) PO_4 level every 8 hours; replace if ≤1 mg/dl
   e) Start dextrose containing IV fluids (usually D_5 ½NS) once BG ≤250 mg/dl
   f) Switch from NS to ½NS (with or without dextrose, depending on BG level) once clinical evidence of dehydration is markedly improved (usually after first 3–4 hr of treatment); also decrease IV fluid rate to 250 ml/hr
   g) Decrease rate of insulin drip to maintain BG level at 150–250 mg/dl; NEVER stop the insulin drip until SQ insulin given; increase rate of dextrose infusion if needed to maintain adequate blood glucose levels once insulin drip at 2–3 units/hr—remember that the hyperglycemia resolves more rapidly than does the acidosis
   h) Treat underlying cause of DKA, if present and requires treatment
5. Post-DKA care
   a) Once the patient is able to drink fluids and the ketoacidosis has resolved (indicated by a decreasing anion gap and a rise in serum bicarbonate level), SQ insulin should be started; it is likely that the patient will continue to have a suppressed serum bicarbonate level due to a hypercholeremic metabolic acidosis after the ketoacidosis has resolved
   b) Give a dose of SQ insulin based on the patient's prior dose of insulin (if patient not previously on insulin, start with 10 units of NPH insulin before breakfast and 5 units of NPH insulin before supper in a lean patient—increase the NPH dose by 5 units in an obese patient; add 2–4 units of regular insulin to each NPH dose, as well); give the insulin at the usual time of day the patient would be taking it (e.g., a dose of NPH and regular insulin before breakfast); discontinue the IV insulin 30 min after the SQ insulin is given

ABG = Arterial blood gases; BG = blood glucose; BUN = blood urea nitrogen; CBC = complete blood count; CXR = chest x-ray; EKG = electrocardiogram; Glu = glucose; IV = intravenous; KCl = potassium chloride; NPH = neutral protamine Hagedorn; NS = normal saline; SQ = subcutaneous; STAT = immediately.

clear, since measured insulin levels tend to be similar in patients with DKA and HNKS. However, in HNKS, levels of free fatty acids are lower; therefore, the formation of ketone bodies and subsequent development of DKA does not occur.

In the absence of elevated serum ketone levels, patients have much less nausea, vomiting, and severe abdominal pain than occurs in patients with DKA. Patients with HNKS often gradually develop hyperglycemia with polyuria and subsequent dehydration. Restricted access to free water is common among patients who develop HNKS; this further aggravates the condition. Many patients present with a depressed mental status, although only 20% are comatose. Focal neurologic abnormalities and seizures may occur, caused by the HNKS. However, it is important to search for other causes of focal neurologic changes and seizures, as such concomitant treatable lesions as subdural hematoma may contribute to the central nervous system abnormalities.

Mixed Syndrome

Patients can also develop a mixed syndrome, somewhere along the spectrum between DKA and HNKS. This is most commonly seen in patients who are developing type II diabetes and develop acute bacterial infections or undergo significant physiologic stress. Severe hyperglycemia along with mild to moderate ketoacidosis can occur. With treatment, the syndrome resolves and often patients can subsequently be treated with oral antidiabetic medication.

TREATMENT. The treatment for DKA and HNKS is similar, although some modifications may be necessary, depending on the clinical status of the patient. (Table 71–9 gives an overview of treatment.) Treatment consists of providing fluid, insulin, potassium, and phosphate (if needed) and managing any precipitating illnesses. Rehydration is the most important step in treating these syndromes—without adequate fluid replacement insulin will not work effectively and blood glucose concentrations will remain elevated. Table 71–10 provides guidelines for choosing intravenous fluids. Initial fluid rates should be 500 to 1000 ml/hr, decreasing to 200 to 500 ml/hr once orthostatic changes in blood pressure resolve. Once blood glucose concentrations fall to <250 to 300 mg/dl, intravenous fluids should be changed to contain 5% dextrose (usually D_5 with 0.45% sodium chloride) to prevent blood glucose levels from falling too rapidly to prevent development of cerebral edema.

TABLE 71–10	Choice of Fluids for Treating Diabetic Ketoacidosis (DKA)			
Serum Sodium (mEq/L)	Orthostatic Hypotension	Assessment of Volume Status	Type of Saline	
130–150	Present	Decreased	Normal	
130–150	Absent	Decreased	Half-normal	
<130	Immaterial	Immaterial	Normal	
>150	Immaterial	Immaterial	Half-normal	

Insulin and potassium replacement must be provided in adequate quantities. If a patient presents with an initially low or even normal serum potassium level, replacement of fluid and insulin can drop potassium levels dangerously low. Therefore, potassium replacement (20 to 40 mEq/L) must be started early and continued vigorously until the patient has recovered from the episode of DKA. The morphology of the T wave on the electrocardiogram can be helpful in managing potassium replacement. T waves will fall as serum potassium levels decrease. If the initial T waves are peaked or the patient is anuric, no potassium should be given until a measured level is obtained. If T waves are low and flat and/or U waves are present, start potassium replacement (30 to 40 mEq/hr) before the laboratory measurement is available.

An insulin infusion should be started at a rate of approximately 5 units/hr. This is usually adequate, although if the patient is not responding (<10% fall in blood glucose levels) after 2 to 3 hours (and hydration is adequate), the infusion rate should be doubled. Initially the fall in blood glucose levels is due to renal losses of glucose rather than to the insulin per se, but eventually insulin is required to stop the acidosis (in DKA) and to normalize blood glucose levels. To prepare an insulin infusion, add 100 units (1 ml) of U-100 regular insulin to 500 ml 0.9% sodium chloride, producing a concentration of 0.2 units insulin/ml fluid. Therefore, a drip at a rate of 5 units/hr = 25 ml/hr. Plastic intravenous tubing will adsorb the insulin that initially passes through it, so 50 ml of the insulin solution needs to be run through the IV tubing and emptied into a sink to saturate the adsorption sites before the insulin drip is begun in the patient.

The occasional use of bicarbonate is predicated on the unusual clinical situation of life-threatening hyperkalemia or cardiac arrhythmias only. Even if pH values are <7.0, bicarbonate therapy has not been shown to be helpful. If administered, it should never be given as an intravenous bolus (unless treating hyperkalemia) since it can drive serum potassium levels down and is hyperosmolar. To give bicarbonate, prepare an intravenous infusion and deliver, gradually over several hours.

Phosphate (PO_4) levels fall with treatment; however, this is generally not clinically significant. If PO_4 levels fall below <1mg/dl, half of the potassium replacement can be given as potassium phosphate. However, use of potassium phosphate may cause a fall in serum calcium levels, so replacement should occur gradually, and calcium levels must be monitored.

Elderly patients with HNKS often have underlying cardiovascular disease and should be treated in an intensive care unit, with judicious use of fluids (including central monitoring, if indicated). It is important to evaluate patients for the presence of myocardial infarction because this can trigger HNKS, and the patient may be asymptomatic (or unable to provide an accurate history).

Chronic Complications

The chronic complications of diabetes include microvascular (retinopathy and nephropathy) and neuropathic changes and macrovascular disease. Table 71–11 lists these complications, potential outcomes if they develop, and strategies for preventing and treating them.

TABLE 71–11	Treatment of Diabetic Complications		
Complication	**Treatment**	**Prevention**	**Outcome if Untreated**
Retinopathy (macular edema or proliferative)	Laser photocoagulation Vitrectomy	Near-euglycemia	Blindness
Nephropathy	ACE inhibitors Meticulous control of hypertension Low-protein diet	Near-euglycemia	Dialysis Renal transplantation
Peripheral neuropathy	Education about daily, careful foot care Symptomatic treatment for pain	Near-euglycemia	Foot ulcer
Hypertension	Antihypertensive agents (ACE inhibitors)	Diet Exercise	Stroke Myocardial infarction Renal failure
Peripheral vascular disease	Vascular surgery Exercise	Gentle walking to improve circulation	Lower extremity amputation*
Dyslipidemia	Low-fat diet Weight loss Exercise Lipid-lowering drugs	Low-fat diet Exercise	Atherosclerotic vascular disease

* At times, in conjunction with neuropathy and foot ulcer.
ACE = Angiotensin-converting enzyme.

Retinopathy

Some degree of diabetic retinopathy will develop in >90% of patients who have diabetes if they live long enough with the disease. Up to 25% of patients with "new-onset" type II diabetes will have retinopathy at the time of diagnosis. However, the DCCT proved that maintaining blood glucose levels that are close to normal can decrease the rate of the development of diabetic retinopathy and progression to clinically significant (vision-threatening) forms of the disease. It must be noted, however, that when a patient's blood glucose levels are rapidly brought under control, retinopathy may transiently worsen. However, if near-euglycemia is maintained over time, the retinopathy regresses and patients have less retinopathy in the long term, compared with that in patients who maintain higher blood glucose levels.

There are five stages in the progression of diabetic retinopathy: (1) dilation of the retinal venules and formation of retinal capillary microaneurysms, (2) increased vascular permeability, (3) vascular occlusion and retinal ischemia, (4) proliferation of new blood vessels on the surface of the retina, and (5) hemorrhage and contraction of the fibrovascular proliferation and the vitreous. Patients with type II diabetes do not develop proliferative retinopathy as frequently as those with type I diabetes.

The first two stages of diabetic retinopathy are known as "background" or nonproliferative retinopathy. Initially there is dilation of the venules in the retina, followed by the appearance of microaneurysms. These are 25 to 100 μm in diameter and appear as tiny red dots on the retina. They cause no visual impairment. However, as the microaneurysms and retinal capillaries become more permeable, hard exudates, reflecting the leakage of plasma proteins, appear. They are sharply defined yellow deposits, composed mostly of lipid material. Hard exudates are often found in partial or complete rings (circinate pattern), which usually include microaneurysms. These rings usually mark an area of edematous retina. Edema of the retina occurring in the region of the macula is known as macular edema.

Macular edema can cause visual loss, although patients may notice no change in visual acuity until the center of the macula is involved with marked edema. Laser therapy is quite effective at decreasing macular edema and preserving vision, but it is less effective at restoring vision once it is lost. Therefore, early referral and treatment is essential.

Preproliferative and proliferative diabetic retinopathy are the next stages in the progression of the disease. Cotton wool spots (ischemia of the retina) can be seen in preproliferative retinopathy due to capillary occlusion. In proliferative retinopathy, neovascularization occurs, which is the development of new networks of fragile vessels in response to retinal ischemia. These vessels undergo cycles of proliferation and regression. During these cycles, hemorrhage occurs and adhesions develop between the vessels and the vitreous, causing traction on the retina and retinal detachment. Contraction also further tears the fragile new vessels, which continue to hemorrhage into the vitreous. Patients may notice a small hemorrhage as a "floater" in their field of vision, although a larger hemorrhage may result in marked visual loss. Patients with preproliferative or proliferative retinopathy must be referred immediately for ophthalmologic evaluation, since laser therapy is also effective for these conditions, hopefully prior to actual hemorrhage.

If any degree of diabetic retinopathy is seen on office fundoscopic examination, it is important to send the patient expeditiously to see an ophthalmologist, because more serious retinopathy is often present. All patients with type II diabetes should be referred annually for a dilated ophthalmologic examination (usually performed by an ophthalmologist). All patients with type I diabetes who have had the diagnosis for more than 5 years should also have a dilated ophthalmoscopic examination yearly.

Nephropathy

End-stage renal disease affects 30 to 35% of patients with type I diabetes diagnosed prior to 1965 (and 10 to 15% of patients diagnosed after 1965) and 15 to 20% of patients with type II diabetes. However, since type II diabetes is much more common, patients with type II diabetes constitute the majority of diabetic patients with end-stage renal disease. The goal in treating patients with diabetes is to prevent the development of diabetic nephropathy, which can be particularly difficult if patients are not diagnosed with diabetes until they have had the disease for a number of years.

There are five phases of diabetic nephropathy. The first is hyperfiltration, with an increased glomerular filtration rate (GFR), albumin excretion rate (AER), and renal hypertrophy. The GFR returns to normal after several weeks to months. This phenomenon is associated with an increase in intraglomerular pressure, which may be instrumental in the development of proteinuria in the future if it persists.

In phase II, albumin excretion remains normal (<20 μg/min or 30 mg/24 hr). Some patients (particularly those with poor glycemic control) may persist in having hyperfiltration, which portends an increased risk for the future development of diabetic nephropathy. During this time, patients may gradually develop glomerulosclerosis, with thickening of the glomerular capillary basement membrane and the expansion of the collagen matrix within the mesangial region. Although this process occurs in many patients with diabetes, progression to end-stage renal disease does not occur in all but is more likely to occur in those patients with higher blood glucose levels.

Patients who are progressing toward end-stage renal disease enter phase III (incipient diabetic nephropathy), in which microalbuminuria is present. Microalbuminuria is defined as an albumin excretion rate of 20 to 200 μg/min (30 to 300 mg/24 hr). During this phase of nephropathy, patients usually initially have a normal GFR, which begins to fall as the microalbuminuria increases. Approximately 80% of patients with sustained microalbuminuria will develop clinical diabetic nephropathy over the next 7 to 14 years, although the decline into renal failure can be slowed by meticulous control of blood glucose levels and hypertension, as well as use of angiotensin-converting enzyme ACE inhibitors.

Dipstick positive proteinuria characterizes phase IV. This correlates with an albumin excretion rate > 200 μg/min or 300 mg/24 hr. During this phase, a progressive fall in GFR occurs and hypertension is common. As described previously, close control of hypertension and use of ACE inhibitors is helpful, as is a low-protein (0.6 to 0.8 g/kg/day) diet. Maintenance of near-euglycemia for prevention of diabetic nephropathy is of less benefit, since diabetic nephropathy is now well established.

Phase V is end-stage renal disease and eventually occurs in most patients who develop clinical proteinuria due to diabetic nephropathy. Dialysis is usually started at a GFR of 15 ml/min. However, it is helpful to refer patients to a nephrologist somewhat in advance of starting dialysis so a discussion regarding options (hemodialysis versus peritoneal dialysis versus transplantation) can occur. In diabetic patients, serum creatinine levels can underestimate the severity in the reduction of the GFR, so consideration of referral to a nephrologist should be made when the serum creatinine rises above 3 mg/dl.

Neuropathy

There are many types of diabetic neuropathy, which can be both peripheral and autonomic. As with the microvascular complications, the risk of developing neuropathy is related to the duration of diabetes and the degree of diabetic control maintained over those years. The most frequent type of neuropathy seen is a distal symmetric sensorimotor polyneuropathy (with a "glove and stocking" distribution). The importance of this type of neuropathy, in addition to the pain often experienced by the patient in its early stages, is the eventual loss of peripheral sensation. This leads to an inability to perceive trauma. Motor involvement can lead to muscle weakness and atrophy. These changes can result in a variety of foot deformities, which can increase the pressure on various areas of the feet not routinely subject to such pressures. The combination of decreased sensation, foot deformities, and peripheral arterial insufficiency often leads to foot ulceration and eventual need for amputation.

The onset of a distal polyneuropathy is gradual and usually begins in the feet. Patients initially have sensory symptoms (burning paresthesias, hyperesthesias) that can be quite painful and disturbing, especially at night. As the neuropathy progresses, the feet become numb, and the patient loses the protective sensation required to avoid trauma to the feet. On physical examination, patients lose their distal reflexes, vibration sense, and sense of touch. An inability to feel a 5.07 monofilament on the sole of the foot indicates that the patient has lost enough sensation to be at risk for the development of foot ulcers.

There are a variety of acute-onset mononeuropathies in diabetes. These include acute cranial mononeuropathies, mononeuropathy multiplex, focal lesions of the brachial or lumbosacral plexus, and radiculopathies. Of cranial neuropathies, the third nerve (oculomotor) is the most commonly affected, followed by the sixth (abducens) and, finally, the fourth (trochlear). Acute cranial nerve mono-

neuropathies usually resolve within 2 to 9 months. These neuropathies are thought to be caused by acute thrombosis or ischemia of the blood vessels supplying the nervous system structure involved.

The types of autonomic dysfunction that can occur are myriad and can involve any part of the sympathetic or parasympathetic chain. They include alterations in heart rate, blood pressure, skin, gastrointestinal motility, and the genitourinary tract (including impotence as well as incontinence). Treatment is symptomatic, and symptoms tend to wax and wane over time. Patients with gastroparesis may benefit from use of metoclopramide, cisapride, or erythromycin. Those with diabetic diarrhea may benefit from a trial of antibiotics. Patients with disabling orthostatic hypotension may be treated with salt tablets, support stockings, or 9α-fluorohydrocortiosone.

Diabetic Foot

Fifty to seventy percent of all nontraumatic lower extremity amputations occur in diabetic patients. This complication can usually be prevented if adequate foot care is provided. At one clinic, the rate of amputation was halved after patients were required to remove their shoes and socks at every visit. It is important to teach patients to examine their own feet daily and to take off their shoes to have their feet examined at every visit to a physician. If patients become involved in this process, they can have a significant impact on lowering their risk of amputation.

Amputation is the end result of a cascade of events, the key to which is distal sensory motor neuropathy compounded by arterial insufficiency. The insensate, poorly perfused foot is at risk for ulcers from pressure necrosis or inflammatory autolysis from repeated moderate skin stress and unnoticed trauma. Either can evolve into cellulitis or the more serious complications of osteomyelitis or nonclostridial gangrene that end in amputation.

Diabetic patients presenting with wounds, infections, or ulcers of the foot should be treated intensively (see Chapter 101). In addition to appropriate use of antibiotics, it is mandatory to prevent further trauma to the healing foot through the use of crutches, wheelchairs, or bed rest. Patients should be treated by a podiatrist or an orthopedist with experience in the care of a diabetic foot. If bone or tendon is visible or osteomyelitis is present, hospitalization for intravenous antibiotics is usually necessary. Many patients need a vascular evaluation in conjunction with local treatment of the foot ulcer, since in some cases a revascularization procedure may be required to provide adequate blood flow for wound healing.

Macrovascular Disease

Macrovascular disease is the leading cause of death in patients with diabetes, causing 75% of the deaths in this population, compared with approximately 35% of deaths in patients without diabetes. The presence of diabetes causes a twofold increase in men and a fourfold increase in women in myocardial infarction that is in addition to the other known risk factors. The risk of stroke is doubled, and the risk of developing peripheral vascular disease is increased fourfold. In the presence of other risk factors for macrovascular disease, such as increased low-density lipoprotein (LDL) cholesterol, hypertension, family history of heart disease, or cigarette smoking, the likelihood of macrovascular disease increases further. Although the disease process itself is the same as in patients without diabetes, atherosclerosis develops earlier and follows a more malignant course in patients with diabetes.

No direct correlation exists between hyperglycemia and macrovascular disease. Abnormalities such as small, dense LDLs (which are more atherogenic), oxidized or glycated LDL, increased platelet aggregation, and increased clotting factors probably contribute to the enhanced risk of atherosclerotic vascular disease. Hypertension is twice as common in patients with type II diabetes; this also increases the risk of atherosclerosis.

Patients with diabetes must therefore have their hypertension and measurable lipid abnormalities treated aggressively to lessen their risk of developing serious atherosclerosis. Ideally, all patients with diabetes should have an LDL cholesterol level <130 mg/dl (<100 mg/dl if coronary artery disease is already present) and a triglyceride level of <250 mg/dl (<150 mg/dl if coronary artery disease is present). The initial approach to therapy is diet, exercise, and attainment of near-euglycemia (which will lower triglyceride levels). If this fails, the patient should be started on a 3-hydroxy-3-methylglutoryl-coenzyme A (HMG Co-A) reductase inhibitor for lowering cholesterol levels or gemfibrozil for lowering triglyceride levels (see Chapter 60). For patients with persistent elevations in both LDL cholesterol and triglyceride levels, a combination of the two drugs may be cautiously tried, recognizing that the risk for developing rhabdomyolysis is increased. If a patient has a persistently elevated LDL cholesterol level on a maximal dose of an HMG Co-A reductase inhibitor and does not have hypertriglyceridemia, a small dose of a resin (cholestyramine, colestid) can be added for further cholesterol lowering.

Hypertension should be treated initially with ACE inhibitors to lower the risk of developing diabetic nephropathy. However, since hypertension accelerates the development of atherosclerosis and nephropathy, it is most important that it is adequately treated. Ideally, the blood pressure should be lowered to <130/85 mm Hg. If ACE inhibitors are not tolerated or are associated with unacceptable hyperkalemia, calcium channel blockers, alpha-adrenergic blockers, or vasodilators, which have no adverse effects on diabetes or lipids, should be used. Beta blockers, which may mask the hyperadrenergic warning signs of hypoglycemia, may be dangerous, especially in insulin-treated patients. Small doses of thiazide diuretics can be used, although it is important to maintain normal serum potassium levels (decreased potassium levels can decrease insulin secretion).

Patients with diabetes have a lifelong struggle to reach and maintain blood glucose levels as close to the normal range as possible. With appropriate glycemic control, the risk of the microvascular and neuropathic complications is markedly decreased. Additionally, if hypertension and hyperlipidemia are aggressively treated, the risk of the macrovascular complications should fall as well. However, these benefits are weighed against the risk of hypoglycemia (especially in patients with type I diabetes) and the cost of providing high-quality preventive care. In the long term, improved diabetic control will reduce the costs associated with the chronic complications of diabetes, but in the short term, it is more expensive. Therefore, it is important that with each physician encounter, patients with diabetes are educated and encouraged to follow an appropriate treatment plan. It is also necessary to ensure that all necessary referrals (e.g., ophthalmology, podiatry), laboratory tests (e.g., quarterly $HgbA_{1c}$ levels, yearly lipid panel, and assessment of renal function), and diabetes-related examinations (e.g., foot and neurologic examinations) are performed.

REFERENCES

American Diabetes Association: Standards of medical care for patients with diabetes mellitus. Diabetes Care 1994; 17:616–623.

Clark CM, Lee DA: Prevention and treatment of the complications of diabetes mellitus. N Engl J Med 1995; 332:1210–1217.

DeFronzo RA, Goodman AM, et al: Efficacy of metformin in patients with non–insulin-dependent diabetes mellitus. N Engl J Med 1995; 333:541–549.

DeFronzo RA, Matsuda M, Barrett EJ: Diabetic ketoacidosis. Diabetes Rev 1994; 2:209–238.

The Diabetes Control and Complications Trial Research Group: The effect of intensive treatment of diabetes on the development and progression of long-term complications in insulin-dependent diabetes mellitus. N Engl J Med 1993; 329:977–986.

72

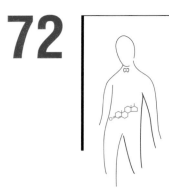

Hypoglycemia

The clinical syndrome of hypoglycemia is defined by a low blood glucose level accompanied by the signs and symptoms of the adrenergic and/or neuroglycopenic symptoms of hypoglycemia that are relieved by the ingestion of carbohydrate and a return of blood glucose levels toward normal. There are many possible causes for the development of hypoglycemia, apart from hypoglycemia associated with the treatment of diabetes mellitus. In some situations, hypoglycemia occurs primarily in a fasted condition, while in others it is more common in the fed state. The clinical situation of the patient is also important in determining the etiology of the disorder. Hospitalized, acutely ill patients have somewhat different reasons for developing hypoglycemia than do otherwise healthy outpatients. It is also important to remember that low blood glucose levels (even < 45 mg/dl) can be found in completely normal women during a fast or oral glucose tolerance test, without symptoms of hypoglycemia. Therefore, biochemical hypoglycemia may not indicate that the patient has clinical hypoglycemia. On the other hand, adrenergic symptoms of "hypoglycemia" may occur in patients without low blood glucose levels. Therefore, the diagnosis of hypoglycemia in an otherwise healthy patient must be based both on the presence of biochemical hypoglycemia and concomitant hypoglycemic symptoms.

DEFINITION OF A LOW BLOOD GLUCOSE LEVEL

When measuring blood glucose levels, it is important to know the circumstances under which the value was obtained. For instance, glucose concentrations in plasma or serum samples are 15% higher than those measured in whole blood samples. A capillary sample produces different results than a venous sample. Fasting values have different normal ranges than do post-prandial values. During insulin-induced hypoglycemia, adrenergic symptoms (Table 72–1) of hypoglycemia start at ~60 mg/dl, and evidence of neuroglycopenia occurs at ~50 mg/dl. In general, hypoglycemia is considered to be present at a fasting plasma glucose concentration of <60 mg/dl or a fasting whole blood (or capillary) glucose concentration of <50 mg/dl. In the fed state, several

hours after eating glucose or food, hypoglycemia is considered present when these values are approximately 10 mg/dl lower.

NORMAL PHYSIOLOGY

In patients who do not have disorders of glucose metabolism, preprandial blood glucose levels are usually 70 to 100 mg/dl, with a small post-prandial increase (blood glucose values rise steadily with age, however). Blood glucose and insulin levels peak 1 hour after eating and return to baseline within 3 to 4 hours. In the fasting state, a balance is maintained between glucose utilization and production, so normal blood glucose levels are maintained. The major glucose-requiring tissues are the brain, red blood cells, and muscle. Glucose production occurs through glycogenolysis (the breakdown of glycogen), which accounts for most of the glucose production during an overnight fast, and gluconeogenesis (the synthesis of new carbohydrate from noncarbohydrate sources), which is an increasingly important source of glucose as glycogen stores are depleted. When a patient is fasting for a prolonged period, glucose levels fall gradually and then stabilize, usually at a level 15 to 20 mg/dl lower than normal. Insulin levels fall until the patient eats.

Response to Hypoglycemia

Glucoreceptors in the hypothalamus sense low blood glucose levels and cause the secretion of counterregulatory hormones. Glucagon is the primary counterregulatory hormone in nondiabetic humans (patients with type 1 diabetes lose their glucagon response to hypoglycemia within the first 5 years of the onset of the disease). Its onset of action is rapid, and it acts by increasing hepatic glycogenolysis as well as gluconeogenesis. If glucagon is not present, epinephrine serves as the major counterregulatory hormone. It has a rapid onset of action. It acts by inhibiting glucose utilization by muscle, increasing gluconeogenesis, and inhibiting insulin secretion. Cortisol and growth hormone are secreted as part of normal hypoglycemic counterregulation, but their release is delayed and they do not contribute to the acute recovery from hypoglycemia.

TABLE 72–1	Signs and Symptoms of Hypoglycemia

Adrenergic*

Weakness
Sweating/warmth
Tachycardia
Palpitations
Tremor
Nervousness
Irritability
Tingling of mouth and fingers
Hunger
Nausea†
Vomiting†

Neuroglucopenic‡

Headache
Hypothermia
Visual disturbances
Mental dullness
Confusion
Amnesia
Seizures
Coma

* Caused by increased activity of the autonomic nervous system—most accurately called autonomic or neurogenic symptoms since the symptoms reflect increased activity of the sympathetic and parasympathetic nervous system.
† Unusual.
‡ Caused by decreased activity of the central nervous system.

Signs and Symptoms of Hypoglycemia

The signs and symptoms of hypoglycemia fall into two categories: adrenergic (those caused by increased activity of the autonomic nervous system) and neuroglycopenic (those caused by depressed activity of the central nervous system) (see Table 72–1). Symptoms of hypoglycemia vary from person to person, but within an individual, the set of hypoglycemic symptoms remains fairly constant from episode to episode. Patients who are chronically hypoglycemic seem to accommodate to the hypoglycemia. These patients may not have an adrenergic response to hypoglycemia until blood glucose levels are ≤50 mg/dl and close to the time when neuroglycopenic symptoms develop. This can occur in patients with hypoglycemia due to any cause—intensively treated patients with type 1 diabetes as well as those with insulinomas. Patients with diabetes have several causes for this syndrome, known as hypoglycemia-associated autonomic failure. Defective glucose counterregulation, lowered glycemic threshold due to intensive insulin therapy, lowered glycemic thresholds following recent hypoglycemia, and hypoglycemia-associated autonomic failure all contribute, in various proportions, to a patient's inability to sense episodes of hypoglycemia. These diabetic patients are left with only the late counterregulatory hormone response, which occurs too late to prevent the development of neuroglycopenic symptoms. Much individual variation exists in patients' responses to hypoglycemia; some patients tolerate low blood glucose levels better than others. Therefore, patients with hypoglycemic disorders may present with unusual symptoms of neuroglycopenia rather than with classic adrenergic symptoms of hypoglycemia.

CAUSES OF HYPOGLYCEMIA

Fasting Hypoglycemia in Healthy-Appearing Individuals

Drugs

The most common cause of hypoglycemia is the use of insulin or sulfonylurea agents (Table 72–2). Usually a patient is under treatment for known diabetes, and the cause of the hypoglycemia is obvious. Occasionally, nondiabetic patients use insulin or sulfonylurea agents to create factitious hypoglycemia. The surreptitious use of medication can be assessed by measurement of sulfonylurea agents in the plasma or by the presence of high insulin levels but suppressed C-peptide levels on a 72-hour fast (see later). Sometimes patients, especially elderly patients, may mistakenly take another's sulfonylurea agent, confusing it with another drug. Alternatively, pharmacy errors may occur. Therefore, it is often useful to have the patient or a family member bring in all of the medications currently being taken to determine if inadvertent ingestion of a sulfonylurea agent is occurring.

Pentamidine may cause destruction of the B cell, with acute release of insulin, which produces hypoglycemia. Later, hyperglycemia develops. Propranolol can cause hypoglycemia by reducing the glycogenolytic response to epinephrine in muscle. It can also mask the

TABLE 72–2	Causes of Hypoglycemia

Fasting

Healthy-appearing individual*
  Drugs
    Exogenous insulin
    Sulfonylurea agents
    Beta-adrenergic blocking agents
    Disopyramide
    Quinine
    Pentamidine
    Salicylates
    Others
  Ethanol
  Non–B cell tumors
  Insulinomas†
  Insulin autoantibodies†
  Insulin receptor autoantibodies†
  Inherited disorders of metabolism
Ill-appearing/hospitalized patient
  Hepatic failure
  Renal failure
  Adrenal insufficiency†
  Sepsis
  Shock
  Malnutrition/anorexia nervosa
  Congestive heart failure

Fed (Reactive)

Alimentary
Impaired glucose tolerance
Idiopathic reactive

* Causes of hypoglycemia under this category can also occur in the ill-appearing patient.
† Can cause fasted and/or fed hypoglycemia.

adrenergic symptoms of hypoglycemia. Salicylates inhibit prostaglandins, which may increase insulin secretion, resulting in hypoglycemia in children. Disopyramide and monoamine oxidase inhibitors occasionally cause hypoglycemia. Quinine treatment of malaria may also cause hypoglycemia. This may be due to drug-induced insulin release or possibly to increased glucose utilization by parasitized red blood cells. A number of other medications may rarely cause hypoglycemia, either alone or in combination with other drugs. If a new medication has been started in a patient who subsequently experiences hypoglycemia, a literature search should be performed to determine if the medication is known to cause hypoglycemia. If not, and if discontinuing the new medication does not relieve the hypoglycemia, a search for other causes for the hypoglycemia must be undertaken.

Ethanol

Excessive ethanol ingestion can cause hypoglycemia. This is due to suppression of hepatic gluconeogenesis, and it is readily reversed by administration of carbohydrate. This occurs both in malnourished chronic alcoholics and in heavy weekend drinkers (or, rarely, social drinkers) who eat inadequate amounts of food while drinking.

Insulinomas (B Cell Tumors)

Insulinomas are rare tumors that occur in 1 per 250,000 individuals. The median age at diagnosis is 50 years (except in multiple endocrine neoplasia I [MEN I] syndrome, in which the median age of onset is in the mid-20s). Most are benign (95%) and solitary (93%). Eight percent are associated with MEN I syndromes. Patients with insulinomas often are undiagnosed for several years, and because they have become so adapted to hypoglycemia, they manifest neuroglycopenic symptoms (e.g., diplopia, blurred vision, weakness, confusion, bizarre behavior, seizures) instead of classic adrenergic symptoms. In at least 20% of patients, these symptoms are initially misdiagnosed as a psychiatric or neurologic disorder. Patients with insulinomas often note weight gain, which occurs because they eat large amounts of food to self-treat the hypoglycemia.

Patients are usually diagnosed with a 72-hour fast (see later). Most patients have predominantly fasting hypoglycemia, although a few may have post-prandial hypoglycemia as well. After the biochemical diagnosis is made, imaging studies are usually performed. However, standard imaging techniques often fail to localize the tumor because many are < 2 cm in size. Computed tomography, ultrasound, magnetic resonance imaging, and celiac-axis angiography are not sufficiently sensitive for localizing the smaller insulinomas. Much depends on the skill and experience of the radiologist. Transhepatic portal venous sampling can often identify the region where the insulinoma is located but is not widely available.

If the biochemical findings are convincing enough, surgery should be performed by an experienced surgeon, even when imaging studies are negative. At surgery, tumors are often found by intraoperative ultrasound, which is the most sensitive method for localization. If no tumor is located at the time of surgery, a distal pancreatectomy can be performed in the hope that the tumor will be found in the section removed.

Although surgical removal is the treatment of choice, some patients refuse surgery, and others need medical therapy while waiting for surgery. Diazoxide is usually the most effective medical form of therapy, although phenytoin, chlorpromazine, propranolol, or verapamil can all be used to raise blood glucose levels. If the tumor is malignant, chemotherapy using streptozotocin is most effective.

Non–B Cell Tumors

A variety of different non–B cell tumors can produce hypoglycemia. These include large mesenchymal tumors (~50%), hepatocellular carcinomas (~25%), adrenal carcinomas (5 to 10%), gastrointestinal tumors (5 to 10%), lymphomas (5 to 10%), and, rarely, other tumors. The mechanism by which these tumors cause hypoglycemia is not clear in many cases. Some tumors secrete insulin-like growth factor II (IGF-II), which can cause hypoglycemia. Hypoglycemia caused by non–B cell tumors is diagnosed in a patient who either has a known tumor or elevated levels of IGF-II (with suppressed IGF-I levels). Some patients undergo a 72-hour fast before the diagnosis is made (Table 72–3). Treatment is linked with treatment of the tumor. If it is impossible to reduce the tumor burden and frequent meals are not effective, some patients benefit from treatment with glucocorticoids.

TABLE 72–3	Protocol for Performing a 72-Hour Fast

1. Patient admitted to hospital.
2. Blood glucose level monitored by bedside glucose meter every 4 hours and when symptoms of hypoglycemia develop.
3. When symptoms of hypoglycemia develop accompanied by a blood glucose (BG) level of ≤50 mg/dl, draw "diagnostic labs." These labs consist of a fasting plasma glucose (FPG) concentration, serum insulin, C-peptide and proinsulin levels, and a serum sample for sulfonylurea agents and insulin-like growth factor (IGF)-I and IGF-II levels (the latter three to be sent only once per fast).
4. The fast is completed when the patient has symptoms of hypoglycemia and a documented blood glucose of <50 mg/dl (or plasma glucose of <45 mg/dl from blood sent for laboratory measurement of glucose) or after 72 hours.
5. The patient is fed a meal and discharged from the hospital.
6. If severe, persistent hypoglycemia is documented, the patient may need to be started on medication, such as diazoxide, to prevent further episodes of hypoglycemia while the work-up is proceeding.

Insulin Autoantibodies/Insulin Receptor Autoantibodies

These are exceedingly rare syndromes in which patients develop antibodies either to the insulin molecule itself or to the insulin receptor. In the former situation, the antibodies can bind insulin, releasing it at inappropriate times, leading to hypoglycemia. Such patients often have other autoimmune disorders. In the latter case, the antibodies usually cause insulin resistance but can stimulate the receptor in some circumstances, leading to hypoglycemia.

Hypoglycemia in the Ill-Appearing/Hospitalized Patient

Hypoglycemia can occur in hospitalized patients. Over 1% of acutely ill, hospitalized patients may have plasma glucose levels < 49 mg/dl on at least one occasion. The primary causes of hypoglycemia in the hospital setting are renal insufficiency, malnutrition, liver disease, infection, and shock. Many patients have more than one risk factor for hypoglycemia. Patients with these causes for hypoglycemia are usually seriously ill, and the diagnosis is fairly straightforward. However, in some cases, adrenal insufficiency, a reversible cause for hypoglycemia, may be present; this possibility should be evaluated if the clinical situation does not explain the hypoglycemia (see Chapter 67).

Hepatic Failure

Hepatic failure sometimes leads to hypoglycemia because the liver loses its capacity to release and store glycogen, as well as to perform gluconeogenesis. Hypoglycemia may occur in cases of fulminant hepatic failure and may also occasionally occur in such disorders as acute viral hepatitis and severe right heart failure.

Renal Failure

The mechanism by which renal failure causes hypoglycemia has not been well defined. Reduced food intake may play a role, as well as the prolonged half-life of potentially hypoglycemia-inducing medications (such as insulin and sulfonylurea agents).

Adrenal Insufficiency

Adrenal insufficiency does not often cause symptomatic hypoglycemia, but must be considered in the differential diagnosis for hypoglycemia. Cortisol is necessary to support gluconeogenesis, and without it glucose levels (especially fasting ones) may fall. To screen for adrenal insufficiency, a cortrosyn stimulation test (0.25 mg IV of cortrosyn; blood samples for cortisol at baseline and 30 and 60 minutes later) can be performed. A cortisol level of ≥ 20 μg/dl following cortrosyn is considered a normal test result. If there is a strong clinical suspicion for secondary adrenal insufficiency, a metyrapone stimulation test can be carried out (see Chapter 67). Treatment of hypoglycemia caused by adrenal insufficiency consists of providing intravenous hydrocortisone (usually 100 mg every 8 hours for at least the first 24 hours) and adequate intravenous glucose.

Miscellaneous Causes

Many other clinical situations are associated with hypoglycemia. The etiology of the hypoglycemia is often multifactorial. The differential diagnosis includes sepsis, shock, congestive heart failure, and states of severe malnutrition, including anorexia nervosa. In children, certain congenital metabolic syndromes can cause hypoglycemia, which persists into adulthood if the patient survives; these syndromes include glycogen storage disease, glucose-6-phosphatase deficiency, galactosemia, hereditary fructose intolerance, and carnitine deficiency. Usually these are diagnosed within the first year of life, and patients must receive lifelong treatment for the disorder.

Fed (Reactive) Hypoglycemia

Alimentary

Alimentary hypoglycemia is hypoglycemia that occurs in patients who have undergone gastrointestinal surgery, usually gastrectomy, or, less commonly, gastrojejunostomy, pyloroplasty, or vagotomy. Patients have symptoms of hypoglycemia that occur 30 to 120 minutes after eating. The hypoglycemia is thought to occur because the relationship between the stomach and small intestine is disturbed, such that gastric contents empty more quickly into the duodenum. This causes rapid absorption of glucose, and the ensuing hyperglycemia triggers an enhanced insulin response. In addition, the release of one or more gastrointestinal hormones that augment glucose-stimulated insulin secretion might occur.

Idiopathic Reactive Hypoglycemia/Idiopathic Postprandial Syndrome

Much attention has been given to this putative form of hypoglycemia. In general, it has been hard to document that the adrenergic symptoms occur simultaneously with the biochemical finding of hypoglycemia. The adrenergic symptoms are often vague and not relieved by food. (If symptoms are relieved by food, it is more likely that they are due to true hypoglycemia.) Part of the reason that this disorder is overdiagnosed is because women with normal glucose tolerance can have blood glucose levels that fall below 45 mg/dl during a 5-hour oral glucose tolerance test (OGTT) (as well as during a 72-hour fast); some interpret this as clinical hypoglycemia, which is not appropriate unless the low glucose value is accompanied by symptoms of hypoglycemia. Moreover, even if symptoms occur during one of these artificial testing situations, the symptoms are often not associated with low blood glucose levels following mixed meals in an ambulatory setting. Therefore, biochemical hypoglycemia can occur during testing when the patient does not have a clinically relevant hypoglycemia disorder.

Impaired Glucose Tolerance (IGT)

Some patients with IGT and 'mild' diabetes experience post-prandial hypoglycemia. This is due to an initially delayed insulin response to food, which is followed by increased insulin secretion that produces post-prandial hypoglycemia. If a patient has risk factors for the development of type II diabetes, a 2-hour OGTT can be performed to diagnose diabetes or impaired tolerance (not to diagnose hypoglycemia).

DIAGNOSTIC WORK-UP FOR HYPOGLYCEMIA

To evaluate a patient for the presence of hypoglycemia, it is important to document that true hypoglycemia is occurring (Fig. 72–1). Ambulatory patients can be trained in

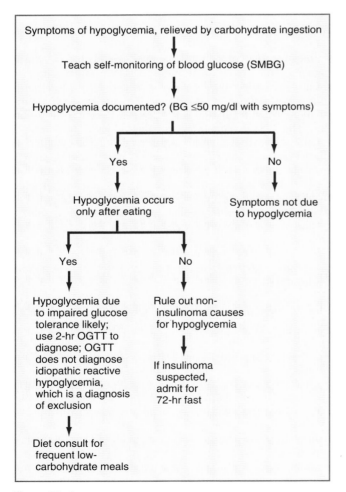

Figure 72–1
Outpatient work-up for suspected hypoglycemia.

self-monitoring of blood glucose (SMBG) and in checking their blood glucose levels when they have symptoms of hypoglycemia. If the blood glucose levels are low and the symptoms resolve when carbohydrate is ingested, it is likely that the patient has bone fide hypoglycemia. If the hypoglycemia occurs in the fed state, it is likely to be caused by impaired glucose tolerance and, in rare cases, by idiopathic reactive hypoglycemia. If reactive hypoglycemia is diagnosed (see Fig. 72–1), the patient should see a dietitian for a diet designed to ameliorate these episodes.

When fasting hypoglycemia occurs, it is more likely to be caused by an organic medical problem, although some of the underlying disorders (such as insulinoma or adrenal insufficiency) can present with both fasting and fed hypoglycemia (see Table 72–2). When patients are hospitalized and acutely ill, the distinction between fasting and fed hypoglycemia is less clear; the work-up should then originate with an understanding of the patient's underlying medical problems and medications and how these might alter blood glucose levels (see Table 72–2).

The standard evaluation for hypoglycemia not attributable to any other underlying cause is to admit the patient to the hospital for a supervised 72-hour fast. During the period of the fast, the patient is allowed to consume noncaloric, noncaffeinated beverages, but nothing else (except for required medications). Table 72–3 describes the procedure for the fast. Blood glucose levels are measured with a reflectance meter every 4 hours; plasma glucose and serum insulin, C-peptide, and proinsulin levels are measured only when the blood glucose level drops below 50 mg/dl *and* the patient experiences symptoms of hypoglycemia. The fast is ended when blood glucose levels (by reflectance meter) fall below 50 mg/dl ($<$45 mg/dl in a plasma sample) *and* the patient has symptoms of hypoglycemia, or when 72 hours has passed. At the end of the fast, all of the specified samples should be sent to the laboratory and the patient fed a meal. Approximately 75% of patients with an insulinoma will develop symptomatic hypoglycemia within the first 24 hours, an additional 10% in the next 24 hours, and only 5% in the final 24 hours. Difficulties in performing the fast arise when blood glucose levels fall below 50 mg/dl and the patient has no symptoms of hypoglycemia, or when the patient develops symptoms at normal blood glucose levels. In the former case, it may be useful to continue to measure blood and blood glucose levels while the patient is under close observation by a physician until blood glucose levels fall to $<$45 mg/dl. In the latter instance, the fast can be continued as long as it seems clinically warranted to convince both patient and physician that the symptoms the patient is experiencing are not associated with hypoglycemia. Table 72–4 summarizes the expected findings in various conditions at the completion of the fast.

TREATMENT

Hypoglycemia should be considered in every unconscious patient, and blood should be obtained for a glucose deter-

TABLE 72–4	Interpretation of Results from a 72-Hour Fast					
Condition	Glucose (mg/dl)	Insulin (μU/ml)	C-Peptide (nmol/L)	Proinsulin (pmol/L)	Plasma Sulfonylurea Level	IGF-II
Normal*	≥40	<6	<0.2	<5	−	−
Insulinoma	≤45	≥6	≥0.2	≥5	−	−
Exogenous insulin	≤45	≥6†	<0.2	<5	−	−
Sulfonylurea agents	≤45	≥6	≥0.2	≥5	+	−
Tumor secreting IGF-II	≤45	≤6	<0.2	<5	−	+ (↓ IGF-I)

* Normal insulin, C-peptide, and proinsulin levels may be higher if blood glucose levels are not <60 mg/dl.
† Insulin levels may be very high (>100 μU/ml) in these patients.
IGF = Insulin-like growth factor; − = absent; + = present or elevated.
Adapted with permission from Service FJ: Hypoglycemic disorders. New Engl J Med 1995; 332:1144–1152.

mination prior to treatment. The initial treatment of a confused or comatose patient is to infuse a bolus of 50 ml of 50% glucose intravenously, after a sample for measuring glucose levels has been obtained. The bolus of glucose should be followed by the continuous infusion of 10% glucose at a rate sufficient to keep the plasma glucose level >100 mg/dl. When the patient is capable of eating, a diet with a minimum of 300 gm/day of carbohydrates should be supplied. In many situations, especially following administration of long-acting insulin or oral hypoglycemic drugs, the hypoglycemia will last for an extended time. It is very important to continue treatment and close observation for an extended period to prevent a relapse.

Longer-term therapy depends on the cause of the hypoglycemia. If the hypoglycemia is a secondary process (such as that due to hepatic or renal failure or sepsis), treatment of the underlying disorder will treat the hypoglycemia. If the hypoglycemia is due to an insulinoma, surgical removal of the tumor is the treatment of choice.

For treatment of all types of reactive hypoglycemia, diet therapy is the cornerstone of therapy. Patients should avoid simple or refined carbohydrates. Some patients also benefit from frequent, small feedings of snacks that con-

tain a mixture of carbohydrate, fat, and protein. Restricting the daily carbohydrate intake to 35 to 40% of total calories can be helpful if avoidance of simple carbohydrates and eating more frequently is ineffective. Drug therapy with propantheline bromide or phenytoin may sometimes be helpful but should be reserved for severe cases. If the disorder is due to alimentary hypoglycemia, diet therapy is usually helpful; in refractory cases (rare), surgery to slow gastric transit time may be successful.

REFERENCES

Charles MA, Hofeldt F, Shackelford A, Waldeck N, Dodson LE, Bunker D, Coggins JT, Eichner H: Comparison of oral glucose tolerance tests and mixed meals in patients with apparent idiopathic postabsorptive hypoglycemia. Diabetes 1981; 30:465–470.

Davidson MB: Hypoglycemia in adults. In Lavin N (ed.): Manual of Endocrinology and Metabolism. Boston, Little Brown & Co, 1994, pp. 459–447.

Service FJ: Hypoglycemic disorders. New Engl J Med 1995; 332:1144–1152.

Service FJ, McMahon MM, O'Brien PC, Ballard DJ: Functioning insulinoma—incidence, recurrence, and long-term survival of patients: A 60-year study. Mayo Clin Proc 1991; 66:711–719.

Diseases of Bone and Bone Mineral Metabolism

Section XI

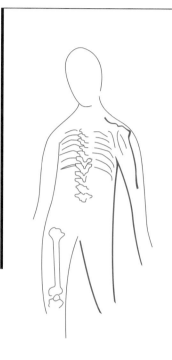

73

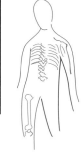

Normal Physiology of Bone and Bone Minerals

BONE STRUCTURE AND METABOLISM

Bone is one of the largest organs in the body. It is superbly designed to carry out several vital functions, including (1) providing support for the body; (2) protecting the hematopoietic system and the structures within the cranium, pelvis, and thorax; (3) allowing for movement by providing levers, articulations, and points of attachment for muscles; and (4) serving as a reservoir for essential ions such as calcium, phosphorus, magnesium, and sodium.

Types of Bone

The skeleton is composed of two types of bone. Cortical bone, sometimes called compact bone, is arranged as circumferential lamellae in the subperiosteal and endosteal layers and as concentric lamellae around a central vascular supply (referred to as osteons or haversian systems) between these two surfaces (Fig. 73–1). Cortical bone constitutes about 80% of the adult skeleton and predominates in the shafts of the long bones. Trabecular bone, sometimes called spongy or cancellous bone, is arranged in microscopically parallel lamellae. It forms a more open pattern than cortical bone and predominates in the vertebral bodies, ribs, pelvis, and ends of the long bones. In general, cortical bone serves the mechanical and protective functions of the skeleton, whereas trabecular bone serves most of the metabolic functions.

Composition of Bone

Cellular Components

Bone is composed of cellular and noncellular components. The three specialized cells necessary for the metabolic activities of bone are the osteoblast, osteoclast, and osteocyte. Osteoblasts are derived from local mesenchymal stem cells and are the bone-forming cells. They are responsible for synthesizing the uncalcified bone matrix, or osteoid, and its subsequent mineralization. Osteoblasts have both parathyroid hormone (PTH) and estrogen receptors. PTH and estrogen, along with other factors in-

cluding insulin-like growth factor–1 and transforming growth factor–β, also stimulate osteoblast activity.

Osteoclasts are multinucleated giant cells that are probably derived from mononuclear phagocytic cells of hematopoietic origin. By creating a localized acidic environment under the ruffled border of the cell, osteoclasts resorb the bone mineral and provide an ideal environment for proteolytic enzymes to degrade the bone matrix. Osteoclasts appear to lack PTH receptors. Thus, stimulation of osteoclasts by PTH appears to be indirect, probably via release of an unidentified paracrine factor from osteoblasts. Osteoclasts do, however, have calcitonin receptors. Osteoclast activity is also stimulated by interleukin-1, prostaglandin E_2, and tumor necrosis factor.

Osteocytes are osteoblasts that have become embedded within the structure of bone and are relatively quiescent. They communicate with each other and with surface osteoblasts through canaliculi and may play a role in mobilizing bone minerals.

Noncellular Components

The noncellular components of bone are the organic matrix and the inorganic matrix. By weight, the organic matrix constitutes about 30 to 35% of bone mass, and the inorganic matrix, about 60 to 65% of bone mass, with the remainder made up of the cellular components. Type I collagen composes 90% of the organic matrix of bone. Other proteins in bone include small amounts of other collagens and noncollagenous proteins, the most abundant of which are osteonectin, osteocalcin, osteopontin, fibronectin, thrombospondin, bone sialoprotein, proteoglycans, and serum proteins. The inorganic matrix of bone is largely composed of hydroxyapatite, a mineral with the formula $Ca_{10}(PO_4)_6(OH)_2$. Its crystals are laid down on the collagen fibrils and in the glycoproteins and proteoglycans (i.e., ground substance) between collagen fibrils. The remaining inorganic components of bone are other calcium phosphates and trace minerals.

CALCIUM METABOLISM

Total body calcium in normal adults is about 1 to 2 kg. Ninety-nine percent of total body calcium is in the skele-

555

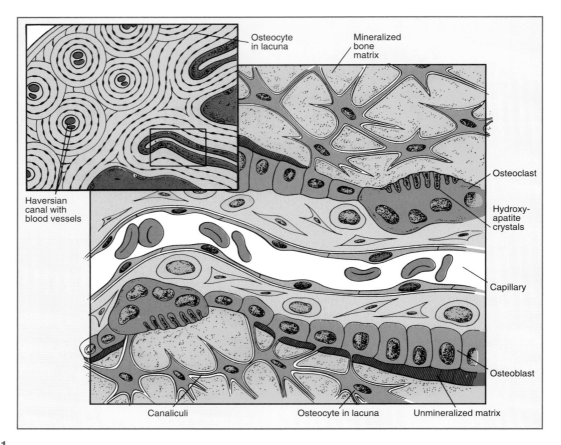

Figure 73–1

The most active bone remodeling occurs around the haversian canals, through which capillaries run. Osteoclasts and osteoblasts in all stages of development are found in greatest density in these areas. *Larger-scale inset drawing* depicts the syncytium-like layer of osteoblasts, connected with lacunar osteocytes via canaliculi, across which substances are exchanged between the modified bone interstitial fluid and the systemic extracellular fluid (ECF). (Reprinted with permission from Levine MM, Kleeman CR: Hypercalcemia: Pathophysiology and treatment. HOSPITAL PRACTICE 1987; 22(7):93. ©1987, The McGraw-Hill Companies. Illustration by Robert Margulies.)

ton, 1% is in the extracellular fluid, and 0.1% is in the cytosol. Calcium has two important physiologic roles. In bone, calcium salts are essential for maintaining the structural integrity of the skeleton. In the extracellular fluid and the cytosol, calcium is essential for a variety of cellular processes. Calcium also acts as an intracellular second messenger for many hormones, paracrine factors, and neurotransmitters.

Extracellular Calcium

Calcium circulates in the plasma in three forms (Fig. 73–2): (1) ionized calcium (approximately 50%), (2) protein-bound calcium (approximately 40%), and (3) calcium that is complexed, mainly to bicarbonate, citrate, and phosphate (about 10%). The free or ionized fraction of blood calcium is physiologically the most important. Albumin accounts for most of the protein binding of calcium; globulins account for the remainder. Acidosis decreases binding of calcium to albumin, thereby increasing ionized calcium, whereas, alkalosis produces the converse situation. Changes in the concentration of albumin in the

blood affect the measurement of the total blood calcium. One frequently used formula for estimating the total blood calcium concentration when blood protein concentrations are altered is

Corrected total calcium concentration (mg/dl)
    = measured total calcium concentration (mg/dl)
  + 0.8 × [4 − measured albumin concentration (gm/dl)]

Because this formula is only a rough approximation, direct measurement of ionized calcium is especially useful in critically ill patients, in those with significant acid-base disturbances, and in those in hypoalbuminemic states.

Intracellular Calcium

The normal cytosolic calcium concentration is about 1/10,000 of extracellular levels. This low concentration is maintained by a system of active transport pumps in the plasma membrane, the inner membrane of the mitochondria, the sarcoplasmic reticulum, and the endoplasmic reticulum.

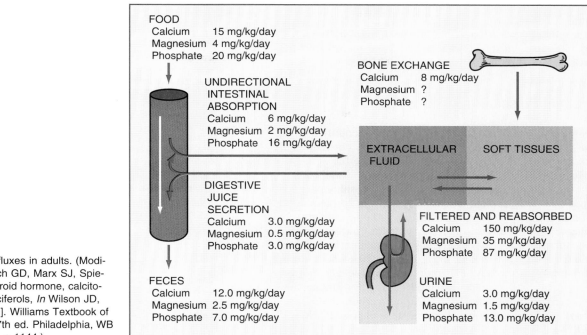

Figure 73–2
Typical mineral fluxes in adults. (Modified from Aurbach GD, Marx SJ, Spiegel AM: Parathyroid hormone, calcitonin, and the calciferols, *In* Wilson JD, Foster DW [eds.]. Williams Textbook of Endocrinology. 7th ed. Philadelphia, WB Saunders, 1985, p 1144.)

Calcium Balance

The level of ionized calcium in the extracellular fluid is homeostatically maintained by an effective balance of bone formation, bone destruction, calcium absorption, and calcium excretion. The principal sites of this regulation are in bone, kidney, and the gastrointestinal tract and are controlled by PTH, 1,25-(OH)$_2$D, and other factors.

Calcium Absorption

The normal dietary intake of healthy adults varies greatly. The average diet of an adult in the United States contains approximately 400 to 1000 mg of calcium, mostly derived from dairy products. The amount of calcium absorbed also varies greatly and is on the order of 25 to 70% of the ingested calcium. On average, adults require daily calcium intakes greater than 400 mg to balance obligate losses in urine, feces, and sweat. When dietary calcium intake exceeds 1000 mg/day, net intestinal calcium absorption tends to increase less steeply in relation to dietary intake than at low intakes. Calcium absorption occurs principally in the duodenum and the jejunum by an active process against an electrochemical gradient. The principal determinant of intestinal absorption of calcium is 1,25-(OH)$_2$D. Calcium absorption is also influenced by dietary intake (at low calcium intakes, fractional calcium absorption is greater than at high calcium intakes), age (calcium absorption declines with advancing age), and underlying medical conditions such as intestinal malabsorption and absorptive idiopathic hypercalciuria.

Calcium Excretion

Calcium is lost in urine, feces, and, to a minor extent, sweat. Fecal calcium excretion consists of both the fraction of the ingested calcium that was not absorbed and the calcium secreted into the gastrointestinal tract in biliary, pancreatic, and gastric juices. The calcium from these intestinal fluids that is not reabsorbed is known as the "endogenous fecal calcium" and accounts for approximately 60 to 150 mg/day of fecal calcium.

The other major route of calcium excretion is the kidneys. Approximately 7 to 10 gm of calcium are filtered by the glomerulus each day, 98% of which is normally reabsorbed. The principal sites of renal calcium reabsorption are the proximal tubule and the loop of Henle. The amount of calcium excreted in the urine of normal individuals varies widely, usually ranging from 50 to 300 mg/day but occasionally being as much as 400 mg/day. Reabsorption of renal tubular calcium is enhanced by PTH, phosphate, metabolic alkalosis, thiazide diuretics, and increased reabsorption of sodium. Renal calcium clearance is enhanced by metabolic acidosis, hypermagnesemia, loop diuretics, saline diuresis, high dietary protein intake, ethanol, severe phosphate depletion, and deficiencies of PTH.

PHOSPHORUS METABOLISM

Phosphate is necessary for a variety of structural and metabolic functions. In the adult, phosphorus constitutes about 10 to 13 gm/kg of body weight, of which 80 to 85% is in the skeleton and 10% is intracellular. In the skeleton, phosphorus is mainly in the form of hydroxyapatite crystals, which are essential for the structural strength of bone. Extracellular phosphorus exists largely as inorganic phosphate ions. Intracellular phosphate is primarily bound or in the form of organic phosphate esters.

Normal Plasma Phosphorus

Normal plasma inorganic phosphate concentration is 0.8 to 1.4 mmol/L (2.5 to 4.5 mg/dl). This is conventionally expressed as elemental phosphorus because the amount of phosphorus in its different forms ($H_2PO_2^-$ and HPO_4^{2-}) varies with pH. In contrast to calcium, phosphorus is 85% free and 15% protein bound. Of the non–protein-bound component, some is complexed to sodium, calcium, and magnesium. The intra- and extracellular concentrations of phosphorus are less closely regulated than those of calcium or magnesium and may vary by 30 to 50% during the course of the day. Plasma phosphorus levels are influenced by age (higher in children and postmenopausal women), diet (levels decrease after carbohydrate ingestion), pH, and a number of hormones, such as PTH, 1,25-$(OH)_2D$, insulin, and growth hormone.

Absorption of Dietary Phosphate

The average diet in the United States contains approximately 600 to 1600 mg of phosphorus per day, 60 to 80% of which is absorbed by passive transport related to the luminal phosphorus concentration and by active transport stimulated by 1,25-$(OH)_2D$. Phosphorus absorption is directly proportional to dietary phosphorus intake. Deficiency in dietary phosphate or an abnormality of absorption is rarely a cause of phosphorus deficiency except in alcoholics or individuals taking large amounts of antacids containing aluminum hydroxide, which binds phosphate and prevents its absorption.

Excretion of Phosphate

Most plasma phosphate is filtered by the glomerulus, after which 80 to 90% is actively reabsorbed, largely in the proximal tubule. In normal adults, urinary phosphate excretion is directly related to dietary phosphate intake. Proximal tubular reabsorption of phosphate is increased by phosphate depletion, hypoparathyroidism, volume contraction, growth hormone, and hypocalcemia. Urinary phosphate excretion is increased by PTH, PTH-related protein, phosphate loading, volume expansion, hypercalcemia, systemic acidosis, hypokalemia, hypomagnesemia, glucocorticoids, calcitonin, carbonic anhydrase inhibitors, thiazides, and furosemide.

Hypophosphatemia

Causes of hypophosphatemia are listed in Table 73–1. Hypophosphatemia does not necessarily indicate a deple-

TABLE 73–1	Causes of Hypophosphatemia

Increased Urinary Losses

Hyperparathyroidism
Humoral hypercalcemia of malignancy
Oncogenic osteomalacia
Extracellular fluid volume expansion
Diabetes mellitus
Acquired renal tubular defects (hypokalemia, hypomagnesemia)
X-linked vitamin D–resistant rickets
Alcohol abuse
Renal tubular acidosis
Hypothyroidism
Drugs: diuretics, glucocorticoids, calcitonin, bicarbonate

Decreased Intestinal Absorption

Vitamin D deficiency
Malabsorption syndromes
Antacid abuse
Starvation
Alcohol abuse

Shifts into Cells

Carbohydrate administration
Acute alkalosis
Nutritional recovery syndrome
Acute gout
Salicylate poisoning
Gram-negative bacteremia
Posthypothermia

Adapted from Favus MJ (ed.): Primer on the Metabolic Bone Diseases and Disorders of Mineral Metabolism. Kelseyville, CA, American Society for Bone and Mineral Research, 1990; with permission.

tion of total body inorganic phosphate because only 1% of total body phosphate is in the extracellular fluid compartment. Conversely, serious phosphate depletion can exist with normal serum inorganic phosphate levels. The pathogenesis and differential diagnosis of hypophosphatemia are discussed in Chapter 75.

Symptoms of hypophosphatemia usually do not occur until serum inorganic phosphate levels fall below 1 mg/dl. The acute effects are listed in Table 73–2. Phosphate depletion is associated with a reduction in erythrocytic 2,3-diphosphoglycerate (2,3-DPG). Because this molecule normally stimulates the dissociation of oxygen from hemoglobin, phosphorus depletion can impair tissue oxygen delivery. In severe phosphate deficiency (serum level < 1.0 mg/dl), erythrocyte membrane integrity may be compromised, with resultant hemolytic anemia and dysfunction of leukocytes and platelets. In muscle, phosphate depletion may produce myalgias and weakness and lead to rhabdomyolysis. Phosphate depletion effects renal function by increasing excretion of urinary calcium, bicarbonate, and magnesium, and increasing synthesis of 1,25-$(OH)_2D$. Central nervous system impairment varies from irritability, fatigue, and weakness to encephalopathy and coma. The consequences of long-term phosphate depletion include osteomalacia and rickets (see Chapter 75).

The metabolic abnormalities associated with phosphate depletion are rapidly reversible by correcting the underlying disorder or using phosphate therapy, although the bone abnormalities may require months or years of

TABLE 73-2	Consequences of Severe Hypophosphatemia

Acute

Hematologic
    Red cell dysfunction and hemolysis
    Leukocyte dysfunction
    Platelet dysfunction
Muscle
    Weakness
    Rhabdomyolysis
    Myocardial dysfunction
Kidney
    Increased 25-OH-D 1α-hydroxylase activity
    Increased calcium, bicarbonate, and magnesium excretion
    Metabolic acidosis
Reduced formation of 2,3-DPG with impaired tissue oxygen delivery
Central nervous system dysfunction

Chronic

Osteomalacia or rickets

Revised from Smith LH Jr: Phosphorus deficiency and hypophosphatemia. *In* Wyngaarden JB, Smith LH Jr, Bennett JC (eds.): Cecil Textbook of Medicine. 19th ed. Philadelphia, WB Saunders, 1992, p 1137.

TABLE 73-3	Causes of Hyperphosphatemia

Decreased Renal Phosphate Excretion

    Renal failure (acute or chronic)
    Hypoparathyroidism
    Pseudohypoparathyroidism
    Acromegaly
    Etidronate
    Tumoral calcinosis

Increased Phosphate Entry into Extracellular Fluid

    Excess phosphate administration (intravenous, oral, or rectal)
    Transcellular shifts
        Rhabdomyolysis
        Acute tumor lysis
        Hemolytic anemia
        Acidosis
        Catabolic states
        Infections
        Hyperthermia
        Fulminant hepatitis
    Vitamin D intoxication

Adapted from Favus MJ (ed.): Primer on Metabolic Bone Diseases and Disorders of Mineral Metabolism. Kelseyville, CA, American Society for Bone and Mineral Research, 1990; with permission.

replacement therapy. Milk is an excellent source of phosphorus, containing about 1000 mg/L. Alternatively, sodium and potassium phosphate tablets (which contain 250 mg of inorganic phosphate) can be given in amounts of up to 3 gm/day in divided doses. Diarrhea is a common side effect of oral phosphate therapy. In rare circumstances, such as with neurologic disturbances, hemolysis, or rhabdomyolysis, intravenous phosphate administration may be indicated.

Hyperphosphatemia

Causes of hyperphosphatemia are listed in Table 73–3. Common causes of hyperphosphatemia include renal insufficiency (acute or chronic), hypoparathyroidism, acromegaly, rhabdomyolysis, acute tumor lysis, hemolytic anemia, vitamin D intoxication, and sodium etidronate administration. In growing children, serum inorganic phosphate is normally elevated compared with the normal adult range. In chronic renal insufficiency, normal serum inorganic phosphate levels are maintained by decreased renal phosphate reabsorption until the glomerular filtration rate falls below 20 to 25 ml/min. The most important acute effects of hyperphosphatemia are hypocalcemia and tetany (see Chapter 74). Hyperphosphatemia lowers serum calcium levels acutely by complexing with calcium and chronically by inhibiting the activity of renal 1α-hydroxylase, thereby diminishing synthesis of 1,25-$(OH)_2$D. This aggravates hypocalcemia both by impairing intestinal calcium absorption and by inducing a state of skeletal resistance to the action of PTH. Acute or chronic hyperphosphatemia can cause metastatic calcifications, particularly in patients with normal or elevated serum calcium levels. Treatment of hyperphosphatemia generally requires restricting dietary phosphorus plus administering phosphate binders such as aluminum hydroxide or calcium carbon-

ate. Because of the risk of aluminum toxicity with long-term aluminum therapy, calcium salts have become the first-line therapy for chronic hyperphosphatemia in renal failure.

MAGNESIUM METABOLISM

In the adult, magnesium constitutes about 0.35 gm/kg of body weight. Slightly more than half of total body magnesium is in bone, and most of the remainder is localized in the intracellular compartment. Magnesium is the second most abundant intracellular cation, after potassium, and the most abundant intracellular divalent cation. Approximately 60% of intracellular magnesium is contained in the mitochondria, and only about 5 to 10% is free in the cytosol. It plays an important structural role in bone crystals and is a cofactor in many vital enzymatic reactions.

Normal adults require about 0.15 to 0.18 mmol/kg/day of magnesium to maintain a positive balance. The average diet contains about 7 to 30 mmol (168 to 720 mg) of magnesium per day, derived mainly from meats and green vegetables. About 40% of ingested magnesium is absorbed in the intestine; the amount varies directly with dietary intake. Magnesium metabolism bears some relationship to that of calcium: (1) these cations compete for renal tubular reabsorption and may compete for intestinal absorption; (2) magnesium and calcium are physiologic antagonists in the central nervous system; (3) magnesium is necessary for the release of PTH and for the action of the hormone on its target tissues.

Magnesium balance is usually assessed by its serum concentration, although this does not parallel its tissue concentration. In the plasma, magnesium circulates at a concentration of 0.75 to 1.05 mmol/L (1.8 to 2.5 mg/dl), of which approximately 30% is protein bound, and the remainder is ionized. The extent of body stores of magnesium can be assessed more sensitively by measuring basal urinary magnesium excretion or the percentage of an intravenous load of magnesium that is excreted in the urine (the Thoren test). Retention of > 25 to 50% is presumed to reflect depleted stores.

The kidney is the main site of magnesium excretion, with $< 2\%$ of endogenous magnesium appearing in the feces. About 2 to 10% of the filtered load of magnesium is normally excreted in the urine; the remainder is reabsorbed primarily in the thick limb of the ascending loop of Henle. Urinary magnesium excretion increases with the inhibition of proximal tubular reabsorption by osmotic diuretics or with extracellular fluid volume expansion. Some drugs, notably furosemide and cisplatin, inhibit magnesium reabsorption in the loop of Henle. PTH and aldosterone both decrease renal magnesium reabsorption. When dietary magnesium is restricted, urinary losses can fall to < 1 mEq/day.

Hypomagnesemia

Magnesium deficiency usually occurs in association with more generalized nutritional and metabolic abnormalities. It can be due to decreased absorption, increased renal or intestinal losses, or redistribution of magnesium. The most common causes of hypomagnesemia are listed in Table 73–4. Clinically, magnesium deficiency is most often encountered in alcoholics (poor dietary intake, vomiting, diminished absorption, and/or increased renal excretion), diabetics, patients with malabsorption, and during prolonged intravenous fluid therapy. Significant depletion of magnesium may result in any or all of the abnormalities listed in Table 73–5, many of which are nonspecific. The most common clinical presentations of hypomagnesemia are caused by associated hypocalcemia (due to interference with the secretion and action of PTH) and hypokalemia (due to an inability of the kidney to preserve potassium). Other clinical manifestations of hypomagnesemia include neuromuscular hyperexcitability and electrocardiographic abnormalities such as prolongation of the PR and QT intervals and arrhythmias.

Treatment of magnesium deficiency is rarely an emergency. A common regimen is to administer 2 gm of $MgSO_4$ (16 mEq Mg) as a 50% solution every 8 hours intramuscularly. Because the injections can be painful, an alternative is to administer 48 mEq/day (preferably as $MgCl_2$ to prevent binding of calcium by sulfate) by continuous intravenous infusion. Either regimen usually produces a normal or slightly elevated serum magnesium level. However, because a normal serum level frequently does not indicate repletion of total body magnesium stores, therapy should be continued for several days, during which time associated abnormalities such as hypocalcemia and hypokalemia should correct themselves. In patients with chronic magnesium loss, magnesium oxide can be given orally in a dose of 300 mg of elemental magnesium per day in divided doses. The most common side effect of oral replacement therapy is diarrhea. Caution should be exercised when administering magnesium to

patients with renal insufficiency in order to prevent hypermagnesemia.

Hypermagnesemia

Hypermagnesemia almost always occurs in the setting of renal insufficiency. In such patients, excessive use of

TABLE 73–4	Causes of Hypomagnesemia

Decreased Absorption

Poor dietary intake
Malabsorption syndromes
Extensive bowel resection
Ethanol effect on absorption

Increased Gastrointestinal Losses

Acute and chronic diarrhea
Intestinal and biliary fistulas
Vomiting or nasogastric suction

Increased Renal Losses

Chronic intravenous fluid therapy
Chronic renal disease (tubular, glomerular, interstitial)
Osmotic diuresis
Diabetes mellitus
Hypercalcemia
Phosphate depletion
Metabolic acidosis
Primary aldosteronism
Drugs
    Diuretics (furosemide, ethacrynic acid)
    Aminoglycosides
    Cisplatin
    Cyclosporine
    Amphotericin B
    Ethanol

Internal Redistribution

Acute pancreatitis
"Hungry bone syndrome"

Revised from Smith LH Jr: Disorders of magnesium metabolism. *In* Wyngaarden JB, Smith LH Jr, Bennett JC (eds.): Cecil Textbook of Medicine. 19th ed. Philadelphia, WB Saunders, 1992, p 1139.

TABLE 73–5	Consequences of Magnesium Deficiency

Neuromuscular

Lethargy, weakness, fatigue, decreased mentation
Neuromuscular irritability (partly due to associated hypocalcemia)

Gastrointestinal

Anorexia, nausea, vomiting
Paralytic ileus

Cardiovascular

Prolongation of PR and QT intervals
Tachyarrhythmias
Increased sensitivity to digitalis

Metabolic

Hypocalcemia (due to decreased parathyroid hormone secretion and action)
Hypokalemia (due to renal potassium wasting)

Revised from Smith LH Jr: Disorders of magnesium metabolism. *In* Wyngaarden JB, Smith LH Jr, Bennett JC (eds.): Cecil Textbook of Medicine. 19th ed. Philadelphia, WB Saunders, 1992, p 1139.

magnesium-containing antacids and cathartics or parenteral magnesium may produce hypermagnesemia. Magnesium is a standard form of therapy for pre-eclampsia and may cause intoxication in both the mother and the neonate. Modest elevations of serum magnesium levels are seen in familial hypocalciuric hypercalcemia, lithium ingestion, and volume depletion.

Neuromuscular symptoms are the most common presenting problem of hypermagnesemia. Somnolence may be seen at concentrations of 3 mEq/L; the deep tendon reflexes generally disappear at serum concentrations of 4 to 7 mEq/L; and respiratory depression and apnea occur at higher concentrations. Moderate hypermagnesemia may result in hypotension. At concentrations above 5 mEq/L, electrocardiographic abnormalities such as prolonged PR and QT intervals and increased QRS duration may occur, and at extremely high levels—above 15 mEq/L—patients may experience complete heart block or cardiac arrest. In most circumstances, the only treatment needed is to discontinue magnesium administration. In patients with renal failure, dialysis against a low magnesium bath lowers magnesium levels. In emergencies, intravenous calcium can be given in a dose of 100 to 200 mg over 5 to 10 minutes to antagonize the toxic effects of magnesium.

VITAMIN D

In terms of its availability, metabolism, and mechanism of action, vitamin D is more properly a steroid hormone than a vitamin. Although there is a dietary necessity for vitamins, no dietary source of vitamin D is needed when there is sufficient exposure to sunlight. Like other steroid hormones, it undergoes several chemical transformations to synthesize the biologically active form. The close regulation of renal 1,25-$(OH)_2$ vitamin D synthesis is typical of hormones. Finally, like other steroid hormones, it exerts its biologic effects by binding to specific, high-affinity receptors in target tissues.

Synthesis of Vitamin D (Fig. 73–3)

The active form of vitamin D is synthesized in three sequential steps in the skin, liver, and kidneys. In the skin, ultraviolet light converts 7-dehydrocholesterol to previtamin D_3, which is then slowly converted nonenzymatically to vitamin D_3 (cholecalciferol). Vitamin D_3, bound to a specific vitamin D–binding protein (DBP), is then transported to the liver, where it is enzymatically hydroxylated to 25-hydroxyvitamin D (calcifidiol or 25-OH-D). This activation step, catalyzed by a cytochrome P-450 mixed-function oxidase in hepatocytes, is not under tight homeostatic regulation. Although 25-OH-D is only weakly biologically active, its circulating level furnishes a good index of the bioavailability of vitamin D because it has a long serum half-life (2 weeks). Then, 25-OH-D, bound to DBP, is transported to the kidney and other organs, where it is either hydroxylated at the 1 position to produce 1,25-dihydroxycholecalciferol (calcitriol or 1,25-

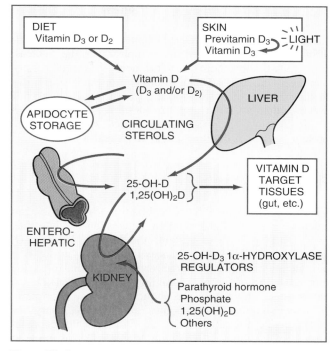

Figure 73–3

The vitamin D endocrine system. Vitamin D_2 (from diet) and vitamin$_3$ (from diet or from conversion of 7-dihydrocholesterol in skin) are progressively hydroxylated in liver and kidney to produce 1,25-$(OH)_2$D (calcitrol). (From Marx SJ: Mineral and bone homeostasis. *In* Wyngaarden JB, Smith LH Jr, Bennett JC [eds.]: Cecil Textbook of Medicine. 19th ed. Philadelphia, WB Saunders, 1992, p 1402.)

$[OH]_2$D), the most biologically active form of vitamin D, or in other positions to produce a variety of other steroids. Renal 1α-hydroxylation is under tight metabolic control and is increased by PTH, hypophosphatemia, hypocalcemia, growth hormone, insulin, estrogens, prolactin, and low levels of 1,25-$(OH)_2$D. Conversely, renal synthesis of 1,25-$(OH)_2$D is diminished by hypercalcemia, hyperphosphatemia, high levels of 1,25-$(OH)_2$D, low levels of PTH, severe renal disease, and in many elderly people.

Absorption of Vitamin D

The dietary source of vitamin D is either vitamin D_2 (ergocalciferol) formed from irradiation of ergosterol (a plant sterol) or vitamin D_3. Ergocalciferol differs from cholecalciferol in the structure of its side chain but is equal in potency, undergoes the same biotransformations, and is measured by the same commonly employed competitive protein-binding assays.

Although the minimal dietary requirement for vitamin D is difficult to establish, the suggested daily intake for adults in the United States is 10 μg (400 International Units) of vitamin D_2 or vitamin D_3. Because it is a fat-soluble vitamin, chronic malabsorption of fat without adequate exposure to ultraviolet light can lead to hypovitaminosis D.

Molecular Mechanism of Action of 1,25-(OH)₂D

In the target cell, 1,25-(OH)₂D binds to a specific, high-affinity receptor in either the cytoplasm or the nucleus. The DNA-binding domain of the hormone-receptor complex then interacts with the hormone-responsive element in the genome of the target cell, producing either up- or downregulation of the gene in question. This interaction results in either increased or decreased synthesis of the protein for which that messenger RNA codes.

Function of Vitamin D

Vitamin D acts with PTH to maintain the level of ionized calcium in extracellular fluid by actions on the intestine, bone, and, to a lesser extent, the kidney. Vitamin D, largely as 1,25-(OH)₂D, enhances the intestinal absorption of calcium and phosphate absorption and enhances the mineralization of osteoid. Vitamin D as 1,25-(OH)₂D also has a direct effect on bone: it increases bone resorption. *In vivo*, vitamin D metabolites are also necessary for normal bone formation. Vitamin D may enhance renal tubular reabsorption of calcium. Vitamin D may play an important role in cellular differentiation and proliferation, such as the differentiation of hematopoietic cells of the monocyte-macrophage line into osteoclasts, and may have an important role in immune function.

Diagnosis of Vitamin D Deficiency

Vitamin D deficiency is generally indicated by a low serum level of 25-OH-D. In many patients with low levels of 25-OH-D, serum 1,25-(OH)₂D levels are normal or increased, particularly if serum PTH levels are high. Other findings that support the diagnosis of vitamin D deficiency include mild hypocalcemia, hypophosphatemia, secondary hyperparathyroidism, and low levels of urinary calcium excretion. Deficiency of 1,25-(OH)₂D secretion is seen most often in patients with severe renal disease but also occurs in patients with hypoparathyroidism or with inherited or acquired defects in 1α hydroxylation of 25-OH-D (see Chapter 75).

Hypervitaminosis D

Hypervitaminosis D occurs from the excessive ingestion of vitamin D or one of its active metabolites or from the abnormal conversion of 25-OH-D to 1,25-(OH)₂D at sites not subject to normal metabolic regulation. The former usually occurs during therapy of hypocalcemia, osteomalacia, or osteoporosis. The latter occurs in granulomatous diseases such as sarcoidosis and tuberculosis and in certain T cell lymphomas in which the 1α-hydroxylase is pathologically expressed in the abnormal tissue. Clinically, hypervitaminosis D presents with hypercalcemia and/or metastatic calcification. The hypercalcemia is due not only to vitamin D's effect on calcium absorption but also to its osteolytic effects. For any level of hypercalcemia, patients with vitamin D intoxication are more likely to have metastatic calcification than are patients with hyperparathyroidism or humoral hypercalcemia of malignancy because serum inorganic phosphate levels are higher. Vitamin D intoxication caused by ingesting ergocalciferol can persist for several weeks after discontinuing therapy, whereas the effects of intoxication with calcitriol generally subside in several days. Treatment of vitamin D intoxication involves discontinuing vitamin D and, in some patients, the usual acute treatment of hypercalcemia (see Chapter 74) or the use of corticosteroids.

Hypovitaminosis D

The clinical picture of hypovitaminosis D is that of hypocalcemia (see Chapter 74), osteomalacia (see Chapter 75), or rickets (see Chapter 75).

CALCITONIN

Calcitonin is a 32-amino acid peptide that is secreted by the parafollicular C cells of the thyroid gland. Its secretion is regulated acutely by the serum calcium concentration (when the blood calcium level rises, calcitonin secretion increases) and chronically by gender and, perhaps, age (women tend to have lower calcitonin levels than men, and some studies report a progressive decline in calcitonin levels with age). The main biologic effect of calcitonin is to inhibit osteoclastic bone resorption. Calciuria, phosphaturia, and analgesia occur at supraphysiologic concentrations.

Hypocalcitoninemia

Patients with calcitonin deficiency do not have any recognized abnormalities. Patients who have undergone a total thyroidectomy do not require calcitonin replacement and do not have a greater incidence of osteoporosis.

Hypercalcitoninemia

Elevated serum calcitonin concentrations are seen in individuals with medullary carcinoma of the thyroid gland, a malignancy of the calcitonin-producing C cells. Despite high calcitonin levels, these patients do not have any associated bone disease or metabolic disorders of calcium or inorganic phosphate. Early stages of the disease may be detected by measuring the calcitonin response to intravenous calcium or pentagastrin administration. Patients with sporadic medullary thyroid carcinoma usually present with a thyroid nodule. Some patients have a secretory diarrhea. Familial medullary thyroid carcinoma occurs as part of multiple endocrine neoplasia types IIA (Sipple's syndrome) and IIB, both of which are inherited in an autosomal dominant fashion. Hypercalcitoninemia may also be seen in patients with small cell lung cancer, carcinoid tumors, islet cell tumors, renal failure, and hypercalciuria.

REFERENCES

Bringhurst FR: Calcium and phosphate distribution, turnover, and metabolic actions. *In* DeGroot LJ (ed): Endocrinology. Philadelphia, WB Saunders, 1995, pp 1015–1043.

Favus MJ (ed.): Primer on the Metabolic Bone Diseases and Disorders of Mineral Metabolism. 2nd ed. New York, Raven Press, 1993.

Holick MF: Vitamin D: Photobiology, metabolism, and clinical applications. *In* DeGroot LJ (ed.): Endocrinology, Philadelphia, WB Saunders, 1995, pp 990–1014.

Levi M, Cronin RE, Knochel JP: Disorders of phosphate and magnesium metabolism. *In* Coe FL, Favus MJ (eds.): Disorders of Bone and Mineral Metabolism, New York, Raven Press, 1992, pp 587–610.

74

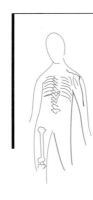

The Parathyroid Glands, Hypercalcemia, and Hypocalcemia

NORMAL PHYSIOLOGY

The four parathyroid glands are found near the thyroid gland. Occasionally one of the glands may be in the thyroid or an aberrant location, usually in the superior mediastinum. Each normal gland weighs approximately 25 mg.

Secretion of Parathyroid Hormone

Parathyroid hormone (PTH) is an 84 amino acid single-chain polypeptide with a molecular weight of 9500. PTH is initially a larger precursor molecule, pre-pro-PTH, consisting of 115 amino acids. This precursor is rapidly converted within the glands to an intermediate form of 90 amino acids, termed pro-PTH, which is subsequently converted to the 84 amino acid hormone. The biologic activity of PTH resides in the first 34 residues. After release into the circulation, the intact hormone is cleaved, primarily in the liver and kidney, to smaller biologically inactive midregion and carboxy-terminal fragments. Biologically active amino-terminal fragments do not seem to circulate.

Parathyroid hormone secretion is controlled primarily by the serum ionized calcium level: when the level falls, PTH secretion is stimulated; when it rises above the normal set point, the secretion of PTH is suppressed. With prolonged hypocalcemia, the parathyroid glands can become markedly hyperplastic.

Actions of Parathyroid Hormone (Fig. 74–1)

The main function of PTH is to defend against hypocalcemia. PTH acts by binding to specific receptors on the cell membrane. Signal transduction occurs by activation of membrane-bound adenylate cyclase with the subsequent intracellular release of cyclic AMP or by increasing inositol phosphate metabolism with release of intracellular calcium. The major actions of PTH are the following:

1. Stimulation of bone resorption by osteoclasts, thereby releasing calcium and phosphate into the extracellular fluid. How PTH works on bone is not well understood. PTH receptors have not been demonstrated on osteoclasts so that, at the present time, the bone-resorbing effect of PTH appears to be indirect. In contrast, osteoblasts do contain PTH receptors. In response to PTH, osteoblasts release a factor (or factors) that stimulates osteoclastic bone resorption. The action of PTH on bone is partially impaired with deficiencies of calcitriol or intracellular magnesium.

2. Stimulation of renal tubular reabsorption of calcium (and magnesium).

3. Inhibition of the renal tubular reabsorption of phosphate and bicarbonate.

4. Stimulation of synthesis of the active form of vitamin D, calcitriol, from 25-OH-D by activating the specific 1α-hydroxylase in the kidney. By virtue of its effect on calcitriol synthesis, PTH indirectly enhances the intestinal absorption of calcium.

Measurement of Parathyroid Hormone

Circulating levels of PTH are measured by radioimmunoassay. In the past, the antibodies used were multivalent and heterogeneous, recognizing fragments of the PTH molecule that were often biologically inert. This problem was particularly noteworthy in patients with renal failure because the biologically inert C-terminal fragments of PTH are normally cleared by the kidney. Currently, double-antibody assays (immunoradiometric assays; IRMA) allow measurement of intact, biologically active PTH.

HYPERCALCEMIA

Hypercalcemia is a common clinical disorder that may develop in the setting of an obvious serious underlying illness or may often be detected by routine laboratory testing in patients without any obvious illness. Overall, primary hyperparathyroidism is the most common cause of hypercalcemia in the adult population, although malignancy remains the most common cause of hypercalcemia among hospitalized patients.

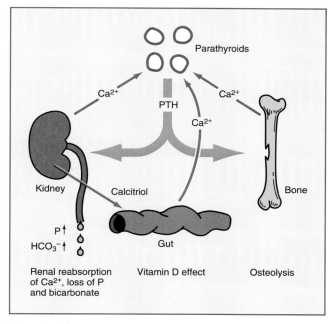

Figure 74–1
Actions of parathyroid hormone (PTH) in calcium homeostasis.

Clinical Manifestations

The clinical manifestations of hypercalcemia are summarized in Table 74–1. In general, the severity of the symptoms tends to parallel the level of ionized calcium in extracellular fluid, but wide variations can occur. Nausea, vomiting, and polyuria, which can produce dehydration and thus decrease renal calcium clearance, can worsen hypercalcemia.

Differential Diagnosis

Causes of hypercalcemia are listed in Table 74–2. More than 90% of patients with hypercalcemia have either primary hyperparathyroidism or a malignancy. With modern immunoradiometric assays, the distinction between these two disorders can generally be made on the basis of the serum PTH level, which is elevated or inappropriately normal in patients with primary hyperparathyroidism and suppressed in patients with hypercalcemia associated with malignancy.

Primary Hyperparathyroidism

In primary hyperparathyroidism, PTH is secreted inappropriately despite an elevation in the ionized calcium level in the extracellular fluid. Although PTH secretion is partially autonomous, negative feedback regulation can be seen (although with an altered set point) because PTH can be partially suppressed by calcium. The peak incidence of primary hyperparathyroidism occurs in the 20s to 40s, and it is more common in women than in men. The annual incidence of primary hyperparathyroidism is

TABLE 74–1	Signs and Symptoms of Primary Hyperparathyroidism

Related to Hypercalcemia

Central nervous system
    Lethargy
    Drowsiness
    Depression
    Impaired ability to concentrate
    Confusion
    Stupor
    Coma
Neuromuscular
    Proximal muscle weakness
    Hyporeflexia
Gastrointestinal
    Nausea
    Vomiting
    Anorexia
    Constipation
    Peptic ulcer disease
    Pancreatitis
Renal
    Polyuria
    Polydipsia
    Decreased concentrating ability
    Impaired renal function
    Nephrocalcinosis
    Nephrolithiasis
Cardiovascular
    Hypertension
    Short QT interval
    Bradycardia
    Increased sensitivity to digitalis

Related to Hypercalciuria

Nephrolithiasis

Related to Parathyroid Hormone Effect on Bone and Joints

Arthralgias
Bone pain
Bone cysts
Gout
Pseudogout

TABLE 74–2	Differential Diagnosis of Hypercalcemia

Primary hyperparathyroidism
Malignant disease
    Osteolytic metastases (e.g., breast cancer, multiple myeloma)
    Humoral hypercalcemia of malignancy (e.g., lung, head and neck, esophagus, renal cell, ovary)
    Hematologic malignancies (e.g., multiple myeloma, lymphoma, leukemia)
Sarcoidosis, tuberculosis, and other granulomatous diseases
Thyrotoxicosis
Drug-induced
    Vitamin D intoxication
    Vitamin A intoxication
    Thiazide diuretics
    Lithium
    Tamoxifen
Immobilization (in setting of high bone turnover)
Milk-alkali syndrome
Familial hypocalciuric hypercalcemia (FHH)
Adrenal insufficiency
Acute and chronic renal failure
Pheochromocytoma

estimated to be 1 in every 1000 men over age 60 and 2 in every 1000 women over age 60. Many patients are identified by multiphasic screening while still asymptomatic.

Etiology

Enlargement of a single parathyroid gland (parathyroid adenoma) is seen in approximately 85% of cases. Many parathyroid adenomas result from the clonal expansion of a single cell. Most of the remaining 15% of patients have hyperplasia of all four glands, although the enlargement is often asymmetric, so that some glands may look grossly like adenomas, whereas others appear indistinguishable from normal parathyroid glands. In some patients, hyperparathyroidism occurs as part of a familial disorder without other endocrinologic abnormalities. In others, it occurs as part of multiple endocrine neoplasia type I (Wermer's syndrome)—hyperparathyroidism, pancreatic islet cell tumors, and anterior pituitary tumors—or multiple endocrine neoplasia type II (Sipple's syndrome)—hyperparathyroidism, medullary carcinoma of the thyroid, and pheochromocytoma. Most patients with familial hyperparathyroidism have parathyroid hyperplasia, and the disorder is inherited in an autosomal dominant fashion. Parathyroid carcinoma occurs rarely in patients with primary hyperparathyroidism, and tends to grow slowly and to spread locally, although it occasionally metastasizes to liver, lungs, or bone. Long-term survival is common. Although serum calcium and PTH levels are usually higher in patients with parathyroid carcinoma than in those with primary hyperparathyroidism, it may be clinically indistinguishable from other forms of primary hyperparathyroidism and difficult to diagnose at the time of initial surgery.

Symptoms and Signs

With the widespread use of multiphasic chemistry screening, most patients with primary hyperparathyroidism today are asymptomatic at presentation or present with vague symptoms, such as fatigue, weakness, arthralgias, mental disturbances, polyuria, constipation, and nausea (see Table 74–1). Although symptoms are usually mild, they may worsen with intercurrent illnesses. On rare occasions, patients may present with life-threatening hypercalcemia and severe symptoms—so-called acute primary hyperparathyroidism, or parathyroid crisis. Approximately 10 to 15% of patients with primary hyperparathyroidism today develop kidney stones, usually composed of calcium oxalate or calcium phosphate, in contrast to a prevalence of 60 to 70% before the advent of routine chemistry screening. Other complications of hyperparathyroidism include pancreatitis, chondrocalcinosis, calcific periarthritis, and perhaps peptic ulcer disease.

Laboratory and Radiologic Manifestations

In primary hyperparathyroidism, serum calcium levels are continuously or intermittently elevated, and serum phosphorus levels tend to be low. The serum calcium level may be normal in the setting of concomitant vitamin D deficiency. In these patients, hypercalcemia develops when correcting the vitamin D deficiency. Serum alkaline phosphatase is usually normal but may be elevated, especially in patients with osteitis fibrosa cystica. Urinary calcium levels may be normal or elevated. Elevated urinary calcium levels help distinguish patients with primary hyperparathyroidism from those with familial hypocalciuric hypercalcemia (see later). A mild hyperchloremic acidosis is often present. Serum PTH levels are frankly elevated in most patients, but a few patients have PTH levels in the normal range. Serum 1,25-(OH)$_2$D levels may be elevated owing to the stimulatory effect of PTH on renal 1α-hydroxylase activity.

Most patients with primary hyperparathyroidism show no radiographic evidence of bone disease. The classic radiographic finding of osteitis fibrosa cystica is uncommon today. The most common radiographic finding in patients with primary hyperparathyroidism is osteopenia. Occasionally, radiographs may show subperiosteal bone resorption of the distal phalanges (Fig. 74–2); resorption of the distal end of the clavicle, or a "salt-and-pepper" appearance of the skull. Bone densitometry measurements often indicate a disproportionate loss of cortical

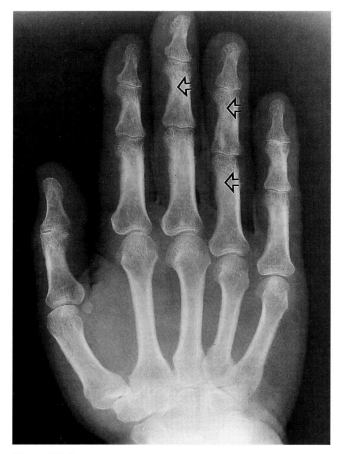

Figure 74–2
Subperiosteal bone resorption in the phalanges of a patient with primary hyperparathyroidism.

bone. Radiographic or ultrasound examination of the kidneys may show renal stones or diffuse deposition of calcium in the renal parenchyma (nephrocalcinosis).

Evaluation and Diagnosis

The diagnosis of primary hyperparathyroidism is based on finding hypercalcemia with an elevated or inappropriately normal PTH level. With the newer immunoradiometric assays that have high specificity for intact PTH, distinguishing primary hyperparathyroidism from non–PTH-mediated causes of hypercalcemia is rarely a problem (Fig. 74–3). A 24-hour urine collection should be made to rule out familial hypocalciuric hypercalcemia (see later). Most of the other causes of hypercalcemia listed in Table 74–2 can be readily identified by other clinical manifestations or by laboratory studies.

Parathyroid ultrasonography is usually reserved to assist the surgeon prior to neck exploration once the diagnosis of primary hyperparathyroidism has been established biochemically. Many masses identified by ultrasound examination of the neck turn out to be thyroid nodules, lymph nodes, or asymmetric parathyroid hyperplasia. A nodule felt in the neck is more likely to be a thyroid nodule than a parathyroid adenoma.

Indications for Treatment

The treatment of choice for symptomatic patients with primary hyperparathyroidism is surgical removal of the abnormal gland or glands. A panel of experts from a National Institutes of Health (NIH) Consensus Conference suggested the following guidelines for surgical treatment of patients with asymptomatic primary hyperparathyroidism:

1. A markedly elevated serum calcium level (i.e., 1.0 to 1.6 mg/dl above the upper limit of normal)
2. A history of prior life-threatening hypercalcemia
3. Kidney stone (or stones) detected by abdominal radiography
4. Creatinine clearance reduced by > 30% compared with age-matched normal subjects
5. Marked hypercalciuria (> 400 mg/24 hr)
6. Substantially reduced bone density, particularly if more than 2 standard deviations (SD) below age- and sex-matched controls
7. Patients in whom medical surveillance is neither desirable nor suitable:
   a. Patient requests surgery
   b. Consistent follow-up is deemed unlikely
   c. Coexistent illness complicates medical management
   d. Patient is ≤ 50 years old

Among those in whom medical surveillance is recommended, it is important to recognize early worsening of hypercalcemia, deteriorating bone or renal status, and typical symptoms of hyperparathyroidism. Patients should be seen on a regular basis and questioned about potential symptoms of hypercalcemia, and blood pressure, serum calcium, and creatinine clearance should be measured. Abdominal radiographs, 24-hour urinary calcium determinations, and bone density measurements, preferably of sites with predominantly cortical bone should be followed. Progression of symptoms requires surgery. Adequate hydration should be maintained. Thiazide diuretics should be avoided because they decrease urinary calcium excretion and may worsen hypercalcemia. Dietary intake of calcium should be moderate because severe restriction could further stimulate PTH secretion. Oral phosphate administration may be beneficial if hypophosphatemia is present. In postmenopausal women, estrogen replacement therapy may lower serum calcium levels, although at the expense of a compensatory rise in PTH secretion.

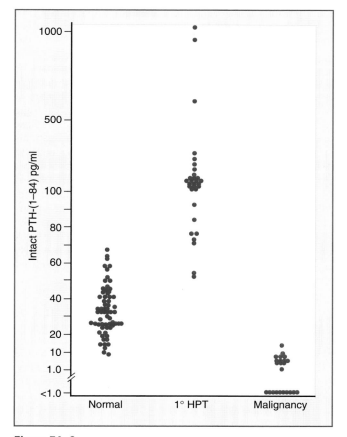

Figure 74–3

Intact parathyroid hormone (PTH) 1-84 levels measured by immunoradiometric assay in sera from 72 normal individuals, 37 patients with surgically proven hyperparathyroidism (HPT), and 24 patients with hypercalcemia associated with malignancy. (From Nussbaum SR, et al: Highly sensitive two-site immunoradiometric assay of parathyrin, and its clinical utility in evaluating patients with hypercalcemia. Clin Chem 1987; 33:1364; with permission.)

Hypercalcemia of Malignancy

Hypercalcemia of malignancy occurs in 10 to 20% of cancer patients during the course of their illness. Hypercalcemia usually occurs late in the course of malignancy, and survival is often limited to weeks or months. Malignancy is rarely the cause of unexplained hypercalcemia.

Hypercalcemia is most frequently seen in patients with breast cancer; squamous carcinomas of the head and neck, lung, and kidney; and hematologic malignancies such as multiple myeloma or lymphoma. In patients with T cell lymphomas associated with the human T cell lymphotrophic virus type I (HTLV-I), the incidence of hypercalcemia approaches 100%.

Localized Bone Destruction

In patients with malignancies, extensive localized bone destruction is often an important cause of hypercalcemia. In these patients, tumor metastases may release bone-resorbing cytokines directly into the skeleton or may stimulate host mononuclear cells to elaborate mediators, which stimulate nearby osteoclasts to resorb bone. Human multiple myeloma cells secrete tumor necrosis factor (TNF)-α and -β (lymphotoxin) and interleukin-1 (IL-1) and -6; breast cancer cells can produce PTH-related protein (PTHrP) and prostaglandin E_2; lymphocytes in lymphomas can elaborate 1,25-$(OH)_2D$ and cytokines; and solid tumors can produce IL-1, IL-6, and tumor-derived growth factors, all of which are potent stimulators of osteoclastic bone resorption. However, even in patients with these malignancies, humoral mechanisms may contribute to hypercalcemia, as evidenced by the diffuse osteoporosis often seen in patients with multiple myeloma, the occurrence of hypercalcemia in some patients with breast cancer in the absence of detectable skeletal metastases, and the enhanced intestinal absorption of calcium in patients with lymphomas that produce 1,25-$(OH)_2D$.

PTHrP

In many patients with malignancy-associated hypercalcemia, the primary mechanism for hypercalcemia is increased osteoclastic bone resorption caused by production of a PTHrP. This syndrome is frequently referred to as humoral hypercalcemia of malignancy (HHM). HHM is most common in patients with squamous cell carcinomas of the lung, esophagus, or head and neck, but it is also seen in patients with renal, bladder, ovarian, breast, and other carcinomas. PTHrP is a 141 amino acid protein in which 9 of the first 13 amino acids are identical to PTH. Like PTH, the full biologic activity of PTHrP on mineral ion homeostasis resides in its first 34 amino acids. PTH and PTHrP bind to the same receptors on bone and kidney, and both peptides increase bone resorption, renal calcium reabsorption, urinary phosphate excretion, and nephrogenous cyclic AMP excretion. Although PTHrP stimulates 1,25-$(OH)_2D$ production in some experimental systems, 1,25-$(OH)_2D$ levels are typically normal in patients with HHM. Immunoassays for PTH do not detect PTHrP, although assays are now available to assess PTHrP levels directly. PTHrP has been identified in many normal tissues, including keratinocytes, breast, nerve cells, and placenta, and thus it may have a normal physiologic role that has not yet been discovered.

Other Causes of Hypercalcemia

Familial hypocalciuric hypercalcemia (FHH, or familial benign hypercalcemia) is a rare genetic disorder transmitted as an autosomal dominant trait. It is characterized by modest hypercalcemia and relative hypocalciuria. Patients are usually asymptomatic and are detected as a result of screening after a family member has been identified or during evaluation of those initially thought to have asymptomatic primary hyperparathyroidism. Hypercalcemia has been detected in family members as early as the first months of life. Immunoactive PTH levels are usually normal but may be mildly elevated, occasionally causing confusion with primary hyperparathyroidism. Serum magnesium levels are higher in FHH than in primary hyperparathyroidism, usually high normal or frankly elevated. Because parathyroid surgery fails to cure the hypercalcemia unless a total parathyroidectomy is performed, surgery is usually contraindicated in FHH. To screen for this disorder, urinary calcium excretion should be determined in patients with asymptomatic hypercalcemia, and serum calcium levels should be measured in their relatives. The diagnosis should be suspected in hypercalcemic patients with normal or elevated PTH levels who present at a young age, have a family history of hypercalcemia or FHH, have hypermagnesemia, and/or have a urinary calcium excretion of < 100 mg/24 hr despite a normal creatinine clearance.

Hypercalcemia due to vitamin D intoxication can be caused by excessive ingestion of vitamin D or endogenous overproduction of 1,25-$(OH)_2D$. The latter occurs in some patients with granulomatous diseases or hematologic malignancies due to extrarenal 25-OH-D 1α-hydroxylase activity. Hypercalcemia occasionally occurs in patients with hyperthyroidism. Immobilization regularly leads to accelerated bone turnover and can produce hypercalcemia in patients whose underlying rate of bone turnover is high, as is seen in young people, and individuals with Paget's disease (see Chapter 77). Other causes of hypercalcemia include adrenal insufficiency, lithium therapy, pheochromocytoma, the milk-alkali syndrome, vitamin A intoxication, and the use of thiazide diuretics, particularly in patients who have some degree of underlying parathyroid autonomy.

Treatment of Hypercalcemia

Whenever possible, the treatment of hypercalcemia should be directed toward reversing the underlying abnormality. For example, severe or symptomatic primary hyperparathyroidism is best treated by surgery.

In patients who have severe hypercalcemia ($\geq$ 13 to 14 mg/dl) or who are symptomatic, medical treatment is indicated. The following approaches, presented briefly, are available and may be used in sequence or concurrently, if indicated by the severity of the hypercalcemia.

1. *Hydration.* Dehydration frequently accompanies severe hypercalcemia. Restoring intravascular volume is the first step in therapy and may significantly reduce hy-

percalcemia. Intravenous isotonic saline is the fluid of choice because renal calcium excretion is directly linked to sodium excretion. Caution must be exercised in administering large volumes of saline, particularly in elderly individuals and those with cardiac or renal disease.

2. *Furosemide* (or ethacrynic acid). Loop diuretics facilitate sodium and calcium excretion. However, they should not be administered until intravascular volume has been restored. Otherwise, further dehydration and worsening hypercalcemia may ensue. Because patients given these diuretics also lose potassium and magnesium, their serum levels must be monitored closely during intensive treatment and the losses replaced. Thiazide diuretics should be avoided because they decrease renal calcium excretion and may worsen hypercalcemia.

3. *Glucocorticoids.* High doses of glucocorticoids (prednisone, 50 to 100 mg/day, or the equivalent of another agent) may lower serum calcium levels, especially in patients with sarcoidosis, vitamin D intoxication, multiple myeloma, or other hematologic malignancies.

4. *Calcitonin.* Calcitonin inhibits osteoclastic bone resorption and increases urinary calcium excretion. When administered subcutaneously or intramuscularly in a dose of 2 to 4 IU/kg every 6 to 12 hours, it decreases the release of calcium from bone. However, tachyphylaxis may develop in several days with a rebound in serum calcium levels.

5. *Mithramycin.* Mithramycin diminishes osteoclastic activity when given intravenously. The usual dose is 15 to 25 μg/kg body weight by slow infusion over 2 to 4 hours. Its utility is often limited by kidney, liver, or bone marrow toxicity. Responsiveness may diminish after several courses of therapy.

6. *Phosphate.* Phosphate must be given with great care when treating severe hypercalcemia because of the danger of metastatic calcification. In the presence of hypophosphatemia and good renal function, oral phosphate can be given in amounts sufficient to return the serum inorganic phosphate level to normal. Diarrhea is a common side effect of therapy. Phosphate should rarely, if ever, be given intravenously now that equally potent but safer alternatives are available.

7. *Bisphosphonates.* Bisphosphonates are structural analogues of pyrophosphate that inhibit osteoclast-mediated bone resorption. Two bisphosphonates are available for treating hypercalcemia in the United States: ethane hydroxy 1,1-diphosphonic acid (etidronate disodium, EHDP, Didronel) and aminohydroxypropylidene bisphosphonate (pamidronate APD, Aredia). EHDP is administered as a daily intravenous infusion for 3 days at a dose of 7.5 mg/kg/day. APD is administered at a dose of 60 to 90 mg intravenously over 24 hours. Fever is a common side effect during APD infusion. Serum calcium levels may remain in the normal range for weeks to months after bisphosphonate therapy.

8. *Gallium nitrate.* In selected patients, gallium nitrate can be used to treat hypercalcemia due to malignancy. The usual dose is 200 mg/m² of body surface daily for five consecutive days.

9. *Dialysis.* On rare occasions, such as in patients with acute hypercalcemia and renal insufficiency, dialysis may be required for the treatment of hypercalcemia.

HYPOCALCEMIA

Hypocalcemia is an abnormal reduction in serum ionized calcium concentration. A reduction in the total serum calcium concentration, as may occur in patients with hypoalbuminemia, does not necessarily reflect a reduction in ionized calcium (see Chapter 73).

Etiology and Pathogenesis

Causes of hypocalcemia are summarized in Table 74–3. Hypocalcemia is usually due to a deficiency in the production, secretion, or action of PTH or 1,25-(OH)$_2$D.

Hypoparathyroidism

The causes of hypoparathyroidism range from surgical removal of the parathyroid glands to resistance to the action of PTH at the tissue level. In hypoparathyroidism, there is reduced mobilization of calcium from bone, reduced renal reabsorption of calcium, reduced renal clear-

TABLE 74–3	Causes of Hypocalcemia

Hypoparathyroidism
  Idiopathic
  Postsurgical
  Hypomagnesemia
  Post–neck irradiation
  Infiltrative; e.g., hemochromatosis, granulomatous diseases
  DiGeorge's syndrome
  MEDAC syndrome
Parathyroid hormone resistance
  Pseudohypoparathyroidism
  Hypomagnesemia
Vitamin D deficiency
  Decreased dietary intake
  Lack of sunlight exposure
  Intestinal malabsorption
  Postgastrectomy
  Anticonvulsant therapy
  Vitamin D–dependent rickets type I
Vitamin D resistance
  Vitamin D–dependent rickets type II
Chronic renal failure
Hyperphosphatemia
  Renal failure
  Tumor lysis
  Rhabdomyolysis
  Excessive phosphate administration
Hungry bone syndromes
Osteoblastic metastases (e.g., prostate)
Acute pancreatitis
Multiple citrated blood transfusions
Gram-negative sepsis
Antiresorptive agents (e.g., bisphosphonates, calcitonin, mithramycin)

MEDAC = Multiple endocrine deficiency with mucocutaneous candidiasis.

ance of inorganic phosphate, and decreased intestinal calcium absorption due to reduced synthesis of 1,25-(OH)$_2$D. The results are hypocalcemia and hyperphosphatemia. Hypoparathyroidism can result from autoimmune destruction of the parathyroid glands, either as a sporadic disorder or as part of an inherited syndrome associated with other hormone deficiencies, including adrenal insufficiency, gonadal failure, and diabetes mellitus (multiple endocrine deficiency with mucocutaneous candidiasis, MEDAC syndrome). Hypoparathyroidism after neck surgery may reflect removal of the parathyroid glands or disruption of their blood supply. Transient hypocalcemia frequently occurs after surgical removal of solitary parathyroid adenomas because of suppression of the remaining parathyroid glands or the rapid movement of calcium and phosphate into bones (e.g., "hungry bones syndrome"). Hypomagnesemia induces a functional state of hypoparathyroidism caused by a combination of impaired PTH secretion and end-organ resistance to the effects of PTH. The causes of hypomagnesemia are listed in Table 73–4. Less common causes of hypoparathyroidism include granulomatous or malignant infiltration of the parathyroid glands, iron overload of the parathyroid glands, the DiGeorge syndrome (congenital abnormality representing absence of the embryologic formation of the parathyroid glands and the thymus with severe immunodeficiency), and neck irradiation.

Pseudohypoparathyroidism

In contrast to patients with hypoparathyroidism in whom PTH levels are inappropriately low for the degree of hypocalcemia, PTH levels are elevated in patients with pseudohypoparathyroidism (PHP) due to end-organ resistance to PTH action. PHP represents a group of disorders that share resistance to PTH action but have variable biochemical abnormalities, end-organ responses to exogenous PTH, and molecular defects in PTH action. Patients with PHP type Ia have a deficient response in urinary cyclic adenosine monophosphate (cAMP) following administration of PTH. These patients also have a more generalized abnormality impairing production of cAMP in other tissues and often have a group of somatic abnormalities referred to as Albright hereditary osteodystrophy (AHO) (short stature, round face, subcutaneous ossifications, short metacarpals and metatarsals, obesity, and basal ganglia calcifications). The molecular defect in patients with PHP Ia is reduced activity of the alpha stimulatory subunit of the guanine nucleotide–binding protein that couples PTH to adenyl cyclase (G$_s\alpha$). Some subjects exhibit the somatic abnormalities of AHO and variable G$_s\alpha$ activity but have a normal serum calcium level and a normal response of urinary cAMP to exogenous PTH. This variant is called pseudopseudohypoparathyroidism (pseudo PHP). Pseudo PHP is genetically related to PHP and may represent a mild variant of PHP type Ia. Patients with PHP type Ib have normal G$_s\alpha$ activity and biochemical abnormalities similar to PHP Ia, but lack the AHO phenotype. A defect in the PTH receptor may be the cause. Patients with PHP type II have a reduced phospha-

turic increase to exogenous PTH despite a normal response in urinary cAMP excretion, suggesting a defect in the ability of cAMP to initiate the metabolic events typical of PTH action. There does not appear to be a genetic basis for PHP type II.

Vitamin D Deficiency and Resistance

Hypocalcemia can also result from vitamin D deficiency, abnormalities in vitamin D metabolism, or resistance to the actions of vitamin D. In these patients, hypocalcemia is usually accompanied by normal or low levels of serum inorganic phosphate and elevated serum PTH concentrations. The causes of vitamin D deficiency and resistance are discussed in Chapter 75.

Chronic Renal Failure

Chronic renal failure is the most common cause of hypocalcemia. The hypocalcemia is due to several factors, including hyperphosphatemia, reduced 1,25-(OH)$_2$D production, and impaired sensitivity of the skeleton to PTH action. Patients develop secondary hyperparathyroidism and parathyroid gland hyperplasia. With long-standing secondary hyperparathyroidism, autonomous parathyroid function and hypercalcemia can occur (e.g., "tertiary hyperparathyroidism").

Other Causes

Other causes of hypocalcemia include hyperphosphatemia, for example, from administering parenteral phosphate, rhabdomyolysis, malignant hyperthermia, or acute tumor lysis; acute pancreatitis, possibly due to chelation of cal-

TABLE 74–4	Signs and Symptoms of Hypocalcemia

Neuromuscular Irritability

Paresthesias—circumoral, fingers, and toes
Carpal pedal spasm—positive Chvostek's and Trousseau's signs
Laryngospasm
Bronchospasm
Blepharospasm
Tetany

Central Nervous System

Seizures
Electroencephalographic abnormalities
Increased intracranial pressure with papilledema
Extrapyramidal disturbances

Cardiovascular

Prolonged QT interval
Heart block
Congestive heart failure

Other

Abnormalities of teeth, fingernails, skin, and hair
Lenticular cataracts

TABLE 74–5	Vitamin D Preparations			
	Ergocalciferol	**Dihydrotachysterol**	**Calcifediol**	**Calcitriol**
Abbreviation	D_2	DHT	$25OHD_3$	$1,25(OH)_2D_3$
Trade Name	Drisdol, Calciferol	Hytakerol	Calderol	Rocaltrol
Physiologic dose (daily)	2.5–10 μg*	25–100 μg	1–5 μg	0.25–0.5 μg
Pharmacologic dose (daily)	0.625–5.0 mg	0.2–1.0 mg	20–200 μg	0.25–2.0 μg
Onset of action (days)	30	15	15	2–3
Duration of action	1–3 mo	1–4 wk	2–6 weeks	2–5 days

* 1 μg = 40 units.

cium by free fatty acids; osteoblastic metastases, as in prostate cancer; citrate administration in people receiving multiple blood transfusions; gram-negative sepsis; and medications that inhibit bone resorption, such as bisphosphonates, calcitonin, and mithramycin.

Signs and Symptoms (Table 74–4)

Hypocalcemia is often asymptomatic. Symptoms depend on the level of blood calcium, the duration of hypocalcemia, and the rate at which hypocalcemia develops. The most frequent symptoms of hypocalcemia are caused by neuromuscular irritability, including paresthesias of the hands and feet and circumoral region, and muscle cramps. Severe hypocalcemia can produce bronchospasm, laryngeal stridor, diplopia, blepharospasm, and seizures. Other central nervous system manifestations include electroencephalographic abnormalities, increased intracranial pressure with papilledema, myelopathy, and extrapyramidal disturbances from calcification of the basal ganglia. Cardiac manifestations of hypocalcemia include prolongation of the QT interval and, rarely, congestive heart failure. Physical examination may reveal a positive Chvostek sign (twitching of the facial muscles following tapping of the facial nerve) and a positive Trousseau sign (carpal spasm following inflation of the blood pressure cuff for 2 minutes above the systolic blood pressure). Cataracts, basal ganglia signs, and abnormalities of the teeth, hair, skin, and fingernails are occasionally seen.

Laboratory and Radiologic Manifestations

Hypocalcemia due to hypoparathyroidism is characterized by hyperphosphatemia and serum PTH levels that are either undetectable or inappropriately low for the levels of serum calcium. In PHP, PTH levels are high owing to end-organ resistance to PTH. The diagnosis of PHP may require determining urinary cAMP and phosphaturic responses to exogenous PTH infusion (the Ellsworth-Howard test). In hypocalcemia caused by malabsorption or deficiency of vitamin D, serum inorganic phosphate levels are generally low or normal, and serum PTH levels are increased. A notable exception is chronic renal failure, which is characterized by secondary hyperparathyroidism and hyperphosphatemia. In patients with hereditary PHP, calcifications in the basal ganglia as well as short fourth

and fifth metacarpals and metatarsals can be seen on radiography.

Treatment

The mainstays of therapy for hypocalcemia are calcium and vitamin D. Patients with acute symptomatic hypocalcemia may require intravenous calcium salt solutions. In such situations, one ampule of 10% calcium gluconate, which contains approximately 90 mg of elemental calcium, can be infused over 5 to 10 minutes. Less acute administration of intravenous calcium gluconate can be achieved by mixing calcium gluconate with dextrose and infusing 500 to 1000 mg of calcium over 24 hours and closely monitoring blood calcium levels. If hypomagnesemia is present, it should be corrected (see Chapter 73).

The management of chronic hypocalcemia depends on its underlying cause. Most patients require a combination of oral calcium and one of several vitamin D preparations (Table 74–5). In mild vitamin D deficiency, a multivitamin containing 400 IU of vitamin D and 800 to 1200 mg of oral calcium may be sufficient. Patients with hypoparathyroidism typically require high doses of vitamin D (e.g., vitamin D_2, 25,000 to 100,000 IU/day or $1,25$-$(OH)_2D$, 0.25 to 2.0 μg/day) plus oral calcium in amounts sufficient to maintain serum calcium levels in the low-normal range. Compared with vitamin D_2, $1,25$-$(OH)_2D$ has the advantages of more rapid onset of action and short half-life but is considerably more expensive. If patients are hyperphosphatemic, administering aluminum-containing antacids may be necessary. Hypercalciuria due largely to the absence of PTH-induced renal calcium reabsorption can be controlled by thiazide diuretics, which may also help maintain normocalcemia. In patients with chronic renal failure, hyperphosphatemia should be controlled with oral calcium supplements alone, if possible, to avoid metabolic bone disease from aluminum toxicity.

REFERENCES

Bilizikian JP, Marcus R, Levine MA: The Parathyroids: Basic and Clinical Concepts. New York, Raven Press, 1994.
Eastell R, Heath H III: The hypocalcemic states: Their differential diag-

nosis and management. *In* Coe FL, Favus MJ, (eds.): Disorders of Bone and Mineral Metabolism. New York, Raven Press, 1992, pp 571–585.

Levine MA, Spiegel AM; Pseudohypoparathyroidism. *In* DeGroot LJ (ed.): Endocrinology. Philadelphia, WB Saunders, 1995, pp 1136–1150.

Potts JT Jr (ed.): Proceedings of the NIH Consensus Development Conference on Diagnosis and Management of Asymptomatic Primary Hyperparathyroidism. J Bone Miner Res 1991;6(Suppl 2): S1–S166.

Stewart AF, Insogna KL, Broadus AE; Malignancy-associated hypercalcemia. *In* DeGroot LJ (ed.): Endocrinology. Philadelphia, WB Saunders, 1995, pp 1061–1674.

75

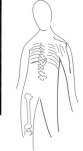

Osteomalacia and Rickets

Osteomalacia and rickets are disorders of calcification. Osteomalacia is a failure to mineralize the newly formed organic matrix (osteoid) normally. In rickets, a disease of children, there is also an abnormality in the zone of provisional calcification related to endochondral skeletal growth at the open epiphyses.

PATHOGENESIS

In forming new bone, the osteoblasts lay down osteoid in an appositional fashion. Bone mineralization, a complex process in which calcium-phosphate bone salts are deposited in the osteoid, begins soon thereafter. Optimal mineralization requires (1) an adequate supply of calcium and phosphate ions from the extracellular fluid, (2) an appropriate pH (approximately 7.6), (3) bone matrix that is normal in composition and rate of synthesis, and (4) control of inhibitors of mineralization. Several metabolites of vitamin D may also play important roles in the process of mineralizing normal bone. Defects in any of these steps can lead to osteomalacia.

SPECIFIC CAUSES

The conditions in which osteomalacia and rickets are most frequently found are listed in Table 75–1. The major categories of diseases that produce osteomalacia or rickets are vitamin D deficiency (due to decreased intake, impaired absorption, impaired activation, increased catabolism, or peripheral resistance to its action), phosphate depletion, systemic acidoses, and inhibitors of mineralization. The major entities associated with osteomalacia are discussed briefly.

Vitamin D Deficiency

Decreased Formation of Vitamin D or Metabolites

As can be seen in Figure 73–3, formation of 1,25-$(OH)_2D$ requires an adequate source of precursors in the form of either vitamin D_3 from ultraviolet light or diet or vitamin D_2 from the diet. These precursors must then be converted to 25-OH-D in the liver and then to 1,25-$(OH)_2D$ in the kidney to produce the biologically active metabolite. Disorders that interfere with any of these processes can lead to vitamin D deficiency and osteomalacia. In elderly people who get little exposure to sun and eat diets deficient in milk, eggs, and fish liver oils, osteomalacia is relatively common. It also occurs in patients with vitamin D malabsorption, particularly if there is inadequate exposure to sunlight. Patients with end-stage liver disease may have impaired 25-hydroxylase activity. Similarly, patients with chronic renal failure frequently have impaired activity of the renal 25-OH-D 1 α-hydroxylase. Patients with vitamin D–dependent rickets type I (VDDR-I) have a congenital defect in the activity of the renal 25-OH-D 1 α-hydroxylase. These children generally present with hypocalcemia, normal or high levels of 25-OH-D, low levels of 1,25-$(OH)_2D$, and elevated levels of parathyroid hormone (PTH) (Table 75–2) and can be treated effectively with physiologic replacement doses of 1,25-$(OH)_2D$.

Decreased Action of 1,25-$(OH)_2D$

Hereditary resistance to 1,25-$(OH)_2D$, often called vitamin D–dependent rickets type II (VDDR-II), is a rare disorder caused by a variety of defects in the vitamin D receptor. These defects include (1) a failure of 1,25-$(OH)_2D$ to bind to its receptor due either to a gene deletion or a mutation in the receptor's hormone-binding domain, (2) a decrease in the number of hormone-binding sites with normal binding affinity, (3) a defect in hormone-binding affinity, (4) a defect in the localization of the hormone-receptor complex to the nucleus, and (5) decreased binding by the hormone-receptor complex to DNA due to mutations in the DNA-binding domain of the vitamin D receptor. Biochemical abnormalities are similar to those of patients with VDDR-I except that serum concentrations of 1,25-$(OH)_2D$ are markedly elevated (see Table 75–2).

Increased Metabolism or Excretion of Vitamin D

Vitamin D metabolism can be accelerated by drugs, notably isoniazid and rifampin and possibly anticonvulsants. Renal excretion of vitamin D is increased in patients with

TABLE 75-1	Causes of Osteomalacia and/or Rickets

A. Vitamin D deficiency
  1. Decreased formation of vitamin D or metabolites: dietary lack, too little sunshine, malabsorption (post gastrectomy, sprue, Crohn's disease, intestinal bypass or resection, pancreatic insufficiency), cirrhosis, renal insufficiency, nephrosis, hypoparathyroidism, VDDR-1, X-linked VDRR
  2. Decreased action of 1,25-$(OH)_2D$: VDDR-II
  3. Increased metabolism or excretion of vitamin D: isoniazid, rifampin, anticonvulsants, nephrotic syndrome, CAPD
B. Chronic phosphate depletion
  1. Alcohol abuse
  2. Vitamin D deficiency (see above), especially with secondary hyperparathyroidism
  3. Aluminum hydroxide overdosage
  4. Selective renal tubular leaks
  5. Fanconi's syndrome
  6. X-linked VDRR and adult-onset VDRR
  7. Oncogenic osteomalacia
C. Systemic acidosis
  1. Distal renal tubular acidosis
  2. Proximal renal tubular acidosis
  3. Ureterosigmoidostomy
  4. Fanconi's syndrome
D. Calcium malabsorption and chronic hypocalcemia
E. Inhibitors of mineralization
  1. Sodium fluoride
  2. Disodium etidronate
  3. Aluminum
  4. Systemic acidosis
F. Miscellaneous
  1. Hypophosphatasia

CAPD = Chronic ambulatory peritoneal dialysis; VDRR = vitamin D-resistant rickets.

phosphaturia. Hypophosphatemia often accompanies vitamin D deficiency, particularly when secondary hyperparathyroidism is present, owing to both decreased intestinal absorption and increased urinary excretion of phosphate. Hypophosphatemia can also be caused by ingestion of large amounts of nonabsorbable antacids, selective defects in renal tubular phosphate reabsorption, and generalized renal tubular disorders (Fanconi's syndrome), in which increased urinary calcium excretion, abnormal vitamin D metabolism, and systemic acidosis may also contribute to the mineralization defect. Patients with X-linked VDRR, also call x-linked hypophosphatemia (XLH), have severe renal phosphate wasting and an abnormality in renal 25-OH-D 1-α-hydroxylase activity. They present as children with severe hypophosphatemia, normal serum calcium concentrations, normal 25-OH-D levels, low-normal 1,25-$(OH)_2D$ levels, lower limb deformities, and impaired growth (Fig. 75–1; also see Table 75–2). Similar biochemical abnormalities have been reported in patients with a variety of mesenchymal tumors, so-called oncogenic osteomalacia. In these individuals, removing the neoplasm normalizes the biochemical abnormalities and cures the bone disease.

Pure Calcium Malabsorption

Malabsorption of calcium, independent from alterations in vitamin D metabolism, may be the primary or a contributing factor in the development of osteomalacia in patients who have undergone partial gastrectomy, intestinal nephrotic syndrome and in chronic ambulatory peritoneal dialysis.

Chronic Phosphate Depletion

The causes of hypophosphatemia are summarized in Table 75–1. Hypophosphatemia can be produced by a dietary deficiency of the element, excessive losses in the urine or stool, or shifts into cells. Whatever the cause, hypophosphatemia may reduce the mineralization potential of bone salts below the critical level for normal deposition in osteoid. Because phosphorus is present in most foods, it is difficult to create a selective phosphorus deficiency by dietary means alone. Alcohol abuse is the most common cause of severe hypophosphatemia, probably due to poor food intake, vomiting, antacid use, and marked

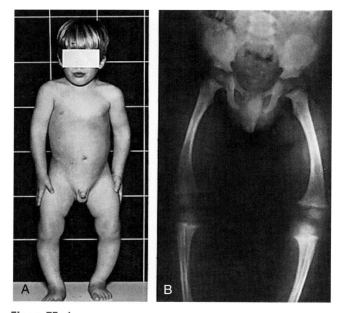

Figure 75–1

The clinical (A) and radiographic (B) appearance of a young boy with X-linked hypophosphatemic rickets. Note the striking bowing of the legs, apparent in both femora and tibiae, with flaring of the ends of the bones at the knee. (Courtesy of Dr. Sara B. Arnaud. From Bikle DB: Osteomalacia and rickets. In Wyngaarden JB, Smith LH Jr, Bennett JB [eds.]: Cecil Textbook of Medicine. 19th ed. Philadelphia, WB Saunders, 1992, p 1408.)

TABLE 75-2	Typical Laboratory Findings in Rickets

	Ca^{2+}	PO_4	25-OH-D	1,25-$(OH)_2D$	iPTH
VDDR-I	D	D	N or I	D	I
VDDR-II	D	D	N or I	I	I
VDRR	N	D	N	N or D	N

D = Decreased; I = increased; iPTH = immunoreactive parathyroid hormone; N = normal; VDDR = vitamin D–resistant rickets.

resection or bypass, or who have generalized intestinal diseases such as regional enteritis or sprue. In these patients, serum calcium levels are usually normal or slightly low, serum inorganic phosphate levels are low, 25-OH-D and 1,25-(OH)$_2$D levels are normal, and serum immunoreactive PTH (iPTH) concentrations are increased.

Systemic Acidosis

Acidosis increases resorption of bone mineral to buffer retained hydrogen ions. A decrease in systemic pH may inhibit mineralization by lowering the pH below the critical level needed for normal mineralization at calcifications sites. Finally, acidosis may alter the response to vitamin D. Conditions that produce chronic acidosis and are associated with rickets and/or osteomalacia include proximal and distal renal tubular acidosis, ureterosigmoidostomy, and Fanconi's syndrome.

Inhibitors of Mineralization

Aluminum-containing antacids or dialysis fluid high in aluminum in patients with chronic renal failure may inhibit mineralization, as may sodium fluoride and etidronate disodium (EHDP).

CLINICAL MANIFESTATIONS

The clinical features of rickets are mainly related to skeletal pain and deformity, fracture of the abnormal bone, slippage of epiphyses, and disturbances in growth. The child is usually listless, weak, and hypotonic, particularly when vitamin D deficiency is also present. Dental eruption is delayed, and enamel defects are common. The epiphyses are enlarged, as are the costochondral junctions, the latter producing the classic "rachitic rosary." Depending on the underlying cause, the child may have symptoms of hypocalcemia. If treated appropriately before age 4, the skeletal deformities are usually reversible.

In adults, osteomalacia is often difficult to diagnose on clinical grounds alone. Diffuse skeletal pain, often prominent around the hips, and proximal muscle weakness are the most common complaints. Physical examination may reveal a waddling gait, muscle weakness, bone tenderness, and hypotonia with preservation of brisk reflexes.

LABORATORY AND RADIOGRAPHIC FEATURES

The laboratory findings depend on the specific cause of the mineralization defect. The most typical findings are slight hypocalcemia, somewhat more profound hypophosphatemia, elevated serum alkaline phosphatase, low-normal urinary calcium excretion, and an elevated level of iPTH. Although some of these values may be normal, it is unusual for all of these values to be normal in a patient with osteomalacia. Serum levels of 25-OH-D are often depressed. Serum 1,25-(OH)$_2$D levels are often elevated,

TABLE 75–3	Typical Laboratory Findings in Serum in Metabolic Bone			
	Ca^{2+}	PO$_4$	Alkaline Phosphatase	iPTH
Osteomalacia	N or D	D	I	I
Primary hyperparathyroidism	I	D	I	I
Osteoporosis	N	N	N	N

D = Decreased; I = increased; iPTH = immunoreactive parathyroid hormone; N = normal.

despite low 25-OH-D levels, in patients with secondary hyperparathyroidism. However, serum 1,25-(OH)$_2$D levels may occasionally be depressed, particularly in patients with renal disease. Bone mineral density may be decreased, normal, or even increased depending on the cause of the mineralization defect. A comparison of the typical laboratory features of osteomalacia, primary hyperparathyroidism, and osteoporosis is given in Table 75–3.

The radiographic findings in osteomalacia are usually nonspecific and show only diffuse osteopenia. Trabeculae are poorly defined, the corticomedullary junction is

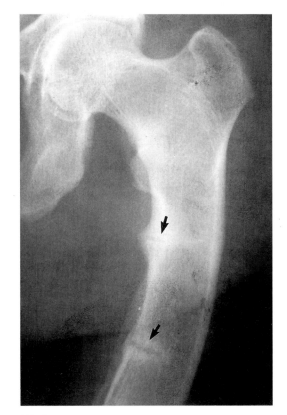

Figure 75–2
Pseudofractures (Looser's zones) of the medial aspect of the femur of a patient with osteomalacia. (Courtesy of Dr. Daniel Rosenthal.)

blurred, and the cortices are thinned. The only specific radiographic manifestation is the pseudofracture, or Looser's zone. Classically, pseudofractures are bilateral and symmetric and oriented perpendicular to the surface of the bone (Fig. 75–2). They are most common on the concave surface of the proximal femur, femoral neck, pubic and ischial rami, pelvis, ribs, and axillary margins of the scapula.

In rickets, the most characteristic alterations occur at the epiphyseal growth plate, which is widened. Enlargement of the growth plate leads to flaring, cupping, and fraying of the metaphyses (see Fig. 75–1). Bowing of long bones, scoliosis, a bell-shaped thorax, basilar invagination of the skull, and acetabular protrusion all may occur in rachitic bones.

DIAGNOSIS

In osteomalacia and rickets, mineralization of osteoid (and of cartilage in rickets) does not keep pace with formation of osteoid. The diagnosis of rickets is usually apparent on clinical and radiographic grounds, whereas the diagnosis of osteomalacia is best established by iliac crest bone biopsy after double tetracycline labeling. In patients with osteomalacia, osteoid seams are wider than normal and cover a greater extent of bone surface, and the rate of bone formation is depressed. A mean osteoid seam width > 15 μm and a mineralization lag time > 100 days are generally considered appropriate kinetic criteria to diagnose osteomalacia; however, some experts also require an absolute increase in the total osteoid volume and an increased number of osteoid lamellae.

TREATMENT

Because of the diverse causes of osteomalacia and rickets, it is difficult to generalize treatment. Most patients require calcium and vitamin D therapy, and some require large supplements of phosphate. In patients with vitamin D deficiency, administering vitamin D produces a rapid increase in levels of serum inorganic phosphate. Serum calcium levels may decrease transiently when therapy is instituted before returning to normal. Normalization of serum alkaline phosphatase and iPTH levels may take several months. In patients with severe hypophosphatemia, as in VDRR, oral phosphate therapy is associated with a rapid rise in serum inorganic phosphate levels, which is often accompanied by a slight fall in serum calcium levels, reduced excretion of urinary calcium, and a transient increase in serum iPTH levels. Combined therapy with vitamin D and phosphate accelerates healing of the bone disease and allows the use of lower doses of oral phosphate supplements in patients with VDRR.

REFERENCES

Favus MJ (ed.): Primer on the Metabolic Bone Diseases and Disorders of Mineral Metabolism. 2nd ed. New York, Raven Press, 1993.
Goldring SR, Krane SM, Avioli, LV: Disorders of calcification: Osteomalacia and rickets. *In* DeGroot LJ (ed.): Endocrinology. Philadelphia, WB Saunders, 1995, pp 1204–1227.

76

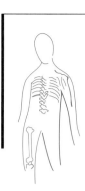

Osteoporosis

GENERAL CONSIDERATIONS

Osteoporosis, the most common type of metabolic bone disease, is characterized by a parallel reduction in bone mineral and bone matrix so that bone is decreased in amount but is of normal composition. Osteoporosis affects 20 million Americans and leads to approximately 1.3 million fractures in the United States each year. During the course of their lifetime, women lose about 50% of their trabecular bone and 30% of their cortical bone, and 30% of all postmenopausal white women eventually will have osteoporotic fractures. By extreme old age, one third of all women and one sixth of all men will have a hip fracture. The annual cost of health care and lost productivity due to osteoporosis exceeds $10 billion in the United States.

ETIOLOGY AND PATHOGENESIS

At any point in time, bone density depends on both the peak bone density achieved during development and the subsequent adult bone loss (Fig. 76-1). Thus, osteopenia can result either from deficient pubertal bone accretion, accelerated adult bone loss, or both.

Determinants of Peak Bone Density

Bone density increases dramatically during puberty in response to gonadal steroids and eventually reaches values in young adults that are nearly double those of children. Other factors that influence peak bone density are listed in Table 76-1. The impact of genetic factors on bone density has been demonstrated in several ways. For example, bone density is lower in the daughters of women with osteoporosis than in those without osteoporosis. Moreover, the concordance of bone density is much higher among monozygotic than dizygotic twins. Recent data suggest that most of the genetic differences in bone density can be accounted for by a gene closely linked to the vitamin D receptor gene, perhaps the receptor gene itself. One large, cross-sectional analysis of white men and women revealed that allelic variations of the vitamin D receptor gene are associated with absolute differences in bone density of 10 to 12%, an effect as large as that

caused by 5 years of estrogen deficiency. However, other studies have not found similar differences in bone density associated with polymorphisms in the vitamin D receptor gene.

Men have higher bone density than women, and blacks have higher bone density than whites. Men with histories of constitutionally delayed puberty have decreased peak bone density, a finding that may be important in the pathogenesis of osteoporosis in some men. Similar findings have been reported in women with delayed menarche. Studies in identical twins suggest that moderate calcium supplementation can enhance prepubertal bone accretion. Associations between peak bone density and physical activity have also been reported.

Physiologic Causes of Adult Bone Loss

After peak bone density is reached, bone density remains stable for years and then declines. Considerable evidence suggests that bone loss begins before menopause in women and in the 20s to 40s in men. Once the menopause is established, the rate of bone loss is accelerated several-fold in women. During the first 5 to 10 years of the menopause, trabecular bone is lost faster than cortical bone, with rates of approximately 2 to 4% and 1 to 2% per year, respectively. A woman can lose 10 to 15% of her cortical bone and 25 to 30% of her trabecular bone during this time, a loss that can prevented by estrogen replacement therapy. Furthermore, rates of bone loss vary considerably between women. A subset of women in whom osteopenia is more severe than expected for their age are said to have type I or "postmenopausal" osteoporosis (Fig. 76-2). Clinically, type I osteoporosis often presents with vertebral "crush" fractures or Colles' fractures. The mechanism whereby estrogen deficiency leads to bone loss is still not established. Recent evidence suggests that estrogen deficiency may increase local production of bone-resorbing cytokines such as interleukin (IL)-1, IL-6, and tumor necrosis factor. Because estrogen also increases local production of growth factors, such as insulin-like growth factor-1 and transforming growth factor-β, that stimulate bone formation, estrogen deficiency might diminish bone formation. Estrogen deficiency increases the skeleton's sensitivity to the resorptive effects of parathyroid hormone. Estrogen deficiency therefore leads to a

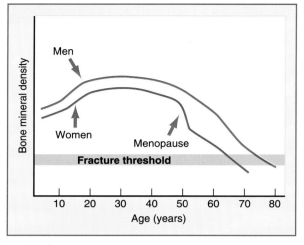

Figure 76-1

Cortical bone mineral density versus age in men and women. Women have lower peak cortical bone density than men and experience a period of rapid bone loss at the time of the menopause, thus reaching the fracture threshold (the level of bone density at which the risk of developing osteoporotic fractures begins to increase) earlier than men.

small increase in serum calcium levels. According to one hypothesis, increased calcium levels suppress parathyroid hormone secretion, thereby decreasing renal 1,25-(OH)$_2$ vitamin D formation, which then limits intestinal calcium absorption (see Fig. 76-2). Finally, the discovery of estrogen receptors on osteoblasts suggests that estrogen deficiency may also alter bone formation directly.

Once the period of rapid postmenopausal bone loss ends, bone loss continues at a more gradual rate throughout life. The osteopenia that results from normal aging, which occurs in both women and men, has been termed type II or "senile" osteoporosis (Fig. 76-3). Because type II osteoporosis is associated with a more balanced decrease in cortical and trabecular bone mass, fractures of the hip, pelvis, wrist, proximal humerus, proximal tibia, and vertebral bodies all occur commonly. Factors that may be important in the pathogenesis of type II osteoporosis include (1) a primary defect in the ability of the kidney to make 1,25-(OH)$_2$ vitamin D and/or decreased intestinal sensitivity to 1,25-(OH)$_2$ vitamin D, leading to diminished calcium absorption and mild secondary hyperparathyroidism; and (2) a decrease in osteoblastic bone

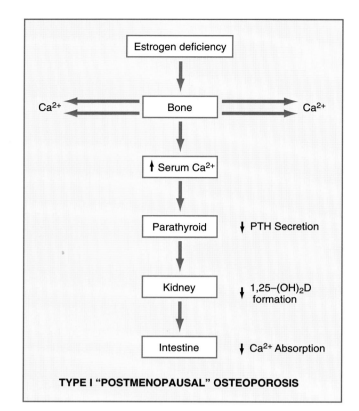

TYPE I "POSTMENOPAUSAL" OSTEOPOROSIS

Figure 76-2

Physiologic alterations in women with type I ("postmenopausal") osteoporosis.

formation with aging. Finally, the distinctions between type I and type II osteoporosis are often quite arbitrary, and there may be considerable overlap between these syndromes.

TABLE 76-1	Factors That May Affect Peak Bone Mass
	Gender
	Race
	Genetic factors
	Gonadal steroids
	Growth hormone
	Timing of puberty
	Calcium intake
	Exercise

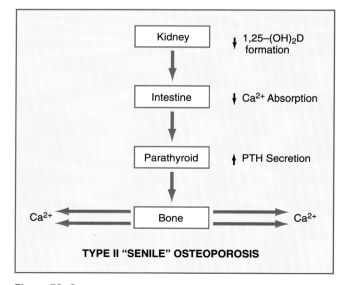

TYPE II "SENILE" OSTEOPOROSIS

Figure 76-3

Physiologic alterations in women with type II ("senile") osteoporosis.

Secondary Causes of Adult Bone Loss

Many of the disorders that can lead to osteoporosis independent from the normal effects of the menopause in women and aging in both women and men are listed in Table 76–2. These conditions should be considered when evaluating patients with osteoporosis and include endogenous and exogenous glucocorticoid excess, hypogonadism, hyperthyroidism, hyperparathyroidism, vitamin D deficiency, gastrointestinal diseases, bone marrow disorders, immobilization, connective tissue diseases, and certain drugs.

CLINICAL MANIFESTATIONS

Osteoporosis is asymptomatic unless it results in a fracture—usually a vertebral compression fracture or a fracture of the wrist, hip, ribs, pelvis, or humerus. Vertebral compression fractures often occur with minimal stress, such as with sneezing, bending, or lifting a light object. The middle and lower thoracic and upper lumbar regions are most frequently involved. Back pain usually begins acutely, often radiates laterally to the flanks and anteriorly, and then subsides gradually over a period of several weeks. Patients with multiple fractures that result in spinal deformity may have a chronic backache that is made worse by standing. Such patients lose height and may develop the characteristic dorsal kyphosis and cervical lordosis known as the "dowager's hump." In some patients, vertebral collapse can occur slowly and without symptoms. Hip fractures are of the femoral neck and intertrochanteric types. Hip fractures are associated with falls, occurring either as a result of modest trauma, or, in some instances, prior to the fall. The likelihood of suffering a hip fracture during a fall is also related to the direction of the fall; fractures are more likely to occur when the person falls to the side. Secondary complications of hip fractures carry a mortality rate of 15 to 20% in elderly patients and lead to severe disability and the need for long-term nursing home care in many others.

RADIOGRAPHIC FINDINGS

A characteristic radiograph of osteoporosis of the spine is shown in Figure 76–4. With the loss of trabecular bone in the vertebral bodies, the vertebral end-plates appear to be accentuated. Vertebral deformity may take the form of collapse (reduction in both anterior and posterior height), anterior wedging (reduction in anterior height), or the so-called codfish deformity (due to weakening of the subchondral plates and expansion of the intervertebral discs). Protrusion of the intervertebral discs in the vertebral bodies produces "Schmorl's nodules." In the absence of fractures, radiographs are insensitive indicators of bone loss, because a substantial reduction in bone mass is required before bone loss is visible on radiographs.

TABLE 76–2	Secondary Causes of Osteoporosis

Endocrine Diseases

Female hypogonadism
   Hyperprolactinemia
   Hypothalamic amenorrhea
   Anorexia nervosa
   Premature and primary ovarian failure
Male hypogonadism
   Primary gonadal failure (e.g., Klinefelter's syndrome)
   Secondary gonadal failure (e.g. idiopathic hypogonadotropic hypogonadism)
   Delayed puberty
Hyperthyroidism
Hyperparathyroidism
Hypercortisolism
Growth hormone deficiency

Gastrointestinal Diseases

Subtotal gastrectomy
Malabsorption syndromes
Chronic obstructive jaundice
Primary biliary cirrhosis and other cirrhoses
Alactasia

Bone Marrow Disorders

Multiple myeloma
Lymphoma
Leukemia
Hemolytic anemias
Systemic mastocytosis
Disseminated carcinoma

Connective Tissue Diseases

Osteogenesis imperfecta
Ehlers-Danlos syndrome
Marfan's syndrome
Homocystinuria

Drugs

Alcohol
Heparin
Glucocorticoids
Thyroxine
Anticonvulsants
Gonadotropin-releasing hormone agonists
Cyclosporine
Chemotherapy

Miscellaneous Causes

Immobilization
Rheumatoid arthritis

DIAGNOSIS

The diagnosis of osteopenia can be made by either documenting a typical fragility fracture or measuring bone mineral density, in which case a bone density value below the lower limit of normal for sex-matched young adults establishes the diagnosis. Most individuals with osteopenia will have osteoporosis, although only a histomorphometric analysis of bone can distinguish osteoporosis from osteomalacia with certainty. Several techniques are available for measuring bone mineral density in the axial and appendicular skeleton (Table 76–3). Large prospective studies have demonstrated that bone density measurements of the distal and proximal radius, os calcis, proximal femur, or spine can predict the development of

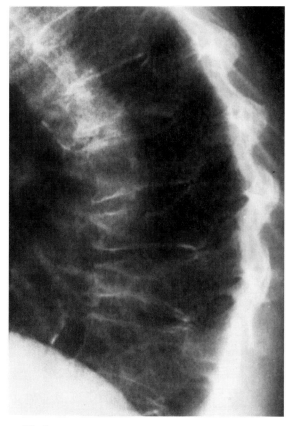

Figure 76–4
Radiograph showing radiolucency, compression fractures, and kyphosis in the spine of a patient with osteoporosis.

the major types of osteoporotic fractures, including hip fractures. Of the available techniques, quantitative computed tomography (QCT) of the spine is the most sensitive method for diagnosing osteopenia because it exclusively measures trabecular bone within the vertebral bodies. However, because the expense and radiation dose of QCT are high and its reproducibility relatively poor, it is not an ideal technique when repeat measurements aimed at detecting small changes in bone density are needed. Single-photon absorptiometry of the proximal forearm has good precision and low radiation exposure but is relatively insensitive for detecting osteopenia because it measures cortical bone, which is lost more slowly than trabecular bone in the early menopause. Dual-photon absorptiometry (DPA), the first technique available for measuring bone density in the spine and hip, is limited by poor reproducibility, long examination times, and artifacts. For most patients, dual-energy x-ray absorptiometry (DXA) of the lumbar spine or hip is the method of choice for measuring bone mineral density. Because DXA scans of the spine in the anterior-posterior projection include both the trabecular-rich vertebral bodies and the cortical-rich posterior spinal elements, DXA is not as sensitive as QCT for detecting early trabecular bone loss. However, its far greater precision, low radiation dose, rapid examination time, and lower cost make DXA preferable to QCT in most situations. Newer DXA scanners can measure spinal bone mineral density in both the anterior-posterior and lateral projections. Lateral spine DXA is more sensitive than anterior-posterior spine DXA for detecting osteoporosis, although its reproducibility is slightly worse.

Secondary causes of osteoporosis should be sought in patients with an established diagnosis of osteoporosis, particularly when the bone density is significantly lower than that of age- and sex-matched individuals. A history and physical examination that focus on the factors that

TABLE 76–3	Techniques for Measuring Bone Mineral Density*			
Sites Measured	**Precision (%)**	**Accuracy (%)**	**Scan Time (min)**	**Radiation Dose (mrems)**
Quantitative computed tomography (QCT) Lumbar spine	2–10	5–20	10–15	100–1000
Single-photon absorptiometry (SPA) Proximal radius Distal radius Calcaneus	1–3	4–6	3–5	10–20
Dual-photon absorptiometry (DPA) Lumbar spine AP Lumbar spine lateral Proximal femur Total body	2–6	4–10	20–45	10–15
Dual-energy x-ray absorptiometry (DEXA) Lumbar spine AP Lumbar spine lateral Proximal radius Distal radius Proximal femur Total body	1–2	3–5	2–8	1–3

*For SPA, numbers refer to measurements of the proximal radius. For DPA and DEXA, numbers refer to AP measurements of the lumbar spine.

may affect peak bone mass (see Table 76–1) and secondary causes of osteoporosis (see Table 76–2) and selected laboratory tests are sufficient in most patients. Levels of serum calcium, inorganic phosphate, and alkaline phosphatase are usually normal in patients with osteoporosis, although the latter may be elevated transiently after a fracture. Other routine chemistries can help exclude renal or hepatic diseases, and a complete blood count may help uncover a hematologic or myeloproliferative disorder. Because multiple myeloma can mimic involutional osteoporosis, it should be considered when evaluating patients with osteoporosis, particularly those with severe disease. Measuring serum parathyroid hormone and 25-OH vitamin D levels is recommended to exclude hyperparathyroidism and vitamin D deficiency. A serum thyroid-stimulating hormone level should be checked when thyrotoxicosis is suspected. In men with unexplained osteoporosis, a serum testosterone level should be measured. The clinical utility of measuring biochemical markers of bone formation (serum osteocalcin, bone-specific alkaline phosphatase, or type-1 procollagen carboxy-terminal propeptide) and bone resorption (urine hydroxyproline, urine pyridinoline cross links, or urine cross-linked N-telopeptides of type 1 collagen) has not been established. These markers may help predict rates of bone loss or the response to therapy. Finally, in selected patients, iliac crest bone biopsy after double tetracycline labeling may be useful, particularly for distinguishing osteoporosis from osteomalacia.

TREATMENT

At present, it is not possible to reverse established osteoporosis. However, early intervention can prevent osteoporosis in most people, and later intervention can halt the progression. If a secondary cause of osteoporosis is present, specific treatment should be aimed at correcting the underlying disorder. During the acute phase of vertebral compression, attention is directed toward relieving pain with analgesics, muscle relaxants, heat, massage, and/or rest. Many patients with discomfort related to osteoporotic fractures or deformity benefit from a well-designed program of physical therapy. Some patients appear to benefit from a corset or an orthopedic back brace. Both weight-bearing and non–weight bearing exercises appear to have beneficial effects on bone mass. For most patients, exercises to strengthen the abdominal and back muscles are appropriate, and referral to a physical therapist with expertise in treating osteoporotic patients is often helpful. Precautions to prevent falls should be taken. Pharmacologic therapy is aimed at preventing further bone loss and decreasing the likelihood of future fracture.

Calcium

Both dietary calcium intake and fractional intestinal calcium absorption decrease with age. Most postmenopausal women consume < 500 mg/day of calcium, far below the United States recommended dietary allowance (RDA) of 800 to 1000 mg/day. It appears that calcium can retard, but not arrest, cortical bone loss from the forearm in women who are within the first several years of the menopause. Most studies have failed to demonstrate a protective effect of calcium on spinal bone loss in early menopausal women. Calcium therapy appears to be more effective in arresting bone loss in late menopausal women, although some studies indicate that administering calcium does not halt their bone loss completely. Most experts recommend that postmenopausal women consume between 1000 and 1500 mg/day of calcium, either in their diet or from supplements. Because calcium may enhance peak bone mass, the RDA for adolescents and young adults in the United States is 1500 mg/day of calcium.

Estrogen

Both oral and transdermal estrogen replacement therapy prevent bone loss in estrogen-deficient women, regardless of when therapy is begun. Because bone loss is most rapid in the first years of the menopause, the benefits of estrogen therapy probably are greater if started before a substantial amount of bone loss has occurred. Case-control studies suggest that estrogen therapy significantly reduces the risk of forearm, vertebral, pelvic, and hip fractures in postmenopausal women. The minimally effective doses of estrogen to prevent bone loss are 0.625 mg/day of conjugated estrogens, 2 mg/day of estradiol, 25 μg/day of ethinyl estradiol, or 50 μg/day of transdermal estrogen, although some studies have shown that lower doses of conjugated estrogens (0.3 mg/day) prevent bone loss when combined with sufficient calcium intake. How long a woman should remain on estrogen replacement therapy has not been established.

The decision to treat with estrogen is influenced by several factors and should be individualized. In some women, estrogen is prescribed to alleviate menopausal symptoms. In others, the prospect of adhering to a treatment program that will produce cyclic menstruation is unacceptable. When given without concomitant progestin, estrogen replacement therapy increases the risk of endometrial carcinoma. Thus, in the woman whose uterus is intact, estrogen replacement therapy should be combined with a progestin, administered either cyclically (e.g., 5 to 10 mg medroxyprogesterone acetate for 12 to 14 days each month) or continuously (e.g., 2.5 mg/day medroxyprogesterone acetate). The latter regimen often eliminates menstrual bleeding after an initial period of 3 to 6 months during which irregular bleeding may occur. In the woman who has had a hysterectomy, unopposed estrogen should be given daily.

The relationship between estrogen replacement therapy and breast cancer or cardiovascular disease has been the subject of many case-control and cohort studies yet remains unclear. Some studies suggest that postmenopausal estrogen use, particularly when continued for more than 5 to 10 years, is associated with an increased risk of breast cancer, although other studies have failed to detect such a relationship. Numerous case-control and cohort studies have reported that estrogen replacement therapy decreases the risk of major coronary disease by approximately 40 to 50%. However, the potential for bias due to patient selection or uneven diagnostic surveillance in these nonrandomized studies cannot be excluded completely. Although estrogen clearly reduces low-density lipoprotein (LDL) cholesterol levels, the beneficial effects of estrogens on coronary heart disease may be related to direct effects on vascular wall function or coagulation factors.

Calcitonin

Calcitonin appears to prevent spinal bone loss both in early and late menopausal women, although appendicular (i.e., cortical) bone loss continues. The effect of calcitonin therapy on the rate of osteoporotic fractures has not been well studied. Calcitonin is now available both for parenteral and intranasal use. The recommended dose is 100 IU subcutaneously or 200 IU intranasally each day, given with adequate calcium and vitamin D, but it is possible that lower doses are equally effective. Side effects such as nausea and flushing are common in patients treated with parenteral calcitonin but are rare with subcutaneous calcitonin. Calcitonin also appears to produce significant analgesic effects. Thus, it may be particularly useful in patients with osteoporosis who have chronic pain related to fractures or skeletal deformity.

Bisphosphonates

Bisphosphonates inhibit osteoclastic bone resorption and have become an important form of therapy for osteoporosis. Until recently, the only bisphosphonate available for oral administration in the United States was etidronate, although it is not approved by the Food and Drug Administration (FDA) for treating osteoporosis. Prospective studies have demonstrated that cyclic etidronate increases spinal bone mineral density slightly and decreases the incidence of vertebral fractures in late menopausal women when given for 2 to 3 years. The effect on fracture rate of continuing etidronate therapy for more than 2 to 3 years is unclear. Recent data suggest that etidronate also prevents bone loss in early menopausal women. The most commonly used dose of etidronate is 400 mg/day for the first 2 weeks of every 3-month period. To ensure adequate absorption, it must be taken on an empty stomach.

Alendronate, a second-generation bisphosphonate that is roughly 50 times as potent as etidronate, was recently approved by the FDA for the treatment of postmenopausal women with osteoporosis. Alendronate therapy increases bone density of the spine and hip and reduces the risk of both spine and nonspine fractures. The recommended dose of alendronate is 10 mg daily, taken after an overnight fast and at least 30 minutes before any food is ingested. Other bisphosphonates, including tiludronate and risedronate, are currently in clinical trials.

Vitamin D and Its Metabolites

Because of low vitamin D intake, insufficient exposure to sunlight, and reduced ability to synthesize vitamin D in the skin, many elderly people are at risk for vitamin D deficiency. Furthermore, the ability to convert 25-OH vitamin D to 1,25-(OH)$_2$ vitamin D is impaired in many elderly people. Decreased vitamin D formation and calcium absorption in the elderly may lead to secondary hyperparathyroidism and accelerated bone loss.

Small doses of vitamin D (800 IU/day) plus calcium dramatically reduce the incidence of hip fractures and other nonspine fractures in elderly women. Because toxicity from such doses of vitamin D has not been reported, this therapy can be recommended to virtually all postmenopausal women. The use of 1,25-(OH)$_2$ vitamin D as a therapy for postmenopausal osteoporosis is more controversial. Although it has been reported that 0.5 μg/day of 1,25-(OH)$_2$ vitamin D plus calcium preserves spinal bone mass and decreases the rate of fractures, it is unclear whether 1,25-(OH)$_2$ vitamin D therapy is superior to treatment with physiologic doses of vitamin D. Because the therapeutic index of 1,25-(OH)$_2$ vitamin D therapy is small, its use should probably be reserved for patients who are not candidates for other forms of pharmacologic therapy.

Future Therapies

Several new types of therapeutic agents are currently in clinical trials. Antiestrogens, such as tamoxifen, can prevent spinal bone loss in postmenopausal women. Raloxifene, an antiestrogen that appears to prevent bone loss without causing endometrial hyperplasia, is being investigated. It is well known that sodium fluoride increases spinal bone density. However, a traditional formulation of sodium fluoride therapy failed to reduce the risk of vertebral fractures and actually increased the incidence of fractures of the appendicular skeleton. Recently it has been reported that lower doses of a slow-release formulation of sodium fluoride increase spinal bone density without accelerating cortical bone loss and reduce the incidence of spine fractures. Parathyroid hormone, when given intermittently in low doses, is a potent stimulator of osteoblastic bone formation. A recent study has demonstrated that parathyroid hormone can prevent bone loss in young women with severe estrogen deficiency. Studies are also in progress to determine whether intermittently administered parathyroid hormone can reverse established osteoporosis.

GLUCOCORTICOID-INDUCED BONE LOSS

Bone loss is a common complication of glucocorticoid excess. The most important adverse effects of glucocorticoids on bone metabolism appear to be suppressed osteoblast activity and a vitamin D–independent inhibition of intestinal calcium absorption. Enhanced osteoclastic activity may also be important. The ability of glucocorticoids to suppress bone formation appears to be mediated, at least in part, by suppression of local secretion of insulin-like growth factor-1 in bone.

The predominant effect on the skeleton of administering glucocorticoids is a loss of trabecular bone, although cortical bone mass also decreases. Bone loss is most rapid in the first 6 to 12 months of therapy, but accelerated bone loss appears to continue as long as therapy is continued.

If it is anticipated that glucocorticoid therapy will be maintained for several months or longer, treatment to prevent bone loss should be strongly considered, particularly in estrogen-deficient women and when a high dosage of glucocorticoids is needed. Small studies have suggested that either subcutaneous or intranasal calcitonin or cyclic etidronate can prevent spinal bone loss in patients receiving long-term glucocorticoid therapy. One controlled study demonstrated that 0.5 to 1.0 μg of calcitriol plus 1000 mg of calcium per day can prevent spinal bone loss for at least 1 year in patients who are starting treatment with glucocorticoids. However, because of the potential for hypercalciuria and/or hypercalcemia, patients receiving calcitriol therapy require careful monitoring. Calcitriol therapy seems most logical in patients with low urinary calcium excretion, suggesting poor intestinal absorption of calcium, and should be avoided in patients with hypercalciuria. Physiologic vitamin D replacement (400 IU/day), can be safely recommended in all patients receiving glucocorticoids and calcium supplementation (1000 mg/day) should be added unless the urinary calcium excretion is excessive.

REFERENCES

Christiansen CC (ed.): Consensus Development Conference on Osteoporosis. Am J Med 1993; 95(5A):1S–78S.

Hahn BH, Mazzaferri EL: Glucocorticoid-induced osteoporosis. Hosp Pract 1995; 30:45–56.

Neer RM: Osteoporosis *In* DeGroot LJ (ed.): Endocrinology. Philadelphia, WB Saunders, 1994, pp 1228–1258.

Riggs BL, Melton III LJ: The prevention and treatment of osteoporosis. N Engl J Med 1992; 327:620–627.

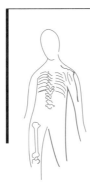

77

Paget's Disease of Bone

Paget's disease is a chronic disorder of bone that may be monostotic or polyostotic. It is characterized by intense osteoclastic bone resorption followed by increased osteoblastic activity, resulting in deposition of woven bone. Paget's disease is commonly asymptomatic, detected incidentally on radiographs or after finding an elevated serum alkaline phosphatase activity. However, it may result in pain, gross skeletal deformity, fracture, or neurologic compression syndromes.

INCIDENCE AND PREVALENCE

After osteoporosis, Paget's disease is the second most common bone disease; it is estimated to affect >3% of persons over age 40 in the United States. Its prevalence varies with geographic location; it is more common in the United States, Great Britain, France, Germany, and Australia and occurs infrequently in Scandinavia, the Middle East, and Asia.

ETIOLOGY

The cause of Paget's disease is unknown. Twenty to thirty percent of affected individuals have a family history of the disorder, and there is an increased frequency of human leukocyte antigen (HLA)-DQW1 in affected individuals. Inclusion bodies that resemble paramyxoviruses are seen in pagetic osteoclasts. Immunohistochemical staining has demonstrated the presence of measles and respiratory syncytial virus antigens, and measles and canine distemper virus sequences have been detected by *in situ* hybridization. These observations suggest that the disorder may result from a slow-activating viral infection, perhaps in genetically susceptible hosts. However, no virus has been cultured from pagetic bone cells, and detection of viral RNA by polymerase chain reaction gene amplification has yielded conflicting results.

PATHOLOGY AND PATHOPHYSIOLOGY

In areas of pagetic bone, osteoclasts are increased in number and size and contain multiple pleomorphic nuclei, increased rough endoplasmic reticulum, and organelles. Osteoblast activity remains coupled to osteoclastic bone resorption so that both bone resorption and formation are increased. However, the resultant bone is woven in appearance and is structurally abnormal. Vascularity of the abnormal bone is increased, and peritrabecular fibrosis may replace the normal cellular marrow. Eventually the processes of resorption and formation may slow, leaving sclerotic "burned out" pagetic bone.

Increased bone resorption may be due to local stimulation of osteoclast proliferation and activation by cytokines such as interleukin-6 (IL-6). Pagetic osteoclasts have receptors for IL-6 and also produce IL-6. IL-6 is detectable in marrow plasma and serum from individuals with Paget's disease but not in normals.

CLINICAL PICTURE (Table 77–1)

Most individuals with Paget's disease are asymptomatic and have only one or a few affected skeletal sites. With more extensive skeletal involvement there can be painless deformity of the skull or other affected bones, and the overlying skin may be warm and erythematous. The most commonly affected sites include the pelvis, femur, spine, skull, and tibia; involvement of the hands or feet is rare. Back pain, headache, and pain in the hips and legs are common complaints. Arthritis is often found in joints near areas involved with Paget's disease, particularly when subchondral bone is affected or the integrity of the joint is compromised by enlarged, distorted bones. Pathologic fractures may occur, but small fissure fractures along the convex surface of long bones are more common. Spinal cord or nerve root compression with associated radicular pain and weakness may result from expanding pagetic bone. Hearing is commonly affected, but other cranial nerves palsies are seen less frequently. Softening of the base of the skull may produce flattening (platybasia) with the development of basilar invagination and may lead to neurologic compression syndromes. Once areas of pagetic involvement have been identified, it is unusual for the disease to involve new bone sites, although local extension along affected areas may occur.

TABLE 77–1	Clinical Manifestations of Paget's Disease

Musculoskeletal pain
Degenerative arthritis in joints near affected areas
Headache
Skeletal deformity
Pathologic fractures
Enlarged skull
Erythema and warmth over pagetic bones
Hearing loss
Platybasia with or without basilar invagination
Neurologic compression syndromes
Angioid streaks in retina
Increased cardiac output—rarely congestive heart failure
Bone tumors
    Osteogenic sarcoma
    Fibrosarcoma
    Chrondrosarcoma
    Reparative granuloma
    Giant cell tumor
Laboratory abnormalities
    Increased serum alkaline phosphatase (bone fraction)
    Increased urinary hydroxyproline
    Hypercalciuria and hypercalcemia during immobilization
    Hyperuricemia
    Characteristic radiographs
    Increased uptake on bone scan

ASSOCIATED CONDITIONS

Secondary arthritis is a common and often debilitating complication of periarticular Paget's disease. Hyperuricemia and gout may occur with increased frequency in affected individuals. Secondary hyperparathyroidism has been noted in 15 to 20% of patients with Paget's disease. The occurence of primary hyperparathyroidism in patients with Paget's disease is currently believed to be a clinical coincidence. The most serious complication of Paget's disease is sarcomatous degeneration, which occurs most commonly in the setting of severe polyostotic disease and may be heralded by a sudden increase in pain, a soft tissue mass, or pathologic fracture. The majority of tumors are osteogenic sarcomas, although fibrosarcomas and chondrosarcomas are also seen. Benign giant cell tumors, most often affecting the skull, are also seen.

LABORATORY ASSESSMENT

Biochemical markers of bone formation, such as serum alkaline phosphatase and osteocalcin, and bone resorption, including urinary excretion of hydroxyproline and pyridinolines, are increased in individuals with active disease. Serum bone-specific alkaline phosphatase activity and urinary pyridinoline excretion appear to be more sensitive markers for assessing disease activity in patients with low levels of disease activity.

A bone scan is the most efficient means for a survey of pagetic sites. Radiographs of affected areas confirm the presence of Paget's disease and are useful for monitoring disease progression as well as for complications. Early in

the course of the disease, osteolysis may be seen as osteoporosis circumscripta in the skull or pelvis (Fig. 77–1*A*) or as an advancing "blade of grass" in long bones (Fig. 77–1*B*). Later, in the mixed phase of the disease, expanded bones with cortical thickening, coarse trabecular markings, and both lytic and sclerotic areas are seen on radiographs (Fig. 77–1*C*). In the late stages of the disease, when bone turnover is quiescent, sclerotic bone predominates (Fig. 77–1*D*). Bone biopsy is rarely needed to diagnose Paget's disease and should be avoided in weight-bearing areas. When done, biopsies show the characteristic histopathology of Paget's disease.

TREATMENT

The two major goals of therapy are to relieve symptoms and prevent complications. Treatment is indicated for individuals with symptoms that cannot be managed with salicylates or nonsteroidal anti-inflammatory drugs (NSAIDs); if the disease involves a weight-bearing bone, the spine, the skull, or bone near a major joint; or when bone deformity, hearing loss, neurologic impairment, or high-output congestive heart failure is present. Treatment may be indicated during periods of immobilization to prevent accelerated bone loss and hypercalciuria. Individuals who are asymptomatic or who have minimal symptoms can often be managed with salicylates or NSAIDs. Antiresorptive agents such as calcitonin or the bisphosphonates form the mainstay of therapy and have largely replaced the use of cytotoxic agents such as plicamycin. Calcitonin, in addition to its antiresorptive action, may have a significant analgesic effect in some individuals. The usual dosage of calcitonin is 50 to 100 units daily by subcutaneous injection. Side effects include nausea and flushing, which usually resolve with continued use. The incidence of side effects can be minimized by gradually increasing the dose and administering the drug before bedtime. Calcitonin therapy can be used to decrease blood flow to pagetic bone prior to surgery.

Bisphosphonates are also well established in the treatment of Paget's disease. Previously, etidronate disodium was the only bisphosphonate available. Although effective, its use was limited by a tendency to induce abnormal mineralization if given at high doses or for more than 6 months at a time. The recommended dose is 5 mg/kg/day for 6 months followed by 6 months without treatment. Its use is contraindicated in patients with lytic disease in weight-bearing bones. The introduction of second-generation bisphosphonates represents a significant advance in the treatment of Paget's disease. These agents may induce a biochemical remission in patients who respond incompletely to treatment with etidronate or calcitonin. Furthermore, they do not produce mineralization defects at the recommended doses. Parental pamidronate, in doses of 30 mg daily for 3 days, often reduces serum alkaline phosphatase and urinary hydroxyproline excretion into the normal range for ≥1 year. Similarly, oral alendronate, given in a dose of 40 mg/day for 6 months, normalizes markers of bone turnover in most patients with Paget's disease. Less than 10% of patients treated

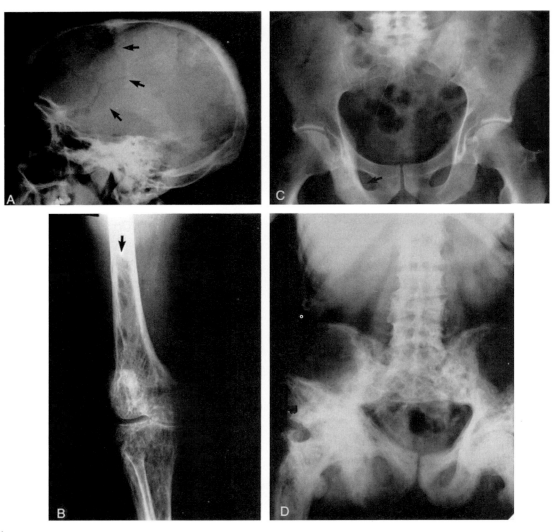

Figure 77–1

Typical radiographic abnormalities in patients with Paget's disease. *A,* Osteoporosis circumscripta of the skull. *B,* Lytic lesions in the femur with the characteristic "blade of grass" or "flamelike" lesion. *C,* Blastic involvement of the right ischial ramus of the pelvis with thickening of the medial cortex. *D,* Mixed lytic and blastic disease involving entire pelvis along with L4 and L5 and both femoral heads. (Courtesy of Dr. Daniel Rosenthal.)

with alendronate have a biochemical recurrence within 12 months. When treating patients with bisphosphonates, it is important to maintain adequate calcium intake (at least 1 gm/day) to prevent the development of secondary hyperparathyroidism. Other oral bisphosphonates, including tiludronate and risedronate, are in advanced stages of clinical testing.

REFERENCES

Singer FR, Wallach S (eds.): Paget's Disease of Bone. Clinical Assessment, Present and Future Therapy. New York, Elsevier, 1991.

Siris ES: Paget's disease of bone. *In* Favus MJ (ed.): Primer on the Metabolic Bone Diseases and Disorders of Mineral Metabolism. 2nd ed. New York, Raven Press, 1993, pp 375–384.

Musculoskeletal and Connective Tissue Disease

Section XII

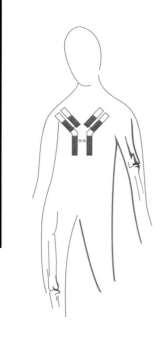

78

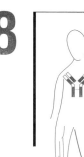

Approach to the Patient with Musculoskeletal Disease

Rheumatology involves the study of diseases affecting joints and periarticular structures. One in six visits to a health professional is for a musculoskeletal complaint; the majority of patient visits to physicians are for nonarticular problems and common musculoskeletal diseases such as osteoarthritis (OA) and rheumatoid arthritis (RA). However, many of the musculoskeletal diseases present major diagnostic and therapeutic challenges. Despite rapid advances in immunology, radiology, and other technologies, *a complete medical history and careful physical examination are the most important steps in the evaluation of the patient with musculoskeletal complaints.* Many musculoskeletal symptoms present with prominent findings that extend to other organ systems. Therefore, the clinician must evaluate the whole patient, even when symptoms appear to be localized. After the complete evaluation, the clinician should be able to classify a patient's problem to direct laboratory and radiographic studies to aid in confirming the clinical diagnosis. On the basis of the initial comprehensive evaluation, the clinician should be able to answer the following questions:

1. Is the condition limited to the musculoskeletal system or is it a systemic process?
2. Is the process articular or nonarticular?
3. Is the process monoarticular or polyarticular?
4. Is the process acute or chronic?
5. Is the condition inflammatory or noninflammatory?
6. Is the arthritis axial, peripheral, or both?
7. Is the process symmetric or asymmetric?
8. Is the pain intermittent or persistent?
9. Is there evidence of muscle or neurologic dysfunction?
10. Is there a family history of a similar process?

A critical decision in the initial evaluation of a patient with musculoskeletal complaints is whether the problem requires immediate evaluation and treatment. For most musculoskeletal complaints, the decision to investigate or treat can wait until the chronicity and severity of the complaints can be fully elucidated. Some clinical situations, however, mandate immediate investigation and treatment:

1. Febrile patient.
2. Single or a few joints involved with acute pain; an acute infectious or crystal arthritis must be excluded or treated immediately.
3. Signs and symptoms suggestive of renal, cardiac, or pulmonary compromise.
4. Symptoms associated with trauma; fracture or internal derangement of joint.
5. Neurologic compromise; bowel or bladder dysfunction; cervical or lumbar cord nerve root compression.
6. Vasculitic process that may result in loss of limb or irreversible organ damage.

A comprehensive physical examination is necessary for evaluating connective tissue disorders, even in a patient with localized symptoms. Many apparent local musculoskeletal complaints have their origin distant from the region of pain. A musculoskeletal examination should include evaluation of specific joints for warmth, swelling, tenderness, crepitus, range of motion (active and passive), and deformity. The evaluation of muscle function requires a simultaneous evaluation of the nervous system in addition to determining the bulk, tone, tenderness, and strength of appropriate muscle groups. Pain and dysfunction in the area of a joint are not necessarily articular in origin; attention should also be directed to the periarticular region. Enthesopathy, bursitis, and tendinitis (Fig. 78–1) are all causes of periarticular pain. The cervical, thoracic, and lumbar spine and sacroiliac joints should be tested for mobility.

Musculoskeletal diseases can be divided into several distinct categories based on pathology (Table 78–1). Identification of the predominant pathophysiologic process (see Fig. 78–1) may suggest different therapeutic decisions.

LABORATORY TESTS

Laboratory tests in patients with musculoskeletal diseases most often provide data to confirm the clinical diagnosis obtained by the detailed history and comprehensive physical examination. Although the majority of patients pre-

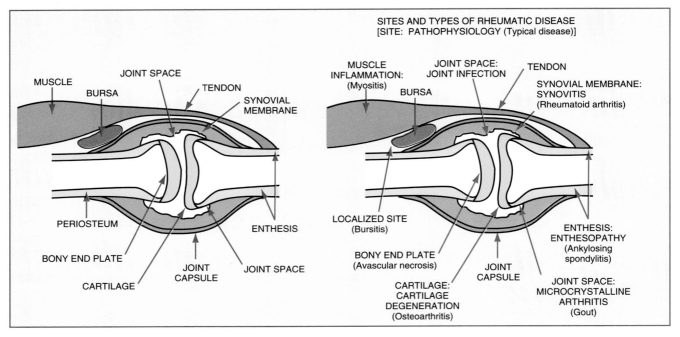

Figure 78-1

Anatomic structures of the musculoskeletal system (*left*). Location of musculoskeletal disease processes (*right*). (From Gordon DA: Approach to the patient with musculoskeletal disease. *In* Bennett JC, Plum F [eds.]: Cecil Textbook of Medicine. 20th ed. Philadelphia, WB Saunders, 1996, pp 1440–1443.)

senting with musculoskeletal problems do not require numerous laboratory tests, complicated or subtle clinical problems may require more extensive testing to assist in diagnosis and to determine therapeutic options.

Synovial Fluid Analysis

Analysis of the synovial fluid is the most useful test in the practice of rheumatology. It should be performed as part of the diagnostic evaluation in any patient with joint disease. Synovial fluid analysis provides the physician with valuable information about processes occurring inside the joint. Many textbooks offer a long list of tests to perform on synovial fluid; however, just a few tests may provide the evidence to establish a specific diagnosis (most commonly gout and infection) (Table 78–2). Gross examination of the fluid plus a leukocyte count may narrow the diagnostic possibilities to diseases causing noninflammatory versus inflammatory joint effusions (Table 78–3). These categories are based on the total synovial fluid white cell count; however, in practice this system is not definitive because disease categories may overlap. For example, a "noninflammatory" synovial fluid does not exclude septic or crystal arthritis.

A macroscopic and microscopic inspection of the fluid may alert the physician to specific diagnoses. The presence of blood in the fluid should suggest a number of disorders (Table 78–4). Lipid droplets may be noted in traumatic arthritis, various inflammatory effusions, and pancreatic fat necrosis. Crystals such as monosodium urate, calcium pyrophosphate dihydrate, oxalate, and cholesterol can be detected in synovial fluid using a polarized

light microscope. Special stains on synovial fluid may be helpful in diagnosing Whipple disease (periodic acid–Schiff stain), hemochromatosis, or pigmented villonodular synovitis (Prussian blue stain for iron), amyloidosis

TABLE 78–1	Categories of Musculoskeletal Diseases	
Pathology or Process	**Disease Example**	**Diagnostic Test(s)**
Infection	Septic arthritis, osteomyelitis	Gram's stain and culture of synovial fluid or tissue
Crystal induced	Gout, pseudogout	Synovial fluid examination for crystals, radiographs for chondrocalcinosis
Autoimmune	Rheumatoid arthritis, systemic lupus erythematosus	Clinical and radiographic evaluation, serologies (rheumatoid factor, antinuclear antibody)
Degenerative	Osteoarthritis	Clinical and radiographic evaluation
Enthesopathy	Ankylosing spondylitis, Reiter's syndrome	Clinical and radiographic evaluation
Vasculitis	Polyarteritis nodosa	Clinical evaluation, biopsy and/or arteriogram
Nonarticular, focal	Bursitis, carpal tunnel syndrome	Clinical evaluation, nerve conduction velocities
Nonarticular, diffuse	Fibromyalgia syndrome	Clinical evaluation
Muscle inflammation	Polymyositis/dermatomyositis	Clinical evaluation, serum muscle enzymes, muscle biopsy
Fibrosis	Scleroderma	Clinical evaluation

TABLE 78–2	Standard Tests to Perform on Synovial Fluid

Volume and gross appearance
Wet preparation
White cell concentration and differential
Polarized light microscopy
Gram's stain and culture (when clinically indicated)

TABLE 78–4	Differential Diagnosis of Hemarthrosis

Trauma with or without fractures
Pigmented villonodular synovitis
Synovioma, other tumors
Hemangioma
Charcot's joint or other severe joint destruction
Von Willebrand's disease
Anticoagulant therapy
Myeloproliferative disease with thrombocytosis
Thrombocytopenia
Scurvy
Ruptured aneurysm
Arteriovenous fistula
Idiopathic

From Schumacher HR: Synovial fluid analysis and synovial biopsy. *In* Kelley WN, Harris ED Jr, Ruddy S, Sledge CB (eds.): Textbook of Rheumatology. 3rd ed. Philadelphia, WB Saunders, 1989, p 638.

(Congo red stain), and systemic lupus erythematosus (SLE) (Wright's stain for LE cells).

Immunologic Testing

Autoantibodies are antibodies directed against self-antigens, including immunoglobulins and cell surfaces as well as nuclear, cytoplasmic, and circulating molecules. Common serologic tests used to detect autoantibodies in evaluating musculoskeletal diseases are listed in Table 78–5. These tests should not be used as "screening" tests for patients with musculoskeletal complaints, because most of these autoantibodies are found in several different connective tissue diseases. For example, serum rheumatoid factors can be demonstrated in a variety of other acute and chronic inflammatory conditions (Table 78–6), as well as in healthy persons. The same lack of specificity of disease associations applies to antinuclear antibodies. However, a few of these serologic tests do appear to be disease-specific: anti-dsDNA and anti-Sm are seen only in patients with SLE; anti-RNP in high titers is found only in mixed connective tissue disease but is found in low titers in other diseases; and antineutrophil cytoplasmic antibody (ANCA) is fairly specific for Wegener's granulomatosis.

Serum protein electrophoresis is used routinely to characterize and quantify serum immunoglobulins. Hypergammaglobulinemia may be seen in several of the autoimmune diseases and vasculitis. Monoclonal immunoglobulin spikes may be indicative of multiple myeloma. A seronegative (for rheumatoid factor) inflammatory arthritis that clinically resembles RA is occasionally seen in persons with hypogammaglobulinemia. Elevated levels of circulating immune complexes occur in many autoimmune diseases as well as in infections and malignancies. Measurement of circulating immune complexes may be useful in following the disease activity of SLE and various systemic vasculitides.

Measurement of total hemolytic complement (CH_{50}) and individual complement components, especially C3 and C4, are often helpful in the diagnosis and management of SLE and vasculitis. The CH_{50} depends on intact and functional classic and alternative pathways, resulting in effective target lysis (Fig. 78–2). CH_{50} measures the ability of serum to lyse antibody-coated erythrocytes and

TABLE 78–3	Classification of Synovial Effusions by Synovial White Cell Count			
Group	Diagnosis (Examples)	Appearance	Synovial Fluid White Cell Count/mm³*	Polymorphonuclear Cells
Normal		Clear, pale yellow	0–200	<10%
I. Noninflammatory	Osteoarthritis Trauma	Clear to slightly turbid	50–2000 (600)	<30%
II. Mildly inflammatory	Systemic lupus erythematosus	Clear to slightly turbid	0–9000 (3000)	<20%
III. Severely inflammatory (noninfectious)	Gout	Turbid	100–160,000 (21,000)	~70%
	Pseudogout	Turbid	50–75,000 (14,000)	~70%
	Rheumatoid arthritis	Turbid	250–80,000 (19,000)	~70%
IV. Severely inflammatory (infectious)	Bacterial infections	Very turbid	150–250,000 (80,000)	~90%
	Tuberculosis	Turbid	2500–100,000 (20,000)	~60%

* Mean values in parentheses.

TABLE 78–5	Common Serologic Tests Used in Musculoskeletal Diseases

Test	Disease Association
Rheumatoid factor	RA, several other diseases
Antinuclear	SLE, scleroderma, RA, myositis, other diseases
Anti-Sm (Smith)	SLE
Anti-ds-DNA	SLE
Anti-histone H_1, H_3-H_4	SLE
Anti-histone H_{2A}, H_{2B}	More common in drug-induced SLE
Anti-RNP (ribonucleoprotein)	MCTD (high titers), SLE
Anti-SSB (anti-La)	Sjögren's syndrome, SLE
Anti-SSA (anti-Ro)	Sjögren's syndrome, SLE, neonatal lupus
Anticentromere	More common in limited scleroderma
Antitopoisomerase I (Scl-70)	More common in diffuse scleroderma
Antineutrophil cytoplasmic (ANCA)	Wegener's granulomatosis, less common in other vasculitides
Anticardiolipin	SLE, antiphospholipid antibody syndrome
Lupus anticoagulant	SLE, antiphospholipid antibody syndrome
Anti-Jo-1	Dermatomyositis/polymyositis with interstitial lung disease

MCTD = Mixed connective tissue disorders; RA = rheumatoid arthritis; SLE = systemic lupus erythematosus.

reflects the activity of all complement components. Decreased CH_{50} levels suggest either depletion of complement proteins by an immune-mediated process or inherited deficiency of an individual protein. Low levels of C3 and C4 are usually seen when a decreased CH_{50} is secondary to an immune mechanism. An extremely low CH_{50} in the presence of relatively normal values of C3 and C4 suggests a genetic complement deficiency, with C2 deficiency being most common. Deficiencies of C1,

TABLE 78–6	Diseases Commonly Associated with Rheumatoid Factor

Rheumatic diseases: rheumatoid arthritis, systemic lupus erythematosus, scleroderma, mixed connective tissue disease, Sjögren's syndrome
Acute viral infections: mononucleosis, hepatitis, influenza, and many others; after vaccination (may yield falsely elevated titers of antiviral antibodies)
Parasitic infections: trypanosomiasis, kala-azar, malaria, schistosomiasis, filariasis, others
Chronic infectious/inflammatory diseases: tuberculosis, leprosy, yaws, syphilis, brucellosis, subacute bacterial endocarditis, salmonellosis
Neoplasms: after irradiation or chemotherapy
Other hyperglobulinemia states: hypergammaglobulinemic purpura, cryoglobulinemia, chronic liver disease, sarcoid, other chronic pulmonary diseases

From Schumacher HR: Synovial fluid analysis and synovial biopsy. *In* Kelley WN, Harris ED Jr, Ruddy S, Sledge CB (eds.): Textbook of Rheumatology. 3rd ed. Philadelphia, WB Saunders, 1989, p 200.

C4, and C2 are associated with SLE, glomerulonephritis, and nonspecific vasculitis. The acquired deficiency of C1 inhibitor is associated with SLE and lymphoid malignancies.

Acute Phase Reactants

The most clinically useful measures of acute phase response are the erythrocyte sedimentation rate (ESR) and C-reactive protein (CRP). Because the ESR is inexpensive and quick and easy to do, it is more commonly used to detect inflammation than is CRP, even though the latter may be more accurate. Although it is a sensitive indicator of inflammation, the ESR lacks specificity but is particularly useful in following the treatment of patients with polymyalgia rheumatica and temporal arteritis.

Other Laboratory Tests

A complete blood count and urinalysis are routinely done in patients with signs and symptoms of a systemic illness. In a small percentage of patients with nonspecific joint complaints, more extensive laboratory testing may be required. In such cases, a chemistry profile, serum iron and ferritin, and thyroid function tests may provide useful clues for certain systemic diseases. Renal and liver function should also be evaluated to monitor for potential toxicity from commonly used medications such as nonsteroidal anti-inflammatory drugs and disease-modifying antirheumatic drugs.

RADIOLOGIC EVALUATION

Radiographs are a vital investigative tool in rheumatology and provide information about the distribution of joint involvement as well as specific diagnoses. Radiographs of the hands and feet may reveal certain "target" joints and changes that are characteristic of specific diseases (e.g., gout—first metatarsophalangeal [MTP] joint erosions; rheumatoid arthritis—fourth and fifth MTP joint erosions). A single anteroposterior view of the pelvis and a lateral view of the lumbar spine and sacroiliac joints are sufficient to evaluate most disorders of the lumbosacral spine and sacroiliac joints. Radiographic changes that show joint space loss with osteophyte formation are diagnostic of OA. Chrondocalcinosis and other soft tissue calcifications can be easily demonstrated using plain radiograph films. Chrondrocalcinosis is detected primarily in the menisci of knees, triangular fibrous cartilage of the wrist, symphysis pubis, acetabular and glenoid labra, and intervertebral discs.

Ultrasonography in rheumatology is used primarily to detect synovial cysts, chiefly in the popliteal area (Baker's cyst). Computed tomography (CT) and magnetic resonance imaging (MRI) are useful in evaluating the spine and sacroiliac joints and in detecting disc hernia-

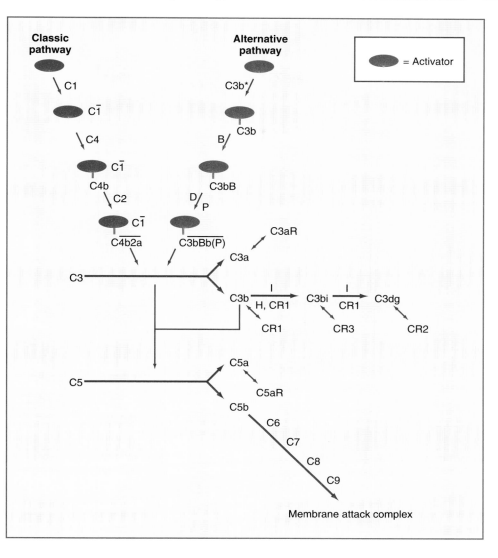

Figure 78-2

Complement activation. Formation of the C3 and C5 convertases in the two pathways of complement activation and the major biologically active fragments generated from C3 and C5 are shown. *Bidirectional arrows* indicate interactions with major receptors. C3b* = metastable C3b; overbars indicate enzymatically active proteins or protein complexes. CR = complement receptor. (From Talal N [ed.]: Molecular Autoimmunity. San Diego, Academic Press Limited, 1991, p 84.)

tions. In addition, they are useful in diagnosing other disorders such as avascular necrosis and osteomyelitis. MRI can also detect damage to the menisci and ligaments of the knee. Bone and joint scans are useful in the diagnosis or exclusion of several musculoskeletal disorders, including osteomyelitis, septic arthritis, avascular necrosis, reflex sympathetic dystrophy, stress fractures, and bone tumors.

REFERENCES

Fries JF: Approach to the patient with musculoskeletal disease. *In* Bennett JC, Plum F (eds.): Cecil Textbook of Medicine. 20th ed. Philadelphia, WB Saunders, 1996, pp 1440–1443.

Schumacher HR: Synovial fluid analysis and synovial biopsy. *In* Kelley WN, Harris ED Jr, Ruddy S, Sledge CB (eds.): Textbook of Rheumatology. 3rd ed. Philadelphia, WB Saunders, 1989, pp 637–648.

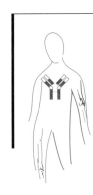

79

Rheumatoid Arthritis

Rheumatoid arthritis (RA) is a chronic inflammatory disease that can affect various organs but predominantly involves the synovial tissues of the diarthrodial joints. It occurs worldwide in all ethnic groups but with significant variations in the prevalence rates among populations. Certain major histocompatibility complex (MHC) class II alleles (and encoded human leukocyte antigen [HLA]) occur with increased frequency in affected individuals. In patients with RA, HLA-DR4 may reach a frequency of 60 to 70%, compared with 25 to 30% in normal individuals. The molecular biology suggests that with HLA-DR4 subtypes Dw4, Dw14, and Dw15, predisposition to RA depends on the binding site for antigen presentation. This information suggests that an unknown antigen may initiate the rheumatoid process. Hence, the infectious origin of RA has been hypothesized and has ranged from various bacteria, including streptococci, mycoplasma, clostridia, and diphtheroids, to a variety of viral infections, including parvovirus, Epstein-Barr virus (EBV), and retroviruses. To date, no conclusive evidence has been presented for any of these as precipitating events. HLA-DR1 is found in most HLA-DR4–negative patients and is most strongly associated with disease in certain ethnic groups (Israelis and Asian Indians).

PATHOGENESIS

A hallmark of the pathology of rheumatoid synovitis is membrane proliferation and ultimate erosion of articular cartilage and subchondral bone (Fig. 79–1). Although the precise initiating event is unknown, it does seem to involve some specific antigenic stimulation of susceptible T lymphocytes bearing the appropriate MHC molecules. This results in both T and B cell proliferation, stimulation of blood vessel proliferation in the synovial membrane, accumulation of inflammatory cells including polymorphonuclear leukocytes, synovial cell proliferation, and development of a rapidly growing and invasive pannus. The last-named grows almost like a benign tumor, to invade cartilage, activate chondrocytes, and release digestive enzymes that degrade cartilage and bone, finally resulting in destructive erosions associated with inflammatory processes surrounding tendons.

CLINICAL MANIFESTATIONS

The articular manifestations of RA are best understood from knowledge of the sequential events that take place in the pathogenetic process (Table 79–1). As indicated, the inflammatory process may be under way for some time before swelling, tissue reaction, and joint destruction are seen. Appreciation of this sequence of events is important in considering therapeutic approaches.

Rheumatoid arthritis affects about 1.5% of most populations, but frequencies as high as 5% have been reported in some Native American tribes. The disease afflicts women in the childbearing years three times more frequently than men. In older age groups, there is a trend toward more equal involvement of men and women.

Rheumatoid arthritis is an idiopathic, symmetric synovitis affecting similar joints bilaterally. The criteria for classification of RA are presented in Table 79–2. Occasionally, the disease presents as a monoarthritis or asymmetric oligoarthritis but eventually assumes a symmetric distribution. Very early in its course, the predominant symptoms may be vague: variable aching, polyarthralgias, and fatigability with little, if any, evidence of synovitis (see Table 79–1). During this early phase, the diagnosis may be unclear, and alternative possibilities, such as fibrositis and polymyalgia rheumatica, are considered. A second, commonly observed onset is frank synovitis in an otherwise healthy individual. The synovitis most commonly affects the metatarsophalangeal (MTP) joints of the feet and the metacarpophalangeal (MCP) and proximal interphalangeal (PIP) joints of the hands, although other joints can be simultaneously involved. A third but uncommon mode of presentation is a rapidly progressive and debilitating polyarticular synovitis. Rarely, one may observe the onset of extra-articular disease before clinical evidence of synovitis (Table 79–3). Although these patterns of onset may not be associated with the early presence of IgM rheumatoid factors, the aggressive/destructive form of RA is often characterized by high titers of these immunoglobulins.

The clinical course of RA is highly variable and can be (1) sporadic, punctuated by intervals of disease inactivity; (2) insidious, with relentless progression of synovitis and periodic, debilitating flares; and (3) aggressive and

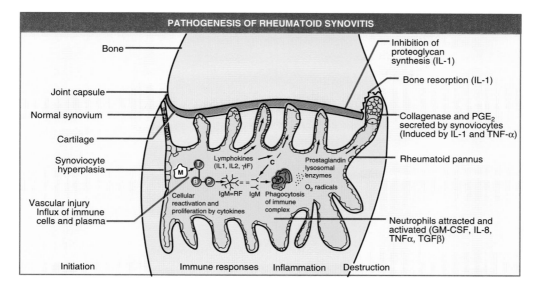

Figure 79–1

Events involved in the pathogenesis of rheumatoid synovitis progress from left to right. M = macrophage; T = T lymphocyte, B = B lymphocyte; P = plasma cell; IL = interleukin; TNFα = tumor necrosis factor alpha; TGFβ = transforming growth factor beta; GM-CSF = granulocyte-macrophage colony stimulating factor; γIf = gamma-interferon; RF = rheumatoid factor; PGE$_2$ = prostaglandin E$_2$; IgM = immunoglobulin M; IgG = immunoglobulin G; C = complement. (From Arnett FC: Rheumatoid arthritis. *In* Bennett JC, Plum F (eds.): Cecil Textbook of Medicine. 20th ed. Philadelphia, WB Saunders, 1996.)

"malignant," with no period of relative remission. The last is characterized by severe polyarticular synovitis, rheumatoid nodules, weight loss, very high titers of rheumatoid factor, and hypocomplementemia. Extra-articular organ involvement (see Table 79–3) is common.

The small joints of the hands and feet are the most common diarthrodial articulations affected. Initially, the synovitis of the PIP joints results in fusiform swelling associated with warmth, erythema, pain, and limitation of motion. MCP joints develop soft tissue swelling, squeeze tenderness, and limitations of motion due to synovitis.

Chronic synovitis of joints and tendon sheaths often leads to permanent deformities. In the feet one commonly sees subluxation of the heads of the MTPs and foreshortening of the extensor tendons, giving rise to "hammer toe" or "cock-up" deformities. A similar process in the

TABLE 79–1	**Stages of Rheumatoid Arthritis**			
Stage	**Pathologic Process**	**Symptoms**	**Physical Signs**	**Radiographic Changes***
1	Presentation of antigen to T cells	Probably none	—	—
2	T cell proliferation B cell proliferation Angiogenesis in synovial membrane	Malaise, mild joint stiffness and swelling	Swelling of small joints of hands or wrists, or pain in hands, wrists, knees, and feet	None
3	Accumulation of neutrophils in synovial fluid Synovial cell proliferation without polarization or invasion of cartilage	Joint pain and swelling, morning stiffness, malaise and weakness	Warm, swollen joints, excess synovial fluid, soft tissue proliferation within joints, pain and limitation of motion, rheumatoid nodules	Soft tissue swelling
4	Polarization of synovitis into a centripetally invasive pannus Activation of chondrocytes Initiation of enzyme (proteinase) degradation of cartilage	Same as stage 3	Same as stage 3, but more pronounced swelling	MRI reveals proliferative pannus; radiographic evidence of periarticular osteopenia
5	Erosion of subchondral bone Invasion of cartilage by pannus Chondrocyte proliferation Stretched ligaments around joints	Same as stage 3, plus loss of function and early deformity (e.g., ulnar deviation at metacarpophalangeal joint)	Same as stage 3, plus instability of joints, flexion contractures, decreased range of motion, extra-articular complications	Early erosions and narrowing of joint spaces

*MRI = Magnetic resonance imaging.
Reprinted, by permission, from the New England Journal of Medicine, Vol 322, pp. 1277–1289, 1990.

TABLE 79–2	Classification Criteria for Rheumatoid Arthritis*

1. Morning stiffness (≥1 hr)
2. Swelling (soft tissue) of three or more joints
3. Swelling (soft tissue) of hand joints (PIP, MCP, or wrist)
4. Symmetric swelling (soft tissue)
5. Subcutaneous nodules
6. Serum rheumatoid factor
7. Erosions and/or periarticular osteopenia, in hand or wrist joints, seen on radiograph

*Criteria 1–4 must have been continuous for 6 wks or longer and must be observed by a physician. A diagnosis of rheumatoid arthritis requires that four of the seven criteria be fulfilled.
MCP = Metacarpophalangeal; PIP = proximal interphalangeal.
From Arnett FC: Rheumatoid arthritis. *In* Bennett JC, Plum F (eds.): Cecil Textbook of Medicine. 20th ed. Philadelphia, WB Saunders, 1996, p 1459.

TABLE 79–3	Extra-Articular Organ System Involvement in Rheumatoid Arthritis

Organ System	Extra-Articular Manifestations
Skin	**Cutaneous vasculitis** **Rheumatoid nodules**
Eye	**Episcleritis** Scleritis Scleromalacia perforans Corneal ulcers/perforation **Uveitis** Retinitis Glaucoma Cataract
Lung	**Pleuritis** Diffuse interstitial fibrosis Vasculitis Rheumatoid nodules Caplan's syndrome Pulmonary hypertension
Heart and blood vessels	**Pericarditis** Myocarditis Coronary arteritis Valvular insufficiency Conduction defects Vasculitis **Felty's syndrome**
Nervous system	**Mononeuritis multiplex** Distal sensory neuropathy

Bold type indicates more commonly seen manifestations.

hands results in volar subluxation of the MCP joints and ulnar deviation of the fingers. An exaggerated inflammatory response of an extensor tendon can result in a spontaneous, often asymptomatic rupture. Hyperextension of a PIP joint and flexion of the distal interphalangeal (DIP) joint produces a swan-neck deformity (Fig. 79–2). The boutonnière deformity is a fixed flexion contracture of a PIP joint and extension of a DIP joint.

The joints of the wrists are frequently affected in RA. There is variable tenosynovitis of the dorsa of the wrists and, ultimately, interosseous muscle atrophy and diminished movement due to articular destruction and/or bony ankylosis. Volar synovitis can lead to a compression neuropathy termed *carpal tunnel syndrome* (see Chapter 90).

Chronic synovitis of the elbows, shoulders, hips, knees, and/or ankles creates special secondary disorders. Destruction of the elbow articulations can lead to flexion contracture, loss of supination and pronation, and/or subluxation. When the shoulder is involved, limitation of shoulder mobility, dislocation, and spontaneous tears of the rotator cuff resulting in chronic pain can occur. A result of long-term synovitis of the knee is hypertrophy of the gastrocnemius-semimembranous bursa (Baker's cyst) of the popliteal fossa. Dissection of the cyst distally into the leg and rupture can mimic acute thrombophlebitis.

Involvement of the cervical spine by RA tends to be

a late occurrence in more advanced disease. Inflammation of the supporting ligaments of C1–C2 eventually produces laxity, sometimes giving rise to atlantoaxial subluxation. Spinal cord compression can result from anterior dislocation of C1 or from vertical subluxation of the odontoid process of C2 into the foramen magnum.

TREATMENT

The objectives of treating RA are to (1) relieve pain, (2) reduce or suppress inflammation, (3) avoid or recognize

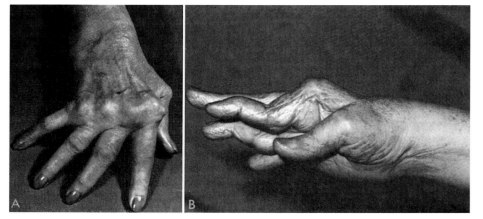

Figure 79–2

Hand deformities characteristic of chronic rheumatoid arthritis. *A*, Subluxation of metacarpophalangeal joints with ulnar deviation of digits. *B*, Hyperextension ("swan-neck") deformities of proximal interphalangeal joints. (From Arnett FC: Rheumatoid arthritis. *In* Bennett JC, Plum F [eds.]: Cecil Textbook of Medicine. 20th ed. Philadelphia, WB Saunders, 1996, p 1511.)

side effects early, (4) preserve or restore function, and (5) maintain lifestyle.

Therapy of RA requires a multifaceted approach. The importance of an ongoing educational program cannot be overstated. The patient's education should emphasize the benefits of a balanced daily program of rest and exercise. Physical and occupational therapy instruction in the appropriate exercises, along with the judicious application of splinting, can prevent and treat deformities, enhance muscle tone and strength, and preserve or improve function.

The pharmacologic therapy of RA often requires a combination of agents. Treatment is usually initiated with either aspirin or another nonsteroidal anti-inflammatory drug (NSAID). The use of aspirin should result in a therapeutic serum salicylate level (20 to 30 mg/dl).

Owing to the potential side effects of acetylated salicylates, such as gastrointestinal hemorrhage secondary to peptic ulcer or gastritis or a bleeding diathesis resulting from aspirin-induced inhibition of platelet aggregation, the use of a nonacetylated derivative (e.g., choline magnesium salicylate) should be considered. Similarly, using NSAIDs requires monitoring for gastrointestinal blood loss. Antimalarials, notably hydroxychloroquine, are also active in early or mild cases. The major toxicity of the antimalarials is their potential to deposit on the cornea, to produce macular pigmentation, or to result in field defects. Although emphasis has been placed upon these potential adverse reactions, the occurrence of visual impairment due to hydroxychloroquine is rare and can be prevented by routine ophthalmologic examinations. If the desired therapeutic response is not obtained within 6 months, the agent is discontinued.

Gold salts are regarded as remitting agents. Although the precise mode (or modes) of action in RA is unknown, these agents appear to alter macrophage function. Two intramuscular forms of the agent are currently available — gold thioglucose and gold sodium thiomalate — and are generally given in doses of 25 to 50 mg/wk. In general, the agents are more efficacious when begun early in the course of seropositive disease. In the absence of significant side effects, the response to therapy should be evaluated after a total of about 1 gram has been given. These agents should be carefully monitored at regular intervals for hematologic, dermatologic, and renal side effects.

Penicillamine has been found useful for treating RA and can sometimes induce remission. However, like gold, its effects are slow in expression, and it can have significant toxicity on the bone marrow and kidneys. Immunosuppressive agents such as azathioprine, cyclophosphamide, chlorambucil, and methotrexate have been used and found effective, particularly in severe RA. At the present time, relatively low doses of oral methotrexate have been found to be very effective and relatively free of toxicity. The oral dose generally begins at 7.5 mg one time per week. Toxic effects of methotrexate target the liver and may rarely produce cirrhosis; it may also cause bone marrow suppression and pneumonitis with pulmonary fibrosis. As with any of these drugs, frequent monitoring at regular intervals is advised.

Corticosteroids are routinely used in both the acute and chronic management of RA. Although the agents are clearly beneficial in the therapy of an acute flare, their long-term use is not warranted because steroids neither cure nor alter the natural course of the disease. Although the prolonged use of corticosteroids, even in small or "maintenance" doses, is fraught with numerous unwanted complications, 5 to 10 mg every other day may be required in some patients in conjunction with other agents. Intra-articular corticosteroids are useful following arthrocentesis to quell synovitis, reduce pain, and improve function.

Specific biologic agents that may block the events depicted in Fig. 79–1 are being evaluated.

REFERENCES

Arnett FC: Rheumatoid arthritis. *In* Bennett JC, Plum F (eds.): Cecil Textbook of Medicine. 20th ed. Philadelphia, WB Saunders, 1996, pp 1459–1466.

Fox DA: Biological therapies: A novel approach to the treatment of autoimmune disease. Am J Med 1995; *99*:82.

Harris ED: Rheumatoid arthritis; pathophysiology and implication for therapy. N Engl J Med 1990; 322:1277.

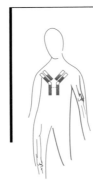

80 | Systemic Lupus Erythematosus

Systemic lupus erythematosus (SLE), a disease of unknown cause, is characterized by the production of autoantibodies that participate in immunologically mediated tissue injury in several organ systems. The clinical course is characterized by periods of remissions and acute or chronic relapse. The clinical spectrum of SLE ranges from the mildest forms of skin rash to fulminant life-threatening internal organ involvement. No one clinical abnormality or one single test definitively establishes the diagnosis. Therefore, criteria developed for epidemiologic and research purposes can be used to identify patients with SLE and differentiate them from patients with other disorders (Table 80–1). Common causes of death in SLE include renal failure, hemorrhage, infection, pulmonary disease, and vasculitis. The 10-year survival rate is approximately 90%.

Systemic lupus erythematosus can occur at any age, with the peak incidence of onset between ages 16 and 55 years. SLE occurs more frequently in women and appears to be more common in certain racial groups, particularly blacks and possibly Chinese and other Asian populations. The risk to a black woman for developing SLE is estimated to be 1 : 250.

ETIOLOGY AND PATHOGENESIS

Essentially every aspect of the immune system has been reported to be abnormal in patients with SLE. Therefore, it is unclear which defects are fundamental to the pathogenesis of SLE. Immune hyperactivity is illustrated by the production of numerous autoantibodies that may result from the interplay of genetic, environmental, and hormonal factors (Fig. 80–1). What triggers this immune overactivity is not fully understood. However, various environmental agents such as drugs or ultraviolet light can trigger the disease. In some persons, the inherited predisposition to SLE may be very important. If a family member has SLE, the likelihood of developing SLE increases by approximately 30% for identical twins and 5% for other first-degree relatives. Several complement deficiencies, the most common being C2 deficiency, have also been associated with SLE.

Systemic lupus erythematosus is classified as an immune complex disorder; it is a disease mediated primarily by antibodies. This process has been well demonstrated in renal disease associated with SLE but has not been as well defined in other organ systems. Antibodies—antinuclear (ANA) and anti–double stranded DNA (anti-dsDNA)—react with antigens in the circulation or the glomerulus, resulting in complement fixation followed by release of chemotactic factors and release of mediators of inflammation from leukocytes. Continued deposition of antibody and induction of inflammation may ultimately lead to irreversible renal damage. Similar processes may occur in other organs or with other cells; autoantibodies may be produced against erythrocytes, platelets, and lymphocytes.

Three histologic lesions are most characteristic of SLE: "*onion-skin lesions*," found in arteries of the spleen, which consist of concentric layers of fibrosis surrounding the vessel; *Libman-Sacks verrucous endocarditis*, vegetations on heart valves; and *hematoxylin bodies*, globular masses of bluish, dense, homogeneous material seen on hematoxylin and eosin stain. The hematoxylin bodies, which can be found in all organs, are identical to the inclusion bodies of lupus erythematosus (LE) cells and probably represent the interaction of antibodies to nucleoprotein.

Specific Subsets of Lupus

Although SLE is a disease of extreme variability in clinical presentation and course, certain subtypes of SLE deserve special mention (Table 80–2). Ninety percent of patients with discoid lupus erythematosus (DLE) have disease limited to the skin. Ten percent of patients with idiopathic SLE have discoid skin lesions at the start of their illness, and 25% may develop these lesions during the course of their illness. The characteristic lesions are erythematous scaly plaques with follicular plugging. Central scarring often results in permanent depigmentation.

Subacute cutaneous lupus erythematosus (SCLE) usually occurs in patients who are negative for ANA and positive for the anti-Ro(SS-A) antibodies. About 10% of patients with SLE have this type of skin lesion. These lesions are small, erythematous, annular, symmetric, superficial, and nonscarring. Patients with SLE-associated complement deficiencies often present with this type of skin lesion. These patients are often markedly photosensitive.

TABLE 80-1	Criteria for Classification of Systemic Lupus Erythematosus*

Criteria	Definition
1. Malar rash	Fixed erythema, flat or raised, over the malar eminences, tending to spare the nasolabial folds
2. Discoid rash	Erythematous raised patches with adherent keratotic scaling and follicular plugging; atrophic scarring may occur in older lesions
3. Photosensitivity	Skin rash as a result of unusual reaction to sunlight, by patient history or physician observation
4. Oral ulcers	Oral or nasopharyngeal ulceration, usually painless, observed by a physician
5. Arthritis	Nonerosive arthritis involving two or more peripheral joints, characterized by tenderness, swelling, or effusion
6. Serositis	a. Pleuritis—convincing history of pleuritic pain or rub heard by a physician or evidence of pleural effusion OR b. Pericarditis—documented by electrocardiogram or rub or evidence of pericardial effusion
7. Renal disorder	a. Persistent proteinuria >0.5 gm/day or >3+ if quantitation not performed OR b. Cellular casts—may be red cell, hemoglobin, granular, tubular, or mixed
8. Neurologic disorder	a. Seizures—in the absence of offending drugs or known metabolic derangements, e.g., uremia, ketoacidosis, or electrolyte imbalance OR b. Psychosis—in the absence of offending drugs or known metabolic derangements, e.g., uremia, ketoacidosis, or electrolyte imbalance
9. Hematologic disorder	a. Hemolytic anemia—with reticulocytosis OR b. Leukopenia—<4000/mm³ total on two or more occasions c. Lymphopenia—<1500/mm³ on two or more occasions OR d. Thrombocytopenia—<100,000/mm³ in the absence of offending drugs
10. Immunologic disorder	a. Positive lupus erythematosus cell preparation OR b. Anti-DNA: antibody to native DNA in abnormal titer OR c. Anti-Sm: presence of antibody to Sm nuclear antigen OR d. False-positive serologic test for syphilis known to be positive for at least 6 months and confirmed by *Treponema pallidum* immobilization or fluorescent treponemal antibody absorption test
11. Antinuclear antibody	An abnormal titer of antinuclear antibody by immunofluorescence or an equivalent assay at any point in time and in the absence of drugs known to be associated with "drug-induced lupus" syndrome

* The classification is based on 11 criteria. For the purpose of identifying patients in clinical studies, a person shall be said to have systemic lupus erythematosus if any 4 or more of the 11 criteria are present, serially or simultaneously, during any interval of observation.
From Schur PH: Systemic lupus erythematosus. *In* Bennett JC, Plum F (eds.): Cecil Textbook of Medicine. 20th ed. Philadelphia, WB Saunders, 1996, pp 1475–1477.

Late-onset SLE, defined as presentation after age 50, accounts for approximately 15% of all cases. These patients have a higher incidence of interstitial lung disease but much less neuropsychiatric or renal involvement. Diagnosing SLE in the older group may be difficult owing to a greater prevalence of autoantibodies in the aging population, a greater exposure to drugs causing the serologic hallmark of SLE, and a higher prevalence of other rheumatic diseases such as Sjögren's syndrome that may present with the same features observed with SLE.

Neonatal lupus, a rare syndrome, appears to be a complication of maternal antibodies to Ro(SS-A) and/or La(SS-B) transferred through the placenta. Shortly after birth, infants develop typical discoid lesions with exposure to ultraviolet light. However, very few of these infants develop SLE later in life. Some infants develop other transient complications such as thrombocytopenia, hemolytic anemia, and, rarely, congenital heart block, which may be fatal. Patients with SLE who have a child with neonatal lupus have a 25% likelihood of having another child with neonatal lupus in a subsequent pregnancy.

Several drugs have been reported to induce features of SLE, but only hydralazine, procainamide, chlorpromazine, methyldopa, and isoniazid are considered to have a definite association. The clinical features of drug-induced lupus are similar to those of idiopathic SLE except for the uncommon involvement of the renal and central nervous systems. In addition, the symptoms are usually mild and reversible when the drug is stopped. However, ANA can remain positive for months or years. A strong association exists between high doses of procainamide, hydralazine, and isoniazid and possessing the slow acetylation phenotype.

CLINICAL FEATURES

The "typical" presentation of SLE occurs in only a few patients. More commonly, patients initially present with one or two symptoms such as fatigue, myalgias, and arthritis and later may develop additional features of SLE (Table 80–3). SLE is characterized by periods of exacerbation followed by remission or inactive disease. Most patients have constitutional symptoms such as fatigue, fever, and weight loss at the time of diagnosis. Fatigue,

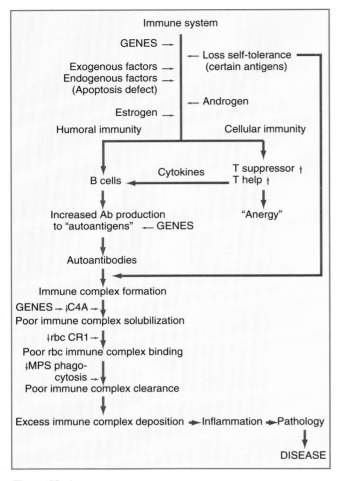

Figure 80–1
Pathogenic events in systemic lupus erythematosus (SLE). MPS = Mononuclear phagocyte system. (From Schur PH: Systemic lupus erythematosus. *In* Bennett JC, Plum F [eds.]: Cecil Textbook of Medicine. 20th ed. Philadelphia, WB Saunders, 1996, pp 1475–1477.)

| TABLE 80–3 | Common Clinical Abnormalities in Patients with SLE |

Manifestation	Approximate Frequency (%)	
	At Onset	At Any Time
Nonspecific		
Fatigue	—	90
Fever	36	80
Weight loss	—	60
Arthralgia/myalgia	69	95
Specific		
Arthritis	—	
Skin		
Butterfly rash	40	50
Discoid LE	6	20
Photosensitivity	29	58
Mucous ulcers	11	30
Alopecia	—	71
Raynaud's	18	30
Purpura	—	15
Urticaria	—	9
Renal	16	50
Nephrosis	—	18
Gastrointestinal	—	38
Pulmonary	3	50
Pleurisy	—	45
Effusions	—	24
Pneumonia	—	29
Cardiac	—	46
Pericarditis	—	48
Murmurs	—	23
ECG changes	—	34
Lymphadenopathy	7	50
Splenomegaly	—	20
Hepatomegaly	—	25
Central nervous system	12	75
Functional	—	Most
Psychosis	—	20
Seizures	—	20
Hematologic	—	90

ECG = Electrocardiogram; LE = lupus erythematosus; SLE = systemic lupus erythematosus.
From Schur PH: Systemic lupus erythematosus. *In* Bennett JC, Plum F (eds.): Cecil Textbook of Medicine. 20th ed. Philadelphia, WB Saunders, 1996, p 1477.

although difficult to evaluate, may be the first sign of an exacerbation of disease.

Arthralgias or arthritis occurs in 95% of patients with SLE. The joint manifestations are usually more transient than in patients with rheumatoid arthritis (RA). The arthritis is typically symmetric and involves small joints of hands, wrists, and feet. Deformities similar to those in RA develop in 10 to 15% of patients; however, bony

| TABLE 80–2 | Subsets of Lupus |

Idiopathic
Systemic
Discoid
Subacute cutaneous (ANA negative)
Late-onset
Neonatal
Drug-induced

ANA = Antinuclear antibodies.

erosions characteristic of RA do not occur. In addition, rheumatoid nodules (7%) and rheumatoid factors (15 to 20%) can be detected in SLE patients. Infectious arthritis and avascular necrosis of bone are two additional causes of joint pain that should be considered in SLE patients.

Abnormalities of the skin, hair, or mucous membranes are the second most common manifestation of SLE, occurring in 85% of patients. Many different types of skin manifestations may appear in SLE. The classic malar butterfly rash, an erythematous rash covering both cheeks and the bridge of the nose, with sparing of the nasolabial folds, may occur in the absence of exposure of the skin to sunlight but may worsen with exposure. The second most common erythematous rash seen in SLE patients is a maculopapular rash that may be located anywhere on the body. In addition to the discoid and SCLE lesions discussed here, other skin manifestations include urticaria, bullae, livedo reticularis, panniculitis (lupus profundus), alopecia, and vasculitic lesions. One fifth of patients have vasculitic skin lesions that are manifested as livedo reticularis, tender nodules, purpuric leg ulcers, or splinter hemorrhages. Mucosal ulcers, often painless, occur on the hard and soft palate. Raynaud's phenomenon may be severe enough to result in digital gangrene.

Conjunctivitis, episcleritis, or keratoconjunctivitis occurs in approximately 20% of patients. Retinal vasculitis is uncommon but may lead to blindness. Cytoid bodies, white exudates adjacent to retinal blood vessels, are associated with active disease of the central nervous system.

Abdominal pain, often a diagnostic problem, may be a manifestation of serositis, mesenteric arteritis, or pancreatitis or may be secondary to visceral perforation (drug-induced peptic ulceration or secondary to vasculitis). Hepatosplenomegaly is noted in about 30% of patients.

Pleuritic chest pain with or without pleural effusions occurs commonly. The presence of pulmonary emboli should be excluded because thrombophlebitis occurs in about 10% of SLE patients. Acute parenchymal lung involvement may present as acute pneumonitis with or without pulmonary hemorrhage. However, the diagnosis of lupus pneumonitis should be made only after a rigorous search for an infectious cause. "Shrinking" lung syndrome, an uncommon entity, results from a myopathy of the diaphragm and usually causes progressive loss of lung volume.

Clinically significant renal involvement occurs in about 50% of patients with SLE, but fortunately only a minority have renal involvement that results in irreversible organ failure. Proteinuria is the most common clinical sign of lupus nephritis; hypertension, hematuria, and red blood cell casts are other clues to active renal disease. The degree of active disease and scarring are factors that significantly affect the patient's prognosis; therefore, a renal biopsy is often done to help guide therapy by determining the activity and chronicity of disease.

Neuropsychiatric manifestations of SLE are frequent and encompass the entire range of neurologic diseases. Depression and psychosis are frequent. Central nervous system involvement may also be manifested by organic brain disease, such as impairment of orientation, memory, or cognition. Abnormal cerebrospinal fluid findings during active neuropsychiatric disease include an elevated protein in about 50% of patients. Nonsteroidal anti-inflammatory drug (NSAID)–induced aseptic meningitis has been reported in several SLE patients. The clinical usefulness of antineuronal or ribosomal P antibodies as an indicator of active disease is controversial.

Pericarditis, the most common cardiac manifestation, occurs in up to 30% of patients; it rarely progresses to tamponade or constrictive pericarditis. LE cells are found frequently in pericardial fluid. Myocarditis, often associated with pericarditis, manifests clinically as tachycardia, ST-T wave changes, congestive heart failure, and cardiomegaly. Severe valvular lesions, primarily of the mitral and aortic valves, may occur. Verrucous endocarditis is present at autopsy in nearly all patients with cardiac involvement; subacute and acute bacterial endocarditis has occurred on valves affected by lupus endocarditis. Myocardial infarctions may result from coronary arteritis, thrombosis, or premature atherosclerosis secondary to chronic corticosteroid use.

One or more hematologic abnormalities are present in nearly all SLE patients with active disease; these include normochromic, normocytic anemia, hemolytic anemia (sometimes Coombs' positive), leukopenia (usually lymphopenia), and thrombocytopenia. Antibodies to several clotting factors have been noted in SLE patients; the most common is the lupus anticoagulant (an antiphospholipid antibody), which is found in up to 25% of patients and is usually recognized by a prolonged partial thromboplastin time (see Chapter 52). However, it is associated with thrombotic disease and not with bleeding. Arterial and venous thrombosis, placental infarction, and thrombocytopenia are all more common in patients with the lupus anticoagulant. Inhibitors that specifically inactivate clotting factors (II, VIII, IX, and XII) are associated with major bleeding episodes. False-positive tests for syphilis have been noted in up to 25% of patients, and there is a strong association between the presence of the circulating lupus anticoagulant and false-positive tests for syphilis.

The use of oral contraceptives containing estrogen derivatives has often been associated with an exacerbation of SLE; thus, they should be avoided in these patients. Current data suggest that SLE patients in remission are not likely to have exacerbations during pregnancy; however, women with active SLE, especially those with renal disease, have an increased frequency of exacerbation of their disease as well as missed abortions, stillbirths, and premature labor and delivery. Pre-eclampsia is a frequent complication of pregnancy that may be difficult to distinguish from a flare of nephritis in a patient with SLE.

LABORATORY EVALUATION

The serologic hallmark of SLE is the production of high-titer autoantibodies directed against a variety of nuclear components (ANA) (Table 80–4). Determination of the ANA level is useful as a screening test, but many patients with other autoimmune diseases and even unrelated diseases may also have positive tests (Table 80–5). Serum antibodies to dsDNA and Sm are detected almost exclusively in patients with SLE.

Anemia is usually present in patients with active disease. Leukopenia is present in half the patients. Leukocytosis may occur but should not be attributed to SLE until there has been a careful search for an infection. Hypergammaglobulinemia and reduced hemolytic complement levels (CH_{50}) are common, especially in active disease.

Proteinuria, casts, and white blood cells are found in the urine of patients with active kidney disease. Pleural effusions are usually exudative. LE cells may be seen in the pleural and pericardial fluid.

TREATMENT

Systemic lupus erythematosus is a disease without a known cure, so treatment is based on relieving symptoms, suppressing inflammation, and preventing future pathology. The risk-to-benefit ratio of potentially toxic drugs must be tailored to the individual patient. The organ sys-

TABLE 80–4	Autoantibodies Found in Patients with SLE

Specificity of Antibody	Comment
Nuclear	
ANA	Present in about 90% of SLE patients, also found in several other disorders
Double-stranded DNA	Restricted to SLE; occurs in 50% of patients
Histones H1, H3-H4	SLE
Histones H2A-H2B	More common in drug-induced SLE
Sm	Restricted to SLE; found in 25–60% of patients
Ribonucleoprotein (RNP)	Highest titers in mixed connective tissue disease, also found in SLE
SS-A (Ro)	Sjögren's syndrome, SLE (30–40%)
SS-B (La)	Sjögren's syndrome, SLE (15%)
Cell membrane determinants	Common in SLE
Red cells	May occur with or without hemolysis
White cells	Granulocytes, T cells, B cells
Platelets	Common with or without thrombocytopenia
Others	
Clotting factors	SLE and other diseases
Phospholipids (cardiolipin; lupus anticoagulant)	SLE, others, without other diseases
Neuronal	Active CNS lupus
Ribosomal P protein	Active CNS lupus

ANA = Antinuclear antibodies; CNS = central nervous system; SLE = systemic lupus erythematosus.
Modified from Steinberg AD: Systemic lupus erythematosus. In Wyngaarden JB, Smith LH Jr, Bennett JC (eds.): Cecil Textbook of Medicine. 19th ed. WB Saunders, 1992, p 1524.

tem (or systems) involved and the severity of disease dictate specific therapy. A patient with skin rash and/or joint symptoms requires different management than a patient with proteinuria, red blood cell casts in urine, and low serum complement levels.

Patients need to be educated about the disease, the

TABLE 80–5	Diseases Associated with ANA

Systemic lupus erythematosus
Sjögren's syndrome
Rheumatoid arthritis
Juvenile arthritis
Leprosy
Infectious mononucleosis
Scleroderma
Liver disease
Primary pulmonary fibrosis
Vasculitis
Dermatomyositis/polymyositis
Mixed connective tissue disease
Mixed cryoglobulinemia
Aging
Medications

ANA = Antinuclear antibodies.
Schur PH: Systemic lupus erythematosus. In Bennett JC, Plum F (eds.): Cecil Textbook of Medicine. 20th ed. Philadelphia, WB Saunders, 1996, pp 1475–1477.

treatments, and the generally good prognosis of SLE. Many of the more serious problems do not affect most patients. Ultraviolet light should be limited or avoided in those patients who are photosensitive. Sunscreens with an SPF of ≥15 are helpful for most persons. Estrogen, unless contraindicated or associated with disease exacerbation, is recommended for its benefit regarding coronary artery disease and osteoporosis. Hypertension should be treated aggressively. Renal disease demands special therapeutic decisions; renal biopsies are done to determine appropriate therapy and prognosis. A biopsy demonstrating active proliferative lesions provides the rationale for use of cytotoxic drugs, whereas histology consistent with membranous nephropathy may lead the clinician to use only corticosteroids.

Specific pharmacologic intervention includes the use of NSAIDs, corticosteroids, antimalarials, and cytotoxic agents. NSAIDs are used to treat arthralgias, mild arthritis, pleurisy, pericarditis, myalgias, and headaches. The potential side effects of NSAIDs include gastrointestinal symptoms, altered renal function, and, rarely, aseptic meningitis. Corticosteroids are frequently given, but the indications for their use are imprecise. The primary objective of corticosteroid therapy is to control the inflammatory response to prevent end-organ damage. High doses (>60 mg/day of prednisone) may be necessary for brief periods, and attempts should be made to taper to every-other-day dosing as quickly as possible because the side effects with steroids given every other day are much less severe than with daily therapy. The long-term toxicities of corticosteroids must continually be weighed against the benefits of continued therapy.

Antimalarials are often used for dermatologic and musculoskeletal manifestations. Retinal toxicity is the major side effect of these drugs, and patients should be seen by an ophthalmologist before starting treatment and every 6 months while receiving therapy. Azathioprine may be useful for patients with moderate renal disease or those with intractable skin disease or arthritis. Daily oral cyclophosphamide or monthly pulse intravenous cyclophosphamide combined with corticosteroids is commonly used to treat proliferative types of nephritis. Current data suggest that renal function can be preserved for long periods with cyclophosphamide therapy.

REFERENCES

Boumpas DT, Austin HA, Fessler BJ, et al.: Systemic lupus erythematosus: Emerging concepts. Part 1: Renal, neuropsychiatric, cardiovascular, pulmonary, and hematologic disease. Ann Intern Med 1995; 122: 940–950.

Boumpas DT, Austin HA, Fessler BJ, et al.: Systemic lupus erythematosus: Emerging concepts. Part 2: Dermatologic and joint disease, the antiphospholipid antibody syndrome, pregnancy and hormonal therapy, morbidity and mortality, and pathogenesis. Ann Intern Med 1995; 122:42–53.

Rothfield NF: Systemic lupus erythematosus: Clinical aspects and treatment. In McCarty DJ, Koopman WJ (eds.): Arthritis and Allied Conditions, 12th ed. Philadelphia, Lea & Febiger, 1993, pp 1155–1178.

Schur PH: Systemic lupus erythematosus. In Bennett JC, Plum F (eds.): Cecil Textbook of Medicine. 20th ed. Philadelphia, WB Saunders, 1996, pp 1475–1483.

81

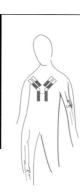

Sjögren's Syndrome

Sjögren's syndrome (SS) is a chronic inflammatory disorder of probable autoimmune nature characterized by infiltration and destruction of the exocrine glands, particularly the salivary and lacrimal glands, by lymphocytes and plasma cells. The spectrum of the disease includes the primary form, referred to as the sicca complex, and the secondary form, which is commonly associated with rheumatoid arthritis, systemic lupus erythematosus (SLE), or, less commonly, other connective tissue disorders and lymphoproliferation, which may be benign or malignant.

CLINICAL FEATURES

Signs and symptoms of SS may be subtle and therefore require a thoughtful history and careful physical examination. Lymphocytic infiltration of the lacrimal and salivary glands results in the sicca complex. Dryness of the eyes and accumulation of thick, ropy secretions along the inner canthus occur because of the decreased and altered tear production, giving the sensations of a "film" across the field of vision and of grittiness or the presence of a foreign body. With time, variable conjunctival injection, reduced visual acuity, and photosensitivity develop. Prolonged desiccation leads to erosions and sloughing of the corneal epithelium (filamentary keratitis), as demonstrated by rose bengal staining and slit-lamp examination. Drying of the mouth, xerostomia, is frequent but variable in severity. Patients may describe difficulty in eating dry foods as being like trying to eat crackers without water. Dental caries are accelerated owing to a decrease in the volume of saliva and the relative loss of its antibacterial factors.

Other mucosal surfaces can also be affected by the same inflammatory response. Epistaxis, hoarseness, bronchitis, or pneumonia can result if the respiratory tract is involved. Inspissation of secretions in eustachian tubes leads to obstruction, chronic otitis media, and conduction deafness. Mucosal gland involvement of the gastrointestinal tract can be associated with dysphagia, reduced gastric acid output, constipation, and pancreatic insufficiency. Vaginal dryness can result in dyspareunia.

Extraglandular features can complicate the course of SS but occur more frequently in patients having primary rather than secondary SS. Renal tubular acidosis results from infiltrative interstitial nephropathy. Both peripheral and cranial neuropathies have been attributed to vasculitis

of the vasa nervorum. Other associated neuromuscular disorders include myopathy, polymyositis, and cranial vasculitis. Dyspnea may be the presenting symptom of underlying diffuse interstitial pneumonitis due to lymphocytic infiltration. An obstructive ventilatory defect has been attributed to lymphocytic infiltration around small airways. Nonthrombocytopenic purpura of the dependent regions is associated with a polyclonal hypergammaglobulinemia. Raynaud's phenomenon occurs in about 20% of patients. Several other chronic disorders have been reported in association with SS (Table 81–1).

Malignant or pseudomalignant lymphoproliferation may be a prominent part of the illness, especially in primary SS. Most of these lymphomas derive from B cell lineage and may develop into monoclonal gammopathies. These include Waldenström's macroglobulinemia, light chain myeloma, and, occasionally, IgG and IgA monoclonal gammopathies. Clinically, one may expect an increased risk of malignancy in patients who have a persistent or greatly increased parotid swelling, splenomegaly, or generalized lymphadenopathy. An elevated serum β-microglobulin level may offer a clue to this clinical subset of SS disease.

DIAGNOSIS

The diagnosis of SS is based upon the results of Schirmer's filter paper test (wetting of < 5 mm in 5 min in an unanesthetized eye), ophthalmologic examination, and minor salivary gland biopsy. The demonstration of superficial corneal erosions by rose bengal staining and filamentory keratitis by slit-lamp examination indicates more advanced keratoconjunctivitis sicca.

Biopsy of the minor salivary glands of the lower lip in SS demonstrates lymphocytic infiltration of the acinar glands and progressive destruction of glandular tissue. The diagnosis of SS requires the presence of two of the following three criteria: (1) a characteristic labial salivary gland biopsy; (2) keratoconjunctivitis sicca; (3) an associated connective tissue or lymphoproliferative disorder.

Autoantibodies are common in SS (see Table 78–5). Multiple organ-specific antibodies can be noted, including those directed against gastric parietal, thyroid microsomal, thyroglobulin, mitochondrial, smooth muscle, and salivary duct antigens. Antibodies to a nuclear protein antigen,

TABLE 81–1	Disorders Associated with Sjögren's Syndrome

Rheumatoid arthritis
Systemic lupus erythematosus
Progressive systemic sclerosis
Overlap syndrome
Polymyositis/dermatomyositis
Graft-versus-host disease
Malignant lymphoma
Chronic Hashimoto's thyroiditis
Chronic active hepatitis
Biliary cirrhosis
Graves' disease
Premature ovarian failure
Celiac disease
Dermatitis herpetiformis
Myasthenia gravis
Pemphigus
Lipodystrophy

SS-B (also termed La), occur in approximately 50 to 70% of patients with primary SS and, to a lesser extent, in patients with SLE. Antibodies to a related antigen SS-A (also termed Ro) are somewhat less specific for SS, may occur in SLE, and are more frequently associated with vasculitis. The B cell hyperreactivity in patients with SS gives rise to hyperglobulinemia and sometimes circulating immune complexes and may be associated with rheumatoid factor activity. Complement is only infrequently low.

TREATMENT

Treatment is directed at alleviating symptoms and the complications of xerophthalmia and xerostomia. Xerophthalmia can be treated with artificial tears or surgical punctal occlusion. The common complication, staphylococcal blepharitis, should be treated immediately with topical or, if necessary, systemic antibiotics. Xerostomia is managed by maintaining oral hydration and the liberal use of sialogogues. Bronchopulmonary infections require both supportive regimens and antibiotics. Dyspareunia is treatable with commercial water-soluble vaginal lubricants. Corticosteroids or immunosuppressive agents should be used only in patients with severe functional disability such as that seen in renal or pulmonary involvement.

REFERENCES

Hochberg MC: Sjögren's Syndrome. *In* Bennett JC, Plum F (eds.): Cecil Textbook of Medicine. 20th ed. Philadelphia, WB Saunders, 1996, p 1488.
Moutsopoulos HM, Youinou P: New developments in Sjögren's syndrome. Curr Opin Rheumatol 1991; 3:815–822.

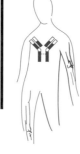

82

Idiopathic Inflammatory Myopathies

The group of idiopathic inflammatory myopathies (IIMs) includes polymyositis (PM) and dermatomyositis (DM) as well as myositis associated with other connective tissue diseases (CTDs), myositis associated with cancer (CAM), and inclusion-body myositis (IBM) (Table 82–1). They are all generally characterized by progressive symmetric muscle weakness, usually associated with elevated serum levels of muscle enzymes, a muscle biopsy showing mononuclear cell inflammation, and characteristic patterns of electromyographic abnormalities. From a clinical perspective, IIM may be viewed as three rather discrete groupings: (1) polymyositis, (2) dermatomyositis, and (3) inclusion-body myositis.

On biopsy (the standard for diagnosis) of these groups, one sees prominent histologic evidence of necrosis and regeneration of muscle fibers. Capillary obliteration and endothelial damage are common. Inflammatory infiltrates in DM are predominantly perivascular or in the septa around, rather than within, fascicles of muscle. In PM and IBM, endomysial inflammation is generally seen, and lymphocytes and macrophages surround or invade individual muscle fibers. In DM, the intramuscular blood vessels also show endothelial hyperplasia, fibrin thrombi, and obliteration of capillaries. IBM is characterized by basophilic granular inclusions around the edge of vacuoles, termed "rimmed" vacuoles, and eosinophilic cytoplasmic inclusions. Electron microscopic studies of biopsies are often required to make the diagnosis because paraffin processing can distort the basophilic granule and rimmed vacuole pattern.

CLINICAL COURSE

Idiopathic inflammatory myopathy has an incidence of approximately 1 per 100,000. Both children and adults can be afflicted with DM (females more than males); PM occurs primarily in adults, generally past the teens; IBM (males more than females) tends to occur past the 40s.

The common presenting manifestation of all of the IIMs is symmetric muscle weakness that develops over weeks to months. Difficulties in climbing stairs, getting up from a chair, and lifting objects are common initial symptoms. Involvement of ocular muscles and facial muscles is extremely rare, except in very advanced cases, and generally fine-motor movements of the hands are preserved. Respiratory muscles also are preserved until very late in the disease. Myalgia and muscle tenderness can be predominant manifestations in some patients, particularly in DM.

Dermatomyositis is distinct by virtue of its accompanying characteristic rash. The so-called heliotrope rash occurs typically on the upper eyelids and generally with edema. Gottron's sign is characterized by erythema of the knuckles of the fingers and often presents as a raised, somewhat scaly eruption. An erythematous rash may also recur on other body surfaces, including knees, elbows, the V-region of the neck and upper chest, and across the back and shoulders. DM in children is notable for its more frequent extramuscular manifestations, generally due to a systemic vasculitis that can involve almost any organ system. PM has no distinguishing clinical manifestations, and the diagnosis is generally made by excluding other muscular and neuromuscular diseases.

Inclusion-body myositis may not be suspected early in the course but generally comes to mind when the patient is observed to respond poorly to therapy. Clinically, there is a greater likelihood of involvement of distal muscles of the fingers and feet. These patients may lose their patellar reflex early because of weakness of the quadriceps muscle and may even give the early impression of a neurologic disease.

As in PM, IBM can also be found in association with a diversity of autoimmune CTD such as systemic lupus erythematosus (SLE) and scleroderma. The association of IIM with other diseases such as scleroderma, SLE, and rheumatoid arthritis constitutes what has been referred to as an overlap syndrome. When this is seen, arthralgias, myalgias, and Raynaud's phenomenon may be quite prominent.

The occurrence of malignancy in the setting of IIM is relatively uncommon (<10%, but may be higher in older age groups). Carcinomas of the breast, lung, ovaries, colon, endometrium, prostate, and stomach are the leading tumors that have been reported to be associated with IIM. In approximately three fourths of CAM patients, the myositis precedes the diagnosis of malignancy by 12 to 24 months. It would, therefore, be appropriate to search for malignancy in patients over 50; that is, those with greater risk for associated cancer.

TABLE 82–1	Classification of Idiopathic Inflammatory Myopathies (IIMs)	

Description	Group Designation
Primary idiopathic polymyositis	PM
Primary idiopathic dermatomyositis	DM
Autoimmune connective tissue diseases with myositis	CTM
Myositis associated with malignancy	CAM
Inclusion-body myositis	IBM

TABLE 82–3	Autoantibodies Found in Patients with Idiopathic Inflammatory Myopathies	

Autoantibody	Clinical Association
Myositis-specific autoantibodies	
Anti-tRNA synthetases	PM with interstitial lung
Anti-Jo-1	disease, arthritis, and
Anti-PL-7	fever; less common
Anti-PL-12	in DM
Anti-OJ	
Anti-EJ	
Anti-SRP	PM with poor prognosis
Anti-MAS	PM after alcoholic rhabdomyolysis
Anti-Mi-2	DM

Anti-SRP = Anti-signal recognition particle; DM = dermatomyositis; PM = polymyositis.
Adapted from Wortmann RL: Idiopathic inflammatory myopathies. *In* Bennett JC, Plum F (eds.): Cecil Textbook of Medicine. 20th ed. Philadelphia, WB Saunders, 1996, p 1501.

The clinical course in these diseases is generally prolonged, with remissions and exacerbations, but can involve fatal complications, including cardiac arrhythmias, probably due to involvement of myocardial muscle, and the development of restrictive lung disease, which may occur in as many as 20% of cases.

DIAGNOSTIC AND LABORATORY FINDINGS

The clinical picture of positive electromyographic findings, elevated muscle enzymes, and distinctive muscle biopsy are the tools necessary for the diagnosis of IIM and its various subgroups (Table 82–2).

Recent work has been directed at examining possible subsets of IIM based on a variety of serologic measurements. These include the myositis-specific antibodies, anti-aminoacyl-tRNA synthetases, and anti-signal recognition particle (anti-SRP) (Table 82–3). The clinical rele-

vance of these subsets, as well as their etiologic significance, remains to be determined.

TREATMENT

Treatment of PM or DM generally involves corticosteroids with supportive physical therapy; if indicated, immunosuppressive agents may be added (Fig. 82–1). It is important to recognize that IBM generally does not respond to corticosteroid therapy. One must also be aware

TABLE 82–2	Diagnostic Criteria for Idiopathic Inflammatory Myopathies				

Criterion	Polymyositis		Dermatomyositis		Inclusion-Body Myositis
	Definite	Probable*	Definite	Mild or Early	Definite
Muscle strength	Myopathic muscle weakness†	Myopathic muscle weakness†	Myopathic muscle weakness†	Seemingly normal strength‡	Myopathic muscle weakness with early involvement of distal muscles†
Electromyographic findings	Myopathic	Myopathic	Myopathic	Myopathic or non-specific	Myopathic with mixed potentials
Muscle enzymes	Elevated (up to 50-fold)	Elevated (up to 50-fold)	Elevated (up to 50-fold) or normal	Elevated (up to 10-fold) or normal	Elevated (up to 10-fold) or normal
Muscle-biopsy findings	Diagnostic for this type of inflammatory myopathy	Nonspecific myopathy without signs of primary inflammation	Diagnostic	Nonspecific or diagnostic	Diagnostic
Rash or calcinosis	Absent	Absent	Present	Present	Absent

* An adequate trial of prednisone or other immunosuppressive drugs is warranted in probable cases. If, in retrospect, the disease is unresponsive to therapy, another muscle biopsy should be considered to exclude other diseases or possible evolution to inclusion-body myositis.
† Myopathic muscle weakness, affecting proximal muscles more than distal ones and sparing eye and facial muscles, is characterized by a subacute onset (weeks to months) and rapid progression in patients who have no family history of neuromuscular disease, no endocrinopathy, no exposure to myotoxic drugs or toxins, and no biochemical muscle disease (excluded on the basis of muscle-biopsy findings).
‡ Although strength is seemingly normal, patients often have new onset of easy fatigue, myalgia, and reduced endurance. Careful muscle testing may reveal mild muscle weakness.
Reprinted, by permission, from the New England Journal of Medicine, Vol 325, p 1487, 1991.

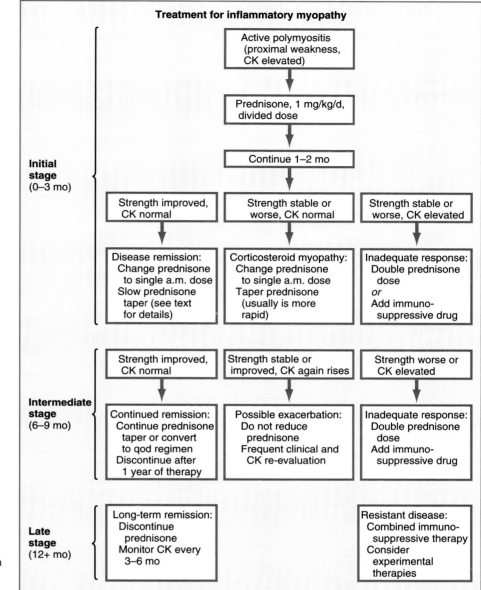

Figure 82–1

Treatment algorithm for inflammatory myopathy. CK = Creatine kinase; qod = every other day. (Modified from Oddis CV: Therapy for myositis. Curr Opin Rheumatol 1991; 3:921, with permission.)

of the entity of corticosteroid myopathy when treating with high-dose corticosteroids for a long period. In that case, reducing the corticosteroid dose may become the appropriate therapy.

The long-term prognosis in the PM and DM groups is extremely good with corticosteroid and immunosuppressive therapy, with 15-year survival rates of 85 to 90%.

REFERENCES

Dalakas MC: Polymyositis, dermatomyositis and inclusion-body myositis. N Engl J Med 1991; 325:1487.

Oddis CV: Therapy for myositis. Curr Opin Rheumatol 1991; 3:919.

Wortmann RL: Idiopathic inflammatory myopathies. *In* Bennett JC, Plum F (eds.): Cecil Textbook of Medicine. 20th ed. Philadelphia, WB Saunders, 1996, p 1500.

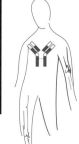

83

Scleroderma (Systemic Sclerosis)

Scleroderma (literally "hard skin") is an uncommon disease with various presentations and, depending on the extent of visceral involvement, varied outcomes. Scleroderma may be classified according to the degree and extent of skin thickening (Table 83–1). Systemic sclerosis (SSc) is seen most commonly in adults, whereas the localized forms of scleroderma (morphea) are seen most often in children. Persons with limited SSc, formerly called CREST syndrome (C = calcinosis, R = Raynaud's phenomenon, E = esophageal disease, S = sclerodactyly, T = telangiectasias), usually do not develop internal organ involvement for several years. In contrast, persons with rapidly progressive, widespread skin thickening (diffuse SSc) that affects the proximal extremities and trunk are at greater risk for developing early, serious visceral involvement.

The clinical hallmarks of SSc are light skin and Raynaud's phenomenon. SSc is a generalized disorder of small arteries and the connective tissue characterized by vascular obliteration and fibrosis in skin and internal organs, including the gastrointestinal tract, lungs, heart, and kidneys. The mechanisms of excessive fibrosis are unknown.

LOCALIZED SCLERODERMA

Localized scleroderma affects primarily children and young adults and is a heterogeneous group of conditions that does not have the typical visceral and serologic manifestations seen with SSc (see Table 83–1). Morphea starts with areas of erythema or violaceous discoloration of the skin, which evolve to sclerotic and waxy or ivory-colored lesions. The plaques may increase in size to several centimeters in diameter and often are surrounded by a violaceous border of inflammation. Lesions may become widespread and confluent, a condition called generalized morphea. Most often, the lesions soften spontaneously over months to years. With the linear form, sclerotic lesions appear as linear streaks or bands, most commonly on the extremities and less frequently on the forehead, trunk, or frontoparietal scalp. When the frontoparietal area is involved, it is termed *en coup de sabre* and may result in disfiguring facial asymmetry with hemiatrophy.

LIMITED SYSTEMIC SCLEROSIS (CREST VARIANT)

The usual age of onset of limited SSc is in the 20s to 30s. The patient may have a history of Raynaud's phenomenon for several years and subsequently presents with skin edema or tightening of hands, face, and feet. Patients with limited SSc have a much lower frequency of serious internal organ involvement (renal, pulmonary); however, pulmonary hypertension and esophageal disease are not uncommon in limited SSc (Table 83–2).

DIFFUSE SYSTEMIC SCLEROSIS

Although diffuse SSc is less common than limited SSc, it has a worse prognosis owing to more frequent renal and pulmonary involvement (see Table 83–2). An abrupt onset of swollen hands, face, and feet associated with Raynaud's phenomenon may occur. These changes may evolve over several weeks or months to include more proximal areas of the extremities as well as the thorax and abdomen. These patients should be followed closely for visceral involvement, especially hypertension and renal involvement.

SCLERODERMA SINE SCLERODERMA

Scleroderma sine scleroderma is an uncommon condition in which there are characteristic internal organ manifestations and vascular and serologic abnormalities but no clinically detectable skin changes.

CLINICAL FEATURES

Virtually all patients with SSc have Raynaud's phenomenon, which is defined as episodic *pallor* of digits following cold exposure or stress associated with *cyanosis*, followed by *erythema*, tingling, and pain. Raynaud's phenomenon, attributable to both vasospasm and structural disease of the blood vessels, primarily affects the hands and feet and less commonly the ears, nose, and tongue. The duration of the triphasic color change can

TABLE 83-1	Classification of Scleroderma

Localized scleroderma
  Morphea
    Circumscribed, guttate
    Generalized
  Linear (with hemiatrophy)
  En coup de sabre (with or without facial hemiatrophy)
Systemic scleroderma (SSc)
  Diffuse SSc
  Limited SSc (formerly called CREST syndrome)
  Systemic sclerosis sine scleroderma
  Overlap with other connective tissue disease
Environmental and drug related
  Vinyl chloride disease
  Pentazocine
  Bleomycin
  Toxic oil syndrome (adulterated rapeseed oil)
  Trichloroethylene
  5-Hydroxytryptophan and L-tryptophan
  Breast augmentation mammoplasty (paraffin, silicone)
Diseases with skin changes mimicking scleroderma
  Eosinophilic fasciitis
  Eosinophilic myalgia syndrome
  Chronic graft-vs-host disease
  Carcinoid syndrome
  Acromegaly
  Diabetic cheiroarthropathy (syndrome of limited joint mobility)
  Scleredema adultorum of Buschke
  Scleromyxedema (papular mucinosis)
  Lichen sclerosis et atrophicus
  Werner's syndrome
  Porphyrias
  Acrodermatitis chronica atrophicans
  Amyloidosis (primary and myeloma associated)
  Progeria
  Phenylketonuria

CREST = Calcinosis, Raynaud's phenomenon, esophageal disease, sclerodactyly, and telangiectasias.

vary from minutes to hours. Severe Raynaud's phenomenon can exhibit a predominant phase of cyanosis and can result in digital pitting scars, frank gangrene, and/or autoamputation of the fingers or toes.

The appearance of the skin is the most distinctive diagnostic feature of SSc; the diagnosis can be made by examining the texture and location of hidebound skin. By definition, patients with diffuse SSc have taut skin in the more proximal parts of extremities, in addition to the thorax and abdomen. However, the skin tightening of SSc begins on the fingers and hands in nearly all cases; therefore, making the distinction between limited and diffuse SSc may be difficult early in the illness. The initial phase of skin involvement is characterized by painless pitting edema followed by gradual loss of edema, leaving thick, indurated, tight skin. These changes may evolve over 12 to 18 months to include more proximal areas of the extremities, as well as the trunk. At later stages of disease, atrophy (thinning) may develop, leading to laxity of the superficial dermis; the clinical observation of improving skin change in late SSc may reflect this atrophic phase. Atrophy is noted primarily over joints at sites of flexion contractures such as the elbow and proximal interphalangeal joints; these areas are prone to the development of ulcerations. Areas of hypo- and hyperpigmentation are

common. Other skin changes include subcutaneous calcifications and telangiectasias of the fingers, face, lips, and forearms.

Involvement of the gastrointestinal tract is the third most common manifestation of SSc, following skin changes and Raynaud's phenomenon. Esophageal hypomotility can be documented in more than 90% of patients having either diffuse or limited SSc. With the loss of lower esophageal sphincter function, reflux of gastric contents occurs, resulting in peptic esophagitis. Substernal burning pain or "heartburn," primarily at night, is a common early symptom. Dysphagia, especially for solid food with food "sticking" in the substernal region, is also common, especially with the development of esophageal strictures. Hypomotility and strictures can be detected with barium contrast and esophageal motility studies. Severe complications such as esophageal stricture and ulcerations can be prevented by early management.

Similar changes (but only in 10 to 20% of patients) occur in the small intestine, resulting in reduced motility, and may cause intermittent diarrhea, bloating and cramping, malabsorption, and weight loss. Colon involvement is an infrequent cause of clinical symptoms, but may present with constipation, obstipation, and pseudo-obstruction. Pathognomonic radiographic findings on barium contrast studies include wide-mouth diverticula of the large bowel (due to atrophy of the muscularis); these may be sites of bleeding or abscess. Primary biliary cirrhosis is well de-

TABLE 83-2	Comparison of Clinical and Laboratory Features of Limited and Diffuse Systemic Sclerosis

	Limited (% Patients)	Diffuse (% Patients)
Demographic		
Age (<40 yr at onset)	50	42
Gender (female)	86	77
Duration of symptoms (years)	12.1	3.4
Organ System Involvement		
Telangiectasis	88	63
Calcinosis	49	15
Raynaud's phenomenon	96	91
Arthralgias or arthritis	26	69
Joint contractures	51	91
Tendon friction rubs	5	62
Myopathy (skeletal)	5	11
Esophageal hypomotility	73	67
Pulmonary fibrosis	35	35
Pulmonary hypertension	11	<1
Congestive heart failure	6	13
"Scleroderma renal crisis"	3	16
Laboratory Data		
Antinuclear antigen positive (1:16+)	90	95
Anticentromere antibody positive (1:40+)	45	2
Anti–Scl-70 antibody positive (any titer)	14	32
Cumulative survival from first diagnosis		
5 yr	82	79
10 yr	69	56

Adapted from Medsger TA: Systemic sclerosis (scleroderma), localized forms of scleroderma, and calcinosis. *In* McCarty DJ, Koopman WJ (eds.): Arthritis & Allied Conditions. 12th ed. Philadelphia, Lea & Febiger, 1993.

scribed in patients with SSc, primarily those with long-standing limited SSc.

"Scleroderma renal crisis," the abrupt onset of accelerated hypertension, oliguria, and microangiopathic hemolysis, once accounted for the majority of deaths in SSc. At present, however, with the early diagnosis and treatment of hypertension with inhibitors of angiotensin-converting enzymes (ACE), renal failure in SSc is less common. Renal involvement is usually observed in an individual with diffuse SSc whose disease is relatively early and at a stage of rapid progression of skin involvement.

The leading cause of mortality in SSc is pulmonary disease. Interstitial lung disease with fibrosis, pulmonary hypertension, pleurisy, and pleural effusions are the pulmonary manifestations of SSc. Patients with diffuse SSc are at a higher risk of developing interstitial fibrotic disease, whereas patients with limited SSc are at a higher risk of developing pulmonary hypertension. Physical findings include fine inspiratory crackles and an audible splitting of S_2 on deep inspiration. Chest radiography is not a sensitive screening test to detect pulmonary abnormalities in early SSc. In long-standing disease, increased interstitial markings, enlarged pulmonary arteries, or pleural effusions may be demonstrated. The single-breath diffusion capacity is the most sensitive pulmonary screening test for SSc pulmonary disease. Reductions in vital capacity or restrictive lung disease can also be detected with pulmonary function testing.

Cardiac involvement in SSc can be manifested clinically as a cardiomyopathy, pericarditis, pericardial effusion, or arrhythmias. Although > 90% of patients with diffuse SSc have some form of cardiac involvement, these features are often not clinically relevant. Physical findings include ventricular gallops, tachycardia, signs of congestive heart failure, and occasional pericardial friction rubs. Pericardial effusions may predispose to renal failure by unknown mechanisms. Echocardiography reveals evidence of pericardial thickening and effusion in 50% of patients, but clinically relevant pericarditis and tamponade are infrequent. The cardiomyopathy is a result of intermittent myocardial ischemia and necrosis with resultant fibrosis. Fibrosis of the conducting pathways can lead to arrhythmias and conduction disturbances.

Musculoskeletal manifestations of SSc include arthralgias, arthritis, and myopathy. Morning stiffness and generalized arthralgias are common. Clinically significant synovitis is uncommon, although 10% of SSc patients present with a symmetric polyarthritis indistinguishable from rheumatoid arthritis. Indolent myopathy in SSc is common. Muscle weakness (proximal or distal) is often secondary to disuse atrophy. Two other forms of myopathy may occur in SSc. First, a bland, nonprogressive myopathy, characterized by proximal weakness, mild elevation of serum creatine kinase, and noninflammatory replacement of muscle tissue, which is refractory to corticosteroids, may occur. Less frequently, an inflammatory myositis indistinguishable from polymyositis occurs that usually responds to glucocorticoids. A muscle biopsy is often needed to distinguish these forms of myopathy. In addition, hypothyroidism is common in SSc patients and

should be investigated in any SSc patient with muscle weakness.

Less common clinical abnormalities in patients with SSc include unilateral or bilateral trigeminal neuralgia, impotence, keratoconjunctivitis sicca, and xerostomia. Hashimoto's thyroiditis and fibrous replacement of thyroid tissue have been observed and are commonly associated with clinical evidence of hypothyroidism.

Antinuclear antibodies are common in SSc (see Table 83–2). The anticentromere antibody (ACA) is most commonly seen in limited SSc, whereas antibodies to topoisomerase I (Scl-70) are fairly specific for diffuse SSc. However, ACA and anti–Scl-70 are detected in the serum of < 50% of all patients with SSc. The clinical and biologic relevance of the ACA and anti–Scl-70 remains to be elucidated; they may be of prognostic value in patients with early signs and symptoms of SSc.

DIFFERENTIAL DIAGNOSIS

Raynaud's Phenomenon

The prevalence of Raynaud's phenomenon is estimated to be 5 to 10% in nonsmokers and up to 22% in premenopausal females. The initial evaluation of a person presenting with Raynaud's phenomenon should include a comprehensive history and physical examination (Table 83–3). A careful history that elicits the patient's drug exposure and occupational history is essential. Useful tests to help identify those persons with Raynaud's who are destined to develop scleroderma include a wide-field nailfold capillary microscopy, in addition to ANA testing. Patients with idiopathic Raynaud's phenomenon should be monitored yearly because surveillance of such persons may permit early recognition of potentially treatable diseases.

Scleroderma-Like Skin Changes

There are several other diseases in which thick or hide-bound skin may occur (see Table 83–1). Raynaud's phenomenon is consistently absent in these disorders. *Eosinophilic fasciitis* is a syndrome that typically manifests as swelling and tightness of the skin of the trunk and proximal extremities, followed by progressive induration of the skin and subcutaneous tissue. The skin is typically shiny with a coarse orange-peel appearance. It is more frequent in young adults, and the onset frequently follows periods of physical exertion and trauma, particularly in males. Deep skin and subcutaneous biopsy confirm inflammatory changes. Although peripheral eosinophilia is present, eosinophils may or may not be present in the skin lesions. Most patients improve spontaneously or with corticosteroids. Eosinophilic fasciitis has been associated with aplastic anemia and myeloproliferative syndromes.

More recently, a syndrome called *eosinophilic myalgia syndrome* (EMS) has been documented in persons

TABLE 83–3	Differential Diagnosis of Raynaud's Phenomenon

Idiopathic Raynaud's phenomenon (Raynaud's disease)
Other connective tissue diseases
    Systemic sclerosis
    Mixed connective tissue disease
    Systemic lupus erythematosus
    Polymyositis/dermatomyositis
    Rheumatoid arthritis
    Vasculitis
    Thromboangiitis obliterans and Takayasu's arteritis
Occupational
    Vibration and physical trauma (e.g., jackhammer operator)
    Cold injury (frostbite)
Chemical exposure
    Vinyl chloride (plastics industry)
    Mining exposure (coal, silicates, gold, heavy metals)
    Organic solvents (trichlorethylene, others)
Environmental and drug-associated
    Toxic oil syndrome
    Arsenic
    Bleomycin
    Vinblastine
    Cisplatin
    Ergotamine
    Beta blockers (high dose)
    5-Hydroxytryptophan and L-tryptophan
Intravascular causes
    Intravascular coagulation
    Cold agglutinin disease
    Cryoglobulinemia
    Cryofibrinogenemia
    Paraproteinemia and hyperviscosity syndromes
    Polycythemia
Structural
    Thoracic outlet syndrome
    Crutch pressure
    Atherosclerosis
Other
    Reflex sympathetic dystrophy

who have ingested L-tryptophan. The putative cause is a contaminant in the preparation of L-tryptophan–containing products. The early phase of EMS is characterized by an acute onset of intense myalgia, skin rashes, dyspnea, fever, and weight loss. Later clinical manifestations include skin induration, myopathy, and a diffuse peripheral neuropathy. The most characteristic laboratory abnormality in EMS is profound eosinophilia. Although treatment with corticosteroids results in prompt amelioration of symptoms, the optimal management and natural history of EMS are not yet known.

Scleroderma-like skin changes occur commonly in patients with diabetes mellitus (see Chapter 89 and Table 83–1).

TREATMENT

No single drug or combination of drugs has been shown to halt the progression of cutaneous or visceral manifestations of SSc in prospective controlled trials. D-Penicillamine, an agent that interferes with the intermolecular cross-linking of mature collagen and also acts as an immunomodulating agent, has been advocated on the basis of retrospective studies that showed minimal skin softening and improved pulmonary function in some patients with SSc. Significant side effects from D-penicillamine occur in 30 to 40% of patients.

A major breakthrough in treating hypertension and preventing renal failure in many patients has been the use of ACE inhibitors. Dialysis and renal transplantation have offered an increased lifespan for those who do develop renal failure. Glucocorticoids are indicated for treatment of inflammatory myositis and pericarditis. Gastrointestinal reflux is successfully treated with raising the head of the bed and using histamine$_2$ (H$_2$)-blockers or proton pump inhibitors. Dilation may be required for esophageal strictures. Bacterial overgrowth in areas of intestinal stasis is often responsive to broad-spectrum antibiotics such as tetracycline. Agents such as metoclopramide, erythromycin and cisapride may be useful for treating gut hypomotility. Glucocorticoids and cyclophosphamide may be used in patients with alveolitis, as detected by high-resolution computed tomographic scan or bronchoalveolar lavage.

Educating the patient regarding measures to prevent exacerbations of Raynaud's phenomenon is one of the most important aspects of treatment. Such measures include avoiding cold exposure and wearing protective clothes, especially gloves. Pharmacologic agents used to treat Raynaud's phenomenon include calcium channel blockers such as verapamil, diltiazem, and nifedipine, as well as nitroglycerin ointments. When digital gangrene occurs, stellate ganglion blockade, epidural blocks, or surgical sympathectomy may prevent autoamputation.

REFERENCES

Gay S, Trabandt A, Moreland LW, Gay RE: Growth factors, extracellular matrix, and oncogenes in scleroderma. Arthritis Rheum 1992; 35: 304–310.
Leroy EC: Systemic sclerosis (scleroderma). *In* Bennett JC, Plum F (eds.): Cecil Textbook of Medicine. 20th ed. Philadelphia, WB Saunders, 1996, pp 1483–1488.
Medsger TA Jr: Systemic sclerosis (scleroderma), localized forms of scleroderma, and calcinosis. *In* McCarty DJ, Koopman WJ (eds.): Arthritis & Allied Conditions. 12th ed. Philadelphia, Lea & Febiger, 1993, pp 1253–1292.

84

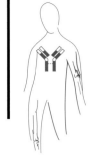

Mixed Connective Tissue Disease, Overlap Syndrome, and Antiphospholipid Antibody Syndrome

MIXED CONNECTIVE TISSUE DISEASE AND OVERLAP SYNDROME

As many as 25% of all patients with features suggestive of a connective tissue disease do not fit into a definite diagnostic category such as systemic lupus erythematosus (SLE), rheumatoid arthritis (RA), scleroderma, or polymyositis. As a result, there has been confusion about the appropriate way to classify these patients' diseases. Three terms used to describe such patients have been *early undifferentiated connective tissue disease* (EUCTD), *mixed connective tissue disease* (MCTD), and *overlap syndrome*.

When a patient has features suggestive of connective tissue disease but not definitively diagnostic of any one disorder, it is best to label the patient as having EUCTD. Most patients with EUCTD have Raynaud's phenomenon; many of them develop definite scleroderma, a few develop SLE, and some remain undifferentiated.

The terms *MCTD* and *overlap syndrome* have often been used interchangeably; however, specific serologic criteria should be applied to make the diagnosis of MCTD. The designation of overlap syndrome is appropriate when a patient exhibits features of one or more established diseases, such as RA or SLE. An example would be a patient with rheumatoid factor–positive, nodular, erosive arthritis who has RA and who subsequently develops high-titer antinuclear antibodies, oral ulcers, malar rash, and antibodies to native DNA. An additional diagnosis of SLE could then be made, and it would be appropriate to label this patient as having an overlap syndrome. Myositis is a frequent component of SLE, scleroderma, and RA, as well as of polymyositis/dermatomyositis; therefore, the finding of myositis in a patient with scleroderma, RA, or SLE does not justify a diagnosis of overlap syndrome.

The diagnosis of MCTD is generally reserved for patients with evidence of very high titers of antibodies to a ribonucleoprotein (RNP) (Table 84–1). The presenting features of MCTD do not differentiate it from other diffuse connective tissue diseases such as SLE, scleroderma,

or polymyositis. Antibodies to RNP constitute the only constant feature in patients with MCTD. An equally important feature in MCTD is the absence of antibodies to double-stranded DNA, Sm antigen, and histones. Many patients (35 to 40%) who fulfill the criteria for a diagnosis of SLE (see Table 80–1) may also have low titers of serum antibodies to RNP, and most do not have myositis or sclerodactyly. Patients with high titers of anti-RNP experience a relatively favorable prognosis and little renal disease.

The pattern of organ system involvement is a useful guide to therapy in patients with MCTD or overlap syndrome. For example, treatment of erosive arthritis should be the same as that for RA. Patients with scleroderma-like features are least likely to improve. Although the prognosis of patients with MCTD is favorable, serious and sometimes fatal complications such as pulmonary hypertension do occur.

ANTIPHOSPHOLIPID ANTIBODY SYNDROME

Antiphospholipid antibodies, those responsible for the *in vitro* lupus anticoagulant test and those directed against negatively charged phospholipids (e.g., cardiolipin), are associated with a variety of clinical manifestations (Table 84–2). Approximately one third of patients with SLE have antiphospholipid antibodies or a lupus anticoagulant.

The specific serologic feature of this syndrome is the production of antibodies that cross-react with cardiolipin and other negatively charged phospholipids. The most useful tests for detecting antiphospholipid antibodies are the lupus anticoagulant and the anticardiolipin antibody tests. Only a minority of patients with antiphospholipid antibodies develop thrombosis, fetal loss, or thrombocytopenia. Approximately 30% of patients with the lupus anticoagulant develop thrombosis. Thrombosis and fetal loss occur more frequently in persons with moderate to high titers of IgG anticardiolipin antibodies. To fulfill the minimum criteria for this syndrome, patients must have both a positive antiphospholipid test and a related clinical complication.

The lupus anticoagulant test relies on the ability of some antiphospholipid antibodies to inhibit *in vitro* clot formation. Antiphospholipid syndrome patients are often first identified by a prolonged partial thromboplastin or prothrombin time, not corrected by the addition of normal plasma. The most sensitive test for antiphospholipid antibodies is the anticardiolipin antibody test. Antiphospholipid antibodies are paradoxically associated with thrombosis rather than hemorrhage. Treatment for the an-

TABLE 84–1	Guidelines for Diagnosing MCTD

General

Clinical features of a diffuse connective tissue disorder

Serologic

1. Positive ANA, speckled pattern, titer >1:1000
2. Antibodies to U1 RNP
3. Absence of antibodies to dsDNA, histones, Sm, Scl-70, and other specificities
4. Commonly: Hypergammaglobulinemia and positive rheumatoid factor

Clinical

1. Sequential evolution of overlap features over course of *several years,* including Raynaud's phenomenon, serositis, gastrointestinal dysmotility, myositis, arthritis, sclerodactyly, skin rashes, and an abnormal DL_{co} on pulmonary function tests
2. Absence of truncal scleroderma, severe renal disease, and severe central nervous system involvement
3. A nail fold capillary pattern identical to that seen in systemic sclerosis (dropout and dilated vessels)

ANA = Antinuclear antibodies; dsDNA = double-stranded DNA; MCTD = mixed connective tissue disease; RNP = ribonucleoprotein.
From Bennett RM: Mixed connective tissue disease and other overlap syndromes. *In* Kelley WN, Harris ED Jr, Ruddy S, Sledge CB (eds.): Textbook of Rheumatology. 3rd ed. Philadelphia, WB Saunders, 1989, p 1150.

TABLE 84–2	Clinical Manifestations of the Antiphospholipid Antibody Syndrome

Common
  Venous thrombosis
  Arterial thrombosis
    Stroke
    Extremity gangrene
    Visceral infarction
  Recurrent fetal loss
  Thrombocytopenia
  Livedo reticularis
Uncommon
  Coombs'-positive hemolysis
  Valvular heart disease
  Chorea
  Nonstroke ischemia syndrome
  Transverse myelopathy

tiphospholipid antibody syndrome has not been clearly defined. Aspirin, corticosteroids, and heparin have been used to prevent fetal loss; however, their efficacy has yet to be determined. Patients with thrombotic events should be treated with anticoagulants. However, because thrombosis occurs only in a minority of patients with antiphospholipid antibodies, prophylactic treatment is not justified in patients who have these antibodies but no history of thrombosis.

REFERENCES

Harris EN, Khamashta MA, Hughes GRV: *In* McCarty DJ, Koopman WJ (eds.): Arthritis & Allied Conditions. 12th ed. Philadelphia, Lea & Febiger, 1993, pp 1201–1212.
Sharp GC, Singsen BH: Mixed connective tissue disease. *In* McCarty DJ, Koopman WJ (eds.): Arthritis & Allied Conditions. 12th ed. Philadelphia, Lea & Febiger, 1993, pp 1213–1224.

85

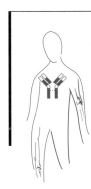

Vasculitides

The vasculitides represent a heterogeneous group of syndromes. They are characterized by inflammation of the blood vessel wall and may involve vessels of any size and in any location. The syndrome may be exclusively an arteritis, exclusively a venulitis, or a combination of the two. The location of the inflammatory process, that is, arteries, or arterioles, postcapillary venules, or veins, determines the diffuse symptoms that may occur in each of these syndromes. Some vasculopathies involve only skin and surface areas, whereas others involve deep tissues, are systemic, and can be rapidly fatal.

CLASSIFICATION

Historically, the vasculitides are classified by the pathologist and reflect the size of the artery involved. However, because extensive overlaps occur with this method, a system of categorization by clinical syndrome has recently grown in popularity among clinicians. Table 85–1 presents a useful classification that combines some of the earlier histopathologic descriptions as well as the more modern understanding of the clinical settings in which these various syndromes occur.

IMMUNOPATHOGENESIS

A precise definition of the immunopathogenic process in the vasculitides remains incomplete. In many of these syndromes, antigen-antibody complexes and complement can be identified and are associated with the endothelial layer of the blood vessel wall. These complexes may be either deposited from the circulation or formed *in situ*.

Definition of the broad spectrum of possible antigens has also proved elusive, although in lupus complexes of DNA and its antibody and in rheumatoid vasculitis, rheumatoid factors can be found. Similarly, in some cases of polyarteritis nodosa, hepatitis B virus, together with its antibody and complement, may be observed. However, it is also clear that antigen-antibody complexes do not account for the entire syndrome. For example, in Wegener's granulomatosis, granulomas consist of T cells and macrophages; presumably, they form at least some part of the pathogenic process above and beyond what is usually seen in a typical immune complex–mediated vasculitis.

HYPERSENSITIVITY ANGIITIS

Hypersensitivity angiitis is the most common form of vasculitis and is usually localized to the small vessels of the skin. The characteristic histopathologic picture is a leukocytoclastic venulitis. Leukocytoclasis refers to nuclear debris derived from infiltrating neutrophils. Red blood cell extravasation, thrombosis of the vessel lumen, and fibrinoid necrosis can also be seen. A variety of cutaneous lesions are associated with this form of vasculitis, but usually they appear first on the lower extremities as erythematous macules that evolve into a relatively specific physical sign, palpable purpura.

Diagnosis of cutaneous vasculitis is usually made by biopsy. Laboratory findings are variable: erythrocyte sedimentation rate (ESR) can be either normal or elevated; complement can be normal or depressed; and immune complexes can be detected, usually in low concentrations.

Certain hypersensitivity vasculitides are seen as discrete clinical syndromes. Henoch-Schönlein purpura is characterized by fever, abdominal pain, nonthrombocytopenic purpura, arthralgia, and renal disease. The classic triad of purpura, arthritis, and abdominal pain occurs in about 80% of patients. Children and young adults are most commonly affected, but the disorder can afflict persons of any age. Although the disease is of limited duration (usually 6 to 16 weeks), 5 to 10% of patients can develop a relapsing renal disease characterized by glomerulonephritis. Involvement of the wall of the gastrointestinal tract can result in colicky abdominal pain, intestinal bleeding, obstruction, infarction, intussusception, or perforation. Immunoglobulin and complement can be demonstrated in involved blood vessels. In Henoch-Schönlein purpura, serum IgA levels can be elevated; complement levels are usually normal, but IgA deposits can be demonstrated in the vessel wall.

Another syndrome of hypersensitivity vasculitis is essential mixed cryoglobulinemia, which is characterized by arthralgia, purpura, weakness, and cryoglobulinemia. There are recurrent bouts of palpable purpura of the lower extremities, hepatosplenomegaly, lymphadenopathy, and polyarthralgias. Renal failure can result from a diffuse proliferative glomerulonephritis. Cryoglobulins containing IgG and IgM, sometimes with rheumatoid factor activity, can be detected. This syndrome may also coexist with other autoimmune disease. Bacterial infections (i.e.,

TABLE 85–1	The Clinical Spectrum of Vasculitis

Polyarteritis Nodosa Group

Classic polyarteritis nodosa
Allergic angiitis and granulomatosis (Churg-Strauss disease)
Overlap syndrome

Hypersensitivity Vasculitis

Henoch-Schönlein purpura
Serum sickness and serum sickness-like reactions
Vasculitis associated with infectious diseases
Vasculitis associated with neoplasms
Vasculitis associated with connective tissue diseases
Vasculitis associated with other underlying diseases
Congenital deficiencies of the complement system

Granulomatous Vasculitides

Wegener's granulomatosis
Angiocentric immunoproliferative lesions (lymphomatoid granulomatosis)
Giant cell arteritides
   Cranial or temporal arteritis
   Takayasu's arteritis

Other Vasculitic Syndromes

Mucocutaneous lymph node syndrome (Kawasaki's disease)
Behçet's disease
Vasculitis isolated to the central nervous system
Thromboangiitis obliterans (Buerger's disease)
Erythema nodosa
Erythema multiforme
Erythema elevatum diutinum
Miscellaneous vasculitides

From Rossenwasser LJ: The vasculitic syndromes. *In* Bennett JC, Plum F (eds.): Cecil Textbook of Medicine. 20th ed. Philadelphia, WB Saunders, 1996, p 1491.

streptococcal), serum sickness, chronic active hepatitis, ulcerative colitis, Sjögren's syndrome, retroperitoneal fibrosis, and Goodpasture's syndrome may be seen in association with the histopathologic picture of hypersensitivity vasculitis.

Treatment of hypersensitivity angiitis includes managing the associated entities (e.g., drug reactions, bacterial infections). Fortunately, this form of vasculitis is usually self-limited, but occasionally patients require nonsteroidal anti-inflammatory agents, corticosteroids, or immunosuppressive agents.

POLYARTERITIS NODOSA

Polyarteritis nodosa involves primarily the medium and small muscular arteries. It can occur in any age group but has a peak incidence in the 40s and 50s. The male to female ratio is approximately 2.5:1.0. Early signs and symptoms are fever, weight loss, abdominal pain, and musculoskeletal pain (Table 85–2).

Renal

The kidneys are the most commonly involved organ system. Inflammation of the arcuate arteries as well as other medium-sized vessels can result in segmental aneurysmal dilatations. A rapidly progressive, necrotizing glomerulonephritis can lead to the sudden onset of severe hypertension, nephrotic syndrome, and renal failure. Spontaneous rupture of aneurysms can result in retroperitoneal hemorrhage or a perinephric hematoma.

Cardiovascular

Coronary arteritis can produce angina pectoris or myocardial infarction. Pericarditis is common but is often diagnosed only post mortem. Approximately 70% of patients eventually have cardiac involvement.

Gastrointestinal

Polyarteritis nodosa also involves the gastrointestinal tract, causing abdominal pain, intestinal bleeding, obstruction, or perforation. Rupture of mesenteric aneurysms can lead to intraperitoneal hemorrhage, hypovolemic shock, and death.

Neurologic

Disorders of the peripheral nervous system are attributable to arteritis of the vasa nervorum. The peripheral neuropathies include mononeuritis multiplex, which is characterized by paresthesia, pain, weakness, and sensory loss. Involving several or many individual nerves at the same time, the neuropathy is asymmetric and has both a sensory and a motor distribution.

Vasculitis of the central nervous system (CNS) in polyarteritis nodosa is estimated to occur in 20 to 40% of cases. Encephalopathy secondary to severe hypertension and/or primary neuronal dysfunction produces a global cognitive disorder. Vasculitis affecting different anatomic structures of the CNS can lead to seizures and hemorrhagic or ischemic events.

TABLE 85–2	Presenting Complaints in Patients with Classic Polyarteritis Nodosa

Presenting Complaint	Patients (%)
Malaise/weakness	13
Abdominal pain	12
Leg pain	12
Neurologic signs/symptoms	10
Fever	8
Cough	8
Myalgias	5
Peripheral neuropathy	5
Headache	5
Arthritis/arthralgia	4
Skin involvement	4
Painful arms	4
Painful feet	4

From Cupps T, Fauci A: The Vasculitides. Philadelphia, WB Saunders, 1981, p 30.

Cutaneous

Polyarteritis nodosa affects the integument in some form in 25% of patients. An uncommon but quite characteristic sign is cutaneous and subcutaneous nodules. These nodules, which measure 0.5 to 1.0 cm, are usually movable and are often transient. Livedo reticularis, peripheral gangrene, and polymorphic lesions with purpura and urticaria also occur.

Diagnosis

The laboratory findings of polyarteritis nodosa often reflect the presence of a severe systemic inflammation. The ESR, serum immunoglobulin levels, C-reactive protein, white blood cell count, and platelet count are all frequently elevated. Anemia is frequently observed and can be due to blood loss or renal failure. Microscopic hematuria, cylindruria, and proteinuria result from glomerulonephritis. Hypocomplementemia may be present, but antinuclear antibodies and rheumatoid factor are absent. As many as 30% of patients exhibit hepatitis B surface antigenemia. The cerebrospinal fluid is normal unless a subarachnoid hemorrhage has occurred.

Biopsy provides the definitive diagnosis. Any affected organ, such as the skin, muscle, testis, sural nerve, liver, or kidney, is an appropriate biopsy site. Angiography of the renal, hepatic, and mesenteric arteries is often performed to seek evidence of aneurysmal formation or other signs of vasculitis. When CNS vasculitis is suspected, angiography is necessary because neither the magnetic resonance nor computed tomography scan provides sufficient evidence to confirm the diagnosis.

Treatment

Effective treatment requires a combination of a corticosteroid and immunosuppressive agents. The current recommended initial therapy is prednisone, 1 to 2 mg/kg/day, and cyclophosphamide, 2 mg/kg/day. These drugs are tapered gradually as the clinical response allows but may be required to maintain remission.

ALLERGIC VASCULITIS OF CHURG AND STRAUSS

The Churg-Strauss syndrome belongs to the polyarteritis nodosa group and is characterized by hypereosinophilia, allergic rhinitis and/or asthma, and evidence of systemic vasculitis.

This syndrome tends to evolve over many years, during which the predominant clinical findings appear to have an allergic basis. Rhinitis usually precedes the onset of extrinsic asthma. Hypereosinophilia and eosinophilic tissue infiltration occur, and with time a systemic necrotizing vasculitis develops. Hypereosinophilia and asthma

are essential criteria for the diagnosis of the Churg-Strauss syndrome.

Vasculitis of the Churg-Strauss syndrome is similar to polyarteritis nodosa and Wegener's granulomatosis in that it involves medium and smaller blood vessels. However, its unique histology distinguishes it from Wegener's disease, and its predominance of respiratory tract allergy-like symptoms and hypereosinophilia distinguishes it from the usual polyarteritis nodosa.

The treatment of Churg-Strauss syndrome is similar to that of the other systemic necrotizing vasculitides. It generally responds readily to high-dose corticosteroids (i.e., prednisone, 60 mg/day), but addition of cyclophosphamide may be required.

WEGENER'S GRANULOMATOSIS

Wegener's granulomatosis is a systemic necrotizing vasculitis characterized by (1) necrotizing granulomatous vasculitis of the upper and lower respiratory tract and (2) a focal necrotizing glomerulonephritis and vasculitis of other organ systems. The disease has a male-to-female ratio of 3 : 2. Although the peak incidence occurs in the 30s and 40s, with an average age of 40 years, the age range varies between 15 and 75 years.

The majority of individuals in whom the diagnosis of Wegener's granulomatosis is eventually made present with symptoms of upper respiratory tract disease (Table 85–3), including nasal ulcers, rhinorrhea, and sinus pain. Ocular inflammation also develops in more than half of

TABLE 85–3	Presenting Signs and Symptoms in Wegener's Granulomatosis
Sign or Symptom	**Occurrence (%)**
Pulmonary infiltrates	71
Sinusitis	67
Joint (arthralgia or arthritis)	44
Fever	34
Otitis	25
Cough	34
Rhinitis or nasal symptoms	22
Hemoptysis	18
Ocular inflammation (conjunctivitis, uveitis, episcleritis, and scleritis)	16
Weight loss	16
Skin rash	13
Epistaxis	11
Renal failure	11
Chest discomfort	8
Anorexia or malaise	8
Proptosis	7
Shortness of breath or dyspnea	7
Oral ulcers	6
Hearing loss	6
Pleuritis or effusion	6
Headache	6

Reproduced with permission from Fauci AS, Haynes BF, Katz P, et al: Wegener's granulomatosis: Prospective clinical and therapeutic experience with 85 patients for 21 years. Ann Intern Med 1983; 98:76–85.

TABLE 85–4	Treatment of Wegener's Granulomatosis			
Drug	**Indications**	**Initial Dose**	**Monitoring**	**Duration**
Cyclophosphamide	Moderate to severe	1–2 mg/kg/day (po)	CBC weekly; keep WBC >3000, PMN >1000 and monitor liver tests; urine cytology and/or cystoscopy if prolonged therapy	Approximately 1 yr beyond clinical remission
	Fulminant	3–4 mg/kg/day IV for 2–3 days, then reduce to 2 mg/kg/day po or IV		
Corticosteroids	Moderate to severe	1 mg/kg/day prednisone equivalent (IV initially or po)	Glucose, lipids, bone density	Taper to low dose (5–10 mg/day) or alternate-day therapy over 2 mo
Methotrexate	Mild to moderate; upper airway; or diffuse disease without significant renal involvement	Up to 15–25 mg once weekly	Monitor CBC and liver tests q 4–8 wk	Taper to lowest dose controlling features; ? trial off 1 yr past clinical remission; close follow-up
Antibiotics	Adjunctive, not primary, to treat secondary bacterial infections; consider chronic suppression in chronic upper airway disease (sulfa may be contraindicated with methotrexate)			Intermittent or chronic low-dose "prophylaxis"
Cyclosporine	Refractory disease; dialysis dependent; patients awaiting renal transplant	3–5 mg/kg/day	BP, chemistries (Cr, Mg)	1 yr beyond clinical remission or until transplant

BP = Blood pressure; CBC = complete blood count; IV = intravenous; PMN = polymorphonuclear neutrophil leukocytes; po = orally; WBC = white blood cells.
From Allen NB: Wegener's granulomatosis. *In* Bennett JC, Plum F (eds.): Cecil Textbook of Medicine. 20th ed. Philadelphia, WB Saunders, 1996, p 1497.

all patients and includes conjunctivitis, episcleritis, scleromalacia, corneal ulcers, and retinal artery thrombosis.

The lungs become involved in most patients. Although variable, the radiographic findings of solitary or multiple infiltrates or nodules and multilocular, irregular cavities can be seen. Biopsy of the lung usually provides documentation of the necrotizing granulomatous process.

The pathologic lesions are a focal or diffuse proliferative glomerulonephritis and interstitial nephritis. The glomerulonephritis often produces a urinary sediment with proteinuria, hematuria, and cylindruria. Nodular skin lesions and purpuric papules can be seen. Active synovitis is rare, but about one half of patients complain of joint pains.

Diagnosis

Laboratory studies usually reveal an elevated ESR; a normochromic, normocytic anemia; and a polyclonal hypergammaglobulinemia. Further, the serum of many patients with Wegener's granulomatosis contains antibodies to a cytoplasmic antigen from polymorphonuclear leukocytes (c-ANCA). Since sensitivity of this antibody test varies from 30 to 90%, it cannot be used as a sole diagnostic criterion. However, detection of antibodies to a more specific antigen, proteinase-3 (PR-3), may prove to be more useful. Definitive diagnosis is made on the basis of the biopsy. Occasionally it may be necessary to distinguish between Wegener's granulomatosis and midline granuloma. The latter consists of destructive granuloma involving the nose, paranasal sinuses, and palate, but vasculitis

is not a prominent feature and does not appear to be part of the underlying process.

Treatment

The current therapy for Wegener's granulomatosis utilizes corticosteroid and cytotoxic agents. Critically ill patients should be treated with intravenous cyclophosphamide until the course of the disease is stabilized and may then be switched to oral therapy. Treatment with corticosteroids alone is insufficient to control disease activity and induce remission (Table 85–4).

POLYMYALGIA RHEUMATICA AND GIANT CELL ARTERITIS

Polymyalgia rheumatica (PMR) and giant cell arteritis are closely related entities, and many believe that they represent the spectrum of a single disease. PMR is characterized by aching and myalgia of the shoulder and pelvic girdle musculature, neck, and proximal extremities. Onset is in the 50s or later, and it is about twice as frequent in women as in men. The yearly incidence is approximately 54 per 100,000 population.

Symptoms of aching, stiffness after rest, and myalgia often begin precipitously, although the disease may progress relatively slowly over time. Polyarthralgias or a true synovitis can be present. Other commonly observed constitutional features include fever, weight loss, malaise, and anorexia.

TABLE 85-5	Polymyalgia Rheumatica: Diagnostic Criteria

>50 yr of age
Aching and morning stiffness in at least two of the following areas:
 Neck
 Shoulder girdle
 Pelvic girdle
Erythrocyte sedimentation rate (ESR) >40 mm in 1 hr
Duration of symptoms for 1 mo
No other disease present

From Hunder G: Polymyalgia rheumatica and giant cell arteritis. *In* Bennett JC, Plum F (eds.): Cecil Textbook of Medicine. 20th ed. Philadelphia, WB Saunders, 1996, p 1498.

The physical examination reveals tender muscles but no weakness or atrophy. Synovitis of the knees with or without small effusions occurs, but synovitis of the small joints of the hands and feet is rare (Table 85–5).

There are no specific laboratory tests to identify PMR, but nearly all patients with PMR have an elevated Westergren sedimentation rate. The absence of rheumatoid factor differentiates PMR from rheumatoid arthritis. The differential diagnosis includes infections, neoplasia (i.e., plasma cell dyscrasia), fibromyalgia, and painful myopathies. Giant cell arteritis can present or be associated with PMR in 20 to 40% of patients (Table 85–6).

Giant cell arteritis (temporal arteritis) usually affects individuals over age 50 years, with an approximate annual incidence of 12 per 100,000 individuals. The onset of giant cell arteritis may be precipitous or insidious. When the disorder coexists with PMR, proximal extremity aching, stiffness, fatigue, and headache are common presenting symptoms. Other constitutional symptoms include recurrent and unexplained fevers, anorexia, weight loss, and malaise (Table 85–7). In addition, confusion, depressive reactions, psychosis, and, rarely, dementia can occur.

TABLE 85-7	Giant Cell Arteritis: Clinical Findings in 94 Patients

Clinical Manifestation	Frequency (%)
Headache	77
Abnormal temporal artery	53
Jaw claudication	51
Scalp tenderness	47
Constitutional symptoms	48
Polymyalgia rheumatica	34
Fever	27
Respiratory symptoms	23
Facial pain	14
Diplopia/blurred vision	12
Transient vision loss	5
Blindness (partical or complete)	13
Hemoglobin <11.0 gm/dl	24
Erythrocyte sedimentation rate >40 mm/hr	97

After Machado EBV, Michet CJ, Ballard DJ, et al: Trends in incidence and clinical presentation of temporal arteritis in Olmsted County, Minnesota, 1950–1985. Arthritis Rheum 1988; 31:745–749. Reprinted from Arthritis and Rheumatism Journal, copyright 1988. Used by permission of the American College of Rheumatology.

The symptoms of headache, vision changes, and scalp tenderness are the result of arteritis. Jaw claudication, a symptom in one third to one half of patients with giant cell arteritis, is a consequence of impaired blood flow in the temporal or maxillary arteries.

The visual alterations of giant cell arteritis include transient blurring, ptosis, diplopia, and transient, permanent, partial, or complete blindness. These symptoms are the result of arteritis affecting the posterior ciliary or ophthalmic vessels or, less commonly, the central retinal artery. Although blindness is usually preceded by other visual changes for weeks or months, it can occur precipitously without warning.

Headache and scalp tenderness, very common early symptoms, are due to arteritis of the temporal or occipital

TABLE 85-6	Differential Features in Polymyalgia Rheumatica and Similar Disorders

	Polymyalgia Rheumatica	Giant Cell Arteritis	Rheumatoid Arthritis	Dermatomyositis	Fibromyalgia
Morning stiffness >30 min	+	±	+*	±	Variable
Headache and/or scalp tenderness	0	+	0	0	Variable
Pain with active joint movement	+	0	+*	0	Inconstant
Tender joints	±	0	+*	0	Tender spots
Swollen joints	±	±	+	0	0
Muscle weakness	±†	0	+*	+	0
Normochromic anemia	+	+	+	0	0
Elevated ESR	+	+	+	±	0
Elevated serum creatine kinase	0	0	0	+	0
Serum rheumatoid factor	0	0	70%	0	0
Distinct electromyographic abnormality	0	0	0	+	0
Response to nonsteroidal anti-inflammatory drug (NSAID)	±	0	+	0	0

0 = Absent; + = present; ± = present in minority of cases; ESR = erythrocyte sedimentation rate.
* = Associated with affected joints.
† = Pain inhibits movement. Disuse atrophy may occur.
From Hunder G: Polymyalgia rheumatica and giant cell arteritis. *In* Bennett JC, Plum F (eds.): Cecil Textbook of Medicine. 20th ed. Philadelphia, WB Saunders, 1996, p 1499.

vessels. The new onset of an ill-defined headache of variable severity in an older person should raise the suspicion of giant cell arteritis.

Diagnosis

There are no specific laboratory abnormalities in giant cell arteritis, but evidence of inflammation may be seen. Leukocytosis of $< 20,000/mm^3$ and a thrombocytosis of $< 1,000,000/mm^3$, elevated fibrinogen, α_2-globulin, IgG, and total hemolytic complement are frequently observed. The elevated ESR remains a *sine qua non* for the diagnosis of giant cell arteritis, just as it does for PMR.

When the diagnosis is suspected, biopsy of a clinically involved or symptomatic portion of the temporal artery should be obtained. If the temporal artery appears clinically uninvolved, a biopsy specimen of a segment several centimeters in length should be taken to obtain sufficient tissue to identify the commonly observed "skip" lesions of temporal arteritis. History of claudication of an extremity and the presence on examination of a bruit implicate large vessel arteritis, which should be confirmed by angiography.

Treatment

The treatment of choice is corticosteroids. The usual initial daily dosage is the equivalent of prednisone, 60 mg.

If there is a moderate to high likelihood of giant cell arteritis, corticosteroid therapy should be instituted immediately, prior to biopsy, to avert the dreaded potential for blindness. The characteristic histologic findings are present if biopsy is performed within 1 week after starting corticosteroid therapy. The response to therapy is monitored clinically by resolution of symptoms as well as by a decrease in the ESR. Upon remission and return of the ESR to normal levels, the corticosteroid dose can be tapered as the ESR is periodically monitored.

REFERENCES

Allen NB: Wegener's granulomatosis. *In* Bennett JC, Plum F (eds.): Cecil Textbook of Medicine, 20th ed. Philadelphia, WB Saunders, 1996.

Haynes BF, Allen NB, Fauci AS: Diagnostic and therapeutic approach to the patient with vasculitis. Med Clin North Am 1986; 70:355.

Hoffman GS, Kerr GS, Leavitt RY, Hallahan CW, Lebovics RS, Travis WD, Rottem M, Fauci AS: Wegener's granulomatosis: An analysis of 158 patients. Ann Intern Med 1992; 116:488.

Hunder G: Polymyalgia rheumatica and giant cell arteritis. *In* Bennett JC, Plum F (eds.): Cecil Textbook of Medicine, 20th ed. Philadelphia, WB Saunders, 1996.

Rosenwasser LJ: Polyarteritis nodosa group. *In* Bennett JC, Plum F (eds.): Cecil Textbook of Medicine, 20th ed. Philadelphia, WB Saunders, 1996.

Rosenwasser LJ: The vasculitic syndromes. *In* Bennett JC, Plum F (eds.): Cecil Textbook of Medicine. 20th ed. Philadelphia, WB Saunders, 1996.

86 | The Spondyloarthropathies

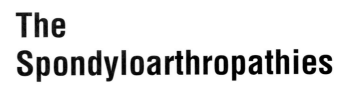

The spondyloarthropathies are a group of interrelated disorders that share certain epidemiologic, pathogenetic, clinical, and pathologic features. They characteristically involve the sacroiliac joints, as well as peripheral inflammatory arthritis, and by definition are not seropositive for rheumatoid factor. They have a tendency to a familial aggregation of cases and demonstrate inflammation of the ligamentous insertion into bone (esthesis). There is extensive overlap among the several diseases that compose this group (Table 86–1).

ANKYLOSING SPONDYLITIS

Ankylosing spondylitis (AS) is the prototype of the spondyloarthropathies. It is characterized by enthesopathy, sacroiliitis, and spondylitis; inflammatory ocular diseases; an asymmetric oligoarthritis predominantly of the large joints of the lower limbs; and an association with human leukocyte antigen (HLA)-B27. The European Spondyloarthropathy Study Group (ESSG) has recently defined criteria for the inclusive diagnosis of all spondyloarthropathies (Fig. 86–1).

Prevalence

The prevalence of AS is about 0.2% of the general population.

Clinical Features

Ankylosing spondylitis usually presents during young adulthood with vague symptoms of mid and low back stiffness and pain. Complaints are radiation of the pain into the buttocks and prominent stiffness in the back after rest. Thoracic cage pain also occurs in AS and can have a pleuritic quality. Dactylitis, Achilles tendinitis, plantar fasciitis, and iliac crest tenderness occur as a result of inflammation at the entheses. The proximal synovial joints, including the shoulders, hips, and knees, are more often involved than the smaller distal joints. Acute ante-

rior uveitis occurs in approximately one quarter of patients with AS and appears as pain, redness, and photophobia that is usually episodic and may be unilateral or bilateral. Examination of the patient with early AS can demonstrate reduced spinal mobility, partial or complete loss of the physiologic lumbar lordosis, and increased thoracic kyphosis. Later findings include restriction of chest wall expansion during deep inspiration (< 2.5 cm), gradual development of a stooped posture, fixation of the spine, and a shuffling gait.

Radiologic Features

The long-standing pathologic changes produce characteristic radiographic features in AS. Inflammation of the sacroiliac joints leads to gradual destruction of cartilage and subchondral erosions, giving the radiographic appearance of "pseudowidening." An osteoblastic response of the affected bone then results in sclerosis of the joint margins. Subsequent fusion of the joint results from the ingrowth of osteoid tissue, calcification, and bony bridging of the joint margins.

Osteitis of subchondral vertebral bone results in the radiographic picture of squaring of the bodies, which can be the earliest radiographic change of AS. Healing of the cartilage and bone inflammation are associated with fibrosis, calcification, new bone formation with replacement of the annulus fibrosus, and development of syndesmophytes that bridge the margins of adjacent vertebral bodies. The gradual ossification of the annulus fibrosus, formation of syndesmophytes, and ossification of the perispinal ligaments give the radiographic appearance of the "bamboo" spine (Fig. 86–2). Extra-articular involvements in AS and the other spondyloarthropathies are compared in Table 86–1.

Treatment

The management of AS is predicated upon a vigorous approach to physical therapy and the judicious use of certain nonsteroidal anti-inflammatory drugs (NSAIDs).

TABLE 86-1	Comparison of the Spondyloarthropathies

	Ankylosing Spondylitis	Posturethral Reactive Arthritis	Postdysenteric Reactive Arthritis	Enteropathic Arthritis	Psoriatic Arthritis
Sacroiliitis	+++++	+++	++	+	++
Spondylitis	++++	+++	++	++	++
Peripheral arthritis	+	++++	++++	+++	++++
Articular course	Chronic	Acute or chronic	Acute > chronic	Acute or chronic	Chronic
HLA-B27	95%	60%	30%	20%	20%
Enthesopathy	++	++++	+++	++	++
Common extra-articular manifestations	Eye Heart	Eye GU Oral/GI Heart	GU Eye	GI Eye	Skin Eye
Other names	Bekhterev's Marie-Strumpell	Reiter's syndrome, SARA, NGU, chlamydial arthritis	Reiter's syndrome	Crohn's disease, ulcerative colitis	

GI = Gastrointestinal; GU = genitourinary; HLA = human leukocyte antigen; NGU = nongonococcal urethritis; SARA = sexually acquired reactive arthritis.
From Cush JJ, Lipsky PE: The spondyloarthropathies. *In* Bennett JC, Plum F (eds.): Cecil Textbook of Medicine. 20th ed. Philadelphia, WB Saunders, 1996.

Although NSAIDs do not alter the course of AS, by providing analgesia they promote function. The long-term objective of the exercise regimen is to halt the insidious development of disabling axial immobility and to preserve maximal motion and function.

REITER'S SYNDROME

Reiter's syndrome is characterized by arthritis, urethritis, conjunctivitis, and mucocutaneous lesions. The disease

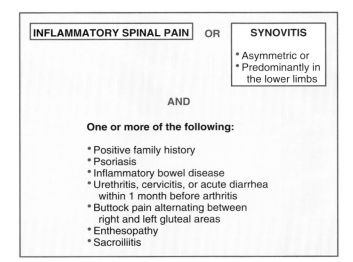

Figure 86-1

European Spondyloarthropathy Study Group (ESSG) criteria for the classification of spondyloarthropathy. (Modified from Dougados M, et al: The European Spondyloarthropathy Study Group: Preliminary criteria for the classification of spondyloarthropathy. Arthritis Rheum 1991; 34:1218. Reprinted from Arthritis and Rheumatism Journal, copyright 1991. Used by permission of the American College of Rheumatology.)

most commonly affects young males (male to female ratio approximates 10 to 15:1) during their 20s and 30s.

Epidemiology and Immunogenetics

The onset of Reiter's syndrome often occurs following venereal infections or dysentery. The venereal relationship appears more frequently in the United States. Chlamydia can be cultured from the urethras of untreated patients in 33 to 47% of cases. Moreover, antichlamydial antibodies can eventually be detected in about one half of patients, and chlamydial antigens have been found in inflamed synovial tissue. The postdysenteric form of Reiter's syndrome, which is found more frequently in Africa, Europe, and the Far and Middle East, usually results from a gastrointestinal infection with *Shigella flexneri* but may also follow enteric infections with *Salmonella* spp., *Yersinia enterocolitica*, or *Campylobacter jejuni*. Joint fluids of Reiter's syndrome patients yield no bacterial growth, and therefore the syndrome has been regarded as a reactive arthritis. In fact, many patients have only arthritis without the full-blown Reiter's syndrome and are classified (see Table 86–1) as having reactive arthritis. However, the pathogenic pathways are considered to be similar.

Human leukocyte antigen-B27 is found by serotyping in 80% of white and 35% of black patients. Although the precise significance of the B27 allotype remains uncertain, this cellular surface antigen may predispose individuals with certain bacterial infections (i.e., *Shigella* species, *Salmonella*, *Y. enterocolitica*) to the eventual development of a reactive arthritis, including Reiter's syndrome.

Clinical Features

Characteristically, Reiter's syndrome develops 1 to 4 weeks following venereal exposure or diarrhea. Urethritis

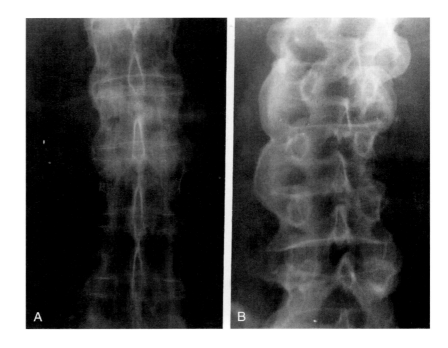

Figure 86-2
A, Lumbar spondylitis in ankylosing spondylitis with symmetric, marginal bridging syndesmophytes and calcification of the spinal ligament. *B,* The bulky, nonmarginal, asymmetric syndesmophytes of Reiter's syndrome with lumbar spondylitis. (From Cush JJ, Lipsky PE: The spondyloarthropathies. *In* Bennett JC, Plum F (eds.): Cecil Textbook of Medicine, 20th ed. Philadelphia, WB Saunders, 1996.)

manifested by burning and frequency is often the earliest symptom. An erosion of the glans penis around the meatus—circinate balanitis—may be found in association with the urethritis. A profuse and watery diarrhea can precede the onset of urethritis in Reiter's syndrome. Following an epidemic of *Shigella* dysentery, approximately 2 of every 1000 affected persons can be expected to develop Reiter's syndrome.

The conjunctivitis of Reiter's syndrome is mild and is characterized by an evanescent irritation with burning usually lasting a few days, or, less commonly, as long as several weeks. The process is ordinarily self-limiting. In contrast, the development of an acute uveitis can be complicated by pain and potential vision loss. Mucocutaneous lesions are commonly observed during Reiter's syndrome. Lesions can be identified on the buccal mucosa, tongue, palate, and pharyngeal mucosa as painless vesicles, elevated erythematous papules, or superficial ulcers. Keratoderma blennorrhagicum, which occurs in 20% of patients and is found most often on the plantar surfaces of the feet, has the appearance of a brown or yellow cone-shaped papule. Coalescence of the papules leads to desquamating lesions.

The arthritis of Reiter's syndrome often presents precipitously and frequently affects the knees and ankles. The distribution of the arthritis is asymmetric and can be monoarticular and pauciarticular. A particularly notable feature of Reiter's syndrome is the enthesopathy. Although enthesopathic signs are present in other forms of spondyloarthritides, these symptoms are present so often, especially during the early phase of the disorder, as to suggest the diagnosis of Reiter's syndrome.

The onset of Reiter's syndrome can be abrupt, occurring over several days or more gradually over several weeks. Patients can appear quite toxic and exhibit high fevers, weight loss, malaise, and debilitation. Although the recognition of Reiter's syndrome presenting in this manner can be difficult, the presence of urethritis and diarrhea, especially if a history of enthesopathy can be elicited, should suggest the diagnosis. Although the course of Reiter's syndrome is variable, nearly two thirds of patients experience only acute self-limited disease.

Laboratory Findings

During active disease, a normocytic, normochromic anemia, leukocytosis ($< 30,000/mm^3$), and elevation of the erythrocyte sedimentation rate are often observed. Urinalysis can show microscopic hematuria and pyuria, but cultures are sterile.

Radiographic Findings

Radiographic changes are notably absent early in the disease course. Juxta-articular osteoporosis can be observed around affected peripheral joints. Periostitis of the os calcis is common. The sacroiliitis associated with Reiter's syndrome tends to be asymmetric (see Fig. 86-2) but becomes symmetric late in the disease. The spondylitis is notable radiographically for nonmarginal syndesmophytes bridging the vertebrae.

Treatment

The management of Reiter's syndrome requires both supportive and preventive measures. Careful ophthalmologic examinations should be performed because failure to diagnose and effectively manage iridocyclitis can lead to significant visual loss. A regimen of bed rest, physical therapy, and NSAIDs is often very effective in the symptomatic management of the arthritis. The local injection of corticosteroids into regions of tendinitis temporarily ameliorates the pain. Low-dose oral methotrexate has been found to be effective in more resistant cases.

PSORIATIC ARTHRITIS

Arthropathy occurs in approximately 20% of individuals with psoriasis, most particularly in those with involvement of the nails. Psoriasis itself is associated with HLA-B13, HLA-Bw17, and HLA-Cw6. HLA-Bw38, HLA-DR4, and HLA-DR7 appear to be genetic markers associated with peripheral arthropathy. The major histocompatibility complex (MHC) marker HLA-B27 occurs in about 20% of individuals with arthropathy but in 50% of those who have psoriatic spondylitis. Psoriatic arthropathy can take several forms, and it is often difficult to separate from Reiter's syndrome, rheumatoid arthritis, and other inflammatory joint diseases. There are at least five clinical subsets:

1. *Asymmetric oligoarthropathy.* This is characterized by asymmetric involvement of both large and small joints, and the appearance of sausage-shaped digits is common. There appears to be little relationship between the joint and skin activity in this group. This form of arthropathy may appear before any evidence of skin disease.
2. *Symmetric polyarthropathy resembling rheumatoid arthritis.* This pattern is rare but when it occurs is indistinguishable from that seen in rheumatoid disease and may, in fact, represent coincidental occurrence of the two diseases.
3. *Arthritis mutilans.* This is a severe destructive arthropathy resulting in mutilation of the joints and telescoping of digits to produce the so-called opera-glass hand.
4. *Psoriatic spondylitis.* Approximately 20% of patients with psoriasis and arthritis have radiographic sacroiliitis. There is a male predominance of 3.5:1.
5. *Psoriatic nail disease and distal interphalangeal joint involvement.* This form is found in association with depressions of the nail, nail splitting, and subungual hyperkeratosis. The direct relationship between destructive lesions on the nail and in the distal interphalangeal joints is striking, but what role this proximity plays in pathogenesis is unclear.

Radiographic Findings

The radiographic features of the peripheral joints include soft tissue swelling, demineralization, loss of cartilage space, erosions, bony ankylosis, subluxation, and subchondral cysts. Several radiographic findings are classically observed in arthritis mutilans. These findings include "whittling," "pencil-in-cup," "la main en lorgnette" (opera-glass hand), and "doigt en lorgnette" (telescope finger).

Treatment

Aspirin and NSAIDs can be used for short-term treatment to give anti-inflammatory action and to reduce synovitis and control pain. Short-term treatment with corticosteroids may be used if the patient fails to respond to the conservative approach.

In the presence of more severe disease with attendant erosive arthritis, a remitting agent should be used. Gold salts, 6-mercaptopurine, and methotrexate have been used with some success. The use of remitting agents may be complicated by dermatoses, bone marrow toxicity, and hepatotoxicity. Care must be taken to follow the clinical course at regular intervals and to obtain appropriate laboratory studies to exclude toxicity.

ARTHRITIS ASSOCIATED WITH INFLAMMATORY BOWEL DISEASE

Inflammatory bowel disease is an idiopathic chronic inflammatory process involving the gastrointestinal tract. Both ulcerative colitis and regional enteritis (Crohn's disease) can be associated with an inflammatory arthritis. Two distinct types are observed in these disorders: a peripheral arthritis and ankylosing spondylitis. These entities are discussed in Chapter 36.

REFERENCES

Cush JJ, Lipsky PE: The spondyloarthropathies. *In* Bennett JC, Plum F (eds.): Cecil Textbook of Medicine. 20th ed. Philadelphia, WB Saunders, 1996.

Dougados M, van der Linden S, Juhlin R, Huitfeldt B, Amor B, Calin A, Cats A, Dijkman B, Olivieri I, Pasero G, Veys E, Zielder H: The European Spondyloarthropathy Study Group: Preliminary criteria for the classification of spondyloarthropathy. Arthritis Rheum 1991; 34: 1218.

Khan MA (ed.): Spondyloarthropathies Curr Opin Rheumatol 1994; 6: 351.

87

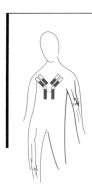

Osteoarthritis

Osteoarthritis (OA), or degenerative joint disease, is the most common musculoskeletal disease. Well over 60 million Americans have pain and limitation of motion as a result of OA. It is characterized as a slowly progressive loss of articular cartilage as well as formation of new bone at the joint surfaces. OA is not a single entity but rather the end result of several mechanical and biologic factors that trigger the processes resulting in cartilage destruction (Fig. 87–1). Almost 100,000 total hip replacements and about as many knee replacements are performed annually in the United States; most of these are for OA.

CLASSIFICATION

Because OA is a "final common pathway" for a variety of conditions, classification is difficult. Table 87–1 represents the latest classification of OA. OA is classified as (1) *primary* (idiopathic), which is the type often referred to as "aging" and is unrelated to known systemic or local diseases; it also includes certain hereditary and erosive subsets; or (2) *secondary*, in which a clearly identifiable underlying cause, such as an inflammatory, metabolic, endocrine, developmental, traumatic, or heritable connective tissue disease, can be identified. These classification criteria are not designed for diagnosis; their primary purpose is to develop standardized reporting and investigation in various subsets of OA.

ETIOLOGY AND PATHOGENESIS

The prevalence of OA increases with age; of all risk factors for primary OA, age is the strongest. At age 60 years, more than 60% of the population have some degree of cartilage abnormality in many of their joints. Certain genetic factors play a role; OA of the distal interphalangeal joints of the hands has an incidence in women 10 times greater than in men. Repetitive trauma causes stiffness of subchondral bone, resulting in increased wear of overlying cartilage. Obesity, with its added mechanical stress, is associated with OA of the knee. Certain occupational or sports-related stress is associated with OA: the lumbar spine is affected in coal miners, and the shoulders in bus drivers, for example.

There is a role for mechanical, biochemical, inflammatory, and immunologic factors in the pathologic changes of OA (see Fig. 87–1). A working hypothesis of the pathogenesis of OA is that the insult (or insults) leads to release of proteolytic and collagenolytic enzymes from chondrocytes, which then degrade collagen and proteoglycans; this is followed by reparative processes with increased bone formation. The role of calcium pyrophosphate dihydrate (CPPD) crystal deposition in the development of OA is not clear. Approximately half of the knees treated surgically in patients over age 65 have evidence of meniscal chondrocalcinosis. Many endocrine and metabolic disorders such as acromegaly, hyperparathyroidism, Wilson's disease, ochronosis, hemochromatosis, and hypothyroidism are associated with secondary OA (see Table 87–1), and their association may be a result of the increased frequency of chondrocalcinosis in these disorders. Repeated shedding of these crystals may result in an inflammatory process with release of proteolytic enzymes from neutrophils with resultant cartilage damage.

Gross pathologic changes in OA include cartilage fibrillation, fissuring, and erosions, which lead to completely bare areas of bone. Spur formation (osteophytes) seen predominantly at joint margins represents the proliferative response. Osteophytes are a cardinal feature of OA. Other pathologic changes include sclerosis and thickening of subchondral bone in addition to juxta-articular bone cyst formation. In more advanced disease, synovitis is common; this may result from crystal-induced synovitis (CPPD or calcium apatite) or from synovial clearance of cartilage breakdown products.

CLINICAL FEATURES

Despite a multiplicity of possible causes and pathogenetic mechanisms, the clinical presentation of the disease is often remarkably stereotypic, which may explain why many clinicians consider OA to be a single distinct entity. OA is generally suspected on the basis of history and physical examination (Table 87–2).

The most commonly affected joints are the hips, knees, spine, and small joints of the hands (first carpometacarpals, proximal and distal interphalangeals) and feet (metatarsophalangeals). The wrist, elbow, shoulder,

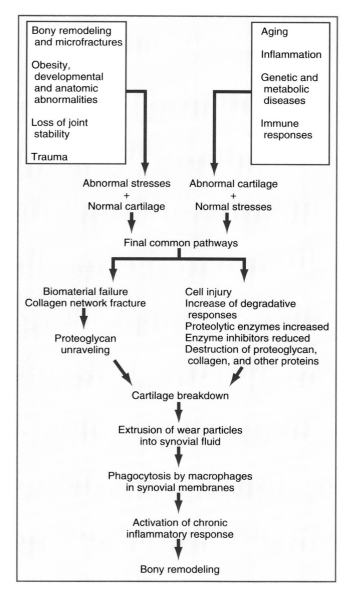

Figure 87–1

Etiopathogenic factors in osteoarthritis. (Modified from McCarty DJ: Arthritis & Allied Conditions. 11th ed. Philadelphia, Lea & Febiger, 1989. Reprinted with permission.)

There may be "stiffness" of the joint after a period of inactivity. With severe disease there may be gradual limitation of motion of the affected joints and nocturnal pain.

Another common complaint is *crepitus*, or "cracking" of the affected joint. This may be painless but often is associated with pain and is more pronounced in the patellofemoral joint. As the OA progresses, a noticeable *deformity* may develop; this most often is manifested as one knee larger than the other or an enlargement of a finger joint. Joint enlargement can be a result of increased bone, increased amounts of synovial fluid, and synovitis. Other deformities include a lateral (varus) or medial (valgus) bowing of a knee. When OA of the hip or knee has progressed to a severe stage, there may be a noticeable limp or an antalgic gait related to the pain associated with weight bearing. Acute inflammatory flares may be precipitated by crystal-induced synovitis in response to shedding of CPPD crystals.

Symptoms of OA in the cervical spine depend upon the neural segment involved; pain often radiates into the supraclavicular and upper trapezius regions and distal upper extremities. A myelopathy may result from overgrowth of bone in the cervical or lumbar spine; neurogenic claudication is an important symptom in lumbar spinal stenosis.

Large synovial effusions are uncommon. *Osteophytes* (spurs) account for most of the enlargement of joints; in the distal interphalangeal joint they are referred to as Heberden's nodes and, if associated with the proximal interphalangeal joints, Bouchard's nodes.

Limitation of motion is the most frequent finding on examination. Early on this may not be present, but it gradually worsens and becomes severe with progressive disease. With advanced disease there often is a *joint contracture*. The degree and nature of the contracture depend on the joint involved. Varus or valgus deformities are often seen in more advanced stages of knee OA. These deformities are due to cartilage loss of the medial and lateral compartments, respectively.

Characteristic radiographic findings of primary OA are summarized in Table 87–2. These radiographic find-

and ankle are usually spared unless there is evidence of trauma, congenital abnormality or metabolic/endocrine disease. OA of the first metatarsophalangeal joints of the feet and distal interphalangeal joints of the hand is most often encountered in women and occurs with high frequency in families. Cervical and lumbar spine OA is common in elderly persons.

Signs and symptoms are usually local, confined to one or a few joints. There are no systemic symptoms. The most common symptom is progressive *pain*; the pain initially is intermittent and mild but becomes constant and more disabling. The pain almost always is partially relieved by rest and exacerbated by movement, especially weight-bearing movement. The pain may be referred; OA of the hip may localize to the medial side of the knee.

TABLE 87–1	Classification of Osteoarthritis

Idiopathic (Primary)

Localized
Generalized—includes three or more areas
Mineral deposition diseases

Secondary

Post-traumatic
Congenital or developmental
Disturbed local tissue structure by primary disease, e.g., ischemic necrosis, tophaceous gout, rheumatoid arthritis
Miscellaneous additional diseases
    Endocrine
    Metabolic
    Neuropathic arthropathies
    Mechanical

Modified from Howell DS: Osteoarthritis (degenerative joint disease). *In* Wyngaarden JB, Smith LH Jr, Bennett JC (eds.): Cecil Textbook of Medicine. 19th ed. Philadelphia, WB Saunders, 1992, p 1555.

TABLE 87–2	Clinical Features of Primary Osteoarthritis

Symptoms

Pain: Progressive pain (months to years), exacerbated by movement and weight bearing, relieved partially with rest; may be referred or radicular

Limitation of motion: Flexion contracture

Crepitus

Deformity: Bony enlargement, bowing of knee, limp

Signs

Limitation of motion: Flexion contracture

Crepitus

Joint enlargement: Heberden's and Bouchard's nodes

Joint effusion

Deformity: Varus, valgus, etc.

Radiographs

Marginal osteophytes

Subchondral sclerosis

Subchondral cysts

Joint space narrowing

Laboratory

Synovial fluid—noninflammatory (white cell count <1500/mm^3)

ings confirm the pathologic findings—loss of cartilage (narrowed joint space) with new bone formation (osteophytes and sclerosis). Conditions associated with secondary OA usually have radiographic findings that are more indicative of the underlying pathology, such as Paget's disease, rheumatoid arthritis, and hyperparathyroidism.

Routine laboratory studies are generally unremarkable in OA and are of little diagnostic help. The synovial fluid is generally clear and noninflammatory. Leukocyte counts in synovial fluid are generally in the range of 150 to 1500/mm^3. CPPD crystals may be seen in many OA joint effusions.

DIFFERENTIAL DIAGNOSIS

Primary OA of a hip or knee can usually be diagnosed rather easily and is not often confused with other types of arthritis. Other diagnoses that should be entertained in someone with suspected OA of the hip include pigmented villonodular synovitis and osteonecrosis. Internal joint derangements, chronic infections, and osteochondritis are among several less common entities that should be considered in the differential diagnosis of someone with knee OA. An erosive inflammatory OA that involves primarily the distal or proximal interphalangeal joints of the hands may be mistaken for rheumatoid arthritis, Reiter's syndrome, or psoriatic arthritis.

TREATMENT

Therapeutic options need to be individualized to fit the severity of the disease. The multidisciplinary components of a treatment program for the patient with OA include education, drugs, physical measures, and surgery. Although no cures are available for OA, much can be done to alleviate pain, maintain mobility, and minimize disability. Early disease with no evidence of joint contracture or instability can often be treated with intermittent analgesics, appropriate joint protection and rest, and, if needed, weight reduction. Appliances such as canes and other physical therapy means such as exercise programs are beneficial in joint protection.

Pharmacologic agents commonly used to provide analgesia include acetaminophen, aspirin, and nonsteroidal anti-inflammatory drugs (NSAIDS). Gastrointestinal side effects such as peptic ulceration are common with the use of NSAIDs, and they should be used cautiously, especially in persons over age 60 years. Oral or parenteral corticosteroids are contraindicated in the treatment of OA. However, intra-articular injections with corticosteroids may provide temporary relief of pain and are usually given no more than twice a year for an involved joint. Topical treatment with capsaicin, a substance-P inhibitor, may benefit some patients.

Hip and knee arthroplasties (replacements) produce significant symptomatic relief and improved range of motion. Surgical procedures are reserved for patients with more severe disease, with persistent pain and impaired function. Arthroscopy with lavage of the joint and removal of free cartilage fragments may prevent joint locking and prevent rapid wear of the joint surfaces. Although abrasion arthroplasty (chondroplasty) has been used widely in patients with knee OA, there are no data demonstrating its efficacy. Spinal surgery is indicated when there is evidence of spinal cord impingement (neurologic deficits, altered bowel or bladder function) or intractable pain unresponsive to medical management.

REFERENCES

Howell DS, Pelletier J-P: Etiopathogenesis of osteoarthritis. *In* McCarty DJ, Koopman WJ (eds.): Arthritis & Allied Conditions. 12th ed. Philadelphia, Lea & Febiger, 1993, pp 1723–1734.

Moskowitz RW: Clinical and laboratory findings in osteoarthritis. *In* McCarty DJ, Koopman WJ (eds.): Arthritis & Allied Conditions. 12th ed. Philadelphia, Lea & Febiger, 1993, pp 1735–1760.

Schnitzer TJ: *In* Bennett JC, Plum F (eds.): Cecil Textbook of Medicine. 20th ed. Philadelphia, WB Saunders, 1996, pp 1517–1521.

88

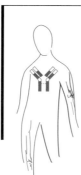

The Crystal-Induced Arthropathies

CHONDROCALCINOSIS AND ASSOCIATED DISORDERS

Several different forms of crystals are known to induce various patterns of arthritis. The most extensively studied of these forms of arthritis is gout, in which urate crystals are associated with acute synovial inflammation. Calcium in various crystalline configurations, including pyrophosphate, oxalate, and apatite, can deposit in articular cartilage, synovium, and periarticular tissues (Table 88–1). Chondrocalcinosis results from the deposition of calcium pyrophosphate dihydrate (CPPD) crystals in cartilage (Fig. 88–1). The resulting clinical disorder, pseudogout, generally begins as a monoarticular or pauciarticular arthritis but may become polyarticular. Most often it is idiopathic, but it can be associated with aging and certain metabolic disorders (Table 88–2). It affects about 5% of the adult population and may exceed 25% in the over-80 population. The acute attacks resemble gout clinically, but as time passes pseudogout may be confused with rheumatoid arthritis (RA), neurotrophic arthritis, or osteoarthritis.

Pseudogout is an acute inflammatory arthritis that results from phagocytosis of IgG-coated CPPD crystals by synovial fluid neutrophils and the subsequent release of inflammatory mediators. Initially monoarticular, the attacks soon become oligoarticular or polyarticular. Frequently, acute attacks are self-limiting, lasting for 1 day to several days, as in gout. However, more severe attacks involving both the peripheral and axial joints can more slowly resolve over weeks. The large joints of the lower extremities are the more likely targets, with the knee joint being involved in more than one half of all cases of pseudogout. The presence of chondrocalcinosis can be identified radiographically by the characteristic punctate or linear radiodensities in hyaline articular cartilage and in the menisci in the knee. Other areas frequently exhibiting these findings include the wrists and pelvis.

The diagnosis of pseudogout should not depend upon the radiographic findings alone because chondrocalcinosis is observed in only 75% of cases of pseudogout. Arthrocentesis is a necessary diagnostic procedure because acute infectious arthritis and gout can clinically resemble pseudogout. The synovial fluid exhibits a leukocytosis with a predominance of neutrophils and has a low viscosity (see Table 78–3). CPPD crystals are rhomboid in shape and produce weakly positive birefringence under compensated polarizing microscopy. The typical crystals are seen in the synovial fluid but can also be observed within neutrophils. It should also be noted that monosodium urate and CPPD crystals can coexist within the same joint.

Chronic CPPD crystal disease can exhibit a symmetric polyarticular distribution and can clinically mimic RA. Patients describe prolonged morning stiffness, fatigability, and malaise, and the course can extend over many months. Although flexion contractures may be seen and the sedimentation rate may be elevated, radiographs show secondary osteoarthritic changes of affected joints, and the synovial fluid contains CPPD crystals and shows none of the inflammatory markers of rheumatoid arthritis.

About half of all cases of CPPD crystal disease develop signs of osteoarthritis (pseudo-osteoarthritis) involving the knees, wrists, metacarpophalangeal joints, hips, shoulders, elbows, and ankles. As expected, CPPD crystals are found in synovial fluid even when radiographs do not demonstrate the punctate or linear calcification of the cartilage. In contrast, asymptomatic persons can inadvertently be found to have CPPD crystal deposits on radiographs.

Clinically symptomatic CPPD disease responds to rest, joint protection, and use of a nonsteroidal anti-inflammatory drug (NSAID). Colchicine is efficacious in acute attacks of pseudogout as well as in gout. The instillation of a corticosteroid preparation may hasten resolution of the inflammatory process but should not be started until arthrocentesis and crystal identification have established the diagnosis. Maintenance therapy with an NSAID is usually satisfactory.

Calcium oxalate deposition is usually seen in patients with renal failure who are on chronic dialysis. Examination of the synovial fluid shows the characteristic bipyramidal crystals. These crystals may also be seen in synovial tissue biopsies of involved joints. It should be noted that vitamin C can potentiate oxalate deposition.

The third calcium crystal–induced rheumatic syndrome is associated with apatite crystals. The spectrum of clinical manifestations ranges from calcific tendinitis to frank arthritis that is typically episodic and monoarticular. Apatite crystals seem to play a causative role in "Milwaukee shoulder," an inflammatory and extremely destructive arthritis that can be associated with rotator cuff tears.

TABLE 88–1	Differential Diagnostic Features for Some of the Crystal-Associated Arthropathies	
	Other Points	**X-ray Findings**
Calcium pyrophosphate dihydrate	Elderly and consider associated metabolic diseases	Chondrocalcinosis, bony sclerosis
Apatite	Clumps stained with Alizarin red S	Soft tissue calcification
Oxalate	Renal failure	Chondrocalcinosis or soft tissue calcification
Monosodium urate	Middle-aged men and elderly women	Cysts and erosions; tophi may calcify
Liquid lipid crystals	Unexplained acute arthritis	
Cholesterol	May complicate RA and OA	
Depot corticosteroids	Can cause iatrogenic inflammation	
Immunoglobulins, other proteins	Cryoglobulinemia	
Charcot-Leyden	Eosinophilic synovitis	

OA = Osteoarthritis; RA = rheumatoid arthritis.
Adapted from Schumacher HR Jr: Other crystal deposition arthropathies. *In* Bennett JC, Plum F (eds.): Cecil Textbook of Medicine. 20th ed. Philadelphia, WB Saunders, 1996.

TABLE 88–2	Metabolic Disorders Associated with CPPD Deposition
	Diabetes mellitus
	Gout
	Hemochromatosis
	Hyperparathyroidism
	Hypomagnesemia
	Hypophosphatasia
	Myxedematous hypothyroidism
	Ochronosis
	Wilson's disease

CPPD = Calcium pyrophosphate dihydrate.

The differentiation of apatite-induced inflammation from acute septic arthritis, gout, or pseudogout is made by synovial fluid examination. Apatite crystals are nonbirefringent globules, and definitive identification can be made only by electron probe elemental analysis or x-ray diffraction. Acute arthritis or periarthritis is treated with NSAIDs. Apatite deposits can be found in soft tissue in chronic renal disease owing to phosphate retention and can be seen in association with repeated depot corticosteroid injection and in scleroderma.

REFERENCES

Gibilisco PA, Schumacher HR, Hollander JL, Soper KA: Synovial fluid crystals in osteoarthritis. Arthritis Rheum 1985; 28:511.
McCarty DJ: Diagnostic mimicry in arthritis—patterns of joint involvement associated with calcium pyrophosphate dihydrate crystal deposits. Bull Rheum Dis 1974–1975; 25:804.
Schumacher HR, Smolyo AP, Tse RL, Maurer K: Arthritis associated with apatite crystals. Ann Intern Med 1977; 87:411.

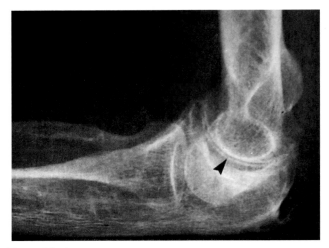

Figure 88–1
Chondrocalcinosis (*arrow*) at the elbow joint. (From Schumacher HR Jr: Crystal deposition arthropathies. *In* Wyngaarden JB, Smith LH Jr, Bennett JC [eds]: Cecil Textbook of Medicine. 19th ed. Philadelphia, WB Saunders, 1992, p 1552.)

89

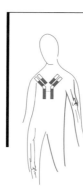

Miscellaneous Forms of Arthritis

Many of the disorders discussed in this chapter have prominent systemic features; however, their musculoskeletal manifestations often provide clues to their initial and perhaps earlier diagnosis. Table 89–1 lists the laboratory studies that may provide helpful clues for diagnosing systemic diseases in which arthralgias may be an early manifestation.

MUSCULOSKELETAL SYNDROMES ASSOCIATED WITH MALIGNANCY

Musculoskeletal manifestations are not prominent features of most malignancies. However, several syndromes may present with features suggestive of gout, rheumatoid arthritis (RA), and other connective tissue diseases. In addition, several musculoskeletal diseases are associated with increased frequencies of malignancy (Table 89–2).

Hypertrophic Osteoarthropathy

Hypertrophic osteoarthropathy is defined as a syndrome of (1) chronic proliferative periostitis of long bones, (2) clubbing of fingers and toes, and (3) synovitis. Although the underlying disease is usually readily apparent, occasionally clinical manifestations may precede symptoms of the associated disease by several months. Hypertrophic osteoarthropathy is often associated with lung carcinoma, most frequently with adenocarcinomas and squamous cell carcinomas; it is rarely seen with small cell carcinoma. It occurs in 5 to 10% of all intrathoracic malignancies, especially those involving the pleura or the periphery of the lung. If associated with a malignancy, the onset may be explosive, with exquisite tenderness resembling acute gout. A bone scan may be abnormal before there is other radiologic evidence of periostitis.

Carcinomatous Polyarthritis

Carcinomatous polyarthritis is an inflammatory polyarthritis of unknown pathogenesis that clinically may resemble RA. Eighty percent of women with this syndrome have breast carcinoma. Prostate and bladder carcinomas are also common.

Metastatic Disease

The arthritis associated with metastatic disease is most commonly monoarticular, usually involving the knee or hip. Breast and lung carcinomas are the most common neoplasms.

Leukemia

Arthritis or arthralgias occur in approximately 12% of adults with chronic leukemia, 13% of adults with acute leukemia, and up to 60% of children with acute lymphoblastic leukemia. Articular symptoms are the result of leukemic infiltrates of the synovium, periosteum, or periarticular bone or of secondary gout or hemarthrosis. In children, acute lymphocytic leukemia may produce fevers as well as arthritis, thereby mimicking Still's disease or acute rheumatic fever.

Lymphoma

Skeletal involvement has been found at autopsy in as many as 50% of patients with Hodgkin's disease; however, these lesions are usually asymptomatic.

Vasculitis

Necrotizing vasculitis has been reported with lymphomas, leukemias, sarcomas, and multiple myeloma. Polyarteritis nodosa has been described in patients with Hodgkin's disease and with hairy cell leukemia.

Reflex Sympathetic Dystrophy

Reflex sympathetic dystrophy has been reported in patients with metastatic ovarian carcinoma and lung and brain tumors. Palmar fasciitis and arthritis have been described in association with ovarian carcinoma and prostate cancer.

TABLE 89-1	Laboratory Tests in Evaluating Nonspecific Joint Pain

Test	Disorder
Serum thyroxine, thyroid-stimulating hormone	Hypo- and hyperparathyroidism
Complete blood count	Sickle cell disease, leukemia
Serum calcium and phosphorus	Hyperparathyroidism
Serum amylase and lipase	Pancreatic-associated arthritis
Serum protein electrophoresis	Primary amyloidosis, hypogammaglobulinemic arthritis
Serum liver enzymes	Primary biliary cirrhosis, hepatitis
Serum iron, total iron-binding capacity, and ferritin	Hemochromatosis
Parvovirus antibodies	Parvovirus arthritis
Hepatitis B and C antibodies	Viral hepatitis–related arthritis, vasculitis and cryoglobulinemia

Polymyositis

Neoplasms are reported in 5 to 10% of all patients with polymyositis or dermatomyositis. In most patients, evidence of myositis precedes discovery of the malignancy by < 2 years; however, 30% have a malignancy diagnosed prior to the development of myositis. The most common malignancies are breast and lung cancer (see Chapter 82).

Panniculitis

Pancreatic panniculitis is a triad consisting of subcutaneous fat necrosis, arthralgia or arthritis, and a pancreatic abnormality such as pancreatitis or pancreatic cancer. The arthropathy, which is secondary to periarticular fat necrosis, may be monoarticular or polyarticular.

Sjögren's Syndrome

The incidence of lymphoma is increased 44-fold in Sjögren's syndrome. Pseudomalignant or malignant lympho-

TABLE 89-2	Musculoskeletal Diseases Associated with Malignancy

Hypertrophic osteoarthropathy
Carcinomatous polyarthritis
Arthritis of metastatic disease
Leukemia
Lymphoma
Vasculitis
Reflex sympathetic dystrophy
Polymyositis
Panniculitis
Scleroderma
Sjögren's syndrome
Rheumatoid arthritis
Paget's disease

proliferation may be present initially or may develop later in the illness.

RA

The incidence of lymphoma and myeloma is increased in RA. Rheumatoid nodules in the lung may mimic neoplastic disease.

Paget's Disease

Osteosarcoma occurs in < 1% of patients with Paget's disease of bone; other less common neoplasms include giant cell tumors and non-neoplastic granulomas.

ARTHROPATHIES ASSOCIATED WITH ENDOCRINE DISEASES

The endocrine diseases are associated with a wide spectrum of musculoskeletal syndromes (Table 89-3). Therefore, endocrine disorders should be included in the differential diagnosis of many musculoskeletal conditions.

TABLE 89-3	Musculoskeletal Manifestations of Endocrine Disease

Endocrine Disease	Musculoskeletal Manifestation
Diabetes mellitus	Carpal tunnel syndrome
	Charcot arthropathy
	Adhesive capsulitis
	Syndrome of limited joint mobility (cheiroarthropathy)
	Scleroderma adultorum of Buschke
Hypothyroidism	Proximal myopathy
	Arthralgias
	Joint effusions
	Carpal tunnel syndrome
	Chondrocalcinosis
Hyperthyroidism	Myopathy
	Osteoporosis
	Thyroid acropachy
Hyperparathyroidism	Myopathy
	Arthralgias
	Erosive arthritis
	Chondrocalcinosis
Hypoparathyroidism	Muscle cramps
	Soft tissue calcifications
	Spondyloarthropathy
Acromegaly	Carpal tunnel syndrome
	Myopathy
	Raynaud's phenomenon
	Back pain
	Premature osteoarthritis
Cushing syndrome	Myopathy
	Osteoporosis
	Avascular necrosis

Diabetes Mellitus

Carpal tunnel syndrome is present in about 5% of diabetic patients. Charcot arthropathy occurs most commonly in the ankle-foot area, but the knee is also frequently involved. This must be differentiated from osteomyelitis, which is also common in the feet of patients with diabetes mellitus. Calcific peritendinitis and bursitis of the shoulder leading to adhesive capsulitis and reflex sympathetic dystrophy have also been associated with diabetes.

Scleroderma diabeticorum, or scleroderma adultorum of Buschke, is a syndrome characterized by thick, hidebound skin over the posterior neck and upper back. Diabetic cheiroarthropathy, or syndrome of limited joint mobility, is a sclerosing cutaneous disorder that occurs in one third of patients with type I diabetes mellitus and less frequently in type II diabetics.

Hypothyroidism

Musculoskeletal symptoms are most likely to occur in patients with fully developed myxedema, and most respond to hormone replacement. Unlike in RA, the joint fluid is highly viscous and the white blood cell count is usually < 1000 cells/mm³. Muscle weakness, usually proximal, may be profound. Elevated serum creatine kinase levels occur in about 90% of cases. Although chondrocalcinosis is found in a large percentage of patients with myxedema, pseudogout is uncommon in untreated patients, but attacks may develop after patients are started on thyroid replacement.

Hyperthyroidism

Although patients with hyperthyroidism can also present with proximal muscle weakness, serum muscle enzyme levels are usually not elevated. Hyperthyroidism, either endogenous or exogenous, results in increased bone turnover and remodeling, the net result being osteoporosis.

Thyroid acropachy, an unusual but very distinctive syndrome, occurs in < 1% of patients with fully developed Graves' disease. Patients can be euthyroid at the time of its recognition, and it has been reported to appear as long as 28 years after successful treatment of the hyperthyroidism. The syndrome is characterized by an insidious onset of diffuse, often painless swelling of the extremities. Radiographically a periosteal reaction involves the diaphyses of the metacarpals, metatarsals, and proximal phalanges.

Hyperparathyroidism

Arthralgias and inflammatory arthritis with erosions are the most common musculoskeletal manifestations of hyperparathyroidism. Chondrocalcinosis, most often asymptomatic, or acute calcium pyrophosphate dihydrate

(CPPD) crystal arthritis has been reported in 18 to 40% of cases.

Hypoparathyroidism

Patients with hypoparathyroidism can have hypocalcemic muscular cramps and carpopedal spasm. Soft tissue calcifications produce symptoms because of their localization in muscles or tendons.

Acromegaly

Musculoskeletal manifestations of acromegaly include myopathy, back pain, carpal tunnel syndrome, and peripheral arthropathy. At least half of the patients with acromegaly complain of nonradiating lumbosacral back pain. Accelerated premature osteoarthritis of the hips and knees can occur.

Cushing Syndrome

A proximal myopathy without elevation of serum muscle enzyme occurs in some patients with Cushing syndrome. Generalized osteoporosis resulting in fractures is characteristic of both excessive endogenous and exogenous steroids.

ADDITIONAL MISCELLANEOUS DISORDERS

A few additional disorders that are not common should be included in the differential diagnosis of many patients with musculoskeletal complaints (Table 89–4).

Pigmented Villonodular Synovitis

This uncommon benign disorder of young adults usually affects the entire synovium of a single joint. The pathology consists of lipid- and hemosiderin-laden cells and multinucleated giant cells with exuberant proliferation of synovial lining cells and the formation of villi and lobulated masses that fuse into nodules. The knee is the joint most commonly involved. Treatment is total synovectomy.

Multicentric Reticulohistiocytosis

Multicentric reticulohistiocytosis, a rare systemic disease, is characterized by infiltration of multinucleated giant cells and histiocyte-like cells into various tissues. Destructive polyarthritis and skin lesions are the most common clinical features. Confluence of nodules over the face and malar areas can give the appearance of leonine facies. Mucosal surfaces are involved in about 50% of cases.

A symmetric polyarthritis affects most commonly the interphalangeal joints of the fingers and may clinically

TABLE 89–4	Additional Miscellaneous Forms of Arthritis
Disorder	**Distinctive Features**
Pigmented villonodular synovitis	Monoarticular indolent arthritis; dark brown synovial fluid
Multicentric reticulohistiocytosis	Reddish-purple skin nodules, symmetric destructive polyarthritis
Charcot arthropathy	Diabetes mellitus, syphilis, syringomyelia
Hemarthrosis	Hemophilia, other bleeding disorders, trauma, scurvy, pigmented villonodular synovitis
Sarcoidosis	Acute arthritis, erythema nodosum, bilateral hilar adenopathy
Amyloidosis	Green birefringence with Congo red staining of affected tissues
Primary biliary cirrhosis	Antimitochondrial antibodies
Familial Mediterranean fever	Triad of recurrent fever, serositis, and arthritis
Whipple's disease	PAS-positive macrophages in bowel or synovial tissue
Sickle cell disease	Acute arthritis, osteomyelitis, avascular necrosis, dactylitis
Hemochromatosis	Chondrocalcinosis, increased serum iron and iron binding capacity

PAS = Periodic acid-Schiff.

resemble RA. Progressive destruction of articular cartilage and underlying bone results in arthritis mutilans in 30 to 45% of cases.

Charcot Arthropathy

Charcot arthropathy, or neuropathic joint disease, is a progressive degenerative arthritis most commonly seen in patients with diabetes mellitus. Other diseases associated with Charcot arthropathy are syphilis and syringomyelia. The knee and hip joints are most often affected in patients with tabetic neuropathic joint disease. In syringomyelia, upper limb involvement is typical. Neuropathic joint disease in diabetes mellitus is more likely to involve the joints of the feet.

Hemarthrosis

Trauma and hemophilia (see Chapter 53) are the most common causes of hemarthrosis (see Chapter 89). The presence of fat globules floating on the surface of bloody synovial fluid usually indicates a fracture.

Sarcoidosis

Sarcoidosis (see Chapter 17) is a multisystem disorder that may involve any organ but has a predilection for lung tissue and thoracic lymph nodes. Acute arthritis of the ankles or knees is the most common musculoskeletal manifestation (15%); this may occur early or late in the

disease. Erythema nodosum often coexists with acute arthritis; when accompanied by bilateral hilar adenopathy, this triad is called *Löfgren's syndrome*.

Amyloidosis

Amyloidosis, characterized by the accumulation of extracellular fibrous protein (amyloid) in connective tissues, can be classified as primary (or associated with multiple myeloma), or secondary to chronic inflammatory or infectious diseases. Carpal tunnel syndrome may result from the local deposition of amyloid around the median nerve. Amyloid may infiltrate the synovium and periarticular tissues, resulting in an arthritis that clinically resembles RA. The joints most frequently involved are the shoulders, wrists, knees, and fingers. Subcutaneous nodules are present in 70% of cases. Most, but not all, patients with amyloid arthropathy eventually develop multiple myeloma. The diagnosis is established by the demonstration of the typical birefringent tissue deposits seen with Congo red staining.

Primary Biliary Cirrhosis

Primary biliary cirrhosis (see Chapter 43), a disease primarily of middle-aged women, is a rare, chronic, immunologically mediated progressive liver disease. Serum autoantibodies, elevated levels of immunoglobulins, and circulating immune complexes are typically observed in this disorder. Musculoskeletal manifestations include polyarthritis with erosive bone lesions, hypertrophic osteoarthropathy, avascular necrosis, osteomalacia, and osteoporosis. Many have identifiable rheumatic diseases such as RA, Sjögren's syndrome, or a limited form of systemic sclerosis.

Familial Mediterranean Fever

The major clinical features of familial Mediterranean fever are serositis, fever, and arthritis. Arthritis, most commonly an acute intermittent monoarthritis of a large joint of the lower extremities, occurs in 70% of patients. Daily oral colchicine decreases the frequency and severity of the febrile attacks, arthritis, as well as amyloidosis.

Whipple's Disease

Arthritis or arthralgias occur in 65 to 90% of patients with Whipple's disease. Fever, diarrhea, and weight loss are other prominent features. Arthritis is intermittent in 60% of patients with acute attacks lasting from days to weeks. Chronic arthritis lasting for several years can occur, although joint destruction is rare. The arthritis may antedate gastrointestinal symptoms by several years, making a diagnosis difficult. Characteristic macrophages with periodic acid-Schiff (PAS)–positive rod-shaped bacilli may be identified in the small bowel or synovial tissue.

Antibiotics, especially penicillin or tetracycline, effectively treat the joint symptoms.

Sickle Cell Disease

Sickle cell crisis is frequently associated with intense periarticular pain and arthritis. The arthritis is secondary to occlusion of small vessels caused by local sickling. Subchondral and interosseous hemorrhages contribute to the destruction of articular cartilage. The knees and elbows are the joints most commonly involved. Osteonecrosis, most commonly of the femoral head, occurs in both SC and SS disease. Sickle cell dactylitis, or hand-foot syndrome, is a condition in young children of transient swelling and tenderness of the hands and feet secondary to periostitis.

Hemochromatosis

Arthritis is often the first sign of hemochromatosis, which typically occurs between ages 40 and 50. Commonly involved joints include metacarpophalangeal, wrists, knees, and hip joints. Radiographic findings include chondrocalcinosis as well as features of osteoarthritis.

REFERENCES

Ball EV: Miscellaneous forms of arthritis. *In* Bennett JC, Plum F (eds.): Cecil Textbook of Medicine. 20th ed. Philadelphia, WB Saunders, 1996, pp 1526–1527.
Ball EV: Systemic diseases in which arthritis is a feature. *In* Bennett JC, Plum F (eds.): Cecil Textbook of Medicine. 20th ed. Philadelphia, WB Saunders, 1996, pp 1525–1526.

90

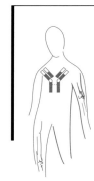

Nonarticular Rheumatism

The term *nonarticular rheumatism* describes a group of common disorders that primarily affect soft tissues or periarticular structures such as bursae, tendons, and fasciae. Many manifest as acute localized pain (bursitis) or chronic diffuse pain (fibromyalgia syndrome).

PAINFUL SHOULDER

Shoulder pain affects approximately 20% of the adult population at some point in their lives and is a common reason for visiting a physician. It is the most common musculoskeletal complaint in individuals over age 40. As illustrated by the numerous causes of shoulder pain (Table 90–1), the clinician needs to understand the anatomy of the shoulder and to recognize that shoulder pain can be referred from several other locations. Pain may be referred from the cervical region (spondylosis), the intra-thoracic region (Pancoast's tumor or myocardial infarction), or the intra-abdominal region (gallbladder disease). Most shoulder problems can be diagnosed by performing a detailed history and physical examination.

BURSITIS

Bursae are synovium-lined, fluid-filled sacs located between tendons, muscles, and bone (Fig. 78–1). Bursitis has many causes, but overuse or strain is commonly implicated; gout and infection may also cause acute bursitis. Commonly involved bursae include the subdeltoid, olecranon, trochanteric, iliopsoas, ischial, anserine, prepatellar, Achilles, and retrocalcaneal.

CARPAL TUNNEL SYNDROME

Carpal tunnel syndrome, the entrapment of the median nerve, is the most common of entrapment neuropathies.

Symptoms include burning pain or tingling in the palmar side of the first three fingers and occasionally the radial half of the fourth finger (Fig. 90–1). These symptoms often occur at night and are relieved by shaking the hand. Weakness and atrophy of the muscles of the thenar eminence may occur. Several disorders are associated with carpal tunnel syndrome, such as rheumatoid arthritis, gout, and amyloidosis and trauma, but often no obvious cause can be found.

TABLE 90–1	Differential Diagnosis of the Painful Shoulder

Periarticular

Bursitis (subdeltoid)
Calcific tendinitis
Rotator cuff rupture
Bicipital tendinitis
Acromioclavicular arthritis
Fibromyalgia
Impingement syndrome
Amyloid arthropathy
Polymyalgia rheumatica

Glenohumeral

Adhesive capsulitis
Osteoarthritis
Milwaukee shoulder
Dislocation/subluxation
Infection
Neoplasia
Inflammatory arthritis
Osteoarthritis
Osteonecrosis

Referred

Cervical nerve root compression
Brachial neuritis
Reflex sympathetic dystrophy
Thoracic outlet syndrome
Gallbladder disease
Subphrenic abscess
Myocardial infarction

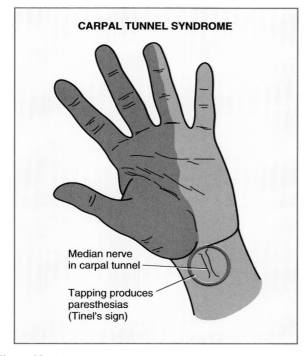

CARPAL TUNNEL SYNDROME

Median nerve
in carpal tunnel

Tapping produces
paresthesias
(Tinel's sign)

Figure 90–1

Distribution of pain and/or paresthesias (*shaded area*) when the median nerve is compressed by swelling in the wrist (carpal tunnel). (From Arnett FC: Rheumatoid arthritis. *In* Bennett JC, Plum F [eds.]: Cecil Textbook of Medicine. 20th ed. Philadelphia, WB Saunders, 1996, p 1462.)

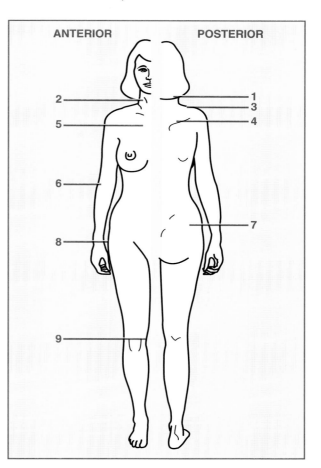

Figure 90–2

Locations of nine bilateral tender point sites for the American College of Rheumatology classification criteria for fibromyalgia. 1, Suboccipital muscle insertions; 2, cervical, at the anterior aspects of the intertransverse spaces at C5-C7; 3, trapezius, at the midpoint of the upper border; 4, supraspinatus, at the origin, above scapular spine near the medial border; 5, second rib, at the costochondral junction; 6, lateral epicondyle, 2 cm distal to the epicondyle; 7, gluteal, in upper outer quadrant of the buttock; 8, greater trochanter, just posterior to the trochanteric prominence; 9, knee at the medial fat pad proximal to the joint line. (From Yunus MB, Masi AT: Fibromyalgia, restless legs syndrome, periodic limb movement disorder, and psychogenic pain. *In* McCarty DJ, Koopman WJ [eds.]: Arthritis & Allied Conditions. 12th ed. Philadelphia, Lea & Febiger, 1993, p 1387.)

FIBROMYALGIA SYNDROME

Fibromyalgia syndrome, previously referred to as fibrositis, is a syndrome characterized by chronic diffuse pain with characteristic tender points (Fig. 90–2) at multiple sites; e.g., at least 11 of 18 specific sites in the criteria of the American College of Rheumatology. It occurs predominantly (80 to 90%) in women of childbearing age; its prevalence in the general population may be as high as 5%. The major complaints are diffuse musculoskeletal pain, stiffness, and fatigue. A sleep disturbance, although usually not a presenting complaint, is a common feature. Patients awaken feeling tired; this has been linked to a disturbance of stage 4 (non–rapid eye movement [non–REM]) sleep. The only abnormal finding on examination is the presence of numerous tender points; these are sought by firm palpation with the thumb.

Common associations with fibromyalgia syndrome are mitral valve prolapse and irritable bowel syndrome. Fibromyalgia syndrome has many of the same clinical characteristics as the chronic fatigue syndrome. Chronic fatigue syndrome, myofascial pain syndrome, and fibromyalgia syndrome probably belong to a spectrum of syndromes with overlapping features (Fig. 90–3). However, the exact relationships of these three common clinical conditions have yet to be determined. The diagnosis of fibromyalgia syndrome is a clinical diagnosis that is made after other numerous causes of diffuse aching and fatigue are excluded.

Education of the patient should emphasize the benign, nondeforming nature of this syndrome and its lack of progression to total disability. Physicians should encourage patients to improve their level of physical fitness, minimize stress, and adopt sound sleeping habits. Medications that help achieve restorative sleep include amitriptyline and cyclobenzaprine at bedtime. Other tricyclic antidepressants can be used but have not been studied in controlled trials. Narcotics and corticosteroids are contraindicated.

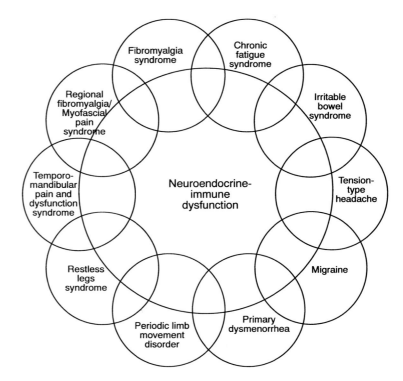

Figure 90-3

A schematic representation of the proposed members of the dysfunctional spectrum syndrome (DSS) family, depicting interrelationships and overlapping features among the members. Neuroendocrine-immune dysfunction is the postulated common biophysiological mechanism for these disorders. (From Yunus MB: Clinical spectrum and epidemiology of fibromyalgia. J Musculoskeletal Pain 1994; 2(3):5–21. Copyright 1994, Haworth Press, Inc.)

REFERENCES

Ball EV: Nonarticular rheumatism. *In* Bennett JC, Plum F (eds.): Cecil Textbook of Medicine. 20th ed. Philadelphia, WB Saunders, 1996, pp 1527–1528.

Wolfe F, Smythe HA, Yunus MB, et al: The American College of Rheumatology, 1990, Criteria for the classification of fibromyalgia. Arthritis Rheum 1990;33:160.

Yunus MB, Masi AT: Fibromyalgia, restless legs syndrome, periodic limb movement disorder, and psychogenic pain. *In* McCarty DJ, Koopman WJ (eds.): Arthritis & Allied Conditions. 12th ed. Philadelphia, Lea & Febiger, 1993, pp 1383–1405.

Infectious Disease

Section XIII

91

Organisms That Infect Humans

Of diseases afflicting humans, most that are curable and preventable are caused by infectious agents. The infectious diseases that capture the attention of physicians and the public periodically shift—for example, from syphilis to tuberculosis to acquired immunodeficiency syndrome (AIDS)—but the challenges of dealing with these processes endure. To the student, an understanding of infectious diseases offers insights into medicine as a whole. Osler's adage (with updating) remains relevant: "He (or she) who knows syphilis (AIDS), knows medicine."

VIRUSES

Viruses produce a wide variety of clinical illnesses. A virus consists of either DNA or RNA (rarely, both) wrapped within a protein nucleocapsid. The nucleocapsid may be covered by an envelope composed of glycoproteins and lipids. Viral genes can code for only a limited number of proteins, and viruses possess no metabolic machinery. They are entirely dependent upon host cells for protein synthesis and replication and are therefore obligate intracellular parasites. Some viruses are dependent upon other viruses to produce active infection. Such is the case with the delta agent, which produces disease only in the presence of hepatitis B infection. All must attach to "receptors" on the host cell and achieve entry into the cell through host-derived mechanisms, including receptor-mediated endocytosis, fusion, and pinocytosis. Once within the cells, the virus uncoats, allowing its nucleic acid to utilize host cellular machinery to reproduce (productive infection) or to integrate into the host cell (latent infection). Some viruses, such as influenza virus, cause disease by lysis of infected cells. Others, such as hepatitis B virus, do not directly cause cell destruction but may involve the host immune responses in the pathogenesis of disease. Still others, such as the human T lymphotropic virus type I, promote neoplastic transformation of infected cells.

Viruses have developed several mechanisms of evading host defense mechanisms. By multiplying within host cells, viruses can avoid neutralizing antibodies and other extracellular host defenses. Some viruses can spread to uninfected cells by intercellular bridges. Some viruses, especially the herpes group, are capable of persisting without multiplication in a metabolically inactive form within host cells for prolonged periods (latency). The influenza virus is capable of extensive gene rearrangements, resulting in significant changes in surface antigen structure. This allows new strains to evade host antibody responses directed at earlier strains.

Some viruses, as they exit the host cell during productive infection, may carry antigens of host cell origin, thus providing another mechanism for evading host defenses.

CHLAMYDIAE

Chlamydiae are also obligate intracellular parasites, but, unlike viruses, they always contain both DNA and RNA, divide by binary fission (rather than multiplying by assembly), can synthesize proteins, and contain ribosomes. They are unable to synthesize ATP and thus depend on energy from the host cell to survive. The three chlamydial species known to cause disease in humans are *Chlamydia trachomatis, Chlamydia psittaci,* and *the TWAR agent, Chlamydia pneumoniae. C. trachomatis* causes trachoma, the major cause of blindness in the developing world, and a variety of sexually transmitted genitourinary disorders, including urethritis, salpingitis, and lymphogranuloma venereum. *C. psittaci,* cause of a common infectious disease of birds, can produce a serious systemic illness, with prominent pulmonary manifestations, in humans. The TWAR agent is a recently described cause of pneumonia. Chlamydiae are susceptible to tetracycline and erythromycin.

RICKETTSIAE

Rickettsiae are also small bacterial organisms that, like chlamydiae, are obligate intracellular parasites. Rickettsiae are primarily animal pathogens that generally produce disease in humans through the bite of an insect vector, such as a tick, flea, louse, or mite. The organisms specifically infect vascular endothelial cells. With the exception of Q fever, rash due to vasculitis is a prominent manifestation of these often disabling febrile illnesses. These organisms are susceptible to tetracyclines and chloramphenicol.

MYCOPLASMAS

Mycoplasmas are the smallest free-living organisms. In contrast to viruses, chlamydiae, and rickettsiae, mycoplasmas can grow on cell-free media and produce disease without intracellular penetration. Like other bacteria, these organisms have a membrane, but, unlike other bacteria, they have no cell walls. Thus, antibiotics that are active against bacterial cell walls have no effect on mycoplasmas. Four major species of mycoplasmas cause disease in humans. *Mycoplasma pneumoniae* is an agent of pharyngitis and pneumonia, whereas *Mycoplasma hominis* and *Ureaplasma urealyticum* are agents of genitourinary disease. *Mycoplasma fermentans* is a possible cause of disseminated disease in normal humans and may also be an opportunistic pathogen in persons with AIDS. Mycoplasmas are sensitive to erythromycin or tetracycline or both.

BACTERIA

Bacteria are a tremendously varied group of organisms that are generally capable of cell-free growth, although some produce disease as intracellular parasites. There are numerous ways of classifying bacteria, including morphology, ability to retain certain dyes, growth in different physical conditions, ability to metabolize various substrates, and antibiotic sensitivities. Although combinations of these methods are used to identify bacteria in clinical bacteriology laboratories, relatedness for taxonomic purposes is established by DNA homology.

Spirochetes

Spirochetes are slender, motile, spiral-shaped organisms that are not readily seen under the microscope unless stained with silver or viewed under darkfield illumination. Many of these organisms cannot yet be cultured on artificial media or in cell culture. Four genera of spirochetes cause disease in humans. *Treponema* species include the pathogens of syphilis and the nonvenereal endemic syphilis-like illnesses of yaws, pinta, and bejel. The illnesses caused by these organisms are chronic and characterized by prolonged latency in the host. Penicillin is active against *Treponema*. *Leptospira* species are the causative agents of leptospirosis, an acute or subacute febrile illness occasionally resulting in aseptic meningitis, jaundice, and (rarely) renal insufficiency. *Borrelia* species are arthropod-borne spirochetes that are the causative agents of Lyme disease (see Chapter 95) and relapsing fever. During afebrile periods in relapsing fever, these organisms reside within host cells and emerge with modified cell surface antigens. These modifications may permit the bacterium to evade host immune responses and produce relapsing fever and recurrent bacteremia. *Spirillum minus* is one of the causative agents of rat-bite fever.

Anaerobic Bacteria

Anaerobes are organisms that cannot grow in atmospheric oxygen tensions. Some are killed by very low oxygen concentrations, whereas others are relatively aerotolerant. As a general rule, anaerobes that are pathogens for humans are not as sensitive to oxygen as nonpathogens. Anaerobic bacteria are primarily commensals. They inhabit the skin, gut, and mucosal surfaces of all healthy individuals. In fact, the presence of anaerobes may inhibit colonization of the gut by virulent, potentially pathogenic bacteria. Anaerobic infections generally occur in two circumstances:

1. Contamination of otherwise sterile sites with anaerobe-laden contents. Examples include (a) aspiration of oral anaerobes into the bronchial tree, producing anaerobic necrotizing pneumonia; (b) peritonitis and intra-abdominal abscesses following bowel perforation; (c) fasciitis and osteomyelitis following odontogenic infections or oral surgery; (d) some instances of pelvic inflammatory disease.
2. Infections of tissue with lowered redox potential as the result of a compromised vascular supply. Examples include (a) foot infections in diabetic patients, in whom vascular disease may produce poor tissue oxygenation; and (b) infections of pressure sores, in which fecal anaerobic flora gain access to tissue whose vascular supply is compromised by pressure.

The pathogenesis of anaerobic infections, that is, soilage by a complex flora, generally results in polymicrobial infections. Thus, the demonstration of one anaerobe in an infected site generally implies the presence of others. Often, facultative organisms (organisms capable of anaerobic and aerobic growths) coexist with anaerobes. Certain anaerobes, such as *Clostridium,* produce toxins that cause well-defined systemic illnesses such as food poisoning, tetanus, and botulism. Other toxins may play a role in the soft tissue infections—cellulitis, fasciitis, and myonecrosis—occasionally produced by *Clostridium* species. *Bacteroides fragilis,* the most numerous bacterial pathogen in the normal human colon, has a polysaccharide capsule that inhibits phagocytosis and promotes abscess formation. Clues to the presence of anaerobic infection include (1) a foul odor (the diagnosis of anaerobic pneumonia can, on occasion, be made from across the room); (2) the presence of gas, which may be seen radiographically or manifested by crepitus on examination (not all gas-forming infections are anaerobic, however); and (3) the presence of mixed gram-positive and gram-negative flora on a Gram stain of purulent exudate, especially when there is little or no growth on plates cultured aerobically. Most pathogenic anaerobes are sensitive to penicillin. Exceptions are strains of *Bacteroides fragilis* (usually sensitive to metronidazole, clindamycin, or ampicillin/sulbactam) and *Clostridium difficile,* which is almost always sensitive to metronidazole and vancomycin. Strains of *Fusobacterium* may also be relatively resistant to penicillin. As a general rule, infections caused by anaerobes originating from sites above the diaphragm are more often penicillin sensitive, whereas infections below the diaphragm are often caused by penicillin-resistant organisms, notably *Bacteroides fragilis.*

Gram-Negative Bacteria

The cell walls of these bacteria, which appear pink on a properly prepared Gram stain, contain lipopolysaccharide, a potent inducer of fever and mediators associated with septic shock, such as tumor necrosis factor (TNF). These organisms cause a wide variety of illnesses. Gram-negative bacteria are the most common cause of cystitis and pyelonephritis. *Haemophilus* species organisms are common pathogens of the respiratory tract causing otitis media, sinusitis, tracheobronchitis, and pneumonia. Lower respiratory tract infections due to these organisms are particularly common in adults with chronic obstructive pulmonary disease. *Haemophilus* is also an important cause of meningitis, particularly in children. Excepting *Haemophilus* species, gram-negative bacteria are uncommon causes of community-acquired pneumonia but common causes of nosocomial pneumonia.

Except for the peculiar risk of *Pseudomonas* infection in intravenous drug users, gram-negative organisms are rare causes of endocarditis on natural heart valves but are occasional pathogens on prosthetic valves. The Enterobacteriaceae include *Escherichia coli, Klebsiella, Enterobacter, Serratia, Salmonella, Shigella,* and *Proteus.* These are large gram-negative rods. Except for the occasional presence of a clear space surrounding some *Klebsiella* (representing a large capsule), these organisms are not readily distinguished from each other on Gram's stain. The Enterobacteriaceae can be thought of as gut-related or genitourinary pathogens. *Salmonella,* a relatively common cause of enteritis, may occasionally infect atherosclerotic plaques or aneurysms. *Shigella* is an agent of bacterial dysentery. *Proteus* species, which split urea, are the agents associated with staghorn calculi of the urinary collecting system.

Gram-negative cocci that cause disease in humans include *Neisseria* and *Moraxella* species. These kidney bean–shaped diplococci are not distinguishable from one another on Gram stain. *Neisseria meningitidis* is an important cause of meningitis, and *Neisseria gonorrhoeae* causes gonorrhea. *Moraxella catarrhalis,* part of the normal oral flora, is a recently recognized cause of lower respiratory tract infection.

Gram-Positive Bacteria

Although these organisms (which appear deep purple on Gram stain) lack endotoxin, infections with gram-positive bacteria also produce fever and cannot be reliably distinguished, on clinical grounds, from infections caused by gram-negative bacteria.

Gram-Positive Rods

Infections due to gram-positive rods are relatively uncommon outside certain specific settings. Diphtheria is rare, but other corynebacteria produce infections in the immunocompromised host and on prosthetic valves and shunts. Because corynebacteria are regular skin colonizers, they often contaminate blood cultures; in the appropriate setting, however, they must be considered potential pathogens. *Listeria monocytogenes* resembles *Corynebacterium* on initial isolation and is an important cause of meningitis and bacteremia in the immunocompromised patient. *Bacillus cereus* is a recognized cause of food poisoning. Serious infections due to this and other *Bacillus* species occur among intravenous drug users. *Clostridium* species are gram-positive rods. Infections due to clostridia are discussed under anaerobes (see previous).

Gram-Positive Cocci

Staphylococcus aureus is a common pathogen that produces a wide spectrum of disease in humans. Staphylococci can infect any organ system. They are common causes of bacteremia and sepsis. The organism often colonizes the anterior nares, particularly among insulin-treated diabetics, hemodialysis patients, and intravenous drug users; these populations also have a greater frequency of infections due to this organism. Hospital workers colonized with *S. aureus* have also been responsible for hospital epidemics of staphylococcal disease.

Generally protected by an antiphagocytic polysaccharide capsule, staphylococci also possess catalase, which inactivates hydrogen peroxide—a mediator of bacterial killing by neutrophils. Staphylococci tend to form abscesses; the low pH within an abscess cavity also limits the effectiveness of host defense cells. Staphylococci elaborate several toxins that mediate certain manifestations of disease. A staphylococcal enterotoxin is responsible for staphylococcal food poisoning. Staphylococcal toxins also mediate the scalded skin syndrome and the multisystem manifestations of toxic shock syndrome. Most staphylococci are penicillinase producing, and some are resistant to penicillinase-resistant penicillin analogues as well. Vancomycin is active against almost all strains. Some staphylococci are "tolerant" to cell wall–active antibiotics such as penicillins or vancomycin; such organisms are inhibited but not killed by these agents. The clinical significance of tolerance is not certain. Other staphylococci are distinguished from *S. aureus* primarily by their inability to produce coagulase. Some of these coagulase-negative staphylococci produce urinary tract infection (*Staphylococcus saprophyticus*). Another, *Staphylococcus epidermidis,* is part of the normal skin flora and an increasingly important cause of infection on foreign bodies such as prosthetic heart valves, ventriculoatrial shunts, and intravascular catheters. Like *Corynebacterium,* *S. epidermidis* may be a contaminant of blood cultures but in the appropriate setting should be considered a potential pathogen. *S. saprophyticus* is sensitive to a variety of antibiotics used in the treatment of urinary tract infection; *S. epidermidis* is often resistant to most antimicrobials but is sensitive to vancomycin.

Streptococci are classified into groups according to the presence of serologically defined carbohydrate capsules (Lancefield typing). Group A streptococci produce skin infections and pharyngitis. These organisms also are associated with the immunologically mediated poststreptococcal disorders — glomerulonephritis and acute rheumatic fever. Group D streptococci include enterococci, which are unique among the streptococci in their uniform resistance to penicillin. Recently, strains of enterococci also resistant to vancomycin have emerged; infections due to these multidrug–resistant organisms have not responded well to available therapies. Streptococci can be classified according to the pattern of hemolysis on blood agar — alpha for incomplete hemolysis (producing a green discoloration on the agar), beta for complete hemolysis, and gamma for nonhemolytic strains. Most Lancefield group strains are beta-hemolytic. An important alpha-hemolytic strain is *Streptococcus pneumoniae* (pneumococcus), the most common cause of bacterial pneumonia and an important cause of meningitis and otitis media. A heterogeneous group of streptococci, often improperly referred to as viridans streptococci (these organisms show alpha- or gamma-hemolysis) includes several species of streptococci that are common oral or gut flora and are important agents of bacterial endocarditis, abscesses, and odontogenic infections.

Mycobacteria

Mycobacteria are a group of rod-shaped bacilli that stain weakly gram-positive. These organisms are rich in lipid content and are recognized in tissue specimens by their ability to retain dye after washing with acid-alcohol (acid-fast). These bacteria are generally slow-growing (some require up to 6 weeks to demonstrate growth on solid media) obligate aerobes. They generally produce chronic disease and manage to survive for years as intracellular parasites of mononuclear phagocytes. Some escape intracellular killing mechanisms by blocking phagosome/lysosome fusion or by disrupting the phagosome. Almost all provoke cell-mediated immune responses in the host, and clinical disease expression may be related in large part to the nature of the host immune response. Tuberculosis is caused by *Mycobacterium tuberculosis*. Other mycobacteria — nontuberculous mycobacteria — can produce diseases resembling tuberculosis. Certain rapid-growing mycobacteria cause infections following surgery or implantations of prostheses, and *Mycobacterium avium complex* (MAC) is an important cause of disseminated infection among patients with AIDS. MAC infections are frequently resistant to drugs usually used in the treatment of tuberculosis but generally respond to combination therapy including clarithromycin or azithromycin and ethambutol (see Chapter 108). Leprosy is a mycobacterial disease of skin and peripheral nerves caused by the noncultivatable *Mycobacterium leprae*.

Actinomycetales

Nocardia and *Actinomyces* are weakly gram-positive filamentous bacteria. *Nocardia* is acid-fast and aerobic; *Actinomyces* is anaerobic and not acid-fast. *Actinomyces* inhabits the mouth, gut, and vagina and produces cervicofacial osteomyelitis and abscess, pneumonia with empyema, and intra-abdominal and pelvic abscess, the last often associated with intrauterine contraceptive devices. *Nocardia* most commonly produces pneumonia and brain abscess. Approximately half of patients with *Nocardia* infection have underlying impairments in cell-mediated immunity. Infections with either of these organisms require long-term treatment. *Actinomyces* is relatively sensitive to most antibiotics; penicillin is the treatment of choice. *Nocardia* infections are best treated with high doses of sulfonamides.

FUNGI

Fungi are larger than bacteria. Unlike bacteria, they have rigid cell walls that contain chitin as well as polysaccharides. They grow and proliferate by budding, by elongation of hyphal forms, and/or by spore formation. Excepting *Candida* and related species, fungi rarely are visible on Gram-stained preparations but can be stained with Gomori's methenamine silver stain or calcofluor white. They also are resistant to potassium hydroxide and can often be visualized on wet mounts of scrapings or secretions to which several drops of a 10% solution of potassium hydroxide have been added. Fungi are resistant to antibiotics used in the treatment of bacterial infections and must be treated with drugs active against their unusual cell wall. Most fungi can exist in a yeast form — round to ovoid cells that may reproduce by budding — and a mold form — a complex of tubular structures (hyphae) that grow by branching or extension.

Candida species are oval yeasts that often colonize the mouth, gastrointestinal tract, and vagina of healthy individuals. They may produce disease by overgrowth and/or invasion. *Candida* stomatitis (thrush) often occurs in individuals who are receiving antibiotic or corticosteroid therapy or who have impairments of cell-mediated immunity. Vulvovaginitis due to *Candida* may occur in these same settings but is also seen among women with diabetes mellitus or with no apparent predisposing factors. *Candida* can also colonize and infect the urinary tract, particularly in the presence of an indwelling urinary catheter. Occasionally, *Candida* species may gain entry into the blood stream and produce sepsis. This may occur in the setting of neutropenia after chemotherapy, where the portal of entry is the gastrointestinal tract, or in individuals receiving intravenous feedings, in whom the catheter is the source of the infection. Mucosal candidiasis can be treated with topical (clotrimazole) or systemic (fluconazole) imidazole drugs; systemic candidiasis is generally treated with amphotericin B.

Histoplasma capsulatum is a fungus endemic to the Ohio and Mississippi River valleys that produces a mild febrile syndrome in most individuals and a self-limited pneumonia in some. Occasionally, patients develop potentially fatal disseminated disease. Some individuals with chronic pulmonary disease may develop chronic pneumonia due to this yeast. Systemic or progressive disease is treated with amphotericin B; itraconazole may also be effective in some cases.

Coccidioides immitis is endemic in the southwestern

TABLE 91–1	Some Protozoal Diseases of Humans		
Protozoan	**Clinical Illness**	**Transmission**	**Diagnosis**
Plasmodium	Malaria: fever, hemolysis	Mosquito, transfusion	Peripheral blood smear
Babesia microti	Fever, hemolysis	Tick, transfusion	Peripheral blood smear
Trichomonas vaginalis	Vaginitis	Sexual contact	Vaginal smear
*Toxoplasma gondii**	Fever, lymph node enlargement; encephalitis, brain abscess in compromised host	Raw meat, cat feces	Serologies, tissue biopsy
*Pneumocystis carinii**†	Pneumonia in immunocompromised host	?Airborne‡	Lung biopsy, bronchial lavage
Entamoeba histolytica	Colitis, hepatic abscess	Fecal-oral	Stool smear, serologies
Giardia lamblia	Diarrhea, malabsorption	Fecal-oral	Stool smear, small bowel aspirate
Cryptosporidium†	Diarrhea	?Fecal-oral	Sugar flotation, acid-fast stain of stool, biopsy
Isospora belli†	Diarrhea, malabsorption	?Fecal-oral	Wet mount or acid-fast stain of stool
Microsporidium†	Diarrhea, malabsorption, dissemination	?Fecal-oral	Small bowel biopsy Electron microscopy

* Morphologically classified as a protozoan, genetically more closely related to fungi.
† Important opportunistic pathogens in persons with acquired immunodeficiency syndrome (see Chapter 108).
‡ Primary infection is presumably airborne, but clinical disease usually results from multiplication of resident microorganisms in an immunocompromised host. Respiratory isolation is not indicated.

United States and, like *H. capsulatum*, produces a self-limited respiratory infection or pneumonia in most infected individuals. Immunocompromised individuals are at greatest risk for fatal systemic dissemination. Fluconazole or amphotericin B is used for progressive or extrapulmonary disease.

Cryptococcus neoformans is a yeast with a large polysaccharide capsule. It produces a self-limited or chronic pneumonia, but the most common clinical manifestation of infection with this fungus is a chronic meningitis. Although patients with impairment in cell-mediated immunity are at risk for cryptococcal meningitis, some patients with this syndrome have no identifiable immunodeficiency. Treatment is with amphotericin B combined with flucytosine. Long-term oral fluconazole therapy is effective in preventing relapse in persons with AIDS.

Blastomyces dermatitidis is a yeast also endemic in the Ohio and Mississippi River basins. Acute self-limited pulmonary infection is followed rarely by disseminated disease. Skin disease is most common, but bones and the genitourinary tract may be involved as well. Amphotericin B is used for treating systemic disease.

Aspergillus is a mold that produces several different clinical illnesses in humans. Acute bronchopulmonary aspergillosis is an IgE-mediated hypersensitivity to *Aspergillus* colonization of the respiratory tract. This condition produces wheezing and fleeting pulmonary infiltrates in patients with asthma. Occasionally, *Aspergillus* will colonize a pre-existent pulmonary cavity and produce a mycetoma or fungus ball. Hemoptysis is the most serious complication of such infection. Invasive pulmonary aspergillosis rarely is a chronic illness of marginally compromised hosts, but more often it is a cause of acute, life-threatening pneumonia in patients with neutropenia or in recipients of organ transplants. Amphotericin B is the drug of choice for invasive aspergillosis.

The zygomycetes (Mucorales) are molds with ribbon-shaped hyphae that produce disease in patients with poorly controlled diabetes mellitus or hematologic malignancy and among recipients of organ transplantation. Invasive disease of the palate and nasal sinuses, which may extend intracranially, is the most common presentation, but pneumonia may be seen as well. These infections are generally treated with surgical excision plus amphotericin B.

PROTOZOANS

The protozoal pathogens listed in Table 91–1 are all important causes of disease within the United States. Infections caused by these organisms are diagnosed as indicated in Table 91–1 and are discussed in the relevant disease-oriented chapters.

HELMINTHS

Diseases due to helminths are among the most prevalent diseases in the developing world but are uncommon causes of illness in North America. In contrast to the pathogens discussed previously, helminths are multicellular parasites. Helminth diseases acquired in the United States include ascariasis (maldigestion, obstruction), hookworm (intestinal blood loss), enterobiasis (pinworm, anal pruritus), and strongyloidiasis (gastroenteritis, dissemination in the immunocompromised host). It is important to recognize the risk of other helminthic diseases in travelers returning from endemic regions (see Chapter 110).

REFERENCES

Mandell GL, Karchmer AW, Diana RJ, et al: Bacterial diseases. *In* Bennett JC, Plum F (eds.): Cecil Textbook of Medicine. 20th ed. Philadelphia, WB Saunders, 1996, pp 1566–1605.
Tyler KL, Fields BN: Introduction to viruses and viral diseases. *In* Mandell GL, Bennett JC, Dolin R (eds.): Principles and Practice of Infectious Diseases. 4th ed. New York, Churchill Livingstone, 1995, pp 1314–1325.

92

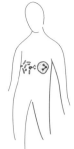

Host Defenses Against Infection

Infectious agents and hosts are engaged in a complex struggle that has evolved over eons. The pathogenic and evasive mechanisms of microbes are countered by multiple and overlapping host immune and nonspecific defense mechanisms. In some cases, the pathogen "wins," with destruction of the host; in others, the host immune response prevails, with eradication of the parasite. Often there is a standoff characterized by latent infection; pathogens capable of a latent phase have the capacity to reactivate as the host ages or as its immune response deteriorates because of superimposed diseases.

A few general statements are germane regarding the roles of the components of the host defense network in the response to infectious diseases. The skin and mucosal surfaces represent the primary interface with the external world and its microbial flora. At these sites, anatomic barriers, the nonspecific inflammatory response, secretory IgA, products of effector cells, and the normal microbial flora defend against the development of invasive disease. Neutrophils are the critical effector cells in defense against infection with organisms constituting the normal microbial flora, such as Enterobacteriaceae, *Staphylococcus aureus*, *Candida*, and *Aspergillus*. Once local barriers are breached, the specific immune response, often acting in concert with nonspecific effector mechanisms, is required to control the infection.

The elements of the host response that are critical in combating many of the more common infectious agents are known; in fact, awareness of infections that occur in the immunocompromised host (see Chapter 109), as well as research in experimental models, provides the basis for this understanding. Antibody, which is the product of the interactions of B cells, antigen, and T helper cells, is critical for defense against encapsulated pathogenic bacteria such as *Streptococcus pneumoniae*, *Haemophilus influenzae*, *Neisseria meningitidis*, or *Salmonella* species. The cellular immune response—specifically T cell–dependent macrophage activation—is the critical effector arm against organisms capable of evading destruction by the effector cell and replicating intracellularly. An example of such an organism is *Mycobacterium tuberculosis*. Antiviral immunity is more difficult to characterize and varies with the agent in question. Neutralizing antibody is sufficient to disturb the life cycle of viruses with an important extracellular phase (such as rubella). Protective mechanisms operant against viruses with a latent intracel-

lular phase in the host, such as herpes simplex virus, are chiefly provided by T cells. In this case, cytotoxic T cells often must destroy the infected host cells to expose the virus to neutralizing factors in the external milieu (antibody, complement).

This chapter is organized as follows. First, local barriers to infection are discussed. Then, the interaction of the components of the immune system is presented, followed by discussion of nonspecific effector mechanisms. Finally, host defenses against representative infectious agents are discussed. As noted, infections in immunocompromised hosts are dealt with in Chapter 109.

LOCAL BARRIERS TO INFECTION

Both nonspecific and specific host defense mechanisms contribute to the prevention of infectious diseases. Since very few microorganisms have the ability to penetrate intact skin, the integument and the mucous membranes provide vital mechanical barriers to infection. The indigenous flora of these surfaces, particularly the anaerobic bacteria, prevent colonization with virulent organisms by competing for nutrients and receptor sites on host cells and by producing factors, termed bacteriocins, that are toxic to other bacteria. The local milieu, chiefly the pH and redox potential, provides an additional barrier to colonization and infection with certain pathogenic organisms. Gastric acid reduces bacterial counts by 10- to 10,000-fold. The normal flow of mucus and other secretions helps to eliminate microorganisms from mucosal surfaces. The mucociliary blanket, for example, transports organisms away from the lungs. In addition, locally produced and active antimicrobial substances prevent infection. Factors contributing to protection of the urinary tract include pH, bladder flushing, prostatic secretions, hypertonicity of the renal medulla, and length of the urethra. In the vagina, estrogens promote the growth of acidogenic bacteria, which produce an environment unfavorable to most pathogens. Lactoperoxidase, lysozyme, and lactoferrin in salivary and vaginal secretions and milk have microbicidal activity. Secretory IgA has a particularly important role in this respect, opsonizing organisms and thereby blocking their ability to adhere to epithelial surfaces and colonize the mucosa.

COMPONENTS OF THE IMMUNE SYSTEM

The principal cells of the immune system are bone marrow–derived (B) and thymus-dependent (T) lymphocytes and mononuclear phagocytes. They are organized as a recirculating pool of lymphocytes and monocytes, bone marrow cells, and organized lymphoid tissue (lymph nodes, spleen, Peyer's patches, and the thymus).

The primary function of the immune system is to destroy foreign organisms and clear foreign antigens without damaging host tissues. Immunity also is important in maintaining certain infectious agents in a latent stage and may play a role in destroying virally infected cells or cells that have undergone malignant transformation. The immune response is characterized by three features—immunologic memory, specificity, and systemic action. The functional organization of the immune response can be considered in six sequential steps: encounter, recognition, activation of lymphocytes, deployment, discrimination, and regulation.

Encounter

Microbes and soluble antigens encounter antigen-presenting cells (APCs) in the tissues and are ingested and catabolized. Monocytes, macrophages, dendritic cells, and Langerhans cells are examples of APCs. The physical form of the antigen and the site of exposure or breaching of tissue determine which type of APC is relevant. Particulates are more readily ingested by active phagocytes such as macrophages; dendritic cells may be critical to the handling of soluble protein antigens. The gastrointestinal and respiratory tracts, important sites for interface of the immune system with the environment, possess well-differentiated APCs in submucosal areas. Some microbes elicit a neutrophilic inflammatory response and are phagocytosed and degraded by neutrophils, thereby bypassing traditional APCs and eliciting inflammation but little detectable immune response. Nonetheless, acute infection almost invariably produces an antibody response and memory for the same, presumably as the result of the processing of soluble microbial products. The disposition of soluble antigen is determined by the likelihood of uptake by APCs; an aggregated form of antigen or antigen bound by specific antibody in immune complexes favors uptake by APCs. Following ingestion by APCs, the foreign antigen is degraded in acidic vesicles and reprocessed to the surface of the cell, where, in close approximation, or bound, to determinants encoded by the class II major histocompatibility complex (MHC), it is accessible to lymphocytes. APCs also produce cytokines such as interleukins (e.g., IL1 and IL6), which amplify immune induction.

Recognition

The immune system has the capability of responding to an almost infinite number of antigens. It appears that B cells and T cells utilize similar mechanisms to generate and express the diversity required for such a broad range of specific antigenic responses.

Five classes of antibodies (isotypes) are recognized (Table 92–1). An IgG1 antibody (Fig. 92–1) consists of two light (kappa or lambda) and two heavy chains. Each antibody has constant regions, which are identical in structure to all antibodies of that class, and distinctive antigen recognition sites whose structures are quite variable. An IgG1 molecule has two such antigen-combining sites. The antigen-combining sites of antibody molecules recognize the three-dimensional structure of an antigen and bind to an antigen in a lock-and-key manner, through multiple weak, noncovalent interactions. The variable regions consist of the approximately 110 N-terminal amino acids of each chain. There are three short, hypervariable regions in each of the light and the heavy chains. The six hypervariable regions form the combining site.

The generation of antibody diversity is understood at the molecular level. The variable portion of the heavy chain is encoded by three different genes—V, D, and J; there are 500 to 1000 different V genes, 10 D genes, and 4 J genes. The variable portions of the light chains are encoded by V and J genes; there are 200 possible V

TABLE 92–1	Properties of Human Immunoglobulins				
	IgG	**IgA**	**IgM**	**IgD**	**IgE**
H chain class	γ	α	μ	δ	ϵ
Molecular weight (approximate)	150,000	170,000	900,000	180,000	190,000
Complement fixation (classic)	++	0	++++	0	0
Opsonic activity (for binding)	++++	++	0	0	0
Reaginic activity	0	0	0	0	++++
Serum concentration (approximate mg/dl)	1500	150–350	100–150	2	2
Serum half-life (days)	23	6	5	3	2.5
Major functions	Recall response; opsonization; transplacental immunity	Secretory immunity	Primary response; complement fixation	?	Allergy; antihelminth immunity

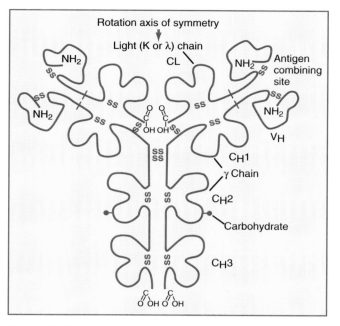

Figure 92–1
Schematic diagram of a molecule of human IgG, showing the two light (κ or λ) chains and two heavy (γ) chains held together by disulfide bonds. The constant regions of the light (CL) and heavy (C_H1, C_H2, and C_H3) chains and the variable region of the heavy chain (V_H) are indicated. Loops in the peptide chain formed by intrachain disulfide bonds (C_H1 and so forth) constitute separate functional domains. (Reprinted, by permission, from the New England Journal of Medicine, Vol 316, p 1320, 1987.)

genes and 6 J genes. During the differentiation of B cells, somatic translocations randomly select the V, D, and J heavy chain genes and the V and J light chain genes that will be transcribed in that cell. The diversity achieved by these means is enormous. Somatic mutations in B cells allow the possibility of improving the fit between antibody and antigen; repeated or sustained exposure to antigen selects B cells capable of producing antibody with the highest binding affinity. These circulate as memory cells.

T lymphocytes can be divided into two subpopulations based on the polypeptide chains constituting the antigen receptor. The $\alpha\beta$ T cells, constituting the larger population (~95%), possess a receptor comprising a heterodimer of α and β polypeptide chains (Fig. 92–2). The variable portion of the $\alpha\beta$ T cell receptor is composed of the approximately 100 N-terminal amino acids. The generation of diversity is by translocation of V, D, and J genes, as is the case for B lymphocytes. The T cell receptor is directed at the foreign antigen associated with MHC determinants. $\alpha\beta$ T cells can be divided by their surface expression of glycoproteins into CD4 and CD8 subpopulations. CD4 and CD8 cells also differ in their genetic restriction and function. Class I MHC products are recognized by CD8 suppressor/cytotoxic T cells, and class II by CD4 helper T cells. The T cell receptor recognizes linear peptides of 5 to 20 amino acids in length. The second subpopulation of T lymphocytes, $\gamma\delta$ T cells, constitutes approximately 5% of circulating and lymphoid

T cells; their T cell receptor contains a heterodimer of γ and δ chains. Activation of $\gamma\delta$ T cells does not require recognition of either the class I or the class II MHC on APCs.

Activation of Lymphocytes

The initial physical apposition of T cells and APCs is stabilized by interactions of so-called accessory molecules on T cells with their respective ligands on APCs. Accessory molecules usually are members of the immunoglobulin or the integrin gene family. For example, leukocyte functional antigen (LFA)–1 on the T cell binds to intercellular adhesion molecule (ICAM)–1 on the APCs, and CD2 on the T cell binds with LFA-3 on APCs. These reciprocal interactions facilitate the initial cell contact and are reinforced during the process of activation. CD4 helper T cells are activated when the T cell receptors are occupied and effectively cross-linked by the antigen–class II MHC complex on the surface of an APC (Fig. 92–3). Activation of the T cell is promoted by IL1 and IL6 released as a consequence of the cellular interactions. The helper T cell enlarges, secretes a variety of lymphokines, and divides to form a clone. The antigen molecule may also form a bridge between T cells and B cells, permitting the targeted delivery of B cell growth and differentiation factors from T cell to B cell. The B cell, which is activated by a combination of signals provided by binding of antigen and by T cells, enlarges, divides, and differentiates into an antibody-producing cell. T cell products also promote an isotype switch from IgM to production of IgG, IgA, or IgE.

The initial exposure of humans to microbial antigens leads to the proliferation of B cells recognizing the antigen and differentiation into antibody-forming plasma cells. T cell help is required for responses to most antigens, although bacterial polysaccharides may directly elicit antibody production. Following the first exposure to

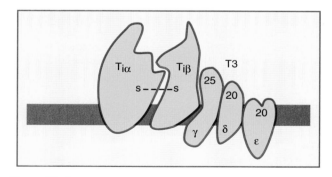

Figure 92–2
Structure of the human T cell receptor and its subunits. This diagram shows subunit composition of the human T cell receptor. The $Ti\alpha$ and $Ti\beta$ subunits are held together by S-S bonds and are anchored in the cell membrane with their transmembrane segments. The T_1 protein of the T cell receptor is most closely associated with the 25-kd γ chain of the T3 molecule. The T3 complex includes two additional subunits (δ and ϵ), with molecular weights of 20,000. (Reprinted, by permission, from the New England Journal of Medicine, Vol 316, p 1320, 1987.)

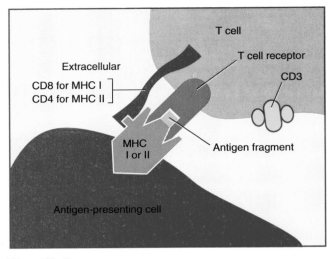

Figure 92-3

The molecular events in antigen presentation. Shown are the interactions between the various molecules, including the major histocompatibility complex (MHC), the T cell receptor, the CD8 or CD4 molecules, and the CD3 complex. (From Bennett JC: Introduction to diseases of the immune system. *In* Wyngaarden JB, Smith LH Jr, Bennett JC [eds.]: Cecil Textbook of Medicine. 19th ed. Philadelphia, WB Saunders, 1992, p 1440.)

example, interferon-gamma activates macrophages to destroy certain facultative intracellular pathogens. By contrast, Th2 cells secrete cytokines that favor B cell growth and differentiation (IL4, IL5, IL6, IL9, IL10, and IL13). Further distinctions concerning the heterogeneity of CD4 cells in humans are not nearly so clear.

Special consideration is warranted concerning cytotoxic mechanisms that destroy parasitized host cells. Certain viruses usurp the machinery of cells that they infect and replicate intracellularly, where they are inaccessible to antibody and complement. The only effective host response requires destruction of the parasitized host cell. This usually is accomplished by class I MHC–restricted CD8 cells that target on virally encoded proteins expressed on the host cell surface. Antibody to the viral products can also bind to the host cell surface, rendering it susceptible to destruction by Fc receptor–bearing effector cells in the process of ADCC. Class II MHC–restricted cytotoxicity mediated by CD4 lymphocytes can be called into play when host cells are heavily parasitized with certain organisms such as mycobacteria, or after ingestion and presentation of viral or other microbial products by APCs. The relative roles of class II as opposed to class I MHC–restricted cytotoxicity and ADCC in the destruction of parasitized host cells vary with the infectious agent. Once the host cell is destroyed, however, the microbe is susceptible to antibody, complement, or the attack of other phagocytes and T lymphocytes.

an antigen, IgM is the main antibody class or isotype produced. An isotype switch then occurs such that IgG predominates. On any re-exposure to the antigen, production of IgG antibody is accelerated, and antibody is produced in high titer and with high avidity for the antigen. Secretory IgA is found in tears, saliva, and bronchial, nasal, vaginal, prostatic, and intestinal secretions. Its primary role is to prevent organisms and antigens from attaching to and breaching mucosal barriers.

Immunoglobulin M accounts for 10% of normal immunoglobulins and is the antibody isotype most efficient at complement fixation. Both IgM and IgG can neutralize the infectivity of viruses and lyse bacteria through complement fixation. Mononuclear phagocytes, neutrophils, and some lymphocytes possess surface receptors for the Fc fragment of IgG and/or the third component of complement. Therefore, IgG antibody or complement can bind to and opsonize bacteria, facilitating their phagocytosis (Fig. 92–4), and IgG antibody can arm host effector cells for preferential destruction of selected targets by the process of antibody-dependent cell-mediated cytotoxicity (ADCC).

Antigen-presenting cells and CD4 cells acting in concert are required for activation of CD8 cells for cytotoxic and suppressor cell activity. The activated CD4 cell also secretes a number of factors important in hematopoiesis, mobilization of bone marrow precursor cells, chemotaxis of mononuclear and other cells to areas of inflammation, and expression of the cellular immune response.

In experimental studies, helper T lymphocytes can be divided into two subpopulations. The Th1 subset secretes IL2, interferon-gamma, and lymphotoxin and is most effective at stimulating cellular immune responses. For

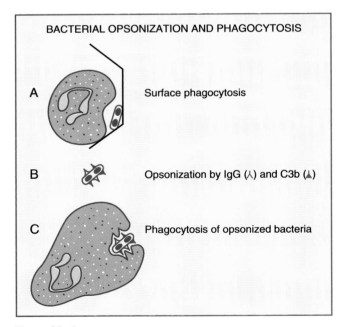

Figure 92-4

Ingestion of pneumococci by the neutrophil. In the absence of opsonins, the slippery pneumococcus must be forced against an alveolar surface to be ingested, the inefficient process of surface phagocytosis. Bacteria are opsonized by C3b and IgG, which interact with receptors on the neutrophil, thereby facilitating phagocytosis.

Deployment

The mobility of lymphocytes is central to the memory and systemic function of the immune response. Some progeny of activated B and T cells return to the resting stage, leaving the peripheral lymphoid tissue to traffic as memory cells in the recirculating pool. These lymphocytes perfuse the tissues of the body and can re-enter the lymph nodes. Reinfection or re-exposure to an antigen at any site can lead to activation of memory lymphocytes.

The events thus far discussed are required for activation of antigen-specific lymphocytes. Neither antibody nor activated lymphocytes are capable of directly destroying pathogenic organisms. Rather, they act in concert with antigen-nonspecific components of the immune response, including phagocytes and the complement and other molecular systems, to destroy pathogenic microbes. For example, one of the key cytokines produced by activated CD4 cells is interferon-gamma; this interferon activates mononuclear phagocytes and thus renders them capable of killing intracellular parasites and tumors.

Discrimination

Tolerance of self-antigens prevents autoimmune disease. Several mechanisms contribute to tolerance. Early in ontogeny, exposure to antigen leads to refractoriness to that antigen. This process has been termed "clonal anergy." Suppressor T cells are activated when soluble antigen is injected intravenously without adjuvant; this resembles exposure to most self-antigens. Moreover, self-antigens are not presented to reactive CD4 cells in combination with class II MHC determinants, so that immune induction fails to occur. The breakdown of tolerance and autoimmune disease may result from a combination of factors: tissue damage exposing new antigens to the immune system and genetic factors that regulate the response to self-antigens and determine end-organ susceptibility to damage.

Cross-reactivity exists between bacterial and mammalian cellular products. For example, the heat shock protein (HSP) 60 of mycobacteria has polypeptide spans with close homology to human HSP60. In fact, synovial fluid T cells from patients with rheumatoid arthritis are reactive with these bacterial peptides. For individuals expressing an autoimmune diathesis, whether on a genetic or some other basis, bacterial infection may trigger autoimmune tissue damage.

Regulation

The immune response must be appropriate to the challenging event; too little may permit unchecked infection, whereas too great a response may damage tissue. Regulatory mechanisms amplify or mute an immune response and may be specific or nonspecific.

Antigen itself regulates the immune response. As antigen is cleared, a process enhanced by specific antibody, only lymphocytes bearing the highest-affinity receptors are activated. Once antigen is cleared entirely, the immune response diminishes, although memory cells continue to provide surveillance for re-exposure to the antigen. Antibody has an additional role in immunoregulation, since immune complexes may directly modulate the response of specific lymphocytes. Antibody may also be directed at the antigen-combining site of antibody itself. Production of "anti-idiotypic antibodies" is stimulated by the immune response and may suppress further production of the relevant antibody.

Activation of the immune response also induces cellular regulatory mechanisms. For example, the activated CD4 cell is an important stimulus for induction of suppression by CD8 cells and mononuclear phagocytes. Cytokines that may mediate suppression of CD4 cell responses include IL4, IL10, transforming growth factor β, and the IL1 receptor antagonist.

NONSPECIFIC EFFECTOR MECHANISMS

Complement

Complement activity results from the sequential interaction of a large number (25 are recognized) of plasma and cell membrane interactive proteins. The classic complement pathway is activated by antibody-coated targets or antigen-antibody complexes. The alternative pathway is activated by bacterial polysaccharides. Complement binds to bacteria, facilitating their attachment by C3b receptors on phagocytes, thus constituting the heat-labile opsonic system (see Fig. 92–4); it directly damages certain bacteria and viruses, and it induces inflammation through chemotactically active fragments. The classic complement pathway is the major effector mechanism for antibody-mediated immune responses. It is the Fc receptor of antigen-activated antibody molecules that binds and activates C1. The alternative pathway is activated in the absence of antibody by constituents of the microbial surface, including polysaccharides, and generates C3 convertase, which catalyzes proteolysis of C3. Both the classic and the alternative pathways converge and result in the formation of the membrane attack complex involving C5 to C9. This complex forms pores in the membrane of microbes, subjecting them to osmotic lysis.

The complement system has several other notable biologic functions. C3b or iC3b deposited on the surface of microbes binds to complement receptors (CR1, CR3, and CR4) on neutrophils and macrophages, promoting phagocytosis. C5a is a chemotaxin for neutrophils and activates oxidative burst activity. C5a and C3a also stimulate histamine release from mast cells, thus promoting inflammation. Finally, C3b promotes clearance of immune complexes by linking them to CR1 on the erythrocyte surface.

Neutrophils

Neutrophils respond rapidly to chemotaxins and are the primary effector cells of the acute inflammatory response. They are activated by cytokines, including interferon-gamma and tumor necrosis factor (TNF); this activation enhances neutrophil adhesion to vascular endothelium near the sites of infection, the first step in local accumulation. The cytokines also activate oxidative metabolism. Neutrophils ingest antibody and complement-opsonized bacteria and destroy so-called "extracellular" bacteria by exposing them to toxic oxygen metabolites in the presence of myeloperoxidase and halide. Neutrophils also possess potent antibacterial peptides termed defensins.

Mononuclear Phagocytes

Macrophages differ from other phagocytic cells in that they have immunoregulatory and secretory properties in addition to their role as effector cells of cell-mediated immunity. Macrophages ingest and kill extracellular bacteria directly and in antibody-dependent reactions. Facultative intracellular pathogens have evolved a variety of means for escaping intracellular destruction. These include disruption and escape from the phagosome, as well as blockage of phagosome-lysosome fusion. It is the process of activation of macrophages by T cells and their products that overcomes the evasive mechanisms to destroy the organism. The macrophage activation factor (MAF) varies according to the microbe in question. For many, including *Toxoplasma gondii* as an example, it is interferon-gamma. Recent data suggest that TNF may have a critical role in activating the killing of *M. tuberculosis*.

Natural Killer (NK) Cells

Natural killer cells are large lymphocytes with cytoplasmic granules, sometimes referred to as large granular lymphocytes. They lack specific antigen receptors but possess the ability to kill certain tumor cells or normal cells infected by virus. NK cells are neither T nor B cells, although they express the CD2 molecule and a low-affinity receptor for the Fc portion of IgG (CD16). They can acquire additional "specificity" by virtue of FcR-dependent attachment to IgG antibody–coated targets, thereby serving as an effector cell of ADCC. They produce and respond to cytokines, which modulate their functions. The mediators of target lysis include porins and other granule contents.

$\gamma\delta$ T Cells

$\gamma\delta$ T cells have excited interest as a potential intermediary between nonspecific inflammatory and specific immune effector cells. They constitute approximately 5% of T cells in circulation and in lymphoid organs. $\gamma\delta$ T cells are not class I or class II MHC restricted and appear to target to broadly cross-reactive HSPs. They may function, therefore, in the initial or innate response to microbes, and possibly in the pathogenesis of autoimmune diseases. $\gamma\delta$ T cells express cytokines and possess cytotoxic function. Their relative role in infection and immunity awaits definition.

Integration of the various host defense mechanisms is apparent as one examines resistance to specific representative infectious agents.

RESISTANCE TO EXTRACELLULAR BACTERIA

Encapsulated Organisms

Streptococcus Pneumoniae

The type-specific polysaccharide capsule is a major virulence factor because of its antiphagocytic properties. Antibody to the polysaccharide is itself capable of preventing pneumococcal disease, as reflected by experimental studies and the efficacy of pneumococcal polysaccharide vaccines.

In the absence of immunity, pneumococci reaching the alveoli are not effectively contained by the host. Their phagocytosis by neutrophils is inefficient, since organisms must be trapped against a surface to be ingested ("surface phagocytosis"—see Fig. 92–4). The pneumococcus does, however, elicit a neutrophilic inflammatory response. The organism activates complement by the alternative pathway and interactions of C-reactive protein in serum with pneumococcal C-polysaccharide. Activated complement fragments (C3a, C5a, C567) and bacterial oligopeptides are chemotactic for neutrophils. Opsonic complement fragments (C3b) coating pneumococci favor their attachment to neutrophils but are less effective in promoting phagocytosis and killing than is specific antibody. Clinical observations also directly support the primal role of antibody in immunity. It is the development of specific antibody on days 5 to 9 of untreated pneumococcal pneumonia that produces a clinical "crisis," with dramatic resolution of symptoms. Opsonization of *S. pneumoniae* by type-specific antipolysaccharide antibody promotes ingestion and oxidative burst activity, with destruction of the organism.

Neisseria Meningitidis

Capsular polysaccharide also represents an important virulence factor for meningococci. In addition, pathogenic *Neisseria* species produce an IgA protease that dissociates the Fc fragment from the Fab portion of secretory and serum IgA, thus interfering with effector properties of the antibody molecule. Antibody-dependent complement-mediated bacterial killing is the critical host defense against meningococci. In illustration of this principle, the age-specific incidence of meningococcal meningitis during the first 12 years of life is inversely proportional to the age-related frequency of serum bactericidal antibody directed against capsular and cell wall bacterial antigens. Therefore, the presence of bactericidal antibody is associated with protection against the meningococcus. In epidemic situations, 40% of individuals who become colonized with the epidemic strain but lack bactericidal antibodies develop disease. Protective serum antibody is elicited by colonization with (1) nonencapsulated and encapsulated strains of meningococci of low virulence, which elicit antibodies cross-reactive with virulent strains, and (2) *Escherichia coli* and *Bacillus* species with cross-reacting capsular polysaccharides. The lack of bactericidal activity in the serum of adolescents and adults manifesting susceptibility to *N. meningitidis* may be due to blocking IgA antibody. Susceptibility of patients lacking C6, C7, or C8 to meningococcal infection provides important evidence that the dominant protective mechanism against this organism involves complement-mediated bacteriolysis. Evaluation of individuals developing meningococcal disease in a nonepidemic setting sometimes reveals underlying abnormalities of the complement system.

Exotoxin-Producing Organisms

Clostridium Tetani

All disease manifestations produced by this organism can be ascribed to the tetanus toxin, tetanospasmin. Antibody to toxin is protective. Survival from tetanus does not, however, lead to immunity to subsequent infection, because the toxin is sufficiently potent to cause disease at subimmunogenic concentrations.

RESISTANCE TO OBLIGATE INTRACELLULAR PARASITES: VIRUSES

Host antiviral defense is characterized by overlap and redundancy, which allow a rapid and effective response to most viral agents. The key element of the response varies with the virus, the site, and the timing. Initially, infection is limited at the local site by type I interferons, which increase the resistance of neighboring cells to spread of the infection. Complement directly neutralizes some enveloped viruses. NK cells destroy infected cells, a process enhanced by the interferons. As specific antibody is produced, IgA neutralizes the virus at mucosal surfaces; IgG neutralizes virus that has spread systemically to extracellular sites and allows uptake and destruction by FcR-bearing effector cells through antibody ADCC. Later effector cells, cytotoxic T lymphocytes (CTLs), are expanded and activated to lyse host cells expressing viral antigens in the context of MHC products. CTLs disrupt parasitized cells, exposing viruses to extracellular neutralization and clearance mechanisms.

The host thus directs several defenses against viral infection. The same humoral and cellular mechanisms that destroy bacteria serve to clear extracellular viruses. The host immune response also is effective against intracellular replicative stages of viruses and may destroy infected host cells that express viral antigens on their surfaces. Clinical and experimental observations indicate the respective roles of humoral and cellular immunity in resistance against certain viruses. In Hodgkin's disease and in T lymphocyte–deficient experimental models, selective defects in cellular immunity lead to reactivation of certain latent Herpesviridae: herpes simplex, varicella-zoster, and cytomegalovirus. The prominent role for cellular immunity against these agents is biologically advantageous because virions spread intercellularly via desmosomes or intercellular bridges; viruses thereby avoid exposure to the antibody-rich extracellular milieu. Destruction of virus-infected cells by specific cytotoxic T cells becomes an essential first step in host defense by allowing extracellular mechanisms to mop up free viral particles.

In contrast, antibody- and complement-dependent mechanisms assume major importance against viruses that themselves lyse host cells and spread by extracellular means; for these agents, passive transfer of antibody confers protection. Nevertheless, the absence of greatly increased susceptibility of hypogammaglobulinemic patients to measles and influenza implies the continued contribution of cellular immunity in protection against these agents and indicates important overlap in antiviral host effector mechanisms.

The major antiviral defenses include humoral mechanisms, cellular immunity, and interferons.

Humoral Defenses

Complement-Independent Neutralization

Specific IgG, IgM, and IgA neutralize infectivity of viruses. The respective antibodies first combine with proteins of the virus coat. Resultant conformational changes may prevent adsorption of viruses to cells and cellular penetration; sometimes, antibody coating of extracellular virus interferes with subsequent intracellular events, such as uncoating. Alternatively, antibody may physically aggregate viral particles.

Immunoglobulin A is the key defender against viral infections that begin on or are confined to respiratory epithelium. For infections such as polio, measles, and rubella, which begin on a mucosal surface and then disseminate hematogenously, local IgA antibody prevents infection, whereas serum IgG antibody prevents disease.

Complement-Facilitated Neutralization

Complement neutralizes some enveloped viruses by direct or antibody-dependent steric changes or aggregation. Infected host cells expressing surface virus antigens also are susceptible to lysis by mechanisms involving the alternate complement pathway and further enhanced by antibody.

Opsonization of extracellular viruses by complement and IgG antibody facilitates phagocytosis by neutrophils and macrophages. This process destroys some viruses (enteroviruses) but aids cellular penetration and replication of others (arboviruses).

Enzyme Inhibition

Antibody may interfere with release of progeny influenza virus by blocking viral neuraminidase. Replication is thereby limited, although the virion is not neutralized.

Cellular Immunity

Cellular Cytotoxicity

These defenses are of chief relevance for viruses that spread by intercellular means.

CTL

These cells appear early in viral infection and are specific for viral antigens expressed on the surface of parasitized cells. Most are CD8 cells that effect class I MHC–restricted killing. Class II MHC–restricted killing by CD4 cells is also important in the immune response to certain viruses. CD4 cells also promote differentiation and activation of CD8 and CTLs.

ADCC

Virus-infected cells that display surface viral antigens are opsonized by IgG antibodies and lysed by ADCC. The effector cells are lymphocytes (killer cells), macrophages, and neutrophils; all bear surface Fc receptors.

NK Cells

Natural killer cells spontaneously lyse virally infected cells; this effector mechanism is activated by interferon-gamma and IL2.

Interferons

The antiviral action of interferons provides a major host defense against viruses. Interferons are a family of proteins produced by lymphocytes, fibroblasts, epithelial cells, and macrophages early in the course of viral infection, before specific antibody develops. Exposure of cells to interferon induces their synthesis of proteins that, in turn, selectively inhibit the production of viral proteins. The immunoregulatory effects of interferon-gamma may also contribute indirectly to antiviral immunity by activating effector cells.

Type I interferons consist of two serologically distinct families of proteins. Interferon-gamma is produced by mononuclear phagocytes and interferon-beta by fibroblasts; other cells can also secrete these factors in response to viral infection. Viral infection induces type I interferon, which protects uninfected neighboring cells by inducing synthesis of enzymes such as 2', 5'-oligoadenylate synthetase that interfere with replication of viral RNA or DNA. Type I interferons have two other functions that promote viral defense: they promote the lytic potential of NK cells, and they increase target expression of class I MHC molecules, thus increasing target susceptibility to lysis by CTLs. Interferon-gamma is a type II interferon, with prominent immunoregulatory activity, produced by activated T lymphocytes.

RESISTANCE TO FACULTATIVE INTRACELLULAR PARASITES: *MYCOBACTERIUM TUBERCULOSIS*

Activation of host phagocytes provides the critical defense mechanism against *M. tuberculosis*. Primary infection progresses locally in the nonhypersensitive host, since ingested organisms persist and multiply within mononuclear phagocytes. The bacteria escape intracellular digestion by virtue of constituents (sulfatides, suramin, poly-D-glutamic acid) that inhibit phagolysosomal fusion. Antibody-coated mycobacteria do not evade phagolysosomal fusion but nonetheless resist degradation, probably because of shielding provided by their rich lipid content. The development of cellular immunity leads to T lymphocyte–dependent macrophage activation and to the killing of the intracellular tubercle bacillus organism. The lesions of primary tuberculosis regress. However, latent foci persist, and delayed reactivation remains a threat throughout the lifetime of the host.

REFERENCES

Abbas AK, Lichtman AH, Pober JS: Cellular and Molecular Immunology. Philadelphia, WB Saunders, 1991.

Holland SM, Gallin JI: Evaluation of the patient with suspected immunodeficiency. *In* Mandel GL, Bennett JE, Dolin R (eds.): Principles and Practices of Infectious Diseases. 4th ed. New York, Churchill Livingstone, 1995, pp 1490–1580.

Nossal GJV: Current concepts: Immunology. The basic components of the immune system. N Engl J Med 1987;316:1320.

Pizzo PA: The compromised host. *In* Bennett JC, Plum F (eds.): Cecil Textbook of Medicine. 20th ed. Philadelphia, WB Saunders, 1996.

Rubin RH, Young LS: Clinical Approach to Infection in the Compromised Host. New York, Plenum Medical Books, 1994.

93

Laboratory Diagnosis of Infectious Diseases

Five basic laboratory techniques can be used in the diagnosis of infectious diseases: (1) direct visualization of the organism; (2) detection of microbial antigen; (3) a search for "clues" produced by the host response to specific microorganisms; (4) detection of specific microbial nucleotide sequences; and (5) isolation of the organism in culture. Each technique has its use and each its pitfalls. The laboratory can usually provide the clinician with prompt, accurate and, if used judiciously, inexpensive diagnosis.

DIAGNOSIS BY DIRECT VISUALIZATION OF THE ORGANISM

In many infectious diseases, pathogenic organisms can be directly visualized by microscopic examination of readily available tissue fluids, such as sputum, urine, pus, and pleural, peritoneal, or cerebrospinal fluid. With the use of Gram's or acid-fast stains, bacteria, mycobacteria, and *Candida* can be readily identified. An India ink preparation can often identify *Cryptococcus,* and potassium hydroxide (KOH) preparations can occasionally identify other fungal pathogens.

Preparation of Specimens for Staining

Sputum and pus are often thick, and thinning is necessary to obtain a helpful preparation. A drop of sputum or pus is placed on a clean glass slide, and another slide is pressed on top of the specimen and pulled away. This step can be repeated as often as necessary (using a clean slide each time) until the specimen has been thinned sufficiently to allow newsprint to be read through it. Unless grossly purulent, fluids such as cerebrospinal fluid (CSF) must be centrifuged to concentrate the organisms and the pellet used for staining. If no organisms are seen upon examining spun CSF, the pellet must then be examined. To prevent the specimen from washing away during the staining procedure, a drop of CSF may be mixed with a drop of fresh serum or other sterile protein source. The

specimen is allowed to air dry and is then gently fixed by being passed quickly through a flame.

Gram's Stain

1. Flood the slide with crystal violet—15 seconds.
2. Rinse with water.
3. Flood with Gram's iodine—15 seconds.
4. Rinse with water.
5. Decolorize with 95% ethyl alcohol.

This step is critical. Rinse with alcohol until blue stain just disappears from the rinse.

6. Immediately rinse with water.
7. Flood with safranin—15 seconds.
8. Rinse with water.
9. Air dry.
10. Examine using oil immersion lens.

Proper decolorization is crucial. A good Gram's stain should show neutrophil nuclei as deep pink in all but the most dense regions, where they may have a touch of blue. Interpretation of the staining of organisms should be based on inspection of the areas in which transition of the coloration of neutrophil nuclei is present, that is, where some nuclei show minimal blue or purple staining. This will avoid areas that are overdecolorized or underdecolorized.

Acid-Fast Stain

The Kinyoun stain for acid-fast bacilli should be examined for at least 10 minutes using an oil immersion lens. Mycobacteria will appear pink, often beaded, and slightly curved. Other bacteria will not retain pink dye. (Exceptions: *Nocardia* and the Pittsburgh agent *Legionella micdadei* may also appear acid-fast.) Experience is necessary to distinguish acid-fast bacilli that may be slightly refractile from debris and other artifacts that may be highly refractile. Microbiology laboratories may be able to stain clinical samples for mycobacteria using the auramine-rhodamine technique. Mycobacteria fluoresce when stained in this way. This feature permits rapid screening of many microscopic fields. A positive auramine-rhodamine stain should be confirmed by a Kinyoun acid-fast stain.

India Ink Preparation

A drop of centrifuged CSF is placed on a microscope slide next to a drop of artist's India ink. A coverslip is placed over the drops, and the area of mixing of CSF and India ink is examined at $100 \times$ magnification. Cryptococci are identified by their large capsules, which exclude the India ink (Fig. 93–1). The entire slide should be examined.

KOH Preparation

A drop of sputum, a skin scraping, or a smear of vaginal or oral exudate is placed on a slide together with 1 drop of 5 to 40% KOH. A coverslip is placed on the specimen, and the slide is heated for 2 to 5 seconds above a flame. The condenser of the microscope is lowered, and the specimen is examined at $100 \times$ magnification when searching for elastin fibers (whose presence in sputum suggests a necrotizing pneumonia) or $400 \times$ when looking for fungal forms. The KOH will partially dissolve host cells and bacteria, sparing fungi and elastin fibers.

Tzanck's Preparation

A vesicle suspected of harboring herpesvirus (zoster or simplex) is unroofed with a scalpel, and the base is gently scraped. The scrapings are placed on a glass slide, air-dried, and stained with Wright's stain, Giemsa's stain, or a rapid stain such as methylene blue. The slide is then examined at low ($100 \times$) power for the presence of multinucleated giant cells; their characteristic appearance is then confirmed at high ($400 \times$) power. Demonstration of giant cells is diagnostic for herpesvirus infection.

These simple bedside techniques provide rapid and inexpensive diagnosis of many infectious diseases. There are other techniques that directly visualize pathogens, but they require more sophisticated techniques. Silver staining using the Gomori methenamine technique can identify most fungi and *Pneumocystis carinii*. Experienced pathologists also can identify *P. carinii* on Giemsa-stained specimens of induced sputum. Immunofluorescence techniques using antibodies directed against the organisms rapidly identify pathogens such as *Legionella pneumophila* and *Bordetella pertussis*. Immunofluorescence also can be used to identify cells infected with influenza virus, respiratory syncytial virus, and adenovirus in respiratory secretions. Darkfield microscopy can identify *Treponema pallidum*, and electron microscopy can often detect viral particles in infected cells.

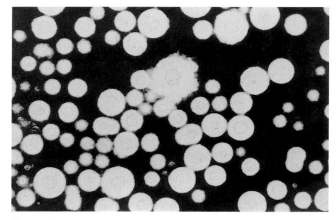

Figure 93–1
India ink preparation of cerebrospinal fluid revealing encapsulated cryptococci. Note the large capsules surrounding the smaller organisms.

DIAGNOSIS BY DETECTION OF MICROBIAL ANTIGENS

Certain pathogens can be detected by examination of specimens for microbial antigens (Table 93–1). These studies can be performed rapidly—often within 1 hour. The diagnosis of meningitis due to *Pneumococcus, Haemophilus*, some strains of meningococci, and *Cryptococcus* can be made rapidly by detection of specific polysaccharide antigen in the CSF using latex agglutination. Although these diagnoses can often be more rapidly made by Gram's stain or India ink preparation, antigen detection is especially helpful when attempts at direct visualization of the pathogen are not diagnostic (e.g., in the patient with partially treated bacterial meningitis). The demonstration of hepatitis B surface antigen in blood establishes the presence of infection by this virus.

TABLE 93–1	Diseases Often Diagnosed by Detection of Microbial Antigens	
Disease	**Assay**	**Agent Detected**
Meningitis	Latex agglutination	*Streptococcus pneumoniae, Haemophilus influenzae, Neisseria meningitidis, Cryptococcus*
Respiratory tract infection	Immunofluorescence	*Bordetella pertussis, Legionella pneumophila*, influenza virus, respiratory syncytial virus, adenovirus
Genitourinary tract infection	Enzyme immunoassay	*Chlamydia* species, herpes simplex virus 1 and 2
Hepatitis	Radioimmunoassay	Hepatitis B surface antigen
Human immunodeficiency virus (HIV) infection	Enzyme immunoassay	HIV p24 core antigen

DIAGNOSIS BY EXAMINATION OF HOST IMMUNE OR INFLAMMATORY RESPONSES

Histopathologic examination of biopsied or excised tissue often reveals patterns of the host inflammatory response that can narrow down diagnostic possibilities. As a general rule, a polymorphonuclear leukocytic infiltrate is compatible with acute infection and suggests a bacterial process. A lymphocytic infiltrate is compatible with a more chronic process and is seen in viral, mycobacterial, fungal, and other nonbacterial infections. Eosinophilia is often seen in helminthic infestations. Granuloma formation suggests mycobacterial and certain fungal infections. Some diseases such as syphilis (obliterative endarteritis), cat-scratch disease (mixed granulomatous, suppurative, and lymphoid hyperplastic changes), and lymphogranuloma venereum (stellate abscesses) have fairly characteristic histologic features. Several viral infections produce characteristic changes in host cells; these may be detected by cytologic examination. Skin or respiratory infection due to herpes viruses, or pneumonia due to cytomegalovirus or measles virus, for example, can be diagnosed with reasonable accuracy by cytologic examination. Similarly, examination of cells and chemistries in infected fluids such as CSF will provide clues to the etiology of the infection. Bacterial infections generally provoke a polymorphonuclear leukocytosis with elevated protein and depressed glucose concentrations. Viral infections most often provoke a lymphocytic pleocytosis; protein elevations are less marked, and glucose levels are usually but not always normal.

Host cell–mediated immune responses can be used to help make certain diagnoses. A positive skin test for delayed-type hypersensitivity to mycobacterial or fungal antigens indicates active or previous infection with these agents. A negative skin test may be seen despite active infection in individuals with depression of cell-mediated immunity (anergy). Therefore, control skin tests using commonly encountered antigens (e.g., *Candida*, mumps, *Trichophyton*) must also be applied to ascertain if the patient can mount a delayed-type hypersensitivity response. Occasionally, the response to disease-related antigens is depressed selectively.

Host humoral responses may be used to diagnose certain infections, particularly those due to organisms whose cultivation is difficult or expensive to perform or hazardous to laboratory personnel (Table 93–2). In general, two sera are obtained at intervals of at least 2 weeks. A fourfold or greater rise (or fall) in antibody titer generally suggests a recent infection. Antibodies of the IgM class also suggest recent infection.

DIAGNOSIS BY DETECTION OF MICROBIAL NUCLEOTIDE SEQUENCES

Detection of microbial nucleotide sequences can provide a sensitive and specific means for identification of pathogens in clinical specimens and rapid speciation of slow growing microbial isolates. Genetic probes are used to rapidly speciate mycobacteria and may be applied soon to

TABLE 93–2	Diseases Often Diagnosed by Measurement of Host Humoral Responses (Antibody Levels)
	Many viral infections
	Mycoplasmal pneumonia
	Rickettsial infections
	Chlamydial infections
	Lyme disease
	Syphilis
	Leptospirosis
	Rheumatic fever
	Legionnaires' disease
	Tularemia
	Brucellosis
	Histoplasmosis
	Coccidioidomycosis
	Amebiasis

identify genetic markers of antimicrobial resistance in bacteria and viruses.

Most standard techniques for detection of microbial antigens cannot reliably detect fewer than 1 million molecules in clinical samples. Gene amplification using the polymerase chain reaction (PCR) can detect as few as three to five molecules in clinical samples. PCR techniques utilize a heat-stable DNA polymerase to amplify microbial nucleotide sequences to levels that are readily detectable. The PCR has been used successfully to diagnose infection with human immunodeficiency virus, cytomegalovirus, herpes simplex virus, *Bartonella henselae*, *Treponema pallidum*, and a variety of other pathogens. It is anticipated that numerous infectious diseases will soon be diagnosed with great sensitivity, using this technique. The exquisite sensitivity of this technique may, however, yield false-positive results unless performed with great care.

DIAGNOSIS BY ISOLATION OF THE ORGANISM IN CULTURE

Isolation of a single microbe from an infected site is generally considered evidence that the infection is due to this organism. However, information obtained from the culture must be interpreted according to the clinical setting. For example, cultures obtained from ordinarily contaminated sites (e.g., vagina, pharynx) may be overgrown with nonpathogenic commensals, and fastidious organisms such as *Neisseria gonorrhoeae* will be difficult to recognize unless cultured on medium that selects for their growth. Similarly, cultures of expectorated "sputum" may also be uninterpretable if heavily contaminated with saliva. The culture of an organism from an infected but ordinarily sterile site is reasonable evidence for infection due to that organism. On the other hand, the failure to culture an organism may simply result from inadequate culture conditions (e.g., "sterile" pus from brain abscess cultured only on aerobic media. Most brain abscesses are caused by anaerobic bacteria that do not grow under the aerobic conditions most commonly utilized.) Thus, when submitting samples for culture, the physician must alert the laboratory to likely pathogens.

Gram's stains of specimens submitted for culture are often invaluable aids to the interpretation of culture results. A Gram's stain of "sputum" will readily detect contamination by saliva if squamous epithelial cells are seen. On the other hand, a Gram's stain revealing bacteria despite negative cultures suggests infection by fastidious organisms. The presence of an organism in high density and within neutrophils also suggests that the corresponding bacterial isolate is causing disease rather than colonizing the patient or contaminating the specimen. Gram staining of the initial clinical specimen may also help determine the relative importance of different isolates when cultures reveal mixed flora.

Viral Isolation

Since all viral pathogens that can be cultured require eukaryotic cells in which to grow, virus isolation is expensive and often laborious. Throat washings, rectal swabs, or cultures of infected sites should be transported immediately to the laboratory or, if this is not possible, placed in virus transport medium—usually an isotonic salt solution containing antibiotics and protein—and refrigerated overnight until they can be cultured in the laboratory. Notifying the laboratory of the suspected pathogens allows selection of the best cell lines for culture. The clinician must be aware of the viruses that the hospital's laboratory can isolate. As the antiviral armamentarium expands, cultivation of viruses will become more routine. A fourfold rise in titer of antibody to the isolated virus suggests that it is causing disease.

Isolation of Rickettsia, Chlamydia, and Mycoplasma

Rickettsiae are cultivated primarily in reference laboratories. Diagnosis of rickettsial illness is generally made on clinical grounds and confirmed serologically. Chlamydiae can be propagated in cell cultures used in most hospital virology laboratories. Mycoplasmas will grow on selective media; the prolonged period of incubation required results in little advantage over serologic diagnosis.

Bacterial Isolation

Isolation of common bacterial pathogens is achieved readily by most hospital laboratories. Specimens should be carried promptly to the laboratory. In instances in which likely isolates may be fastidious (e.g., bacterial meningitis) and laboratories are closed, the specimen should be placed directly onto the culture medium, with careful attention to sterile technique. The specimen is placed onto the culture plate. A loop is sterilized in a flame until it is red, then allowed to cool. The specimen is then streaked on bacteriologic medium. This practice allows separation of different bacterial colonies and rough quantitation of bacterial growth.

Isolation of anaerobic bacteria is often critically important for clinical diagnosis. When anaerobes are suspected, the specimen, if pus or liquid, can be drawn into a syringe, the air expelled, and the syringe capped before transport to the laboratory. Otherwise, specimens must be taken immediately to the laboratory or placed in an anaerobic transport medium appropriate for survival of pathogens. Alternatively, the specimen may be placed in a vial containing thioglycolate broth. This practice will permit anaerobic growth but will not allow quantification of growth. Because of contamination by oral anaerobes, sputum should not be cultured anaerobically unless the sample was obtained by transtracheal or percutaneous lung aspiration.

Isolation of Fungi and Mycobacteria

Specimens for fungal and mycobacterial culture must be processed and cultured by the microbiology laboratory. Although some fungi and rapid-growing mycobacteria grow readily on standard agars used for routine isolation of bacteria, others, such as *Mycobacterium tuberculosis* and *Histoplasma capsulatum*, must be cultured on special media for as long as several weeks.

REFERENCES

Woods GL, Washington JA: The clinician and the microbiology laboratory. *In* Mandell GL, Bennett JC, Dolin R (eds.): Principles and Practice of Infectious Diseases. 4th ed. New York, Churchill Livingstone, 1995, pp 169–198.

Lakeman FD, Whitley RJ, National Institute of Allergy and Infectious Diseases Collaborative Antiviral Study Group: Diagnosis of herpes simplex encephalitis: Application of polymerase chain reaction to cerebrospinal fluid from brain-biopsied patients and correlation with disease. J Infect Dis 1995;171:857–863.

94

Antimicrobial Therapy

The advent of antimicrobial therapy has been the most dramatic advance in medical practice in this century. Antimicrobials are agents that interfere with microbial metabolism, resulting in inhibition of growth or death of bacteria, viruses, fungi, protozoa, or helminths. Some, like penicillin, are natural products of other microbes. Others, such as sulfa drugs, are chemical agents synthesized in the laboratory. Still others are semisynthetic—chemical modifications of naturally occurring substances that result in enhanced activity (e.g., nafcillin) and/or diminished toxicity.

The most effective antimicrobials are characterized by their relatively selective activity against microbes. Some, such as penicillins and amphotericin B, interfere with the synthesis of microbial cell walls that are absent in human cells. Others, such as trimethoprim and sulfa drugs, inhibit obligate microbial synthesis of essential nucleic acid intermediates, pathways not required by human cells. Still others, such as acyclovir, an antiviral agent, are relatively inactive until metabolized by pathogen-derived enzymes. Nonetheless, these agents, although relatively selective in activity against microbes, have variable degrees of toxicity for human cells. Thus, monitoring for toxicity during antimicrobial therapy is important.

In the selection of an antimicrobial agent for a patient, the following factors must be considered.

THE PATHOGEN

If the pathogen has been clearly identified (Chapter 93), a drug with a narrow spectrum of activity (i.e., highly selective for the particular pathogen) is usually the most reasonable choice. If the pathogen responsible for the patient's illness has not been identified, then the physician must choose a drug or combination of drugs active against the most likely pathogens in the specific setting. In either instance, the physician must be guided by patterns of antimicrobial resistance common in the community and in the specific hospital. Some pathogens (e.g., group A streptococci) are almost always sensitive to narrow-spectrum antimicrobials such as penicillin. Other pathogens such as staphylococci are variably resistant to penicillins but almost always susceptible to vancomycin. Resistance patterns, particularly among hospital-acquired bacteria, may vary widely and are important in devising antimicrobial strategies. Broad-spectrum antimicrobial coverage for all febrile patients ("shotgunning") must not be substituted for carefully evaluating the clinical problem and pinpointing therapy directed toward the most likely pathogen or pathogens. Widespread use of broad-spectrum antimicrobials almost invariably leads to emergence of resistant strains. On the other hand, the more sick a patient appears and the less certain the physician is of the responsible pathogen, the more important initial empiric broad-spectrum coverage becomes. Initial empiric treatment is also frequently indicated in the immunocompromised febrile patient (e.g., the patient with severe neutropenia secondary to chemotherapy). Once the pathogen is isolated and its antimicrobial sensitivities are known, empiric therapy must be scaled down to a definitive regimen with narrow and optimal activity against the specific microorganism.

SITE OF INFECTION

The location of the infection is also important in determining the selection and dosage of an antimicrobial. Deep-seated infections and bacteremic infections generally require higher doses of antimicrobials than, for example, superficial infections of the skin, upper respiratory tract, or lower urinary tract. Penetration of various antimicrobials into sites such as meninges, eye, and prostate is quite variable. Thus, treatment of infections at these sites involves selection of an antimicrobial agent that penetrates these tissues in concentrations sufficient to inhibit or kill the pathogen. The meninges are relatively resistant to penetration by most antimicrobials; inflammation renders the meninges somewhat more permeable. Therefore, high doses of antibiotics are the rule when treating meningitis. Bacterial infections of certain sites such as the heart valves or meninges must be treated with antibiotics that kill the microbe (bactericidal) as opposed to simply inhibiting its growth (bacteriostatic). This is so because local host defenses at these sites are inadequate to rid the host of infecting organisms. Infections involving foreign bodies are often difficult to eradicate without removing the foreign material.

Antimicrobials alone are often insufficient in the treatment of large abscesses. Although many drugs achieve reasonable concentrations in abscess walls, the

TABLE 94–1	Characteristics of Commonly Used Antimicrobial Agents

Drug Class	Site of Action	CNS Penetration	Excretion	Uses/Activity
Antibacterials				
Beta-lactams				
Penicillins	Cell wall	+/−	Renal	Streptococci, *Neisseria,* oral anaerobes
Beta-lactamase–resistant penicillins, e.g., nafcillin	Cell wall	+/−	Renal and/or hepatic	Methicillin-sensitive staphylococci
Amino penicillins, e.g., ampicillin	Cell wall	+/−	Renal	Gram-positive organisms, not staphylococci, some gram-negative organisms
Extended-spectrum penicillins, e.g., mezlocillin	Cell wall	+/−	Renal	Broad-spectrum gram-positive organisms; gram-negative organisms, including *Pseudomonas,* not *Staphylococcus*
Beta-lactamase inhibitors, e.g., clavulanic acid	Inactivates beta-lactamase	−	Renal/metabolic	Used with ampicillin or ticarcillin, expands activity to include anaerobes, many gram-negative organisms, and methicillin-sensitive staphylococci
Cephalosporins*	Cell wall			
First generation, e.g., cefazolin		−	Renal	Broad spectrum
Second generation, e.g., cefuroxime		+/−	Renal	Some with anaerobic activity, e.g., cefoxitin
Third generation, e.g., ceftriaxone		+	Renal or hepatic	Some active against *Pseudomonas,* e.g., ceftazidime
Monobactams				
Aztreonam	Cell wall	+/−	Renal	Aerobic gram-negative bacilli
Carbapenems				
Imipenem/cilastatin	Cell wall	+/−	Renal	Very broad-spectrum, some enterococci, and methicillin-sensitive staphylococci
Vancomycin	Cell wall	+/−	Renal	Coagulase-positive and -negative staphylococci, other gram-positive bacteria
Sulfonamides/trimethoprim	Inhibit nucleic acid synthesis	+	Renal	Gram-negative bacilli, *Salmonella, Pneumocystis carinii, Nocardia*
Quinolones	DNA gyrase	+/−	Some hepatic metabolism	Very broad spectrum, not including streptococci or anaerobes
Metronidazole	DNA disruption	+	Hepatic metabolism	Anaerobes, *Clostridium difficile,* amebas, *Trichomonas*
Rifampin	Transcription	+	Hepatic metabolism/renal	*Mycobacterium tuberculosis;* meningococcal and *Haemophilus influenzae* prophylaxis
Aminoglycosides	Ribosome	−	Renal	Gram-negative bacilli; no activity in anaerobic conditions
Chloramphenicol	Ribosome	+	Hepatic metabolism/renal	Broad spectrum; especially useful for *Salmonella,* anaerobes, *Rickettsia*
Clindamycin	Ribosome	−	Hepatic metabolism/renal	Anaerobes; gram-positive cocci
Tetracyclines	Ribosome	+/−	Renal/hepatic metabolism	Broad spectrum; especially useful for spirochetes, *Rickettsia*
Macrolides/Azalides				
Erythromycin	Ribosome	−	Hepatic	Gram-positive cocci, *Legionella, Mycoplasma*
Azithromycin Clarithromycin	Ribosome	+	Hepatic	High intracellular levels have enhanced activity against mycobacteria, *Toxoplasma*
Antifungals				
Polyenes				
Amphotericin B	Binds membrane ergosterol	+/−	?	Most fungi
Nystatin	Binds membrane ergosterol	−	Fecal	Mucosal candidiasis
Flucytosine	Blocks DNA synthesis	−	Renal	Candidiasis; *Cryptococcus* with amphotericin B
Azoles	Block ergosterol biosynthesis	+	Renal	
Ketoconazole		−	Hepatic	Mucosal candidiasis, pulmonary histoplasmosis (nonmeningeal)
Itraconazole		−	Hepatic	Histoplasmosis, blastomycosis
Fluconazole		+	Renal	Candidiasis, cryptococcosis, coccidioidomycosis

TABLE 94–1	Characteristics of Commonly Used Antimicrobial Agents *Continued*

Drug Class	Site of Action	CNS Penetration	Excretion	Uses/Activity
Antivirals				
Acyclovir	DNA polymerase	+	Renal	Herpes simplex, including encephalitis; herpes zoster in immunosuppressed hosts
Ganciclovir	DNA polymerase	+	Renal	Cytomegalovirus, herpesviruses
Foscarnet	DNA polymerase	+	Renal	Cytomegalovirus, herpesviruses, ?HIV
Amantadine/rimantadine	?Uncoating	+	Renal	Influenza A treatment and prophylaxis
Vidarabine	DNA polymerase	+	Renal	Neonatal herpes simplex
Zidovudine (AZT)	Reverse transcriptase	+	Hepatic glucuronidation/renal	HIV
Didanosine (ddl)	Reverse transcriptase	+/−	Renal	HIV
Zalcitabine (ddC)	Reverse transcriptase	?	Renal	HIV
Lamivudine (3TC)	Reverse transcriptase	−	Renal	HIV, hepatitis B
Stavudine (d4T)	Reverse transcriptase	−	Renal/?	HIV
Nevirapine	Reverse transcriptase	−	Hepatic/renal	HIV
Saquinavir	Protease	−	Hepatic	HIV
Indinavir	Protease	−	Hepatic/renal	HIV
Ritonavir	Protease	−	Hepatic	HIV
Ribavirin	?RNA synthesis	+	Hepatic/renal	RSV, ?influenza, ?hemorrhagic fever, ?Lassa fever

* As a rule, first-generation cephalosporins have better activity against gram-positive cocci and minimal CNS penetration. Second-generation cephalosporins have somewhat better activity against gram-negative bacteria and may penetrate the CNS. Third-generation cephalosporins have the broadest activity against gram-negative bacteria and generally penetrate the CNS, but they are relatively less active against gram-positive cocci.
CNS = Central nervous system; HIV = human immunodeficiency virus; RSV = respiratory syncytial virus.

low pH antagonizes the activity of some drugs (e.g., aminoglycosides), and some drugs bind to and are inactivated by white blood cells or their products. The large number of organisms, their depressed metabolism in this unfavorable milieu, and the frequent polymicrobial nature of certain abscesses increase the likelihood that some organisms present may be resistant to antimicrobial therapy. Most extracranial abscesses should be drained whenever anatomically possible.

CHARACTERISTICS OF THE ANTIMICROBIAL

The physician must know the pharmacokinetics of the drug (i.e., its absorption, its penetration into various sites, its metabolism and excretion) and its toxicity, as well as its spectrum of antimicrobial activity, before selecting it for use (Table 94–1).

Distribution and Excretion

Lipid-soluble drugs, such as chloramphenicol and rifampin, penetrate most membranes, including the meninges, more readily than do more ionized compounds, such as the aminoglycosides. The physician must be certain that the drug concentration achievable at the site of infection is sufficient to inhibit or kill the pathogen. Understanding a drug's distribution, rate and site of metabolism, and route of excretion is essential in selecting the appropriate drug and dose. Drugs excreted unchanged in the urine may be particularly good for the treatment of lower urinary tract infection or for the treatment of systemic infection in the presence of renal insufficiency. Some antimicrobials are metabolized in the liver and must be adjusted appropriately in the presence of hepatic insufficiency.

Activity of the Drug

The physician must understand both the spectrum of activity of the drug against microbial isolates and the mechanism of activity of the agent and whether it is bactericidal or bacteriostatic in achievable concentrations. As a general rule, cell wall–active drugs are likely to be bactericidal. Bactericidal drugs are necessary for treatment of infections sequestered from an effective host inflammatory response such as meningitis and endocarditis. With the exception of aminoglycosides and certain azalide and macrolide antibiotics, agents inhibiting protein synthesis at ribosomal sites are generally bacteriostatic.

Toxicity of the Drug

The physician must have a thorough understanding of the contraindications of the drug, as well as the major toxicities of the drug and their general frequency. This will help in evaluating the risks of treatment and also will assist in advising the patient about the drug's effects and in anticipating possible adverse reactions. History of drug hypersensitivity must be sought before prescribing any antimicrobials. The presence or absence of previous reactions to penicillin should be documented for every patient. Patients with a history suggestive of immediate hypersensitivity to penicillin, such as hives, wheezing, hypotension, laryngospasm, or angioedema at any site, must be considered at risk for anaphylaxis. These patients should not receive penicillins or related drugs (cephalosporins) if adequate alternatives are available. The major and minor determinants of penicillin allergy (breakdown products that bind to serum proteins to form haptens) can be used to detect most persons at risk for serious immediate hypersensitivity. If skin test reactivity to these determinants is present and there are no reasonable alternatives to therapy with a penicillin or related compound, these patients may be desensitized to penicillin using a graduated protocol of intracutaneous penicillin administration. Desensitization should be done only in consultation with an experienced allergist. Patients with a history of an uncomplicated morbilliform or delayed rash after penicillin therapy are not likely to be at risk for immediate hypersensitivity and may be treated with cephalosporins, for which the risk of cross-hypersensitivity to penicillins is likely to be in the range of 5%. Patients with immediate hypersensitivity reactions to penicillin are also at risk for anaphylactic reactions to cephalosporins and imipenem. Evidence to date suggests that cross-hypersensitivity to aztreonam is less common.

ROUTE OF ADMINISTRATION

Oral administration of antimicrobials can often prevent the morbidity and expense associated with parenteral (intravenous or intramuscular) administration. Although some antimicrobials (e.g., amoxicillin and the fluoroquinolones) are very well absorbed after oral administration, most patients hospitalized with severe infections should, at least initially, be treated with intravenous antibiotics. Gut absorption of antimicrobials can be unpredictable, and the intravenous route often permits administration of greater amounts of drug than can be tolerated orally. Intramuscular administration of some antimicrobials can result in excellent drug absorption but should be avoided in the presence of hypotension (erratic absorption) and coagulation disorders (hematomas). Repeated intramuscular injections are uncomfortable and also can result in the formation of sterile abscesses (e.g., pentamidine).

Duration of Therapy

Antimicrobial therapy should be initiated as part of a treatment plan of defined duration. In some settings, the duration of optimal antimicrobial therapy is established (e.g., 10 days but not 7 days of oral penicillin will prevent rheumatic fever after streptococcal pharyngitis); in many others, the duration of treatment is empiric and sometimes can be based on the clinical and bacteriologic course. Blood stream infections without endocarditis or other focal infections can generally be treated for 10 to 14 days. Pneumococcal pneumonia can be effectively treated in 7 to 10 days. The duration of therapy for endocarditis is largely dictated by the characteristics of the culpable microorganism but generally is at least 4 weeks.

Combinations

Combinations of antimicrobials are indicated in serious infection when they provide more effective activity against a pathogen than any single agent. In some instances, combinations of drugs are used to prevent the emergence of resistance (e.g., infections due to *Mycobacterium tuberculosis*). In others, combinations are used because they provide synergistic action against the pathogen (e.g., penicillin, a cell wall–activity antibiotic, facilitates uptake of aminoglycosides by enterococci). In still other instances, drug combinations are used in empiric therapies to cover a wide spectrum of potential pathogens when the causative agent is unidentified or when infection is likely to be due to a mixture of organisms (e.g., fecal soilage of the peritoneum). Use of more than one drug increases the likelihood of toxicity, increases costs, and often increases the risk of superinfection.

MONITORING OF ANTIMICROBIAL THERAPY

The physician (and patient) should be alert to potential toxicities and should be prepared to halt the drug in the event of serious toxicity. For some antimicrobials, such as aminoglycosides, the ratio of effective to toxic drug levels is low. Thus, serum levels of the drug must be monitored to ensure appropriate dosing. For some infections (e.g., infective endocarditis due to relatively resistant organisms), monitoring of antimicrobial activity in serum shortly after (peak) and just before (trough) drug administration may help guide antimicrobial choices and usage. Although these techniques are not well standardized, clinicians often adjust drugs and doses to maintain serum bactericidal titers of at least 1:8 in treating certain forms of endocarditis (e.g., enterococcal) in which the antimicrobial resistance pattern of the microorganism may be quite variable.

ANTIVIRAL AGENTS

As obligate intracellular pathogens, viruses depend upon interactions with host cellular machinery for completion of the life cycle. Thus, many potential antiviral treatment strategies are limited by toxicities to host cells. Specificity for viruses or virus-infected cells can be obtained by interfering with the function of unique viral elements, such as the M2 protein of influenza virus that is the target of amantadine and rimantadine, or by developing drugs such as acyclovir that must be processed by viral enzymes (in this instance, phosphorylated by herpesvirus thymidine kinase) before becoming active. Recent years have seen a dramatic increase in the numbers and types of drugs effective in the treatment of viral infections. In contrast to antibacterial drugs, however, antiviral agents generally have a limited spectrum of activity, with each agent useful against a small number of viruses (see Chapter 108).

ANTIFUNGAL AGENTS

A number of drugs are useful in the treatment of fungal diseases. Most target the ergosterol-containing cell membrane either by inhibiting ergosterol synthesis (azoles) or by aggregating in proximity to ergosterol and increasing membrane permeability (polyenes). Flucytosine inhibits fungal DNA synthesis. Increasing resistance to azoles and flucytosine among clinically relevant fungal isolates is limiting the utility of these agents in patients requiring chronic therapy.

REFERENCES

Moellering RC: Principles of antiinfective therapy. *In* Mandell GL, Bennett JC, Dolin R (eds.): Principles and Practice of Infectious Diseases. 4th ed. New York, Churchill Livingstone, 1995, pp 199–212.
Whitley RJ: Antiviral therapy (non-AIDS). *In* Bennett JC, Plum F (eds.): Cecil Textbook of Medicine. 20th ed. Philadelphia, WB Saunders, 1996, pp 1742–1747.

95

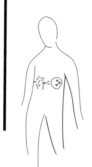

Fever and Febrile Syndromes

REGULATION OF BODY TEMPERATURE

Although "normal" body temperature ranges vary considerably, oral temperature readings in excess of 37.8°C (100.2°F) are generally abnormal. In healthy humans, core body temperature is maintained within a narrow range, so that for each individual, daily temperature variations greater than 1 to 1.5°C are distinctly unusual. This homeostasis is controlled by hypothalamic nuclei that establish "set points" for body temperature. Homeostasis is effected by a complex balance between heat-generating and heat-conserving mechanisms that raise body temperature, on the one hand, and mechanisms that dissipate heat and lower body temperature, on the other (Table 95–1). Heat is regularly generated as a by-product of obligate energy utilization (e.g., cellular metabolism, myocardial contraction, breathing). When an increase in body temperature is needed, shivering—nondirected muscular contraction—generates large amounts of heat. Peripheral vessels constrict to diminish heat lost to the environment. At the same time, the person feels cold; this heat preference promotes heat-conserving behavior, such as wrapping up in a blanket.

Obligate heat loss to the environment occurs through the skin and by evaporation of water through sweat and respiration. When the body must cool down, heat loss is promoted. Vasodilation flushes the skin capillaries, temporarily raising skin temperature but ultimately lowering core body temperature by increasing heat loss through the skin to the cooler environment. Sweating promotes rapid heat loss via evaporation, and at the same time, the subject feels warm and sheds blankets or initiates other activities to promote heat loss.

FEVER AND HYPERTHERMIA

Fever is an elevated body temperature that is mediated by an increase in the hypothalamic heat-regulating set point. Thus, although fever may be precipitated by exogenous substances such as bacterial products, the increase in body temperature is achieved through physiologic mechanisms. In contrast, hyperthermia is an increase in body temperature that overrides or bypasses the normal homeostatic mechanisms. As a general rule, body temperatures

in excess of 41°C are rarely physiologically mediated and suggest hyperthermia. Hyperthermia may be seen after vigorous exercise, in patients with heat stroke, as a heritable reaction to anesthetics (malignant hyperthermia), as a response to phenothiazines (neuroleptic malignant syndrome), and occasionally in patients with central nervous system disorders such as paraplegia (see also Chapter 113). Some patients with severe dermatoses are also unable to dissipate heat and therefore experience hyperthermia.

Fever usually is a physiologic response to infection or inflammation. Monocytes or tissue macrophages are activated by various stimuli to liberate various cytokines with pyrogenic activity (Fig. 95–1). Interleukin (IL)-1 is also an essential cofactor in initiation of the immune response. Another pyrogenic cytokine, tumor necrosis factor (TNF) α, or cachectin, activates lipoprotein lipase and also may play a role in immune cytolysis. Another cytokine, TNFβ, or lymphotoxin, has similar properties. A fourth, interferon-alpha, has antiviral activity (see Chapter 92). IL6, a cytokine that potentiates B cell immunoglobulin synthesis, also has pyrogenic activity. Endogenous pyrogens activate the anterior preoptic nuclei of the hypothalamus to raise the set point for body temperature by the mechanisms shown in Table 95–1. A list of classes of disorders that can cause fever is shown in Table 95–2. Infection by all types of microorganisms can be associated with fever. Tissue injury with resultant inflammation, as is seen in myocardial or pulmonary infarction or after trauma, can produce fever. Certain malignancies such as lymphoma, renal carcinoma, and hepatic carcinoma are also associated with fever; in some instances, this is related to liberation of endogenous pyrogen by monocytes in the inflammatory response surrounding the tumor, and in other cases, the malignant cell may release an endogenous pyrogen. Many immunologically mediated disorders, such as connective tissue diseases, serum sickness, and some drug reactions, are characterized by fever. In most cases of drug-induced fevers, the mechanisms of fever are unknown. Virtually any disorder associated with an inflammatory response (e.g., gouty arthritis) can be associated with fever. Certain endocrine disorders such as thyrotoxicosis, adrenal insufficiency, and pheochromocytoma also can produce fever.

The association of fever with infections or inflammatory disorders raises the question of whether fever is

TABLE 95-1	Mechanisms of Heat Regulation

To Raise Body Temperature

Heat generation
    Obligate heat production
    Muscular work
    Shivering
Heat conservation
    Vasoconstriction
    Heat preference

To Lower Body Temperature

Heat loss
    Obligate heat loss
    Vasodilatation
    Sweating
    Cold preference

TABLE 95-2	Causes of Fever

Infection
Tissue injury—infarction, trauma
Malignancy
Drugs
Immune-mediated disorders
Other inflammatory disorders
Endocrine disorders

beneficial to the host. For example, IL1 (an endogenous pyrogen) is critical for initiation of the immune response, certain *in vitro* immune responses are marginally enhanced by elevated temperatures, and some infectious organisms prefer cooler temperatures. It is not certain, however, that fever is helpful to humans in any infectious disease with the possible exception of neurosyphilis. Fever is deleterious in certain situations. Among individuals with underlying brain disease, and even in the healthy elderly, fever can produce disorientation and confusion. Fever and associated tachycardia may compromise patients, especially the elderly, with significant cardiopulmonary disease. In young children, fever can result in seizures. Fever should be controlled if the patient is particularly uncomfortable or whenever it poses a specific risk to the patient. Fever in children with a history of febrile seizures and in patients with severe congestive heart failure or recent myocardial infarction should be treated with antipyretics, such as salicylates or acetaminophen. Acetaminophen or nonsteroidal anti-inflammatory drugs (NSAIDs) are preferred for children because of the association of salicylates with Reye's syndrome.

Heat stroke almost always results from prolonged exposure to high environmental temperature and humidity, usually associated, in otherwise healthy individuals, with strenuous exercise. It is characterized by a body temperature greater than 40.6°C and is associated with

altered sensorium or coma and with cessation of sweating. Rapid cooling is critical to the patient's survival. Covering the patient with cold (11°C), wet compresses until core temperature reaches 39°C is the most effective initial therapeutic approach and should be followed by intravenous infusions of fluids appropriate to correct the antecedent fluid and electrolyte losses.

Fever Patterns

The normal diurnal variation in body temperature results in a peak temperature in the late afternoon or early evening. This variation often persists when patients have fever. In certain instances, fever patterns may be helpful in suggesting the cause of fever. Rigors—true shaking chills—often herald a bacterial process (especially blood stream infection), although they may occur in cases of viral infection, as well as in drug or transfusion reactions. Hectic fevers, characterized by wide swings in temperature, may indicate the presence of an abscess, disseminated tuberculosis, or collagen vascular diseases. Patients with malaria may have a relapsing fever with episodes of shaking chills and high fever, separated by 1 to 3 days of normal body temperature and relative well-being. Patients with tuberculosis may be relatively comfortable and unaware of a markedly elevated body temperature. Patients with uremia, diabetic ketoacidosis, or hepatic failure generally have a lowered body temperature, and "normal" temperature readings in these settings may indicate infection. Similarly, elderly patients with infection often fail to mount a febrile response and may present instead with loss of appetite, confusion, or even hypotension without

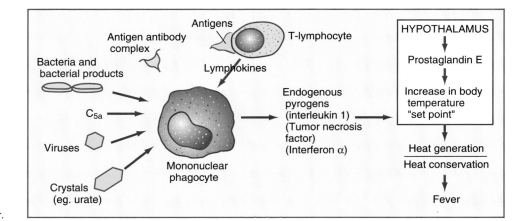

Figure 95-1
Pathogenesis of fever.

fever. The administration of anti-inflammatory drugs (aspirin, NSAIDs, corticosteroids) also blunts or ablates the febrile response.

ACUTE FEBRILE SYNDROMES

Fever is one of the most common complaints that brings patients to a physician. The challenge is in discerning the few individuals who require specific therapy from among the many with self-limited benign illness. The approach is simplified by considering patients in three groups: (1) those with fever without localizing symptoms and signs, (2) those with fever and rash, and (3) those with fever and lymphadenopathy. This chapter deals only with fever caused by microbial agents. Clearly, autoimmune, neoplastic, and other disease processes may cause fever as well (see Table 95–2).

Fever Only

Most patients with fever as their sole complaint defervesce spontaneously or present with localizing clinical or laboratory findings within 2 to 3 weeks of onset of illness (Table 95–3). Beyond 3 weeks, the patient can be considered to have a fever of unexplained or unknown origin (FUO), a designation with its own circumscribed group of management considerations, as discussed here.

Viral Infections

In young, healthy individuals, acute febrile illnesses generally represent viral infections. The causative agent is rarely established, largely because establishing the precise diagnosis seldom has major therapeutic implications. Rhinovirus, parainfluenza, or adenovirus infections usually, but not invariably, are associated with symptoms of coryza or upper respiratory tract infection (rhinorrhea, sore throat, cough, hoarseness). Enterovirus and enteric cytopathogenic human orphan (ECHO) virus infections occur predominantly in summer, usually in an epidemic setting. Undifferentiated febrile syndromes account for the majority of enteroviral infections, but the etiology is more likely to be established definitively when a macular rash, aseptic meningitis, or a characteristic syndrome such as herpangina (vesicular pharyngitis due to coxsackievirus A) or acute pleurodynia (fever, chest wall pain, and tenderness due to coxsackievirus B) is present. Serologic surveys also indicate that many arthropod-borne viruses (California encephalitis virus; eastern, western, and Venezuelan equine encephalitis; St. Louis encephalitis) usually produce mild, self-limited febrile illnesses. Influenza causes myalgias, arthralgias, and headache in addition to fever; it most often occurs in an epidemic pattern during the winter months. It is unusual, however, for fever to persist beyond 5 days in uncomplicated influenza.

The mononucleosis syndromes caused by Epstein-Barr virus, cytomegalovirus, and (rarely) *Toxoplasma gondii* may present in a typhoidal manner—that is, with fever but little or no lymphadenopathy. Diagnosis and management are discussed later under "Generalized Lymphadenopathy," the more typical presentation of these processes.

Colorado tick fever is a disease caused by arbovirus and transmitted by tick bite. Viremia is prolonged, lasting about 4 weeks. The illness is biphasic—2 to 3 days of fever followed by a similar period of remission, then a second febrile episode. Some patients have rash, pericarditis, or aseptic meningitis.

The syndromes just described are self-limited and untreatable. The impetus for establishing a specific diagnosis, therefore, is small. The differentiation between viral and other causes of febrile illnesses is, on the other hand, of critical importance. Viral cultures of throat and rectum and virus-specific antibodies in acute and convalescent serum samples may allow retrospective diagnosis of viral etiology. Usually, however, the fever is gone long before results of serologies become available.

Bacterial Infections

Bacterial disease may cause septicemia, which dominates the clinical presentation (see Chapter 96). *Staphylococcus aureus* frequently causes sepsis, sometimes without an obvious primary site of infection. Fever may be the predominant clinical manifestation of the illness. *S. aureus* sepsis should be considered in patients undergoing intravenous therapy with a plastic cannula, hemodialysis patients, intravenous drug users, and patients with severe chronic dermatoses. In the patient with *S. aureus* bacteremia, the question of whether intravascular infection exists is key in determining the length of therapy. The following are more typical of endocarditis: community-acquired infection, long duration of symptoms, absence of removable focus of infection (e.g., intravenous cannula, soft tissue abscess), metastatic sites of infection (e.g., septic pulmonary emboli, arthritis, meningitis), and new heart murmur. *Listeria monocytogenes* septicemia is seen predominantly in patients with depressed cell-mediated immunity. One half of patients with *Listeria* sepsis have meningitis. Occasionally, a relatively indolent clinical syndrome belies the bacterial etiology of *S. aureus* and *L. monocytogenes* bacteremia.

Enteric fevers also may present in a subacute fashion despite the presence of bacteremia. The major species producing this syndrome are *Salmonella typhi,* which has a human reservoir, and *Salmonella paratyphi* A, B, and C. The paratyphoid strains also have their major reservoir in humans but produce less severe disease than *S. typhi. S. typhi* is acquired by ingestion of food or water contaminated with fecal material from a chronic carrier or a patient with typhoid fever. A large number of bacteria (10^6 to 10^8) must be ingested to cause disease in the normal host. Major host risk factors are achlorhydria, malnutrition, malignancy (particularly lymphomas and leukemias), sickle cell anemia, and other defects in cellular and humoral immunity. Major protective mechanisms are gastric acidity and fatty acid products of bacteria composing the normal gut flora. *S. typhi* penetrates the gut wall and enters the lymphoid follicles (Peyer's patches), where it multiplies within mononuclear phago-

TABLE 95–3	Infections Presenting as Fever Without Localizing Signs or Symptoms		
Infectious Agent	**Epidemiology/Exposure History**	**Distinctive Clinical and Laboratory Findings**	**Diagnosis**
Viral			
Rhinovirus, adenovirus, parainfluenza	None (adenovirus in epidemics)	Often URI symptoms	Throat and rectal cultures, serologies
Enterovirus, ECHO virus	Summer, epidemic	Occasionally, aseptic meningitis, rash, pleurodynia, herpangina	Throat and rectal cultures, serologies
Influenza	Winter, epidemic	Headache, myalgias, arthralgias	Throat cultures, serologies
EBV, CMV	(See text)		
Colorado tick fever	Southwest, Northwest, tick exposure	Biphasic illness, leukopenia	Blood, CSF cultures, erythrocyte-associated viral antigen (indirect immunofluorescence)
Bacterial			
Staphylococcus aureus	IV drug users, patients with IV plastic cannulas, hemodialysis, dermatitis	Must exclude endocarditis	Blood cultures
Listeria monocytogenes	Depressed cell-mediated immunity	One half have meningitis	Blood, CSF cultures
Salmonella typhi, Salmonella paratyphi	Food or water contaminated by carrier or patient	Headache, myalgias, diarrhea or constipation, transient rose spots	Early blood, bone marrow cultures; late stool culture
Streptococci	Valvular heart disease	Low-grade fever, fatigue, anemia	Blood cultures
Post Animal Exposure			
Coxiella burnetii (Q fever)	Infected livestock	Retrobulbar headache, occasionally pneumonitis, hepatitis, culture-negative endocarditis	Serologies
Leptospira interrogans	Water contaminated by urine from dogs, cats, rodents, small mammals	Headache, myalgias, conjunctival suffusion Biphasic illness Aseptic meningitis	Serologies
Brucella species	Exposure to cattle or contaminated dairy products	Occasionally epididymitis	Blood cultures, serologies
Ehrlichia chaffeensis	South and Southeast, deer or dog tick exposure	Acute onset of headache, fever, myalgias; leukopenia and thrombocytopenia	PCR, serologies
Granulomatous Infection			
Mycobacterium tuberculosis	Exposure to patient with tuberculosis, known positive tuberculin skin test	Back pain suggests vertebral infection; sterile pyuria or hematuria suggests renal infection	Liver, bone marrow histology, cultures
Histoplasma capsulatum	Mississippi and Ohio River valleys	Pneumonitis, oropharyngeal lesions	Serologies; histology and cultures on liver, bone marrow, oral lesions

CMV = Cytomegalovirus; CSF = cerebrospinal fluid; EBV = Epstein-Barr virus; ECHO = enteric cytopathogenic human orphan; IV = intravenous; PCR = polymerase chain reaction; URI = upper respiratory infection.

cytes and produces local ulceration. Primary bacteremia occurs with spread to the reticuloendothelial system (liver, spleen, and bone marrow). After further multiplication at those sites, a secondary bacteremia occurs and can localize to lesions such as tumors, aneurysms, and bone infarcts. Infection of the gallbladder, particularly in the presence of gallstones, leads to the chronic carrier state. Approximately 2 weeks after exposure, patients develop prolonged fever with chills, headache, and myalgias. Diarrhea or constipation may be present but usually does not dominate the clinical picture. Occasionally, crops of rose spots (2- to 4-mm erythematous maculopapular le-

sions) appear on the upper abdomen but are evanescent. Untreated, typhoid fever usually resolves in about 1 month. However, complication rates are high owing to bowel perforation, metastatic infection, and general debility of patients. *S. typhi* may be isolated from blood or stool to confirm the diagnosis. Culture of the bone marrow often is positive early in the course of disease. Typhoid fever should be treated with chloramphenicol, 50 mg/kg/day given intravenously or orally, for 2 weeks. Chloramphenicol-resistant strains of *S. typhi* have appeared in Mexico, India, and Vietnam and should be treated with third-generation cephalosporins or fluoroquinolones. Bactericidal agents become the drug of choice in endocarditis or infected aneurysms and in patients with sickle cell anemia, in whom the dose-related bone marrow suppression by chloramphenicol is unacceptable.

Localized bacterial infection can be clinically occult and present as an undifferentiated febrile syndrome. Intraabdominal abscess, vertebral osteomyelitis due to *S. aureus* or *Pseudomonas aeruginosa,* streptococcal pharyngitis, urinary tract infection, infective endocarditis, and early pneumonia may all cause fever with surprisingly few clinical clues to the location of the infection. Therefore, urinalysis, throat and blood cultures, and chest radiography should be performed in the febrile patient presenting with features suggestive of a bacterial infection.

Febrile Syndromes Associated with Animal Exposure

Q fever, brucellosis, and leptospirosis are diseases associated with exposure to fluids from infected animals and may have similar clinical presentations.

Q FEVER. Q fever is an underrecognized cause of acute febrile illness. *Coxiella burnetii,* the causative agent, produces mild infection in livestock. Humans are infected by inhalation of aerosolized particles or by contact with placental and amniotic fluids from infected animals. The source of animal exposure may go unnoticed. For example, in an outbreak of Q fever at the University of Colorado Medical School, 70% of infected individuals lacked direct exposure to infected sheep.

Q fever characteristically begins explosively with severe, often retrobulbar headache, high fever, chills, and myalgias. Pneumonitis and hepatitis may occur but are seldom severe. Diagnosis usually is based on a fourfold rise in titer of complement-fixing antibodies. Untreated, Q fever lasts 2 to 14 days. *C. burnetii* is sensitive to tetracycline, which should be used in its treatment (2 gm/day orally for 14 days). Q fever may cause endocarditis, apparently as a form of reactivation of infection. The occurrence of hepatomegaly and thrombocytopenia in a patient with apparently culture-negative endocarditis may be a clue to this diagnosis.

LEPTOSPIROSIS. Humans are infected with *Leptospira interrogans* by exposure to urine from infected dogs, cats, wild mammals, and rodents. Exposure on the farm, in the slaughterhouse, on camping trips, or during swims in contaminated water is frequent. After an incubation period of about 1 week, patients develop chills, high fever, headache, and myalgias. The illness often pursues a biphasic course. During the second phase of illness, fever is less prominent, but headache and myalgias are excruciating, and nausea, vomiting, and abdominal pain become prominent complaints. Aseptic meningitis is the most important manifestation of the second or immune phase of the illness. Suffusion of the bulbar conjunctivae, with visible corkscrew vessels surrounding the limbus, is a useful early sign, suggesting the diagnosis of leptospirosis. Lymphadenopathy, hepatomegaly, and splenomegaly may occur. Leptospirosis also may pursue a more severe clinical course characterized by renal and hepatic dysfunction

and hemorrhagic diathesis. Although darkfield examination will reveal leptospires in body fluids, most laboratories do not have the expertise to identify the organisms. The diagnosis is made, rather, by a fourfold rise in indirect hemagglutination antibody titer. Antibiotic treatment shortens the duration of fever and may reduce complications. However, to be effective, antibiotics must be initiated presumptively, before serologic confirmation. Penicillin G, 2.4 to 3.6 million units/day, or tetracycline, 2.0 gm/day given orally, is effective therapy.

BRUCELLOSIS. *Brucella* species infect the genitourinary tract of cattle *(Brucella abortus),* pigs *(Brucella suis),* and goats *(Brucella mellitensis).* Humans are exposed occupationally or by ingestion of unpasteurized dairy products. Acute disease is characterized by chills, fever, headache, arthralgias, and sometimes lymphadenopathy, hepatomegaly, and splenomegaly. During the associated bacteremia, any organ may be seeded. Epididymo-orchitis is one of the more characteristic findings. With or without antibiotic treatment of the acute infection, brucellosis may relapse or enter a chronic phase. *Brucella* species can be isolated from blood or other normally sterile fluids. However, the laboratory should be alerted to the suspicion of this infection, since the organism requires special conditions for growth. Otherwise, diagnosis must be made serologically. Treatment consists of doxycycline, 100 mg bid, and rifampin, 600 mg qd given orally for 21 days. Trimethoprim, 480 mg/day, with sulfamethoxazole, 2400 mg/day given orally, is an acceptable alternative regimen, but relapses may be more frequent.

CAT-SCRATCH DISEASE. Tender enlargement of a regional lymph node, sometimes associated with low-grade fever, is the major manifestation of this illness, which is caused by a small bacillus, *Bartonella henselae,* usually introduced by the scratch of a domestic cat. In most instances, a papule or small pustule develops at the inoculation site, distal to the painful lymph node, within 2 weeks after the scratch. Although the painful lymph node enlargement usually persists for 2 to 4 months, sometimes longer, resolution almost always occurs without specific antimicrobial therapy in the immunocompetent host.

Granulomatous Infection

TUBERCULOSIS. Extrapulmonary and miliary tuberculosis may present as febrile syndromes. In disseminated tuberculosis, initial chest radiographs may be normal, and tuberculin skin tests often are nonreactive. This is particularly true in elderly patients. Protracted fevers of uncertain origin should always suggest this possibility. Liver biopsy and bone marrow biopsy should be performed and have a high yield in miliary disease. Genitourinary and vertebral tuberculosis may present as unexplained fever. However, careful history, urinalysis, intravenous pyelography, and radiographs of the spine should reveal the site of tissue involvement. Extrapulmonary tuberculosis should be treated with isoniazid, 300 mg orally, rifampin, 600 mg orally, ethambutol, 15 mg/kg/day, and pyrazinamide, 15 to 30 mg/kg (maximum, 2 gm/

day), given orally, for the first 2 months. Thereafter, isoniazid and rifampin are continued for 7 months (longer in cases of skeletal tuberculosis). The ethambutol can be discontinued once the organism is shown to be sensitive to isoniazid. Corticosteroids may be a useful adjunctive measure in the patient with severe systemic toxicity or central nervous system involvement (see Chapter 97). Steroids should be tapered as soon as the patient shows symptomatic improvement.

HISTOPLASMOSIS. Most individuals living in endemic areas in the Mississippi and Ohio River valleys have a subclinical, self-limited febrile illness as a manifestation of acute pulmonary histoplasmosis. Although patients may complain of chest pain or cough, physical examination of the chest usually is unremarkable despite radiographic findings of infiltrates and mediastinal and hilar adenopathy. Therefore, in the absence of chest radiographs, the lower respiratory tract component of the illness is easily overlooked. A complement fixation titer of at least 1:32 or a fourfold rise in titer is suggestive of the diagnosis of acute histoplasmosis. Although spontaneous resolution of symptoms is the norm, unusually prolonged illness (more than 2 to 3 weeks) may require antifungal treatment with amphotericin B or itraconazole.

Progressive disseminated histoplasmosis may occur as a consequence of reactivation of latent infection in immunosuppressed individuals (e.g., acquired immunodeficiency syndrome [AIDS] patients) or may reflect an uncontained or poorly contained primary infection. The febrile illness in such patients is protracted, and the differential diagnosis is that of FUO. Oropharyngeal nodules and ulcerative lesions are commonly found in disseminated histoplasmosis. Biopsy of such lesions permits rapid diagnosis. Serologies are less helpful in disseminated histoplasmosis, as they are positive in only one third of cases; cultures and methenamine silver stains of bone marrow biopsy specimens, however, should establish the diagnosis. In AIDS patients, *Histoplasma* urine antigen detection is a sensitive predictor of disseminated infection. Disseminated histoplasmosis is treated with amphotericin B, 0.5 to 0.6 mg/kg/day administered intravenously for a total dose of 2 to 3 gm. Itraconazole, 400 to 600 mg/day for 6 to 12 months, appears to be an effective alternative for patients who are unable to tolerate amphotericin B and who do not have meningeal disease.

OTHER. Malaria produces febrile paroxysms that in some cases occur every 48 to 72 hours. The diagnosis should be suspected in travelers who have returned from endemic areas, intravenous drug users, and recipients of blood transfusions. *Plasmodium falciparum* causes a high level of parasitemia and is associated with a high mortality rate unless recognized and treated promptly. Daily fevers may be seen in the course of this form of malaria. Although *Plasmodium vivax* and *Plasmodium malariae* may cause relapse long after primary infection, owing to latent extraerythrocytic infection, the course is milder. Demonstration of parasites in blood smears establishes the diagnosis of malaria.

Many, if not most, infectious diseases may present with fever as an early finding, with subclinical or eventual clinical involvement of specific organ systems. Examples include cryptococcosis, coccidioidomycosis, psittacosis, infection with *Legionella* species, and *Mycoplasma pneumoniae* infections. Pulmonary involvement by these infectious agents tends to produce few signs on physical examination; chest radiographs often reveal more prominent abnormalities than are suspected clinically.

Fever and Rash

Some of the febrile syndromes already discussed may occasionally be associated with a skin rash (Table 95–4). This section, however, considers diseases in which rash is a prominent feature of the presentation. The most life-

TABLE 95–4	Differential Diagnosis of Infectious Agents Producing Fever and Rash

Maculopapular Erythematous

Enterovirus
EBV, CMV, *Toxoplasma gondii*
HIV
Colorado tick fever virus
Salmonella typhi
Leptospira interrogans
Measles virus
Rubella virus
Hepatitis B virus
Treponema pallidum
Parvovirus B19
Human herpesvirus 6

Vesicular

Varicella-zoster
Herpes simplex virus
Coxsackie A virus
Vibrio vulnificus

Cutaneous Petechiae

Neisseria gonorrhoeae
Neisseria meningitidis
Rickettsia rickettsii (RMSF)
Rickettsia typhi (murine typhus)
Ehrlichia chaffeensis
Echoviruses
Viridans streptococci (endocarditis)

Diffuse Erythroderma

Group A streptococci (scarlet fever, toxic shock syndrome)
Staphylococcus aureus (toxic shock syndrome)

Distinctive Rash

Ecthyma gangrenosum—*Pseudomonas aeruginosa*
Erythema chronicum migrans—Lyme disease

Mucous Membrane Lesions

Vesicular pharyngitis—Coxsackie A virus
Palatal petechiae—rubella, EBV, scarlet fever (group A streptococci)
Erythema—toxic shock syndrome *(Staphylococcus aureus* and group A streptococci)
Oral ulceronodular lesion—*Histoplasma capsulatum*
Koplik's spots—measles virus

CMV = Cytomegalovirus; EBV = Epstein-Barr virus; HIV = human immunodeficiency virus; RMSF = Rocky Mountain spotted fever.

threatening infections associated with fever and rash include meningococcemia, staphylococcal bacteremia, and Rocky Mountain spotted fever (RMSF).

Bacterial Diseases

Petechial lesions, purpura, and ecthyma gangrenosum are lesions associated with bacteremia (see Chapter 96). Disseminated gonococcemia causes sparse vesiculopustular, hemorrhagic, or necrotic lesions on an erythematous base, typically on the extremities, particularly their dorsal surfaces (see Chapter 107). Meningococcemia is also an important cause of fever and a petechial skin rash that may be sparse.

Bacterial toxins produce characteristic clinical syndromes. Pharyngitis or other infections with an erythrogenic toxin-producing *Streptococcus* may lead to scarlet fever. Diffuse erythema begins on the upper part of the chest and spreads rapidly, although sparing palms and soles. Small red petechial lesions are found on the palate, and the skin has a sandpaper texture caused by occlusion of the sweat glands. The tongue at first shows a yellowish coating and then becomes beefy red. The rash of scarlet fever heals with desquamation. *Corynebacterium hemolyticum* also produces pharyngitis and skin rash.

Toxic shock syndrome (TSS) was first recognized as a distinct entity in 1978 and became epidemic in 1980 and 1981, probably because of the marketing of hyperabsorbable tampons. *S. aureus* strains producing toxic shock syndrome toxin (TSST-1) or other closely related exotoxins cause the syndrome. TSST-1 is a potent stimulus of IL1 production by mononuclear phagocytes and enhances the effects of endotoxin; these properties may be important in the pathogenesis of this syndrome. Most cases have occurred in 15- to 25-year-old girls and women using tampons. Other settings include prolonged use of contraceptive diaphragms, vaginal or cesarean deliveries, and nasal surgery. TSS in men usually is caused by superficial staphylococcal infections and abscesses. Patients with TSS develop the abrupt onset of high fever (temperature > 40°C), hypotension, nausea and vomiting, severe watery diarrhea and myalgias, followed in severe cases by confusion and oliguria. Characteristically, diffuse erythroderma (a sunburn-like rash) with erythematous mucosal surfaces is apparent. Later, intense scaling and desquamation of skin, particularly of the palms and soles, occurs. Laboratory abnormalities include elevated liver and muscle enzyme levels, thrombocytopenia, and hypocalcemia. Diagnosis is based on the clinical findings and requires specific exclusion of RMSF, meningococcemia, leptospirosis, and measles. Management of the patient consists of restoring an adequate circulatory blood volume by administration of intravenous fluids, removal of tampons if present, and treatment of the staphylococcal infection with nafcillin, 12 gm/day intravenously. Vancomycin is the alternative therapy for nafcillin-resistant staphylococci. Patients must be advised against using tampons in the future, as TSS often recurs within 4 months of the initial episode if tampon use continues.

A streptococcal toxic shock–like syndrome associated with scarlet fever toxin A has recently been documented as a complication of group A streptococcal soft tissue infections and occasionally following cases of influenza. Major manifestations include cellulitis and/or fasciitis with septicemia, shock, acute respiratory distress syndrome, renal failure, hypocalcemia, and thrombocytopenia. Treatment consists of high-dose penicillin and supportive measures. The mortality remains high (>30%) with optimal current therapy.

Viral Infections (Table 95–5)

The rashes associated with viral infections may be so typical as to establish unequivocally the cause of the febrile syndrome. Varicella-zoster requires special consideration because of the availability of an effective antiviral drug, acyclovir. In the normal host, neither chickenpox nor herpes zoster confined within specific dermatomes requires treatment with antiviral agents. Ophthalmic zoster demands antiviral treatment, since it is associated with potentially severe complications, including orbital compression syndromes and intracranial extension. Acyclovir is also effective in decreasing the severity of chickenpox in immunocompromised children and in limiting the extradermatomal spread of zoster in immunocompromised adults.

Rickettsial Diseases

In the United States, three rickettsial diseases are endemic: RMSF, Q fever, and murine typhus. Rash is not a characteristic of Q fever. RMSF is a misnomer, as most cases occur in the southeastern United States. The causative organism, *Rickettsia rickettsii,* is transmitted from dogs (or small wild animals) to ticks to humans. Infection occurs primarily during warmer months, periods of greatest tick activity. About two thirds of patients cite a history of tick exposure. After 2 to 14 days, there is the fulminant onset of severe frontal headache, chills, fever, myalgias, conjunctivitis, and, in one fourth, cough and shortness of breath. At this point, the diagnosis may be particularly obscure. Rash characteristically begins on the third to fifth day of illness as 1- to 4-mm erythematous macules on hands, wrists, feet, and ankles. Palms and soles may be involved. The rash spreads to the trunk and may become petechial. Intravascular coagulopathy develops in some severely ill patients. Diagnosis and institution of appropriate therapy should be based on the clinical findings. The specific complement fixation test shows a rise in titers and allows retrospective confirmation of the diagnosis. Treatment is with chloramphenicol, 50 mg/kg given orally or parenterally, or tetracycline, 25 to 50 mg/kg/day administered orally for 7 days.

Human Ehrlichiosis

Human ehrlichiosis is a recently recognized acute, febrile illness caused most frequently by *Ehrlichia chaffeensis. E.*

TABLE 95–5	Fever and Rash in Viral Infection	
Coxsackie/ECHO virus	Maculopapular "rubelliform": 1–3 mm, faint pink, begins on face, spreading to chest and extremities. "Herpetiform": vesicular stomatitis with peripheral exanthem (papules and clear vesicles on an erythematous base), including palms and soles (hand, foot, and mouth disease).	Summertime, no itching or lymphadenopathy; multiple cases in household, or community-wide epidemic; mostly diseases of children.
Measles	Erythematous, maculopapular rash begins on upper face and spreads down to involve extremities, including palms and soles; Koplik's spots are bluish-gray specks on a red base found on buccal mucosa near second molars; atypical measles occurs in individuals who received killed vaccine, then are exposed to measles; the rash begins peripherally and is urticarial, vesicular, or hemorrhagic.	Incubation period, 10–14 days; first, severe upper respiratory symptoms, coryza, cough, conjunctivitis; then Koplik's spots, then rash.
Rubella	Maculopapular rash beginning on face and moving downward; petechiae on soft palate.	Incubation, 12–35 days; adenopathy: posterior auricular, posterior cervical, and suboccipital.
Varicella	Generalized vesicular eruption; lesions in different stages from erythematous macules to vesicles to crusted; spread from trunk centrifugally. Zoster—see text.	Incubation, 14–15 days; late winter, early spring.
Herpes simplex virus	Oral primary: small vesicles on pharynx, oral mucosa, which ulcerate; painful and tender. Recurrent: vermillion border, one or few lesions. Genital: see Chapter 107.	Incubation, 2–12 days.
Hepatitis B	Prodrome in one fifth: erythematous maculopapular rash, urticaria.	Arthralgias, arthritis; abnormal liver function tests; hepatitis B antigenemia.
EBV	Erythematous, maculopapular rash on trunk and proximal extremities; occasionally urticarial or hemorrhagic.	Transiently occurs in 5–10% of patients during first week of illness.
HIV	Maculopapular truncal rash may occur as early manifestation of infection.	Associated fever, sore throat, and lymph node enlargement may persist for 2 or more wk.

EBV = Epstein-Barr virus; ECHO = enteric cytopathogenic human orphan; HIV = human immunodeficiency virus.

chaffeensis, like *R. rickettsii,* is transmitted by woodland exposure to deer or dog ticks and causes illness, with peak incidence in the summer months. Since first recognized in 1986, cases of ehrlichiosis have been identified in 21 contiguous southeastern states, from Maryland to Texas. The illness characteristically begins with fever, chills, headache, and myalgias, with a maculopapular rash occurring in less than a third of cases. Although there is a wide spectrum of illness, roughly half of clinically recognized cases are associated with pulmonary infiltrates; acute respiratory distress syndrome, often associated with renal failure, may develop, most often in elderly patients. In untreated patients, the mortality rate may exceed 10% in hospitalized cases.

Presumptive diagnosis is made on clinical grounds in patients with acute febrile illnesses, generally associated with decreasing leukocyte and platelet counts, following tick exposure. Treatment with tetracycline, 500 mg qid for 7 days, is effective in decreasing both duration and severity of illness.

Major clinical distinctions between human ehrlichiosis and RMSF include the earlier, more frequent, and more severe cutaneous manifestations of RMSF and the more common pulmonary manifestations and the characteristically decreasing leukocyte counts in ehrlichiosis. Rapid laboratory confirmation can be made by polymerase chain reaction.

At least one other *Ehrlichia* species has been associated with acute febrile illness in Wisconsin and Minnesota, and the full extent of human ehrlichiosis has not yet been defined.

Lyme Disease

Lyme disease is a common, multisystem spirochetal infection caused by *Borrelia burgdorferi* and transmitted by the tick *Ixodes dammini.* Initial case reports were clustered in several major foci (the Northeast, Wisconsin and Minnesota, California, and Oregon), but it is now clear that this infection is distributed broadly throughout North America and Western Europe. Three days to 3 weeks after the tick bite, of which most individuals are unaware, patients develop a febrile illness, usually associated with headache, stiff neck, myalgias, arthralgias, and erythema chronicum migrans (ECM). ECM begins as a red macule or papule at the site of the tick bite; the surrounding bright red patch expands to a diameter of up to 15 cm. Partial central clearing often is seen. The centers of lesions may become indurated, vesicular, or necrotic. Several red rings may be found within the outer border. Smaller secondary lesions may appear within several days. Lesions are warm but nontender. Enlargement of regional lymph nodes is common. The skin rash usually fades in about 1 month.

Several weeks after the onset of symptoms, important neurologic manifestations occur in more than 15% of patients. Most characteristic is meningoencephalitis with cranial nerve involvement and peripheral radiculoneuropathy. Bell's palsy may occur as an isolated phenomenon; when associated with fever, this finding is strongly suggestive of Lyme disease. The cerebrospinal fluid (CSF) at this time shows about 100 lymphocytes per milliliter. Heart involvement also may become manifest as atrioventricular block, myopericarditis, or cardiomegaly.

Joint involvement eventually occurs in 60% of patients. Early in the course, arthralgias and myalgias may be quite severe. Months later, arthritis often develops, with marked swelling and little pain in one or two large joints, typically the knee. Episodes of arthritis may recur for months or years; in about 10% of patients, the arthritis becomes chronic, and erosion of cartilage and bone occurs. Diagnosis is suspected on clinical grounds and confirmed by demonstration of IgM antibody to the spirochete, which peaks by the third to sixth week. Total serum IgM is increased, as are IgM-containing immune complexes and cryoglobulins. The level of IgM is reflective of disease activity and predictive of neurologic, cardiac, and joint involvement. However, serologic studies are not precise. Antibody titers may be negative in early disease, and early antibiotic therapy may blunt the antibody response. Synovial fluid contains an average of 25,000 cells per milliliter, most of them neutrophils.

Treatment of the early manifestations of Lyme disease with doxycycline, 100 mg twice daily for 14 to 21 days, usually prevents late complications. Meningitis, cardiac involvement, or arthritis should be treated with aqueous penicillin G, 20 million units, or intravenous ceftriaxone, 4 gm/day for 14 to 21 days. Repeated courses may be necessary if relapses occur.

Fever and Lymphadenopathy

Many infectious diseases are associated with some degree of lymphadenopathy (Table 95–6). However, in some, lymphadenopathy is a major manifestation of the disease. These can be further divided according to whether lymphadenopathy is generalized or regional.

Generalized Lymphadenopathy

The mononucleosis syndromes are important causes of fever and generalized lymphadenopathy.

TABLE 95–6	Infectious Disease Associated with Generalized Lymphadenopathy but with Other Dominant Features
Viral	Measles, rubella, hepatitis B
Bacterial	Scarlet fever, brucellosis, leptospirosis, tuberculosis, syphilis, Lyme disease

MONONUCLEOSIS SYNDROMES

Epstein-Barr Virus (EBV). Approximately 90% of American adults have serologic evidence of EBV infection; most infections are subclinical and occur before the age of 5 years or midway through adolescence.

Clinically manifest infectious mononucleosis usually develops late in adolescence after intimate contact with asymptomatic oropharyngeal shedders of EBV. Patients develop sore throat, fever, and generalized lymphadenopathy and sometimes experience headache and myalgias. Five to 10% of patients have a transient rash that may be macular, petechial, or urticarial. Palatal petechiae often are present, as is pharyngitis, which may be exudative. Cervical lymphadenopathy, particularly involving the posterior lymphatic chains, is prominent, although some involvement elsewhere is common. The spleen is minimally enlarged in about 50% of patients. Although rare, autoimmune hemolytic anemia, thrombocytopenia, encephalitis or aseptic meningitis, Guillain-Barré syndrome, hepatitis, or splenic rupture may dominate the clinical presentation. Three fourths of patients present with an absolute lymphocytosis. At least one third of their lymphocytes are atypical in appearance: large, with vacuolated basophilic cytoplasm, rolled edges often deformed by contact with other cells, and lobulated, eccentric nuclei. Immunologic studies indicate that some circulating B cells are infected with EBV and that the cells involved in the lymphocytosis are mainly cytotoxic T cells capable of damaging EBV-containing lymphocytes. Atypical lymphocytes are not restricted to infectious mononucleosis but may be seen in other viral illnesses.

B cell infection with EBV is a stimulus to production of polyclonal antibodies. Antibodies to foreign red cells (heterophile) can be helpful in the diagnosis. However, rapid diagnostic tests, such as the Monospot test, have largely replaced the need for heterophile determination. The Monospot test is sensitive and specific; false-positive results occur rarely in patients with lymphoma or hepatitis. Some patients with EBV infection show delayed development of heterophile antibodies. Recourse to determination of antibodies to EBV is necessary only in atypical, heterophile-negative cases. The presence of IgM antibody to viral capsid antigen is diagnostic of acute infectious mononucleosis. The appearance of antibody to EBV nuclear antigen also is indicative of EBV infection.

Infectious mononucleosis pursues a surprisingly benign course even in patients with neurologic involvement. The fever resolves after 1 to 2 weeks, although residual fatigue may be protracted. Occasional patients have a persistent or recurrent syndrome with fever, headaches, pharyngitis, lymphadenopathy, arthralgias, and serologic evidence of chronic active EBV infection. Patients should be managed symptomatically. Acetaminophen may be useful for sore throat. Antibiotics, particularly ampicillin, should be avoided. The use of ampicillin causes a skin rash in almost all patients with EBV infection, and this phenomenon can also be a diagnostic clue to the occurrence of EBV infection. Corticosteroids are indicated in the rare individual with serious hematologic involvement (i.e., thrombocytopenia, hemolytic anemia) or impending airway obstruction.

Acute bacterial superinfections of the pharynx and peritonsillar abscesses should be considered when the course is unusually septic.

The differential diagnosis of heterophile-negative mononucleosis is shown in Table 95–7.

Cytomegalovirus (CMV). Serologic surveys indicate that most adults have been infected with CMV. The ages of peak incidence of CMV infection are in the perinatal period (transmission by breast milk) and during the second to fourth decades. CMV shares with the other Herpesviridae the propensity to reactivate, particularly in immunosuppressed patients.

Two modes of transmission of CMV are particularly important in the development of lymphadenopathy in otherwise healthy adults. CMV can be transmitted sexually. Semen is an excellent source for viral isolation. The frequency of antibody to CMV and active viral excretion is particularly high in male homosexuals. Blood transfusions carry a risk of approximately 3% per unit of blood for transmitting CMV infection. This risk becomes substantial in the setting of open heart surgery or multiple transfusions for other indications.

Primary infection with CMV causes about 50% of cases of heterophile-negative mononucleosis. The distinction between CMV and EBV may be impossible on clinical grounds alone. However, CMV tends to involve older patients (mean age, 29) and produce milder disease, and it may be typhoidal in its presentation; that is, it causes fever with little or no adenopathy. The infrequent but serious forms of neurologic and hematologic involvement that occur in EBV infection also can occur with CMV. In addition, pneumonitis and hepatitis (which may be granulomatous) may be found. Isolation of CMV from urine or semen and demonstration of conversion of serologies (indirect fluorescent antibody test or complement fixation) from negative to positive are useful in establishing etiology. However, in groups such as male homosexuals, in whom asymptomatic excretion of CMV is found frequently, viral isolation alone is inadequate for determining the etiology of lymphadenopathy. CMV mononucleosis is a self-limited disease that does not require or respond to specific therapy. CMV infection in the immunocompromised host may be life threatening; in this setting, it often responds to long-term therapy with ganciclovir or foscarnet.

TABLE 95–7	Differential Diagnosis of Heterophile-Negative Mononucleosis

EBV mononucleosis (particularly in children)
CMV
Acute toxoplasmosis
Streptococcal pharyngitis
Hepatitis B
Acute HIV infection

CMV = Cytomegalovirus; EBV = Epstein-Barr virus; HIV = human immunodeficiency virus.

Acute Acquired Toxoplasmosis. *T. gondii* is acquired by ingesting oocysts contaminating meat and other foods or by exposure to cat feces. In certain geographic areas, such as France, 90% of individuals have serologic evidence of *Toxoplasma* infection. In the United States, the figure is close to 50% by age 50. Ten to twenty percent of infections in normal adult hosts are symptomatic. Presentation may take the form of a mononucleosis-like syndrome, although maculopapular skin rash, abdominal pain due to mesenteric and retroperitoneal lymphadenopathy, and chorioretinitis also may occur. Striking lymph node enlargement and involvement of unusual chains (occipital, lumbar) may necessitate lymph node biopsy to exclude lymphoma. More commonly, cervical adenopathy is observed in symptomatic cases. Overall, however, toxoplasmosis accounts for less than 1% of mononucleosis-like illnesses. Histologically, focal distention of sinuses with mononuclear phagocytes, histiocytes blurring the margins of germinal centers, and reactive follicular hyperplasia indicate *Toxoplasma* infection. Acute acquired toxoplasmosis is suggested by conversion of the indirect fluorescent antibody test from negative to positive or a fourfold increase in titer. Usually the titer is $> 1:1000$ and is associated with increased specific IgM antibody. Acute acquired toxoplasmosis generally is self-limited in the immunologically intact host and does not require specific therapy. Significant involvement of the eye is an indication for treatment with pyrimethamine plus sulfadiazine.

Granulomatous Disease. Disseminated tuberculosis, histoplasmosis, and sarcoidosis may be associated with generalized lymphadenopathy, although involvement of certain lymph node chains can predominate. Lymph node biopsy shows granulomas or nonspecific hyperplasia.

Persistent Generalized Lymphadenopathy (PGL). Patients infected by the human immunodeficiency virus (HIV) (see Chapter 108) may develop lymph node enlargement in at least two extrainguinal sites, persisting for at least 3 months, thereby fulfilling the standard diagnostic criteria for PGL. Additional symptoms such as fever, night sweats, fatigue, diarrhea, and weight loss may develop as the severity of immunodeficiency increases. Among individuals belonging to groups at increased risk for AIDS, the presence of generalized lymphadenopathy also could represent Kaposi's sarcoma, CMV infection, toxoplasmosis, tuberculosis, cryptococcosis, B cell lymphoma, or syphilis. Lymph node biopsy in a patient with HIV-related PGL is rarely necessary. A serum Venereal Disease Research Laboratories test should be performed to exclude secondary syphilis. A tuberculin skin test should also be performed.

Regional Lymphadenopathy

PYOGENIC INFECTION. *S. aureus* and group A streptococcal infections produce acute suppurative lymphadenitis. The most frequently affected lymph nodes are submandibular, cervical, inguinal, and axillary, in that order. Involved nodes are large (> 3 cm), tender, and firm or fluctuant.

Pyoderma, pharyngitis, or periodontal infection may be present at the presumed primary site of infection. Patients are febrile and have a leukocytosis. Fluctuant nodes should be aspirated. Otherwise, antibiotic therapy should be directed toward the most common pathogens. Penicillin G therapy is appropriate if pharyngeal or periodontal origin implicates a streptococcal or mixed anaerobic infection. Skin involvement suggests possible staphylococcal infection and is an indication for nafcillin (or dicloxacillin) therapy. The dosage and route of administration of the drug should be determined by the severity of the infection.

TUBERCULOSIS. Scrofula, or tuberculous cervical adenitis, presents in a subacute to chronic fashion. Fever, if present, is low grade. A large mass of matted lymph nodes is palpable in the neck. If *Mycobacterium tuberculosis* is the causative organism, other sites of active infection usually are present. The most common causative agent in children in the United States is *Mycobacterium scrofulaceum*. Infection with this and other drug-resistant nontuberculous mycobacteria usually requires surgical excision.

CAT-SCRATCH DISEASE. Chronic regional lymphadenopathy following exposure to cats or cat scratch should suggest the diagnosis. Histopathologic studies indicate a gram-negative bacterial origin of this syndrome. About 1 week after contact with the cat, a local papule or pustule may develop. One week later, regional adenopathy appears. Lymph nodes may be tender (sometimes exquisitely so) or just enlarged (1 to 7 cm). Fever is low grade if present at all. Lymph node enlargement usually persists for several months. Lymph node biopsy shows necrotic granulomas with giant cells and stellate abscesses surrounded by epithelial cells. Pleomorphic gram-negative bacilli ("cat-scratch bacilli") can be identified by the Warthin-Starry silver stain in lymph node biopsies during the first 4 weeks of illness. The diagnosis can usually be established on clinical grounds. Serologic testing is now available through the Centers for Disease Control and Prevention to detect antibodies to *Bartonella*. The course usually is self-limited and benign in immunocompetent individuals but may be life threatening in persons with severe immunodeficiency. The best approach to treatment of cat-scratch disease in the immunocompromised patient is not known; apparent responses to erythromycin, doxycycline, or antimycobacterial drugs have been described in small numbers of patients.

ULCEROGLANDULAR FEVER. Tularemia is the classic cause of ulceroglandular fever. The syndrome is acquired by contact with tissues or fluids from an infected rabbit or the bite of an infected tick. Patients have chills, fever, an ulcerated skin lesion at the site of inoculation, and painful regional adenopathy. When infection is acquired by contact with rabbits, the skin lesion usually is on the fingers or hand, and lymph node involvement is epitrochlear or axillary. In tick-borne transmission, the ulcer is on the lower extremities, perianal region, or trunk, and the adenopathy is inguinal or femoral. Most cases are diagnosed serologically, as Gram-stained preparations usually are negative, and culture of the causative organism, *Francisella tularensis,* is hazardous. A fourfold rise in agglutination titer is diagnostic. Patients should be treated presumptively with streptomycin, 15 to 20 mg/kg/day for 7 to 10 days.

OCULOGLANDULAR FEVER. Conjunctivitis with preauricular lymphadenopathy can occur in tularemia, cat-scratch disease, sporotrichosis, lymphogranuloma venereum infection, listeriosis, and epidemic keratoconjunctivitis due to adenovirus.

INGUINAL LYMPHADENOPATHY. Inguinal lymphadenopathy associated with sexually transmitted diseases (see Chapter 107) may be bilateral or unilateral. In primary syphilis, enlarged nodes are discrete, firm, and nontender. Early lymphogranuloma venereum causes tender lymphadenopathy with later matting of involved nodes, and sometimes fixation to overlying skin, which assumes a purplish hue. The lymphadenopathy of chancroid is most often unilateral, very painful, and composed of fused lymph nodes. Tender inguinal lymphadenopathy also occurs in primary genital herpes simplex virus infection.

PLAGUE. Bubonic plague usually presents as fever, headache, and a large mat of inguinal or axillary lymph nodes, which go on to suppurate and drain spontaneously. Plague is an important consideration in the acutely ill patient with possible exposure to fleas and rodents in the southwestern United States. If plague is suspected, blood cultures and aspirates of the buboes should be obtained, and tetracycline, 30 to 50 mg/kg/day, plus streptomycin, 20 to 30 mg/kg/day, instituted. Gram-stained preparations of the aspirate reveal gram-negative rods in two thirds of cases. A fluorescent antibody test allows rapid specific diagnosis and is available through the Centers for Disease Control and Prevention.

FUO

Fever of undetermined origin is the term applied to febrile illnesses with temperatures exceeding 101°F that are of at least 3 weeks' duration and remain undiagnosed after 3 days in the hospital or after three outpatient visits. Improvements in noninvasive diagnostic testing have resulted in newly proposed categories of FUO. They include (1) classic FUO, for which the common etiologies are infections, malignancy, inflammatory diseases, and drug fever; (2) neutropenic ($\leq$ 500 neutrophils per cubic millimeter) FUO, with perianal and periodontal infections, candidemia, and aspergillosis as major causes; (3) HIV-associated FUO, with *Mycobacterium avium* complex infections, tuberculosis, non-Hodgkin's lymphoma, drug fever, and CMV as important etiologies; and (4) nosocomial FUO, with septic thrombophlebitis, *Clostridium difficile* colitis, and drug fever as the major diagnostic possibilities. The evaluation of an FUO remains among the most challenging problems facing the physician. The majority of illnesses that cause FUO are treatable, making pursuit of the diagnosis particularly rewarding. There is no substitute for a meticulous history and physical examination. These should be repeated frequently during the patient's hospital course, as frequent questioning of the patient may jar an important historical clue from the patient, and important physical findings may develop while the patient is in the hospital. These clues may direct the next series of diagnostic studies. Patients with unexplained fevers should be offered HIV testing if at risk or if ancillary clinical or laboratory findings (e.g., generalized lymph node enlargement, lymphocytopenia) are suggestive of HIV infection. Directed biopsies of lesions should be stained and cultured for pathogenic microbes. In many instances, however, localizing clues are not present or fail to yield rewarding information. In these cases, bone marrow biopsy can reveal granulomatous or neoplastic disease, even in the absence of clinical evidence of bone marrow involvement. Similarly, liver biopsy may also reveal the etiology of an FUO but seldom in the absence of any clinical or laboratory evidence of liver disease. Exploratory laparotomy is generally not helpful unless signs, symptoms, or laboratory data point to abdominal pathology. Recent refinements in computed tomography (CT) may assist in determining the need for laparotomy in cases of FUO. If tuberculosis remains a reasonable possibility after careful work-up fails to establish a diagnosis, an empirical trial of antituberculous therapy may be initiated while awaiting results of bone marrow, liver, and urine cultures.

Table 95–8 indicates the final diagnoses in a study

TABLE 95–8	Fever of Undetermined Origin*

Infections
Intra-abdominal abscesses
  Subphrenic
  Splenic
  Diverticular
  Liver and biliary tract
  Pelvic
Mycobacterial
Cytomegalovirus
Infection of the urinary tract
Sinusitis
Osteomyelitis
Catheter infections
Other infections
Neoplastic Diseases
Hematologic neoplasms
  Non-Hodgkin's lymphoma
  Leukemia
  Hodgkin's disease
  Other
Solid tumors
Collagen Diseases
Granulomatous Diseases
Miscellaneous
Factitious Fever
Undiagnosed

*Adapted from Larson EB, Featherstone HJ, Petersdorf RG: Fever of undetermined origin: Diagnosis and follow-up of 105 cases, 1970–1980. Medicine 61:269–292, 1982. ©1982, The Williams & Wilkins Company, Baltimore.

of over 100 cases of FUO observed in the decade from 1970 to 1980. More recent series of FUO cases have emphasized an increasing occurrence of malignancy-associated FUO, some decreases in intra-abdominal abscesses because of the increasing sensitivity of CT imaging, and the more frequent identification of prolonged viral illnesses, especially CMV, in adolescents and young adults. Table 95–8 simply emphasizes the range of diagnostic possibilities to be considered. Numbers in each category are not presented, as regional and temporal variations in the frequency of specific diagnoses are great. Infectious diseases were the cause of about one third of these cases; another third were due to neoplasms; and the remainder were due to connective tissue disorders, granulomatous diseases, and other illnesses.

Causes of FUO

Infections

Abscesses account for as many as one third of infectious causes of FUO. Most of these abscesses are intra-abdominal or pelvic, as abscesses elsewhere (e.g., lung, brain, or superficial abscesses) are readily identifiable radiographically or as a result of the signs or symptoms they produce.

Intra-abdominal abscesses generally occur as a complication of surgery or leakage of visceral contents, as might be seen with perforation of a colonic diverticulum. Surprisingly, large abdominal abscesses may be present with few localizing symptoms. This is especially so in the elderly or immunocompromised host. Abscesses of the liver (see Chapter 102) occur as a consequence of inflammatory disease of the biliary tract or of the bowel; in the latter instance, bacteria reach the liver via portal blood flow. Occasionally, blunt trauma predisposes to abscesses of the liver or spleen. Hepatic, splenic, or subdiaphragmatic abscesses are generally readily detected by ultrasonography or CT scan. However, diagnosis of intra-abdominal abscess may be challenging, since even large abscesses in the pericolonic spaces may be difficult to distinguish from fluid-filled loops of bowel on CT scan. Gallium or tagged white blood cell scanning, ultrasonography, or barium enemas may assist if the diagnosis is suspected and CT scans are not definitive.

Endovascular infections (infective endocarditis, mycotic aneurysms, infected atherosclerotic plaques) are uncommon causes of FUO, since blood cultures are generally positive unless the patient has received antibiotics within the preceding 2 weeks. Infections of intravascular catheter sites generally are also associated with bacteremia unless the infection is limited to the insertion site. Diagnosis of endovascular infection is more difficult to make when blood cultures are negative and infection is due to slow-growing or fastidious organisms, such as *Brucella* species, *C. burnetii* (Q fever), or *Haemophilus* species. It is especially difficult among patients who have been treated with antimicrobials. If endocarditis is suspected, blood cultures should be repeated for at least 1 week after antimicrobials are discontinued, the bacteriology laboratory should be alerted to the possibility of infection due to a fastidious organism, and evidence of valvular vegetations should be sought by two-dimensional echocardiography. A transesophageal echocardiogram may be helpful if the two-dimensional study is equivocal. Occasionally, the suspicion of valvular infection is strong enough to warrant empirical antibiotic treatment of a presumed culture-negative endocarditis.

Although most patients with osteomyelitis have pain at the site of infection, localizing symptoms are occasionally absent and patients present only with fever. Technetium pyrophosphate bone scans and gallium scans demonstrate uptake at sites of osteomyelitis, but positive scans are not always specific for infection. Magnetic resonance imaging can be especially useful in differentiating between bone and soft tissue infection.

Mycobacterial infections, generally due to *M. tuberculosis,* are important causes of FUO. Patients with impaired cell-mediated immunity are at particular risk for disseminated tuberculosis, and occult infection with this organism is seen with particular frequency among elderly patients or those with renal failure who are undergoing hemodialysis. Fever may be the only sign of this infection. Both among immunocompromised patients and previously well persons with disseminated tuberculosis, purified protein derivative (PPD) skin tests are often negative. In some patients, careful review of chest radiographs reveals apical calcifications or upper lobe scars suggestive of remote tuberculous infection. A diffuse, often subtle, radiographic pattern of "millet seed" densities, best appreciated on the lateral chest views, is highly suggestive of disseminated tuberculosis. In this setting, transbronchial or open lung biopsy will establish the diagnosis. Similar radiographic patterns may be seen in sarcoidosis, disseminated fungal infection (e.g., histoplasmosis), and some malignancies. Bone marrow or liver biopsy often reveals granulomas, and cultures of these sites are positive in 50 to 90% of cases of disseminated tuberculosis.

Viral infections such as those caused by CMV or EBV can produce prolonged fevers. Both infections may be seen in young, healthy adults. Recipients of blood are at risk for acute post-transfusion CMV infection. Recipients of organ transplantation and other immunosuppressed patients may experience reactivation of latent CMV infection producing fever, leukopenia, and pulmonary and hepatic disease. Lymph nodes are often enlarged in EBV infection, and peripheral blood smear usually reveals a lymphocytosis with increased numbers of atypical lymphocytes. Occasionally, the atypical lymphocytosis is delayed several weeks after the onset of fever. A positive Monospot test may clarify the diagnosis. Unexplained fever may be a complication of infection with HIV; most such fevers are attributable to complicating opportunistic pathogens (see Chapter 108).

Simple lower urinary tract infections are readily diagnosed by symptoms and urinalysis. Complicated infections such as perirenal or prostatic abscess may be occult and present as FUO. Generally there is a history of antecedent urinary tract infection or disorder of the urinary tract. In prostatic abscess the prostate is usually tender on rectal examination. In suspected cases of perirenal and prostatic abscess, the urinalysis should be repeated if it is initially normal, as abnormalities of the sediment may be intermittent. Ultrasonography or CT scan will detect most of these lesions.

Although most patients with sinusitis have localizing symptoms, infections of the paranasal sinuses may occasionally present with fever only, particularly among hospitalized patients who have had nasotracheal and/or nasogastric intubation. Sinus films reveal fluid in the sinuses. Infection of the sphenoid sinus may be difficult to detect unless special views or CT scans are obtained.

Neoplastic Diseases

Neoplasms account for approximately one third of cases of FUO. Some tumors, particularly those of hematologic origin and hypernephromas, release endogenous pyrogens. In others, the mechanism of fever is less clear but may result from pyrogen release by infiltrating or surrounding inflammatory cells. Lymphomas can present as FUO; usually there is enlargement of lymph nodes or spleen. Some lymphomas present with intra-abdominal disease only. CT scan may be helpful in detecting these tumors. Leukemia also may present as FUO, sometimes with a normal peripheral blood smear. Bone marrow examination reveals an increased number of blast forms. Renal cell carcinoma, atrial myxoma, primary hepatocellular carcinoma, and tumor metastatic to the liver also may present as FUO. Liver function abnormalities (predominantly alkaline phosphatase) are common in all these tumors except atrial myxoma. Myxoma can be suspected in the presence of heart murmur and multisystem embolization (mimicking endocarditis) and is readily diagnosed by echocardiogram. Radiographic studies of the abdomen and retroperitoneum (CT scan or ultrasonography) generally detect the other tumors. Colon carcinoma also must be considered in the differential diagnosis, since a third or more of patients with this diagnosis may present with low-grade fever, and in some this is the only sign of disease.

Other Causes of FUO

Collagen vascular diseases account for approximately 10% of cases of FUO. Systemic lupus erythematosus is readily diagnosed serologically and thus accounts for a small proportion of cases of FUO. Vasculitis remains an important cause of FUO and should be suspected in febrile patients with "embolization/infarctions" or with "multisystem disease." Giant cell arteritis should be considered in older patients with FUO, particularly in the presence of polymyalgia rheumatica symptoms (see Chapter 85). Juvenile rheumatoid arthritis, or Still's disease, can present as FUO with joint symptoms. An evanescent rash, sore throat, adenopathy, and leukocytosis may occur in this disorder, which is diagnosed on the basis of clinical criteria in the absence of other potential causes of fever.

Granulomatous diseases without a defined etiology have been associated with FUO. Sarcoidosis is a multisystem granulomatous disorder often involving the lungs, skin, and lymph nodes. The majority of patients are anergic to skin test antigens. Diagnosis is based upon the demonstration of discrete, noncaseating granulomas on biopsy of bone marrow, liver, lung, or other tissues. Granulomatous hepatitis can present with prolonged fevers, occasionally lasting for years. Serum alkaline phosphatase levels are generally elevated; liver biopsy reveals granulomas, and no underlying etiology can be demonstrated.

A number of miscellaneous disorders, including Crohn's disease, familial Mediterranean fever, and hypertriglyceridemia, make up the remainder of FUO cases. Drug-related fevers and recurrent pulmonary emboli always demand consideration in the differential diagnosis. A significant minority of FUOs (approximately 10%) remain undiagnosed after careful evaluation. The majority of these patients have experienced an undefinable but self-limited illness, with fewer than 10% of these patients developing an underlying serious disorder after several years' follow-up.

FACTITIOUS OR SELF-INDUCED FEVER. Patients with factitious or self-induced illness present unique ethical and therapeutic problems. Once the possibility of factitious or self-induced illness is considered, the doctor-patient relationship is changed. Typically, the physician can rely on the good faith of the patient's history. In the case of factitious or self-induced illness, the physician must assume a more detached role to establish the diagnosis. Patients with factitious fever are typically young, often female. Many have been or are employed in health-related professions. Usually articulate and well-educated, these patients are adept at manipulating their family, friends, and physicians. In these instances, a consultant new to the patient may provide a detached and helpful perspective on the problem.

Clues to factitious fever include the absence of a toxic appearance despite high temperature readings, lack of an appropriate rise in pulse rate with fever, and absence of the physiologic diurnal variation in temperature. Suspected factitious readings can be evaluated by immediately repeating the reading with the nurse or physician in attendance. Use of electronic thermometers allows rapid and accurate recording of a patient's temperature (see also Chapter 112).

Self-injection of pyrogen-containing substances, usually bacteria-laden culture medium, urine, or feces, can produce bacteremia and high fever; usually these bacteremic episodes are polymicrobial and intermittent, often suggesting a diagnosis of intra-abdominal abscess. However, patients with self-induced bacteremia may appear remarkably well between episodes of fever, in contrast to most patients with abscesses. The occurrence of polymicrobial bacteremia in an otherwise healthy person should suggest the possibility of self-induced infection. Illicit ingestion of medications known by the patient to produce fever can also present a very difficult diagnostic problem. Clues to the presence of self-induced illness are subtle. The patients are often emotionally immature; some exaggerate their importance and fabricate unrelated aspects of their history. Some are surprisingly stoic about the apparent seriousness of their illness and the procedures employed to diagnose or treat them. In some instances, interview of family members can elicit clues to the possibility of factitious or self-induced illness. Confirming the diagnosis is crucial and, in many instances, requires search of the patient's hospital room. Although most will deny their role in inducing or feigning illness, the diagnosis must be explained, and psychiatric care is essential. These complicated patients are at risk for inducing life-threatening disease; some respond to psychiatric counseling.

REFERENCES

Dinarello CA, Cannon JG, Wolff S: New concepts of the pathogenesis of fever. Rev Infect Dis 1988; 10:168–169.

Durack D, Street A: Fever of unknown origin—reexamined and redefined. *In* Remington J, Swartz M (eds.): Current Clinical Topics in Infectious Diseases. St. Louis, Mosby-Year Book, 1991, pp 35–51.

Knockaert D, Vanneste LJ, Vanneste SB, Bobbaers HJ: Fever of unknown origin in the 1980s. An update of the diagnostic spectrum. Arch Intern Med 1992; 152:51–55.

96

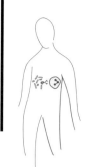

Bacteremia

Sepsis syndrome, the systemic response to an infectious process, is a leading cause of morbidity and mortality in hospitalized patients. A major advance over the past decade has been the growing understanding of the pathophysiology of sepsis. Novel therapeutic approaches now being tested in the sepsis syndrome are a direct result of the elucidation of the molecular mechanisms of sepsis and the practical application of modern techniques of biochemistry and molecular biology to rational drug design.

The bases for current definitions of sepsis syndrome and related disorders are presented in Table 96–1 and Figure 96–1. Infection, defined by the presence of microbial pathogens in normally sterile sites, can be symptomatic or inapparent. Bacteremia implies the presence of organisms that can be cultured from blood. Septicemia implies bacteremia with greater severity. Sepsis indicates clinical settings in which there is evidence of infection as well as a systemic response to infection (fever/hypothermia, tachycardia, tachypnea, or leukocytosis/leukopenia). Sepsis syndrome emphasizes an increased degree of severity with evidence of altered organ perfusion with one of the following: hypoxemia, oliguria, altered mentation, or elevated serum lactate level. Severe sepsis represents a more advanced degree of organ compromise. Septic shock indicates sepsis plus hypotension despite adequate intravenous fluid challenge. Refractory septic shock is defined as shock lasting more than 1 hour unresponsive to fluids and/or vasopressors. Noninfectious insults (e.g., thermal burns, severe trauma, severe pancreatitis, certain toxins, therapy with monoclonal antibodies for solid organ transplant rejection) can also be associated with a severe systemic reaction simulating the sepsis syndrome. The term *systemic inflammatory response syndrome* (SIRS) encompasses both infectious and noninfectious causes of a profound host inflammatory response with systemic symptoms and signs; sepsis syndrome is the predominant cause of SIRS.

EPIDEMIOLOGY

The incidence of sepsis and associated deaths has increased dramatically in the United States. The National Hospital Discharge Survey demonstrated an increase in the diagnosis of septicemia from 164,000 cases in 1979 to 425,000 cases in 1987. Septicemia was associated with a 25.3% mortality in 1987 and ranked thirteenth among the causes of death in the United States from 1979 to 1987.

The National Nosocomial Infection System indicates marked increases in the frequency of septicemia caused by gram-positive infections over the past 15 years. Highest rates for hospital-acquired septicemias occur in oncology patients and burn/trauma victims and in high-risk nurseries. Hospital-acquired blood stream infections are associated with 7.4 extra days of hospitalization and $4000 of extra hospital charges per occurrence. The most commonly identified blood stream pathogens include staphylococci, streptococci, *Escherichia coli*, *Enterobacter* species, and *Pseudomonas aeruginosa*. Fungal blood stream isolates are less frequent. Major epidemiologic factors that have contributed to the increased occurrence of sepsis include the growing number of immunocompro-

TABLE 96–1	Definitions of Sepsis and Related Disorders
Disorder	**Definition**
Infection	Microorganisms in a normally sterile site; subclinical or symptomatic
Bacteremia	Bacteria present in blood stream; may be transient
Septicemia	Same as bacteremia but greater severity
Sepsis	Clinical evidence of infection plus systemic response to infection (fever/hypothermia, tachycardia, tachypnea, leukocytosis/leukopenia)
Sepsis syndrome	Sepsis plus altered organ perfusion (hypoxemia, oliguria, altered mentation)
Severe sepsis	Sepsis syndrome plus hypotension/hypoperfusion
Septic shock	Sepsis with hypotension despite adequate fluid resuscitation; patients on vasopressors may not be hypotensive at the time hypoperfusion abnormalities are evident
Refractory septic shock	Shock lasting more than 1 hr unresponsive to fluid administration and/or vasopressors
Systemic inflammatory response syndrome (SIRS)	Wide variety of insults (infectious and noninfectious) that initiate profound systemic responses; sepsis syndrome is a subset of SIRS

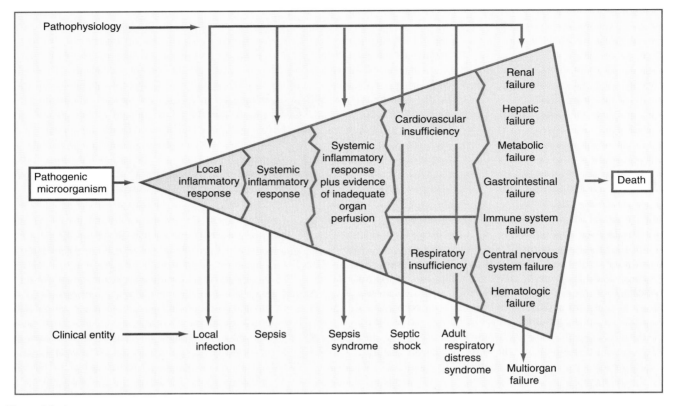

Figure 96-1
Natural history of the sepsis process.

mised hosts resulting from more intense chemotherapy regimens, an aging population, and the aggressive employment of more invasive procedures and complex surgery.

Table 96-2 lists organisms important in the sepsis syndrome as they relate to host factors. Factors that have

TABLE 96-2	Microorganisms Involved in Sepsis Syndrome in Relation to Host Factors
Host Factors	**Organisms of Particular Importance**
Asplenia	Encapsulated organisms: *Streptococcus pneumoniae, Haemophilus influenzae, Neisseria meningitidis,* bacillus (DF-2)
Cirrhosis	*Vibrio, Yersinia,* and *Salmonella* spp, other gram-negative rods (GNRs), encapsulated organisms
Alcoholism	*Klebsiella* spp, *Streptococcus pneumoniae*
Diabetes	Mucormycosis and *Pseudomonas* spp, *Escherichia coli*
Steroids	Tuberculosis, fungi, herpes viruses
Neutropenia	Enteric GNRs, *Pseudomonas, Aspergillus, Candida,* and *Mucor* spp, *Staphylococcus aureus*
T cell dysfunction	*Listeria, Salmonella,* and *Mycobacterium* spp, herpesvirus group (herpes simplex virus, cytomegalovirus, varicella-zoster virus)

negatively influenced survival in the setting of bacteremia have included severity of underlying disease, delayed initiation of appropriate antimicrobial therapy, virulence of the pathogen (e.g., *P. aeruginosa*), extremes of age, site of infection (respiratory > abdominal > urinary), nosocomial acquisition, polymicrobial infection, and development of end-organ complications (adult respiratory distress syndrome [ARDS], anuria, disseminated intravascular coagulation [DIC], coma). When there is evidence of dysfunction in two or more systems, the diagnosis of multiorgan system failure can be made. Mortality rises in proportion to the number of organ systems involved and is near 100% when four or more systems are dysfunctional.

PATHOGENESIS

The pathogenesis of sepsis is shaped largely by the infected host's complex response to the invading pathogen (Fig. 96-2). Gram-negative bacterial lipopolysaccharide (LPS), or endotoxin, is representative of a larger class of bacterial products causally linked to the septic shock syndrome. Cell wall products of gram-positive bacteria, such as techoic acid and peptidoglycan, induce inflammatory responses similar to those produced by LPS. Indeed, the sepsis syndrome may complicate infections with bacteria, viruses, fungi, rickettsiae, mycobacteria, and parasites. The pathogenesis of shock involves a series of events

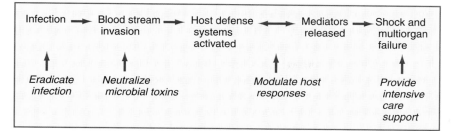

Figure 96-2
The pathogenesis and treatment of sepsis syndrome.

initiated by the invading pathogen or its products and is effected through a causally related sequence of host responses. Endotoxin, for example, activates the clotting, fibrinolytic, and complement pathways both directly and indirectly through its effects on platelets, macrophages, polymorphonuclear leukocytes, and hepatocytes.

Endotoxin induces macrophages to produce a number of proinflammatory cytokines including tumor necrosis factor (TNF)-alpha, interleukin (IL)-1, IL6, IL8, gamma-interferon, and granulocyte colony-stimulating factor (G-CSF). Each of these cytokines exerts multiple effects related directly or indirectly to the development of septic shock, and each cytokine modulates its own production and that of other mediators and, in some cases, acts synergistically with one or more of the cytokines. These macrophage-associated cytokines can also stimulate B and T lymphocytes, natural killer cells, and bone marrow cells. Mediators released from macrophages can stimulate T lymphocytes to generate IL2, IL4, and IL10 and granulocyte-macrophage colony-stimulating factor (GM-CSF).

Endotoxin stimulates membrane phospholipid metabolism, leading to the generation of platelet-activating factor and other bioactive metabolites of arachidonic acid, including prostaglandins and leukotrienes. These compounds, in turn, exert a variety of synergistic and antagonistic effects on vascular endothelium, smooth muscle, platelets, and leukocytes and thus contribute to or modulate pathophysiologic events associated with septic shock. Endotoxin may also serve as a cofactor to prime granulocytes to produce toxic oxidative radicals. Lastly, endotoxin induces the production of β-endorphins (which have been implicated in the pathogenesis of sepsis) as well as counterregulatory hormones such as cortisol, glucagon, and catecholamines, which may oppose certain of the shock-producing actions of endorphins and other mediators.

CLINICAL MANIFESTATIONS

The clinical manifestations of the sepsis syndrome are multiple and often do not point to the specific etiology (Table 96-3). The clinician is faced with the challenge of early recognition and sorting through the various possible etiologies of the SIRS so that appropriate therapy can be initiated. Patients presenting with the clinical picture of sepsis of uncertain etiology should be presumed to have bacteremic infection and treated accordingly. Prompt careful cultures of blood and suspicious local sites should be followed immediately by initiation of antibiotics appropriate for the most likely pathogens.

Fever and chills are usually present, but elderly or debilitated patients (especially with renal or liver failure) may not develop fever. Hypothermia may occur and is associated with a poor prognosis. One of the early clues to a systemic infectious process is hyperventilation and respiratory alkalosis.

Skin manifestations in sepsis can occur with any infectious agent and at times may represent the earliest sign of the sepsis syndrome. Staphylococci and streptococci can be associated with cellulitis or diffuse erythroderma in association with toxin-producing strains. Blood stream infection with gram-negative bacteria can be associated with a skin lesion called ecthyma gangrenosum (round/oval 1- to 15-cm lesions with a halo of erythema and usually a vesicular or necrotic central area). Although ecthyma gangrenosum is most commonly associated with *P. aeruginosa, Aeromonas, Klebsiella, E. coli,* and *Serratia* may also cause ecthyma gangrenosum (see also Chapter 101). *Neisseria meningitidis* bacteremia is often heralded by petechial and hemorrhagic skin lesions and followed by rapidly progressive shock.

The sepsis syndrome is characteristically associated with hypotension and oliguria. In many patients, hypotension will initially respond to intravenous fluids. Other patients progress from an initial stage of hypotension, tachycardia, and vasodilatation (warm shock) to deep pallor, vasoconstriction, and anuria (cold shock). Of all infectious causes of the sepsis syndrome, gram-negative bacilli most often cause shock; up to 35% of patients with gram-negative sepsis develop shock, often with mortality rates between 40 and 70%.

As the sepsis syndrome progresses, myocardial function becomes profoundly depressed. This greatly complicates fluid management and necessitates continuous cardiopulmonary monitoring in an intensive care setting.

TABLE 96-3	**Signs and Symptoms Indicative of the Sepsis Syndrome**
	Fever, chills
	Hyperventilation
	Hypothermia
	Mental status changes
	Hypotension
	Leukopenia, thrombocytopenia
	End-organ failure: lung, kidney, liver, heart, disseminated intravascular coagulation

Pulmonary complications of the sepsis syndrome are frequent. ARDS, characterized by $Pa_{O_2} < 50$ mm Hg despite $FIO_2 > 50\%$, diffuse alveolar infiltrates, and pulmonary capillary wedge pressure < 15 mm Hg, occurs in 10 to 40% of sepsis syndrome patients and is most frequent in conjunction with gram-negative organisms. ARDS may be worsened by the injudicious administration of intravenous fluids in an attempt to improve cardiac output. Failure of respiratory muscles can also complicate sepsis and contribute significantly to morbidity and mortality.

Most patients with sepsis have a neutrophilic leukocytosis. Leukopenia may occur, most often with overwhelming bacteremias, but also with severe systemic viral infections. Alcoholics and the elderly are at greater risk for sepsis-associated neutropenia. A low platelet count and evidence of coagulopathy occur in up to 75% of patients with gram-negative bacillary bacteremia. DIC occurs in roughly 10% of septic patients.

Renal insufficiency in the sepsis syndrome is multifactorial and depends to varying degrees on the host, the microbe, and the therapy administered. Most often in sepsis, acute tubular necrosis is the basis for renal dysfunction and may be secondary to hypotension, volume depletion, or cytokines elaborated in the sepsis syndrome. Tubulointerstitial disease caused by specific pathogens and/or antimicrobial therapy may also occur.

Upper gastrointestinal tract bleeding may be a life-threatening complication in septic patients with coagulopathy and thrombocytopenia. Liver dysfunction may occur, with evidence of cholestatic jaundice or of hepatocellular injury. With bacteremia related to gram-negative bacilli, "hyperbilirubinemia of sepsis" often occurs, with little change in other liver enzymes. Large increases in transaminases usually indicate shock liver; these abnormalities usually resolve rapidly with restoration of blood pressure.

Hypoglycemia may complicate sepsis syndrome and can be a correctable cause of mental status change or seizures. Hypoglycemia occurs more frequently in individuals with underlying liver disease.

DIAGNOSIS

The initial evaluation of the patient with possible sepsis syndrome ideally begins with a careful history. However, in patients with the fully developed sepsis syndrome, the working diagnosis is made on the basis of physical findings, and the detailed history must necessarily follow correction of hemodynamic problems, obtaining appropriate microbial cultures, and empirical initiation of antimicrobial therapy. Attention should be focused upon underlying diseases or predispositions to sepsis, previous infections and antimicrobial therapy, available microbiologic information, and symptoms suggesting localization of infection. A history of travel, environmental exposure, and any contact with infectious agents should be carefully obtained. Information on the complications of previous treatment (e.g., drug toxicities or allergies) can be critical in the selection of therapy.

Physical examination should focus upon discovering clues to infection and localizing sites thereof. Appropriate specimens for microbiologic evaluation must be obtained.

Two or three sets of blood cultures from bacteremic patients will yield the organism 89% and 99% of the time, respectively.

The selection of additional laboratory studies should be based upon the clinical manifestations. Obtaining appropriate diagnostic studies expeditiously is critical. These studies are usually aimed at delineating the focus of infection (e.g., cerebrospinal fluid examination, computed tomography scans) and determining whether adjunctive surgical therapy (e.g., abscess drainage, foreign body removal) is indicated.

THERAPY

Time does not allow holding antimicrobial therapy until bacteremia or an infectious source is proven in patients with the sepsis syndrome. The key to management of sepsis is the early recognition of the systemic response and initiation of therapy before hypotension and complications ensue.

Patients with sepsis syndrome, especially if hypotensive, are probably best managed in the intensive care unit. The essential therapies of the sepsis syndrome and septic shock include antibiotics, adequate fluid administration, oxygen, and vasopressors. Antibiotic choices should reflect epidemiologic concerns (see Table 96–2), antibiotic resistance patterns, and potential sites of infection. Until culture results and other diagnostic studies are completed, empirical broad spectrum antimicrobial therapy, covering both gram-positive and gram-negative pathogens, is necessary in sepsis patients. Initiation of appropriate empirical antimicrobial therapy has a major impact on survival of these patients. As soon as a specific microbial etiology has been established by culture, antibiotics should be changed, if necessary, to target the etiologic agent.

The limitations of currently available therapy for sepsis and septic shock are evidenced by the continued high mortality rates associated with this disease, despite improvement in antibiotic therapy and critical care techniques. Standard approaches to therapy of sepsis and septic shock are crucial. If various steps in the pathogenesis of septic shock are recognized, beginning with tissue invasion by the offending organism and culminating in pathophysiologic phenomena associated with the septic shock syndrome, current therapy addresses only the initial and final stages of this process (see Figs. 96–1 and 96–2). Few currently employed therapies target intermediate steps in the pathogenesis of septic shock even though these steps dominate the disease process in the fully developed sepsis syndrome. Newer strategies entail attempts to amplify selectively or modulate the host responses to the invading pathogen or its pathogenic products. Targets include the bacterium, endotoxin (or other bacterial products), host cells that respond to endotoxin, mediators produced by these cells in response to endotoxin, and cells injured by endotoxin-induced mediators (see Fig. 96–2).

A multicenter evaluation of monoclonal antibodies against endotoxin showed modest benefit in survival of patients with documented bacteremia caused by gram-negative bacilli but no benefit in other patients with the sepsis syndrome. New strategies employing antibody against TNF are now being evaluated.

REFERENCES

Bone RG: The pathogenesis of sepsis. Ann Intern Med 1991;115: 457–469.

Hoffman WD: Anti-endotoxin therapies in septic shock. Ann Intern Med 1994;120:771–783.

Parrillo JE: Pathogenetic mechanisms of septic shock. N Engl J Med 1993;328:1471–1477.

Young L: Sepsis syndrome. *In* Mandell GM, Bennett JE, Dolin R (eds.): Principles and Practice of Infectious Diseases. 4th ed. New York, Churchill-Livingstone, 1995, pp 690–705.

Ziegler EJ, Fisher CJ, Sprung CL, et al.: Treatment of gram-negative bacteremia and septic shock with human monoclonal antibody against endotoxin. A randomized, double-blind, placebo-controlled trial. N Engl J Med 1991;324:429–436.

97

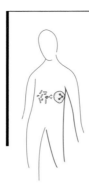

Infections of the Nervous System

Infections of the central nervous system (CNS) range from fulminating, readily diagnosed septic processes to indolent illnesses requiring exhaustive searches to identify their presence and define their cause. Neurologic outcome and survival depend largely on the extent of CNS damage present before effective treatment begins. Accordingly, it is essential that the physician move quickly to achieve a specific diagnosis and institute appropriate therapy. The initial evaluation must, however, take into account both the urgency of beginning antibiotic treatment in bacterial meningitis and the potential hazard of performing a lumbar puncture in the presence of focal neurologic infection or mass lesions.

Patients with CNS infection usually present with some combination of fever, headache, altered mental status, depressed sensorium, seizures, focal neurologic signs, and stiff neck. The history and physical examination, results of lumbar puncture (Table 97–1), and neuroradiographic procedures provide the mainstays of diagnosis. The order in which the last two procedures are performed is critical. A subacute history, evolving over 7 days to 2 months, of unilateral headache with focal neurologic signs and/or seizures implies a mass lesion that may or may not be infectious. A brain-imaging procedure should be performed first; lumbar puncture is potentially dangerous, as it may precipitate cerebral herniation, even in the absence of overt papilledema. By contrast, patients admitted with fulminating symptoms of fever, headache, lethargy, confusion, and stiff neck should have an immediate lumbar puncture and, if this test proves abnormal, antibiotics should be instituted for presumed bacterial meningitis. If the distinction between focal and diffuse CNS infection is unclear or not adequately evaluable, as in the comatose patient, cultures of blood, throat, and nasopharynx should be obtained, antibiotic therapy started, and an emergency scanning procedure performed. If the last is unavailable, lumbar puncture should be delayed pending evidence that no danger of herniation exists. Inevitably, this approach means that some patients will receive parenteral antibiotics several hours before a lumbar puncture is performed. In acute bacterial meningitis, 50% of cerebrospinal fluid (CSF) cultures will be negative by 4 to 12 hours after institution of antibiotics; negative CSF cultures are even more likely if the causative organism is a sensitive pneumococcus. Should the CNS infection actually represent acute bacterial meningitis, however, the characteristics of the CSF still would

suggest the diagnosis, since neutrophilic pleocytosis and hypoglycorrhachia (low CSF sugar) usually persist for at least 12 to 24 hours after antibiotics are instituted. Furthermore, Gram-stained preparation (or assay for microbial antigen in the CSF by latex agglutination) should indicate the causative organism even after antibiotics have rendered the CSF culture negative. Blood and nasopharyngeal cultures obtained before therapy also are likely to be positive in view of the high frequency of isolation of causative organisms from these sites. The approach of treating suspected CNS infections promptly ("shoot first, tap later") is often life saving and does not significantly compromise management. This approach to the use of scanning procedures is germane only for adults with community-acquired CNS infection. In children, technically adequate computed tomography (CT) scans require heavy sedation; therefore, scanning procedures must be reserved for more stringent indications.

Armed with the clinical presentation and the results of the lumbar puncture and CT scan, the clinician must decide on a probable cause and develop a plan for initial management and definitive evaluation. The task is simplified by addressing the following issues:

1. Is the host normal? The spectrum of CNS diseases and their causes shifts dramatically in the immunocompromised host (Table 97–2). The possibility of human immunodeficiency virus (HIV) infection must be determined expeditiously by serologies. Primary HIV infection may cause CNS signs and symptoms prior to seroconversion, requiring additional testing (e.g., p24 antigen or HIV polymerase chain reaction [PCR] assay) if the suspicion is sufficiently high (see Chapter 108).

2. Are there relevant exposures? Exposure to persons with syphilis, tuberculosis, or HIV may be associated with acquisition of same. Ticks may transmit Lyme disease or spotted fever, and mosquitoes, arboviral encephalitis. Exposure to livestock or unpasteurized dairy products suggests brucellosis. Residence in the Ohio and Mississippi River valleys increases the risk of histoplasmosis and blastomycosis; coccidioidomycosis is endemic to semiarid regions of the Southwest. Travel and particularly residence in developing countries may suggest cysticercosis, echinococcal cyst disease, and cerebral malaria.

3. Does the patient have meningitis, encephalitis, or me-

TABLE 97–1	Typical CSF Findings in CNS Infection				
Infection	**Cells**	**Neutrophils**	**Glucose**	**Protein**
Bacterial meningitis	500–10,000/μl	>90%	<40 mg/dl	>150 mg/dl
Aseptic meningitis	10–500/μl	Early > 50%; late < 20%	Normal	<100 mg/dl
Herpes simplex virus encephalitis	0–1000/μl	<50%	Normal	<100 mg/dl
Tuberculosus meningitis	50–500/μl	Early > 50%; late < 50%	<30 mg/dl	>150 mg/dl
Syphilitic meningitis	50–500/μl	<10%	<40 mg/dl	<100 mg/dl

CNS = Central nervous system; CSF = cerebrospinal fluid.

ningoencephalitis? Is the disease acute, subacute, or chronic? These distinctions narrow the differential diagnosis considerably and form the basis for organization of the sections that follow. The meningitis syndrome consists of fever, headache, and stiff neck. Confusion and a depressed level of consciousness may occur as part of the metabolic encephalopathy in patients with acute bacterial meningitis. Seizures are rare and may indicate complicating processes such as cortical vein thrombosis. In contrast, encephalitis characteristically causes confusion, bizarre behavior, depressed levels of consciousness, focal signs, and seizures (grand mal or focal). A presentation suggestive of encephalitis raises a variety of issues quite different from those surrounding a patient with bacterial meningitis.

MENINGITIS

Meningitis is an inflammation of the leptomeninges caused by infectious or noninfectious processes. The most common types of infectious meningitis are bacterial, viral, tuberculous, and fungal. The most common noninfectious causes are subarachnoid hemorrhage, cancer, and sarcoidosis. Infectious meningitis is considered in three categories: acute bacterial meningitis, aseptic meningitis, and subacute to chronic meningitis.

TABLE 97–2	Meningitis and Meningoencephalitis in the Immunocompromised Host
Abnormality	**Infectious Agent**
Complement deficiencies (C6–C8)	*Neisseria meningitidis*
Splenectomy and/or antibody defect	*Streptococcus pneumoniae*
	Haemophilus influenzae
	Enterovirus
	Neisseria meningitidis
Sickle cell disease	*Streptococcus pneumoniae*
	Haemophilus influenzae
Impaired cellular immunity	*Listeria monocytogenes*
	Cryptococcus neoformans
	Toxoplasma gondii
	Histoplasma capsulatum
	Coccidioides immitis
	Mycobacterium tuberculosis
	Treponema pallidum
	JC virus
	Cytomegalovirus

Acute Bacterial Meningitis

Epidemiology

Three fourths of cases of acute bacterial meningitis occur before the age of 15 years. *Neisseria meningitidis* causes sporadic disease or epidemics in closed populations. Most cases occur in winter and spring and involve children younger than 5 years of age. *Haemophilus influenzae* meningitis is even more selectively a disease of childhood, with most cases developing by the age of 10 years. Infections are sporadic, although secondary cases may occur in close contacts. The incidence of *H. influenzae* meningitis has significantly declined with the widespread use of effective conjugated vaccines. In contrast, pneumococcal meningitis is a disease seen in all age groups. Extensive clinical series of adults hospitalized 20 years ago showed a relative frequency of 68% pneumococcal, 18% meningococcal, and 10% *H. influenzae* meningitis. At University Hospitals of Cleveland in the period from 1972 to 1981, the relative frequencies were 40%, 30%, and 20%, respectively, in keeping with the general experience that serious *H. influenzae* (nontypable) infections are increasingly common in adults.

Close contact with a patient with meningococcal or *H. influenzae* disease is particularly important in the development of secondary cases of meningitis and other severe disease manifestations (sepsis, epiglottitis) as well. For example, the risk of meningococcal disease is 500 to 800 times greater in a close contact of a patient with meningococcal meningitis than in a noncontact. Asymptomatic pharyngeal carriers of *H. influenzae* also can spread infection to their contacts.

Pathogenesis and Pathophysiology

The bacteria that cause most community-acquired meningitis transiently colonize the oropharynx and nasopharynx of healthy individuals. Meningitis may occur in nonimmune hosts following bacteremia from an upper respiratory site (meningococcus or *H. influenzae*) or pneumonia and by direct spread from contiguous foci of infection (nasal sinuses, mastoids).

The pathogenesis of acute bacterial meningitis is best understood for meningococcal disease. The carrier state occurs when meningococci adhere to pharyngeal epithelial cells via specialized filamentous structures termed pili. The production of IgA protease by pathogenic *Neisseria* species favors adherence by inactivating IgA, a major host barrier to colonization. Organisms enter and pass through epithelial cells to subepithelial tissues, where they multiply in the nonimmune individual and produce bacteremia. The localization of organisms to the CSF is not well understood but presumably depends on invasive properties of the capsular polysaccharide, which permit penetration of the blood-brain barrier. Immunity is conferred by bactericidal antibody and presumably is acquired by earlier colonization of the pharynx with nonpathogenic meningococci and cross-reacting bacteria. The presence of blocking IgA antibody may increase susceptibility transiently in some individuals.

Table 97–2 summarizes host factors conferring a particular risk of meningitis. Bacterial meningitis remains confined to the leptomeninges and does not spread to adjacent parenchymal tissue. Focal and global neurologic deficits develop because of involvement of blood vessels coursing in the meninges and through the subarachnoid space; in addition, cranial nerves and cerebral tissue can be affected by the attendant inflammation, edema, and scarring as well as by the development of obstructive hydrocephalus.

Gram-negative enteric meningitis occurs mainly in severely debilitated persons or individuals whose meninges have been breached or damaged by head trauma, a neurosurgical procedure, or a parameningeal infection.

Clinical Presentation

Patients with bacterial meningitis may present with fever, headache, lethargy, confusion, irritability, and stiff neck. There are three principal modes of onset. About 25% of cases begin abruptly with fulminant illness; mortality is high in this setting. More often, meningeal symptoms progress over 1 to 7 days. Finally, meningitis may superimpose itself on 1 to 3 weeks of an upper respiratory–type illness; diagnosis is most difficult in this group. Occasionally, no more than a single additional neurologic symptom or sign hints at disease more serious than a routine upper respiratory infection. Stiff neck is absent in about one fifth of all patients with meningitis, notably in the very young, the old, and the comatose. A petechial or purpuric rash is found in one half of patients with meningococcemia; although not pathognomonic, palpable purpura is very suggestive of *N. meningitidis* infection. About 20% of patients with acute bacterial meningitis have seizures, and a similar fraction have focal neurologic findings.

Laboratory Diagnosis

The CSF in acute bacterial meningitis usually contains 1000 to 10,000 cells per microliter, mostly neutrophils (see Table 97–1). Glucose content falls below 40 mg/dl, and the protein level rises above 150 mg/dl in most patients. The Gram-stained preparation of CSF is positive in 80 to 88% of cases. However, certain cautionary notes are appropriate. Cell counts can be lower (occasionally zero) early in the course of meningococcal and pneumo-

TABLE 97–3	**Presentations of Bacterial Meningitis Without Polymorphonuclear Neutrophil Predominance**

Antecedent antimicrobial therapy
Listeria monocytogenes meningitis
Tuberculous meningitis
Syphilitic meningitis

coccal meningitis. Also, predominantly mononuclear cell pleocytosis may occur in patients who have received antibiotics before the lumbar puncture (Table 97–3). A similar mononuclear pleocytosis may be seen in *Listeria monocytogenes* meningitis, tuberculous meningitis, and acute syphilitic meningitis. Gram-stained preparations of CSF may be negative or misinterpreted when meningitis is caused by *H. influenzae, N. meningitidis,* or *L. monocytogenes*; the presence of gram-negative diplococci and coccobacilli may be difficult to appreciate, particularly when the background consists of amorphous pink material. In addition, bacteria tend to be pleomorphic in CSF and may assume atypical forms. In the case of *Listeria*, CSF colony counts are low ($10^3/\mu l$). *If* interpretation of the Gram-stained CSF is not clear-cut, broad-spectrum antibiotics should be instituted while the results of cultures are being awaited. If the initial Gram-stained preparation does not contain organisms, examining the stained sediment prepared by concentrating up to 5 ml of CSF with a cytocentrifuge may reveal the causative organism.

Cultures of CSF, blood, fluid expressed from purpuric lesions, and nasopharyngeal swabs have a high yield. The last mentioned is particularly valuable in patients who have received antibiotic therapy before hospitalization, since most such drugs do not achieve substantial levels in nasopharyngeal secretions.

Recognition of meningitis may be difficult following head trauma or neurosurgery, since the symptoms, signs, and laboratory findings of infection can be difficult to separate from those of trauma. A low CSF glucose level usually indicates infection but can also be seen after subarachnoid hemorrhage. The causative organism, characteristically an enteric gram-negative rod, may already have been cultured from an extraneural site, such as a wound or urine. The known antibiotic sensitivities of such isolates, therefore, may provide a valuable guide to the initial treatment of meningitis.

All patients with meningitis caused by *Streptococcus pneumoniae, H. influenzae,* and unusual agents or mixed infections should undergo radiography of nasal sinuses and mastoids to exclude a parameningeal focus of infection.

Differential Diagnosis

Classic acute bacterial meningitis resembles few other diseases. Ruptured brain abscess should be considered, particularly if the CSF white blood cell count is unusually high and focal neurologic signs are present. Parameningeal foci of infection usually cause fever, headache, and local signs. CSF characteristically shows modest neutrophilic pleocytosis and moderately increased protein, but CSF glucose is usually normal. In patients with bacterial meningitis who have already been given antibiotic treatment, the CSF may be sterile, but neutrophils commonly are present in CSF and the glucose level is depressed. Early in the evolution of viral or tuberculous meningitis, the pleocytosis may be predominantly neutrophilic. Serial examinations, however, will show a progressive shift to a mononuclear cell predominance. Acute viral meningoencephalitis may be difficult to distinguish clinically from bacterial meningitis; the evolution of CSF findings and the clinical course usually decide the matter.

Treatment and Outcome

Bacterial meningitis requires the prompt institution of appropriate antibiotics. If the Gram-stained smear of CSF indicates pneumococcal or meningococcal disease, penicillin G should be administered intravenously in a dose of 25,000 units/kg every 2 hours (up to 24 million units/day). The alternative drug for patients with severe penicillin allergy is chloramphenicol, 25 mg/kg given intravenously every 6 hours. Given the increasing occurrence of penicillin-resistant *S. pneumoniae*, alternative therapy with vancomycin (pending cultures and sensitivity testing) is indicated if penicillin resistance is high in clinical isolates in the locale. Suspected cases of *H. influenzae* meningitis should be treated with cefotaxime, 2 gm given intravenously every 4 hours, or ceftriaxone, 2 gm given intravenously every 12 hours. In a case of suspected community-acquired meningitis, if the Gram-stained preparation of CSF is negative but clinical and laboratory findings suggest bacterial meningitis, penicillin and cefotaxime therapy should be started. Third-generation cephalosporins are the indicated choice for treating sensitive gram-negative enteric organisms causing meningitis. Agents such as ceftazidime, 2 gm given intravenously every 6 to 8 hours, may be effective against *Pseudomonas aeruginosa*. If the organism is resistant to cephalosporins, the patient should be treated with a combination of intraventricular plus parenteral aminoglycoside and a beta-lactam antibiotic selected on the basis of the sensitivity of the isolate (e.g., mezlocillin or piperacillin). The placement of an intraventricular reservoir facilitates treatment of such patients. Regardless of the results of sensitivity testing, chloramphenicol is not an adequate drug for treatment of gram-negative bacillary meningitis; its use has been associated with unacceptably high mortality rates.

The management of bacterial meningitis extends beyond the patient. Contacts must be protected, as they are at substantial risk of developing meningococcal meningitis or serious *H. influenzae* disease. At the time one first suspects bacterial meningitis, respiratory isolation procedures should be initiated. One should begin antibiotic prophylaxis of contacts when the clinical course or Gram-stained preparation of CSF suggests meningococcal or *H. influenzae* meningitis. The recommended drug for household and other intimate contacts of patients with meningococcal meningitis is rifampin, 10 mg/kg (up to 600 mg) twice daily for 2 days. The goal of prophylaxis of contacts of *H. influenzae* type B meningitis is to protect children younger than 4 years of age. Since the organism may be passed from patient to asymptomatic adults to at-risk child, rifampin, 20 mg/kg (up to 600 mg) daily for 4 days, should be given to all members of the household and day care center of the index case who have contact with children younger than 4 years old. Despite parenteral antibiotic therapy, patients with *N. meningitidis* or *H. influenzae* meningitis may have persistent nasopharyngeal carriage and should also receive rifampin treatment before discharge from the hospital.

Although hospital contacts of patients with meningococcal meningitis are at low risk of acquiring the carrier state and disease, occasional secondary cases do occur. Thus, personnel in close contact with the patient's respiratory secretions should receive prophylactic antibiotics. All persons receiving rifampin prophylaxis should be warned that their urine and tears will turn orange and that oral contraceptives will be inactivated temporarily by the antiestrogen effects of the drug.

About 30% of adults with bacterial meningitis die of the infection. In the survivors, deafness (6 to 10%) and other serious neurologic sequelae (1 to 18%) are common. The prognosis in individual cases depends largely on the level of consciousness and extent of CNS damage at the time of the first treatment. Misdiagnosis (> 50% of patients) and attendant delays in starting antibiotics are factors in morbidity that the physician must try to offset. Patients with fulminant meningitis should be treated with antibiotics within 30 minutes of reaching medical care. Even after antibiotic therapy and presumed cure, bacterial meningitis may recur. The pattern of recurrence usually suggests a parameningeal infective focus or dural defect (Table 97–4).

The most common types of bacterial meningitis can be prevented by vaccinating susceptible individuals. Effective polysaccharide vaccines are available for some strains of *N. meningitidis*, *S. pneumoniae*, and *H. influenzae* type B.

Aseptic Meningitis

Leptomeningitis associated with negative Gram's stains of CSF and negative cultures for bacteria has been designated aseptic meningitis, a somewhat unfortunate designa-

TABLE 97–4	"Three R's" of CNS Infection	
R	Deterioration	Possibilities
Recrudescence Relapse	During Rx, same bacteria 3–14 days after stopping treatment, same bacteria	Wrong Rx Parameningeal focus
Recurrence	Delayed, same or other bacteria	Congenital or acquired dural defects

CNS = Central nervous system; Rx = therapy.

tion that implies a benign illness that resolves spontaneously. It is important, however, to assume a high level of vigilance in this group of patients, as they may have a potentially treatable but progressive illness.

Epidemiology

Viral infections are the most frequent cause of aseptic meningitis. Of those cases in which a specific causal agent can be established, 97% are due to enteroviruses (particularly coxsackievirus B and enteric cytopathogenic human orphan [ECHO] virus), mumps, lymphocytic choriomeningitis virus (LCM), herpes simplex virus (HSV), and leptospirosis. Viral meningitis is a disease mainly of children and young adults (70% of patients are younger than 20 years of age). Seasonal variation reflects the predominance of enteroviral infection, so that most cases occur in summer or early fall. Mumps usually occurs in winter, and LCM, in fall or winter.

Pathogenesis and Pathophysiology

Localization to the meninges occurs during systemic viremia. The basis for the meningotropism of those viruses that cause aseptic meningitis is not understood. Herpes simplex virus type 2 may cause meningitis during the course of primary genital herpes.

Clinical Presentation

The syndrome of aseptic meningitis of viral origin begins with the acute onset of headache, fever, and meningismus associated with CSF pleocytosis. The headache often is described as the worst ever experienced and is exacerbated by sitting, standing, or coughing. In typical cases, the course is benign. The development of changes in sensorium, seizures, or focal neurologic signs shifts the diagnosis to encephalitis or meningoencephalitis. Additional clinical features may suggest a particular infectious agent. Patients with mumps may have or may develop parotitis or orchitis and usually give a history of appropriate contact. LCM infection often follows exposure to mice, guinea pigs, or hamsters and causes severe myalgias; an infectious mononucleosis–like illness can ensue, with rash and orchitis. Leptospirosis often follows exposure to rats or mice or swimming in water contaminated by their urine; aseptic meningitis occurs in the second phase of the illness. Aseptic meningitis also can be seen in persons with HIV infection, either as a manifestation of primary infection by the virus or as a later complication. The pleocytosis generally is modest, the protein level is only slightly elevated, and the glucose concentration is normal or slightly depressed. HIV serology may be negative with early infection and should therefore be repeated if suspicion is high (see Chapter 108).

Laboratory Diagnosis

In viral meningitis, the CSF shows a pleocytosis of 10 to 2000 white blood cells per microliter. Two thirds of patients have mainly neutrophils in the initial CSF specimen. However, serial lumbar punctures reveal a rapid shift (within 6 to 8 hours) in the CSF differential count toward a mononuclear cell predominance. CSF protein is normal in one third of cases and almost always less than 100 mg/dl. The CSF glucose level characteristically is normal, although minimal depression occurs in mumps (30% of cases), in LCM (60%), and less frequently in ECHO virus and HSV meningitis. Serial lumbar punctures show a 95% reduction in cell count by 2 weeks. Stool cultures have the highest yield for enterovirus isolation (40 to 50%); CSF and throat cultures are positive in about 15% of cases. Serologies also may indicate a specific causative agent; a fourfold rise in antibody titer is helpful in confirming the significance of a virus isolated from the throat or stool. However, serologic studies are seldom useful in acute diagnosis.

Differential Diagnosis

Partially treated bacterial meningitis and a parameningeal focus of infection may be particularly difficult to distinguish from aseptic meningitis. Serial lumbar punctures may be helpful in establishing the former, and x-ray films of paranasal sinuses and mastoids, the latter. Also in the differential diagnosis are infectious agents that are not cultured on routine bacterial media and are considered to be causes of subacute meningitis (see later). Infective endocarditis may cause aseptic meningitis and is an important diagnostic consideration in the appropriate setting (see Chapter 100).

Treatment and Course

Viral meningitis is generally benign and self-limited. HSV meningitis associated with primary genital herpes occasionally causes sufficient symptoms to warrant treatment with acyclovir.

Subacute and Chronic Meningitis

Certain infectious and noninfectious diseases can present as a subacute or chronic meningitis. Chronic meningitis refers to a clinical syndrome of at least 4 weeks' duration and is discussed in Chapter 120. More germane to the differential diagnosis of aseptic meningitis is a neurologic disease that develops over a course of several days to weeks, clinically takes the form of meningitis or meningoencephalitis, and is associated with a predominantly mononuclear pleocytosis in the CSF. The infectious causes of this syndrome may present as a subacute to chronic meningitis (Table 97–5).

At the outset it is important to consider the possible role of HIV as directly causing this syndrome or predis-

TABLE 97–5	Subacute to Chronic Meningitis

Causative Agent	Association
Human immunodeficiency virus (HIV)	Direct involvement or opportunistic infection
Mycobacterium tuberculosis	May have extraneural tuberculosis
Cryptococcus neoformans	Compromised host
Coccidioides immitis	Southwestern United States
Histoplasma capsulatum	Ohio and Mississippi River valleys
Treponema pallidum	Acute syphilitic meningitis, secondary meningovascular syphilis
Lyme disease	Tick bite, rash, seasonal occurrence

posing to specific opportunistic infections, such as cryptococcosis or toxoplasmosis, which frequently present as subacute meningitis. The patient in a high-risk category for the acquired immunodeficiency syndrome (AIDS) requires special consideration in this regard (see Chapter 108).

Tuberculous meningitis results from the rupture of a parameningeal focus into the subarachnoid space. The presentation is generally one of semiacute or subacute meningitis, with a neurologic syndrome being present for less than 2 weeks in over half of patients. Headache, fever, meningismus, and altered mental status are characteristic, with papilledema, cranial nerve palsies (II, III, IV, VI, or VII), and extensor plantar reflexes each occurring in about one fourth of cases. The initial CSF sample may show predominance of neutrophils, but the differential shifts to mononuclear cells within the next 7 to 10 days. Acid-fast bacilli are identified in the CSF of 10 to 20% of patients; the intermediate-strength tuberculin skin test is positive in 65%. Since delay in institution of treatment is associated with increased mortality, therapy is initiated before confirmation of the diagnosis in most cases. The clinical suspicion of tuberculosis is heightened by a history of remote tuberculosis in one half of patients; concurrent pulmonary disease occurs in about one third, so that the diagnosis may be supported by smears or culture of pulmonary secretions. Appropriate therapy consists of isoniazid, rifampin, ethambutol, and pyrazinamide. "Vasculitis" related to entrapment of cerebral vessels in inflammatory exudate may lead to stroke syndromes. This has been offered as a rationale for the use of corticosteroids as adjunctive therapy. Although evidence of their advantage remains unproved, some authorities believe that corticosteroids should be given, in tapering doses, for 4 weeks when the diagnosis of tuberculosis is established, particularly if cranial palsies appear or stupor or coma supervenes.

Cryptococcal meningitis is the most common fungal meningitis and can occur in apparently normal as well as immunocompromised hosts. The presentation is of insidious onset followed by weeks to months of progressive meningoencephalitis, sometimes clinically indistinguishable from the course of tuberculosis. Certain associations are useful in this differential diagnosis. The presence of immunosuppression suggests cryptococcosis, whereas chronic debilitating disease, miliary infiltrates on chest radiograph, or the syndrome of inappropriate antidiuretic hormone suggests tuberculosis. An India ink preparation of CSF reveals encapsulated yeast in 50% of cases. More than 90% have cryptococcal polysaccharide antigen in CSF or serum. Fungal cultures of urine, stool, sputum, and blood should be obtained; they may be positive in the absence of clinically apparent extraneural disease. Treatment of cryptococcal meningitis requires amphotericin B. Addition of flucytosine allows use of less amphotericin B. Fluconazole is also effective but causes less rapid sterilization of the CSF. Daily fluconazole is effective for life-long maintenance therapy to prevent relapses in persons with AIDS.

Coccidioides immitis is a major cause of granulomatous meningitis in semiarid areas of the southwestern United States; *Histoplasma capsulatum* may cause a similar syndrome in endemic areas (Ohio and Mississippi River valleys).

Neurosyphilis reflects the fact that the spirochete causing syphilis invades the CNS in most instances of systemic infection. The organism then may either be cleared by host defenses or persist to produce a more chronic infection expressed symptomatically only years later. The most common form of neurosyphilis is asymptomatic; patients harbor in the CSF a few white cells and have a positive serologic test for syphilis. Symptomatic neurosyphilis can appear as acute or subacute meningitis (meningitic form) resembling that of other bacterial infections and usually occurring during the stage of secondary syphilis when there are cutaneous changes as well. Hydrocephalus and cranial nerve (VII and VIII) abnormalities may develop. CSF and serum serologies usually are strongly positive, and the disease is responsive to penicillin.

Vascular syphilis begins 2 to 10 years after the primary lesion. The disorder is characterized by both meningeal inflammation and a vasculitis of small arterial vessels, the latter leading to arterial occlusion. Clinically, the disorder produces few signs of meningitis but results in monofocal or multifocal cerebral or spinal infarction. The disorder may be mistaken for an autoimmune vasculitis or even arteriosclerotic cerebrovascular disease. The early and prominent spinal cord signs should lead one to expect syphilis, whereas the findings in the CSF of pleocytosis, elevated gamma globulin, and a positive serologic test for syphilis establish the diagnosis. Patients respond to antibiotic therapy, although recovery from focal abnormalities may be incomplete. Syphilis is more difficult to diagnose and may have an accelerated course in the HIV-infected individual. Meningovascular syphilis may develop within months of primary infection, despite treatment with intramuscular benzathine penicillin (see Chapter 107).

General paresis, once a common cause of admission to mental institutions, is now rare. The disorder results from syphilitic invasion of the parenchyma of the brain and begins clinically 10 to 20 years after the primary infection. Paresis is characterized by progressive dementia, sometimes with manic symptoms and megalomania and often with coarse tremors affecting facial muscles and tongue. The diagnostic clue is the presence of Argyll Robertson pupils (p. 829). The CSF is always abnormal. The diagnosis is made by serologic tests. Early treatment with antibiotics usually leads to improvement but not complete recovery.

Tabes dorsalis is a chronic infective process of the dorsal roots that appears 10 to 20 years after primary syphilitic infection. The disorder is characterized by lightning-like pains and a progressive sensory neuropathy affecting predominantly large fibers supplying the lower extremities. There is profound loss of vibration and position sense as well as areflexia. Autonomic fibers are also affected, causing postural hypotension, trophic ulcers of the feet, and traumatic arthropathy of joints. Argyll Robertson pupils are usually present. CSF serologic tests are usually positive. The disorder responds only partially to treatment with antibiotics.

Rare complications of syphilis include progressive optic atrophy, gumma (a mass lesion in the brain), congenital neurosyphilis, and syphilitic infection of the auditory and vestibular system. Descriptions can be found in appropriate texts.

Lyme disease, a tick-borne spirochetosis (see Chapter 95), is associated in 15% of clinically affected individuals with meningitis, encephalitis, or cranial or radicular neuropathies. Characteristically, the neurologic disease begins several weeks after the typical skin rash, erythema chronicum migrans. Furthermore, the skin rash may have been so mild as to go unnoticed and usually has faded by the time neurologic manifestations appear. The diagnosis should be suspected when a patient develops subacute or chronic meningitis during late summer or early fall, with CSF changes consisting of a modest mononuclear pleocytosis, protein values below 100 mg/dl, and normal glucose levels. The diagnosis is established serologically. Patients with early Lyme disease usually respond to oral doxycycline. Patients with later, or disseminated, Lyme disease respond less predictably to prolonged (14 to 21 days) courses of intravenous ceftriaxone.

Several noninfectious diseases may manifest as a subacute or chronic meningitis. Typical of this group is a CSF containing 10 to 100 lymphocytes, elevated protein levels, and a mild to severely lowered glucose content. Meningeal carcinomatosis represents diffuse involvement of the leptomeninges by metastatic adenocarcinoma, lymphoma, or melanoma. Cytologic analysis often identifies malignant cells. Sarcoidosis may cause a basilar meningitis and asymmetric cranial nerve involvement, as well as a low-grade pleocytosis, sometimes associated with borderline low CSF glucose levels. Granulomatous angiitis and Behçet's disease also belong in this category.

Approach to Diagnosis

Diagnosing the specific cause of subacute or chronic meningitis may be quite difficult. In patients with tuberculous or fungal meningitis, cultures may not become positive for 4 to 6 weeks or longer; moreover, meningitis caused by some fungi (e.g., *H. capsulatum*) is often associated with negative cultures of the CSF.

Because of the uncertainties involved in establishing the diagnosis of infectious cases, and even the question of whether a particular patient has an infectious or noninfectious disease, an organized approach must be taken. In addition to routine laboratory tests (on multiple samples of CSF), including India ink and cultures for bacteria, mycobacteria, and fungi, the patient with chronic meningitis of unknown cause should have the following: Venereal Disease Research Laboratories (VDRL) testing and cryptococcal antigens (and, when appropriate, antibody to *Borrelia burgdorferi*) determined on blood and CSF; fluorescent treponemal antibody (FTA)–absorbed, antinuclear antibody, *Histoplasma* antigen detection in urine and CSF, and antibody to HIV and *H. capsulatum* (and, where appropriate, *C. immitis*) on serum; and cytologies (×3) on CSF. A tuberculin skin test (intermediate strength, 5 TU) should be done, along with anergy skin testing (mumps, *Candida*, tetanus). Diagnosis by polymerase chain reaction (PCR) of specific pathogens in CSF should greatly expedite evaluation of patients with chronic meningitis in the future.

The appropriate management is decided by the patient's clinical status and the results of these tests. If the CSF pleocytosis consists of more than 50 to 100 cells per microliter, then an infectious disease is likely. Empirical therapy for tuberculous meningitis is appropriate. If the tuberculin skin test is negative, however, fungal meningitis becomes more likely. Repeated cytologic and microbiologic studies of the CSF may reveal the diagnosis. If the pleocytosis is low grade, fewer than 50 to 100 cells per microliter, a noninfectious cause becomes more likely; the condition even may be self-limited, the so-called chronic benign lymphocytic meningitis. The approach to treating such patients must be individualized. Only rarely is brain or meningeal biopsy necessary or helpful. If all CSF studies are nondiagnostic and the patient's clinical condition is stable, a period of careful observation is almost always preferable to an invasive diagnostic procedure.

ENCEPHALITIS

Acute viral and other infectious causes of encephalitis usually produce fever, headache, stiff neck, confusion, alterations in consciousness, focal neurologic signs, and seizures.

Epidemiology

A large number of viral and nonviral agents can cause encephalitis (Table 97–6). Seasonal occurrence may help to limit the differential diagnosis. Arthropod-borne viruses peak in the summer (California encephalitis [La Crosse virus] and western equine encephalitis in August, St. Louis encephalitis slightly later). The tick-borne infections (Rocky Mountain spotted fever) occur in early summer, enterovirus infections in later summer and fall, and mumps in the winter and spring. Geographic distribution is also helpful. Eastern equine encephalitis is confined to the coastal states. Serologic surveys indicate that infections by encephalitis viruses are most often subclinical. It

TABLE 97–6	Infectious Agents Causing Encephalitis and Meningoencephalitis

Viral

Herpes simplex
Epstein-Barr
Varicella-zoster
Cytomegalovirus
Mumps
Measles
La Crosse virus
St. Louis encephalitis
Eastern equine encephalitis
Western equine encephalitis
Coxsackie
ECHO
Rabies
HIV

Nonviral

Rickettsia rickettsii
Rickettsia typhi
Mycoplasma pneumoniae
Leptospira species
Brucella species
Mycobacterium tuberculosis
Histoplasma capsulatum
Cryptococcus neoformans
Naegleria species
Acanthamoeba species
Toxoplasma gondii
Trypanosoma species
Plasmodium falciparum
Borrelia burgdorferi

ECHO = Enteric cytopathogenic human orphan; HIV = human immunodeficiency virus.

is not clear why so few among the many infected subjects develop encephalitis.

Herpes simplex virus is the most frequent and devastating cause of sporadic, severe focal encephalitis; overall it is implicated in 10% of all cases of encephalitis in North America. There is no age, sex, seasonal, or geographic preference.

Pathogenesis

Viruses reach the CNS by the blood stream or peripheral nerves. HSV presumably reaches the brain by cell-to-cell spread along recurrent branches of the trigeminal nerve, which innervate the meninges of the anterior and middle fossae. Although this would explain the characteristic localization of necrotic lesions to the inferomedial portions of the temporal and frontal lobes, it is not clear why such spread is so rare, with one case of HSV encephalitis occurring per million in the population per annum.

Clinical Features

The course of HSV encephalitis is considered here in detail because of the importance of establishing the diag-

nosis of this treatable entity. Patients affected by HSV commonly describe a prodrome of 1 to 7 days of upper respiratory tract symptoms followed by the sudden onset of headache and fever. The headache and fever may be associated with acute loss of recent memory, behavioral abnormalities, delirium, difficulty with speech, and seizures, often focal. Disorders of the sensorium are not, however, always apparent at the time of presentation and are not essential for the working diagnosis of this eminently treatable, but potentially lethal, infection of the CNS.

Laboratory Diagnosis

In HSV encephalitis, the CSF can contain 0 to 1000 white blood cells per microliter, predominantly lymphocytes. Protein is moderately high (median, 80 mg/dl). CSF glucose is reduced in only 5% of individuals within 3 days of onset but becomes abnormal in additional patients later in the course. In about 5% the CSF is normal. Other laboratory findings at onset are of little help, although focal abnormalities may be present in the electroencephalogram and develop in CT or magnetic resonance imaging (MRI) brain scan by the third day in most patients. Acyclovir offers such high likelihood of therapeutic benefit in HSV encephalitis, with so little risk in this highly fatal and neurologically damaging disease, that brain biopsy should not be performed unless an alternative, treatable diagnosis seems very likely. A low CSF glucose level should increase suspicion that a granulomatous infection is present (tuberculosis, cryptococcosis). If the initial CSF shows a low glucose level, roughly one third of individuals will have an alternative treatable infection. If CSF studies and brain imaging remain inconclusive in such circumstances, biopsy may be appropriate.

Viral cultures of stool, throat, buffy coat, CSF, and brain biopsy specimens and indirect immunofluorescence or immunoperoxidase staining of tissues may provide a specific diagnosis, but both viral isolation and serologic evidence of a rise in antibody titer usually come too late to guide initial treatment. In the case of HSV encephalitis, serologies are particularly helpful in the 30% of individuals with a primary infection. Also, CSF titers of antibody to HSV, which reflect intrathecal production of antibody, may show a diagnostic fourfold rise.

Differential Diagnosis

Acute (demyelinating) encephalomyelitis, infective endocarditis producing brain embolization, meningoencephalitis caused by *Cryptococcus neoformans, Mycobacterium tuberculosis*, or the La Crosse virus, acute bacterial abscess, acute thrombotic thrombocytopenic purpura, cerebral venous thrombosis, vascular disease, and primary and metastatic tumors may all simulate HSV encephalitis.

Treatment and Outcome

The course of viral encephalitis depends on the etiologic agent. Untreated HSV encephalitis has a high mortality

(70%), and survival is associated with severe neurologic residua. Acyclovir therapy improves survival and greatly lessens morbidity in patients if initiated early, before deterioration to coma. Prognosis is particularly favorable in patients younger than 30 years old.

Rabies

Rabies encephalitis is always fatal, requiring one to place major attention on prevention. Currently, zero to six cases of rabies occur each year in the United States, and approximately 20,000 people receive postexposure prophylaxis.

The incubation period for rabies is generally 20 to 90 days, during which the rabies virus replicates locally and then migrates along nerves to the spinal cord and brain. Rabies begins with fever, headache, fatigue, and pain or paresthesias at the site of inoculation; confusion, seizures, paralysis, and stiff neck follow. Periods of violent agitation are characteristic of rabies encephalitis. Attempts at drinking produce laryngospasm, gagging, and apprehension. Paralysis, coma, and death supervene. When rabies is suspected, protective isolation procedures should be instituted to avoid additional exposure of the hospital staff to saliva and other infected secretions. Confirmation of the diagnosis is possible by assaying rabies-neutralizing antibody or isolating virus from saliva, CSF, and urine sediment. Immunofluorescent rabies antibody staining of a skin biopsy specimen taken from the posterior neck is a rapid means of establishing the diagnosis.

Indications for prophylaxis are based on the following principles. (1) The patient must have been exposed. Nonbite exposure is possible if mucous membranes or open wounds are contaminated with animal saliva; exposure to bat urine in heavily contaminated caves has been followed by rabies. (2) Small rodents (rats, mice, chipmunks, squirrels) and rabbits rarely are infected with rabies and have not been associated with human disease. Consultation with local or state health authorities is essential, since certain areas of the United States are considered rabies free. In other areas, if rabies is present in wild animals, dogs and cats have the potential to transmit rabies. Domestic dogs and cats should be quarantined for 10 days after biting someone; if they develop no signs of illness, there is no risk of transmission by their earlier bite. Nondomestic animals should be destroyed and their brains examined for rabies virus by direct fluorescent antibody testing. If the biting animal escapes, postexposure prophylaxis is usually indicated. Bites of bat, skunk, and racoon require treatment unless the animal is caught. Unusual behavior of animals and truly unprovoked attacks (as opposed to those incurred during handling or feeding) can be signs of rabies.

Currently, postexposure management consists of (1) thorough wound cleansing; (2) human rabies immune globulin, 20 IU/kg, one half infiltrated locally in the area of the bite and one half intramuscularly; and (3) human diploid cell rabies vaccine, 1.0 ml given intramuscularly five times during a 1-month period. Individuals at high risk of exposure to rabies should be vaccinated. Veterinarians, laboratory workers, and those who frequent caves belong in this category.

SPECTRUM OF TUBERCULOUS, FUNGAL, AND PARASITIC INFECTIONS

The approach to the beginning of the chapter was syndromic. Now the spectrum of tuberculous, fungal, and parasitic infections of the CNS is briefly considered. Many, but not all, of these infections are increasing in incidence as the direct result of the increasing prevalence of HIV infection in the population (see Chapter 108).

Tuberculosis

Central nervous system tuberculosis can occur in several forms, sometimes without evidence of active infection elsewhere in the body. The most common form is *tuberculous meningitis*. This disorder is characterized by the subacute onset of headache, stiff neck, and fever. After a few days, affected patients become confused and disoriented. They often develop abnormalities of cranial nerve function, particularly hearing loss due to marked inflammation at the base of the brain. Most patients, if untreated, lapse into coma and die within 3 to 4 weeks of onset. An accompanying arteritis may produce focal signs, including hemiplegia, during the course of the disorder. Tuberculous meningitis must be distinguished from other causes of acute and subacute meningeal infection, a process that often is not easy even after examination of the CSF. The pressure and cell count are elevated with up to a few hundred cells, a mixture of leukocytes and lymphocytes. The protein level is elevated, usually above 100 mg/dl and often to very high levels, and the glucose concentration is depressed. Smears for acid-fast bacilli are positive in only about 10 to 20% of samples. Tuberculosis organisms grow on culture but only after several weeks. Pending complete availability and accuracy of such measures, patients with subacutely developing meningitis suspected of having tuberculosis should be treated with antituberculous agents prior to definitive diagnosis. Large samples of CSF should be sent for culture, and a careful search should be made for tuberculosis elsewhere in the body. Seventy-five percent of such patients have a positive tuberculin skin test, and a careful search may yield evidence of systemic tuberculosis.

Tuberculomas of the brain produce symptoms and signs either of the mass lesion or of meningitis, with the tuberculomas being found incidentally. One or multiple lesions are identified on CT scan, but the scan itself does not distinguish tuberculomas from brain tumor or other brain abscesses. In the absence of evidence of meningeal or systemic tuberculosis, biopsy is necessary for diagnosis. Patients with tuberculomas, like those with tuberculous meningitis, respond to antituberculous therapy, but brain lesions may remain visible in the CT scan long after the patient has improved clinically; the clinical course, not the scan, predicts the outcome.

Less common manifestations of CNS tuberculosis include *chronic arachnoiditis* characterized by a low-grade inflammatory response in the CSF and progressive pain with signs of either cauda equina or spinal cord dysfunction. The diagnosis of arachnoiditis is suggested by a myelogram showing evidence of fibrosis and compartmentalization instead of the usually smooth subarachnoid lining. The disorder responds poorly to treatment. *Tuberculous myelopathy* probably results from direct invasion of the organism from the subarachnoid space. Patients present with a subacutely developing myelopathy characterized by sensory loss either in the legs or in all four extremities, depending on the site of the spinal cord invasion. Many patients have additional signs of meningitis, including fever, headache, and stiff neck. The CSF usually contains cells and tuberculous organisms. The myelogram may show evidence of arachnoiditis and frequently demonstrates an enlarged spinal cord or complete block to the passage of contrast material in the thoracic or cervical region.

Fungal and Parasitic Infections

Fungal and parasitic infections of the CNS are less common than viral and bacterial infections and often affect immunosuppressed patients. Table 97–7 lists the more common of these infections. Like bacterial infections, fungal and parasitic infections may cause either meningitis or parenchymal abscesses. The meningitides, when they occur, manifest with clinical symptoms that, while similar, are usually less severe and abrupt than those of acute bacterial meningitis. The common fungal causes of meningitis include cryptococcosis, coccidioidomycosis, and histoplasmosis. *Cryptococcal meningitis* is a sporadic infection that affects both immunosuppressed patients

TABLE 97–7	Some Fungal and Parasitic Causes of CNS Infections

Fungal Infection

Cryptococcosis
Coccidioidomycosis
Aspergillosis
Mucormycosis
Actinomycosis
Histoplasmosis
Blastomycosis
Candidiasis

Helminthic Infection

Trichinosis
Cysticercosis
Echinococcosis
Schistosomiasis
Angiostrongyliasis
Ascariasis

Protozoan Infection

Toxoplasmosis
Amebiasis
Malaria
Chagas' disease
Trypanosomiasis (African)

CNS = Central nervous system.

(50%) and nonimmunosuppressed patients. The disorder is characterized by headache and sometimes fever and stiff neck. The clinical symptoms may evolve for periods as long as weeks or months; diagnosis can be made only by identifying the organism or its antigen in the CSF. *Histoplasma* and coccidioidomycosis meningitides occur in endemic areas and often affect nonimmunosuppressed individuals. The diagnosis is suggested by a history of residence in the appropriate geographic area and is con-

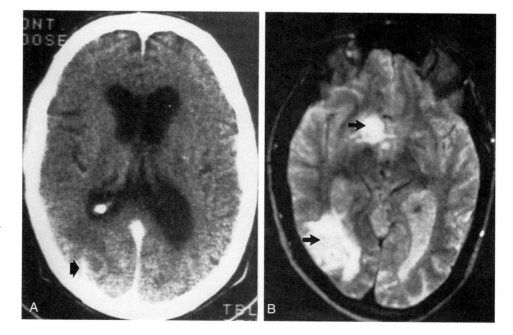

Figure 97–1

Toxoplasma abscesses in a patient with acquired immunodeficiency syndrome. *A,* Computed tomography (CT) scan shows a contrast-enhanced mass *(arrow). B,* Magnetic resonance image reveals multiple masses *(arrows)* not seen on CT scan, leading physicians to suspect abscesses rather than tumor.

firmed by CSF and serologic evaluation. Antifungal treatment, particularly in the nonimmunosuppressed patient, is usually effective.

Parasitic infections of the nervous system usually produce focal abscesses rather than diffuse meningitis. The most common to affect the nonimmunosuppressed host is cysticercosis, a disorder caused by the larval form of the *Taenia solium* tapeworm and contracted by ingesting food or water contaminated with parasite eggs. The disorder is common in the underdeveloped world and parts of the United States having a large Hispanic population. The brain may be invaded in as many as 60% of infected persons. Invasion of the brain leads to formation of either single or multiple cysts, which often lie in the parenchyma but sometimes reside in the ventricles or subarachnoid space. Seizures and increased intracranial pressure are the most common clinical symptoms. CT scanning identifies small intracranial calcifications and hypodense cysts. Serum indirect hemagglutination tests are usually positive and confirm the diagnosis. Where cysts obstruct the ventricular system to cause symptoms, shunting procedures may be necessary. The anthelmintic praziquantel is effective therapy.

Toxoplasmosis of the brain, when it occurs in the adult, is a manifestation of immunosuppression. Patients with abnormal cellular immunity may develop single or multiple abscesses, which appear usually as ring-enhancing lesions on CT scan (Fig. 97–1). The diagnosis and treatment of toxoplasmosis of the brain are discussed in Chapter 108.

REFERENCES

Bacterial Meningitis

Gripshover BM, Ellner JJ: Chronic meningitis. *In* Mandel GL, Bennett JE, Dolin R (eds.): Principles and Practice of Infectious Diseases. 4th ed. New York, Churchill Livingstone, 1995, pp 865–874.
Quagliarello VJ, Scheld WM: New perspectives on bacterial meningitis. Clin Infect Dis 1993;17:603–610.
Swartz MN, Apicella MA, Simberhaff MS: Bacterial meningitis. *In* Bennett JC, Plum F (eds.): Cecil Textbook of Medicine. 20th ed. Philadelphia, WB Saunders Co, 1996, pp 1619–1624.

Aseptic Meningitis

Lepow ML, Carver DH, Wright HT, et al: A clinical, laboratory and epidemiologic investigation of aseptic meningitis during the 4-year period 1955–1958. N Engl J Med 1962;266:1181.

Encephalitis

Johnson R: Viral Infections of the Nervous System. New York, Raven Press, 1982.
Nahmias AJ, Whitley RJ, Visintine AN, Takei Y, Alford CA Jr: HSV encephalitis; Laboratory evaluations and their diagnostic significance. J Infect Dis 1982;145:829.
Whitley RJ: Viral encephalitis. N Engl J Med 1990;323:242–250.

98

Infections of the Head and Neck

INFECTIONS OF THE EAR

Otitis externa is an infection of the external auditory canal. The process may begin as a folliculitis or pustule within the canal. Staphylococci, streptococci, and other skin flora are the most common pathogens. Some cases of otitis externa have been associated with the use of hot tubs. This infection (swimmer's ear) is usually due to *Pseudomonas aeruginosa.*

Patients with otitis externa complain of ear pain that is often quite severe, and they may also complain of itching. Examination reveals an inflamed external canal; the tympanic membrane may be uninvolved. (Patients with otitis media, in contrast, will not have involvement of the external canal unless the tympanic membrane is perforated.) Otitis externa with cellulitis can be treated with systemic antibiotics such as dicloxacillin or erythromycin and local heat. In the absence of cellulitis, irrigation and administration of topical antibiotics such as neomycin and polymyxin are sufficient. Patients with diabetes mellitus are at risk for an invasive external otitis (malignant otitis) due to *P. aeruginosa.* In malignant otitis externa, pain is a presenting complaint, and infection rapidly invades the bones of the skull and may result in cranial nerve palsies, invasion of the brain, and death. Treatment must include debridement of as much necrotic tissue as is feasible and at least 4 to 6 weeks of treatment with an aminoglycoside plus a penicillin derivative active against *Pseudomonas* (e.g., ticarcillin). Ceftazidime, imipenem, or ciprofloxacin may also be effective for this infection.

Otitis media is an infection of the middle ear seen primarily among preschool children but occasionally in adults as well. Infection caused by upper respiratory tract pathogens is promoted by obstruction to drainage through edematous, congested eustachian tubes. *Streptococcus pneumoniae, Haemophilus influenzae,* and *Moraxella catarrhalis* are the most common pathogens, and viral infection with serous otitis may predispose to acute otitis media. Fever, ear pain, diminished hearing, vertigo, or tinnitus may be seen. In young children, however, localizing symptoms may not be appreciated. The tympanic membrane may appear inflamed, but to diagnose otitis media with certainty, either fluid must be seen behind the membrane or diminished mobility of the membrane must

be demonstrated by tympanometry or after air insufflation into the external canal.

Treatment with amoxicillin–clavulanic acid, trimethoprim-sulfamethoxazole, or cefaclor is generally effective; addition of decongestants is of no proven value. Complications of otitis media are uncommon but include infection of the mastoid air cells (mastoiditis), bacterial meningitis, brain abscess, and subdural empyema.

INFECTIONS OF THE NOSE AND SINUSES

Rhinitis is a common manifestation of numerous respiratory virus infections. It is characterized by mucopurulent or watery nasal discharge that may be profuse. When rhinitis is due to respiratory virus infection, pharyngitis, conjunctival suffusion, and fever may be associated. Rhinitis can also be caused by hypersensitivity responses to airborne allergens. Patients with allergic rhinitis often have a transverse skin crease on the bridge of the nose a few millimeters from the tip. The demonstration of eosinophils in a wet preparation of nasal secretions readily distinguishes allergic rhinitis from rhinitis of infectious origin. (Eosinophils can be identified in wet preparations by the presence of large refractile cytoplasmic granules.) Occasionally, following head trauma or neurosurgery, cerebrospinal fluid (CSF) may leak through the nose. "CSF rhinorrhea" places patients at risk for bacterial meningitis. CSF is readily distinguished from nasal secretions by its low protein and relatively high glucose concentrations.

Sinusitis is an infection of the air-filled paranasal sinuses that may complicate viral upper respiratory infections. Allergic rhinitis and structural abnormalities of the nose that interfere with sinus drainage also predispose to sinusitis. Acute sinusitis is primarily caused by upper respiratory tract bacterial pathogens, *Streptococcus pneumoniae* and *Haemophilus influenzae,* and less often by anaerobes and staphylococci.

Sinusitis may be difficult to distinguish from a viral upper respiratory illness that in many instances precedes sinus infection. Patients may complain of headache, "stuffiness," and purulent nasal discharge. Headache may be exacerbated by bending over. There may be tenderness over the involved sinus, and pus may be seen in the turbinates of the nose. Failure of a sinus to light up on transillumination may suggest the diagnosis; sinus radiographs revealing opacification, mucosal thickening, or air-fluid levels establish the diagnosis of sinusitis. Most patients with sinusitis can be treated with a 10-day course of ampicillin, amoxicillin, or trimethoprim-sulfamethoxazole, along with nasal decongestants. Patients who appear toxic or otherwise are severely ill should undergo sinus puncture for drainage, Gram's stain, and culture. Sinusitis may be complicated by bacterial meningitis, brain abscess, or subdural empyema. Therefore, patients with sinusitis and neurologic abnormalities must be evaluated carefully for these complications by computed tomography (CT) scan if a space-occupying lesion is suspected or by CSF examination if meningitis is suspected (see Chapter 97).

Rhinocerebral mucormycosis is an invasive infection arising from the nose or sinuses caused by fungi of the order *Mucorales*. This infection can result in progressive bony destruction and invasion of the brain. Rhinocerebral mucormycosis is seen primarily among poorly controlled diabetics with ketoacidosis, recipients of organ transplants, and patients with hematologic malignancy. Black necrotic lesions of the palate or nasal mucosa are characteristic. Most patients have a depressed sensorium at presentation. Vascular thrombosis and cranial nerve palsies are common. Diagnosis is made by demonstration of the broad, ribbon-shaped, nonseptate hyphae on histologic examination of a scraping or biopsy specimen. Differential diagnosis includes infection due to *Pseudomonas aeruginosa* or to other fungi such as *Aspergillus* species, and cavernous sinus thrombosis. Rhinocerebral mucormycosis is a surgical emergency. Treatment involves correction of the underlying process if possible, broad surgical debridement, and administration of amphotericin B.

INFECTIONS OF THE MOUTH AND PHARYNX

Stomatitis

Stomatitis, or inflammation of the mouth, can be caused by a wide variety of processes. Patients with stomatitis may complain of diffuse or localized pain in the mouth, difficulty in swallowing, and difficulty in managing oral secretions. Various nutritional deficiencies (vitamins B_{12} and C, folic acid, and niacin) and cytotoxic chemotherapies can produce stomatitis and soreness of the mouth.

Thrush is an infection of the oral mucosa by *Candida* species. Thrush may be seen among infants and also in patients receiving broad-spectrum antibiotics or corticosteroids (systemic or inhaled), among patients with leukopenia (e.g., acute leukemia), and among patients with impairments in cell-mediated immunity (e.g., acquired immunodeficiency syndrome [AIDS]). In its milder form, thrush is manifested by an asymptomatic white, "cheesy" exudate on the buccal mucosa and pharynx, which, when scraped, leaves a raw surface. In more severe cases, there may be pain and also erythema surrounding the exudate. The diagnosis is suggested by the characteristic appearance of the lesions and is confirmed by microscopic examination of a KOH preparation of the exudate, which

reveals yeast and the pseudohyphae characteristic of *Candida*. Thrush related to administration of antibiotics and corticosteroids should resolve after the drugs are withdrawn. Otherwise, thrush can be managed with clotrimazole troches. Refractory thrush or candidal infection involving the esophagus should be treated with ketoconazole or fluconazole.

Oral Ulcers and Vesicles (Table 98–1)

Aphthous Stomatitis

Aphthae are discrete, shallow, painful ulcers on erythematous bases; they may be single or multiple and are usually present on the labial or buccal mucosa. Attacks of aphthous stomatitis may be recurrent and quite debilitating. Symptoms may last for several days to 2 weeks. The cause of these ulcerations is unknown, and treatment is symptomatic with saline mouth wash or topical anesthetics. Giant aphthous ulcers may occur in persons with AIDS; they may respond to topical or systemic steroids or to thalidomide.

Herpes Simplex Virus Infection

Although most recurrences of oral herpes simplex infections occur on or near the vermillion border of the lips, the primary attack usually involves the mouth and pharynx. Generalized symptoms of fever, headache, and malaise often precede the appearance of oral lesions by as much as 24 to 48 hours. The involved regions are swollen and erythematous. Small vesicles soon appear; these rupture, leaving shallow, discrete ulcers that may coalesce. The diagnosis can be made by scraping the base of an ulcer. Wright's or Giemsa's stain of this material may reveal the intranuclear inclusions and multinucleated giant cells characteristic of herpes simplex infection. Viral cultures are more sensitive but more expensive. Diagnosis may also be established by immunoassay for viral antigen in the scraping. Treatment of primary infection with acyclovir will decrease the duration of symptoms but has no effect on the frequency of recurrence.

TABLE 98–1	Oral Vesicles and Ulcers
	Aphthous stomatitis
	Primary herpes simplex infection
	Vincent's stomatitis
	Syphilis
	Coxsackievirus A (herpangina)
	Fungi (histoplasmosis)
	Behçet's syndrome
	Systemic lupus erythematosus
	Reiter's syndrome
	Crohn's disease
	Erythema multiforme
	Pemphigus
	Pemphigoid

Vincent's Stomatitis

This is an ulcerative infection of the gingival mucosa due to anaerobic fusobacteria and spirochetes. Breath is often foul, and the ulcerations are covered with a purulent, dirty-appearing, gray exudate. Gram stain of the exudate reveals the characteristic gram-negative fusobacteria and spirochetes. Treatment with penicillin is curative. Untreated, the infection may extend to the peritonsillar space (quinsy) and even involve vascular structures in the lateral neck (see later).

Syphilis

Syphilis may produce a painless primary chancre in the mouth or a painful mucous patch that is a manifestation of secondary disease. The diagnosis should be considered in the sexually active patient with a large (>1 cm) oral ulceration and should be confirmed serologically, since darkfield examination may be confounded by the presence of nonsyphilitic oral spirochetes.

Herpangina

This is a childhood disease that causes tiny, discrete ulcerations of the soft palate and is due to infection with coxsackievirus A.

Fungal Disease

Occasionally, an oral ulcer or nodule may be a manifestation of disseminated infection due to histoplasmosis. These ulcers are generally mildly or minimally symptomatic and are overshadowed by the constitutional symptoms of disseminated fungal illness.

Systemic Illnesses Causing Ulcerative or Vesicular Lesions of the Mouth

Recurrent aphthous oral ulcerations may be part of Behçet's syndrome. Oral ulcerations have been associated with connective tissue diseases, such as systemic lupus erythematosus and Reiter's syndrome, and with Crohn's disease. Although isolated oral bullae and ulcerations may be seen in patients with erythema multiforme, pemphigus, and pemphigoid, almost all patients have an associated skin rash. The "iris" or "target" lesion of erythema multiforme is diagnostic. Otherwise, biopsy will establish the diagnosis. Corticosteroids may be life-saving for pemphigus. Corticosteroids are also used in the treatment of erythema multiforme majorum (Stevens-Johnson syndrome), although proof of their efficacy is not available.

Approach to the Patient with "Sore Throat"

This section discusses the clinical approach to patients with sore throat and also discusses several less common but serious illnesses that can manifest as a "sore throat." When evaluating a patient with a sore throat, it is first important to distinguish between the relatively common and benign sore throat syndromes (viral or streptococcal pharyngitis) and the less common but more dangerous causes of sore throat. Patients with viral or streptococcal pharyngitis often give a history of exposure to individuals with upper respiratory tract infections. Symptoms of cough, rhinitis, and hoarseness (indicating involvement of the larynx) suggest a viral upper respiratory tract infection, although it is important to remember that hoarseness may also be seen with more serious infections, such as epiglottitis.

Examination of the Throat

Two points regarding examination of the throat need emphasis. The first is that complete examination of the oral cavity is important. Not only will a thorough examination give clues to the cause of the complaint, but it may also provide early diagnosis of an asymptomatic malignancy at a time when cure is feasible. The second point is that the normal tonsils and mucosal rim of the anterior fauces are generally a deeper red than the rest of the pharynx in healthy subjects. This should not be mistaken for inflammation. Patients with pharyngitis often have a red, inflamed posterior pharynx. The tonsils are often enlarged and red and may be covered with a punctate or diffuse white exudate. Lymph nodes of the anterior neck are often enlarged.

If any of the seven *danger signs* listed in Table 98–2 is present, the clinician must suspect an illness other than viral or streptococcal pharyngitis. Symptoms persisting longer than 1 week are rarely due to streptococci or viruses and should prompt consideration of other processes (see "Persistent or Penicillin-Unresponsive Pharyngitis"). Respiratory difficulty, particularly stridor, difficulty in handling oral secretions, or difficulty in swallowing should suggest the possibility of epiglottitis or soft tissue space infection. Severe pain in the absence of erythema of the pharynx may be seen with some of the "extrarespiratory" causes of sore throat, as well as in some cases of epiglottitis or retropharyngeal abscess. A *palpable mass* in the pharynx or neck suggests a soft tissue space infection, and *blood in the ear or pharynx* may be an early indication of a lateral pharyngeal space abscess eroding into the carotid artery.

A good history and careful examination will distin-

TABLE 98–2	Seven Danger Signs in Patients with "Sore Throat"

1. Persistence of symptoms longer than 1 week without improvement
2. Respiratory difficulty, particularly stridor
3. Difficulty in handling secretions
4. Difficulty in swallowing
5. Severe pain in the absence of erythema
6. A palpable mass
7. Blood, even in small amounts, in the pharynx or ear

guish between the common and benign causes of a sore throat, and the unusual but often more serious causes.

Pharyngitis

A list of agents that have been associated with pharyngitis is presented in Table 98–3. More than half of all cases are due to respiratory viruses or group A streptococci. Most of the remainder of the cases are without defined etiology. Most cases occur during the winter months. In practice, once a diagnosis of pharyngitis is established clinically, it is most important to distinguish between group A streptococcal infections, which should be treated with penicillin, and viral infections, which should be treated symptomatically (e.g., salicylates, saline gargles). Since clinical criteria do not reliably distinguish streptococcal from nonstreptococcal pharyngitis, all patients with presumed bacterial pharyngitis should have a throat swab for rapid streptococcal antigen test. This test is highly specific, so that a positive test result establishes the diagnosis of streptococcal pharyngitis. The test is less sensitive, so that a negative test result should be followed by culture on sheep blood agar.

PHARYNGITIS AND RESPIRATORY VIRUS INFECTIONS. Many patients with common colds due to rhinovirus, coronavirus, adenovirus or influenza have an associated pharyngitis. Other cold symptoms—rhinorrhea, conjunctival suffusion, and cough—suggest a cold virus; fevers and myalgias suggest influenza. Symptoms generally resolve in a few days without treatment.

Infectious mononucleosis due to Epstein-Barr virus is often associated with pharyngitis. Patients often also complain of malaise and fever. On examination, the pharynx may be inflamed and the tonsils hypertrophied and covered by a white exudate. Cervical lymph node enlargement is often prominent, and generalized lymph node enlargement and splenomegaly are common. Examination of a peripheral blood smear reveals atypical lymphocytes, and the presence of heterophile antibodies (e.g., Monospot test) or a rise in antibodies to Epstein-Barr virus viral capsid antigen will confirm the diagnosis.

Primary HIV seroconversion illness is often manifested by fever, pharyngitis, and lymph node enlargement, sometimes associated with a generalized maculopapular rash (see Chapter 108).

STREPTOCOCCAL PHARYNGITIS. Streptococcal pharyngitis may produce mild or severe symptoms. The pharynx is generally inflamed, and exudative tonsillitis is common but not universal. Fever may be present, and cervical lymph nodes may be enlarged and tender. Clinical distinction between streptococcal and nonstreptococcal pharyngitis is inaccurate, and patients with pharyngitis should therefore have a swab of the posterior pharynx tested for streptococcal infection (see previous). The growth of group A beta-hemolytic streptococci or detection of group A streptococcal antigen is an indication for treatment with penicillin (or erythromycin if the patient is penicillin-allergic). Antibiotics may shorten the duration of symptoms due to this infection but are given primarily to decrease the frequency of rheumatic fever, which may follow untreated streptococcal pharyngitis.

PHARYNGITIS CAUSED BY OTHER BACTERIA. Diphtheria, caused by *Corynebacterium diphtheriae,* is a rare disease in the United States, with five or fewer cases recognized annually since 1980. The grey pseudomembrane bleeds when removed and rarely may cause death via airway obstruction. Most morbidity and mortality in diphtheria are related to the elaboration of a toxin with neurologic and cardiac effects. Treatment consists of antitoxin plus erythromycin. A self-limited pharyngitis, often associated with a diffuse scarlatiniform rash, may be caused by *Arcanobacterium* (formerly *Corynebacterium*) *hemolyticum.* This infection can be treated with penicillin or erythromycin.

Epiglottitis

Epiglottitis, usually an aggressive disease of young children, occurs in adults as well. Early recognition of this entity is critical, because delay in diagnosis or treatment frequently results in death, which may occur abruptly, within hours after the onset of symptoms. This diagnosis must be considered in any patient with a sore throat and any of the following key symptoms or signs: (1) difficulty in swallowing; (2) copious oral secretions; (3) severe pain in the absence of pharyngeal erythema (the pharynx of patients with epiglottitis may be normal or inflamed); and (4) respiratory difficulty, particularly stridor.

Patients with epiglottitis often display a characteristic posture; they lean forward to prevent the swollen epiglottis from completely obstructing the airway and resist any attempt at placement in the supine position. The diagnosis can be confirmed by lateral radiographs of the neck or by indirect laryngoscopy with visualization of the

TABLE 98–3	Causes of Pharyngitis

Viral
Respiratory viruses*
Adenovirus
Herpes simplex
Epstein-Barr virus
Coxsackievirus A (herpangina)
HIV

Mycoplasma pneumoniae

Bacterial
Group A streptococcus*
Group C streptococcus
Vincent's fusospirochetes
Corynebacterium diphtheriae
Arcanobacterium hemolyticum
Neisseria gonorrhoeae

Fungal
Candida (thrush)

*Most frequent identifiable causes of pharyngitis.
HIV = Human immunodeficiency virus.

swollen erythematous epiglottis. This examination should be performed with the patient in the sitting position to minimize the risk of laryngeal spasm. Furthermore, the physician must be prepared to perform emergency tracheostomy should spasm occur. Therapy has two major objectives: protecting the airway and providing appropriate antimicrobial coverage. Prophylactic endotracheal intubation or tracheotomy is often indicated if respiratory distress increases under observation. As the most likely pathogen is *Haemophilus influenzae,* which may be beta-lactamase producing, good antibiotic choices are a second- or third-generation cephalosporin or ampicillin-sulbactam. Corticosteroids may relieve some inflammatory edema; however, their role in this disease remains unproven. Patients with respiratory difficulty should have their airway protected by endotracheal intubation or tracheostomy. Patients without respiratory complaints may be monitored continuously in an intensive care setting and intubated at the first sign of respiratory difficulty. Young children who are close contacts of patients with invasive disease due to *H. influenzae* are themselves at particular risk of serious infection. Children younger than 4 years of age who are close contacts of the index patient and all family members in a household with children younger than 4 years of age should receive prophylaxis with rifampin (20 mg/kg given orally, up to 600 mg twice daily for four doses).

Soft Tissue Space Infections

QUINSY. Quinsy is a unilateral peritonsillar abscess or phlegmon that is an unusual complication of tonsillitis. The patient has pain and difficulty in swallowing and often trouble in handling oral secretions. Trismus (inability to open the mouth due to muscle spasm) may be present. Examination reveals swelling of the peritonsillar tissues and lateral displacement of the uvula. Digital examination may reveal a mass. In the phlegmon stage, penicillin therapy may be adequate; abscess can be identified by CT scan and requires surgical drainage (Table 98–4). Untreated, quinsy may result in glottic edema and respiratory compromise or lateral pharyngeal space abscess.

SEPTIC JUGULAR VEIN THROMBOPHLEBITIS. An uncommon complication of bacterial pharyngitis or quinsy is septic

jugular vein thrombophlebitis (syndrome of postanginal sepsis). Several days following a "sore throat," the patient (generally a teenager or young adult) will note increasing pain and tenderness in the neck. Often there is swelling at the angle of the jaw. The patient will experience high fevers; bacteremia, usually with *Fusobacterium* species; and often septic pulmonary emboli. Treatment is intravenous penicillin, 10 million units/day, plus metronidazole, 500 mg every 6 hours. Patients with persistent fevers may require surgical excision of the jugular vein.

LATERAL PHARYNGEAL SPACE ABSCESS. This rare infection is associated with serious morbidity because of its proximity to vascular structures. Extension to the jugular vein may result in thrombophlebitis with septic pulmonary emboli and bacteremia (syndrome of "postanginal sepsis"), discussed earlier. Erosion of the carotid artery may also complicate this infection, with resultant exsanguination. This may be preceded by small amounts of blood in the ear or pharynx. This infection is generally associated with tenderness and a mass at the angle of the jaw. Prompt surgical intervention may be life-saving.

RETROPHARYNGEAL SPACE ABSCESS. This complication of tonsillitis is rare in adults, since by adulthood the lymph nodes that give rise to this infection are generally atrophied. Most cases in adults are secondary to trauma (e.g., endoscopic) or to extension of a cervical osteomyelitis. The patient often has difficulty in swallowing and may complain of dyspnea, particularly when sitting upright. Diagnosis may be suspected by the presence of a posterior pharyngeal mass and confirmed by lateral neck films.

LUDWIG'S ANGINA. This cellulitis/phlegmon of the floor of the mouth generally is secondary to an odontogenic infection. The tongue is pushed upward, and there is often firm induration of the submandibular space and neck. Laryngeal edema and respiratory compromise may also occur and necessitate protection of the airway. Penicillin is the antibiotic of choice; broad guillotine incision across the submandibular space may sometimes be indicated to provide decompression and adequate drainage, although incision may be unnecessary if the airway can be protected.

Extrarespiratory Causes of Sore Throat

Several extrarespiratory causes of sore throat should be kept in mind. The older patient who complains of soreness in the throat when climbing stairs or when upset may be suffering from angina pectoris with an unusual radiation. The hypertensive patient who presents with an abrupt onset of a "tearing pain" in the throat may have a dissecting aortic aneurysm. In these patients, swallowing is generally unaffected. Patients with deQuervain's subacute thyroiditis may present with fever and pain in the neck radiating to the ears. In patients with thyroiditis, the thyroid is generally tender and the sedimentation rate is increased. Patients with vitamin deficiencies may complain of soreness in the mouth and throat (see Table

TABLE 98–4	Indications for Surgical Drainage: Parapharyngeal Soft Tissue Space Infections

Infection	Indications for Surgery
Quinsy	Abscess or respiratory compromise
Lateral pharyngeal space abscess	Abscess
Jugular vein septic thrombophlebitis	Febrile after 5–6 days of medical therapy
Retropharyngeal abscess	Abscess or respiratory compromise
Ludwig's angina	Abscess or respiratory compromise

98–1). Examination may reveal a red "beefy" tongue with flattened papillae, resulting in a smooth appearance.

Persistent or Penicillin-Unresponsive Pharyngitis

Most cases of viral or streptococcal pharyngitis are self-limited, and symptoms generally resolve within 3 to 4 days. Persistent sore throat should prompt consideration of the following possibilities.

SOFT TISSUE ABSCESS OR PHLEGMON. Rarely, tonsillitis extends to the soft tissues of the pharynx, producing a potentially life-threatening infection (see previous).

PHARYNGEAL GONORRHEA. Although most cases of pharyngeal gonorrhea are asymptomatic, mild pharyngitis may be seen occasionally. This infection will not respond to doses of penicillin used for pharyngitis; moreover, the gonococcus is relatively resistant to phenoxymethyl penicillin (PenV). The gonococcus will not likely be identified on routine culture medium; isolation generally requires culture of a fresh throat swab on a selective medium such as Thayer-Martin (see Chapter 107).

INFECTIOUS MONONUCLEOSIS. One virus that can produce a more protracted exudative pharyngitis is the Epstein-Barr virus, causative agent of infectious mononucleosis. Adenopathy, splenomegaly, generalized malaise, and rash may accompany this illness. Peripheral blood smear usually reveals numerous atypical lymphocytes. The patient should be advised to abstain from contact sports, as traumatic rupture of the enlarged spleen may be fatal.

ACUTE LYMPHOBLASTIC LEUKEMIA. Persistent exudative tonsillitis may be a presentation of acute lymphoblastic leukemia (ALL). Diagnosis can be suspected by examination of the peripheral blood smear; however, some experience may be required to distinguish between the blasts of ALL and the atypical lymphocytes of infectious mononucleosis.

OTHER LEUKOPENIC STATES. Stomatitis or pharyngitis may be the presenting complaint of patients with *aplastic anemia* or *agranulocytosis*. As some of these cases are drug-induced (e.g., propylthiouracil, phenytoin), a complete medication history on initial presentation may suggest this possibility. Prompt discontinuation of the offending drug may be life saving.

Although sore throat is a common complaint of patients with relatively benign illness, rarely it is the presenting complaint of a patient with a serious or life-threatening disease. Any of the key signs or symptoms shown in Table 98–2 should alert the clinician to the possibility of an extraordinary process.

REFERENCES

Gwaltney JM: Pharyngitis. *In* Mandell GL, Bennett JC, Dolin R (eds.): Principles and Practice of Infectious Diseases. 4th ed. New York, Churchill Livingstone, 1995, pp 566–572.

Stevens DL: Streptococcal infections. *In* Bennett JC, Plum F (eds.): Cecil Textbook of Medicine. 20th ed. Philadelphia, WB Saunders, 1996, pp 1585–1590.

Mayo-Smith MF, Spinale JW, Donsky CJ, et al: Acute epiglottitis: An 18-year experience in Rhode Island. Chest 1995;108:1640–1647.

Mufson MA: Viral Pharyngitis, Laryngitis, Croup, and Bronchitis. *In* Bennett JC, Plum F (eds.): Cecil Textbook of Medicine. 20th ed. Philadelphia, WB Saunders, 1996, pp 1749–1751.

99

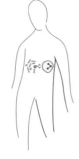

Infections of the Lower Respiratory Tract

Pneumonia currently accounts for about 10% of admissions to adult medical services in North America and is one of the leading causes of death during the productive years of life. Although pneumonia ranks sixth among the causes of death in the United States today, it is first among the potentially lethal illnesses that are readily reversible by the alert physician. Every physician must therefore be adept at the *rapid* diagnosis and management of the patient with pneumonia. Viruses, chlamydiae, rickettsiae, mycoplasmas, bacteria, protozoans, and parasites can all produce serious infection of the lower respiratory tract. Careful history and physical examination can provide clues to the likely cause of infection. The clinical spectra of pneumonias caused by different pathogens overlap considerably, however. Microscopic examination of respiratory secretions provides a rapid and essential step in the differential diagnosis of pneumonia.

PATHOGENESIS OF PNEUMONIA

Microbes can enter the lung to produce infection by hematogenous spread, by spread from a contiguous focus of infection, by inhalation of aerosolized particles, or, most commonly, by aspiration of oropharyngeal secretions. In the last instance, the organisms colonizing the oropharynx will determine the flora of the aspirated secretions and presumably the nature of the resultant pneumonia. Some organisms like *Streptococcus pneumoniae* may transiently colonize the oropharynx in healthy individuals. Others, such as gram-negative bacilli, are more prevalent in the upper respiratory tract of debilitated and hospitalized patients. Aspiration of normal oropharyngeal flora may lead to necrotizing pneumonia caused by mixtures of oral anaerobic bacteria.

Inoculum size (the number of bacteria aspirated) may be an important factor in the development of pneumonia. Studies using radioisotopes have demonstrated that up to 45% of healthy men aspirate some oropharyngeal contents during sleep. In most instances, the bacteria aspirated are relatively avirulent, and back-up defenses, including cough and mucociliary clearance, are adequate to prevent the development of pneumonia. Individuals with structural disease of the oropharynx or patients with impaired cough reflexes due to drugs, alcohol, or neuromuscular disease are at particular risk for the development of

pneumonia due to aspiration. The specialized ciliated cells of the bronchial mucosa are covered by a layer of mucus that traps foreign particles, which are propelled upward by rhythmic beating of the cilia to a point where a cough can expel the particles. Impaired mucociliary transport, as may be seen in persons with chronic obstructive pulmonary disease, may predispose to bacterial infection. Denuding of the respiratory epithelium by infection with the influenza virus may be one mechanism whereby influenza predisposes to bacterial pneumonia. Within the alveoli and smaller airways, alveolar macrophages and humoral opsonins, including antibody and complement, serve as host defenses against infection.

Infection by *Mycobacterium tuberculosis* is usually acquired through inhalation of aerosolized contaminated droplet nuclei. A primary infection is established in the parenchyma of the lungs and in the draining lymph nodes, which may result in a progressive primary infection, but in most instances it resolves after producing a mild respiratory illness. The organism remains alive, sequestered within host macrophages, and contained by host cell-mediated defenses. Reactivation of infection may never occur or may occur without apparent precipitating events or at times when host cell-mediated immune responses are impaired. Examples of these impairments include starvation, intercurrent viral infections, administration of corticosteroids or cytotoxic drugs, and illnesses associated with immunosuppression such as Hodgkin's disease and human immunodeficiency virus (HIV) infection.

EPIDEMIOLOGY

Common pathogens of community-acquired and nosocomial pneumonia are shown in Table 99–1. As a general rule, the pneumococcus is an important pathogen in all age groups, and influenza and tuberculosis become more frequent with increasing age. Although *Mycoplasma* occasionally produces pneumonia in the elderly, it is primarily a pathogen of the young. Certain systemic disorders appear to be associated with pneumonias due to particular organisms (Table 99–2). The exposure history may be helpful in suggesting specific causative agents (Table 99–3). Pneumonias associated with bone marrow suppression and malignant disorders are discussed in Chapter 109.

TABLE 99–1	Important Pathogens Causing Pneumonia
Population	**Pathogens**
Young, healthy adult	*Streptococcus pneumoniae, Mycoplasma pneumoniae, Chlamydia pneumoniae*, respiratory viruses
Elderly	*S. pneumoniae*, influenza virus, *Mycobacterium tuberculosis*
Debilitated	*S. pneumoniae*, influenza virus, oral flora, *M. tuberculosis*, gram-negative bacilli
Hospitalized	Oral flora, *Staphylococcus aureus*, gram-negative bacilli, *Legionella* spp

TABLE 99–3	Exposures Associated with Pneumonia
Source/Location	**Pneumonia**
Cattle, goats, sheep	Q fever, brucellosis
Rabbits	Tularemia
Birds	Psittacosis, histoplasmosis*
Rodents	Hantavirus
Dog ticks	Ehrlichiosis
Southwestern United States	Coccidioidomycosis
Mississippi and Ohio River valleys	Histoplasmosis, blastomycosis
Developing countries	Tuberculosis

* Exposure to bird and bat droppings.

DIAGNOSTIC APPROACH TO THE PATIENT

A critical historical point in the differential diagnosis of pneumonia is the duration of symptoms. Pneumonia due to the pneumococcus, *Mycoplasma,* or virus is usually an acute illness. Symptoms are measured in hours to a few days, although there may occasionally be a longer viral prodrome before bacterial superinfection. In contrast, symptoms of pneumonia lasting 10 days or more are rarely due to the common bacterial pathogens and should raise suspicion of mycobacterial, fungal, or anaerobic pneumonia (anaerobes can produce acute or chronic infection) or the presence of an anatomic defect such as an endobronchial mass.

Occupational exposure and travel history often provide clues to the etiology of some less common pneumonias (see Table 99–3). Although these pneumonias are uncommon, they should be considered in the appropriate setting because, if improperly treated, some may be fatal.

A history of rhinitis or pharyngitis suggests respiratory virus or *Mycoplasma* pneumonia. Diarrhea has been associated with *Legionella* pneumonia in some, but not all, outbreaks. A persistent hacking, nonproductive cough characterizes some *Mycoplasma* infections; symptoms of grippe—malaise and myalgias—are common in influenza and may also be seen with *Mycoplasma* pneumonia. A true rigor is very suggestive of a bacterial (often pneumococcal) pneumonia. Whereas small pleural effusions may be seen in nonbacterial pneumonias, severe pleuritic pain

TABLE 99–2	Specific Disorders and Associated Pneumonias
Disorder	**Pneumonia**
Seizures	Aspiration (mixed anaerobes)
Alcoholism	Aspiration, *Streptococcus pneumoniae*, gram-negative bacilli
Diabetes mellitus	Gram-negative bacilli, *Mycobacterium tuberculosis*
Sickle cell disease	*S. pneumoniae, Mycoplasma pneumoniae*
Chronic lung disease	*S. pneumoniae, Haemophilus influenzae, Moraxella catarrhalis*, gram-negative bacilli, *Legionella pneumophila*
Chronic renal failure	*S. pneumoniae, M. tuberculosis, L. pneumophila*

in a patient with pneumonia is suggestive of bacterial infection. Night sweats are seen in chronic pneumonias and suggest tuberculous or fungal disease.

Most patients with pneumonia have cough, fever, tachypnea, and tachycardia. Fever without a concomitant rise in pulse rate may be seen in legionellosis, *Mycoplasma* infections, and other "nonbacterial" pneumonias. Patients with pulmonary tuberculosis often maintain high fevers in relative comfort when compared with patients with acute bacterial pneumonia. Respirations may be shallow in the presence of pleurisy. Increasing tachypnea, cyanosis, and the use of accessory muscles for respiration indicate serious illness. Foul breath suggests anaerobic infection. Mental confusion in a patient with pneumonia should immediately raise the suspicion of meningeal involvement, which occurs most commonly in patients with pneumococcal pneumonia. Confusion may, however, be the most prominent clinical feature of pneumonia in elderly patients in the absence of associated meningitis. Nonetheless, patients with pneumonia who are confused must be evaluated by examination of cerebrospinal fluid.

Physical evidence of consolidation—dullness to percussion, bronchial breath sounds, rales, increased fremitus, and whispered pectoriloquy—suggest bacterial pneumonia. Early in the course of pneumonia, however, the physical examination may be normal.

RADIOGRAPHIC PATTERNS IN PATIENTS WITH PNEUMONIA

Clinical-radiographic dissociation is seen often in patients with *M. pneumoniae* or viral pneumonia. Chest radiographs of patients with *Mycoplasma* infection often suggest a more serious infection than does the appearance of the patient or the physical examination. The converse is true in patients with *Pneumocystis carinii* infection, who may appear quite ill despite normal or nearly normal chest radiographs. This may also be true early in the course of acute bacterial pneumonias, when pleuritic chest pain, cough, purulent sputum, and inspiratory rales may precede specific radiographic findings by many hours. A "negative" radiograph can never "rule out" the possibility of acute bacterial pneumonia when the patient's symptoms and signs point to this diagnosis. A lobar consolidation suggests a bacterial pneumonia; however, patients

TABLE 99–4	Necrotizing Pneumonias

Common

Tuberculosis
Staphylococcus
Gram-negative bacilli
Anaerobes
Fungi

Rare

Streptococcus pneumoniae
Legionella
Pneumocystis carinii
Virus

? Never

Mycoplasma pneumoniae

with chronic lung disease often fail to manifest clinical or radiographic evidence of consolidation during the course of bacterial pneumonia. Interstitial infiltrates suggest a nonbacterial process but may also be seen in early staphylococcal pneumonia. Enlarged hilar lymph nodes suggest a concomitant lung tumor but may also be seen in primary tuberculous, viral, or fungal pneumonias. Large pleural effusions should suggest streptococcal pneumonia or tuberculosis. Pneumatoceles are seen in patients after respirator-mediated barotrauma but occur frequently in the evolution of staphylococcal pneumonia, particularly among children and also in patients with *P. carinii* pneumonia. The presence of cavitation identifies the pneumonia as necrotizing. This finding virtually excludes viruses and *Mycoplasma* and makes pneumococcal infection unlikely (Table 99–4).

OTHER LABORATORY FINDINGS

In patients with bacterial pneumonia, the white blood cell (WBC) count is often (but not invariably) elevated. Among patients with pneumococcal infection, WBC counts of 20,000 to 30,000/μl or more may be seen. A left shift with immature forms is common. Patients with nonbacterial pneumonias tend to have lower WBC counts. Modest elevations of serum bilirubin (conjugated) may be seen in many bacterial infections but are particularly common in patients with pneumococcal pneumonia.

DIAGNOSIS AND MANAGEMENT OF THE PATIENT WITH PNEUMONIA

When the patient presents with abrupt onset of shaking chills, followed by cough, pleuritic chest pain, fever, rusty or yellow sputum, and shortness of breath, and the physical examination reveals tachypnea and even minimal signs of alveolar inflammation (e.g., harsh breath sounds at one lung base), the presumptive diagnosis of bacterial pneumonia should be made, sputum should be examined, and appropriate therapy should be begun regardless of radiographic findings. The radiographic abnormalities may

lag for several hours after the clinical onset of pneumonia.

Empiric treatment for community-acquired pneumonia without laboratory examination of sputum may be successful in the management of many patients. However, this practice promotes indiscriminate use of broad-spectrum antibiotics with attendant increases in antibiotic resistance. This approach also will result in occasional misdiagnoses and may place nonresponding patients at risk for increased morbidity and death.

Examination of Respiratory Secretions

Examination of respiratory secretions is essential for accurate diagnosis and proper treatment of pneumonia. When the history and physical examination suggest pneumonia, a specimen of sputum must be Gram-stained and examined immediately. The adequacy of the specimen can be ascertained by (1) the absence of squamous epithelial cells and (2) the presence of polymorphonuclear leukocytes (10 to 15 per high-power field). The presence of alveolar macrophages and bronchial epithelial cells confirms the lower respiratory tract origin of the specimen. A specimen with many (more than five per high-power field) squamous epithelial cells is of no value for either culture or Gram's stain, since it is contaminated with upper respiratory tract secretions.

In some cases, the patient cannot produce an adequate sputum sample, despite vigorous attempts at sputum induction using an aerosolized solution of 3% hypertonic saline. The sicker the patient and the greater the likelihood of a penicillin-resistant pathogen, the more important it is to get an adequate sample of sputum for examination and culture. This can often be achieved by nasotracheal aspiration, which is done by placing the patient supine, hyperextending the neck, and passing a well-lubricated, clear, flexible plastic catheter from the nose to the posterior pharynx. During inspiration, the tube is then passed swiftly past the glottis into the trachea, suction is applied, and secretions are collected in a Lugen trap. The vigorous coughing stimulated by this procedure often produces an additional excellent expectorated specimen. (*Note:* Expectorated sputum and sputum obtained through nasotracheal aspiration cannot be cultured anaerobically because of universal contamination with oral flora.)

If nasotracheal aspiration still fails to provide a good specimen for analysis, transtracheal aspiration should be considered *only* if the physician is experienced in this technique and bronchoscopy is not available.

The Gram-stained specimen should be examined using an oil immersion lens. The presence of a predominant organism, particularly if found within WBCs, suggests that this is the pathogen. In cases of aspiration of mouth flora, a mixture of oral streptococci, gram-positive rods, and gram-negative organisms is found. In some cases, there may be inflammatory cells and no organisms seen on Gram's stain. This finding suggests a number of possibilities, many of which are nonbacterial pneumonias (Table 99–5). Unless the diagnosis of acute bacterial pneumonia is clear, an acid-fast stain or fluorescent auramine-rhodamine stain of sputum for mycobacteria

TABLE 99–5	Sputum Gram's Stain Revealing Inflammatory Cells and No Organisms		
Possibilities	**Clinical Setting**	**Confirmation of Diagnosis**	**Treatment**
Prior antibiotic treatment			
Viral pneumonia	Winter months—influenza, may be mild or life threatening	Serologies, virus culture, antigen detection	Rimantadine for influenza A, ribavirin for respiratory syncytial virus
Mycoplasma pneumoniae infection	Hacking, nonproductive cough	Cold agglutinins, serologies	Erythromycin, tetracycline
Legionella pneumophila infection	Chronic lung disease—hospital acquired, summer predominance	DFA of sputum, bronchial brush biopsy, or pleural fluid, culture, serologies	Erythromycin
Chlamydia psittaci infection	Exposure to birds, e.g., parrots, turkeys	Serologies	Tetracycline
Chlamydia pneumoniae infection	Hacking cough, sinusitis	Serologies, antigen detection	Tetracycline
Q fever	Exposure to cattle, South Africa	Serologies	Tetracycline or chloramphenicol

DFA = Direct immunofluorescence assay.

should be performed. If legionellosis is suspected, immunofluorescence stains for *Legionella* can be used, although the yield on expectorated sputum is low. The demonstration of elastin fibers in a potassium hydroxide (KOH) preparation of sputum establishes a diagnosis of necrotizing pneumonia (see Table 99–4). Importantly, this test can be positive in the absence of radiographic evidence of cavitation. Blood cultures should be obtained and may be positive in approximately 20 to 30% of patients with bacterial pneumonia.

Results of sputum cultures must be interpreted with caution, since pathogens causing pneumonia may fail to grow, and sputum isolates may not be the pathogens responsible for infection. Careful screening of sputum specimens using Gram's stain (see previous) will increase the accuracy of culture results. A tuberculin skin test and control skin tests such as for mumps, *Candida,* and *Trichophyton* should be applied in all cases of pneumonia of uncertain etiology. If the tuberculin is negative but tuberculosis remains a diagnostic possibility, the tuberculin test should be repeated in 2 weeks.

SPECIFIC PATHOGENIC ORGANISMS

Viral Agents

Viral infection is usually limited to the upper respiratory tract, and only a small proportion of infected adults develop pneumonia. In children, viruses are the most common cause of pneumonia, and respiratory syncytial virus is the most frequent organism. In adults, viruses are estimated to account for fewer than 10% of pneumonias, and the influenza virus is the most common organism. Patients at increased risk of influenzal pneumonia include the aged; patients with chronic disease of the heart, lung, or kidney; and women in the last trimester of pregnancy. Cytomegalovirus has developed prominence as a cause of pneumonia in immunosuppressed patients, particularly in the acquired immunodeficiency syndrome (AIDS) and the post-transplantation state, in which it has a mortality rate of about 50%. When varicella occurs in adults, some 10 to 20% develop pneumonia, which commonly leaves a pattern of diffuse punctate calcification on chest radiograph. Measles is occasionally complicated by pneumonia. Recently, cases of pneumonia and adult respiratory distress syndrome due to *Hantavirus* have been reported primarily among persons residing in the southwestern United States. This severe, rapidly progressive and often fatal infection occurs largely among otherwise healthy young adults who have been exposed to mouse droppings. Hemoconcentration caused by a generalized increase in capillary permeability appears to be the most critical pathophysiologic defect. Treatment is supportive. Although ribavirin has been used in the treatment of this infection, its value is unproven.

Other viral pneumonias, of which influenza is the prototype in adults, typically occur in community epidemics and usually develop 1 to 2 days after the onset of "flu-like" symptoms. Major features include a dry cough, dyspnea, generalized discomfort, unremarkable physical examination, and an interstitial pattern on the chest radiograph. Influenza-induced necrosis of respiratory epithelial cells predisposes to bacterial colonization. This may result in superimposed bacterial pneumonia, most often caused by *Streptococcus pneumoniae* or *Staphylococcus aureus.* A presumptive diagnosis may be made on the basis of the clinical presentation and the epidemiologic setting. Gram's stain of sputum reveals inflammatory cells and rare bacteria. When available, detection of viral antigens in sputum can confirm the diagnosis rapidly. Viral isolation or serology also can establish the diagnosis but not in time to guide management decisions.

Bacterial Agents

Streptococcus Pneumoniae

The pneumococcus is still the most common bacterial cause of pneumonia in the community. The organism colonizes the oropharynx in up to 25% of healthy adults. An increased predisposition to pneumococcal pneumonia is observed in persons with sickle cell disease, prior splenectomy, chronic lung disease, hematologic malignancy, alcoholism, HIV infection, and renal failure. Clinical features include fever, rigors, chills, cough, respiratory distress, signs of pulmonary consolidation, confusion, and herpes labialis. By the second or third day of illness, the chest radiograph typically shows lobar consolidation with air bronchograms, but a patchy bronchopneumonic pattern may also be found. Abscess or cavitation rarely occurs. Sterile pleural effusions occur in up to 25% of cases and empyema in 1%. Typically, a leukocytosis of 15,000 to 30,000 cells/μl with neutrophilia is found, but leukopenia may be observed with fulminant infection and among alcoholics and persons with HIV infection. Demonstration of gram-positive diplococci on Gram's stain of sputum is helpful in the rapid diagnosis of pneumonia but may fail to demonstrate organisms in some cases of pneumococcal pneumonia. Positive blood cultures are found in 20 to 25% of patients. In most regions, penicillin G remains the treatment of choice; if penicillin-resistant pneumococci are suspected on the basis of regional antibiotic sensitivity patterns, vancomycin therapy is indicated.

Staphylococcus Aureus

Staphylococcus aureus accounts for 2 to 5% of community-acquired pneumonias, 11% of hospital-acquired pneumonias, and up to 26% of pneumonias following a viral infection. Persistent nasal colonization is observed in 15 to 30% of adults, and 90% of adults display intermittent colonization. Presentation is similar to that of pneumococcal pneumonia, but contrasting features include the development of parenchymal necrosis and abscess formation in up to 25% of patients and empyema in 10%. A hematogenous source of infection, such as septic thrombophlebitis, infective endocarditis, or an infected intravascular device, should be suspected in cases of staphylococcal pneumonia, particularly if the chest radiograph reveals multiple or expanding nodular or wedge-shaped infiltrates. Early in staphylococcal pneumonia of hematogenous origin, sputum is rarely available. Blood cultures are usually positive, and associated skin lesions occur in 20 to 40%. When sputum is available, Gram's stain reveals grapelike clusters of gram-positive cocci. *S. aureus* is recovered very easily from mixed culture samples, so that its absence in a purulent specimen usually excludes it as a cause of the pneumonia. Treatment requires a penicillinase-resistant agent, such as nafcillin or vancomycin. In hospital-acquired infections or in communities with endemic methicillin-resistant *S. aureus,* vancomycin should be used until sensitivity studies indicate that the isolate is sensitive to semisynthetic penicillins.

Streptococcus Pyogenes

Streptococcus pyogenes is now a rare cause of pneumonia, probably accounting for less than 1% of all cases. Carriage rate in the pharynx, about 3% in adults, is less than with the other gram-positive cocci. Presentation is similar to that observed with *S. pneumoniae* and *S. aureus,* except that empyema, often massive, is found in 30 to 40% of cases, and the illness may show very rapid progression. Gram's stain reveals gram-positive cocci in pairs or chains. Penicillin G is the treatment of choice.

Haemophilus Influenzae

Haemophilus influenzae is a gram-negative coccobacillus often present in the upper respiratory tract, particularly among patients with chronic obstructive pulmonary disease. Its isolation from sputum in these patients is to be expected. Confirmation of its role in the pathogenesis of pneumonia depends on isolating the organism in the blood, pleural fluid, or lung tissue. Nevertheless, many cases of pneumonia due to this organism will not be confirmed using these rigid criteria, and in a patient with pneumonia the demonstration of gram-negative coccobacilli on Gram's stain of sputum should prompt institution of treatment with ampicillin plus a beta-lactamase inhibitor or a second- or third-generation cephalosporin.

Gram-Negative Bacilli

These have emerged as pathogens of major importance with the introduction of potent antibiotics and the proliferation of intensive care units. They are frequently encountered in patients with debilitating diseases such as chronic alcoholism, cystic fibrosis, neutropenia, diabetes mellitus, malignancy, and chronic diseases of the lungs, heart, or kidney. They are ubiquitous throughout the hospital, contaminating equipment and instruments, and are the major source of nosocomial pneumonia.

Specific organisms are associated with certain situations; for example, *Klebsiella pneumoniae* is particularly common in chronic alcoholics, *Escherichia coli* pneumonia is associated with bacteremias arising from the intestinal or urinary tract, and *Pseudomonas* species commonly infect the lungs of patients with cystic fibrosis. Precise etiologic diagnosis is confounded by the frequency with which these organisms colonize the upper airways in predisposed patients. Treatment in this situation generally includes the use of a penicillinase-resistant penicillin or a cephalosporin and an aminoglycoside.

Other Causes of Acute Pneumonia

Mycoplasma Pneumoniae

Not only is this a common cause of pneumonia in young adults, but it also produces a wide range of extrapulmonary features that may be the only findings. Fewer than 10% of infected patients develop symptoms of lower respiratory tract infection. Respiratory findings resemble those of viral pneumonia. Hacking, nonproductive cough is characteristic. Nonpulmonary features include myalgias, arthralgias, skin lesions (rashes, erythema nodosum and multiforme, Stevens-Johnson syndrome), and neurologic complications (meningitis, encephalitis, transverse myelitis, cranial nerve or peripheral neuritis). The occurrence of acute, multifocal neurologic abnormalities may be helpful in distinguishing *Mycoplasma* pneumonia from that caused by *Chlamydia* or *Legionella*. The neurologic abnormalities characteristically resolve completely as the acute illness subsides.

Cold agglutinins can be demonstrated at the bedside by observing red blood cell clumping on the walls of a glass tube containing anticoagulated blood incubated on ice for at least 10 minutes; they are also occasionally positive in other respiratory infections. A specific complement fixation test or demonstration of *Mycoplasma* antigens in the sputum allows confirmation of the diagnosis. Tetracycline or erythromycin decreases the duration of symptoms and hastens radiographic resolution but does not eradicate the organism from the respiratory tract.

Chlamydia Pneumoniae

Approximately 5 to 10% of cases of community acquired pneumonia may be due to *Chlamydia pneumoniae* (formerly called the TWAR agent). Infection is spread, presumably via the respiratory route, from person to person, and onset of disease is generally subacute, often manifested by pharyngitis, sinusitis, bronchitis and pneumonia. The radiographic appearance of pneumonia due to *C. pneumoniae* resembles that of *Mycoplasma* infection. Illness is relatively mild and often prolonged. Diagnosis of this infection is difficult and requires cultivation of the organism in special cell lines or polymerase chain reaction–based detection of microbial nucleotide sequences. Although the organism is sensitive to erythromycin and tetracyclines, treatment may have little effect on the course of disease.

Legionella Species

Legionella species are fastidious gram-negative bacilli that were responsible for respiratory infections long before the well-publicized outbreak of legionnaires' disease in 1976, which led to the recognition of this distinct disease entity and to the identification of the responsible bacillus. (The high mortality rate from this outbreak of a hitherto unrecognized disease among participants in a legionnaires' convention destroyed the reputation of one of Philadelphia's finest hotels.) These organisms are distributed widely in water, and outbreaks have been related to their presence in water towers, air conditioners, condensers, potable water, and even hospital shower heads. Infection may occur sporadically or in outbreaks. Although healthy subjects are affected, there is an increased risk in patients with chronic diseases of the heart, lungs, or kidneys; malignancy; and impairment of cell-mediated immunity. After an incubation period of 2 to 10 days, the illness usually begins gradually with a dry cough, respiratory distress, fever, rigors, malaise, weakness, headache, confusion, and gastrointestinal disturbance. The chest radiograph shows alveolar shadowing that may have a lobar or patchy distribution, with or without pleural effusions. The diagnosis is suggested clinically by the combination of a rapidly progressive pneumonia, dry cough, and multiorgan involvement. Gram's stain of sputum shows neutrophils and no organisms.

Diagnosis can be made by three methods. (1) Indirect fluorescent antibody testing of serum is positive in 75% of patients, but up to 8 weeks are required for seroconversion. (2) Direct fluorescence antibody testing of respiratory secretions is the most rapid method of establishing the diagnosis and has a specificity of 95%. Sensitivity of this method is greater in specimens obtained from bronchoscopy or transtracheal aspirate than expectorated sputum. (3) The organism can be cultured on charcoal yeast extract medium, but up to 10 days are required for growth.

Erythromycin is the treatment of choice. Prompt treatment results in fourfold to fivefold reduction in mortality. Patients usually respond within 12 to 48 hours, and it is very unusual for fever, leukocytosis, and confusion to persist beyond 4 days of therapy. In severe cases, rifampin may be added. Ciprofloxacin may also be effective, but clinical experience is limited to date.

Community-Acquired Pneumonia of Uncertain Etiology

There are instances in which, because of difficulty in obtaining adequate sputum specimens or lack of laboratory facilities, empiric treatment of acute community-acquired pneumonia may be necessary. In such instances, the recommended initial therapy is cefuroxime and erythromycin.

Tuberculosis

Approximately 25,000 new cases of tuberculosis occur in the United States each year, with a worldwide incidence of 7 to 10 million. These figures will increase because tuberculosis is the major communicable complication of AIDS. In North America, a disproportionately high number of cases occur among the foreign born, the racial and ethnic minorities, and the poor. *Mycobacterium tuberculosis* is transmitted by the respiratory route from an infected patient with cavitary pulmonary tuberculosis to a susceptible host not previously infected with the organism. Primary infection usually is manifested only by development of a positive tuberculin skin test. Occasionally, the patient develops sufficient symptoms of fever and nonproductive cough to visit a physician, and a chest radiograph is taken; patchy or lobular infiltrates are noted in the anterior segment of the upper lobes or in the middle or lower lobes, often with associated hilar adenopathy. Pleurisy with effusion is a less common manifestation of primary tuberculosis. Primary infection usually is self-limited, but hematogenous dissemination seeds multiple organs, and latent foci are established and become niduses for delayed reactivation. Overall, 5 to 15% of infected individuals develop disease. Factors associated with progression to clinical disease are age (the periods of greatest biologic vulnerability to tuberculosis being infancy, childhood, adolescence, and old age); underlying diseases that depress the cellular immune response (see Chapter 109); diabetes mellitus, gastrectomy, silicosis, and sarcoidosis; and the interval since primary infection, with disease progression most likely in the first few years after infection.

Early progression of infection to disease is known as progressive primary tuberculosis and may manifest as miliary tuberculosis, sometimes with meningitis, or as pulmonary disease of the apical and posterior segments of the upper lobes or lower lobe disease.

Most commonly, tuberculosis represents delayed reactivation. Symptoms begin insidiously with night sweats or chills and fatigue; fever is noted by fewer than 50% of patients, and hemoptysis by fewer than 25%. Physical examination may be unremarkable or may show dullness and rales in the upper lung fields, occasionally with amphoric breath sounds. The chest radiograph may show cavitary disease with infiltrates in the posterior segment of the upper lobes or apical segments of the lower lobes.

Extrapulmonary tuberculosis also reflects reactivation of latent foci and accounts for approximately 15% of cases. Miliary tuberculosis is discussed in Chapter 95, meningeal tuberculosis in Chapter 97, and tuberculosis of bones and joints in Chapter 104.

Because of the growing proportion of elderly individuals in our society and the growing prevalence of HIV infection, "atypical" presentations of tuberculosis are increasingly common. The elderly and patients with diabetes mellitus are more likely to have lower lobe tuberculosis. In HIV-infected patients, involvement of the lower lobes is frequent, extrapulmonary tuberculosis is almost as common as pulmonary involvement, and tuberculin skin tests are likely to be negative. The index of suspicion must be high in these settings.

Before starting antituberculosis drug treatment, two or three sputum samples should be obtained for cultures; bronchoscopy and bronchial washing are indicated only if sputum smears are negative for acid-fast bacilli. It is important to obtain baseline evaluation of liver function for individuals who are to receive potentially hepatotoxic drugs (isoniazid, rifampin, pyrazinamide); color vision, visual fields, and acuity when ethambutol will be used; and audiometry for patients who are to receive streptomycin.

The main principle of chemotherapy for tuberculosis is to avoid resistance by treating with at least two drugs to which the organism is likely to be sensitive. Pulmonary tuberculosis assumed to be caused by sensitive organisms should be treated with daily isoniazid (5 mg/kg up to 300 mg), rifampin (10 mg/kg up to 600 mg), and pyrazinamide (15 to 30 mg/kg/day) for 2 months, followed by isoniazid and rifampin for 4 more months. Additional or alternative drugs are necessary if the patient has life-threatening disease as assurance against unsuspected drug resistance, or when the likelihood of resistance is deemed high (Asians, Hispanics, individuals acquiring infection in an area with high levels of resistance, or persons exposed to a patient known to harbor drug-resistant bacilli). In such instances, ethambutol (15 to 25 mg/kg) or streptomycin (15 mg/kg, intramuscular) should be added to the regimen until drug sensitivities are known. At that point, the regimen can be tailored to include at least two drugs to which the organism is sensi-

tive. One of these drugs must be bactericidal. Close monitoring during treatment is mandatory to maximize compliance and minimize side effects.

Contact tracing is critical, as recent infection or additional cases of tuberculosis are likely in some household contacts. Preventive therapy with isoniazid is discussed later.

TREATMENT AND OUTCOME

Bacterial Pneumonia

As soon as the causative organism is identified on Gram's stain, antibiotics must be administered without delay. If the pathogen is readily identified, the antibiotic choices are straightforward (Table 99–6). Patients with *Mycoplasma* and viral pneumonia can generally be treated on an ambulatory basis. An occasional young patient with no underlying disease can also be managed at home, provided that the patient is reliably attended by friends or family and has ready access to a physician or hospital. Otherwise, patients with bacterial pneumonia should be hospitalized.

Supplemental oxygen should be provided if the patient is tachypneic or hypoxemic. Patients at risk for the development of respiratory insufficiency should be monitored in a critical care setting. Patients who are not capable of adequately coughing up respiratory secretions should have frequent clapping and drainage; meticulous attention must be paid to suctioning of oral secretions. Patients with suspected pulmonary tuberculosis should be placed in isolation rooms with negative pressure, frequent

TABLE 99–6	Initial Antibiotics for Treatment of Pneumonia
Pathogen	**Treatment**
Streptococcus pneumoniae	Penicillin G, 1.2 million units/day*
Mycoplasma pneumoniae	Erythromycin, 500 mg po qid
Chlamydia pneumoniae	Erythromycin, 500 mg po qid
Haemophilus influenzae	Ampicillin/sulbactam, 500 mg q8h IV or cefuroxime, 1 gm q8h IV
Staphylococcus aureus	Nafcillin, 3 gm IV q6h, or vancomycin, 1 gm IV q12h
Legionella pneumophila	Erythromycin, 750 mg q6h
Ehrlichia chaffeensis	Doxycycline, 100 mg bid
Mixed oral flora (anaerobes)	Ampicillin/sulbactam, 500 mg q8h†
Gram-negative rods	Aminoglycoside (e.g., gentamicin, 1.7 mg/kg IV q8h) plus third-generation cephalosporin (e.g., ceftazidime, 6 gm/day)‡
Tuberculosis	Isoniazid, 300 mg/day, plus rifampin, 600 mg/day, and pyrazinamide, 1500 mg/day

* Erythromycin, 500 mg q6h for penicillin-allergic patients. Vancomycin, 1 gm IV q12h for penicillin-resistant isolates.
† Clindamycin, 600 mg q6h, if patient fails to respond to penicillin.
‡ Add beta-lactam antibiotic active against *Pseudomonas aeruginosa* (e.g., ceftazidime, 2 gm q8h) if *Pseudomonas* is a possibility. Antibiotics can be adjusted when sensitivity data are available.
IV = Intravenously.

air exchange, and germicidal lamps to prevent nosocomial transmission of infection.

Patients treated for pneumococcal pneumonia should begin to improve within 48 hours after institution of antibiotics; patients with pneumonia caused by gram-negative bacilli, staphylococci, and oral anaerobes may remain ill for longer periods after initiation of treatment. Several possibilities should be considered among patients who fail to improve or who deteriorate while on treatment.

Endobronchial Obstruction

Physical examination may fail to reveal sounds of consolidation, and radiographs may show evidence of lobar collapse. Bronchoscopy can establish the diagnosis.

Undrained Empyema

Radiographs may not always distinguish between fluid and consolidation; ultrasonography and computed tomographic (CT) scans can identify the fluid and provide direction for its drainage.

Purulent Pericarditis

This should be suspected in a very ill patient with pneumonia involving a lobe adjacent to the pericardium. Chest pain and electrocardiographic evidence of pericarditis are usually absent. Distended neck veins and pericardial friction rubs are present in a minority of cases. Echocardiography or chest ultrasonography reveals fluid in the pericardium. If purulent pericarditis is suspected, emergency pericardiocentesis can be life saving (see Chapter 9).

TABLE 99–7	Prevention of Pneumonia: Candidates for Pneumococcal and Influenza Vaccines	
	Pneumococcal Vaccine (One Time Only)	**Influenza Vaccine (Yearly)**
Patients ≥65 years	Yes	Yes
Chronic lung or heart disease	Yes	Yes
Sickle cell disease	Yes	Consider
Asplenic patients	Yes	No
Hodgkin's disease	Yes	Consider
Multiple myeloma	Yes	Consider
Cirrhosis	Yes	Consider
Chronic alcoholism	Yes	Consider
Chronic renal failure	Yes	Consider
Cerebrospinal fluid leaks	Yes	No
Residents of chronic care facilities	Consider	Yes
Diabetes mellitus	Yes	Yes
HIV infection	Yes	Consider

HIV = Human immunodeficiency virus.

TABLE 99–8	Indications for Prophylaxis with Isoniazid (INH)

Documented new skin test conversion to tuberculin over past 2 yr
Tuberculin-positive contacts of patients with active tuberculosis (TB)
Tuberculin-negative contacts of patients with active TB*
Tuberculin-positive persons with HIV infection
Anergic HIV-infected patients at high risk for tuberculosis
Positive tuberculin skin test of unknown duration in patients younger than 35 years of age
Patients with radiographic evidence of inactive TB who have never received an adequate course of antituberculosis drugs
Consider INH prophylaxis for patients with positive tuberculin skin tests and gastrectomy, diabetes mellitus, organ transplantation, silicosis, and prolonged (>1 mo) administration of corticosteroids or immunosuppressive drugs

* These individuals should have repeat skin tests 3 mo after INH is begun. If the repeat test is negative, INH may be discontinued.
HIV = Human immunodeficiency virus.

Incorrect Diagnosis or Treatment

In cases in which clinical response is poor, the patient's hospital course and admission sputum stains should be reviewed by a clinician with expertise in the diagnosis and treatment of pneumonia. Pulmonary embolism with infarction, a treatable disease, can prove fatal if misdiagnosed as bacterial pneumonia. Misinterpretation of sputum Gram-stained preparations—either failure to recognize an important pathogen or a treatment decision based upon examination of an inadequate specimen—is an avoidable pitfall of medical practice. Bronchoscopy should be considered, both to obtain better specimens for diagnosis and to exclude underlying endobronchial obstruction.

The Patient with Pleural Effusion and Fever

The approach to such patients is quite straightforward; the fluid must be examined. If a bacterium other than *S. pneumoniae* is seen on Gram's stain of pleural fluid or grown in culture, chest tube drainage is required. A pleural effusion infected with the pneumococcus can often be treated with simple needle aspiration and antibiotics. Among patients with pneumonia, even fluids that do not reveal organisms on Gram's stain but have a pH of less than 7 and/or a glucose concentration below 40 mg/dl may require chest tube drainage for satisfactory resolution. Patients with empyema complicating an aggressive bacterial pneumonia such as that due to Group A streptococci may benefit from early surgical debridement of the pleural space (decortication).

Pleurisy caused by *M. tuberculosis* is often an acute illness. In most cases, a pneumonia is not present or readily appreciated. Inflammatory cells—polymorphonuclear leukocytes, mononuclear leukocytes, or both—are present in the pleural fluid. Mesothelial cells are usually sparse (<0.5% of the total cell count). Pleural fluid glucose levels are often low but may be normal. Mycobacteria are rarely seen on stains of pleural fluid. As many as one third of patients do not have positive tuberculin skin tests. Other causes of pleural effusion in this setting may be pulmonary infarction (fewer than half of patients produce a hemorrhagic exudate), malignancy (most do not have fever), and connective tissue diseases such as systemic lupus erythematosus and rheumatoid arthritis. If the cause of the effusion is not evident, a biopsy of the pleura is needed.

PREVENTION

Pneumococcal pneumonia may be preventable by immunizing patients at high risk with polyvalent pneumococcal polysaccharide vaccine. The current polyvalent vaccine is 60 to 80% effective in individuals with normal immune responses. Booster immunizations should not be given to immunologically competent patients because of the possibility of serious reactions. Yearly immunization with influenza vaccine is also advised for many of these patients; by decreasing the attack rate of influenza, immunization also decreases morbidity and mortality due to secondary bacterial pneumonia (Table 99–7).

Patients without active tuberculosis but with skin test reactivity to purified protein derivative are at risk for reactivating their infection. The development of active tuberculosis can be prevented in most instances by treatment for 6 to 12 months with isoniazid, 300 mg/day. Indications for prophylaxis are shown in Table 99–8.

REFERENCES

Bartlett JG, Mundy LM. Current Concepts: Community acquired pneumonia. N Engl J Med 1995; 333:1618–24.

Duma RJ: Pneumococcal pneumonia. *In* Bennett JC, Plum F (eds.): Cecil Textbook of Medicine. 20th ed. Philadelphia, WB Saunders, 1996, pp 1569–1576.

Yu VL: Legionella pneumophila (legionnaires' disease). *In* Mandell GL, Bennett JE, Dolin R (eds.): Principles and Practice of Infectious Diseases. 4th ed. New York, Churchill Livingstone, 1995, pp 2087–2097.

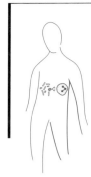

100

Infections of the Heart and Vessels

INFECTIVE ENDOCARDITIS (IE)

Infective endocarditis ranges from an indolent illness with few systemic manifestations, readily responsive to antibiotic therapy, to a fulminant septicemic disease with malignant destruction of heart valves and life-threatening systemic embolization. The varied features of endocarditis relate in large measure to the different infecting organisms. Viridans streptococci are the prototype of bacteria that originate in the oral flora, infect previously abnormal heart valves, and may cause minimal symptomatology despite progressive valvular damage. *Staphylococcus aureus,* in contrast, can invade previously normal valves and destroy them rapidly.

Epidemiology

The average age of patients with endocarditis has increased in the antibiotic era to the current mean of 54 years. This change can be attributed to the decreasing prevalence of rheumatic heart disease, the increasing prevalence of underlying degenerative heart disease, and the increasing frequency of procedures and practices predisposing older patients to bacteremia (genitourinary instrumentation, intravenous catheters, hemodialysis shunts). Rheumatic heart disease remains a predisposing factor in 20 to 30% of patients with IE. About 15% of patients have congenital heart disease (exclusive of mitral valve prolapse). The propensity to develop endocarditis varies with the congenital lesion. For example, infection of a bicuspid aortic valve accounts for one fifth of cases of IE occurring over the age of 60; a secundum atrial septal defect, however, rarely becomes infected. Mitral valve prolapse is the predisposing condition in more than one third of cases of endocarditis of the mitral valve. Intravenous drug users have a unique propensity to develop IE of the tricuspid valve; infection of the mitral or aortic valve is less common. Patients with prosthetic heart valves have a 5 to 10% lifetime risk of infective endocarditis.

Pathogenesis

Endocarditis ensues when bacteria entering the blood stream from an oral or other source lodge on heart valves that may already bear platelet-fibrin thrombi. The frequency of bacteremia is quite high after dental extraction (18 to 85%) or periodontal surgery (32 to 88%) but also is significant following everyday activities such as tooth brushing (0 to 26%) and chewing candy (17 to 51%). The production of extracellular dextran by some streptococcal strains promotes their adherence to dental enamel and also is a factor in the entrapment of circulating organisms on damaged valves and platelet-fibrin thrombi. The localization of infection is partly determined by the production of turbulent flow, with left-sided infection more common than right-sided infection, except among intravenous drug users. Vegetations usually are found on the valve surface facing the lower pressure chamber (i.e., atrial surface of the mitral valve), a relative haven for deposition of bacteria from the swift blood stream. Occasionally, "jet lesions" develop in which the regurgitant stream strikes the heart wall or the chordae tendineae. Once infection begins, bacteria proliferate freely within the interstices of the enlarging vegetation; in this relatively avascular site, they are protected from serum bactericidal factors and leukocytes.

The infection may cause rupture of the valve tissue itself or of its chordal structures, leading to either gradual or acute valvular regurgitation. Some virulent bacteria (e.g., *S. aureus*) or fungal vegetations may become large enough to obstruct the valve orifice or create a large embolus. Aneurysms of the sinus of Valsalva may occur and can rupture into the pericardial space. The conducting system may be affected by valve ring or myocardial abscesses. The infection may invade the interventricular septum, causing intramyocardial abscesses or septal rupture that can also damage the conduction system of the heart. Systemic septic embolization may occur with left-sided endocarditis, and septic pulmonary emboli with right-sided endocarditis.

Clinical Features

Some cases of streptococcal endocarditis become clinically manifest within 2 weeks of initiating events, such as dental extraction. However, diagnosis usually is delayed an additional 4 to 5 weeks or more because of the paucity of symptoms. If the causative organism is slow growing and produces an indolent syndrome, symptoms may be extremely protracted (6 months or longer) before definitive diagnosis. The symptoms and signs of IE relate to systemic infection, emboli (bland or septic), metastatic infective foci, congestive heart failure, or immune complex–associated lesions. The most common complaints in patients with IE are fever, chills, weakness, shortness of breath, night sweats, loss of appetite, and weight loss. Musculoskeletal symptoms develop in nearly one half of patients and may dominate the presentation. Proximal arthralgias are typical and are frequently accompanied by oligoarticular arthritis of the lower extremities. Fever is present in 90% of patients. Fever is more often absent in elderly or debilitated patients or in the setting of underlying congestive heart failure, renal dysfunction, or previous antibiotic treatment. Heart murmurs are frequent (85%); changing murmurs (5 to 10%) and new cardiac murmurs (5%) are unusual but suggest the diagnosis of IE. With endocarditis involving the aortic or the mitral valve, congestive heart failure occurs in two thirds of patients and may begin precipitously, for example, with perforation of a valve or rupture of chordae tendineae. At least one of the peripheral manifestations of endocarditis occurs in one half of patients (Table 100–1). Splenomegaly (25 to 60%) is more likely when symptoms have been prolonged. Clubbing occurs in 10 to 15% of patients.

The clinical syndrome of IE differs in users of intravenous drugs. Tricuspid valve infection is most common; this may be related to scarring of the tricuspid valve by injected particulate matter. Patients most often present with fever and chills but may present with pleuritic chest pain caused by septic pulmonary emboli. Round, cavitating infiltrates may be found on the chest radiograph. The infective foci are initially centered in blood vessels; only after they erode into the bronchial system does cough develop, productive of bloody or purulent sputum.

Serious systemic emboli may cause dramatic findings, at times masking the systemic nature of IE. Embolism to the splenic artery may lead to left upper quadrant pain, sometimes radiating to the left shoulder, a friction rub, and/or left pleural effusion. Renal, coronary, and mesenteric arteries are frequent sites of clinically important emboli. Central nervous system (CNS) embolization is one of the most serious complications of IE, since it may produce irreversible and disabling neurologic deficits. Infective endocarditis must be considered in the differential diagnosis of stroke in young adults, as well as in all patients with valvular heart disease.

Overall, neurologic manifestations occur in one third of patients with IE. The diagnosis is easily missed when CNS signs and symptoms are the presenting features of IE, as occurs in approximately 10% of cases. Patients with IE may complain of headache or may develop seizures. The pathophysiologic explanation for these symptoms is not always apparent. In addition, stroke due to vascular occlusion by an embolus, toxic encephalopathy, which may mimic psychosis, and meningoencephalitis also occur. The aseptic meningitis or meningoencephalitis seen in such patients is not readily distinguished from viral and other etiologies of a similar syndrome.

Clinical syndromes caused by CNS emboli may be more distinctive. The consequences of embolization depend on the site of lodging and the bacterial pathogen. Organisms such as viridans streptococci initially produce a syndrome entirely attributable to the vascular occlusion; however, damage to the blood vessel can result in formation of a mycotic aneurysm that may leak or burst at a later date. Resolution of aneurysms may occur after antimicrobial therapy. In many patients, however, surgical clipping is necessary to prevent recurrent hemorrhage. Single aneurysms in accessible areas should be considered for prompt surgical clipping. *S. aureus,* in contrast, produces progressive infection extending from the site of embolization; brain abscess and purulent meningitis are occasional sequelae.

The kidney can be the site of abscess formation, multiple infarcts, or immune complex glomerulonephritis. When renal dysfunction develops during antibiotic therapy, drug toxicity is an additional consideration.

Laboratory Findings

Nonspecific laboratory abnormalities occur in IE and reflect chronic infection. These include anemia, reticulocytopenia, increased erythrocyte sedimentation rate, hypergammaglobulinemia, circulating immune complexes, false-positive serologic tests for syphilis, and rheumatoid factor. The presence of rheumatoid factor may be a helpful clue to diagnosis in patients with culture-negative endocarditis. Urinalysis frequently shows proteinuria (50 to 60%) and microscopic hematuria (30 to 50%). The presence of red blood cell casts is indicative of immune complex–mediated glomerulonephritis. The finding of

TABLE 100–1	Peripheral Manifestations of Infective Endocarditis (IE)	
Physical Finding (Frequency)	**Pathogenesis**	**Most Common Organisms**
Petechiae (20–40%) (red, nonblanching lesions in crops on conjunctivae, buccal mucosa, palate, extremities)	Vasculitis or emboli	*Streptococcus, Staphylococcus*
Splinter hemorrhages (15%) (linear, red-brown streaks most suggestive of IE when proximal in nail beds)	Vasculitis or emboli	*Staphylococcus, Streptococcus*
Osler's nodes (10–25%) (2- to 5-mm painful nodules on pads of fingers or toes)	Vasculitis	*Streptococcus*
Janeway's lesions (<10%) (macular, red or hemorrhagic, painless patches on palms or soles)	Emboli	*Staphylococcus*
Roth's spots (<5%) (oval, pale retinal lesions surrounded by hemorrhage)	Vasculitis	*Streptococcus*

gram-positive cocci in the urine of a febrile patient with microscopic hematuria should always prompt consideration of the possibility of infective endocarditis.

The bacteremia of IE is continuous and low grade (often 1 to 100 bacteria per milliliter in subacute cases). Three sets of blood cultures should be obtained in the first 24 hours of hospitalization. Two or three additional blood cultures are important if the patient has received antibiotic therapy in the preceding 1 to 2 weeks and if initial blood cultures are negative at 48 to 72 hours. Five to ten percent of patients with the clinical diagnosis of IE have negative blood cultures, usually because of previous antibiotic therapy.

Echocardiography is a useful technique for identifying vegetations in endocarditis. The finding of vegetations is helpful diagnostically and also indicates an increased risk of valvular destruction with congestive heart failure, systemic embolization, and death. Roughly 95% of patients with infective endocarditis have valvular vegetations demonstrable by transesophageal echocardiography. Transesophageal echocardiography also provides improved resolution of bacterial vegetations and valve ring abscesses and may be helpful in difficult determinations concerning the need for surgery. Magnetic resonance imaging (MRI) of the heart similarly may demonstrate myocardial, septal, or valve ring abscesses.

Differential Diagnosis

The diagnosis of IE usually is firmly established on the basis of the clinical findings and the results of blood cultures. In some instances, the distinction between IE and nonendocarditis bacteremia may be difficult. Since the bacteremia is usually continuous in IE and intermittent in other bacteremias, the fraction of blood cultures that are positive may be helpful in distinguishing between these entities. The more frequent causative agents of infective endocarditis are shown in Table 100–2. In streptococcal infection, the speciation of the blood culture isolate may provide circumstantial evidence for or against infection of the heart valves (Table 100–3). The identity of the causative organism may be helpful for other bacteria as well; the ratio of IE to non-IE bacteremias is approximately 1:1 for *S. aureus,* 1:7 for group B strepto-

TABLE 100–3	Relative Frequency of Infective Endocarditis (IE) and Non-IE Bacteremias for Various Streptococci
Species	**IE/Non-IE**
Streptococcus mutans	14:1
Streptococcus bovis	6:1
Streptococcus faecalis	1:1
Group B streptococci	1:7
Group A streptococci	1:32

Modified from Parker MT, Ball LC: Streptococci and aerococci associated with systemic infection in man. J Med Microbiol 1976; 9:275.

cocci, and 1:200 for *Escherichia coli. Streptococcus bovis* bacteremia and endocarditis are often (>50%) associated with colonic carcinomas or polyps. Isolation of this organism warrants thorough evaluation of the lower gastrointestinal tract.

The initial presentation of IE can be misleading: the young adult may present with a stroke, pneumonia, or meningitis; the elderly patient may present with confusion or simply with fatigue or malaise without fever. The index of suspicion for IE, therefore, must be high, and blood cultures should be obtained in these varied settings, particularly if antibiotic use is contemplated.

Major problems in diagnosis arise if antibiotics have been administered before blood is cultured or if blood cultures are negative. Attempts to culture slow-growing organisms, including those with particular nutritional requirements, should be planned by discussion with a clinical microbiologist. The differential diagnosis of culture-negative endocarditis includes acute rheumatic fever, multiple pulmonary emboli, atrial myxoma, and nonbacterial thrombotic endocarditis (NBTE). NBTE (sometimes called marantic endocarditis) occurs in patients with severe wasting, whether due to malignancy or other conditions. Also, patients with systemic lupus erythematosus may develop sterile valvular vegetations, termed Libman-Sacks' lesions, on the undersurfaces of the valve leaflets. These diagnoses should be considered and excluded, if possible, before beginning a prolonged course of therapy for presumed culture-negative IE.

| TABLE 100–2 | Frequency of Infecting Microorganisms in Endocarditis |

Native Valve (%)		PVE (%)			Endocarditis in IVDU	
			Early	**Late**		
Streptococci	50	Coagulase-negative staphylococci	33	29	*S. aureus*	60
Enterococci	10	*S. aureus*	15	11	Streptococci	13
Staphylococcus aureus	20	Gram-negative bacilli	17	11	Gram-negative bacilli	8
HACEK	5	Fungi	13	5	Enterococci	7
Culture negative	5	Streptococci	9	36	Fungi	5
		Diphtheroids	9	3	Polymicrobial	5
					Culture negative	5

HACEK = *Haemophilus, Actinobacillus, Cardiobacterium, Eikenella, Kingella;* IVDU = intravenous drug user; PVE = prosthetic valve endocarditis.
From Levison ME: Infective endocarditis. *In* Bennett JC, Plum F (eds.): Cecil Textbook of Medicine. 20th ed. Philadelphia, WB Saunders, 1996, pp 1596–1605.

Management and Outcome

The outcome of endocarditis is determined by the extent of valvular destruction, the size and friability of vegetations, and the choice of antibiotics. These factors, in turn, are influenced by the nature of the causative organism and delays in diagnosis. The goal of antibiotic therapy is to halt further valvular damage and to cure the infection. Surgery may be necessary for hemodynamic stabilization, prevention of embolization, or control of drug-resistant infection.

Antibiotics should be selected on the basis of the clinical setting (Table 100–4) and started as soon as blood cultures are obtained if the diagnosis of IE appears highly likely and the course is suggestive of active valvular destruction or systemic embolization. The antibiotics can be adjusted later on the basis of culture and sensitivity data.

Antibiotics

A number of different regimens have been advocated for the treatment of IE due to each of the causative organisms. Since few have been subjected to valid comparative trials, the selection of drugs, dosages, and duration is somewhat empiric. Similarly, although sophisticated laboratory tests such as serum bactericidal activity are used to monitor and adjust drug regimens, they have not been standardized or validated adequately. Nonetheless, each regimen must be capable of bactericidal activity against the offending pathogen and must be of sufficient duration—usually 4 to 6 weeks in left-sided endocarditis—to sterilize the affected heart valves.

Most viridans streptococci and nonenterococcal group

TABLE 100–4	Syndromes Suggesting Specific Bacteria Causing Infective Endocarditis

Indolent Course

Viridans streptococci
Streptococcus bovis
Streptococcus faecalis
Fastidious gram-negative rods

Aggressive Course

Staphylococcus aureus
Streptococcus pneumoniae
Streptococcus pyogenes
Neisseria gonorrhoeae

Drug Users

S. aureus
Pseudomonas aeruginosa
S. faecalis
Candida sp.
Bacillus sp.

Frequent Major Emboli

Haemophilus sp.
Bacteroides sp.
Candida sp.

D streptococci, such as *S. bovis,* are exquisitely sensitive to penicillin. The penicillin concentration inhibiting growth of such organisms is less than 0.1 μg/ml, and they are killed by similar concentrations of penicillin. A variety of antibiotic regimens have been advocated to treat this form of IE, and several appear to be equally effective. Aqueous penicillin G, 12 million units/day given intravenously for 4 weeks, is curative in almost all patients, as is a 2-week course of penicillin G plus gentamicin in younger patients with uncomplicated disease. In the stable patient at low risk of complications, some of the antibiotic course can be administered on an outpatient basis.

Treatment of enterococcal endocarditis and IE caused by other penicillin-resistant streptococci is much less satisfactory because of frequent relapses and high mortality. The recommended regimen is intravenous aqueous penicillin G, 20 million units/day, plus intravenous gentamicin, 3 mg/kg/day. This relatively low dose of aminoglycoside is associated with less nephrotoxicity. The aminoglycoside dose should be adjusted according to measured serum levels and the bactericidal activity of serum. Streptomycin, 0.5 gm administered intramuscularly every 12 hours, can be substituted as the aminoglycoside if the organism is sensitive; however, streptomycin may be associated with irreversible vestibular and auditory toxicity in some patients.

Although the value of serum bactericidal determinations has not been firmly established, most experts rely on them as a general guide to the adequacy of antibiotic regimens for enterococcal endocarditis. A drug regimen is considered adequate for treatment of IE if trough serum bactericidal activity is present at dilutions of 1:8 or greater. In view of the high frequency of relapses, regimens to treat enterococcal infection should be continued for 4 to 6 weeks. Culture-negative endocarditis should be treated similarly.

S. aureus endocarditis should be treated with intravenous nafcillin, 12 gm/day, unless the isolate is penicillin-sensitive, in which case penicillin, 12 million units daily, is the treatment of choice. Infection with a methicillin-resistant species of *Staphylococcus* necessitates the use of vancomycin. The addition of an aminoglycoside hastens clearance of bacteremia and is indicated in the patient with a fulminant septic presentation and in the initial treatment of left-sided endocarditis. Once sepsis is controlled, the aminoglycoside should be discontinued. Minimal bactericidal concentrations of antibiotic should be determined. If the bactericidal concentration is more than 32 times the bacteriostatic concentration, the organism can be considered drug tolerant. Patients with IE caused by tolerant staphylococci may have a more complicated clinical course. If the organism fulfills the criteria for tolerance, determination of serum bactericidal activity is appropriate; if this proves inadequate (i.e., bactericidal activity < 1:8 dilution of serum), *and* the patient shows signs of persistent infection, addition of an aminoglycoside or rifampin should be considered. The duration of antibiotic therapy for staphylococcal endocarditis of the mitral or aortic valve is a minimum of 6 weeks.

In the patient with streptococcal or staphylococcal IE

and a history of serious penicillin allergy, vancomycin can be substituted for penicillin. Among patients at risk for complicated disease, consideration should be given to penicillin desensitization.

Pseudomonas endocarditis is a particular problem in intravenous drug users. Therapy should be initiated with tobramycin, 8 mg/kg/day given intravenously, and mezlocillin, 4 gm given intravenously every 8 hours. The unusually high doses of aminoglycosides have improved the outcome of medical therapy of *Pseudomonas* infection of the tricuspid valve with surprisingly few side effects such as nephrotoxicity. Left-sided *Pseudomonas aeruginosa* infections, however, generally require surgery for cure. Although third-generation cephalosporins have attractive in vitro efficacy against *Pseudomonas* species, *in vivo* development of resistance and clinical failure have limited their usefulness, especially as single agents, in this setting. Some young adults have rapid clearance of aminoglycosides, so it is particularly critical to measure serum drug levels and adjust dosages as appropriate when these agents are employed.

Fungal endocarditis is refractory to antibiotics and requires surgery for management. Amphotericin B generally is administered to such patients but is not in itself curative.

Surgery

The indications for early surgery in IE need to be individualized and forged by discussions with the cardiac surgeon. Refractory infection is a clear indication for surgery; as noted, the requirement for surgery is predictable in IE caused by certain organisms. Persistence of bacteremia for longer than 7 to 10 days, despite the administration of appropriate antibiotics, frequently reflects paravalvular extension of infection with development of valve ring abscess or myocardial abscesses. Medical cure is not likely in this setting. Intravenous drug users are more likely to have IE due to organisms refractory to medical therapy (*Candida, Pseudomonas*). Refractory tricuspid endocarditis may be amenable to valve debridement or excision without immediate placement of a prosthetic valve. Valvulectomy may, however, be associated with the eventual onset of right-sided congestive heart failure.

Protracted fever is not unusual in patients undergoing treatment of endocarditis and should not automatically be equated with refractory infection. In fact, 10% of patients remain febrile for more than 2 weeks, and persistent fever is not an independent indication for surgery, particularly when tricuspid endocarditis is complicated by multiple septic pulmonary emboli with necrotizing pneumonia. Delayed defervescence also is common, despite appropriate antimicrobial therapy, with endocarditis due to *S. aureus* and enteric bacteria.

Congestive heart failure refractory to medical therapy is the most frequent indication for early cardiac surgery. The extent of valvular dysfunction may be difficult to gauge clinically, particularly in patients with acute aortic regurgitation (AR); in the absence of compensatory ventricular dilatation, classic physical signs associated with AR, such as wide pulse pressure, may not be present.

Echocardiography, fluoroscopy, and cardiac catheterization may be necessary to evaluate the extent of aortic regurgitation in some instances. However, when congestive heart failure develops in the patient with *S. aureus* IE, aortic valvular destruction usually is extensive, necessitating early surgery. Delaying surgery to prolong the course of antibiotic therapy is never appropriate if the patient is hemodynamically unstable or fulfills other criteria for surgical intervention. Prosthetic valve endocarditis seldom occurs after cardiac valve replacement for IE, and its incidence is not influenced by duration of preoperative antibiotics.

Recurrent major systemic embolization is another indication for surgery. If valvular function is preserved, vegetations sometimes can be removed without valve replacement. Septal abscess, although often difficult to recognize clinically, and aneurysms of the sinus of Valsalva are absolute indications for surgery.

PROSTHETIC VALVE ENDOCARDITIS (PVE)

Prosthetic valve endocarditis complicates approximately 3% of cardiac valve replacements. Two separate clinical syndromes have been identified. Early PVE occurs within 60 days of surgery and most often is caused by *Staphylococcus epidermidis,* gram-negative enteric bacilli, *S. aureus,* or diphtheroids. The prosthesis may be contaminated at the time of surgery or seeded by bacteremia from extracardiac sites (intravenous cannula, indwelling urinary bladder catheter, wound infection, pneumonia). In addition to forming vegetations, which may be quite bulky and cause obstruction, particularly of mitral valve prostheses, circumferential spread of infection often causes dehiscence and paravalvular leak at the site of an aortic prosthesis. The combination of intravenous vancomycin, 2 gm/day, and intravenous tobramycin, 3 to 5 mg/kg/day, plus oral rifampin, 600 mg/day, is indicated to treat *S. epidermidis* infection. Other infections should be treated with synergistic bactericidal combinations of antibiotics based on *in vitro* sensitivity testing. Surgery is mandatory in the presence of moderate to severe congestive heart failure. The mortality of early PVE is approximately 75%.

Late PVE is most frequently caused by viridans streptococcal bacteremia from an oral site that seeds a re-endothelialized valve surface. Treatment with intravenous aqueous penicillin G, 12 to 20 million units/day, plus intravenous tobramycin, 3 to 5 mg/kg/day, is appropriate. The prognosis for cure with antibiotic therapy alone is better in patients infected with penicillin-sensitive streptococci. Moderate to severe congestive heart failure is the main indication for surgery. The mortality of late PVE is approximately 40%.

PROPHYLAXIS OF INFECTIVE ENDOCARDITIS

Patients with prosthetic heart valves or mitral or aortic valvular heart disease are at relatively high risk of developing IE. Mitral valve prolapse associated with a systolic murmur is another risk factor. Neither the value of antibi-

TABLE 100-5	Prophylaxis of Infective Endocarditis	
Indications	**Regimen***

Oral

| Aortic or mitral valve disease in patients undergoing dental procedure with bleeding gums
As above for penicillin-allergic patient or when chronic penicillin prophylaxis has been used to prevent rheumatic fever | 1. Amoxicillin, 3.0 gm orally 1 hr before and 1.5 gm 6 hr after procedure
2. Clindamycin, 300 mg orally 1 hr before and 150 mg orally 6 hr after procedure |

Parenteral

Patient with prosthetic heart valve undergoing dental, gastrointestinal, or genitourinary procedure. Patient with aortic or mitral valve disease undergoing gastrointestinal surgery or genitourinary instrumentation or surgery	1. Ampicillin, 2.0 gm IM or IV, plus gentamicin, 1.5 mg/kg IM or IV, 30 min before procedure May repeat parenteral antibiotics 8 hours after procedure
Penicillin-allergic patient with prosthetic heart valve undergoing dental procedure	2. Vancomycin, 1.0 gm IV over a 1-hr period beginning 1 hr before procedure
Penicillin-allergic patient with aortic or mitral valve disease undergoing gastrointestinal surgery or genitourinary instrumentation or surgery; penicillin-allergic patient with prosthetic valve undergoing gastrointestinal or genitourinary procedure	3. Vancomycin, 1.0 gm IV, plus gentamicin, 1.5 mg/kg IV, beginning 1 hr before procedure. May repeat parenteral antibiotics 8 hours after procedure

* These are empiric suggestions. Additional doses of antibiotic may be given if there is risk of prolonged bacteremia.
IM = Intramuscular; IV = intravenous.

otic prophylaxis nor the optimal regimens have been definitively established. Recommended regimens are presented in Table 100–5.

Administration of antibiotics has become an accepted practice for patients undergoing open heart surgery, including valve replacement. Intravenous cefazolin, 2.0 gm at induction of anesthesia, repeated 8 and 16 hours later, or intravenous vancomycin, 1.0 gm at induction and 0.5 gm 8 and 16 hours later, is an appropriate regimen. Cardiac diagnostic procedures (catheterization), pacemaker placement, and coronary artery bypass do not pose sufficient risk to warrant the use of prophylactic antibiotics for IE or prosthetic valve endocarditis.

Devices that are associated with high rates of infection and bacteremia (intravenous cannulas, indwelling urinary bladder catheters) should be avoided in hospitalized patients at risk for IE if at all possible; established local infections should be treated promptly and vigorously.

BACTERIAL ENDARTERITIS AND SUPPURATIVE PHLEBITIS

Bacterial endarteritis usually develops by one of three mechanisms. (1) Arteries, particularly those with intimal abnormalities, may become infected as a consequence of transient bacteremia. (2) During the course of IE, septic emboli to vasa vasorum may lead to mycotic aneurysms. (3) Blood vessels also may be infected by direct extension from contiguous foci and trauma.

A septic presentation is characteristic of endarteritis due to organisms such as *S. aureus*. Besides sepsis, the major problem caused by endarteritis is hemorrhage. About 3 to 4% of patients with IE develop intracranial mycotic aneurysms. Mycotic aneurysms in IE typically are situated peripherally and in the distribution of the middle cerebral artery. Focal seizures, focal neurologic signs, or aseptic meningitis may herald catastrophic rupture of such aneurysms. These premonitory findings, therefore, indicate the need for evaluation with arteriography; neurosurgical intervention should be contemplated if accessible lesions are demonstrated. Infection of an atherosclerotic plaque can occur as a complication of bacteremia, particularly in elderly patients with bacteremia due to *Salmonella* species. Traumatic endarteritis with pseudoaneurysm often complicates arterial injection of illicit drugs and rarely complicates arterial catheterizations. Treatment often requires combined medical and surgical management; antibiotic selection should be based on the results of *in vitro* sensitivity testing.

Suppurative thrombophlebitis usually is a complication of the use of intravenous plastic cannulas. Burn patients, especially those with lower extremity catheterization, are at particular risk. Typically, intravenous cannulas have been left in place 5 days or more. Often the vein is sclerosed and tender, and the surrounding skin is erythematous. The vein should be milked to identify pus. If pus is present or if bacteremia and fever persist despite antibiotic therapy, involved segments of vein must be excised. Antibiotics should be selected to ensure coverage of the most common pathogens, *Staphylococcus* species (vancomycin, 2 gm/day IV) and Enterobacteriaceae (gentamicin, 5 mg/kg/day IV). When infection of an intravenous cannula is suspected, the catheter should be removed and 2-inch segments rolled across a blood agar plate. The growth of more than 15 colonies suggests infection. The infusate also should be cultured. (See also Chapter 106.)

Suppurative phlebitis is preventable. Peripheral intravenous cannulas should be inserted aseptically and replaced at least every 72 hours by well-trained personnel.

REFERENCES

Levison ME: Infective endocarditis. *In* Bennett JC, Plum F (eds.): Cecil Textbook of Medicine. 20th ed. Philadelphia, WB Saunders, 1996; pp 1596–1605.

Lederman MM, Sprague L, Wallis RS, Ellner JJ: Duration of fever during infective endocarditis. Medicine 1992;71:52.

Wilson WR, Sleckelberg JM (eds.): Infective endocarditis. Infect Dis Clin North Am 1993;7:1.

101

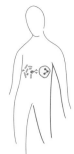

Skin and Soft Tissue Infections

Normal skin is remarkably resistant to infection. Most common infections of the skin are initiated by breaks in the epithelium. Hematogenous seeding of the skin by pathogens is less frequent.

Some superficial infections, such as folliculitis and furuncles, may be treated with local measures. Other superficial infections (e.g., impetigo and cellulitis) require systemic antibiotics. Deeper soft tissue infections, such as fasciitis and myonecrosis, require surgical debridement. As a general rule, infections of the face and hand should be treated particularly aggressively because of the risks of intracranial spread in the former and the potential loss of function due to closed-space infection in the latter.

SUPERFICIAL INFECTIONS OF THE SKIN

Circumscribed Infections of the Skin

Vesicles, pustules, nodules, and ulcerations are the lesions in this category (Table 101–1).

Folliculitis is a superficial infection of hair follicles. The lesions are crops of red papules or pustules; careful examination using a hand lens reveals hair in the center of most papules. Staphylococci, yeast, and, occasionally, *Pseudomonas* species are the responsible pathogens. Local treatment with cleansing and hot compresses is usually sufficient. The skin lesions of disseminated candidiasis seen in neutropenic patients may resemble folliculitis. In this setting, skin biopsy readily distinguishes these two processes; in disseminated disease, yeast are found within blood vessels and not simply surrounding the hair follicle.

Furuncles and *carbuncles* are subcutaneous abscesses due to *Staphylococcus aureus*. The lesions are red, tender nodules that may have a surrounding cellulitis and occur most prominently on the face and back of the neck. They often drain spontaneously. Furuncles may be treated with local compresses. If fluctuant, the larger carbuncles require incision and drainage. Antistaphylococcal antibiotics should be given if the patient has systemic symptoms, such as fever or malaise, if there is accompanying cellulitis, or if the lesions are on the head.

Impetigo is a superficial infection of the skin due to group A streptococci, although *S. aureus* may also be found in the lesions. Impetigo is seen primarily among children, who initially develop a vesicle on the skin surface; this rapidly becomes pustular and breaks down, leaving the characteristic dry, golden crust. This pruritic lesion is highly contagious—usually spread by the child's hands to other sites on the body or to other children. Gram's stain reveals gram-positive cocci in chains (streptococci); occasionally, clusters of staphylococci are also seen. Certain strains of streptococci causing impetigo have been associated with the later development of poststreptococcal glomerulonephritis. The differential diagnosis of impetigo includes herpes simplex infection and varicella. These viral lesions may become pustular; Gram's stain of an unruptured viral vesicle or pustule should not, however, contain bacteria. A Tzanck preparation (see Chapter 93) (or assay for viral antigens for optimal sensitivity) can establish the diagnosis of herpes simplex or varicella if the differential diagnosis is uncertain. Penicillin is the treatment of choice for impetigo, since staphylococci represent secondary infection and will disappear when the streptococci are eradicated. Antibiotics do not appear to affect the development of poststreptococcal glomerulonephritis but will prevent the spread of infection to others.

Ecthyma gangrenosum is a cutaneous manifestation of disseminated gram-negative rod infection, usually due to *Pseudomonas aeruginosa* in neutropenic patients. The initial lesion is a vesicle or papule with an erythematous halo. Although generally small (<2 cm), the initial lesion may exceed 20 cm in diameter. In a short time, the vesicle ulcerates, leaving a necrotic ulcer with surrounding erythema or a violaceous rim. Gram's stain of an aspirate may reveal gram-negative rods; cultures of the aspirate are generally positive. Biopsy of the lesion shows venous thrombosis, often with bacteria demonstrable within the blood vessel walls. Since these lesions are manifestations of gram-negative rod bacteremia, treatment should be instituted immediately with an aminoglycoside plus a third-generation cephalosporin with good activity against *P. aeruginosa* (e.g., ceftazidime) until the results of culture and sensitivity studies are known (see also Chapter 96).

Herpes Simplex Virus. Oral infections due to this virus are discussed in Chapter 98, and genital infections in Chapter 107. On occasion, infection with this virus occurs on extraoral or extragenital sites, usually on the hands. This is most often the case in health care workers but also may result from sexual contact or from autoinoculation.

TABLE 101-1	Circumscribed Cutaneous Infections
Description	**Predominant Organism**
Folliculitis	*Staphylococcus aureus, Candida* sp.
Furuncles, carbuncles	*Staphylococcus aureus*
Impetigo	Group A streptococci, *Staphylococcus aureus*
Ecthyma gangrenosum	Gram-negative bacilli (systemic infection)

Vesicular or Vesiculopustular Lesions of the Skin

Impetigo
Folliculitis
Herpes simplex virus infection
Varicella-zoster virus infection
Rickettsialpox

Ulcerative Lesions of the Skin

Pressure sores
Stasis ulcerations
Diabetic ulcerations
Sickle cell ulcers
Mycobacterial infection
Fungal infection
Ecthyma gangrenosum
Syphilis chancroid

The virus may produce a painful erythema, usually at the junction of the nail bed and skin (whitlow). This progresses to a vesiculopustular lesion. At both stages of infection, herpetic whitlow can resemble a bacterial infection—paronychia. When more than one digit is involved, herpes is much more likely. It is important to distinguish between herpetic and bacterial infections, since incision and drainage of a herpetic whitlow are contraindicated. Puncture of the purulent center of a paronychia and Gram's stain of the exudate allow prompt and accurate diagnosis. In the case of herpetic whitlow, bacteria are not present unless the lesion has already drained and become superinfected. In the case of a bacterial paronychia, bacteria are readily seen. Recurrences of herpetic whitlow may be seen but are generally less severe than the primary infection. Treatment with oral acyclovir may shorten the duration of symptoms.

Varicella-Zoster Virus (see also Chapter 95)

Primary infection with varicella-zoster virus (chickenpox) is thought to occur via the respiratory route but may also occur through contact with infected skin lesions. Viremia results in crops of papules that progress to vesicles, then pustules followed by crustling. The lesions are most prominent on the trunk. This is almost always a disease of childhood. Systemic symptoms may precede development of the characteristic rash by 1 or 2 days but are mild except in the case of an immunocompromised patient or primary infection in the adult. In the immunocompromised, chickenpox can produce a fatal systemic illness. In otherwise healthy adults, chickenpox can be a serious illness with life-threatening pneumonia. Clinical diagnosis is based on the characteristic appearance of the rash. Impetigo and folliculitis are readily distinguished clinically or by Gram's stain or Tzanck preparation of the pustule contents. Disseminated herpes simplex virus infection is seen only in the immunocompromised host or in patients with eczema. Viral culture or viral antigen detection will distinguish herpes simplex from herpes zoster in these settings. Most patients with rickettsialpox, which is confused with chickenpox rarely, also have an ulcer or eschar that precedes the generalized rash by 3 to 7 days and represents the bite of the infected mouse mite, which transmits the disease.

Immunocompromised children exposed to varicella should receive prophylaxis with zoster immune globulin. Immunocompromised persons and seriously ill elderly patients with varicella should be treated with acyclovir.

After primary infection, the varicella-zoster virus persists in a latent state within sensory neurons of the dorsal root ganglia. The infection may reactivate, producing the syndrome of zoster (shingles). Pain in the distribution of the affected nerve root precedes the rash by a few days. Depending upon the dermatome, the pain may mimic pleurisy, myocardial infarction, or gallbladder disease. A clue to the presence of early zoster infection is the finding of dysesthesia—an unpleasant sensation when the involved dermatome is gently stroked by the examiner's hand. The appearance of papules and vesicles in a dermatomal distribution confirms the diagnosis. Herpes zoster infections of certain dermatomes merit special attention. The Ramsay Hunt syndrome can be caused by infection involving the geniculate ganglia and presents with painful eruption of the ear canal and tympanic membrane, often associated with an ipsilateral seventh cranial nerve (facial nerve) palsy. Infection involving the second branch of the fifth cranial nerve (trigeminal nerve) often produces lesions of the cornea. This infection should be treated promptly with systemic acyclovir to prevent loss of visual acuity. A clue to possible ophthalmic involvement is the presence of vesicles on the tip of the nose (see also Chapter 114).

In most instances, dermatomal zoster is a disease of the otherwise healthy adult. However, immunocompromised patients (e.g., persons with HIV infection) are at greater risk for reactivation of this virus. Patients with zoster should receive a careful history and physical evaluation; in the absence of specific suggestive findings or recurrent episodes of zoster, these patients do not require an exhaustive evaluation for a malignancy or immunodeficiency.

In older, nonimmunocompromised patients, postherpetic neuralgia (severe, prolonged burning pain, with occasional lightning-like stabs in the involved dermatomes) may persist for 1 to 2 years and become disabling. A brief course of corticosteroids (40–60 mg of prednisone, tapered over 3–4 weeks) during the acute episode of zoster shortens the duration of acute neuritic pain, but does not consistently prevent postherpetic neuralgia. The constant burning pain may be diminished by tricyclic antidepressants. When this fails, an anesthetic approach, with either subcutaneous local injection or sympathetic blockage, is sometimes helpful.

Cutaneous Mycobacterial and Fungal Diseases. Mycobacteria and fungi can produce cutaneous infection, manifesting generally as papules, nodules, ulcers, crusting lesions, or lesions with a combination of these features. *Mycobacterium marinum,* for example, can produce inflammatory nodules that ascend via lymphatic channels of the arm among individuals who keep or are exposed to fish; similar lesions due to *Sporothrix schenckii* may be seen among gardeners. *Blastomyces dermatitidis* and *Coccidioides immitis* are other fungi that produce skin nodules or ulcerations.

As a general rule, a biopsy should be done on a chronic inflammatory nodule, crusted lesion, or nonhealing ulceration that is not readily attributable to pressure, vascular insufficiency, or venous stasis. Mycobacteria and fungi should be carefully sought, using acid-fast and silver stains and appropriate cultures.

Ulcerative Lesions of the Skin. A common factor in the pathogenesis of many skin ulcers is the presence of vascular insufficiency. Microbial infection of these lesions is secondary but often extends into soft tissue and bone.

Pressure sores occur at weight-bearing sites among individuals incapable of moving. Patients with strokes, quadriplegia, or paraplegia or patients in a coma who remain supine rapidly develop skin necrosis at the sacrum, spine, and heels, since pressures at these weight-bearing sites can exceed local perfusion pressure. Patients kept immobile on their sides will ulcerate over the greater trochanter of the femur. As the skin sloughs, bacteria colonize the necrotic tissues; abetted by further pressure-induced necrosis, the infection extends to deeper structures. Infected pressure sores are common causes of fever and occasional causes of bacteremia in debilitated patients. Not infrequently, a necrotic membrane hides a deep infection. The physician should probe the extent of a pressure sore with a sterile glove; potential sites of deeper infection should be probed with a sterile needle. Necrotic material must be debrided, and the ulceration may be treated with topical antiseptics and relief of pressure. Systemic antibiotics are indicated when bacteremia, osteomyelitis, or significant cellulitis is present. Anaerobes and gram-negative rods are the most frequent isolates. Skin grafting can be used to repair extensive ulceration in patients who can eventually be mobilized. Prevention of pressure sores by frequent turning and by inspection of pressure sites among immobilized patients is far more effective than treatment. The use of specialized beds that distribute pressure more evenly may be of particular value among these patients.

Stasis Ulceration. Patients with lower extremity edema are at risk for skin breakdown and formation of stasis ulcers. These may become secondarily infected but unless cellulitis is present systemic antibiotics are not necessary, and treatment is aimed at reducing the edema.

Diabetic Ulcers. Patients with diabetes mellitus often develop foot ulcers. Peripheral neuropathy may result in the distribution of stress to sites on the foot not suited to weight bearing and may also result in failure to sense foreign objects stepped on or caught within the shoe. The resulting ulceration heals poorly. This may be related to vascular disease, poor metabolic control, or both. Secondary infection with anaerobes and gram-negative bacilli progresses rapidly to involve bone and soft tissue. Prevention of these events requires meticulous foot care, avoidance of walking barefoot, the use of properly fitting shoes, and checking the inside of the shoe before use. Once an ulcer develops, the physician should evaluate the patient promptly. Bed rest and topical antiseptics are always indicated. Systemic antibiotics active against anaerobes and gram-negative bacilli should be employed for all but the most superficial and clean wounds. In most instances, this treatment requires admission to the hospital. Aggressive management is indicated since, if the ulcer is left untreated or improperly treated, the proximate bones and soft tissues of the entire foot may become involved. Once this involvement occurs, eradication of infection without amputation may be difficult.

Other Ulcerative Lesions of the Skin

Ulcerative lesions of the skin, particularly in the genital region, may be due to *Treponema pallidum,* the agent of syphilis, or to *Haemophlilus ducreyi,* the agent of chancroid (see Chapter 107).

More Diffuse Lesions of Skin (Table 101–2)

Erysipelas. Erysipelas is an infection of the superficial layers of the skin; it is almost always caused by group A streptococci. This infection, seen primarily among children and the elderly, most commonly occurs on the face. Erysipelas is a bright red to violaceous raised lesion with sharply demarcated edges. This sharp demarcation distinguishes erysipelas from the deeper tissue infection—cellulitis—the margins of which are not raised and merge more smoothly with uninvolved areas of skin. Fever is generally present but bacteremia is uncommon; rarely, the pathogen can be isolated by aspiration or biopsy of the leading edge of the erythema (clysis culture). Penicillin, 2 to 6 million units/day, is curative, but defervescence is gradual.

TABLE 101–2	**Diffuse Cutaneous and Subcutaneous Bacterial Infections**
Description	**Predominant Organisms**
Erysipelas	Group A streptococci
Cellulitis	Group A streptococci, *Staphylococcus aureus, Haemophilus influenzae, Clostridium perfringens,* other anaerobic organisms, gram-negative bacilli
Fasciitis	Group A streptococci, *Clostridium perfringens,* other anaerobic organisms, enterobacteriaceae
Myonecrosis	*Clostridium perfringens,* other anaerobic organisms

TABLE 101–3	Processes That May Resemble Cellulitis
Process	**Diagnosis**
Thrombophlebitis	Tender cord, no lymphangitis, ultrasound
Arthritis	Pain on passive joint movement, joint effusion, joint aspiration
Ruptured Baker's cyst	History of arthritis, joint effusion, arthrogram
Brown recluse spider bite	Exposure history
Fasciitis	MRI, surgical exploration
Myositis	Muscle tenderness, less prominent skin involvement, ultrasound, MRI, aspiration; surgical exploration

MRI = Magnetic resonance imaging.

Cellulitis. Cellulitis is an infection of the deeper layers of the skin. Cellulitis has a particular predilection for the lower extremities, where venous stasis predisposes to infection. Cellulitis predisposes to recurrent infection, perhaps by impairing lymphatic drainage. A breakdown in normal skin barriers almost always precedes this infection. Lacerations, small abscesses, or even tiny fissures between the toes due to minor fungal infection antedate the onset of pain, swelling, and fever. Although shaking chills often occur, bacteremia is infrequently documented. Linear streaks of erythema and tenderness indicate lymphatic spread. Regional lymph node enlargement and tenderness are common. Patches of erythema and tenderness may occur a few centimeters proximal to the edge of infection; this is probably due to spread through subcutaneous lymphatics. Cellulitis of the calf is often difficult to distinguish from thrombophlebitis. Rupture of a Baker cyst or inflammatory arthritis may also mimic cellulitis (Table 101–3). Pain within the joint on passive motion suggests arthritis, but after a Baker cyst rupture, examination of the joint may be relatively benign. Lymph node enlargement and lymphatic streaking virtually confirm the diagnosis of cellulitis. Most cases of lower extremity cellulitis are due to group A beta-hemolytic streptococci, but on occasion *Staphylococcus aureus* is responsible. Gram-negative bacilli often cause cellulitis in neutropenic and other immunosuppressed patients. Cellulitis of the face or upper extremities, particularly among children, may be due to *Haemophilus influenzae*. Among patients with diabetes mellitus, streptococci and staphylococci are the predominant pathogens of cellulitis. However, if the cellulitis is associated with an infected ulceration of the skin, there is a good chance that anaerobic bacteria and gram-negative rods are also involved.

Occupational exposures are often associated with painful cellulitis of the hands. Erysipeloid cellulitis (caused by *Erysipelothrix rhusiopathiae*) most often occurs in fish or meat handlers, and responds to high doses of penicillin (12 to 20 million units daily). Freshwater exposures are associated with cellulitis caused by *Aeromonas* species, and saltwater exposures may result in aggressive cellulitis caused by *Vibrio* species; third-generation cephalosporious are usually effective in the treatment of these potentially lethal infections.

As in the case of erysipelas, cultures of blood and clysis cultures of the leading edge of infection rarely yield the pathogen. Patients with cellulitis who appear toxic or who have underlying diseases causing impaired immune response should be hospitalized. Cellulitis should be treated with a semisynthetic penicillin active against *Staphylococcus aureus* such as nafcillin (or in regions where methicillin resistance among *Staphylococcus aureus* is high, vancomycin). If *Haemophilus* is suspected, ampicillin/sulbactam is usually effective. Diabetics with foot ulcers complicated by cellulitis should be treated with agents active against anaerobes and enteric gram negative rods (e.g., ampicillin/sulbactam). Radiologic studies should be performed on patients with ulcers to determine if osteomyelitis is present (see Chapter 104). Prevention of cellulitis can be achieved by institution of measures aimed at reducing venous stasis and edema. Patients with recurrent cellulitis may benefit from eradication of fungal infection of toes or interdigital regions if present. Repeated attacks of cellulitis may be prevented by monthly 1-week courses of an oral antibiotic such as erythromycin.

Soft Tissue Gas. Crepitus on palpation of the skin indicates the presence of gas in the soft tissues. Although this often reflects anaerobic bacterial metabolism, subcutaneous gas can also be found after respirator-induced barotrauma or after application of hydrogen peroxide to open wounds.

In the setting of soft tissue infection, crepitus suggests the presence of gas-forming anaerobes. Roentgenograms will occasionally demonstrate gas before crepitus is appreciated (Fig. 101–1). The presence of gas requires emergency surgical incision to determine the extent of necrosis and requirements for debridement. Involvement of the muscle establishes the diagnosis of myonecrosis (see below) and mandates extensive debridement. Despite the often extensive crepitus seen in clostridial cellulitis, exploration reveals the muscles to be uninvolved, and proper treatment is limited to debridement of necrotic tissue, open drainage, and antibiotics, usually penicillin G, 10 to 20 million units/day, and metronidazole, 500 mg every 6 hours. Thus, the principles of treatment for anaerobic soft tissue infections are (1) removal of necrotic tissue, (2) drainage, and (3) appropriate antibiotics. These apply to superficial anaerobic infections (clostridial cellulitis), deeper anaerobic infections (anaerobic fasciitis—

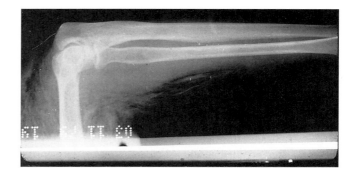

Figure 101–1
Radiograph in a case of clostridial myonecrosis showing gas within tissues. Courtesy of Dr. J. W. Tomford.)

see below), and deepest infections (anaerobic myonecrosis—see below).

DEEPER INFECTIONS OF THE SKIN AND SOFT TISSUE

Fasciitis

This is a deep infection of the subcutaneous tissues that generally occurs following trauma, sometimes minor, or surgery. Most cases are caused by beta-hemolytic streptococci with or without staphylococci; some, especially among diabetics, are due to mixtures of anaerobic organisms and gram-negative bacilli. Because fasciitis involves subcutaneous tissues, the skin may appear normal or may have a red or dusky hue. The clue to this diagnosis is the presence of subcutaneous swelling. In some instances, crepitus is present. The patient appears more toxic than one would expect from the superficial appearance of the skin. Radiographs may reveal gas within tissues; its absence does not exclude the diagnosis. Men with diabetes mellitus, urethral trauma, or obstruction may develop an aggressive fasciitis of the perineum called Fournier's gangrene. Perineal pain and swelling may antedate the characteristic discoloration of the scrotum and perineum. Prompt debridement of all necrotic tissue is critical to the cure of these infections. Once the diagnosis is suspected, the patient must be taken to the operating room, where incision and exploration will determine if fasciitis is present. Gram's stain of necrotic material will guide antibiotic choice.

Infections of Muscle

Pyomyositis. Pyomyositis is a deep infection of muscle usually caused by Staphylococcus aureus and occasionally by group A beta-hemolytic streptococci or enteric bacilli. Most cases occur in warm or tropical regions, and most occur among children. Nonpenetrating trauma may antedate the onset of symptoms, suggesting that infection of a minor hematoma during incidental bacteremia may be causative. Patients present with fever and tender swelling of the muscle; the skin is uninvolved or minimally involved. In older patients, myositis may mimic phlebitis. Diagnosis can be readily made, if suspected, by needle aspiration or ultrasonography. Early aggressive debridement and appropriate antibiotics are usually curative.

Clostridial Myonecrosis (Gas Gangrene). This anaerobic infection generally occurs following a contaminated injury to muscle. Within a day or two of injury, the involved extremity becomes painful and begins to swell. The patient appears toxic and is often delirious. The skin may appear uninvolved at first but eventually may develop a bronzed-blue discoloration. Crepitus may be present but is not as prominent as in patients with clostridial cellulitis (a more benign lesion). Rarely, clostridial myonecrosis occurs spontaneously in the absence of trauma; most of these patients have an underlying malignancy, usually involving the bowel. Regardless of etiology, this illness progresses rapidly, producing extensive necrosis of muscle. Hypotension, hemolytic anemia caused by bacterial lecithinase, and renal failure can complicate this illness. Gram's stain of the thin and watery wound exudate reveals large gram-positive rods and very few inflammatory cells. Emergency surgery with wide debridement is essential if the patient is to survive. Large doses of penicillin (10 to 20 million units/day) may prevent further spread of the bacilli. Chloramphenicol may be used in patients with hypersensitivity to penicillin. Hyperbaric oxygen therapy is of uncertain value.

REFERENCES

Stevens DL: Clostridial myonecrosis and other clostridial diseases. *In* Bennett JC, Plum F (eds.): Cecil Textbook of Medicine. 20th Philadelphia, WB Saunders, 1996, pp 1630–1633.

Swartz MN: Skin and soft tissue infections. *In* Mandell GL, Douglas RG, Bennett JE (eds.): Principles and Practice of Infections Diseases. 4th ed. New York, Churchill Livingstone, 1995, pp 909–929.

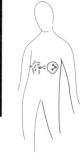

102

Intra-Abdominal Abscess and Peritonitis

INTRA-ABDOMINAL ABSCESS

There are two general categories of intra-abdominal abscess. The first is an infection of a solid intra-abdominal viscus, generally arising as a consequence of hematogenous or enteral spread. The second includes extravisceral abscesses, which are localized collections of pus within the peritoneal or retroperitoneal space. These abscesses usually follow peritonitis or contamination by rupture or leakage from the bowel. Most patients with intra-abdominal abscess are febrile. The fever may be recurrent and may be associated with rigors, suggesting intermittent bacteremia. Nausea, vomiting, and paralytic ileus are common with extravisceral abscesses. Clues to the presence of intra-abdominal abscess may be subtle and may include extravisceral gas or air-fluid levels on plain radiographs. The availability of computed tomography (CT) has simplified both the diagnosis and the management of these potentially life-threatening infections.

With the exception of amebic abscess or multiple microabscesses of the liver, antibiotic therapy alone is rarely curative. Failure of the antibiotic to penetrate the abscess cavities, inactivation of antibiotics within the abscess by bacterial enzymes, low pH, and low redox potential all contribute to the failure of medical management. Drainage is essential; antibiotics are important primarily to prevent bacteremia and seeding of other organs.

ABSCESSES OF SOLID ORGANS

Hepatic Abscess

Pyogenic liver abscess is a disease that occurs predominantly among individuals with other underlying disorders, most commonly biliary tract disease. Obstruction to biliary drainage allows infected bile to produce ascending infection of the liver. Inflammatory diseases of the bowel, such as appendicitis and diverticulitis, may also lead to hepatic abscess via spread of infection through portal veins (Table 102–1). Penetrating or nonpenetrating trauma may also result in pyogenic liver abscess.

Clinical findings in patients with pyogenic hepatic abscess are often nonspecific. Most are febrile, but only about half have abdominal pain and tenderness. Two thirds have palpable hepatomegaly, but less than one in four is clinically jaundiced.

The chest roentgenogram may reveal an elevated right hemidiaphragm and atelectasis or effusion at the right lung base. The diagnosis is best achieved by contrast-enhanced CT of the abdomen or ultrasonography of the right upper quadrant. Pyogenic abscesses may be single or multiple; multiple abscesses often arise from a biliary source of infection.

Anaerobic bacilli, microaerophilic streptococci, and gram-negative bacilli are the predominant microorganisms in pyogenic liver abscess. Occasionally, *Staphylococcus aureus* causes hepatic abscesses during the course of bacteremic seeding of multiple organs. Positive blood cultures are obtained from about half the patients with pyogenic liver abscess.

Clinical laboratory studies generally show a moderate elevation of the alkaline phosphatase level, which is disproportionate to the modest elevation in bilirubin level that occurs in roughly half the patients. (In contrast, patients with the nonspecific jaundice that occasionally accompanies bacterial infection at other sites generally have elevated bilirubin levels—as much as 5 to 10 mg/dl or more—and only slightly elevated alkaline phosphatase levels.) In patients with leukemia, multiple hepatic abscesses caused by *Candida* species may present with fever and poorly localized abdominal pain, and an elevated serum alkaline phosphatase may be the only abnormality pointing to the hepatic origin (see Chapter 109).

Hepatic abscess due to *Entamöeba histolytica* is rare in North America, though it should be suspected in a patient with fever and right upper quadrant pain who has traveled to or emigrated from the developing world. Amebic abscesses are generally single and are usually located in the right lobe of the liver. Only a minority of patients with amebic liver abscess have concurrent intestinal amebiasis. Antibody titers against *E. histolytica* are almost always positive.

The Fitz-Hugh–Curtis syndrome, or gonococcal periphepatitis, may share some clinical manifestations suggestive of hepatic abscess and should be suspected in young, sexually active women with fever and right upper-quadrant tenderness. Tumors involving the liver may produce fever and a clinical and radiologic picture that may mimic hepatic abscess. This is complicated by the occasional

TABLE 102–1	Intra-Abdominal Abscesses			
Site	**Predisposing Factors**	**Likely Pathogens**	**Diagnosis**	**Empiric Treatment***
Solid Organs				
Hepatic	GI or biliary sepsis, trauma	Gram-negative bacilli, anaerobes, streptococci, amebae	CT, MRI, ultrasound	Ampicillin/sulbactam, drainage; metronidazole for amebic abscess
Splenic	Trauma, hemoglobinopathy, endocarditis	Staphylococci, streptococci, gram-negative bacilli	CT	Ampicillin/sulbactam or vancomycin/tobramycin, splenectomy
Pancreatic	Pancreatitis, pseudocyst	Gram-negative bacilli, streptococci	CT	Ampicillin/sulbactam or clindamycin/tobramycin, drainage
Extravisceral				
Subphrenic	Abdominal surgery, peritonitis	Gram-negative bacilli, streptococci, anaerobes	CT	Ampicillin/sulbactam or clindamycin/tobramycin, drainage
Pelvic	Abdominal surgery, peritonitis, pelvic or GI inflammatory disease	Gram-negative bacilli, streptococci, anaerobes	CT	Ampicillin/sulbactam or clindamycin/tobramycin, drainage
Perinephrenic	Renal infection/obstruction, hematogenous	Gram-negative bacilli, staphylococci	CT	Ampicillin/sulbactam or vancomycin/tobramycin, drainage
Psoas	Vertebral osteomyelitis, hematogenous	Staphylococci, gram-negative bacilli, mycobacteria	CT	Ampicillin/sulbactam or vancomycin/tobramycin, drainage

* Ampicillin/sulbactam, 2 gm/1 gm given intravenously (IV) q8h; vancomycin, 1 gm IV q12h; tobramycin, 1.7 mg/kg IV q8h; clindamycin, 600 mg IV q8h.
CT = Computed tomography; GI = gastrointestinal; MRI = magnetic resonance imaging.

concurrence of malignancy and hepatic abscess. Patients with hepatic abscesses generally present with a less acute illness than patients with cholecystitis or cholangitis. Ultrasonography, CT scan, and magnetic resonance imaging (MRI) are all useful in defining liver abscesses; MRI is most effective when the abscesses are less than 1 cm in diameter.

If pyogenic abscess is suspected, needle aspiration is indicated. With the guidance of ultrasonography or CT, a percutaneous catheter can be inserted into the abscess cavity for both diagnostic and therapeutic purposes. The pus should be Gram-stained and cultured aerobically and anaerobically. Unless the Gram stain indicates otherwise, initial therapy for pyogenic liver abscess should include drugs active against enteric aerobic and anaerobic bacteria (see Table 102–1). Antibiotics should be continued for at least 4 to 6 weeks. Patients with multiple hepatic abscess caused by *Candida* species require long-term therapy with either amphotericin B or fluconazole. Duration of therapy may be guided by serial CT scans. Surgery is required to relieve biliary tract obstruction and to drain abscesses that do not respond to percutaneous drainage and antibiotics. Patients with pyogenic liver abscess should be evaluated for a primary intra-abdominal source of infection.

If epidemiologic features strongly suggest an amebic abscess, metronidazole is the drug of choice. Needle aspiration is necessary only to exclude pyogenic infection or, if the abscess is large or close to other viscera, to prevent rupture. In the case of amebic abscess, the anchovy paste material obtained by needle drainage is not pus but necrotic liver tissue. Large numbers of white cells suggest pyogenic abscess or bacterial superinfection. Trophozoites

of *E. histolytica* are infrequently seen on aspiration of abscesses but are often seen on biopsy of the abscess capsule.

Splenic Abscess

Splenic abscesses are generally the result of hematogenous seeding of the spleen. In the preantibiotic era, splenic infarction and abscess were common complications of infective endocarditis. Now the most common predisposing factors are trauma and (in children) sickle cell disease. Patients with splenic abscess most often present with left upper-quadrant abdominal pain, which may be pleuritic. The left hemidiaphragm may be elevated, and there may be an associated pleural rub or effusion. The diagnostic approach, most likely etiologic agents, and initial antimicrobial therapy are outlined in Table 102–1. Splenectomy is usually the definitive treatment, but CT-guided percutaneous drainage of large, solitary abscesses may also be successful in selected cases.

Pancreatic Abscess

Pancreatic abscess is an uncommon complication of pancreatitis. The symptoms of pancreatic abscess, fever, nausea, vomiting, and abdominal pain radiating to the back resemble those of pancreatitis. Thus, abscess should be suspected in cases of persistent recurrent fever following pancreatitis. The inflamed organ becomes colonized and infected with microbes inhabiting the upper gastrointestinal tract. Enterobacteriaceae, anaerobes, and streptococci (including the pneumococcus) are likely pathogens. The diagnosis may be made by CT scanning; however, radiographic definition of the pancreatic bed is often difficult. Initial antibiotic therapy (see Table 102–1) should be followed by surgical drainage of the abscess as soon as the patient is stable. The mortality exceeds 30% even with optimal management.

EXTRAVISCERAL ABSCESSES

Extravisceral abscesses most often arise following peritonitis, after intra-abdominal surgery, as a consequence of rupture of the bowel, or after extension of infection of a viscus, such as diverticulitis or appendicitis. Abscesses may occur in the subphrenic, pelvic, or retroperitoneal spaces. Fever, nausea, vomiting, and paralytic ileus are common. Although fever is almost always present, localizing symptoms may be very subtle, making the diagnosis difficult. Predisposing factors, most likely etiologic pathogens, and appropriate initial antimicrobial therapy are outlined in Table 102–1.

When an abscess is suspected, CT or ultrasound scans should be obtained. CT can identify abscesses in the retroperitoneal and abdominal spaces and guide percutaneous drainage. Ultrasonography may be more helpful in the identification of pelvic fluid collections. Fluid-filled abscesses may be difficult to distinguish from loops of viscera on CT or ultrasound; review of such studies by an experienced radiologist is essential before they are considered negative. Drainage of an abscess either by radiologic guidance or by surgery in conjunction with antibiotics is the mainstay of treatment.

PERITONITIS

Peritonitis may occur spontaneously (primary peritonitis) or as a consequence of trauma, surgery, or peritoneal soilage by bowel contents (secondary peritonitis). Peritonitis also may be caused by chemical irritation. Patients with peritonitis generally complain of diffuse abdominal pain. They may have nausea and vomiting; some have diarrhea, others paralytic ileus. Patients are usually febrile and uncomfortable and prefer to lie quietly in the supine position. Physical examination may reveal diffuse tenderness, diminished bowel sounds, and evidence of peritoneal inflammation, including rebound tenderness and involuntary guarding. In patients with underlying ascites, the signs and symptoms of peritonitis may be more subtle, with fever as the only manifestation of infection.

Primary Peritonitis

Primary or spontaneous peritonitis occurs principally among persons with ascites associated with chronic liver disease or the nephrotic syndrome. Bacteria may infect ascitic fluid via bacteremic spread, transmural migration through the bowel or through the fallopian tubes. In cirrhotic patients, clearance of portal bacteremia by hepatic

TABLE 102–2	Causes, Diagnosis, and Treatment of Peritonitis			
Site	Predisposing Factors	Causative Agent	Clues to Diagnosis	Empiric Treatment*
Primary				
Spontaneous	Cirrhosis, nephrotic syndrome	Gram-negative bacilli, streptococci	>300 neutrophils per ml of ascites	Ampicillin/sulbactam or clindamycin/tobramycin
Secondary				
Postoperative	Hemorrhage, visceral rupture	Gram-negative bacilli, streptococci, staphylococci, anaerobes	Postoperative fever, pain, prolonged ileus	Ampicillin/sulbactam or metronidazole/tobramycin
Chemical	Abdominal surgery	Bile, starch, talc	Postoperative fever, pain	Biliary drainage when indicated
Visceral rupture	Perforating ulcer, ruptured appendix, bowel infarction	Gram-negative bacilli, anaerobes, streptococci	Polymicrobial Gram's stain or culture	Ampicillin/sulbactam or metronidazole/tobramycin
Peritoneal dialysis	—	Staphylococci, gram-negative bacilli	Pain, fever, neutrophilic pleocytosis	Vancomycin/tobramycin; consider catheter removal
Periodic peritonitis	Familial	—	Recurrent, familial	Colchicine prophylaxis, 0.6 mg 2–3 times daily
Tuberculous	Infection of fallopian tubes or ileum	*Mycobacterium tuberculosis*	Lymphocytic pleocytosis, high protein level (>3 gm/dl) in ascitic fluid	Isoniazid, rifampin, pyrazinamide

* Ampicillin/sulbactam, 2 gm/1 gm intravenously (IV) q8h; vancomycin, 1 gm IV q12h; tobramycin, 1.7 mg/kg IV q8h; clindamycin, 600 mg IV q8h; isoniazid, 300 mg qd; rifampin, 600 mg qd; pyrazinamide, 1.5 gm qd, metronidazole, 500 mg IV q8h.

reticuloendothelial cells may be impaired by intrahepatic portosystemic shunting. Not surprisingly, therefore, gram-negative rods, especially *Escherichia coli,* are the predominant pathogens in spontaneous bacterial peritonitis; enteric streptococci are isolated in approximately one third of cases. Staphylococci, *Streptococcus pneumoniae,* or anaerobic bacilli are isolated in fewer than 10% of cases (Table 102–2).

In patients with underlying ascites, the presenting symptoms may be nonspecific abdominal pain, nausea, vomiting, diarrhea, or altered mental status. Thus, febrile patients with ascites should undergo paracentesis unless there is another certain explanation for fever. A white blood cell count in the fluid that exceeds 300 to 500/μl is suggestive of infection. Gram's stain may reveal the responsible pathogen. Antibiotic penetration into the peritoneum is excellent, and medical therapy is the treatment of choice (Table 102–2). If Gram's stain or culture reveals a mixed flora with anaerobes, secondary peritonitis due to leakage of bowel contents should be suspected. Among patients with cirrhosis and ascites, prophylactic administration of norfloxacin or trimethoprim-sulfamethoxazole decreases the risk of spontaneous peritonitis.

Secondary Peritonitis

Secondary peritonitis may follow penetrating abdominal trauma or surgery or may result from contamination of the peritoneum with bowel contents. This syndrome may be heralded by the sudden presentation of visceral rupture (e.g., perforated duodenal ulcer or appendix) or visceral infarction. In the postoperative setting, secondary peritonitis should be suspected in the patient whose abdominal discomfort and fever do not resolve, or even worsen, after the first few postoperative days. If peritonitis is secondary to the leakage of bowel contents, immediate surgical intervention is mandatory. Despite the use of appropriate antibiotics (Table 102–2) and intensive support systems, the mortality of generalized peritonitis approaches 50%.

Tuberculous Peritonitis

Tuberculous peritonitis may occur as a result of hematogenous or local extension of tuberculous infection into the peritoneal cavity. Fever, abdominal pain, and weight loss are common. In patients with underlying ascites, a lymphocytic pleocytosis in the peritoneal fluid should suggest the diagnosis. Laparoscopy, with biopsy of the granulomatous peritoneal nodules, is the most effective approach to diagnosis. Antituberculous therapy is generally curative (see Table 102–2).

REFERENCES

Levison ME, Bush LM: Peritonitis and other intra-abdominal infections, *In* Mandell GL, Bennett JE, Dolin R (eds.): Principles and Practice of Infectious Diseases. 4th ed. New York, Churchill Livingstone, 1995, pp 705–740.
Singh N, Gayowski T, Yu VL, Wagene MM: Trimethoprim-sulfamethoxazole for the prevention of spontaneous bacterial peritonitis in cirrhosis: A randomized trial. Ann Intern Med 1995; 122:595–598.
Wilcox CM, Dismukes WE: Spontaneous bacterial peritonitis, a review of pathogenesis diagnosis and treatment. Medicine 1967; 66:447–450.
Wright TL: Parasitic, bacterial, fungal and granulomatous liver disease. *In* Bennett JC (ed.): Cecil Textbook of Medicine. 20th ed. Philadelphia, WB Saunders, 1996.

103

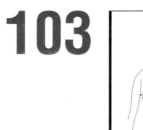

Acute Infectious Diarrhea

Acute diarrheal illnesses caused by bacterial, viral, or protozoal pathogens vary from mild bowel dysfunction to fulminant, life-threatening diseases. Worldwide, acute diarrheal illnesses are the most common cause of death in childhood. With the best techniques available, a specific causative agent can be identified in 70 to 80% of cases (Table 103–1).

PATHOGENESIS AND PATHOPHYSIOLOGY: GENERAL CONCEPTS

In general, pathogens or microbial toxins that produce acute diarrhea must be ingested. Therefore, socioeconomic conditions that result in crowding, poor sanitation, and contaminated water sources lead to increased risk of acute diarrheal illnesses. Normally, the low pH of the stomach, the rapid transit time of the small bowel, and antibody produced by cells in the lamina propria of the small bowel are adequate to keep the jejunum and proximal ileum relatively free of microorganisms (although not sterile). Furthermore, the ileocecal valve inhibits proximal migration of the huge numbers of bacteria that reside in the large bowel.

Pathogenic microorganisms are able to pass through the hostile environment of the stomach if (1) they are acid-resistant (e.g., *Shigella*). (2) they are ingested in sufficiently large numbers that allow for a few survivors (e.g., *Vibrio cholerae* or *Escherichia coli*), or (3) they are ingested with food and therefore partially protected in the neutralized environment. People with decreased gastric acidity, either natural or surgically induced, are at increased risk of acute diarrheal disease.

Once in the small bowel, the organisms either must colonize (e.g., *V. cholerae, E. coli*) or invade (e.g., rotavirus, Norwalk agent) the local mucosa or must pass through into the terminal ileum (*Salmonella*) or colon (*Shigella*) to colonize and invade the mucosa in those sites. Active peristalsis of the small bowel is an effective deterrent to the successful colonization of most organisms. The organisms (e.g., *V. cholerae, E. coli*) that are able to colonize this area have developed special colonization factors such as fimbria (hairlike projections from the cell wall) or lectins (special proteins that attach to specific carbohydrate binding sites) that allow them to adhere tightly to the mucosal cell surface.

Organisms that do not have special colonization properties pass into the terminal ileum and colon, where they compete with the established flora. The normal fecal flora produce substances that serve to prevent most newly introduced bacterial species from proliferating. (*Bacteroides,* for example, produces fatty acids; certain other enteric bacteria produce specific colicins). The ability of the colonic enteropathogens to invade intestinal mucosa allows these microorganisms (e.g., *Shigella*) to multiply preferentially.

TYPES OF MICROBIAL DIARRHEAL DISEASES

Microbes can cause diarrhea either directly by invasion of the gut mucosa or indirectly through elaboration of one of three classes of microbial toxins: secretory enterotoxins, cytotoxins, or neurotoxins.

Toxin-Induced Diarrheas

In secretory enterotoxin-induced diarrheas, the patient seldom has fever or other major systemic symptoms, and there is little or no inflammatory response. The diarrhea is watery, often voluminous, with a low protein concentration and an electrolyte content, isosmotic with plasma, that reflects its source. Rapid loss of this diarrheal fluid results in predictable saline depletion, base-deficit acidosis, and potassium deficiency. The amount and rate of fluid loss determine the severity of the illness. Certain of the secretory diarrheas, such as those caused by *V. cholerae* or *E. coli* enterotoxins, can result in massive intestinal fluid losses, exceeding 1 L/hr in adults.

Characteristically, large numbers of bacteria (10^5 to 10^8) must be ingested with grossly contaminated food or water (although a small inoculum may produce disease in individuals with achlorhydria). The enterotoxin-producing bacteria then colonize, but do not invade, the small bowel mucosal cells. After multiplying to large numbers (10^8 to 10^9 organisms per milliliter of fluid), the bacteria produce enterotoxins that bind to mucosal cells, causing hypersecretion of isotonic fluid at a rate that overwhelms the reabsorptive capacity of the colon. The *V. cholerae* enterotoxin rapidly binds to monosialogangliosides of the gut mucosa and causes sustained stimulation of cell-bound

TABLE 103–1	Major Etiologic Agents in Acute Diarrheal Illnesses

Invasive/Destructive Pathogens

*Shigella**
Salmonella
Campylobacter jejuni
*Vibrio parahaemolyticus**
Yersinia enterocolitica
Enterohemorrhagic *E. coli* (EHEC)*
Clostridium difficile‡
Rotavirus
Other viruses
Entamoeba histolytica

Noninvasive Pathogens

Enterotoxigenic *Escherichia coli†* (ETEC)
Vibrio cholerae†
Giardia lamblia
Isospora belli
Cryptosporidium parvum

Bacterial Toxins (Food Poisoning)

Staphylococcus aureus
Clostridium perfringens
Bacillus cereus

*Destruction mediated, at least in part, by toxin.
†Diarrhea mediated by a secretory enterotoxin.
‡Destruction mediated by toxin.

adenylate cyclase. This results, via both increased secretion and decreased absorption of electrolytes, in net movement of large quantities of isotonic fluid into the gut lumen. The disease runs its course in 2 to 7 days, during which time continued fluid and electrolyte repletion is of critical importance.

E. coli, probably the major cause of traveler's diarrhea worldwide, produces two major types of plasmid-encoded bacterial enterotoxins. The labile toxin (LT) of *E. coli* is similar in structure and nearly identical in mode of action to cholera enterotoxin.

The *E. coli* stable toxins (ST) include STa, which causes gut fluid secretion via activation of guanylate cyclase, and STb, which causes gut fluid secretion by an as yet unknown mechanism. Both STa and STb have a more rapid onset and shorter duration of action than *E. coli* LT. Secretory enterotoxins may also be produced by other enteropathogenic bacteria that cause diarrhea primarily via direct invasion (e.g., *Salmonella typhimurium, Shigella dysenteriae*).

Certain bacteria elaborate cytotoxins, soluble factors that directly destroy mucosal epithelial cells and are associated with diarrhea. *Shigella dysenteriae* elaborates such a toxin; this Shiga toxin plays an important role in the destructive colitis seen in patients with shigellosis. A closely related cytotoxin is produced by enterohemorrhagic *E. coli* strains that are associated with hemorrhagic colitis and hemolytic uremic syndrome. Other bacteria that can produce cytotoxins include *Clostridium perfringens* and *Vibrio parahaemolyticus*. *C. perfringens,* often ingested in contaminated meat or poultry, replicates within the small bowel and elaborates a secretory enterotoxin with cytotoxin activity. Toxin-induced diarrhea due

to *C. perfringens,* like that due to *Staphylococcus aureus* and *Bacillus cereus,* has a short incubation period and brief (< 36 hours) duration. *Clostridium difficile* can colonize the large bowel and, in the presence of antibiotic therapy that limits the growth of microorganisms, can overgrow and elaborate cytotoxins that can cause severe mucosal damage, producing a colitis that in some instances has a pseudomembranous appearance and in other instances resembles the diffuse colitis seen in shigellosis.

Some toxins are ingested directly in food, as with staphylococcal and *Bacillus cereus* food poisoning. These organisms grow to high concentration in the food rather than the small intestine and often cannot be recovered from the stool. Distinctive features of staphyloccal food poisoning include a short incubation period (2 to 6 hours), high attack rates (up to 75% of the population at risk), and prominent vomiting (probably due to the effect of absorbed enterotoxins(s) on the central nervous system). *B. cereus* produces two distinct toxins, one of which is similar to *E. coli* LT and the other to staphylococcal enterotoxins; therefore, two different clinical syndromes may be produced, one indistinguishable from staphylococcal food poisoning and the other similar to the diarrhea caused by enterotoxigenic *E. coli* (ETEC). The former syndrome is often associated with ingestion of contaminated rice.

Diarrheas Caused by Invasive Pathogens

Diarrheas caused by mucosal invasion by microorganisms are often accompanied by fever and other systemic symptoms, including headache and myalgias. Cramping abdominal pain may be prominent, and small amounts of stool are passed at frequent intervals, often associated with tenesmus. These microorganisms often induce a marked inflammatory response, so that the stool contains pus cells, large amounts of protein, and often gross blood. Significant dehydration rarely results from this kind of diarrhea, since the diarrheal fluid volume is small relative to that caused by the secretory enterotoxins, seldom exceeding 750 ml/day in adults. Although certain clinical features are statistically more frequent in invasive diarrheas caused by specific enteropathogens (e.g., more severe myalgias with shigellosis, higher temperature spikes with salmonellosis), epidemiologic characteristics are more helpful than signs or symptoms in determining the etiologic agent in invasive diarrheal illnesses. (Table 103–2).

Acute shigellosis occurs when susceptible individuals ingest fecally contaminated water or food. Shigellosis can occur after ingestion of only 10 to 100 microorganisms. Largely for this reason, direct person-to-person transmission (e.g., in day care centers) is more common with shigellosis than with other bacterial enteric infections. The organism multiplies in the small intestine, during which time a watery, noninflammatory diarrhea may occur. Later, the organisms invade the colonic epithelium, causing the characteristic bloody stool. Unlike *Salmonella, Shigella* rarely causes bacteremia. The disease usually resolves spontaneously after 3 to 6 days, but the

TABLE 103–2	Epidemiologic Characteristics of Common Invasive Enteric Pathogens	
Microorganisms	**Epidemiologic Features**	**Antibiotics**
Shigella	Outbreaks in child care centers or custodial institutions; person-to-person transmission	Yes
Salmonella enteritidis	Zoonosis; survives dessication in processed dairy, poultry, and meat products	Rarely
Campylobacter jejuni	Zoonosis; worldwide distribution; transmitted in dairy products	Maybe
Yersinia enterocolitica	Zoonosis; occasionally transmitted in dairy products	Maybe
Vibrio parahaemolyticus	Coastal salt waters; transmitted by inadequately cooked shrimp and shellfish	No
Clostridium difficile	Almost always follows antimicrobial therapy	Yes
Rotavirus	Outbreaks among children; worldwide distribution; unusual and mild in adults	No
Norwalk virus	Microepidemic pattern; no specific age predilection	No
Entamoeba histolytica	Person-to-person transmission; very rare in United States, Canada, and Western Europe	Yes

clinical course can be shortened by antimicrobials (see Table 103–2).

Acute salmonellosis usually results from ingestion of contaminated meat, dairy, or poultry products. In the industrialized world, *Salmonella* is often transmitted via commercially prepared dried, processed foodstuffs. Unlike *Shigella*, *Salmonella* is remarkably resistant to dessication. The nontyphoidal salmonellae invade primarily the distal ileum. The organism typically causes a short-lived (2 to 3 days) illness characterized by fever, nausea, vomiting, and diarrhea. (This is in marked contrast to the 3- to 4-week febrile illness, usually not associated with diarrhea, that is caused by *Salmonella typhi*.)

Campylobacter jejuni may be responsible for up to 10% of acute diarrheal illnesses worldwide. This organism may invade both the small intestine, most commonly the terminal ileum, and the colon, which may account for the broad spectrum of symptoms, ranging from an acute shigella-type syndrome to a milder, but more protracted, diarrheal illness.

In addition to *Shigella, Salmonella,* and *Campylobacter,* three other organisms—*Yersinia enterocolitica, Vibrio parahaemolyticus,* and enteroinvasive *E. coli* (EIEC—distinct from ETEC)—also cause tissue invasion and acute diarrheal illnesses that may be clinically indistinguishable from those caused by the more commonly recognized invasive bacterial enteropathogens (see Table 103–2). Another distinct *E. coli* strain, enterohemorrhagic *E. coli,* produces bloody diarrhea without evidence of mucosal inflammation (i.e., grossly bloody stool with few or no leukocytes).

Viruses must grow in host cells; by definition, therefore, both the rotavirus and the Norwalk agent produce invasive diarrheal disease. Both these organisms damage the villous epithelial cells, with the degree of injury ranging from modest distortion of epithelial cells to sloughing of villi. Presumably, both the rotavirus and the Norwalk agent cause diarrhea by interfering with the absorption of normal intestinal secretions. This may occur through selective destruction of absorptive villous tip cells with sparing of secretory crypt cells. Affected patients may have low-grade fever and mild to moderate cramping abdominal pain. The stool is usually watery, and its contents resemble those of a noninvasive process, with few inflammatory cells, probably because of lack of damage to the colon.

Protozoa also can cause acute diarrheal illness. In North America, Rocky Mountain water sources are frequent origins of *Giardia lamblia* microepidemics. As is the case in shigellosis, ingestion of only a few organisms is required to establish infection. The organisms multiply in the small bowel, attach to and occasionally invade the mucosa, but do not cause gross damage to the mucosal cells. Clinical manifestations span the spectrum from an acute, febrile diarrheal illness to chronic diarrhea with associated malabsorption and weight loss. Diagnosis may be made by identification of the organism in either the stool or the duodenal mucus or by small bowel biopsy. *Entamoeba histolytica* may cause intestinal syndromes ranging from mild diarrhea to fulminant amebic colitis with multiple bloody stools, fever, and severe abdominal pain. Although *E. histolytica* has a worldwide distribution, it is an uncommon cause of diarrhea in the United States. Two other protozoa, *Cryptosporidium parvum* and *Isospora belli,* occasionally cause self-limited acute diarrheal illness in otherwise healthy individuals and may cause voluminous, life-threatening diarrheal disease in patients with acquired immunodeficiency syndrome (AIDS). Stool examination will distinguish *Giardia, Entamoeba, Isospora,* and *Cryptosporidium.*

Although most diarrheogenic pathogens produce either invasive (cytopathic) or enterotoxic (secretory) diarrhea, both processes contribute to the illness in some situations. Certain strains of *Shigella,* nontyphoidal *Salmonella, Y. enterocolitica,* and *C. jejuni* both invade and possess the capacity to produce secretory enterotoxins *in vitro.* Such enterotoxins may play a contributory role in the acute disease process. The invasive capacity of these organisms is, however, of paramount importance in their ability to produce disease.

GENERAL EPIDEMIOLOGIC CONSIDERATIONS

In developing countries, where sanitation is generally inadequate, young children (up to 2 years of age) contract multiple episodes of diarrhea (often four to eight per year), a process that engenders intestinal immunity to the majority of enteropathogens in their immediate environment. Most of these diarrheal episodes are mild, but some are life-threatening. In these areas, ETEC and rotavirus together cause the large majority of diarrheal illnesses.

Shigella infections are far less common during this period.

In the industrialized world, infants and small children have fewer episodes of diarrhea, and the most common etiologic agent is the rotavirus. Most episodes are mild. ETEC and *Shigella* infections infrequently occur except in a few defined population groups (e.g., individuals in custodial institutions). On the other hand, throughout the world, clinically significant diarrhea in adults is relatively unusual except in specific defined epidemics or common-source outbreaks due to contaminated food or water. The same etiologic agents are largely responsible for the acute diarrheas of both adults and children. This is made apparent by immunologically inexperienced adults from the developed world who visit developing countries. Such tourists have an extremely high incidence of diarrheal disease (traveler's diarrhea), and the organisms responsible are the same ones as those causing most childhood diarrhea in the country visited.

Certain pathogens responsible for acute diarrheal illnesses among sexually active gay males (see Chapter 107) differ from those that most commonly occur in the general population.

DIAGNOSIS

In managing life-threatening diarrheal illnesses, determining the specific etiologic agent is much less important than promptly repleting lost electrolytes. All pathogens that cause serious diarrheal disease produce similar electrolyte losses. The fluid losses represent the chief cause of serious morbidity and mortality. Determination of the specific cause is less important, since antimicrobial therapy has proven value in only a minority of cases (see Table 103–2). Discerning the epidemiology of the illness is often more helpful than laboratory techniques in identifying cases in which antimicrobial therapy is likely to be helpful! Figure 103–1 provides a useful schematic approach to diagnosis and management.

The examination of a methylene blue–stained stool preparation for erythrocytes and pus cells may be helpful in distinguishing between acute diarrheal illnesses caused by invasive pathogens and those caused by noninvasive pathogens. This is easily accomplished by adding one drop of methylene blue dye to one drop of liquid stool or mucus, allowing the preparation to air dry, and examining under the high dry microscope lens. Few, if any, leukocytes or red cells are seen in the stools of patients with diarrhea caused by noninvasive organisms (e.g., ETEC). Variable numbers of leukocytes and red cells are present in diarrheas secondary to invasive bacteria (e.g., *Shigella*) or cytopathic toxins (*C. difficile* toxin).

The precise diagnosis of any diarrheal illness lasting longer than 4 to 5 days is important, as specific antimicrobial therapy may be helpful, as with giardiasis. Furthermore, among patients with negative stool examinations and cultures, endoscopy may yield a diagnosis of a noninfectious disease (e.g., ulcerative colitis or Crohn's disease).

MANAGEMENT: GENERAL PRINCIPLES OF ELECTROLYTE REPLETION THERAPY

Intravenous Fluids

All acute diarrheal disease respond to a similar fluid repletion regimen. Voluminous infectious diarrhea in adults consistently produces the same pattern of fecal electrolyte loss. The electrolyte characteristics differ somewhat in diarrhea in young children in that the mean sodium and chloride concentrations are 15 to 20 mEq/L less than those in adults. Sodium and chloride concentrations in stool may be even less with diarrheal diseases of viral etiology, in which massive fluid loss seldom occurs.

The fluid losses of massive diarrhea can rapidly be corrected by infusing fluids intravenously that approximate those that have been lost. Lactated Ringer's solution is readily available and provides uniformly good results. With patients who are hypotensive, the intravenous fluids should initially be infused rapidly, at a rate of up to 100 ml/min, until a strong radial pulse is restored. The rate can then be slowed until skin turgor has returned to normal. Subsequent maintenance fluid administration can be guided by the patient's clinical appearance, including the vital signs, the appearance of neck veins, and skin turgor. Clinical evaluation alone provides an adequate guide to fluid replacement in most acute diarrheal illnesses. If intravenous fluids are administered in adequate quantities throughout the diarrheal illness, virtually every patient with diarrhea caused by toxigenic bacteria should be restored to health. Complications (e.g., acute renal failure secondary to hypotension) are exceedingly rare if these principles are followed.

Oral Fluids

In most patients with acute diarrheal illness, fluid repletion can also be achieved via the oral route, using isotonic glucose-containing electrolyte solutions. Oral therapy is based on the principle that glucose facilitates sodium absorption by the small bowel and that glucose-facilitated sodium absorption remains intact during enterotoxigenic diarrheal illnesses. A uniformly effective solution can be prepared by the addition of 20 gm of glucose, 3.5 gm of sodium chloride, 2.5 gm of sodium bicarbonate, and 1.5 gm of potassium chloride to a liter of drinking water (Table 103–3). Such fluids should be administered initially in large quantities, 250 ml every 15 minutes in adults, until clinical observations indicate that fluid balance has been restored. Thereafter, one administers fluids in quantities sufficient to maintain normal balance; if stool output is measured, roughly 1.5 L of glucose-electrolyte solution should be given orally for each liter of stool. The oral fluid regimen does not decrease the volume of fluid lost via the intestinal tract but rather facilitates absorption of adequate fluid to counterbalance the toxin-induced fluid secretion.

Since a similar pattern of fluid loss occurs in diarrheal illnesses caused by other intestinal pathogens, pa-

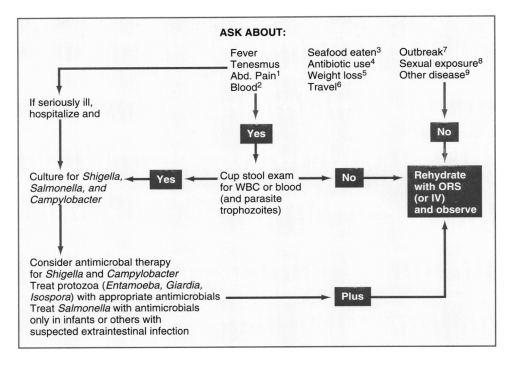

Figure 103–1

Approach to the diagnosis and management of acute infectious diarrhea.

1. If unexplained abdominal pain and fever suggest an appendicitis-like syndrome, culture for *Yersinia enterocolitica*.
2. Bloody diarrhea, in the absence of fecal leukocytes, suggests enterohemorrhagic *Escherichia coli* or amebiasis (where leukocytes are destroyed by the parasite).
3. Ingestion of inadequately cooked seafood prompts consideration of *Vibrio* infections or Norwalk-like viruses.
4. Associated antibiotics should be stopped and *Clostridium difficile* considered.
5. Persistence of diarrhea (>10 days) with weight loss prompts consideration of giardiasis or cryptosporidiosis or inflammatory bowel disease.
6. Travel to tropical areas increases the chance of enterotoxic *E. coli* (ETEC) as well as viral, protozoal (*Giardia, Entamoeba, Cryptosporidium*), and, if focal leukocytes are present, invasive bacterial pathogens.
7. Outbreaks should prompt consideration of *Staphylococcus aureus, Bacillus cereus, Clostridium perfringens*, ETEC, *Vibrio, Salmonella, Campylobacter,* or *Shigella* infection.
8. Sigmoidoscopy in symptomatic homosexual males should distinguish proctitis in the distal 15 cm (caused by herpesvirus, gonococcal, chlamydial, or syphilitic infection) from colitis (*Campylobacter, Shigella,* or *C. difficile* infections).
9. Immunocompromised hosts should have a wide range of viral (e.g., cytomegalovirus [CMV], herpes simplex virus [HSV], rotavirus), bacterial (e.g., *Salmonella, Mycobacterium avium* complex), and protozoal (e.g., *Cryptosporidium, Isospora, Microsporidia, Entamoeba,* and *Giardia*) agents considered. IV = Intravenous; ORS = oral rehydration solution; WBC = white blood cell. (Adapted from Guerrant RL, Shields DS, Thorson SM, et al: Evaluation and diagnosis of acute infectious diarrhea. Am J Med 1985; 78:91–98, with permission.)

tients with fluid depletion caused by invasive microbial agents (e.g., rotavirus, *Salmonella*) also respond well to oral glucose-electrolyte therapy. Although the pathogenesis of diarrheal disease caused by the rotavirus is quite different from that caused by enterotoxigenic bacteria, patients with rotavirus illness consistently respond well to oral glucose-electrolyte replacement.

Antimicrobial Therapy

Most acute infectious diarrheas do not require antibiotic therapy (see Table 103–2). Of the noninvasive bacterial diarrheas, only in cholera do antibiotics dramatically decrease the volume of diarrhea. Oral tetracycline, 40 mg/kg in four divided doses daily for 48 hours, is the drug of choice.

Of the invasive bacterial diarrheas, short-term antimicrobial treatment significantly decreases the duration and severity of shigellosis. In North America, trimethoprim-sulfamethoxazole, twice daily for 5 days, is the drug of

TABLE 103–3	Oral Rehydration Fluid	
Constituents (gm/L)	**Electrolyte Content (mmol/L)**
NaCl—3.5 gm	Na—90
NaHCO₃—2.5 gm	Cl—80
KCl—1.5 gm	K—20
Glucose—20 gm	HCO₃—30
	glucose—110

choice. Because of the increasing frequency of plasmid-mediated antimicrobial resistance, sensitivity testing is necessary to determine the appropriate antibiotic in many other areas of the world.

Antimicrobial therapy may be helpful in decreasing the duration and severity of enteritis caused by *Yersinia* and *Campylobacter*. Oral erythromycin appears to be the drug of choice for *Campylobacter jejuni,* and trimethoprim-sulfamethoxazole or intravenous gentamicin is the preferred treatment for *Yersinia enterocolitica*. Antimicrobials are of no known value in *V. parahaemolyticus* infections. In uncomplicated nontyphoidal *Salmonella* enteritis, antibiotics may prolong the fecal shedding of salmonellae. Treatment of nontyphoidal salmonella gastroenteritis may, however, be indicated in certain settings in order to prevent bacteremia and its complications (e.g., meningitis, endovascular infection, or infections of bone joints or prostheses). Treatment until defervescence with a third generation cephalosporin or a quinoline is therefore indicated for immunocompromised patients, patients with advanced atherosclerotic disease, with sickle cell disease, and those with bone or vascular prostheses.

Antimicrobial therapy is, paradoxically, indicated for treatment of antibiotic-associated diarrhea (AAC). AAC develops in 1 to 15% of patients who receive broad-spectrum antimicrobials and is caused by cytotoxins produced by *C. difficile,* which proliferate in the colonic mucosa when the normal flora is disturbed. Although generally characterized by mild diarrhea, AAC may result in a potentially lethal pseudomembranous colitis. In all cases, the responsible antibiotic should be stopped. In moderate to severe cases (fever, mucosal ulceration, and/or pseudomembranes), vancomycin (250 mg q6h orally for 7 days) or metronidazole (500 mg q8h for 7 days) may be initiated on the basis of strong clinical suspicion, before the diagnosis is confirmed by stool assay for *C. difficile* toxins. Empiric treatment with these agents should be avoided in patients with mild diarrhea since this may result in the emergence of antibiotic-resistant bacteria such as vancomycin-resistant enterococci.

Antimicrobials decrease the duration and severity of giardiasis. In adults, metronidazole, given 750 mg every 8 hours for 3 days, and quinacrine, 300 mg/day for 7 days, appear to be equally effective in adults. Acute intestinal amebiasis demands antimicrobial therapy. Metronidazole, 750 mg every 8 hours for 5 days, is the drug of choice in adults. The duration of diarrhea caused by *Isospora belli* is significantly shortened by administration of trimethoprim-sulfamethoxazole twice daily for 5 days. Cryptosporidiasis in AIDS patients may respond to treatment with paromomycin 4 times daily for 14 to 21 days, but this is unproven.

Antimicrobial Prophylaxis

Prophylactic antimicrobials are effective in preventing traveler's diarrhea, a generally self-limited illness caused most often by ETEC. Doxycycline, trimethoprim-sulfamethoxazole, and norfloxacin are each effective when taken once daily for up to 3 weeks. However, because of the rapid response of most patients to early treatment with any of these three agents, the advantages of prophylactic drugs are, in most instances, outweighed by their potential risks (adverse reactions).

Symptomatic Therapy

Adjuvant symptomatic therapy is not essential but may provide modest symptomatic relief in acute infectious diarrheas associated with cramping abdominal pain. Bismuth subsalicylate, 0.6 gm every 6 hours, may ameliorate symptoms of traveler's diarrhea. Agents that decrease intestinal motility (e.g., codeine, diphenoxylate, loperamide) also relieve the cramping abdominal pain associated with many acute diarrheal illnesses but are potentially hazardous because they may enhance severity of illness in shigellosis, the prototype of invasive bacterial diarrheas.

REFERENCES

Greenough WB: Cholera. *In* Bennett JC, Plum F (eds.): Cecil Textbook of Medicine. 20th ed. Philadelphia, WB Saunders, 1991, pp 1652–1654.

Guerrant RL: Enteric *Escherichia coli* infections. Idem, pp 1554–1557.

Guerrant RL: Principles and syndromes of enteric infections. *In* Mandell GL, Bennett JE, Dolin R: Principles and Practice of Infectious Diseases. 4th ed. New York, Churchill Livingstone, 1995, pp 945–962.

104

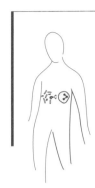

Infections Involving Bones and Joints

ARTHRITIS

In adults, almost all cases of infective arthritis of natural joints occur via hematogenous seeding of the joint. Rarely, intra-articular trauma results in septic arthritis. Bacteria, viruses, mycobacteria, and fungi can all produce an arthritis by infection of the joint. In addition, certain viruses such as hepatitis B virus can produce a polyarthritis via immune complex deposition. Immune mechanisms also underlie arthritis syndromes seen after diarrhea due to *Salmonella, Shigella,* and *Yersinia* infections; the majority of individuals with postdysentery arthritis syndrome share the human leukocyte antigen HLA-B27 (see Chapter 86).

Acute Arthritis

Underlying joint disease, particularly rheumatoid arthritis, predisposes to septic arthritis. Many patients with septic arthritis give a history of joint trauma antedating symptoms of infection. Conceivably, disruption of capillaries during an unrecognized and transient bacteremia allows bacteria to spill into hemorrhagic and traumatized synovium or joint fluid, resulting in the initiation of infection.

Microbiology of Acute Infective Arthritis (Table 104–1)

Staphylococcus aureus is the most common cause of septic arthritis. Patients with underlying joint disease and intravenous drug users are at particular risk for infection with this organism. *Pseudomonas aeruginosa* is another important cause of septic arthritis among intravenous drug users.

Other gram-negative bacilli are infrequent causes of septic arthritis and are seen primarily among elderly debilitated patients with chronic arthritis. In adults under 30, *Neisseria gonorrhoeae* is the most likely pathogen. Isolates causing disseminated gonococcal infection (DGI) with arthritis are generally resistant to killing by normal serum.

Clinical Presentation

Symptoms of septic arthritis are generally present for only a few days before the patient seeks medical attention. Fever is usual; shaking chills may occur. The knee is the most commonly affected joint and is generally painful and swollen. Fluid can be demonstrated in most infected joints, and limitation of motion is marked. In some cases, however, particularly among patients with underlying rheumatoid arthritis who are receiving corticosteroids, physical findings indicating infection may be subtle. In these individuals, who are at particular risk for septic arthritis, superimposed infection may be difficult to distinguish from a flare-up of underlying disease. Symmetric symptoms in multiple joints are more indicative of a rheumatoid flare-up. Approximately 10% of cases of septic arthritis, however, involve more than one joint.

Differential Diagnosis of Acute Monoarticular or Oligoarticular Arthritis

Crystal deposition (uric acid—gout; calcium pyrophosphate—pseudogout), rheumatoid arthritis, systemic lupus erythematosus, and degenerative joint disease can also produce an acute monoarticular arthritis. Radiographs

TABLE 104–1	Infective Arthritis—Acute	
	Etiologic Agent	**Characteristics**
Bacterial	*Staphylococcus aureus*	Most common overall; usually monoarticular, large joint involvement
	Neisseria gonorrhoeae	Most common in young, sexually active adults; commonly polyarticular in onset; often associated with skin lesions
	Pseudomonas aeruginosa	Largely restricted to intravenous drug users; often involves sternoclavicular joint
Viral	Hepatitis B, rubella, mumps, parvovirus	Usually polyarticular, with minimal joint effusions, normal peripheral white blood cell count

may show evidence of osteoarthritis, gouty tophi, or the linear densities of chondrocalcinosis, which are characteristic of pseudogout. All red, warm, tender joints must be aspirated. The synovial fluid should be cultured anaerobically and aerobically. A Gram-stained preparation should be examined; a wet mount of fluid should be examined using a polarized microscope to look for crystals. Synovial fluid leukocyte counts and chemistries are of limited value in the differential diagnosis of a suspected septic joint. As a general rule, however, synovial fluid white blood cell (WBC) counts in excess of $100,000/\mu l$ suggest either infection or crystal-induced disease (see Table 78–3). Blood cultures should be obtained in all cases of suspected septic arthritis.

Treatment of Acute Infective Arthritis

The two major modalities for treatment of acute septic arthritis are drainage and antibiotics. The first needle aspiration of a septic joint should remove as much fluid as possible. Initial antibiotic choice should be based upon the clinical presentation and the results of the Gram stain. Staphylococcal infection can be treated with penicillinase-resistant penicillin or vancomycin. Gonococcal infections should be treated with ceftriaxone, 1 gm every 24 hours for 10 days. Arthritis due to gram-negative rods should be treated with an aminoglycoside plus another drug active against gram-negative bacilli, such as a cephalosporin. In intravenous drug users, the second drug should be active against *Pseudomonas;* therefore, an extended-spectrum penicillin, such as mezlocillin, or a third-generation cephalosporin, such as ceftazidime, is indicated. Arthritis due to *S. aureus* or gram-negative bacilli should be treated with antibiotics for 4 to 6 weeks. Otherwise, 2 to 3 weeks of antibiotic treatment is sufficient to eradicate infection.

Septic joints (with the notable exception of joints infected with the gonococcus) generally reaccumulate fluid after treatment is initiated. These reaccumulations must be removed by repeated needle aspirations as often as necessary. Indications for open surgical drainage of the joint include failure of the synovial fluid WBC count to fall after 5 days of antibiotic treatment and repeated needle aspirations, and the presence of loculated fluid within the joint. Septic arthritis of the hip is generally drained surgically because of the difficulty and potential hazard of repeated needle aspirations of this joint. Early surgical drainage also should be considered for joint infections due to gram-negative rods and to *S. aureus*. Osteomyelitis is an uncommon complication of untreated or inadequately treated septic arthritis. In instances in which the diagnosis and treatment have been delayed, radiographs of the involved joint should be obtained at the beginning and termination of treatment.

Polyarticular Arthritis

Arthritis involving multiple joints is infrequently attributable to direct microbial invasion. In many instances, a polyarticular arthritis represents an immunologically me-

diated process. *Acute rheumatic fever,* a delayed immune-mediated response to group A streptococcal infection, may manifest with a migratory, asymmetric arthritis of the knees, ankles, elbows, and wrists. Heart involvement, subcutaneous nodules, or erythema marginatum is present in a minority of cases. Most patients have serologic evidence of recent streptococcal infection. Antistreptolysin-O, anti-DNase, and antihyaluronidase antibodies are usually present. The importance of making this diagnosis lies primarily in the requirement for long-term prophylaxis against streptococcal infection and the clinical response of this process to salicylates.

Viral infections including hepatitis B, rubella, parvovirus, and mumps may be associated with polyarthritis. In mumps, the arthritis results from direct infection of articular tissue; with rubella and hepatitis B, the joint inflammation is a secondary result of the host immune response to the virus. These processes are self-limited. Serum sickness, polyarticular gout, sarcoidosis, rheumatoid arthritis, and other connective tissue disorders must be considered in the differential diagnosis. Since 10% of cases of septic arthritis involve more than one joint, all acutely inflamed joints containing fluid should be tapped to exclude bacterial infection.

Disseminated gonococcal infection (see Chapter 107) may manifest with fever, tenosynovitis, or arthritis involving several joints and a characteristic rash. The rash may be petechial but usually consists of a few to a few dozen pustules on an erythematous base. Cultures of the joint fluid are usually negative at this stage, but blood cultures are often positive; Gram's stain of a pustule may reveal the pathogen. Ceftriaxone, 1 gm/day for 10 days, is curative.

Chronic Arthritis (Table 104–2)

Mycobacteria and fungi may produce an indolent, slowly progressive arthritis, usually involving only one joint or contiguous joints, such as those of the wrist and hand. Fever may be low-grade or absent. Cultures of joint fluid may be negative. Some patients with tuberculous arthritis have no evidence of active disease in the lungs. As a general rule, patients with inflammatory chronic monoarticular arthritis should have a synovial biopsy for culture and histology. Granulomas indicate the likelihood of fungal or mycobacterial infection. Cultures should confirm the diagnosis.

Fungal arthritis is treated with amphotericin B. Mycobacterial arthritis must be treated for 18 months with at least two drugs active against the isolate. Since some mycobacterial isolates causing joint disease are nontuber-

TABLE 104–2	Causes of Infective Arthritis—Chronic

Tuberculosis
Nontuberculous mycobacteria
Fungi
Lyme disease (oligoarticular)

culous, extensive susceptibility testing may be needed to guide antimicrobial therapy.

A spirochete, *Borrelia burgdorferi* is the pathogen responsible for Lyme disease. Several months to 2 years after the bite of the ixodid tick and the characteristic rash of erythema chronicum migrans, some patients develop an intermittent arthritis involving one or more joints—usually including the knees. This chronic arthritis may result in joint destruction, but fever is unusual. Treatment with intravenous ceftriaxone, 2 gm/day for 14 to 21 days, will halt the progression of disease in the majority of cases (see Chapter 95).

SEPTIC BURSITIS

Septic bursitis is almost always due to *Staphylococcus aureus* and involves either the olecranon or the prepatellar bursa. In most instances, there is a history of antecedent infection or irritation of the skin overlying the bursa. On examination, the skin over the bursa is red and often peeling. The bursa has a doughy consistency and may reveal fluid on careful examination. Needle aspiration and antistaphylococcal antibiotics are generally curative. Occasionally, long courses of antibiotics (> 4 weeks) may be required for cure.

OSTEOMYELITIS

Infections of the bone occur either as a result of hematogenous spread or via extension of local infection.

Hematogenous Osteomyelitis (Table 104–3)

This infection occurs most commonly in the long bones or vertebral bodies. The peak age distributions are in childhood and old age. Individuals predisposed to hematogenous osteomyelitis include intravenous drug users, who are at risk for infections with *S. aureus* and *P. aeruginosa,* and patients with hemoglobinopathy, in whom nontyphoidal salmonellae often infect infarcted regions of bone. Recently, *Staphylococcus epidermidis* has emerged as an important nosocomial pathogen among patients with infected intravenous catheters. Like patients with septic arthritis, patients with hematogenous osteomyelitis often give a history of trauma antedating symptoms of infection, suggesting that transient, unrecognized bacteremia might result in infection of traumatized tissue.

Patients with acute hematogenous osteomyelitis generally present with acute onset of pain, tenderness, and fever; there may also be soft tissue swelling over the affected bone. In most instances, physical examination distinguishes acute osteomyelitis from septic arthritis, since range of joint motion is preserved in osteomyelitis. In the first 2 weeks of illness, roentgenograms may be negative or show only soft tissue swelling; technetium scans or gallium scans are almost always positive, but technetium scans may also be positive in the setting of increased vascularity or increased bone formation of any etiology. Magnetic resonance imaging (MRI) may demon-

TABLE 104–3	Factors Predisposing to Hematogenous Osteomyelitis

Setting	Likely Pathogens
Intravenous drug use	*Staphylococcus aureus*
	Pseudomonas aeruginosa
Intravenous catheters	*Staphylococcus aureus*
	Staphylococcus epidermidis
	Candida species

strate bony erosion before it is apparent on plain films. After 2 weeks of infection, plain radiographs generally show some abnormality, and untreated osteomyelitis may produce areas of periosteal elevation or erosion followed by increased bone formation (sclerosis). The erythrocyte sedimentation rate is generally elevated, as is the WBC count.

A patient with back pain and fever must be considered to have a serious infection until proven otherwise. Spasm of the paravertebral muscles is common in patients with vertebral osteomyelitis, but nonspecific. Point tenderness over bone suggests the presence of local infection. A good history should be obtained and a careful neurologic examination performed. Abnormalities of bowel or bladder or of strength or sensation in the lower extremities suggest the possibility of spinal cord involvement via spinal epidural abscess with or without osteomyelitis. Acute spinal epidural abscess is a *surgical emergency.* The challenge is to make the diagnosis before neurologic signs appear (see Chapter 121). Demonstration of an epidural abscess mandates prompt surgical decompression to avoid disastrous neurologic sequelae. MRI provides excellent definition of epidural or paravertebral abscess and is the diagnostic procedure of choice when available. As an alternative, emergency myelogram can confirm the diagnosis.

Although most cases of hematogenous osteomyelitis have an acute presentation, some cases, particularly those involving the vertebral bodies among intravenous drug users, may have an indolent course. These patients may have an illness of more than 1 year's duration characterized by pain and low-grade fever. Radiographs are abnormal but may reveal only collapse of a vertebral body. This most often occurs in infections due to *P. aeruginosa,* but *Candida* species and *S. aureus* may also occasionally present in this manner.

Blood cultures are positive in about half of acute cases of osteomyelitis. Patients with acute osteomyelitis should have a needle biopsy and culture of the involved bone unless blood culture results are known beforehand. Antibiotic treatment should be continued for 4 to 6 weeks, using agents active against the pathogen.

Osteomyelitis Secondary to Extension of Local Infection

Local infection predisposes to osteomyelitis in several major settings (Table 104–4). The first is after penetrat-

TABLE 104–4	Osteomyelitis Secondary to Contiguous Spread
Setting	**Likely Microorganisms**
Surgery, trauma	*Staphylococcus aureus,* aerobic gram-negative bacilli
Cat or dog bites	*Pasteurella multocida*
Human bites	Penicillin-sensitive anaerobes
Periodontal infections	Penicillin-sensitive anaerobes
Cutaneous ulcers	Mixed aerobic and anaerobic organisms

ing trauma or surgery where local infection gains access to traumatized bone. In postsurgical infections, staphylococci and gram-negative bacilli predominate. Generally, there is evidence of wound infection with erythema, swelling, increased postoperative tenderness, and drainage. A traumatic incident often associated with osteomyelitis is a bite—either human or animal. Human bites, if deep enough, may result in osteomyelitis due to anaerobic mouth flora. Cat bites notoriously result in the development of osteomyelitis because the thin, sharp, long cat's teeth often penetrate the periosteum. *Pasteurella multocida* is a frequent pathogen in this setting. A 4- to 6-week course of penicillin G, 10 million units/day, is indicated.

The intimate relationship of the teeth and periodontal tissues to the bones of the maxilla and mandible may predispose to osteomyelitis following local infection. Debridement of necrotic tissue and penicillin constitute the treatment of choice, since penicillin-sensitive anaerobes are the usual agents of these infections.

The third setting in which local infection predisposes to osteomyelitis is that of an infected sore or ulcer. Pressure sores of the sacrum or femoral region may erode into contiguous bone and produce an osteomyelitis (see Chapter 101) due to a mixed flora containing anaerobic organisms. Patients with diabetes mellitus often develop ulcerations of their toes and feet, with eventual development of osteomyelitis. Anaerobes, streptococci, staphylococci, and gram-negative bacilli are often involved in these infections (see Chapter 101). Treatment involves debridement (often amputation in the case of diabetics) and antibiotics active against the pathogens involved.

Chronic Osteomyelitis

Untreated or inadequately treated osteomyelitis results in avascular necrosis of bone and the formation of islands of nonvascularized and infected bone called sequestra. Patients with chronic osteomyelitis may tolerate their infection reasonably well, with intermittent episodes of disease activity manifested by increased local pain and the development of drainage of infected material through a sinus tract. Some patients have tolerated chronic osteomyelitis for decades. A normochromic normocytic anemia of chronic disease is common in this setting, and occasionally amyloidosis and rarely osteogenic sarcoma complicate this disorder.

S. aureus is responsible for the great majority of cases of chronic osteomyelitis; the major exception is among patients with sickle cell anemia, in whom nontyphoidal salmonellae may cause chronic infection of the long bones.

Cultures of sinus tract drainage do not reliably reflect the pathogens involved in the infection. Diagnosis and cure are best effected by surgical debridement of necrotic material followed by long-term administration of antibiotics active against the organism found in the surgical specimens.

Mycobacteria, especially *Mycobacterium tuberculosis,* can produce a chronic osteomyelitis. The anterior portions of vertebral bodies are the most common sites of infection. Hematogenous dissemination and lymphatic spread are the most likely routes of infection. Paravertebral abscess (often termed *cold abscess* because of lack of signs of acute inflammation) may complicate this infection. Diagnosis is usually confirmed by histologic examination and culture of biopsy material. Treatment with antituberculous drugs is usually curative.

REFERENCES

Baker DG, Shumacher HR: Acute monoarthritis. N Engl J Med 1995; 329:1013–20.

Brause BD: Osteomyelitis. *In* Bennett JC, Plum F (eds.): Cecil Textbook of Medicine. 20th ed. Philadelphia, WB Saunders, 1996; pp 2689–2693.

Goldenberg DL, Reed JI: Bacterial arthritis. N Engl J Med 1985; 312: 764–770.

105

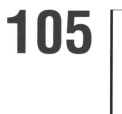

Infections of the Urinary Tract

The urethra, bladder, kidneys, and prostate are all susceptible to infection. Most urinary tract infections (UTIs) cause local symptoms, yet clinical manifestations do not always pinpoint the site of infection. In addition, the criteria used by different clinical laboratories to confirm infection of the urinary tract are variable. This chapter will attempt to simplify the clinical and laboratory approach to diagnosis and treatment of UTIs. Infections associated with indwelling urinary catheters are discussed in Chapter 106.

URETHRITIS

Urethritis is predominantly an infection of sexually active individuals, usually males. The symptoms are pain and burning of the urethra during urination, and there is generally some discharge at the urethral meatus. Urethritis may be gonococcal in origin. However, nongonococcal urethritis (NGU) is now more frequent in North America. NGU may be due to *Chlamydia trachomatis* or *Ureaplasma urealyticum* and less, commonly to *Trichomonas vaginalis* or to herpes viruses. Diagnosis and management of urethritis are considered in Chapter 107.

CYSTITIS AND PYELONEPHRITIS

Epidemiology

Bacterial infection of the bladder (cystitis) and kidney (pyelonephritis) is more frequent in females, and the incidence of infection increases with age. Factors that predispose to UTI include instrumentation (e.g., catheterization, cystoscopy), pregnancy, and diabetes mellitus.

Pathogenesis

Although some infections of the kidney may arise as the result of hematogenous dissemination, most UTIs ascend via a portal of entry in the urethra. Most pathogens responsible for community-acquired UTIs are part of the subject's normal bowel flora. *Escherichia coli* is the most common isolate, and in the female, colonization of the vaginal and periurethral mucosa may antedate infection of the urinary tract. Bacteria capable of adherence to epithelial cells are more likely to cause UTIs. The longer and protected male urethra may account for the lower incidence of UTI in men. Motile bacteria may swim upstream, and reflux of urine from the bladder into the ureters may predispose to the development of kidney infection. Congenital anomalies or obstruction of urine flow at any level also predisposes to infection.

Clinical Features

Suprapubic pain, discomfort, or burning sensation on urination and frequency of urination are common symptoms of infection of the urinary tract. Back or flank pain or the occurrence of fever suggests that infection is not limited to the bladder (cystitis) but involves the kidney (pyelonephritis) or prostate as well. However, clinical presentation often fails to distinguish between simple cystitis and pyelonephritis. Approximately one half of infections that appear clinically to involve the bladder can be shown only by instrumentation and other specialized techniques to actually affect the kidneys. Elderly or debilitated patients with infection of the urinary tract may have no symptoms referable to the urinary tract and may present only with fever, altered mental status, or hypotension.

Laboratory Diagnosis of Urinary Tract Infection

Analysis of a midstream urine sample obtained from patients with infection of the bladder or kidney should reveal white blood cells (WBCs) and may also have red cells and slightly increased amounts of protein. The presence of an increased number of WBCs (pyuria) in a midstream urine sample indicates the likelihood of a UTI. However, since most laboratories count WBCs by examining the sediment of a centrifuged urine sample, and since the urinary WBC count may vary according to the degree of urine concentration, quantitation of pyuria is imprecise. As a general rule, more than 5 to 10 WBCs per high-power field on a centrifuged specimen of urine is abnormal. Resuspending a sedimented urine should be done gently using a Pasteur pipette so that casts are not disrupted. The presence of WBC casts in an infected urine sample indicates the presence of pyelonephritis.

Bacteria may be seen in sedimented urine and can be readily identified using Gram's stain.

At present, most clinical laboratories consider bacterial growth of greater than 10^5 colony-forming units/ml to be indicative of infection. Recent studies indicate that smaller numbers of bacteria can produce UTIs. A hazard in interpreting results of urine culture is that if the sample is allowed to stand at room temperature for a few hours before planting on culture plates, bacteria can multiply. This results in spuriously high bacterial counts. For this reason, urine for culture should not be obtained from a catheter bag. Specimens that are not plated immediately should be refrigerated. Biochemical tests to detect bacteriuria are not reliable.

Treatment and Outcome

Most patients with cystitis are cured by a single high dose of antibiotic (e.g., one double-strength trimethoprim-sulfamethoxazole tablet or 800 mg norfloxacin). Culture and sensitivity confirm the diagnosis and ascertain if the antibiotic is active against the pathogen. Because of the difficulty in clinical distinction between cystitis and upper-tract disease, some patients treated for cystitis with a single dose of an antibiotic may relapse because of unrecognized upper-tract disease.

Occasionally, urine cultures obtained from a patient with symptoms of UTI and pyuria are reported as exhibiting "no growth" or "insignificant growth." This situation has been labeled the "urethral syndrome." Low numbers of bacteria (as few as 100/ml of urine) may produce such infections of the urinary tract. In other instances, the urethral syndrome may be caused by *Chlamydia* or *Ureaplasma,* which will not grow on routine culture media. Thus, if a patient with the urethral syndrome has responded to antibiotics, the course should be completed; otherwise, if symptoms and pyuria persist, the patient should receive a 7- to 10-day course of tetracycline, which is active against *Chlamydia* and *Ureaplasma.* Other considerations for patients with lower urinary tract symptoms and no or "insignificant" growth on cultures of urine include vaginitis, herpes simplex infection, and gonococcal infection. (*Neisseria gonorrhoeae* will not grow on routine media used for urine culture.) Thus, a pelvic examination and culture for gonococci may be indicated in this setting if the patient is sexually active. Men with urethral discomfort and discharge should be evaluated for urethritis (see Chapter 107). Men with suprapubic pain, frequency, and urgency should be evaluated for cystitis, as discussed above.

The presence of fever suggests that infection involves more than just the bladder. Young, otherwise healthy, febrile patients with UTI may be treated on an ambulatory basis with trimethoprim-sulfamethoxazole for 2 weeks, provided that (1) they do not appear toxic, (2) they have friends or family at home, (3) they have good provisions for follow-up, and (4) they have no potentially complicating features, such as diabetes mellitus, history of renal stones, history of obstructive disease of the urinary tract, or sickle cell disease. Gram's stain of urine in patients hospitalized for pyelonephritis will guide initial therapy. Gram-negative rod infection may be treated initially with an aminoglycoside plus ampicillin or a cephalosporin. The aminoglycoside should be promptly discontinued if antibiotic sensitivity studies indicate that it is not essential. The finding of gram-positive cocci in chains suggests that enterococci are the pathogens. This infection should be treated, at least initially, with ampicillin plus an aminoglycoside. Gram-positive cocci in clusters may indicate staphylococci. *Staphylococcus saprophyticus* is a likely agent in otherwise healthy women and is sensitive to most antibiotics used in the treatment of UTI. In the older patient, *Staphylococcus aureus* should be considered, and this infection may be treated with a penicillinase-resistant penicillin, such as nafcillin. Gram-positive cocci in the urine may represent a case of endocarditis with septic embolization to the kidney.

Therapy should be simplified when reports of antimicrobial susceptibility are available. Repeat urine culture after 2 days of effective treatment should show sterilization or a marked decrease in the urinary bacterial count. If the patient fails to demonstrate some clinical improvement after 2 to 3 days of treatment or if the patient presents with the clinical picture of sepsis or has been febrile for more than 1 week, a complicating feature should be suspected. Intranephric or perinephric abscess or obstruction due to a stone or an enlarged prostate may underlie this presentation. Plain films of the abdomen may occasionally reveal a radio-opaque stone, but ultrasonography is a good first diagnostic procedure in this setting. This will generally detect obstruction and collections of pus and may also detect stones greater than 3 mm in diameter. Obstruction must be relieved and abscesses drained to result in cure. Computerized tomographic–guided percutaneous drainage is the procedure of choice whenever possible.

All patients with UTI should have repeat urine cultures 1 to 2 weeks after treatment is completed to check for relapse. If relapse occurs, the patient may have pyelonephritis, prostatitis, or neuropathic or structural disease of the urinary tract. If a 6-week course of antibiotics active against the bacterial isolate is not effective in eradicating infection, the possibility of structural abnormalities or prostatic infection should be investigated. Urologic evaluation should be performed for all males with UTI (excepting urethritis) because of the high frequency of correctable anatomic lesions in this population.

Some women have frequent episodes of UTI due to different bacterial isolates. In some instances, these reinfections are related to sexual activity. Prompt voiding and a single dose of an active antibiotic such as cephalexin just after sexual contact can decrease reinfection rate in these women. In other women, in whom no precipitating factor can be found and infections are frequent, prophylaxis with one half of a tablet of trimethoprim-sulfamethoxazole nightly has been effective.

On occasion, urine cultures reveal bacterial growth in the absence of symptoms. If the sample has been obtained properly and repeat culture reveals the same organism, this is termed *asymptomatic bacteriuria.* This condition is generally observed in elderly or middle-aged individuals and, in the absence of structural disease of the urinary tract or diabetes mellitus, may not require treatment. Asymptomatic bacteriuria occurring during pregnancy should be treated because of the high risk of pyelonephritis in this setting.

The occurrence of pyuria in the absence of bacterial growth on culture of urine ($< 10^2$ colonies/ml) may be termed "sterile pyuria". If this occurs in the patient with lower urinary tract symptoms, chlamydial or gonococcal infection, vaginitis, or herpes simplex infection should be considered. In the absence of lower urinary tract symptoms, sterile pyuria may be seen among patients with interstitial nephritis of numerous causes or with tuberculosis of the urinary tract. Patients with renal tuberculosis often have nocturia and polyuria. More than half of male patients also have involvement of the genital tract, most commonly the epididymis. Diagnosis can be made by biopsy of genital masses, when present, and by three morning cultures of urine for mycobacteria.

PROSTATITIS

Although prostatic fluid has antibacterial properties, the prostate can become infected, usually by direct invasion through the urethra. Symptoms of UTI, back or perineal pain, and fever are common. Some patients experience pain with ejaculation. Rectal examination usually reveals a tender prostate. Patients with acute prostatitis generally have an abnormal urinary sediment and pathogenic bacteria (usually gram-negative enteric rods) in cultures of urine.

Acute prostatitis may be due to the gonococcus but is most often due to gram-negative bacilli. Treatment is directed against the pathogen observed on Gram's stain of urine and is generally effective. Chronic prostatitis may be asymptomatic and should be suspected in males with recurrent UTI. The urine sediment may be relatively benign in patients with chronic prostatitis. In this instance, comparison of the first part of the urine sample, midstream urine, excretions expressed by massage of the prostate, and postmassage urine should reveal bacterial counts more than 10-fold greater in the prostatic secretions and postmassage urine samples than in first-void and midstream samples. Treatment of chronic prostatitis is hampered by poor penetration of the prostate by most antimicrobials. Long-term (4 to 12 weeks) treatment with trimethoprim-sulfamethoxazole has cured approximately one third of patients and prevented symptomatic relapse in another third. Ciprofloxacin also is effective in this setting.

REFERENCES

Kunin CM: Urinary tract infections and pyelonephritis. *In* Bennett JC, Plum F (eds): Cecil Textbook of Medicine. 20th ed. Philadelphia, WB Saunders, 1996, pp 602–605.
Komaroff AL: Acute dysuria in women. N Engl J Med 1984;310: 368–374.

106

Nosocomial Infections

A nosocomial or hospital-acquired infection is an infection not present on admission to the hospital that first appears 72 hours or more after hospitalization. A patient admitted to a hospital in the United States has an approximately 5 to 10% chance of developing a nosocomial infection. These infections result in significant morbidity and mortality (approximately 1% of these infections are fatal, and an additional 4% contribute to death) and greatly increased medical costs (approximately 10 billion dollars per year).

Numerous factors are associated with a greater risk of acquiring a nosocomial infection. These include factors that are not avoidable by optimal medical practice, such as age and severity of underlying illness. Contributing factors that can be minimized by thoughtful management of the patient include prolonged duration of hospitalization, the inappropriate use of broad-spectrum antibiotics, the use of indwelling catheters, and the failure of health care personnel to wash their hands.

APPROACH TO THE HOSPITALIZED PATIENT WITH SUSPECTED NOSOCOMIAL INFECTION

The first clue to the presence of a nosocomial infection is often a rise in temperature. The only sign of infection, particularly in the elderly or demented patient, may be a change in mental status (Table 106-1). Some patients with serious infection do not initially develop fever but instead become tachypneic or confused for no apparent reason. Analysis of arterial blood gases may reveal at first a respiratory alkalosis, followed by a metabolic acidosis due to increased levels of lactate. Arterial oxygen content may be normal or depressed.

When evaluating a hospitalized patient for a new fever (Table 106-2) or suspected nosocomial infection, the physician should first assess the stability of the patient. Hypotension, tachypnea, or new obtundation mandates rapid evaluation and treatment. The patient's problem list must be reviewed; the physician must ascertain if the patient was recently subjected to a potentially hazardous intervention (e.g., genitourinary tract instrumentation or administration of blood products). If the patient can cooperate, the physician should elicit a history directed at possible causes of the fever. Often the patient has a specific complaint that helps identify the source of the fever.

The skin must be examined carefully. Maculopapular rashes often accompany drug fevers; ecthyma gangrenosum can be a sign of gram-negative sepsis (see Chapter 96). Surgical wounds should be examined for the presence of infection. Among debilitated patients, pressure sores located near the sacrum or over the greater trochanters may become infected and produce fever. Abscesses at these sites may be covered by a necrotic membrane, so that exploration with a gloved finger or sterile needle may be required to demonstrate a focus of pus. Patients receiving multiple intramuscular injections may develop fever as a result of the development of sterile abscesses at the injection sites. Headache or sinus tenderness may be present in patients with sinusitis—this may be a problem among patients after nasogastric or nasotracheal intubation. Nuchal rigidity may be a sign of nosocomial meningitis, although it may be absent in some cases, particularly following neurosurgery or head trauma. Furthermore, generalized rigidity is often seen in elderly demented patients without central nervous system infection. The physician should examine the nose and oropharynx and attempt to elicit symptoms of viral upper respiratory tract infections. These do occur in hospitals. A pleural friction rub may indicate a recent pulmonary thromboembolism as a cause of fever; rales or other evidence of consolidation may indicate a nosocomial pneumonia; basilar rales and even egophony and bronchial breath sounds may also be due to atelectasis in debilitated patients. A new S_4 gallop or pericardial friction rub may be the only clinical manifestation of a myocardial infarction.

The abdomen may also be a source of fever in the hospitalized patient. The patient with antibiotic-induced colitis generally has fever, diarrhea, and abdominal pain. Patients with indwelling urinary catheters are at particular risk of infection. These patients should have a careful

TABLE 106-1	Signs of Infection in the Hospitalized Patient

Fever
Change in mental status
Tachypnea
Hypotension
Oliguria
Leukocytosis

TABLE 106–2	Common Causes of Fever in the Hospitalized Patient

Pneumonia
Catheter-related infection
Surgical wound infection
Urinary tract infection
Drugs
Pulmonary emboli
Infected pressure sores

examination of the prostate—looking for abscess or tenderness—and of the urine—looking for white blood cells and bacteria.

The extremities must be examined carefully, particularly the sites of current and old intravenous catheter placements, for evidence of phlebitis. If no other source of fever is found and an intravenous catheter has been in place, it should be replaced and a segment of the catheter should be rolled on an agar plate for culture.

Deep vein thrombophlebitis and pulmonary thromboemboli are life-threatening complications of hospitalization whose only clinical manifestations may be fever. The lower extremities should be examined and measured carefully. An asymmetry in leg or calf circumference, which may not be obvious without a measurement, may be an important clue to an underlying thrombosis. A crystal-induced arthritis is another potential source of fever in a hospitalized patient. Gout and pseudogout may be precipitated by acute infections.

The patient's medication list should be reviewed for drugs likely to produce fever. In this regard antimicrobial agents (particularly penicillins, sulfa drugs, and cephalosporins) are among the most common causes of drug-induced fevers. A drug fever can occur at any time but usually occurs during the second week of drug administration. A review of the peripheral blood smear can give important clues to the cause of the fever. Eosinophilia may suggest drug reaction and lymphocytosis a viral process. A left shift and vacuolization within neutrophils suggest a bacterial infection. Unless the etiology of the fever is apparent, cultures of blood and urine and a chest radiograph should be obtained.

NOSOCOMIAL PNEUMONIA

Although some hospital-acquired pneumonias occur as a result of bacteremic spread, the vast majority occur via aspiration of oropharyngeal contents. The oropharynx of the patient admitted to the hospital rapidly becomes colonized with aerobic gram-negative bacilli and often staphylococci. The administration of broad-spectrum antibiotics, severe underlying illness (e.g., chronic lung disease), respiratory intubation, advanced age, and prolonged duration of hospitalization predispose to colonization.

Sedation, loss of consciousness, and other factors that depress the gag and cough reflexes place the colonized patient at greater risk for aspiration and the development of nosocomial pneumonia. The development of a new pulmonary infiltrate in a hospitalized patient may represent pneumonia, atelectasis, aspiration of gastric contents, drug reaction, or pulmonary infarction. If pneumonia is suspected, prompt definition of the pathogen and appropriate treatment are critical, since nosocomial pneumonia carries a 20 to 50% mortality. If the patient cannot produce good-quality sputum, nasotracheal aspiration should be performed (see Chapter 99). Antibiotic therapy is guided by the results of Gram's stain of the sputum or of the tracheal aspirate. Gram-negative rods are the predominant pathogens in this setting; these infections should be treated with an aminoglycoside plus an extended-spectrum penicillin or cephalosporin until results of culture and sensitivity testing are known. If gram-positive cocci in clusters are seen, vancomycin should be administered; a mixed flora suggestive of aspiration of oral anaerobes should prompt treatment with clindamycin or a penicillin/beta lactamase inhibitor combination such as piperacillin-tazobactam. In certain hospitals, nosocomial pneumonia due to *Legionella* species is frequent, and erythromycin should be included in the initial treatment regimen. (*Legionella* species are rarely detectable on Gram's stain.) Patients with nosocomial pneumonia should also receive respiratory therapy consisting of clapping, postural drainage, and promotion of coughing to assist in bringing up secretions.

The patient in the intensive care unit with an endotracheal tube in place is at particular risk for nosocomial pneumonia. This patient has an ineffective gag reflex and often a depressed cough as well. Many are paralyzed to facilitate ventilator-dependent respiration. The patient is therefore entirely dependent upon suctioning by the staff to clear secretions from the airways. The airways of these patients become rapidly colonized with bacteria. Epidemics of nosocomial pneumonia have sometimes been associated with contamination of tubing and machinery used for ventilation or respiratory therapy, but infection is often due to transmission of pathogens on the hands of medical personnel. Large-volume nebulizers, when contaminated, are also capable of delivering droplets containing bacteria to the lower respiratory tract. Patients whose airways are simply colonized but whose lower respiratory tracts are not infected should not be treated with antibiotics, despite positive sputum cultures. Premature treatment of colonization results in replacement of the initial colonists by more resistant organisms, whereas delay in treatment of nosocomial pneumonia can result in death from overwhelming infection. The physician must therefore be able to distinguish accurately between colonization and infection. The development of new fever, leukocytosis, pulmonary infiltrate, or deterioration of respiratory status as ascertained by blood gas determinations suggests infection (pneumonia) rather than colonization. A Gram stain of sputum should be performed to identify the predominant organism (or organisms). The appearance of elastin fibers in potassium hydroxide preparations of sputum is a very specific indicator of bacterial infection in this setting (see Chapter 93). The appearance of these fibers may actually precede the development of infiltrates on chest radiograph. This test, however, detects fewer than one half of nosocomial pneumonias in the intensive care unit.

Nosocomial pneumonias are best prevented by (1)

avoiding excessive sedation, (2) providing frequent suctioning and respiratory therapy—drainage and clapping—to patients who have difficulty managing secretions, (3) avoiding the use of large-volume reservoir nebulizers, (4) avoiding the injudicious use of broad-spectrum or high-dose antibiotic therapy, (5) frequent handwashing by medical and nursing personnel, and (6) weaning the patient from mechanical respiratory support as soon as possible.

INTRAVASCULAR CATHETER-RELATED INFECTIONS

Infections related to intravascular catheters may occur via bacteremic seeding or through infusion of contaminated material, but the vast majority of these infections occur via bacterial invasion at the site of catheter insertion.

Intravenous catheters may produce a sterile phlebitis. Certain drugs such as tetracycline or erythromycin, when administered intravenously, are particularly likely to produce phlebitis. Bacteria migrating through the catheter insertion site may colonize the catheter and then produce a septic phlebitis or bacteremia without evidence of local infection. Factors associated with a greater risk of intravenous catheter-related infection are shown in Table 106–3. *Staphylococcus epidermidis* and *Staphylococcus aureus* are the predominant pathogens in this setting, followed by the enteric gram-negative rods. A peripheral catheter (and all readily removable foreign bodies) should be replaced if bacteremia occurs and no other primary site of infection is found. The catheter should also be removed if fever without an obvious source occurs or if local phlebitis develops. The value of culturing a peripheral catheter tip is uncertain unless semiquantitative techniques are used (i.e., rolling the catheter across an agar plate). During the evaluation of a hospital-acquired fever, an inflamed vein should be examined carefully, and after the catheter is removed, the inflamed portion of the vein should be compressed in an attempt to express pus through the catheter entry site. If pus can be expressed or the patient remains febrile or bacteremic while on appropriate antibiotics, the vein should be surgically explored and excised if septic phlebitis is found.

Central venous catheters remain in place longer than peripheral catheters and are therefore associated with a greater overall infection rate. This is particularly true if

TABLE 106–3	Factors Associated with Greater Risks of Intravenous Catheter-Related Infection

Failure of staff to wash hands
Duration of catheterization > 72 hr
Plastic catheter > steel needle
Lower extremities and groin > upper extremity
Cutdown > percutaneous insertion
Emergency > elective insertion
Breakdown in skin integrity (e.g., burns)
Inserted by physician > intravenous therapy teams

TABLE 106–4	Factors Predisposing to Nosocomial Urinary Tract Infection

Indwelling catheters
Duration of catheterization
Open drainage (versus closed-bag drainage)
Interruption of closed drainage system
Use of broad-spectrum antibiotics *(Candida)*

total parenteral nutrition is provided by this route. Patients receiving parenteral nutrition are at particular risk for systemic infection with *Candida* species and gram-negative bacilli as well as with staphylococci. Pus at the catheter insertion site or positive blood cultures without another source are indications for catheter removal. In an attempt to decrease percutaneous spread of bacteria to intravascular sites, most centers are now placing long Silastic catheters into the subclavian vein after subcutaneous tunneling. These catheters may be kept in place for prolonged periods with a lower infection risk. As a general rule, persistent bacteremia while the patient is taking appropriate antibiotics, recurrent bacteremia, and fungemia with *Candida* or related yeasts are indications for removal of these catheters.

PRESSURE SORES

See Chapter 101.

NOSOCOMIAL URINARY TRACT INFECTION

Urinary tract infections are the most common nosocomial infections, and infection of the urinary tract accounts for 15% of nosocomial bacteremias. Placement of an indwelling catheter into the urethra of a hospitalized patient facilitates access of pathogens to an ordinarily sterile site. Factors that predispose to infection are shown in Table 106–4. The most common pathogens are enteric gram-negative rods; however, among immunocompromised patients and patients receiving broad-spectrum antibiotics, *Candida* species are also important causes of infection. Prophylactic antibiotics, irrigation, urinary acidification, and use of antiseptics are of no value in prevention of infection in this setting. Nosocomial urinary tract infections can be best prevented by adherence to the following guidelines:

1. Catheterize only when necessary. (Monitoring of intake and output and urinary incontinence are generally not appropriate indications for catheterization.)
2. Remember that repeated straight ("in-and-out") catheterizations are less likely to produce infection than indwelling catheters. Many patients with dysfunctional bladders (e.g., those with multiple sclerosis) have used this technique for years without developing significant urinary tract infections. Thrice-daily straight catheterization, using sterile technique, is preferable to a chronic indwelling catheter.

3. If an indwelling catheter is unavoidable, observe the following guidelines:
   a. Remove the catheter as soon as possible.
   b. Emphasize handwashing.
   c. Maintain a closed and unobstructed drainage system. (Urine specimens for culture and analysis may be obtained by inserting a 22-gauge needle aseptically through the distal end of the catheter wall.) Do not disconnect the catheter from the drainage bag.
   d. Secure the catheter in place.
   e. Keep the catheter bag below the level of the bladder.
   f. Irrigate the catheter only if it is obstructed.

Asymptomatic bacterial colonization of the catheterized bladder need not be treated. If the patient has fever or local symptoms, antibiotic treatment is indicated. *Candida* infection of the bladder often resolves once broad-spec-trum antibiotics are discontinued. If *Candida* infection persists, the catheter may be changed; if infection still persists, twice-daily irrigation of the bladder with amphotericin B or oral fluconazole will often eradicate the organism.

The best way to prevent catheter-related infections of the urinary tract is to avoid catheterization unless absolutely necessary.

REFERENCES

Kunin CM: Detection, Prevention and Management of Urinary Tract Infections. 4th ed. Philadelphia, Lea & Febiger, 1986.

Salata RA, Lederman MM, Shlaes DM, et al: Diagnosis of nosocomial pneumonia in intubated, intensive-care unit patients. Am Rev Resp Dis 1987;135:426–432.

Schaffner W: Prevention and treatment of hospital-acquired infections. *In* Bennett JC, Plum F (eds): Cecil Textbook of Medicine. 20th ed. Philadelphia, WB Saunders, 1996, pp 1548–1553.

107

Sexually Transmitted Diseases

Sexually transmitted diseases (STDs) are a diverse group of infections caused by multiple microbial pathogens. These infections are grouped because of common epidemiologic and clinical features. During the past 15 years, the field of STDs has evolved from one emphasizing the traditional venereal diseases of gonorrhea and syphilis to one concerned also with infections associated with *Chlamydia trachomatis,* herpes simplex virus, and human papillomavirus. More recently, the field has become focused upon the human immunodeficiency virus (HIV).

Changes in sexual attitudes and practices have contributed to a resurgence of all venereal infections. Gonorrhea, for example, has tripled in incidence in the United States since 1963; approximately 3 million cases now occur each year. The number of new cases of syphilis has increased each year since 1986. The incidence of syphilis began to decrease in homosexual males in the same period, in association with safer sex practices. The increase in cases is predominantly due to heterosexual spread and results in part from the widespread exchange of sex for drugs.

At the outset, two common errors in approaching the patient with STD should be avoided. The first is to fail to consider that an individual is at risk for STD. All sexually active persons are at risk, not just because of their own sexual behavior, but that of their sexual partners as well. Failure to consider risk factors often results in mistakes in diagnosis, inappropriate treatment, poor follow-up of infected sexual contacts, and, ultimately, recurrent or persistent infection. A second problem with STDs is the failure to recognize and diagnose coinfection. The most serious coinfection is with HIV. The worldwide epidemic of STDs fuels the global spread of HIV. STDs, many of which can be readily diagnosed and treated, may greatly enhance the transmission of HIV infection. HIV, in turn, may alter the natural history of other STDs.

Sexually transmitted diseases can be considered in broad groups according to whether major initial manifestations are (1) genital ulcers; (2) urethritis, cervicitis, and pelvic inflammatory disease; or (3) vaginitis. All patients with any STD should be strongly encouraged to undergo screening for HIV infection. HIV infection is discussed in Chapter 108.

GENITAL SORES

Six infectious agents cause most genital lesions (Table 107–1). The appearance of the lesions, natural history, and laboratory findings allow a clear-cut distinction among the possible causes in most instances. The two most common and significant infections in North America are herpes simplex virus infection and syphilis.

Herpes Simplex Virus (HSV) Infection

Genital herpes infection has reached epidemic proportions, causing a corresponding increase in public awareness and concern. Genital herpes differs from other STDs in its tendency for spontaneous recurrence. Its importance stems from the morbidity, both physical and psychological, of the recurrent genital lesions, and the danger of transmission of a fulminant, often fatal, disease to newborn infants.

Epidemiology

Herpes simplex virus has a worldwide distribution. Humans are the only known reservoir of infection, which is spread by direct contact with infected secretions. Of the two types of HSV, HSV-2 is the more frequent cause of genital infection. The major risk of infection is in the 14- to 29-year-old cohort and varies with sexual activity. Prevalence rates for HSV-2 infection are as high as 40 to 50% in some North American populations.

After exposure, HSV replicates within epithelial cells and lyses them, producing a thin-walled vesicle. Multinucleated cells are formed with characteristic intranuclear inclusions. Regional lymph nodes become enlarged and tender. HSV also migrates along sensory neurons to sensory ganglia, where it assumes a latent state. Inside the sacral ganglia, HSV DNA can be demonstrated, but the virus does not replicate and is inactive metabolically. Just how viral reactivation occurs is uncertain. During reactivation, the virus appears to migrate back to skin along sensory nerves.

TABLE 107–1	Differentiation of Diseases Causing Genital Sores

Disease	Primary Lesion	Adenopathy	Systemic Features	Diagnosis/Rx
Herpes genitalis, primary 20% sexually active adults, due to HSV-2	Incubation 2–7 days; multiple painful vesicles on erythematous base; persist 7–14 days	Tender, soft adenopathy, often bilateral	Fever	Tzanck smear positive; tissue culture isolation, HSV-2 antigen, fourfold rise in antibodies to HSV-2; Rx: acyclovir
Recurrent	Grouped vesicles on erythematous base, painful; last 3–10 days	None	None	Tzanck, HSV-2 antigen, tissue culture positive; titers not helpful; Rx: acyclovir
Syphilis, 90,000 cases in US per year, caused by *Treponema pallidum*	Incubation 10–90 days (m. 21); chancre: papule that ulcerates; painless, border raised, firm, ulcer indurated, base smooth; usually single; may be genital or almost anywhere; persists 3–6 wk, leaving thin, atrophic scar	1 wk after chancre appears; bilateral or unilateral; firm, discrete, moveable, no overlying skin changes, painless, nonsuppurative; may persist for months	Later stages	Cannot be cultured; positive darkfield; VDRL positive, 77%; FTA–ABS positive, 86% (see Table 107–2)
Chancroid, 2000 cases in US per year caused by *Haemophilus ducreyi*	Incubation 3–5 days; vesicle or papule to pustule to ulcer; soft, not indurated; very painful	1 wk after primary in 50%; painful, unilateral (two thirds), suppurative	None	Organism in Gram's stain of pus; can be cultured (75%) but direct yields highest from lymph node; Rx: ceftriaxone, 250 mg once intramuscularly, or ciprofloxacin, 500 mg bid times 3 days
Lymphogranuloma venereum, 600–1000 cases per year in US due to *Chlamydia trachomatis*	Incubation 5–21 days; painless papule, vesicle, ulcer, evanescent (2–3 days), noted in only 10–40%	5–21 days post primary, one third bilateral, tender, matted iliac/femoral "groove sign"; multiple abscesses; coalescent, caseating, suppurative, sinus tracts; thick yellow pus; fistulas; strictures; genital ulcerations	Fever, arthritis, pericarditis, proctitis, meningoencephalitis, keratoconjunctivitis, preauricular adenopathy, edema of eyelids, erythema nodosum	LGV CF positive 85–90% (1–3 wk); must have high titer (>1:16), as cross-reacts with other *Chlamydia;* also positive STS, rheumatoid factor, cryoglobulins; Rx: doxycycline, 100 mg bid times 7 days
Granuloma inguinale, 50 cases in US per year caused by *Calymmatobacterium granulomatis*	Incubation 9–50 days; at least one painless papule that gradually ulcerates; ulcers are large (1–4 cm), irregular, nontender, with thickened, rolled margins and beefy red tissue at base; older portions of ulcer show depigmented scarring, while advancing edge contains new papules	No true adenopathy; in one fifth, subcutaneous spread via lymphatics leads to indurated swelling or abscesses of groin—"pseudobuboes"	Metastatic infection of bones, joints, liver	Scraping or deep curetting at actively extending border—Wright's or Giemsa's stain reveals short, plump, bipolar staining "Donovan's bodies" in macrophage vacuoles; Rx: tetracycline, 2 gm/day times 21 days
Condyloma acuminatum (genital warts), frequent, due to human papillomavirus (HPV)	Characteristic large, soft, fleshy, cauliflower-like excrescences around vulva, glans, urethral orifice, anus, perineum	None	None per se; association with cervical dysplasia/neoplasia	Chief importance is distinction from syphilis and chancroid; Rx: topical podophyllin ± cryosurgery, laser resection

CF = Complement fixation; FTA–ABS = fluorescent treponemal antibody absorption; HSV = herpes simplex virus; LGV = lymphogranuloma venereum; Rx = prescription; STS = serologic test for syphilis; VDRL = Venereal Disease Research Laboratory.

Clinical Presentation

Primary genital lesions develop 2 to 7 days after contact with infected secretions. In males, painful vesicles appear on the glans or penile shaft; in females, they occur on the vulva, perineum, buttocks, cervix, or vagina. A vaginal discharge frequently is present, usually accompanied by inguinal adenopathy, fever, and malaise. Sacroradiculo-myelitis or aseptic meningitis can complicate primary infection. Perianal and anal HSV infections are common, particularly in male homosexuals; tenesmus and rectal discharge often are the main complaints.

The precipitating events associated with genital relapse of HSV infection are poorly understood. In individual cases, stress or menstruation may be implicated. Overall, genital recurrences develop in about 60% of

HSV-infected patients. Clinically apparent recurrences are more frequent in males with HSV-2 infection. The frequency of asymptomatic cervical recurrence in women is not known. Many patients describe a characteristic prodrome of tingling or burning for 18 to 36 hours before the appearance of lesions. Recurring HSV genital lesions are fewer in number, are usually stereotyped in location, are often restricted to the genital region, heal more quickly, and are associated with few systemic complaints.

Laboratory Diagnosis

The appearance of the characteristic vesicles is strongly suggestive of HSV infection. However, diagnosis should be confirmed by a Tzanck smear (see Chapter 93), Papanicolaou smear, immunofluorescent assay for viral antigen, or viral isolation. Serologies for HSV may be useful in the diagnosis of primary infection. Culture remains the gold standard for diagnosis. Direct antigen detection, using an enzyme immunoassay test, shows greater sensitivity than culture for later stage HSV lesions and is equivalent to culture for early stages.

Treatment

Acyclovir, topical or oral, shortens the course of primary genital HSV infection. Intravenous or oral administration is recommended for severe cases with fever, systemic symptoms, and extensive local disease. Antiviral agents do not, however, prevent the latent stage of virus and cannot prevent recurrent infections. Prophylactic oral acyclovir decreases the frequency of symptomatic recurrences by 60 to 80% when used over a 4- to 6-year period, but asymptomatic viral shedding may occur despite prophylaxis. Oral acyclovir also hastens recovery from severe recurrent episodes. Cervical shedding of HSV from active lesions late in pregnancy, near the time of parturition, is an indication for cesarean section. This is especially true in primary HSV infection, which carries the greatest risk of neonatal infection. The risk to neonates exposed to asymptomatic shedding of HSV during parturition is uncertain.

Syphilis

Syphilis is of unique importance among the venereal diseases because early lesions heal without specific therapy; however, serious systemic sequelae pose a major risk to the patient, and transplacental infections can occur.

Epidemiology

Primary syphilis occurs mostly in sexually active 15- to 30-year-olds, and the incidence of primary syphilis has increased sharply in North America during the past decade. Approximately 50% of the sexual contacts of a patient with primary syphilis become infected. The long incubation period of syphilis becomes a key factor in designing strategies for contact tracing and management. Unless successful follow-up seems certain, contacts of proven cases must be treated with penicillin. Unfortunately, the most rapid increase in syphilis has occurred in groups of individuals at increased risk of HIV infection. This poses a serious problem, since the mucosal lesions of primary syphilis facilitate transmission of HIV infection (see Chapter 108). In turn, HIV appears to accelerate the course of syphilis with more rapid and frequent involvement of the neurologic system.

Pathogenesis

Treponema pallidum penetrates intact mucous membranes or abraded skin, reaches the blood stream via the lymphatics, and disseminates. The incubation period for the primary lesion depends on inoculum size, with a range of 3 to 90 days.

Natural History and Clinical Presentation

Primary syphilis is considered in Table 107–1.

Secondary syphilis develops 6 to 8 weeks after the chancre, if it has not been treated. This time period can be accelerated in HIV-infected persons. Skin, mucous membranes, and lymph nodes are involved. Skin lesions may be macular, papular, papulosquamous, pustular, follicular, or nodular. Most commonly, they are generalized, symmetric, and of like size, and they appear as discrete, erythematous, macular lesions of the thorax or as red-brown hyperpigmented macules on the palms and soles. In moist intertriginous areas, large, pale, flat-topped papules coalesce to form highly infectious plaques or condylomata lata; darkfield microscopy reveals that they are teeming with spirochetes. Mucous patches are painless, dull erythematous patches or grayish-white erosions. They, too, are infectious and darkfield-positive. Systemic manifestations of secondary syphilis include malaise, anorexia, weight loss, fever, sore throat, arthralgias, and generalized, nontender, discrete adenopathy. Specific organ involvement also may develop: gastritis (superficial, erosive); hepatitis; nephritis or nephrosis (immune complex–mediated, remits spontaneously or with treatment of syphilis); and symptomatic or asymptomatic meningitis. One fourth of patients have relapses of the mucocutaneous syndrome within 2 years of onset. Thereafter, infected patients become asymptomatic and noninfectious except via blood transfusions or transplacental spread.

Late syphilis develops after 1 to 10 years in 15% of untreated patients. The skin gumma is a superficial nodule or deep granulomatous lesion that may develop punched-out ulcers. Superficial gummas respond dramatically to therapy. Gummas also may involve bone, liver, and the cardiovascular or central nervous system. Deep-seated gummas may have serious pathophysiologic consequences; treatment of the infection often does not reverse organ dysfunction.

Gradually progressive cardiovascular syphilis begins within 10 years in more than 10% of untreated patients, most frequently men. Patients develop aortitis with medial necrosis secondary to an obliterative endarteritis of the vasa vasorum. There may be asymptomatic linear calcifications of the ascending aorta or (in decreasing frequency) aortic regurgitation, aortic aneurysms (saccular or fusiform, most commonly thoracic), or obstruction of coronary ostia.

Central nervous system (CNS) syphilis develops in 8% of untreated patients 5 to 35 years following primary infection and includes meningovascular syphilis, tabes dorsalis, and general paresis (see Chapter 120). Although general paresis and tabes are classified as separate neurologic syndromes, many patients show elements of both. Late CNS syphilis also may be asymptomatic despite cerebrospinal fluid (CSF) abnormalities indicating active inflammation. The natural history of syphilis may be dramatically altered by coinfection with HIV. Patients with dual infections may develop signs and symptoms of secondary syphilis more rapidly, sometimes even before healing of the primary chancre (see Chapter 108).

Diagnosis and Treatment

The clinical diagnosis of syphilis must be confirmed by darkfield examination and/or serologies. Spirochetes are seen in darkfield preparations of chancres or moist lesions of secondary syphilis. Saprophytic treponemes confuse darkfield diagnosis of oral lesions. Serologic diagnosis is considered in Table 107–2. The differential diagnosis of primary syphilis consists of herpes simplex and three conditions that are relatively rare in the United States: chancroid, lymphogranuloma venereum, and granuloma inguinale. The characteristics of these diseases are presented in Table 107–1.

The presence of neurosyphilis requires modifying the standard antibiotic treatment of syphilis. For this reason, a lumbar puncture should be considered in all patients with latent syphilis (positive Venereal Disease Research Laboratory [VDRL] test at least 1 year after primary syphilis) or syphilis of unknown duration. An elevated CSF white blood cell count, elevated protein, and positive VDRL test on diluted samples of CSF establish the diagnosis of neurosyphilis. A patient with persistent positive blood VDRL and a positive CSF VDRL should be considered to have neurosyphilis and treated accordingly. However, the sensitivity of CSF VDRL in proven cases of neurosyphilis is only 40 to 50%. Treatment for neurosyphilis is therefore indicated in patients with a consistent neurologic syndrome, characteristic CSF changes, and a positive serum VDRL. Because the VDRL may be negative in late syphilis, the presence of a positive serum fluorescent treponemal antibody absorption (FTA-ABS) test in a patient with a neurologic syndrome consistent with syphilis is a sufficient indication for treatment. A small proportion (2 to 3%) of patients with neurosyphilis may undergo abrupt deterioration following treatment with penicillin; this Jarisch-Herxheimer reaction, thought to represent a systemic response to penicillin-induced lysis of spirochetes, may be ameliorated by concomitant treatment with corticosteroids. This is especially important in secondary syphilis with meningeal involvement. After treatment of neurosyphilis, lumbar puncture should be repeated at 6-month intervals

TABLE 107–2	Serologies in Syphilis	
	VDRL	**FTA–ABS**
Technique	Standard nontreponemal test; antibody to cardiolipin-lecithin	Standard treponemal test; antibody to Nichol's strain of *Treponema pallidum* after absorption on nontreponemal spirochetes
Indications	Screening and assessing response to therapy; should be quantified by diluting serum	Confirmation of specificity of positive VDRL; remains reactive longer than VDRL; useful for late syphilis, particularly neurosyphilis
Percent positive in syphilis		
Primary	77%	86%
Secondary	98%	100%
Early latent	95%	99%
Late latent and late	73%	96%
False positives	Weakly reactive VDRL is common (ca. 30% of normals); positive VDRL should be repeated and, if confirmed, FTA–ABS performed; relative frequency of false positives determined by prevalence of syphilis in the population	Borderline positive is frequent (80%) in pregnancy; should be repeated

FTA–ABS = Fluorescent treponemal antibody absorption; VDRL = Venereal Disease Research Laboratory.

for 3 years to ensure adequacy of treatment, as reflected by normalization of CSF and progressive decline in CSF VDRL titer. Retreatment may be necessary if CSF abnormalities persist or recur. Treatment protocols are shown in Table 107–3.

TABLE 107–3	Treatment for Syphilis in the Normal Host	
Clinical Category	**Regimen of Choice**	**History of Penicillin Allergy**
Primary Secondary Early latent Healthy contact*	Benzathine penicillin, 2.4 MU IM	Tetracycline or erythromycin, 2 gm/day times 15 days
Late latent or late	Benzathine penicillin, 2.4 MU IM q week times 3	No regimen adequately evaluated; ? tetracycline or erythromycin, 2 gm/day times 30 days
Neurosyphilis	Aqueous penicillin G, 20 MU IV qd times 10 days	Same as for late latent or late

* Contact of patient with active skin or mucous membrane lesions.
IM = Intramuscularly; IV = intravenously; MU = million units.

Syphilis serologies must be followed after treatment. With the recommended treatment schedules, 1 to 5% of patients with primary syphilis will develop relapse or be reinfected. In adequately treated primary syphilis, the VDRL should become negative by 2 years after therapy (usually by 6 to 12 months). The FTA-ABS, however, often remains positive for life. Seventy-five percent of adequately treated patients with secondary syphilis will have a negative serum VDRL by 2 years. If the VDRL does not become negative or achieve a low fixed titer, lumbar puncture should be performed to evaluate the possibility of asymptomatic neurosyphilis, and the patient should be retreated with penicillin. Two to ten percent of patients with CNS syphilis will relapse following treatment. However, it is rare for asymptomatic patients to develop symptomatic disease after penicillin therapy; the only major exception is the HIV-infected patient, in whom meningovascular syphilis can develop within months of the standard treatment for primary syphilis. Every patient who is treated for syphilis should be seronegative or *serofast* with a low fixed titer before termination of follow-up. If not, therapy should be repeated.

Because of the documented progression to neurosyphilis in some HIV-infected individuals who have received treatment for primary syphilis, the following approach is suggested. All patients with syphilis should be tested for HIV infection. All HIV-infected individuals should be tested for syphilis. If dual infection is likely or documented, a lumbar puncture is indicated regardless of the stage or activity of the syphilis. Any CSF abnormality warrants a 10- to 14-day course of intravenous penicillin to treat neurosyphilis. If the CSF is unremarkable, three weekly doses of benzathine penicillin plus a 10-day course of amoxicillin may be appropriate. In any event, careful clinical and laboratory follow-up is essential.

URETHRITIS, CERVICITIS, AND PELVIC INFLAMMATORY DISEASE (PID)

These syndromes can be considered broadly as gonococcal and nongonococcal in etiology.

Gonorrhea

Neisseria gonorrhoeae is second only to *C. trachomatis* as a cause of sexually transmitted diseases in the United States, and the incidence of gonorrhea has risen sharply in the past decade. An estimated 2 million cases now occur annually in the United States.

Epidemiology

The incidence of gonorrhea reached a plateau in the United States between 1975 and 1980, possibly reflective of a decrease in the size of the at-risk cohort. Reinfection is common, and it is not unusual for one sexually active patient to have 20 or more discrete infections. Particular risk factors are urban habitat, low socioeconomic status, unmarried status, and large numbers of unprotected sexual contacts. Fifty percent of females having intercourse with a male with gonococcal urethritis will develop symptomatic infection. The risk for males is 20% after a single sexual contact with an infected female. Orogenital contact and anal intercourse also transmit infection. Asymptomatic infection of males is an important factor in transmission. Forty percent of male contacts of symptomatic women have asymptomatic urethritis. If untreated, about one quarter develop symptomatic infection within 7 days; a like number spontaneously become culture-negative within this period. The rest remain culture-positive and asymptomatic but capable of transmitting infection for periods of up to 6 months. Coinfection with *C. trachomatis* is observed in up to 30 to 40% of patients with gonorrhea.

Pathogenesis

Neisseria gonorrhoeae is a gram-negative, kidney bean–shaped diplococcus. Specialized projections from the organism, pili, aid in attachment to mucosal surfaces, contribute to resistance to killing by neutrophils, and constitute an important virulence factor. Production of an IgA protease by the organism contributes to pathogenicity. In females, several factors alter susceptibility to infection. Group B blood type increases susceptibility, whereas diverse factors such as vaginal colonization with normal flora, IgA content of vaginal secretions, and high progesterone levels may be protective. Spread from the cervix to the upper genital tract is associated with menstruation because changes in the pH and biochemical constituents of cervical mucus lead to increased shedding of gonococci; cervical dilation, reflux of menses, and binding of the gonococcus to spermatozoa may be additional factors in ascending genital infection and dissemination. Intrauterine contraceptive devices increase the risk of endometrial spread of infection twofold to ninefold (oral contraceptives are associated with a twofold decrease).

Clinical Presentation

In males who develop symptomatic urethritis, disturbing symptoms of spontaneous purulent discharge and severe dysuria usually develop 2 to 7 days after sexual contact. Prompt treatment usually follows, so that more extensive genital involvement is uncommon.

In females, cervicitis is the most frequent manifestation and results in a copious yellow vaginal discharge. Overall, 20% of females with gonococcal cervicitis develop PID, usually beginning at a time close to the onset of menstruation. PID is manifest as endometritis (abnormal menses, midline abdominal pain), salpingitis (bilateral lower abdominal pain and tenderness), or pelvic peritonitis. Salpingitis can cause tubal occlusion and sterility. Gonococcal perihepatitis (Fitz-Hugh–Curtis syndrome) also may complicate PID and present as right upper-quadrant pain.

Females also may develop urethritis with dysuria and frequency. In certain populations of sexually active women, one fourth of women complaining of urinary tract symptoms and 60% of those with symptoms but no bacteriuria have urethral cultures positive for *N. gonorrhoeae.*

Anorectal gonorrhea occurs in homosexual males and heterosexual females who practice receptive anal intercourse. In males, the resultant rectal pain, tenesmus, mucopurulent discharge, and bleeding may represent the only site of infection. Anorectal infection may be recognized only by cultures of asymptomatic contacts of patients with gonorrhea. In females, asymptomatic anorectal involvement is a frequent complication of symptomatic genitourinary disease even in the absence of anal intercourse (44%); isolated anorectal infection (4%) as well as acute or chronic proctitis (2 to 5%) is rare. Treatment failures are frequent in anorectal gonorrhea (7 to 35%).

Because of the frequency of asymptomatic infection in each of the potential sites, patients with symptoms suggestive of gonococcal infection should have cultures from the urethra, anus, pharynx, and (when applicable) cervix.

Pharyngeal gonorrhea occurs in homosexual males or heterosexual females following fellatio and less frequently in heterosexual males. Symptoms of pharyngitis occurring in this setting may be due to associated trauma or to gonococcal pharyngitis. Pharyngeal gonorrhea rarely is the sole site of gonococcal infection (5 to 8%). Infection of the pharynx is important, however, as a source of dissemination, particularly in males.

Extragenital dissemination occurs in approximately 1% of males and 3% of females with gonorrhea. Strains of *N. gonorrhoeae* causing dissemination differ from other gonococci in several respects. They are generally more penicillin-sensitive and resist the normal bactericidal activity of antibody and complement. The latter finding may be due to their binding of a naturally occurring blocking antibody. Complement deficiency states can predispose infected patients to disseminated gonorrhea. Dissemination of gonococcal infection may take the form of the *arthritis-dermatitis syndrome,* with 3 to 20 papular, petechial, pustular, necrotic, or hemorrhagic skin lesions, usually found on the extensor surfaces of the distal extremities. An associated finding is an asymmetric polytenosynovitis, with or without arthritis, which predominantly involves wrists, fingers, knees, and ankles. Joint fluid cultures usually are negative in the arthritis-dermatitis syndrome, leading to speculation that circulating immune complexes, demonstrable in most patients, are important in its pathogenesis. Synovial biopsies may yield positive cultures. Biopsy of skin lesions reveals gonococcal antigens (by immunofluorescent antibody staining) in two thirds of cases. Blood cultures are positive in 50%. Septic arthritis is another manifestation of dissemination; *N. gonorrhoeae* is the most frequent cause of septic arthritis in 16- to 50-year-olds. Sometimes the history indicates an antecedent syndrome suggestive of bacteremia. The joint fluid cultures usually are positive (particularly when the leukocyte count in joint fluid exceeds 80,000/μl), and blood cultures are usually negative. Gonococcemia rarely may lead to endocarditis, meningitis, myopericarditis, or toxic hepatitis.

Laboratory Diagnosis and Management

Gram's stain of the urethral discharge will determine the cause of urethritis in most males with gonorrhea, since typical intracellular diplococci are diagnostic (Fig. 107–1). The finding of only extracellular gram-negative diplococci is equivocal. The absence of gonococci on a smear of urethral discharge from a male virtually excludes the diagnosis. Diagnosis by Gram's staining of cervical exudates is relatively specific but insensitive (<60%). Modified Thayer-Martin medium contains antibiotics that inhibit the growth of other organisms and increase the yield of gonococci from samples likely to be contaminated; it is not necessary for culture of normally sterile fluids, such as joint fluid, blood, and CSF. Specimens from these sites should be cultured on chocolate agar. The addition of 3% trimethoprim to Thayer-Martin medium inhibits fecal *Proteus* and is useful for anorectal cultures. Other important considerations for the isolation of gonococci include the use of synthetic swabs (unsaturated fatty acids in cotton may be inhibitory), the introduction of a very thin calcium alginate swab or a loop 2 cm into the male urethra, and the avoidance of vaginal douching (12 hours), urination (2 hours), and vaginal speculum lubricants before culture. In all suspected cases of gonorrhea, the urethra, anus, and pharynx should be cultured. In females, 20% of cases in which initial cervical cultures were negative yield *N. gonorrhoeae* when cultures are repeated. Gene probes may also detect gono-

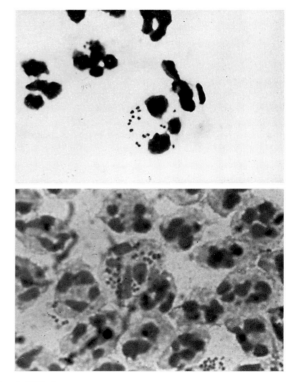

Figure 107–1
Gram's stain of urethral discharge showing typical intracellular diplococci associated with neutrophils.

coccal DNA but are less sensitive than culture in diagnosis.

Gonococcal resistance to penicillin is increasing worldwide. The current recommendation for the treatment of uncomplicated gonorrhea is ceftriaxone, 250 mg given intramuscularly once. This should be followed by a course of doxycycline (100 mg po twice daily for 7 days) to treat concurrent chlamydial infection. Alternative therapies include cefixime, 400 mg once orally, ciprofloxacin, 500 mg once orally, or ofloxacin, 400 mg once. Quinolones are contraindicated in pregnancy. In patients with severe beta-lactam allergies, spectinomycin, 2 gm intramuscularly, can be utilized; this is inadequate therapy for pharyngeal infection. PID should be treated with cefoxitin, 2 gm given intramuscularly, followed by doxycycline, 100 mg twice daily administered orally for 10 days. Seriously ill females with PID should be hospitalized. If they appear toxic, the initial antibiotic regimens should be broad-spectrum. Evaluation by ultrasonography for the presence of a pelvic abscess or peritonitis usually is warranted in this setting. Surgery may be indicated to drain a tubo-ovarian or pelvic abscess.

Disseminated gonococcal infection should be treated with ceftriaxone, 1 gm every 24 hours for 10 days. Cephalosporins should not be used, however, if the history suggests an IgE-mediated allergy to penicillin (anaphylactoid reaction, angioedema, urticaria). In such a case, ciprofloxacin, 500 mg twice daily for 7 days, is an effective alternative.

A VDRL should be obtained in all patients with gonorrhea. If negative, no further follow-up is necessary, since ceftriaxone in the dosage used is probably effective in treating incubating syphilis. This is not true of therapy with all alternative drugs; if they are used, the VDRL should be repeated after 4 weeks. Anal cultures should be part of the routine follow-up of females, since persistent anorectal carriage may be the source of relapse. Postgonococcal urethritis occurs in 30 to 50% of males 2 to 3 weeks after penicillin therapy, if it is not followed by tetracycline. It usually is caused by *C. trachomatis* or *Ureaplasma urealyticum.*

Nongonococcal Urethritis, Cervicitis, and PID

The diagnosis of nongonococcal urethritis (NGU) requires the exclusion of gonorrhea, since considerable overlap exists in the clinical syndromes.

Epidemiology

At least as many cases of urethritis are nongonococcal as gonococcal. Typically, NGU predominates in higher socioeconomic groups. *C. trachomatis* causes 30 to 50% of NGU and can be isolated from 0 to 11% of asymptomatic, sexually active males. *C. trachomatis* also can be isolated from 30% of males with gonorrhea and presumably represents a concurrent infection. Some cases of *Chlamydia*-negative NGU are due to *U. urealyticum* or *Trichomonas vaginalis.*

Clinical Syndromes

Nongonococcal urethritis is less contagious than gonococcal infection. The incubation period is 7 to 14 days. Characteristically, patients complain of urethral discharge, itching, and dysuria. Importantly, the discharge is not spontaneous but becomes apparent after milking the urethra in the morning. The mucopurulent discharge consists of thin, cloudy fluid with purulent specks; these characteristics do not always allow clear distinction from gonococcal disease. *T. vaginalis* causes a typically scanty discharge.

C. trachomatis also is a common cause of epididymitis in males under 35 years of age and can produce proctitis in men and women who practice receptive anal intercourse.

Chlamydial infections are also more common than gonococcal infections in females but frequently escape detection. Two thirds of women with mucopurulent cervicitis have chlamydial infection. Similarly, many females with the acute onset of dysuria, frequency, and pyuria, but sterile bladder urine, have *C. trachomatis* infection. *C. trachomatis* is at least as common a cause of salpingitis as is the gonococcus.

Laboratory Diagnosis

Ordinarily, the distinction between gonococcal and nongonococcal infections relies mainly on Gram-stained preparations of exudate and cultures. In a male with urethritis and typical gram-negative diplococci associated with neutrophils, the diagnosis of gonococcal urethritis is clear-cut and the culture is unnecessary. Coincident NGU cannot be excluded, however. Whenever interpretation of the Gram stain is not straightforward in males, and in all females, culture on Thayer-Martin medium is appropriate. Techniques for isolation and detection of chlamydiae are widely available and should be used routinely in evaluating genital infections.

Treatment

The patient and all sexual contacts should be treated with a 7-day course of tetracycline, 500 mg 4 times a day, or doxycycline, 100 mg twice a day, given orally. Recur-

TABLE 107–4	Organisms Causing Proctocolitis in Male Homosexuals
	Neisseria gonorrhoeae
	Chlamydia trachomatis
	Herpesvirus hominis
	Treponema pallidum
	Shigella species
	Salmonella species
	Campylobacter species
	Entamoeba histolytica
	Giardia lamblia
	Strongyloides stercoralis

| TABLE 107–5 | Vaginitis | | | |

Disease	Epidemiology/ Pathogenesis	Clinical Findings	Laboratory Diagnosis	Treatment
Candidiasis	Yeast are part of normal flora; overgrowth favored by broad-spectrum antibiotics, high estrogen levels (pregnancy, before menses, oral contraceptives), diabetes mellitus, may be early clue to HIV infection	Itching, little or no urethral discharge, occasional dysuria; labia pale or erythematous with satellite lesions; vaginal discharge thick, adherent, with white curds; balanitis in 10% of male contacts	Vaginal pH = 4.5 (normal), negative whiff test, yeast seen on wet mount in 50%, culture positive	Miconazole, butoconazole, or clotrimazole cream or suppositories for 3–7 days
Trichomonas vaginalis infection	STD; incubation 5–28 days; symptoms begin or exacerbate with menses	Discharge, soreness, irritation, mild dysuria, dyspareunia; copious loose discharge, one fifth yellow/green, one third bubbly	Elevated pH; wet mount shows large numbers of WBCs, trichomonads; positive whiff test (10% KOH causes fishy odor)	Metronidazole, 2 gm as single dose; treat sexual contacts
Bacterial vaginosis	Synergistic infection, *Gardnerella vaginalis* and anaerobes (*Mobiluncus* sp.)	Vaginal odor, mild discharge, little inflammation; grayish, thin, homogeneous discharge with small bubbles	Elevated pH; positive whiff test; wet prep contains clue cells (vaginal epithelial cells with intracellular coccobacilli), few WBCs	Metronidazole, 500 mg bid times 7 days; do not treat contacts unless recurrent vaginitis

HIV = Human immunodeficiency virus; KOH = potassium hydroxide; STD = sexually transmitted disease; WBCs = white blood cells.

rence may occur and requires longer periods (2 to 3 weeks) of treatment. Azithromycin given as a single oral dose of 1 gm is highly effective and associated with markedly improved compliance.

Proctocolitis in Homosexual Males

Male homosexuals who practice receptive anal intercourse may present with proctitis/proctocolitis causing anorectal pain, mucoid or bloody discharge, tenesmus, diarrhea, or abdominal pain. Sigmoidoscopy should be performed with culture and Gram's stain of the discharge. Potential causative organisms are shown in Table 107–4. The diarrheal syndromes are considered in Chapter 103. Ten percent of patients harbor two or more pathogens. Proctitis also may occur in male homosexuals without a definable pathogen (42%). Diarrhea in the patient infected with HIV has an entirely different set of implications, as will be discussed in Chapter 108.

Vaginitis

Table 107–5 considers salient features in the diagnosis and management of patients with vaginitis.

REFERENCES

Centers for Disease Control and Prevention: STD treatment guideline project, 1993 sexually transmitted diseases treatment guideline. MMWR 1993; 42:(RR-14):1–103.
Cohen MS, Hook EW III, Hitchcock PJ: Sexually transmitted diseases in the AIDS era. Infect Dis Clin North Am 1993; 7:739–914, and 1994; 8:751–925.
Sparling PF, Hook EW: Sexually transmitted diseases. *In* Bennett JC, Plum F (eds.): Cecil Textbook of Medicine. 20th ed. Philadelphia, WB Saunders Co, 1995, pp 1696–1713.

108

HIV Infection and the Acquired Immunodeficiency Syndrome

The acquired immunodeficiency syndrome (AIDS) is the expression of a spectrum of disorders caused by cellular and humoral immune dysfunction resulting from infection by the human immunodeficiency virus (HIV-1). Since the reports in 1981 of multiple cases of *Pneumocystis carinii* pneumonia and Kaposi's sarcoma in homosexual men in California and New York, epidemiologic, virologic, and clinical investigations have clearly demonstrated that the AIDS pandemic is attributable to sexual, parenteral, and perinatal transmission of HIV-1. By 1996 more than 20 million persons had been infected worldwide, and the World Health Organization estimates that this number will increase to 40 to 100 million by the year 2000.

EPIDEMIOLOGY

Acquired immunodeficiency syndrome was first recognized as a distinct clinical syndrome in previously healthy men who had serious infections with unusual opportunistic pathogens, most frequently *Pneumocystis carinii* pneumonia, previously seen only among patients with severe cellular immunodeficiency. Laboratory studies confirmed profound cell-mediated immunodeficiency in these individuals, leading to the name acquired immunodeficiency syndrome.

As similar opportunistic infections were subsequently observed in injecting drug users and men with hemophilia and their female sexual partners, it became clear that this syndrome was caused by an agent transmissible via sexual contact or through parenteral infusion of contaminated blood or blood products. Since HIV-1 was identified in 1983–84 as the causative agent of AIDS, recognition of a wide spectrum of disease has emerged, ranging from asymptomatic viremia to severe immunocompromise with life-threatening opportunistic infections and/or neoplasms.

The Centers for Disease Control and Prevention (CDC) surveillance criteria for the diagnosis of AIDS, as modified in 1987, included a large number of opportunistic infections (Table 108–1) indicative of a defect in cellular immunity as well as certain neoplasms and other conditions associated with advanced HIV-1 infection (Table 108–2). The occurrence of any one of these condi-

tions in an individual with no other cause of immunosuppression constituted the diagnosis of AIDS. In 1992, the CDC broadened the surveillance definition of AIDS to include all HIV-infected persons with severely depressed levels of cell-mediated immunity as indicated by CD4+ T helper lymphocyte counts (CD4 counts) less than 200/mm^3; the CDC also added invasive carcinoma of the cervix, active pulmonary tuberculosis, and recurrent bacterial pneumonia as AIDS-indicating diagnoses in HIV-1 infected individuals. By 1993, AIDS had become the leading cause of death of American adults aged 25 to 44 (Fig. 108–1). By the end of 1996, over one-half million HIV-1 infected persons in the United States had met the CDC criteria for the diagnosis of AIDS.

Once HIV-1 was identified as the causative agent of AIDS, retrospective studies of stored serum specimens revealed that HIV-1 had been present in parts of Central Africa for two decades prior to the recognition of the clinical syndrome of AIDS. During the 1980s and 1990s, the HIV-1 epidemic spread widely and became a worldwide pandemic. Seroprevalence studies indicate that HIV-1 infection continues to spread, albeit at strikingly different rates, throughout all continents. Exceptionally rapid transmission occurred from 1988 through 1996 in several areas of South Asia, particularly in India and Thailand. By 1996, no nation in the world was free of AIDS.

Although AIDS was initially recognized among sexually active homosexual males and intravenous drug users in the United States, heterosexual contact has been the dominant mode of HIV-1 transmission throughout most of the world, accounting for more than 90% of infections recognized since 1990. The virus is present in both semen and cervicovaginal secretions and can be transmitted both from man to woman and from woman to man during vaginal intercourse. The concurrent presence of other sexually transmissible diseases (STDs), especially those associated with genital ulcerations, strongly facilitates sexual transmission of HIV-1.

Free and cell-associated virus is present in the blood of infected patients. Thus, prior to the nationwide implementation of a blood screening test in late 1985, infection via transfusion of contaminated blood or blood products

TABLE 108–1	Opportunistic Infections Indicative of a Defect in Cellular Immune Function Associated with Acquired Immunodeficiency Syndrome (AIDS)

Protozoan Infection

Pneumocystis carinii pneumonia
Disseminated toxoplasmosis, or Toxoplasma encephalitis, excluding congenital infection
Chronic Cryptosporidium enteritis (>1 mo)
Chronic Isospora belli enteritis (>1 mo)

Fungal Infection

Candida esophagitis
Cryptococcal meningitis or disseminated infection
Disseminated histoplasmosis*
Disseminated coccidioidomycosis*

Bacterial Infection

Disseminated Mycobacterium avium-intracellulare or Mycobacterium kansasii
Extrapulmonary Mycobacterium tuberculosis*
Active pulmonary tuberculosis*
Recurrent Salmonella septicemia*
Recurrent bacterial pneumonia*

Viral Infection

Chronic (>1 mo) mucocutaneous herpes simplex or bronchial or esophageal herpes simplex
Histologically evident cytomegalovirus infection of any organ except liver, spleen, or lymph nodes
Progressive multifocal leukoencephalopathy secondary to JC virus

Helminthic Infection

Strongyloidiasis (disseminated beyond the gastrointestinal tract)

---

* Requires laboratory evidence of human immunodeficiency virus (HIV) infection.

group in which HIV infection is increasing most rapidly in the United States; 20% of new AIDS cases in 1996 occurred in women. In some Northeastern cities, as well as in several rural areas in the Southeast, women accounted for over one third of new cases in 1996.

The sharing of needles used for drug injection transmits the virus efficiently and continues to be a major mode of spread of HIV-1 infection in North America and Western Europe. Because of the concentration of injecting drug users in impoverished inner-city areas, a disproportionate number of North American women infected by HIV-1 are African-American or Latina. Differences in regional patterns of intravenous drug use largely explain the greater than one hundredfold regional variation in prevalence of AIDS cases in the United States (Fig. 108–2).

Heterosexual transmission has played a large role in the rapid rise of neonatal HIV-1 infection. HIV-1 transmission may occur in utero, during labor, or, less frequently, after birth through breast-feeding. Twenty-five to thirty percent of infants born to HIV-1 seropositive mothers who are not receiving antiretroviral therapy are infected by HIV-1. Seroprevalence surveys at prenatal clinics in several North American cities have indicated that up to 3% of pregnant women are HIV-1 infected. Of particular concern, more than half of these women were not aware that they were at risk for HIV infection.

HIV-1 infection also has occurred after accidental parenteral exposures of health care workers to the blood of HIV-1 infected patients. After injury by a needle exposed to the blood of an HIV-1 infected patient, the risk of infection is approximately 0.3%. The possibility that

(e.g., Factors VIII and IX for hemophiliacs) accounted for nearly 3% of AIDS cases in the United States. Since 1985, all blood products in North America have been screened for evidence of antibodies to HIV-1 prior to administration. Factor VIII and Factor IX concentrates are also now heat-treated to inactivate HIV. The risk of transfusion-acquired HIV-1 infection in North America and Western Europe is now extremely small, but not absent. Persons recently infected with HIV-1 may still donate blood during the weeks before they develop detectable HIV-1 antibodies, resulting in false-negative screening tests; these instances are rare.

Because of the long latency between HIV-1 infection and AIDS-associated illnesses, the clinically recognized epidemic of AIDS has lagged 8 to 10 years behind the spread of the virus into new populations. Homosexual and bisexual men accounted for approximately three quarters of the cases of AIDS in North America through 1985; by 1996 this group accounted for a minority of AIDS cases in the United States. Through 1985, fewer than 1% of the cases of AIDS in the United States were acquired through heterosexual contact; by 1996, heterosexual transmission accounted for more than 20% of the cases of AIDS and a considerably higher proportion of persons with asymptomatic HIV infection. From 1981 through 1985, fewer than 4% of AIDS cases in the United States occurred in women. Women are now the

TABLE 108–2	Other Conditions Fulfilling Criteria for AIDS

Condition	Comments
Neoplasm	
Kaposi's sarcoma (in a person <60 yr old)	Most commonly present in homosexual males in US; uncommon among other risk groups
High-grade, B-cell non-Hodgkin's lymphoma* (e.g., Burkitt's lymphoma) Undifferentiated non-Hodgkin's lymphoma* Immunoblastic sarcoma* Primary brain lymphoma*	Limited to brain; may be multicentric
Invasive carcinoma of the cervix*	Recognized as AIDS-defining condition in 1992
Systemic Illness	
HIV wasting syndrome*	Unintentional loss of >10% of body weight
Neurologic Impairment	
HIV encephalopathy*	Variety of symptoms, dementia most common (see text)

---

* Requires laboratory evidence of HIV infection.
AIDS = Acquired immunodeficiency syndrome; HIV = human immunodeficiency virus.

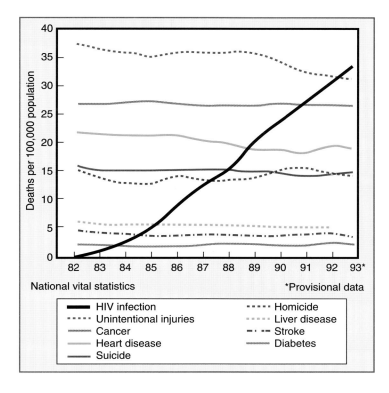

Figure 108-1

Death rates from leading causes in persons aged 25 to 44 years, United States, 1982–1993. Since 1993, acquired immunodeficiency syndrome (AIDS) has been the leading cause of death of Americans aged 25 to 44. HIV = Human immunodeficiency virus.

HIV-infected health care workers who perform invasive procedures may transmit HIV to patients has been carefully investigated; this risk, if present, is extremely small, as not one of several thousand systematically evaluated patients of HIV-infected dentists and surgeons has acquired HIV-1 infection this way.

A second human immunodeficiency virus (HIV-2) was identified in West Africa in the mid-1980s. Although HIV-2 infection also results in AIDS, the majority of known HIV-2-seropositive persons are asymptomatic. Current data support the concept that HIV-2 infection is less aggressive, with a considerably longer clinically latent period than HIV-1. Although HIV-2 shares many biologic and genetic characteristics with HIV-1, each of the two viruses also has regulatory and structural genes that are unique. HIV-2 is more closely related to the simian immunodeficiency virus (SIV) than to HIV-1. The rare HIV-2 infections in the United States to date have been of West African origin. Throughout the remainder of this chapter, the term HIV refers to the HIV-1 virus.

PATHOPHYSIOLOGY

Human immunodeficiency virus is a member of the lentivirus family of retroviruses which includes the agents of visna, equine infectious anemia virus, and the simian immunodeficiency virus (SIV). The core of HIV contains two single-stranded copies of the viral RNA genome, together with a virus-encoded enzyme reverse transcriptase (Fig. 108–3). Surrounding the core (p24) and matrix (p18) proteins is a lipid bilayer derived from the host cell, through which protrude the transmembrane (gp41) and surface (gp120) envelope glycoproteins.

The HIV envelope glycoproteins have a high affinity for the CD4 molecule on the surface of T helper lymphocytes and other cells of the monocyte/macrophage lineage. After HIV binds to cellular CD4, the viral and cellular membranes fuse, and the HIV nucleoprotein complex enters the cytoplasm. The RNA viral genome undergoes transcription by a virally encoded reverse transcriptase. The double-stranded proviral DNA gains entry into the nucleus, where integration of the DNA provirus into the host chromosome is catalyzed by another retroviral enzyme, integrase (Fig. 108–4). Within the host genome the provirus may remain in a latent state without appreciable transcription of RNA or synthesis of viral protein.

When a T helper lymphocyte containing integrated provirus is activated (e.g., by recognition of antigenic peptides or by binding of proinflammatory cytokines to their receptors), increased expression of HIV messenger RNA (mRNA) occurs. Virus-encoded regulatory proteins tat and rev facilitate mRNA expression and cytoplasmic transport, respectively. Core proteins, viral enzymes, and envelope proteins are encoded by the *gag, pol,* and *env* genes of HIV, respectively. Viral polyproteins are cleaved by viral-encoded proteases, and the envelope protein is glycosylated by host glycosylases. Viral particles are assembled, each containing two copies of unspliced mRNA within the core as the viral genome, and virions then are released from the cell by budding. Productive viral replication is lytic to infected T cells. A number of other host cells, including macrophages, dendritic cells, and Langerhans' cells also are infected by HIV, but these cells do not appear to be lysed by the virus. Infected macrophages may play a major role in the spread of HIV infection to other tissues, particularly the central nervous system.

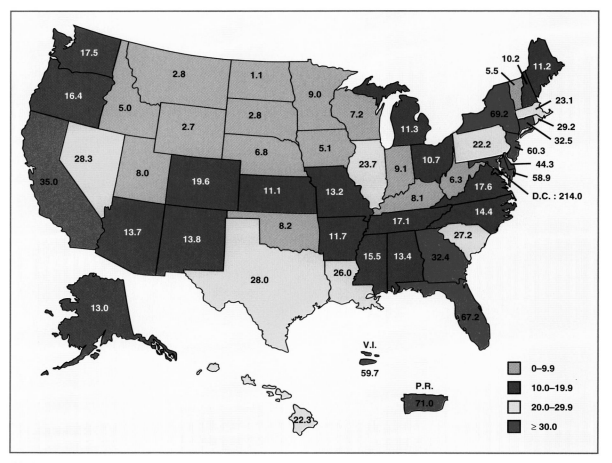

Figure 108–2

The number of acquired immunodeficiency syndrome (AIDS) cases per 100,000 population in the United States, July 1994 to June 1995, shows tremendous regional variation, from 214.0 in the District of Columbia to 1.1 in North Dakota. (From AIDS map. Morbid Mortal Weekly Rep: 1995; 44(38):719.)

Immune Deficiency in HIV Infection

During the first several years of HIV infection, the patient may feel entirely well, and may have only a modest fall in the peripheral CD4 lymphocyte count. During this period of clinical latency, however, rapid viral multiplication occurs. In the asymptomatic infected individual, over one billion new virions may be produced daily, while an equal number are removed from circulation through mechanisms not well understood. Rapid production and turnover of circulating CD4+ T helper cells (CD4 cells) also occur throughout the course of HIV infection. Although a highly dynamic complex equilibrium between HIV and CD4 cells may be maintained for several years, eventually circulating CD4 cells decline in the great majority of individuals; this is accompanied (or preceeded) by an increase in the plasma HIV viral load.

An HIV-1 specific immune response may contribute to stabilization of the rate of viral multiplication following the burst of plasma viremia during the initial weeks after primary HIV-1 infection (Fig. 108–5). During the subsequent months to years of clinical latency, virions are present in large numbers in the follicular dendritic pro-

cesses of the germinal centers of lymph nodes and spleen, which undergo intense hyperplasia. As HIV disease progresses over several years, the architecture of the lymphatic tissues is disrupted and plasma viremia intensifies. In later-stage HIV disease, there is virtual destruction of the host lymphoid tissue and persistent high-level viremia (see Fig. 108–5).

As HIV disease progresses, the decline in the number of CD4 cells is accompanied by a profound functional impairment of the remaining lymphocyte populations. Anergy—the failure to demonstrate delayed hypersensitivity to recall antigens—often develops early in HIV infection and eventually occurs in virtually all persons with AIDS. With development of anergy, T helper lymphocyte proliferation in response to antigenic stimuli is dramatically impaired, as is production of several lymphokines, including interleukin-2, interleukin-12, and interferon-gamma. T cell cytotoxic responses are diminished, and natural killer cell activity against virus-infected cells and tumor cells is impaired, despite normal or increased numbers of these cells. Despite a polyclonal or oligoclonal hypergammaglobulinemia, B lymphocyte function is also diminished, as measured by impaired ca-

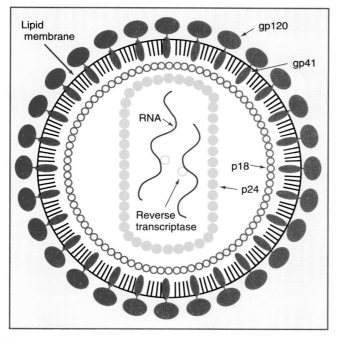

Figure 108-3
Structure of human immunodeficiency virus (HIV) (Adapted from "The AIDS virus," copyright © 1987 by Scientific American, Inc., George V. Kelvin, all rights reserved.)

pacity to synthesize antibody in response to new antigens. This immune dysfunction may be the result of decreases in both the number and function of CD4+ T helper lymphocytes. Although the precise mechanisms of immune deficiency in HIV disease are not completely understood, profound impairment of multiple arms of the immune system underlies the enhanced risk to HIV-infected persons of the opportunistic infections that are characteristic of AIDS.

Inadequacy of Host Defense Mechanisms

A characteristic feature of HIV infection is the ability of the virus to continue to multiply despite brisk host immune responses to the virus. Humoral responses to viral proteins are readily demonstrable in all infected persons. Neutralizing antibodies develop rapidly, but generally in relatively low titer when compared to neutralizing antibodies generated in response to other viral infections. Cell-mediated immune responses to several HIV-derived proteins are also readily demonstrated and are temporally associated with decreases in plasma viremia following acute HIV infection.

There are several possible explanations for the inability of host responses to control HIV infection. The viral replication cycle allows integrated provirus to persist in the host genome in a transcriptionally latent state, in which it is not recognizable by either humoral or cellular immune mechanisms (see Fig. 108–4). The CD4 binding domain of the HIV envelope, a relatively conserved natural target of neutralizing antibody, is apparently recessed

and relatively inaccessible. Other envelope regions are not conserved and vary among different isolates. HIV has tremendous potential for genetic alteration; in fact, genetic diversity of envelope epitopes is consistently observed among different viral isolates obtained from the same patient. Errors in retroviral reverse transcription underlie this high degree of genetic variability. One can easily envision how a selective pressure—for example, the development of antibodies against a nonconserved region of the envelope—can result in the emergence of viral mutants with altered envelope sequences resistant to the neutralizing activity of a specific antibody species. Genetic variability may prove the chief obstacle to both the development of an effective vaccine and long-term antiviral therapy.

DIAGNOSIS AND TESTING FOR HIV INFECTION

Since HIV transmission is preventable, antiretroviral therapy is increasingly effective, and prophylaxis against major opportunistic infections can be achieved, it is important that persons at risk for HIV infection undergo serologic testing. Testing should not be confined only to individuals at highest risk (e.g., injecting drug users) but should be encouraged in sexually active persons with any risk, including all persons with a history of STD and non-monogamous heterosexuals with current or past partners whose HIV status is unknown. Testing must be provided in an environment of confidentiality consistent with relevant state laws. Pretest and post-test counseling is essential to ensure that persons appreciate the importance and consequences of the test results, and are offered appropriate help. Regardless of the outcome of the test, all patients should be counseled regarding safer sexual practices. Injecting drug users should be advised not to share needles. HIV-infected persons must be encouraged to notify their sexual partners and persons with whom they have shared needles. This is often difficult; regional health authorities may be of great assistance in confidential notification of persons at risk.

Diagnosis of HIV infection is established by detection of serum antibody to HIV by enzyme-linked immunosorbent assay (ELISA), and is confirmed by Western blot. These techniques are very sensitive in detecting HIV antibody, but individuals who are recently infected may be antibody-negative. For recently exposed individuals whose initial ELISA test is negative, retesting at 6 weeks, 3 months, and 6 months is indicated. False-positive ELISA tests are rare. When they occur, they are most frequent among patients with autoimmune disorders. Western blot reactivity with at least two different HIV proteins confirms infection. In a person at high risk for HIV-1 exposure, an indeterminate Western blot reaction pattern often represents early seroconversion; in such cases, ELISA and Western blot testing should be repeated after 6 to 8 weeks.

Infants born to HIV-infected mothers who are not receiving antiretroviral therapy have a 25 to 30% risk of acquiring HIV infection, but all such babies have positive ELISA tests because of circulating maternal anti-HIV antibodies. Maternal antibodies disappear by age 6 months.

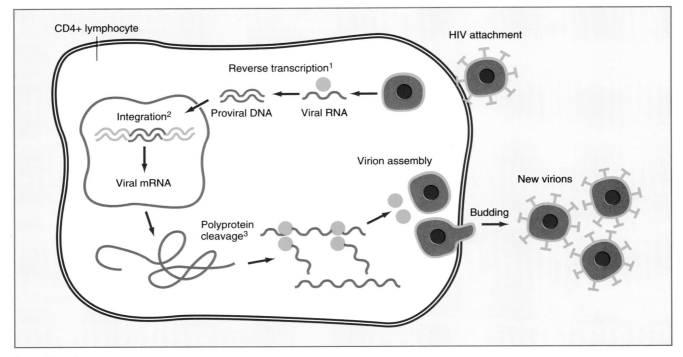

Figure 108–4

Elements of human immunodeficiency virus (HIV) replication cycle and sites of antiretroviral drugs. After attachment and entry into the host cell, HIV viral RNA is transcribed by HIV reverse transcriptase to double-stranded proviral DNA. Catalyzed by HIV integrase, the proviral DNA is integrated into the host genome. Proviral DNA, upon activation, is transcribed to produce genomic and messenger RNA (mRNA), which is translated into polyproteins. The polyproteins are cleaved by HIV protease. The resulting smaller proteins (p17, p24, etc. . . .) are assembled into virions at the host cell membrane, and complete the retroviral life cycle by budding.

[1]Site of action of reverse transcriptase inhibitors (see text).
[2]Site of action of integrase inhibitors (not yet in clinical trials).
[3]Site of action of protease inhibitors (see text).

Figure 108–5

Natural history of human immunodeficiency virus (HIV-1) infection in the adult. Note the long period of clinical latency following primary infection, the erratic but inexorable decline in CD4+ T lymphocyte count, and the uncertain progression of symptoms once profound immunodeficiency has occurred. (Modified from Fauci AS: Multifactorial nature of human immunodeficiency virus disease: implications for therapy. Science 1993; 262:1011, with permission.)

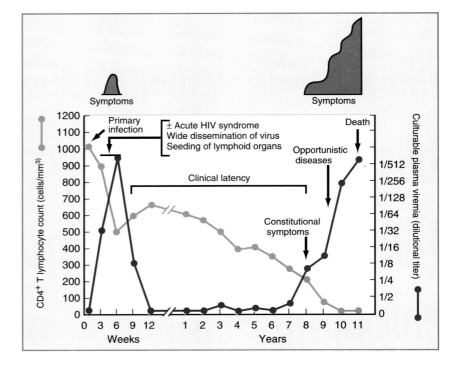

Early diagnosis of HIV-1 infection in this setting may be achieved by sensitive plasma HIV RNA assays or by detection of circulating HIV p24 antigen.

SEQUENTIAL CLINICAL MANIFESTATIONS OF HIV-1 INFECTION

Acute Retroviral Syndrome

Acute symptomatic illness may follow initial infection with HIV. Twenty to sixty percent of HIV-infected persons experience a mononucleosis-like syndrome from 2 to 8 weeks after initial infection (see Fig. 108–5). Acute symptoms of fever, sore throat, lymph node enlargement, arthralgias, and headache usually predominate and last 3 days to 3 weeks (Table 108–3). A maculopapular rash is common, short-lived, and usually affects the trunk or face. Neurologic involvement, documented by cerebrospinal-fluid (CSF) pleocytosis and isolation of HIV from CSF, may occur. Acute, self-limited aseptic meningitis is the most common clinical neurologic presentation, although meningoencephalitis, peripheral neuropathy, myelopathy, and Guillain-Barré syndrome may all occur during the acute retroviral illness.

During the acute retroviral syndrome, HIV antibody is generally not detectable, but HIV infection can be demonstrated by direct cultivation of HIV from blood, by plasma HIV RNA assays, or by detection of HIV p24 antigen in serum. Following HIV infection, within 4 to 12 weeks specific antibodies develop that are directed against the three main gene products of HIV: gag (p55, p24, p15), pol (p34, p68), and env (gp160, gp120, gp41).

Asymptomatic Phase

Human immunodeficiency virus infection usually results in a slow, often erratic, progression to severe immunodeficiency marked by progressive depletion of CD4 cells. Approximately 50% of individuals develop AIDS within 10 years after HIV infection (see Fig. 108–5); an additional 30% have milder symptoms related to immunodeficiency, and only 20% are entirely asymptomatic 10 years after infection. Progression of disease varies greatly among individuals and is also related to age at time of

TABLE 108–3	Acute HIV Retroviral Syndrome: Common Signs and Symptoms
Sign/Symptom	**Frequency (%)**
Fever	98
Lymph node enlargement	75
Sore throat	70
Rash	60
Myalgia or arthralgia	60
Headache	35

HIV = Human immunodeficiency virus.

infection. Adolescents with HIV progress to AIDS at a slower rate than older persons, with fewer than 30% developing AIDS within 10 years after HIV infection. In general, the rate of progression of immunodeficiency is not influenced by the route of HIV transmission. The plasma viral load (HIV RNA copies per ml of plasma) obtained 6 to 12 months after primary infection predicts the subsequent rate of disease progression.

The majority of individuals living with HIV infection, most of whom are unaware of their infection, are asymptomatic, with CD4 counts greater than 200 per mm³. Major life-threatening opportunistic infections seldom occur until the CD4 count is less than 200 per mm³. During the longest phase of the illness, when CD4 counts are greater than 200, dysregulation of the immune system is commonly manifested by increased polyclonal production of antibody (manifested as elevated gamma globulins). Despite the abundance of antibody, patients with HIV infection demonstrate a diminished antibody response to protein and polysaccharide antigens. This is manifest clinically by a three-fold to four-fold increase in incidence of bacterial pneumonias caused by common pulmonary pathogens such as *Streptococcus pneumoniae* and *Haemophilus influenzae*. Acute bacterial pneumonias are even more frequent in HIV-infected individuals who continue to inject heroin and/or cocaine.

Clinically recognized generalized lymph node enlargement occurs in 35 to 60% of asymptomatic HIV-infected persons, may persist for years, and is not associated with either the rate of progression of immunodeficiency or with development of lymphoma. During the early years of HIV infection, thrombocytopenia, probably due to autoimmune platelet destruction, is common. Mucocutaneous manifestations of immune dysfunction are frequent, especially recurrent oral or genital herpes simplex virus (HSV) infections (which are responsive to acyclovir therapy but may recur frequently), polydermatomal varicella-zoster infection, and oral hairy leukoplakia. Certain of these mucocutaneous manifestations (e.g., genital HSV infections) may become more frequent and severe as immune function deteriorates. Clinical manifestations of infection by *Mycobacterium tuberculosis* (which may be pulmonary, extrapulmonary, or disseminated) often occur with CD4 counts over 200.

Symptomatic Phase: Severe Immunosuppression

When the CD4 count drops below 200, patients are at high risk of developing multiple opportunistic infections (Table 108–4). For example, in the absence of specific prophylaxis, 60% of HIV-infected North American men develop *Pneumocystis carinii* pneumonia. Local or disseminated fungal infections with *Cryptococcus neoformans, Histoplasma capsulatum,* or *Coccidioides immitis* may occur. (The incidence of each infection varies, depending on geographic locale.) Protozoal infections with *Toxoplasma gondii* (encephalitis) or with *Cryptosporidium parvum* or *Isospora belli* (enteritis) may prove lethal.

TABLE 108–4	Relation of CD4 Lymphocyte Counts to the Onset of Certain HIV-Associated Infections and Neoplasms in North America	

CD4 Count Cells/mm³*	Opportunistic Infection or Neoplasm	Frequency (%)†
>500	Herpes zoster, polydermatomal	5–10
200–500	*Mycobacterium tuberculosis* infection, pulmonary and extrapulmonary	2–20
	Oral hairy leukoplakia	40–70
	Candida pharyngitis (thrush)	40–70
	Recurrent *Candida* vaginitis	15–30 (F)
	Kaposi's sarcoma, mucocutaneous	15–30 (M)
	Bacterial pneumonia, recurrent	15–20
	Cervical neoplasia	1–2 (F)
100–200	*Pneumocystis carinii* pneumonia	15–60
	Herpes simplex, chronic, ulcerative	5–10
	Histoplasmosis capsulatum infection, disseminated	0–20
	Kaposi's sarcoma, visceral	3–8 (M)
	Progressive multifocal leukoencephalopathy	2–3
	Lymphoma, non-Hodgkin's	2–5
<100	Candida esophagitis	15–20
	Mycobacterium avium-intracellulare, disseminated	25–40
	Toxoplasma gondii encephalitis	5–25
	Cryptosporidium enteritis	2–10
	Cytomegalovirus (CMV) retinitis	20–35
	Cryptococcus neoformans encephalitis	2–5
	CMV esophagitis or colitis	6–12
	Lymphoma, central nervous system (CNS)	4–8

* Table indicates CD4 count at which specific infections or neoplasms generally begin to appear. Each infection may recur or progress during the subsequent course of HIV disease.

† Even within the US, great regional differences in the incidence of specific opportunistic infections are apparent. For example, disseminated histoplasmosis is common in the Mississippi River drainage area, but very rare in individuals who have lived exclusively on the East or West Coast.

F = Exclusively in women; HIV = human immunodeficiency virus; M = almost exclusively in men.

Severe Immunodeficiency

CD4 counts under 50 indicate profound immunosuppression and are associated with a high mortality within the subsequent 24 to 36 months. Cytomegalovirus (CMV) infection of the retina or the gastrointestinal (GI) tract, disseminated *Mycobacterium avium-complex* (MAC) infection, and lymphoma occur frequently and usually respond only transiently to specific therapy.

Sex-Specific Manifestations

Several sex-specific-manifestations are relevant to the management of HIV infection in women. Recognition of sex-specific manifestations is especially important because they are rapidly responsive to specific therapy, if recognized early; each manifestation may serve as the signal for HIV testing in a person with no prior clinical manifestations of immunodeficiency.

1. The earliest clinical manifestation of HIV infection in women may be the new onset, or frequent recurrence, of *Candida* vaginitis in the absence of other predisposing factors. Since recurrent *Candida* vaginitis may develop at a time of moderate immunodeficiency (CD4 count above 200), it may serve as a trigger to discuss HIV testing and lead to earlier diagnosis in otherwise asymptomatic women.

2. Recurrent large painful genital, perianal, or perineal ulcers, caused by HSV-2, appear to be more frequent in women than in men. Occurring at a time of more advanced immunodeficiency, such lesions should always prompt HIV testing, as well as specific antiviral therapy (see Chapter 107).

3. A potentially life-threatening consequence of HIV infection in women may be early development of cervical dysplasia/neoplasia, which may result from impaired host defenses against the human papillomavirus (HPV). HIV-infected women who have had multiple sexual partners show an increased prevalence of high-grade squamous intracellular lesions (SIL) on cervicovaginal examination. Women with HIV infection should therefore obtain two Papanicolaou (Pap) smears at a 6-month interval; if the initial two Pap smears are both normal, repeat Pap smears should be done once a year. Conversely, women with high-grade SIL on Pap smear should be encouraged to undergo testing for HIV infection, in addition to the specific management of these lesions.

MANAGEMENT OF HIV INFECTION

Since patients are asymptomatic during most of the course of HIV-1 infection (see Fig. 108–5), and even seriously immunocompromised individuals often function productively between bouts of opportunistic infections, the ambulatory management of persons with HIV infection deserves major emphasis.

Initial Ambulatory Evaluation

Once an individual is found to be HIV-infected, the physician should discuss, in an unhurried manner, the manifestations of HIV infection and the use of immunologic and virologic studies (e.g., CD4 counts, viral load assays) to guide therapy. Perhaps most important, the physician should emphasize the fact that most patients, even without antiviral therapy, survive for 10 to 12 years after acquiring HIV infection and are asymptomatic during most of that time. The physician should also stress that the asymptomatic period can be extended by prophylaxis against opportunistic infections and by currently available antiviral drugs, and that additional promising new drugs are being evaluated in clinical trials.

Prevention of further transmission through unprotected sex and sharing of needles must be discussed not only at the first visit but also periodically thereafter. In this regard a complete history of STDs is important.

Initial evaluation should include both an HIV-oriented review of symptoms and a complete physical examination (Table 108–5). In particular, the skin must be examined for HIV-associated rashes and Kaposi's sarcoma. Examination of the oral cavity may reveal thrush, gingivitis, hairy leukoplakia, superficial ulcers caused by HSV, aphthous ulcers, or lesions characteristic of Kaposi's sarcoma. The optic fundi may reveal hemorrhagic lesions characteristic of CMV retinitis. Lymph node enlargement, hepatomegaly, splenomegaly, and any genital lesions should all be carefully noted. Neurologic examination for both peripheral neuropathy and decreased global cognition deserves close attention. Pelvic examination with Pap smear should be routine for women.

Purified protein derivative (PPD) testing, in conjunction with baseline chest radiograph, is mandatory. HIV-infected individuals who are PPD-positive are at high risk for developing active tuberculosis and require antituberculous prophylaxis. PPD skin testing should be performed as early in the course of HIV infection as possible, in association with testing cutaneous reactivity to other antigens, usually mumps, *Candida,* and tetanus toxoid. Induration of 5 mm or more should be considered positive. Any patient with a positive PPD should be evaluated for the presence of active tuberculosis; if no active disease is present, the patient should receive 1 year of prophylaxis with isoniazid. If active tuberculosis is identified, multidrug therapy should be initiated, as described in Chapter 99.

Serologic testing for *T. gondii* infection is important in the event that a person subsequently develops an intracerebral lesion (see below). Serologic testing for syphilis should be done at the first visit and followed by prompt treatment if positive (see Chapter 107). Antibody responses to pneumococcal polysaccharides are better among patients with higher CD4 counts; therefore, the pneumococcal vaccine should be administered as soon as the diagnosis of HIV infection is established.

Since the most helpful laboratory guides to the degree of immunodeficiency and to appropriate therapy are the CD4 count and the plasma viral load assay, one of these determinations should be obtained at the first visit and repeated at intervals of 3 to 6 months. The patient

should understand that the CD4 count and the plasma viral load are only rough guides to the degree of immunodeficiency, that modest fluctuations in these measurements may not be indicative of a change in clinical course, and finally, that many persons continue to function well with very low CD4 counts (<50 per mm³).

Antiretroviral Therapy

Elucidation of the mechanisms of HIV replication has identified several potential sites at which retroviral replication might be limited or blocked (see Fig. 108–4). To date five nucleoside analogues that inhibit HIV reverse transcriptase, zidovudine (AZT), didanosine (ddI), zalcitabine (ddc), stavudine (d4T), and lamivudine (3TC), one non-nucleoside reverse transcriptase inhibitor (nevirapine), and four drugs that inhibit HIV protease (saquinavir, indinavir, nelfinavir and ritonavir), have been approved by the United States Food and Drug Administration for treatment of HIV infection. Current research is evaluating the effectiveness of other approaches to disrupting the HIV life cycle.

Recent clinical investigations have resulted in rapid advances in both the evaluation and treatment of HIV disease. Plasma viral load (PVL) assays provide more helpful guides than CD4 counts for the initiation, evaluation, and change of antiviral treatment regimens. The PVL reflects the magnitude of viral replication in the patient; immune dysfunction and HIV disease progression are directly related to the viral load. Protease inhibitors represent a new class of potent antiretroviral agents, which, taken in combination with reverse transcriptase inhibitors (RTIs), give promise of greatly improving treatment of HIV infection. Whereas monotherapy with any of the available RTIs generally causes a less than 10-fold decrease in PVL, monotherapy with the more potent protease inhibitors causes a roughly 100-fold decrease in PVL. Greater decrease in PVL (up to 1000-fold) can be achieved by combinations of a protease inhibitor and one or more RTIs (e.g., indinavir/zidovudine/lamivudine). Such combination therapy can cause marked and sustained decreases in PVL to levels below current limits of detection in the majority of patients for at least 24 months.

The ensuing discussion provides recommendations based on controlled clinical trials. A number of additional studies are in progress, and it is certain that recommendations on when to initiate antiviral treatment, what drug combinations to utilize, and when to change therapeutic regimens will change rapidly over the next few years.

The optimal time to initiate antiretroviral therapy remains uncertain; clinical trials currently in progress should have a major impact on this issue. Current recommendations are to initiate antiretroviral treatment for all patients with CD4 counts <500 and also for patients with CD4 counts >500 when PVL exceeds 30,000 to 50,000 HIV RNA copies/ml. Since the PVL is directly correlated with the risk of disease progression in all phases of HIV infection, the objective of antiviral therapy is maximal viral suppression. A strong rationale can therefore be made for initiating antiretroviral therapy as

TABLE 108–5	Ambulatory Management of Early HIV Disease

Monitoring

Complete baseline history and physical exam; directed interval interview and exam every 6 mo

Laboratory Evaluation

Baseline complete blood count and absolute CD4 cell count with repetition every 3–6 mo

Baseline purified protein derivative (PPD) and anergy panel

Baseline syphilis serology, liver function tests, *Toxoplasma* antibody, CMV antibody, and chest x-ray

Health Care Maintenance

Assessment for ongoing counseling needs and referral for significant psychiatric or social problems

Pneumococcal vaccine

Yearly influenza vaccine (value uncertain)

CMV = Cytomegalovirus.

TABLE 108-6	Examples of Three-Drug Antiretroviral Regimens Appropriate for Initial Treatment of HIV Infection*

1. Indinavir, 800 mg q8h plus zidovudine, 300 mg q12h plus lamivudine, 150 mg q12h
2. Ritonavir, 600 mg q12h plus stavudine, 40 mg q12h plus lamivudine, 150 mg q12h

* Other combinations using one of the four available protease inhibitors and two of the five available nucleoside reverse transcriptase inhibitors may also be appropriate for initial therapy. Three-drug combinations using the non-nucleoside reverse transcriptase inhibitor nevirapine plus two of the five nucleoside reverse transcriptase inhibitors also appear promising and are currently in clinical trials.

soon as the diagnosis is established, with the objective of preventing any significant immunologic damage. No data are yet available, however, on the relative value of very early initiation of antiretroviral therapy.

The current goal of antiretroviral therapy should be to maintain the lowest PVL for as long as possible. Adequate reduction of PVL results in gradual recovery of the damaged immune system (demonstrated by increasing CD4 counts) and significantly delays development of antiretroviral-resistant strains of HIV.

Treatment with a single antiretroviral agent has only a transient effect on PVL and HIV progression and predictably results in development of HIV resistance against the drug. Monotherapy with any of the available antiretroviral drugs should therefore not be used for established HIV disease. Therapy with two nucleoside RTIs (e.g., zidovudine/lamivudine), although more effective in delaying HIV progression than monotherapy, inevitably results in viral resistance to both agents, usually within 8 to 12 months, and is therefore significantly less effective than three-drug combinations in preventing progression to AIDS and/or death. Therefore, three-drug combinations are currently recommended for the initiation of treatment in all patients.

The three-drug regimens that currently provide the most profound, durable suppression of viral replication include a potent protease inhibitor and two reverse transcriptase inhibitors (Table 108–6). Such regimens can maintain PVL below currently detectable limits (400 RNA copies/ml) for up to 2 years in over 80% of patients who adhere closely to the regimen. However, interruptions in the regimen can lead to development of HIV resistance to the antiviral agents, reflected by increasing PVL, decreasing CD4 counts, and risk of disease progression. It is best for the patient to be fully committed to an optimal treatment plan rather than, for example, to attempt to gain patient acceptance by serial addition of single antiretroviral agents. Drug resistance eventually occurs with even the most effective antiviral regimens. Therefore, PVL assays should be repeated at 3- to 4-month intervals during therapy. A change to another regimen is usually indicated when the PVL increases by threefold to fivefold (documented by two PVL assays at least 2 weeks apart) or there is evidence of clinical progression of HIV. The new regimen should include a combination of antiviral drugs that the patient has not previously received, ideally another protease inhibitor and two nucleoside RTIs. If therapeutic options are severely limited, a combination of two protease inhibitors (ritonavir, 400 mg q12h, and saquinavir, 400 mg q12h) has proved very effective in suppressing viral replication in some patients with advanced HIV disease.

Although a number of factors (e.g., adverse drug reactions, development of viral resistance to multiple drugs, suboptimal compliance with complicated regimens) will make it difficult to achieve maximal suppression of PVL in all patients, every effort should be made to achieve this goal.

Prophylaxis Against Opportunistic Infections

During the first 15 years of the HIV pandemic, the most effective medical intervention for persons with HIV infection has been prophylactic measures against opportunistic infections (OIs). The greatest success has been the prevention of *P. carinii* pneumonia for individuals with CD4 counts less than 200 (Table 108–7); routine use of prophylaxis has resulted in a greater than three-fold (from 60% to <20%) decrease in the frequency of *P. carinii* pneumonia as the initial OI in men with HIV infection. Specific antimicrobial prophylaxis (see Table 108–7) is also effective and strongly recommended for the prevention of *T. gondii* encephalitis in all patients with anti-

TABLE 108-7	Prophylaxis Against First Episode of Opportunistic Disease in HIV-Infected Adults

Pathogen	Indication	First Choice	Alternatives
*Pneumocystis carinii**	CD4 count <200	Trimethoprim-sulfamethoxazole, 1 double-strength tablet qd	Dapsone, 100 mg qd Pentamidine, aerosolized, 300 mg qmo Atovaquone, 750 mg qd
*Mycobacterium tuberculosis** Isoniazid-sensitive	TST(t) reaction >5 mm, or prior positive TST without treatment, or contact with case of active tuberculosis	Isoniazid, 300 mg po plus pyridoxine, 50 mg po qd × 12 mo	Rifampin, 600 mg qd × 12 mo
Isoniazid-resistant	Same as above	Rifampin, 600 mg qd × 12 mo	Rifabutin, 300 mg qd × 12 mo
*Toxoplasma gondii**	IgG antibody to toxoplasma and CD4 count <100	TMP-SMZ, 1 double-strength tablet qd	Dapsone 50 mg po qd plus pyrimethimine, 50 mg po qw plus leucovorin, 25 mg po qw
Mycobacterium avium complex†	CD4 count <75	Azithromycin, 1200 mg qw	Clarithromycin, 500 mg po bid

* Strongly recommended as standard of care in all patients.
† Recommended for consideration in all patients.
TST(t) = Tuberculin skin test.

toxoplasma antibodies, and for prevention of active tuberculosis in all patients with positive tuberculin skin tests (see Table 108–7). Prophylaxis is also moderately effective against disseminated MAC infection and the onset of CMV retinitis; in both instances, the value of prophylaxis must be carefully weighed against the potential toxicities of the prophylactic agents and the potential for emergence of resistant isolates. Prophylaxis is very effective against recurrent HSV-2 infection (acyclovir) and against recurrent *Candida* esophagitis (fluconazole), but should generally be reserved for those patients in whom these microorganisms cause recurrent disease.

MANAGEMENT OF SPECIFIC CLINICAL MANIFESTATIONS OF IMMUNODEFICIENCY: A PROBLEM-ORIENTED APPROACH

Opportunistic infections that occur in persons with HIV infection vary considerably in time of onset (see Table 108–4). For example, some patients may develop multidermatomal herpes zoster with CD4 counts greater than 500, and then have no other OIs until they develop *P. carinii* pneumonia with a CD4 count less than 100. On the other hand, occasional patients may remain entirely asymptomatic until their CD4 counts are well below 50, at which time they may develop a major life-threatening OI, such as *T. gondii* encephalitis. In general, life-threatening OIs do not occur with CD4 counts greater than 200 (see Table 108–4). Although the onset of certain infections, such as thrush, is sometimes regarded as a harbinger of rapidly advancing illness, this is not necessarily the case. Some patients may have a severe opportunistic infection, such as *P. carinii* pneumonia and, following successful therapy, enjoy a relatively normal life for several years before developing another major OI.

In general, OIs that occur with CD4 counts greater than 200 respond to routine therapy for the specific infection (e.g., penicillin for pneumococcal pneumonia, standard multidrug therapy for pulmonary tuberculosis) whereas OIs occurring with CD4 counts less than 200 require chronic suppressive therapy following treatment of acute infection (e.g., *P. carinii* pneumonia, CMV retinitis, *Cryptococcus neoformans* meningitis).

An important principle in the management of OIs is recognition that the great majority respond to appropriate antimicrobial therapy, and many patients have years of productive life after the successful treatment of life-threatening opportunistic infections.

Constitutional Symptoms

Nonspecific symptoms may be the initial clinical manifestation of severe immunodeficiency. Patients may develop unexplained fever, night sweats, anorexia, weight loss, or diarrhea. These symptoms may last for weeks or months before the development of identifiable OIs. These constitutional symptoms may represent the earliest manifestations of specific, but unidentified, OIs.

MUCOCUTANEOUS DISEASES

Disorders of the skin and mucosa are among the most common clinical manifestations of HIV disease (Table 108–8).

Oral Disease

Candida stomatitis, or thrush, is often the earliest recognized OI. Thrush may be precipitated by use of broad-spectrum antibiotics. Early thrush may be entirely asymp-

Condition	Description	Treatment
Herpes simplex	Clear or crusted vesicles with an erythematous base; ulceration common when chronic; location; oral or genital mucous membranes, face, and hands	Acyclovir, 200 mg 5 times day
Herpes zoster (shingles)	Cluster of vesicles in a dermatomal distribution; may involve adjacent dermatomes or may disseminate	Acyclovir, 800 mg 5 times day; if disseminated or involvement of ophthalamic branch of trigeminal nerve, IV acyclovir 10 mg/kg q8h
Staphylococcal folliculitis	Erythematous pustules on face, trunk, and groin, often pruritic	Dicloxacillin, 500 mg qid or erythromycin, 500 mg qid
Bacillary angiomatosis	Friable vascular papules or subcutaneous nodules on skin; may involve liver, spleen, and lymph nodes	Clarithromycin 500 mg bid, or doxycycline, 200 mg qd
Molluscum contagiosum	Chronic, flesh-colored papules, often umbilicated, on face or anogenital area	Cryotherapy and curettage
Seborrheic dermatitis	White scaling or erythematous patches on scalp, eyebrows, face, trunk, axilla, and groin	Hydrocortisone cream, 2.5%, and ketoconazole cream
Psoriasis	Scaling, marginated patches on elbows, knees, and lumbosacral areas	Triamcinolone acetonide cream, 0.1%
Candidal rash	Urticarial scaling or erythematous patches on face, trunk, axilla, and groin	Hydrocortisone cream, 1%, and azole cream
Candida infection (thrush)	White or erythematous patches on mucous membranes of mouth	Clotrimazole troches, 5 times day; refractory cases: fluconazole, 100 mg qd

TABLE 108–8 — Dermatologic Conditions Common in HIV Infection

tomatic; as infection becomes more extensive, it causes pain and discomfort upon eating. The cheesy white exudate on the mucous membranes can easily be scraped off. The underlying mucosa may be normal or inflamed. A saline or potassium hydroxide preparation reveals the budding yeast or pseudohyphae typical of *Candida* species.

Oral hairy leukoplakia is a white, lichenified, plaque-like lesion, most commonly seen on the lateral surfaces of the tongue (less commonly on the buccal mucosa). It may be an early manifestation of immunodeficiency. Hairy leukoplakia is painless and may remit and relapse spontaneously.

Patients may develop painful ulcers in the mouth. These may be caused by HSV, but more often represent aphthous lesions of uncertain etiology.

Kaposi's sarcoma, a malignant proliferative disorder seen most often in HIV-infected homosexual men, has a predilection for the oral cavity and skin. Oral lesions may be purple, red, or blue, and may be raised or flat. Usually painless, these lesions cause symptoms when they enlarge, bleed, or ulcerate.

Esophageal Disease

Symptomatic esophageal disease seldom occurs with CD4 counts greater than 50. Pain on swallowing and substernal burning are common and may indicate *Candida* esophagitis, particularly when associated with oral thrush. Esophagoscopy with biopsy, cytology, and culture should be performed if symptoms do not rapidly respond (within 3 to 5 days) to antifungal therapy. If esophagoscopy shows ulcerative lesions, they are usually caused by CMV (50%), aphthae (45%), or HSV (5%). Since each of these lesions is responsive to appropriate therapy, definitive etiologic diagnosis is mandatory (Table 108–9).

Genital Disease

Recurrent genital ulcers are most often due to HSV. Tzanck preparation reveals multinucleated giant cells, and culture or specific immunofluorescence of ulcer scrapings confirms the diagnosis; biopsy is rarely indicated. Primary

TABLE 108–9	HIV-Associated Esophagitis	
Condition	Characteristics	Treatment
Candida infection	Thrush usual, esophageal plaques	Fluconazole, 200 mg/day
CMV infection	Large shallow esophageal ulcers on endoscopy	Ganciclovir, 5 mg/kg bid
Herpes simplex	Deep ulceration on endoscopy	Acyclovir, 200–800 mg 5 times day
Aphthae	Giant ulcers on endoscopy; no virus on biposy	Prednisone, 40–60 mg/day or thalidomide, 200 mg/day*

* Thalidomide must *never* be given during pregnancy.
CMV = Cytomegalovirus; HIV = human immunodeficiency virus.

syphilis also occurs with increased frequency (see Chapter 107). Chancroid is unusual in North America.

Vaginal and Cervical Disease

Candida species, most often *Candida albicans,* can cause an irritating vulvovaginitis in women with HIV infection as well as among healthy HIV-seronegative women. The cheesy white exudate can be examined under light microscopy for budding yeast or pseudohyphae.

Infection with human papilloma virus (HPV) is associated not only with rapid proliferation of genital warts but also with a greater frequency of cervical dysplasia in HIV-infected women. Pap smears indicative of cervical dysplasia should be followed by prompt colposcopy, biopsy when indicted, and appropriate treatment of any dysplastic lesions.

Cutaneous Disease

HIV-infected patients may have a variety of dermatologic ailments; many of these are readily treatable (see Table 108–8). HIV-infected persons have increased frequency of cutaneous and systemic reactions to a variety of medications, particularly sulfa-containing drugs. Severe seborrheic dermatitis, often manifested as a scaly eruption between the eyebrows and the nasolabial fold, often occurs. Psoriasis, a scaling eruption usually most prominent on the elbows, also occurs more frequently.

Herpes zoster, manifested by crops of vesicular lesions on erythematous bases in a dermatomal or polydermatomal distribution, is often preceded by unexplained pain in the involved dermatome(s). Molluscum contagiosum, umbilicated pearly papules due to poxvirus infection, may occur in crops on the face, neck, abdomen, and genitalia of HIV-infected persons. Facial and genital warts due to HPV infection also occur with increased frequency. Generalized pruritus may be a drug reaction but also may be due to dry skin or to "pruritic papules," a syndrome of undefined etiology that is frequent in this population.

Cutaneous lesions of Kaposi's sarcoma may be flat or raised; may be red, brown, or blue in color; and may resemble insect bites, nevi, or cutaneous ecchymoses. On examination, Kaposi's sarcoma lesions often have a firm texture when rolled between the fingers, whereas many benign lesions like ecchymoses are not distinguishable from normal skin by this maneuver. Definitive diagnosis is established by biopsy.

Treatment

Many of the minor mucocutaneous problems can be readily treated, but recurrence is frequent (see Table 108–8). Thrush and *Candida* vaginitis usually respond to topical therapy. Fungal skin infections usually respond to antifungal creams. Esophageal candidiasis necessitates treatment with systemic therapy (fluconazole, 200 mg daily for 10 days).

Recurrent or chronic ulcerative perioral, perianal, or genital herpes simplex usually responds rapidly to oral acyclovir (400 mg administered 5 times per day for 10 days), but chronic acyclovir therapy may be required to prevent frequent relapses. Acyclovir-resistant strains of HSV occasionally develop, necessitating treatment with intravenous foscarnet. Although the effectiveness of therapy of uncomplicated multidermatomal herpes zoster is uncertain, most clinicians prescribe high-dose acyclovir in this setting (800 mg given orally five times per day for 5 to 7 days).

Aphthous ulcers are difficult to treat. Oral ulcers may respond to topical corticosteroids, whereas giant oral or esophageal ulcers require systemic treatment with thalidomide or corticosteroids. Thalidomide should be used only if birth control can be assured, if at all, in women with childbearing potential because of its well-documented adverse effects on fetal development. It is important to obtain cultures for HSV and CMV to be sure that the ulcers are not viral in origin before initiating corticosteroid or thalidomide therapy. CMV esophageal ulcers respond well to intravenous gancyclovir or foscarnet therapy for 2 to 3 weeks, or until resolution is confirmed endoscopically. Esophageal ulcerations caused by HSV usually respond well to intravenous acyclovir (see Table 108–9).

Seborrheic dermatitis often responds to hydrocortisone cream. Warts due to HPV, as well as lesions of molluscum contagiosum, may be treated with ablative procedures (e.g., cryotherapy, laser).

NERVOUS SYSTEM DISEASES

Nervous system complications ultimately occur in the majority of HIV-infected persons and range from mild cognitive disturbances or peripheral neuropathy to severe dementia or life-threatening CNS infections. The physician must be alert to the development of early signs of treatable neurologic complications of HIV disease. As is often the case with other lentiviruses, HIV enters microglial cells of the CNS very early in the course of HIV infection. This process may be associated with neuronal cell loss, vacuolization, and occasional lymphocytic infiltration. The mechanism whereby HIV infection itself results in neurologic disease is not understood, but direct neuronal destruction and effects of viral proteins on neuronal cell function are two of the postulated mechanisms of nervous system disease in AIDS.

Cognitive Dysfunction

Intellectual impairment rarely occurs early in the course of HIV infection, but is common among persons with advanced immunodeficiency (CD4 count less than 50). AIDS dementia complex (ADC) often begins insidiously and progresses over months to years, although occasionally the disorder may be acute in onset (Table 108–10). ADC is characterized by poor concentration, diminished memory, slowing of thought processes, motor dysfunc-

TABLE 108–10	Major Clinical Manifestations of AIDS Dementia Complex	
Cognition	Inattention, reduced concentration, forgetfulness, impaired memory	Global dementia
Motor performance	Slowed movements, clumsiness, ataxia	Paraplegia
Behavior	Apathy, altered personality, agitation	Mutism

tion, and occasionally behavioral abnormalities characterized by social withdrawal and apathy.

Some patients become agitated, confused, or overtly psychotic. Motor abnormalities may include a progressive gait ataxia. As ADC progresses, patients may become demented or develop focal neurologic complications characterized by spastic weakness of the lower extremities and incontinence secondary to vacuolar myelopathy.

The symptoms of clinical depression overlap with many of the characteristics of early ADC and must be considered carefully in differential diagnosis and therapy. ADC must be distinguished from opportunistic complications of HIV infection. Computed tomographic (CT) scan of the head in ADC reveals only atrophy, with enlarged sulci and ventricles. Examination of cerebrospinal fluid (CSF) is most often normal but may show mild elevations of protein and a few lymphocytes.

A large variety of neurologic problems may complicate the later stages of HIV infection. A neuroanatomic classification of these manifestations is presented in Table 108–11, and certain of the more frequent or treatable problems are discussed below.

Focal Lesions of the CNS

Several opportunistic complications of HIV infection produce focal CNS lesions. Patients with focal neurologic signs, seizures of new onset, or the recent onset of rapidly progressive cognitive impairment should undergo CT scanning with contrast or magnetic resonance imaging (MRI) of the brain.

Toxoplasmosis, CNS lymphoma, and progressive multifocal leukoencephalopathy (PML) are the most common causes of CNS focal lesions in this setting (Table 108–12).

Toxoplasma encephalitis occurs in up to one third of HIV-1 infected patients who have serological evidence of *T. gondii* infection, but is very rare in individuals who have no antibodies to *Toxoplasma*. Fewer than 30% of young adults born in the continental United States have antibodies to *T. gondii*, but more than 80% of young adults in Puerto Rico have evidence of antecedent infection. Thus, the importance of toxoplasmosis as an opportunistic infection varies according to region. Patients with CNS toxoplasmosis often present with progressive headache and focal neurologic abnormalities; they are usually, but not always, febrile. CT scan with contrast dye usually demonstrates multiple ring-enhancing lesions, but may

TABLE 108–11	Neuroanatomic Classification of the Common Complications of HIV-1 Infection

Meningitis and Headache

Aseptic meningitis
Cryptococcal meningitis
Tuberculous meningitis
Syphilitic meningitis

Diffuse Brain Diseases

With preservation of consciousness
  AIDS dementia complex
With concomitant depression of arousal
  Toxoplasma encephalitis
Cytomegalovirus encephalitis

Focal Brain Diseases

Cerebral toxoplasmosis
Primary CNS lymphoma
Progressive multifocal leukoencephalopathy
Tuberculous brain abscess *(M. tuberculosis)*
Cryptococcoma

Myelopathies

Subacute/chronic, progressive
  Vacuolar myelopathy
Subacute with polyradiculopathy
  Cytomegalovirus myelopathy

Peripheral Neuropathies

Predominantly sensory polyneuropathy
Toxic neuropathies (zalcitabine, didanosine, stavudine)
Autonomic neuropathy
Cytomegalovirus polyradiculopathy

Myopathies

Polymyositis
Noninflammatory myopathy
Zidovudine myopathy

AIDS = Acquired immunodeficiency syndrome; CNS = central nervous system; HIV = human immunodeficiency virus.

show only focal edema. Management of symptomatic, ring-enhancing brain lesions in persons with AIDS includes initiation of empiric therapy with pyrimethamine, sulfadiazine, and folinic acid. Brain biopsy should be reserved for patients with atypical presentations, those with no serum antibodies to *T. gondii,* or those whose lesions do not respond after 10 to 14 days of antiprotozoal treatment. Because cyst forms of toxoplasmosis are

not eradicated with current therapy, patients must remain on chronic suppressive therapy.

Primary CNS lymphoma complicates HIV infection in 4 to 8% of cases. On CT or MRI scan, lesions are characteristically located in the periventricular space, are often single but may be oligofocal, and usually enhance weakly with contrast (see Table 108–12). Irradiation often provides remission, but most persons with CNS lymphoma survive less than 6 months after diagnosis.

PML is a demyelinating disease due to a papovavirus. Presenting symptoms may include progressive dementia, visual impairment, seizures, and hemiparesis. MRI scan usually reveals multiple lesions predominantly involving white matter. These lesions are often not visible on CT scan, which helps to distinguish PML from other mass lesions of the CNS in AIDS patients. There is no effective specific treatment for PML, but symptoms may improve with effective antiretroviral therapy.

CNS Diseases Without Prominent Focal Signs

Evaluation of the HIV-infected patient who presents with fever and headache is complicated by the often subtle manifestations of serious CNS lesions in immunocompromised patients. Patients with bacterial meningitis (see Chapter 97) are managed as noncompromised patients. Meningeal diseases in most HIV-infected patients, however, fall into the broad categories of aseptic meningitis, chronic meningitis, and meningoencephalitis.

Aseptic Meningitis

Patients with aseptic meningitis complain most often of headache; the sensorium is generally intact and the neurologic examination is normal (see Chapter 97). HIV infection can itself cause aseptic meningitis, most often as a manifestation of the acute retroviral syndrome.

In the HIV-infected person with aseptic meningitis, particular consideration must be given to potentially treatable causes of this syndrome (see Chapter 97). Syphilitic meningitis may be particularly difficult to diagnose in HIV-infected patients (see Chapters 97 and 107), as false-negative serological tests may occur in this setting. If the serum Venereal Disease Research Laboratory (VDRL) or

TABLE 108–12	Comparative Clinical and Radiologic Features of Cerebral Toxoplasmosis, Primary CNS Lymphoma, and Progressive Multifocal Leukoencephalopathy					
	Clinical Onset			**Neuroradiologic Features**		
Condition	**Temporal Profile**	**Level of Alertness**	**Fever**	**Number of Lesions**	**Lesions on CT Scan**	**Location of Lesions**
Cerebral toxoplasmosis	Days	Reduced	Common	Often multiple	Spherical, ring-enhancing	Basal ganglia, cortex
Primary CNS lymphoma	Days to weeks	Variable	Absent	One or few	Irregular, weakly enhancing	Periventricular
Progressive multifocal leukoencephalopathy	Days to weeks	Variable	Absent	Usually multiple	Nonenhancing	White matter

CNS = Central nervous system; CT = computed tomography.

fluorescent treponemal antibody (FTA) test is positive or there is a history of inadequately treated syphilis in the past, the physician may elect to treat for CNS syphilis (see Chapter 107).

HIV-infected patients with early cryptococcal meningitis may present with a headache but no intellectual dysfunction, and the CSF exam may show only a mild CSF pleocytosis, with glucose and protein levels consistent with aseptic meningitis. The presence of cryptococcal antigen in CSF or a positive India ink preparation establishes the diagnosis of cryptococcal infection (see Chapter 97). Treatment with amphotericin B for at least 2 weeks followed by lifelong suppression with fluconazole is indicated.

Chronic Meningitis

Patients with chronic meningitis present with a history of headache, fever, difficulty in concentrating, or changes in sensorium. CSF examination reveals a low glucose concentration, an elevated protein level, and a mild to modest lymphocytic pleocytosis. Cryptococcal meningitis is the most common etiology for this presentation.

Mycobacterium tuberculosis is an eminently treatable cause of subacute to chronic meningitis in the HIV-infected patient, although rare to date in North America. Antituberculosis therapy should be considered in the setting of chronic meningitis if the cryptococcal antigen test is negative (see Chapter 97).

Coccidioidomycosis and histoplasmosis are possible causes of chronic meningitis in patients residing in, or with a travel history to, endemic regions (desert Southwest and Ohio and Mississippi River drainage areas, respectively) (see Chapter 97).

Meningoencephalitis

Patients with meningoencephalitis present with alterations in sensorium varying from mild lethargy to coma. Patients are usually febrile, and neurologic examination often reveals evidence of diffuse CNS involvement. CT or MRI scanning shows only nonspecific abnormalities,

whereas electroencephalography (EEG) often shows diffuse disease of the brain.

CMV encephalitis is difficult to diagnose. Patients may present with confusion, cranial nerve abnormalities, or long tract signs. CSF findings, as well as MRI and CT scanning, may be nonspecific. Many patients have CMV disease elsewhere, most often retinitis. PCR detection of CMV antigens in CSF appears to be a sensitive and specific method for diagnosing CMV encephalitis and polyradiculopathy.

Meningoencephalitis due to HSV, although unusual in HIV infection, generally responds well to treatment with acyclovir and should therefore be suspected with an illness of acute onset characterized by fever, headache, and alteration in sensorium, especially if there is EEG or CT evidence of temporal lobe disease (see Chapter 97).

PULMONARY DISEASES

Pulmonary manifestations of HIV infection are common, and range from nonspecific interstitial pneumonitis to life-threatening pneumonias (Table 108–13). Pneumonia is the most frequent serious infectious complication of HIV infection.

Human immunodeficiency virus-infected patients have a 3- to 4-fold increased risk of bacterial pneumonia, which is generally caused by encapsulated bacteria, including *S. pneumoniae* and *H. influenzae*. The increased risk begins with modest degrees of immunodeficiency (CD4 counts of 200 to 500). The intracellular bacterium *Legionella pneumophila* also causes pneumonia with increased frequency. The onset of bacterial pneumonia is usually abrupt; patients may have rigors and cough productive of purulent sputum. Physical examination and chest radiographs often reveal evidence of consolidation. The response to prompt initiation of therapy is usually good, but delay in appropriate antimicrobial therapy often results in a fulminant downhill course. Initial therapy is guided by the results of Gram's stain of sputum (see Chapter 99).

Pneumocystis carinii pneumonia (PCP) was the most common life-threatening infection in North American persons with AIDS until prophylaxis against PCP became

TABLE 108–13	**Pulmonary Disease Associated with HIV Infection**			
Condition	**Characteristic**	**Chest X-Ray**	**Diagnosis**	**Treatment**
Pneumocystis carinii pneumonia	Subacute onset, dry cough, dyspnea	Interstitial infiltrate most common	Sputum or bronchoalveolar lavage for organism by stain	Trimethoprim-sulfamethoxazole, pentamidine
Bacterial (pneumococcus, *Haemophilus* most common)	Acute productive cough, fever, chest pain	Lobar or localized infiltrate	Sputum Gram's stain and culture, blood culture	Penicillin or cefuroxime
Mycobacterial (*Mycobacterium tuberculosis* or *M. kansasii*)	Chronic cough, weight loss, fever	Localized infiltrate, lymphadenopathy	Sputum acid-fast stain and mycobacterial culture	Isoniazid, rifampin, pyrazinamide
Kaposi's sarcoma	Asymptomatic or mild cough	Pulmonary nodules, pleural effusion	Open lung biopsy	Chemotherapy

HIV = Human immunodeficiency virus.

routine. In developing countries, where tuberculosis and other opportunistic infections are more prevalent, PCP is less frequently diagnosed. Patients with PCP frequently complain of gradual onset of nonproductive cough, fever, and shortness of breath with exertion; a productive cough suggests another process. Patients with PCP often experience an end-inspiratory substernal catch or pain sensation that is unusual with other illnesses. In contrast to the acute onset of PCP in other immunocompromised patients, AIDS patients with PCP may have pulmonary symptoms for weeks before presentation to a physician. Arterial hypoxemia is usual; the chest radiograph generally reveals a subtle interstitial pattern but may be entirely normal. The patient usually appears more sick than the radiograph would suggest. The presence of pleural effusions is suggestive of an etiology other than PCP.

If PCP is suspected clinically, therapy should be started immediately; treatment for several days does not interfere with the ability to make a specific diagnosis. Confirmation of a diagnosis of PCP is essential, since treatment is often complicated by drug reactions. In addition, delay in establishing a correct diagnosis of another treatable condition may be lethal. The diagnosis may often be made by examination of induced sputum. If this fails, bronchoalveolar lavage, with silver staining or immunofluorescence of specimens, is adequate to diagnose PCP in more than 95% of patients.

Treatment with high-dose intravenous trimethoprim-sulfamethoxazole for 3 weeks is effective therapy; this drug combination, however, frequently produces side effects (rash, fever, and granulocytopenia are most common) that limit its effectiveness. Intravenous pentamidine is comparably effective but has more serious side effects; azotemia and pancreatitis presenting with hypoglycemia may occur and persist for days after the drug is stopped. Alternative therapies include atovoquone, trimethoprim plus dapsone, or primaquine plus clindamycin. Aerosolized pentamidine may be effective for milder cases of PCP and has few systemic toxicities. Patients with advanced PCP and arterial hypoxemia ($PO_2 \leq 75$ mm on breathing room air) benefit from administration of corticosteroids (40 mg of prednisone twice daily), utilizing a taper over a period of 2 to 3 weeks.

On occasion, bronchoscopically obtained specimens yield CMV or MAC. Interpretation of these findings is difficult. Evidence of active CMV retinitis or invasive disease elsewhere, or histologic demonstration of intracellular CMV inclusions obtained from bronchoalveolar lavage, often leads to treatment with gancyclovir or foscarnet; there is, however, no evidence that any treatment is effective against CMV pneumonia. MAC is an unusual cause of clinical pneumonia in AIDS.

Some AIDS patients (most often children) with interstitial pneumonitis may have no pathogen identified on transbronchial biopsy.

Mycobacterium tuberculosis infection occurs with greater frequency in regions having a high prevalence of tuberculosis. Active pulmonary tuberculosis may develop at a time when the CD4 count remains well above 200 (see Table 108–4). Chest radiographs in HIV-infected patients may demonstrate features of primary tuberculosis, including hilar adenopathy, lower or middle lobe infiltrates, miliary pattern, or pleural effusions, as well as classic patterns of reactivation. Extrapulmonary *M. tuberculosis* infection also occurs with increased frequency in persons with HIV infection. Blood cultures often yield *M. tuberculosis* in the severely immunocompromised patient.

Both pulmonary and extrapulmonary tuberculosis generally respond promptly to standard antituberculosis therapy, although several outbreaks of multidrug-resistant (MDR) *M. tuberculosis* have occurred in people with HIV infection and are associated with high case-fatality rates. Treatment therefore should begin with four antituberculosis drugs (see Chapter 99).

Because HIV-infected patients may be at risk for relapse once initial therapy is completed, long-term monitoring for reactivation is critical. Since nosocomial transmission of multidrug-resistant *M. tuberculosis* may occur both in hospitals and in ambulatory care centers, physicians must take adequate precautions to prevent spread of *M. tuberculosis,* especially in the health care setting.

The disseminated fungal infections histoplasmosis and coccidioidomycosis occur with much greater frequency in persons with HIV infection. Either fungal infection may present with nodular infiltrates or with a miliary pattern on chest radiograph. Histoplasmosis usually involves bone marrow as well as skin; bone marrow examination often demonstrates the organism. The standard treatment of disseminated mycoses in AIDS patients is high-dose amphotericin. Since relapse is common, oral azole therapy (fluconazole for coccidioidomycosis, itraconazole for histoplasmosis) must be continued following resolution of signs and symptoms.

Nodular pulmonary disease or isolated pleural effusions in AIDS patients may represent Kaposi's sarcoma. Hilar or mediastinal lymphadenopathy is seldom a part of the generalized, HIV-associated lymphadenopathy syndrome; enlargement of these nodes usually represents either an opportunistic infection or a neoplasm.

Prevention of Pulmonary Infections

Some of the serious pulmonary complications of HIV infection are preventable. Immunization against *S. pneumoniae* should be performed as early in the course of HIV disease as possible.

Among persons with a CD4 cell count lower than 200/mm^3, prophylaxis, using trimethoprim-sulfamethoxazole (1 double-strength tablet daily), dapsone (100 mg/day), or aerosolized pentamidine (300 mg/month), is effective in preventing PCP.

All HIV-infected patients should undergo routine PPD skin testing, with follow-up and treatment when indicated.

GASTROINTESTINAL DISEASES

Gastrointestinal (GI) disease presenting as dysphagia, diarrhea, or colitis is common. Each of these processes often contributes to inadequate nutrition, compounding the weight loss associated with advanced HIV disease. Dysphagia is discussed above.

Nausea and Vomiting

Nausea and vomiting are frequent in advanced HIV disease. Often these symptoms are related to medications; these must be reviewed and the likely offending drug (or drugs) withheld as a therapeutic trial. If symptoms of nausea and vomiting remain undefined and do not respond to empiric therapy with histamine (H$_2$) antagonists or an antiemetic, endoscopy should be performed. Biopsy may show a lymphoma or Kaposi's sarcoma, or conditions not directly attributable to HIV disease.

Abnormalities of liver function tests are common in HIV disease and often are nonspecific. Elevations of serum aminotransferases (ALT and AST) often represent chronic active hepatitis B or C, but may reflect hepatic inflammation due to medications such as trimethoprim-sulfamethoxazole or antiretroviral agents. Marked elevations in serum alkaline phosphatase levels may reflect infiltrative disease of the liver (e.g., MAC or CMV) but also can be seen in patients with acalculous cholecystitis, cryptosporidiosis, or AIDS-associated sclerosing cholangitis.

Diarrhea

Diarrhea occurs, at least intermittently, in more than half of persons with AIDS and may be due to a variety of microorganisms (Table 108–14). In many cases no clear etiology is found, and the diarrhea is attributed to HIV-associated enteropathy.

As in other patients with persistent diarrhea, profuse watery diarrhea suggests a secretory diarrhea, and bloody diarrhea with mucus is consistent with colitis (see Chapter 103). Stool specimens should be cultured for the common bacterial pathogens. *Salmonella, Campylobacter,* and *Yersinia* species frequently cause diarrhea in HIV-infected persons. Although bacteremia is common, patients usually respond to standard antimicrobial therapy. AIDS patients may also have recurrent episodes of diarrhea associated with *Clostridium difficile* toxin. Whether this reflects the frequent use of broad-spectrum antibiotics or is attributable to some other factor in HIV disease is unknown.

In cases of persistent diarrhea, a fresh stool specimen also should be examined for parasites, using a modified acid-fast stain for *C. parvum* and *I. belli. C. parvum* and *I. belli* are the most common enteric protozoal infections in AIDS patients throughout the world. Although cryptosporidiosis may be self-limited, massive diarrhea (up to 15 L/day) may occur. Clinical responses to oral paromomycin, a poorly absorbed aminoglycoside, are usually transient. Isosporiasis frequently responds to oral trimethoprim-sulfamethoxazole, but relapse is frequent and chronic therapy may be necessary.

If diagnostic studies are negative and diarrhea persists, patients should undergo endoscopy (see Chapter 33). Biopsy of the duodenum or small bowel may show histologic evidence of cryptosporidial, microsporidial, MAC, or CMV infection. Nonspecific inflammation and villous atrophy are present in patients with HIV-associated enteropathy. Electron microscopy or special stains of small bowel biopsy specimens or stool may reveal evidence of protozoan or microsporidial infection. Biopsy of the colon may show histologic abnormalities indicative of HSV proctitis, CMV colitis, or MAC infection.

For patients with refractory diarrhea, a variety of nonspecific approaches may improve the quality of life. Patients with chronic diarrhea often have an acquired mucosal disaccharidase deficiency; a trial of a lactose-free diet may provide symptomatic improvement. Agents that alter motility (e.g., loperamide hydrochloride) may provide symptomatic relief for many patients with diarrhea of uncertain etiology. Parenteral hyperalimentation may improve both the quality and the duration of life in patients with refractory AIDS-related diarrheal diseases.

TABLE 108–14	Diarrhea in Advanced HIV Infection		
Condition	**Characteristic**	**Diagnosis**	**Treatment**
Frequent			
Cytomegalovirus	Small bowel movements with blood or mucus (colitis)	Colonscopy and biopsy	Ganciclovir, 5 mg/kg bid
Cryptosporidium	Varies from increased frequency to large-volume diarrhea	Acid-fast stain of stool	Paromomycin, 500 mg qid
Mycobacterium avium complex	Abdominal pain, fever, retroperitoneal lymphadenopathy	Blood culture or endoscopy with biopsy	Multidrug regimen, including clarithromycin; ethambutol, nifabutin, clofazamine
Clostridium difficile	Abdominal pain, fever common	*Clostridium difficile* toxin in stool or endoscopy	Metronidazole or vancomycin po
Less Frequent			
Salmonella or *Campylobacter*	Blood or mucus in bowel movements (colitis)	Stool culture	Norfloxacin (check sensitivities)
Isospora belli	Watery diarrhea	Acid-fast stain of stool	Trimethoprim-sulfamethoxazole

HIV = Human immunodeficiency virus.

Unexplained Fever

Fever without localizing signs may be part of the HIV acute retroviral syndrome. However most, if not all, persistent fever late in the course of HIV infection reflects a definable underlying process.

Mycobacterium avium complex (MAC) infection may manifest with nonspecific findings, including persistent fever, anorexia, weight loss, abdominal pain, or diarrhea. Clues to MAC include isolated elevation of serum alkaline phosphatase or splenomegaly in a patient with CD4 count under 50/mm³. This organism may cause extensive disease, involving bone marrow, liver, and GI tract. Rapid diagnosis may often be made by histologic examination of bone marrow specimens, although blood cultures will also eventually yield the organism. Unlike *M. tuberculosis,* MAC uncommonly causes pulmonary disease or meningitis, and aerosolization does not place immunocompetent persons at risk. MAC is resistant to conventional antituberculosis chemotherapy and is treated with combinations of three or more agents that should include either clarithromycin or azithromycin, ethambutol, and rifabutin. Treatment often results in resolution of fevers and weight gain.

Unexplained fever also may be due to disseminated CMV infection. The hemorrhagic exudates that characterize CMV retinitis support the diagnosis. In the absence of retinitis, esophagitis, or colitis, isolation of CMV from the blood is not considered a definite indication for treatment.

Aggressive non-Hodgkin's lymphoma may cause unexplained fever and weight loss. A rapidly enlarging spleen or asymmetric lymph node enlargement may suggest the diagnosis. The lymphomas often have an intra-abdominal presentation. CT-guided biopsy of enlarged intra-abdominal nodes may provide the diagnosis.

Weight Loss and Anorexia

Cachexia is often a prominent feature of advanced HIV disease. In some instances, the wasting is due to an intercurrent infectious process. In many instances, however, no opportunistic process is identified and the cachexia is attributed to progressive HIV disease. Heightened production of tumor necrosis factor/cachectin may contribute to the fever, cachexia, and hypertriglyceridemia in advanced HIV disease.

If orthostatic hypotension occurs, especially if associated with hyperkalemia, an adrenocorticotropin (ACTH) stimulation test should investigate the possibility of adrenal insufficiency, which may result from CMV infection.

Many patients with AIDS-associated cachexia gain weight and achieve a sense of well-being after initiation of antiretroviral therapy. Some also gain weight after administration of either androgens or the appetite-stimulating drug dronabinol. Administration of recombinant growth hormone (GH), of nonmethylated androgens, and of megesterol have each been associated with weight gain and an improved sense of well-being among patients with the AIDS-wasting syndrome.

AIDS-Associated Malignancies

In the United States, Kaposi's sarcoma (KS) occurs primarily among homosexual and bisexual men. Among HIV-infected gay men, the frequency of KS has fallen from 40% at the outset of the epidemic to less than 20% in 1995. Current data, consistent with the occasional observation of KS in HIV-seronegative homosexual men, suggest that this KS results from infection by a newly recognized herpes virus, tentatively called human herpes-virus-8 (HHV-8), and that tumor growth is facilitated by HIV-associated immunodeficiency.

Kaposi's sarcoma is primarily a tumor of the skin and mucosal surfaces that can involve the GI tract, lungs, and lymph nodes. Symptomatic or rapidly progressive disease should be treated. Systemic chemotherapy can provide remissions in many patients with disseminated disease or symptomatic visceral disease. Occasionally, the cutaneous and mucosal lesions may respond to treatment with interferon-alpha.

Non-Hodgkin's B-cell lymphomas may also complicate HIV-1 infection. Most AIDS-associated lymphomas are of small noncleaved or immunoblastic histology. Extranodal presentation of these tumors is the rule with a high frequency of GI or intracranial presentation. These malignancies usually occur late in the course of HIV disease. Chemotherapy for systemic disease or radiation therapy for CNS disease can provide brief clinical responses, but few patients survive more than 6 months after diagnosis.

OTHER COMPLICATIONS OF HIV INFECTION

Cardiac

Whereas subclinical cardiac abnormalities are common in HIV-infected persons, a small proportion of HIV-infected patients develop congestive cardiomyopathy, usually in association with advanced HIV disease.

Renal

Renal insufficiency in AIDS patients may be a consequence of nephrotoxic drug administration, acute tubular necrosis following hypotension, heroin injection, or HIV-associated nephropathy (HIV AN). HIV AN occurs most commonly among African-American patients; certain histologic features such as focal and segmental glomerulosclerosis may distinguish HIV AN from renal failure associated with intravenous heroin use. The disease usually presents with heavy proteinuria, nephrotic syndrome, and progressive renal insufficiency. Without treatment, most patients develop end-stage renal disease within several months. Short-term, high-dose steroid therapy often arrests the progression of renal disease in persons with HIV AN. Renal biopsy may be helpful in excluding other potentially treatable causes of renal failure.

Rheumatologic

Musculoskeletal complaints are common; the relationship of circulating autoantibodies to these manifestations is unknown. Muscle weakness may reflect generalized debilitation, or, if localized, myelopathy-neuropathy (see Table 108–11). When weakness is proximal or is associated with myalgia and tenderness, myopathy should be suspected. The myopathy may be HIV-associated or may, rarely, represent zidovudine toxicity. Muscle biopsy may distinguish between these two processes, with inflammation most prominent in AIDS-associated myopathy and mitochondrial abnormalities in zidovudine-related myopathy. Arthralgias are frequent, and both a Reiter-like syndrome and a Sjögren-like syndrome occur with increased frequency.

PREVENTION OF HIV INFECTION

Three approaches, behavioral modification, aggressive, community-wide treatment of sexually transmitted diseases (STDs), and antiretroviral therapy of seropositive pregnant women have been shown to have a major impact on HIV transmission.

In several communities at increased risk for HIV (e.g., homosexually active men in the United States and Western Europe), adaptation of safer sexual practices has been associated with a decrease in incidence of HIV infection. Sustaining these behavioral changes over long periods is difficult, and thus behavioral reinforcement is important. Moreover, negative attitudes regarding condom use enhance the continuing risk of HIV transmission. Counseling regarding risk behaviors, particularly unprotected sexual intercourse without condoms and sharing of needles, must be part of routine health care.

Studies in Central Africa have clearly demonstrated that periodic community-wide STD-treatment programs may result in a nearly 50% reduction in HIV transmission. Such programs may show considerable regional variations in effectiveness.

Treatment of HIV-infected women with zidovudine during the third trimester of pregnancy and during delivery, followed by zidovudine treatment of the infant for 6 weeks, has been shown to decrease maternal–fetal transmission by 67% (from 25% to 8%) without apparent harm to the newborn child. Studies are now in progress to determine whether administration of combination antiretroviral therapy will further decrease HIV infection in children born to HIV-infected mothers.

Infection control procedures that are routinely recommended to protect health care workers (HCWs) involve the use of universal blood and body fluid precautions. Meticulous attention to the utilization and disposal of sharp instruments is most important, since most nosocomial acquisition of HIV infection has occurred through accidental needlestick. In particular, needles should never be recapped. Health care workers who have had accidental parenteral HIV exposure have an overall 0.3% risk of HIV seroconversion. Most exposures that result in HIV transmission involve accidental deep penetration. Prompt administration of zidovudine has been shown to significantly decrease the likelihood of HIV infection in HCWs following needlestick injuries. Current provisional recommendations by the United States Public Health Service for prophylaxis following high-risk occupational exposure include a combination regimen of indinavir, zidovudine, and lamivudine, initiated as soon as possible after exposure and continuing for 4 weeks. Optimal postexposure prophylaxis is an area of intense study at the present time.

The development of an effective vaccine is the target of active research. Early clinical trials of vaccine candidates are currently under way.

REFERENCES

Carpenter CCJ, Fischl M, Hammer SM, Jacobsen DM, Katzenstein DA, Montaner JSD, et al: Antiretroviral therapy for HIV infection in 1996: Recommendations of an international panel. JAMA 1996; 276:146–154.

Centers for Disease Control and Prevention: Update: Provisional recommendations for chemoprophylaxis after occupational exposure to human immunodeficiency virus. MMWR Morbid Mortal Wkly Rep 1996; 45:468–472.

Fauci AS: AIDS: Newer concepts in the immunopathogenic mechanisms of human immunodeficiency virus disease. Proc Assoc Amer Physicians 1995; 107:1–7.

HIV and the acquired immunodeficiency syndrome. *In* Bennett JC, Plum F (eds): Cecil Textbook of Medicine. 20th ed. Philadelphia, WB Saunders, 1996, pp 1837–1891.

Ho DD, Newman AU, Perelson AS, Chen W, Leonard JM, Markowitz M: Rapid turnover of plasma virions and CD4 lymphocytes in HIV-1 infection. Nature 1995; 362:355–358.

Nadler JP: Early initiation of antiretroviral therapy for infection with human immunodeficiency virus: Considerations in 1996. Clin Infect Dis 1996; 23:227–230.

Saag M, Holodniy M, Kuritzkes DR, et al: HIV viral load markers in clinical practice: Recommendations of an International AIDS Society–USA expert panel. Nature Med 1996; 2:625–629.

Wei X, Ghosh SK, Taylor ME, Johnson VA, Emini EA, Deutsch P, et al: Viral dynamics in human immunodeficiency virus type I infection. Nature 1995; 373:123–126.

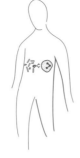

109

Infections in the Immunocompromised Host

Immunosuppression is an increasingly common by-product of diseases and modern approaches to their treatment. The immunocompromised host suffers from increased susceptibility to opportunistic infection, defined as infection caused by organisms of low virulence that compose normal mucosal and skin flora or by pathogenic microbial agents usually maintained in a latent state. Until the 1980s, compromised hosts mainly included patients with congenital immunodeficiencies or those who became immunocompromised as a consequence of cancer and its treatment, bone marrow failure, or treatment with steroids and cytotoxic therapy. The advent of the human immunodeficiency virus (HIV) has brought new meaning and relevance to the term "immunocompromised" host.

Immunocompromise is not an all-or-none phenomenon. The extent of immunosuppression varies with the underlying cause and must exceed a threshold to predispose to opportunistic infections. Importantly, the type of immunosuppression predicts the spectrum of agents likely to cause infections. Accordingly, opportunistic infections can best be considered in categories that reflect the nature of the immune deficiency.

DISORDERS OF CELL-MEDIATED IMMUNITY

Cell-mediated immunity is the major host defense against facultative and some obligate intracellular parasites, as discussed in Chapter 92. A partial list of diseases and situations that produce impaired cell-mediated immunity is presented in Table 109–1. However, only certain of these result in increased susceptibility to infection with intracellular parasites. Foremost among acquired immunodeficiencies are HIV infection (see Chapter 108), Hodgkin's disease and other lymphomas, hairy-cell leukemia, and advanced solid tumors. Severe malnutrition, as well as treatment with high-dose corticosteroids, cytotoxic drugs, or radiotherapy, can produce a similar predilection to infections. Congenital immunodeficiencies are associated with severe infections early in childhood and will not be considered here. Patients with impaired cell-mediated immunity are especially susceptible to the organisms shown in Table 109–2. The relative frequency of occurrence varies with the underlying disease (e.g., *Mycobacterium avium* complex is frequent in HIV infection, *Listeria* is not); geographic area (*Mycobacterium tuberculosis* is

more frequent in developing countries); and the extent of immunosuppression (*M. tuberculosis* is an early, and *M. avium* complex a late, complication of HIV infection).

Thus, with depression of cell-mediated immunity, organisms ordinarily constituting the normal flora, such as *Candida* species, act as virulent opportunistic pathogens capable of causing aggressive infections. Latent viruses, fungi, mycobacteria, and parasites reactivate to cause locally progressive or disseminated disease. Often the signs, symptoms, and laboratory abnormalities suggesting the diagnosis are subtle and nonspecific.

The association between defective cell-mediated immunity and disease produced by the infectious agents listed in Table 109–2 is clear-cut. Sometimes, treatment of the underlying disease causing immunodeficiency or progression of this disease produces a more severe and generalized compromised state, which predisposes to infection by additional microorganisms. For example, during chemotherapy for lymphoma, bacterial infections predominate. Disease progression also results in local factors favoring bacterial infections such as mucosal breakdown and tumor masses obstructing bronchi, ureters, or biliary tract. The result is a marked increase in severe bacterial infection and septicemia late in the course of many diseases associated with impaired cell-mediated immunity.

DISORDERS OF HUMORAL IMMUNITY

The acquired disorders of antibody production associated with increased frequency of infection in adults are common variable immunodeficiency, chronic lymphocytic leu-

TABLE 109–1	Conditions Causing Impaired Cell-Mediated Immunity

Infectious diseases—measles, chickenpox, typhoid fever, tuberculosis, leprosy, histoplasmosis, human immunodeficiency virus infection
Vaccinations—measles, mumps, rubella
Malignancies—Hodgkin's disease, lymphomas, advanced solid tumors
Drugs—corticosteroids, cytotoxic drugs
Miscellaneous—congenital immunodeficiency states, sarcoidosis, uremia, diabetes mellitus, malnutrition, old age

TABLE 109–2	Infections in Patients with Impaired Cell-Mediated Immunity

Viruses—varicella-zoster, herpes simplex, cytomegalovirus, JC virus, human herpesvirus 6
Fungi—pathogenic: *Histoplasma, Coccidioides;* saprophytic: *Cryptococcus, Candida;* less commonly, *Aspergillus, Zygomycetes*
Bacteria—*Listeria monocytogenes, Nocardia, Mycobacterium tuberculosis, Legionella pneumophila,* nontuberculous mycobacteria, *Salmonella* species
Protozoa—*Pneumocystis carinii, Toxoplasma gondii, Cryptosporidium parvum, Leishmania donovani, Giardia lamblia*
Helminths—*Strongyloides stercoralis*

kemia, lymphosarcoma, multiple myeloma, nephrotic syndrome, major burns, and protein-losing enteropathy. The paraproteinemic states belong in this category because of secondary decreases in levels of functioning antibody. Therapy with cytotoxic drugs may produce similar immunocompromise.

Infections due to the pneumococcus, *Haemophilus influenzae*, streptococci, and staphylococci predominate early in the course of the humoral immunodeficiency. As the underlying disease itself progresses, infections due to gram-negative bacilli become more frequent. Treatment of the underlying condition with corticosteroids and cytotoxic drugs causes additional defects in cell-mediated immunity, providing susceptibility to infections with the group of pathogens presented in Table 109–2.

In sickle cell anemia, heat-labile opsonic activity is abnormal. Complement depletion by erythrocyte stroma causes impairment of opsonization of pneumococci and *Salmonella* species, leading to frequent infections with these organisms. Impaired reticuloendothelial system function due to erythrophagocytosis and functional asplenia also may predispose patients with sickle cell disease to serious bacterial infections. The predisposition to infection is age related; once children with sickle cell disease develop antibodies to pneumococcal capsular polysaccharide, they lose their thousandfold increased susceptibility to severe pneumococcal infection.

Splenectomy results in a loss of mechanisms for the clearing of opsonized organisms. Over a period of years, the liver compensates in regard to this filtration function. The splenic tissue also represents a major source of production of antibody as well as other opsonic factors, such as tuftsin, which opsonizes staphylococci. Splenectomy therefore predisposes to fulminant infections caused by encapsulated bacteria. The risk of infection is greater soon after splenectomy and when the spleen is removed for indications other than trauma.

IMPAIRED NEUTROPHIL FUNCTION

Many inherited and acquired diseases impair neutrophil function. The defect may be extrinsic or intrinsic to the neutrophil. Impaired chemotaxis is a significant factor predisposing patients with inherited C3 and C5 deficiencies to frequent bacterial infections (see Chapter 92). Corticosteroid therapy also interferes with chemotaxis.

Whereas circulating neutrophil counts may be normal or increased in patients treated with corticosteroids, these cells are dysfunctional, since they do not localize normally to the site of infection. Defective cell-mediated immunity also contributes to the spectrum of infections associated with corticosteroid therapy. Other conditions associated with impaired neutrophil function include myelodysplasia, paroxysmal nocturnal hemoglobinuria, and radiation and cytotoxic drug therapy.

Intrinsic defects in neutrophils are rare but provide insights into the microbicidal mechanisms of these cells. Neutrophils from patients with chronic granulomatous disease (CGD) cannot develop an oxidative burst. Catalase-negative organisms produce sufficient hydrogen peroxide to facilitate their own killing by CGD neutrophils through the myeloperoxidase pathway. Catalase-producing organisms such as staphylococci, *Serratia, Nocardia,* and *Aspergillus* scavenge the hydrogen peroxide that they produce; these infectious agents, therefore, cannot be killed by CGD neutrophils and produce serious recurrent, deep-seated infections.

The most severe intrinsic neutrophil defects occur in the Chédiak-Higashi syndrome. Patients have giant granules in their leukocytes and defective microtubule assembly. The result is impaired chemotaxis, abnormal phagolysosomal fusion, delayed bacterial killing, and recurrent infections. Diagnosis of this rare syndrome is aided by phenotypic abnormalities: partial albinism, depigmentation of the iris, peripheral neuropathies, and nystagmus.

NEUTROPENIA

Neutropenia is among the most important risk factors for serious infection in the compromised host. Very frequently, other alterations in host defense mechanisms coexist with granulocytopenia; these alterations further increase risk for infection and determine the types of infectious complications. As the neutrophil count falls below $500/\mu l$, an exponential increase occurs in the frequency and severity of infections. Most reliable data derive from patients with acute leukemia. For example, in one study, neutrophil counts of 100 to $500/\mu l$ were associated with infections during 35% of hospitalized days, whereas at counts below $100/\mu l$ infections increased to 55% of days. However, granulocytopenia of other causes, when sustained, may result in a comparable risk of infection. In patients with chronic and cyclic neutropenias, the susceptibility to infection varies inversely with the monocyte count; the mononuclear phagocytes provide some of

TABLE 109–3	Infectious Agents that Frequently Cause Infections in Neutropenic Patients

Bacteria—*Pseudomonas, Klebsiella, Serratia, Escherichia coli, Staphylococcus aureus,* coagulase-negative staphylococci, *Corynebacterium* group JK, streptococci (alpha-hemolytic)
Fungi—*Candida, Aspergillus, Zygomycetes*
Viruses—cytomegalovirus, herpesviruses
Protozoa—*Pneumocystis carinii*

the antibacterial capacity of the missing neutrophils. Following chemotherapy of acute leukemia, neutropenia usually is sustained and associated with damage to mucosal barriers to infection. Patients become susceptible to organisms that are ubiquitous in the environment and ordinarily compose the normal flora (Table 109–3).

DIAGNOSTIC PROBLEMS IN THE COMPROMISED HOST

Pulmonary Infiltrates

The immunocompromised patient with pulmonary infiltrates presents a particularly vexing diagnostic problem. The pulmonary infiltrates could represent infection, extension of underlying tumor, complication of chemotherapy, fluid overload, pulmonary infarction, hemorrhage, or some combination of these. Specific diagnosis is necessary. Unfortunately, noninvasive serodiagnostic tests rarely are helpful in this setting, yet concomitant thrombocytopenia too often increases the risk of lung biopsy.

The clinical setting and radiographic appearance of the pulmonary infiltrate influence the probable yield of lung biopsy and the decision about whether to proceed. For example, in patients with leukemia, parenchymal infiltrates occurring before or within 3 days of initiating chemotherapy usually are bacterial, as are focal infiltrates developing later in the course. Major efforts should be directed at obtaining adequate sputum samples for Gram's stain and culture (see Chapter 99); the evolution of the pneumonitis during antibiotic therapy becomes a useful factor in deciding whether to proceed with lung biopsy.

In contrast, diffuse infiltrates occurring *after* treatment of leukemia are more suggestive of opportunistic infection. *Pneumocystis carinii* is an important preventable, treatable cause of diffuse infiltrates and occurs most often after treatment of acute lymphocytic leukemia or in patients with an acquired deficiency of cell-mediated immunity (see also Chapter 108). In these settings, the diagnosis should be established by examination of induced sputum, by bronchoalveolar lavage, or, less commonly, by transbronchial biopsy. If these diagnostic approaches are not helpful, empirical therapy with trimethoprim-sulfamethoxazole may be initiated.

The indications and timing of lung biopsy, when needed, must be individualized. Delay in proceeding with biopsy, to a point at which the patient is severely hypoxic, reduces the chances of affecting the outcome with therapy, even if the biopsy shows a potentially treatable disease.

Once the decision has been made to perform a biopsy, the next question is which procedure to use. Fiberoptic transbronchial biopsy has provided a good diagnostic yield, particularly in the evaluation of diffuse pulmonary lesions. This technique should not be performed in the thrombocytopenic patient. It is imperative that the tissue obtained be processed and examined quickly. Open lung biopsy has an additional yield of 50 to 75% in the patient with a nondiagnostic transbronchial biopsy and should be performed without delay if the

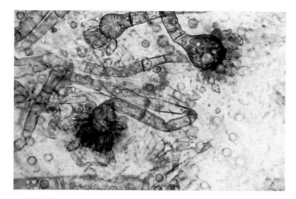

Figure 109–1
Fruiting head of *Aspergillus fumigatus* on lung biopsy. Aspergillosis usually causes an expanding perihilar pulmonary infiltrate. Prompt institution of amphotericin B therapy may lead to a good clinical response.

tempo of progression of the patient's illness mandates immediate diagnosis. Open lung biopsy can generally be performed in thrombocytopenic patients if prophylactic transfusions can achieve an increment in the platelet count and diminish the bleeding time.

Early treatment of most pulmonary infections in immunocompromised hosts, even aspergillosis (Fig. 109–1), is associated with an initially favorable outcome. The long-term result, however, is dependent on the natural history of the underlying disease process.

Disseminated Mycoses

Disseminated mycoses represent another major diagnostic problem in the immunocompromised host. Fungal infections are found post mortem in more than one half of patients with leukemia and lymphoma; usually, the nature of the infection has not been established ante mortem. Culture of a saprophytic organism such as *Candida* from superficial sites does not establish pathogenicity. Even in patients with widespread infection, however, detectable fungemia is a late event.

How, then, can the diagnosis of fungal infection be established early, at a time when the infection is potentially curable? It is important to search for superficial lesions accessible to scraping, aspiration, or biopsy (Fig. 109–2). Dissemination of *Candida tropicalis* frequently causes hyperpigmented macular or pustular skin lesions that show the organism within blood vessel walls on biopsy. Hepatosplenic candidiasis is most frequently encountered in patients with fever following recovery from neutropenia. The presence of "bull's-eye" lesions on computed tomographic scan of the liver and spleen suggests hepatosplenic candidiasis. Cryptococcal polysaccharide antigen may be present in the serum or cerebrospinal fluid of the patient with disseminated cryptococcosis. Serodiagnosis for other fungi has, in general, been disappointing. Acute invasive pulmonary aspergillosis occurs most often in patients with prolonged, profound neutropenia who present with fever and pleuritic chest pain during or following broad-spectrum antibacterial therapy.

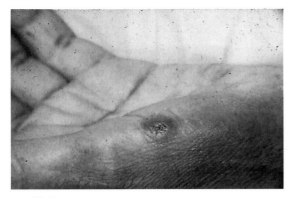

Figure 109-2

Skin lesion in a 76-year-old woman treated with corticosteroids and cytotoxic drugs for chronic lymphocytic leukemia and presenting with nodular pulmonary infiltrates and lymphocytic meningitis. Fluid expressed from the lesion contained encapsulated yeast seen on India ink preparation and yielded *Cryptococcus neoformans* on culture.

In the absence of adequate diagnostic procedures, empirical use of antifungal drugs is often indicated in the immunocompromised host when there is appropriate clinical suspicion of disseminated mycoses (e.g., in the neutropenic patient with fever for more than 7 days despite broad-spectrum antibiotic therapy).

PREVENTION AND TREATMENT OF INFECTIONS IN THE NEUTROPENIC PATIENT

Prevention

Acute bacterial infections and septicemia arising from organisms composing the gut flora occur frequently in granulocytopenic patients and may have fever as their sole manifestation. Prophylactic nonabsorbable antibiotics and protective isolation have generally failed to prevent such infection. Trimethoprim-sulfamethoxazole, given prophylactically, may decrease the number of infections and bacteremic episodes in some neutropenic patients, in addition to preventing the development of *P. carinii* pneumonia. However, its bone marrow toxicity and selection of resistant organisms make it unsuitable for widespread use as a prophylactic agent in neutropenic patients. Quinolones, such as ciprofloxacin, may be at least as effective in preventing bacterial infections and are less toxic; quinolones lack activity, however, against *P. carinii*. Prophylactic administration of imidazoles to prevent systemic fungal infections is of uncertain value in this setting.

Prophylactic granulocyte transfusions decrease the occurrence of bacterial sepsis in patients with acute myelogenous leukemia but are costly and do not affect overall remission rate and duration of survival.

Treatment

Empirical antibiotic therapy is indicated in febrile granulocytopenic patients, since up to two thirds have an underlying infection. Selection of two drugs with activity against *Pseudomonas aeruginosa*, such as tobramycin and mezlocillin, is essential. This two-drug regimen also provides adequate initial antibiotic coverage of staphylococcal infections, although clinical experience favors the use of other drugs (e.g., vancomycin) for their definitive therapy. Despite the early empirical use of antibiotics, the outcome of bacterial infections is poor unless the initial neutrophil count exceeds $500/\mu l$, the count rises during treatment, or the pathogen is a gram-positive organism. Treatment with granulocyte colony-stimulating factors may result in shorter duration of neutropenia and fewer infectious complications.

The appropriate duration of antimicrobial therapy of febrile neutropenic patients is uncertain. Many physicians continue antibiotics until neutropenia resolves. The empirical addition of amphotericin B therapy is indicated in the neutropenic patient who remains febrile for at least 1 week despite broad-spectrum antibiotics. In this setting, it often is best to continue broad-spectrum antibiotics for the duration of the neutropenia unless the cause of the fever can be clearly defined.

REFERENCES

Pizzo PA: The compromised host. *In* Bennett JC, Plum F (eds.): Cecil Textbook of Medicine. 20th ed. Philadelphia, WB Saunders, 1996, pp 1537–1548.
Rubin RH, Young LS (eds.): Clinical Approach to Infection in the Compromised Host. 3rd ed. New York, Plenum Medical Book Company, 1994, pp 1–752.

110

Infectious Diseases of Travelers; Protozoal and Helminthic Infections

This chapter reviews the medical preparation of patients for overseas travel, some common clinical symptoms that may develop on return, and the diagnosis and treatment of common parasitic diseases endemic in the United States and abroad.

PREPARATION OF TRAVELERS

More than 10 million Americans travel to developing countries each year. Major increases in international travel and the resurgence of malaria and other infectious diseases worldwide bring the issues of prevention and management of health problems in travelers into the office of every physician.

Risks associated with international travel are dependent upon the destination, duration of the trip, underlying health and age of the traveler, and activities while abroad. In general, destinations within the industrialized world require no specific health precautions. In contrast, travelers to developing areas, especially the tropics, can be exposed to life-threatening infections. Major issues to be addressed in the pretravel period include immunizations, malaria prophylaxis, traveler's diarrhea, and other problems that can be avoided or prevented. Information about health risks in specific geographic areas, updated weekly, can be obtained from the Centers for Disease Control and Prevention (CDC) through its publications or by calling the International Traveler's Hotline (404-332-4559).

Immunizations

In general, only yellow fever and cholera vaccinations may be required by law for international travel. On occasion, however, both polio and meningococcal meningitis vaccinations have been required during outbreak situations. Although some immunizations are not generally considered "travel" immunizations, many Americans have allowed routine diphtheria-tetanus immunizations to lapse or may not have been fully immunized against measles and polio in their youth. Finally, other immunizations are often strongly recommended, depending on the type and

duration of travel. With a few exceptions, vaccines can be given simultaneously. Before immunization, a careful history should be obtained to determine allergies to eggs or chicken embryo cells. Pregnant women and individuals immunocompromised by human immunodeficiency virus (HIV), malignancy, or chemotherapy pose specific and important challenges; most live virus vaccines are contraindicated in these patients.

Yellow Fever

This live attenuated virus vaccine is highly effective and recommended for travel to areas in South America and Africa where yellow fever is endemic. Vaccination is highly effective and lasts for 10 years but must be given at designated vaccination centers.

Cholera

Cholera is not a common disease of tourists but has recently returned to South and Central America, where it is a major concern to travelers. The vaccine available is not very effective and is therefore not recommended for travel into endemic areas. Health education on likely sources of transmission (e.g., food, water) is far more effective in preventing disease than vaccine. Cholera vaccination is, however, still a legal requirement for travel between some developing countries. In these circumstances, one dose of the vaccine is adequate.

Measles and Mumps

Up to 20% of first-year college students have no serologic evidence of prior measles or mumps infection or immunization and must be presumed to be susceptible. Individuals with no physician-documented record of immunization born after 1956 are at greatest risk for measles, and after 1970, for mumps. In addition, a single immunization with measles vaccine at 15 months of age may permit breakthrough infection as a young adult. As a result, a second measles vaccine is now recommended for international travel for individuals who have never experienced the clinical illness. The same considerations apply to mumps, but this is not yet an official recommendation. All live virus vaccines should be given at least 2 weeks before gamma globulin administration.

Diphtheria-Tetanus

Tetanus is a ubiquitous problem and is most prevalent in tropical countries. A booster within the past 5 years is recommended. This eliminates the need for a tetanus booster if the traveler sustains a tetanus-prone injury overseas. This recommendation is made primarily because of the uncertainty of obtaining sterile, disposable needles in many overseas locations. Given the resurgence of diphtheria in countries of the former Soviet Union and the occurrence of disease in travelers to these areas, diphtheria toxoid should be coadministered with tetanus toxoid.

Polio

Polio remains endemic in many regions of the developing world. Most young adults have been immunized with at least 4 doses of trivalent oral polio vaccine (OPV); an additional booster dose is recommended for international travel. Many adults (>18 years of age) cannot remember, however, whether they received all serotypes of OPV; such individuals should be given inactivated polio vaccine (IPV). IPV should be boosted every 5 years for international travel.

Hepatitis A

Hepatitis A is a major risk for travelers to areas of poor sanitation, affecting an estimated 1 in 1000 travelers per 2- to 3-week trip in some areas. As such, hepatitis A is the most important vaccine-preventable infection for travelers. Hepatitis A vaccine should be given at least 2 weeks before departure. This vaccine is safe and immunogenic.

Meningococcal Meningitis

Meningococcal meningitis is a worldwide disease but cases in international travelers are infrequent except with prolonged contact with the local population. Vaccination with the quadrivalent polysaccharide vaccine (A, C, Y, +W135) is recommended for travel to northern India, Nepal, Saudi Arabia during the Moslem Hajj, certain parts of sub-Saharan Africa, and other locations where travel advisories have been issued.

Typhoid

American international travelers are at greatest risk of contracting typhoid in the Indian subcontinent, Mexico, western South America, and sub-Saharan Africa. Vaccination is recommended for travel to endemic areas where exposure to contaminated food and water is likely or in areas where *Salmonella typhi* is resistant to multiple antibiotics. Vaccination is also strongly indicated for travelers with achlorhydria, immunosuppression, or sickle cell anemia and for those taking broad-spectrum antibiotics. Adequate vaccination with the injectable vaccine takes time (2 injections 1 month apart for those without prior immunizations) and is associated with significant side effects (frequently a sore arm and a flu-like reaction), but it does provide partial protection. An oral vaccine (four enteric-coated capsules given over 7 days) is equally efficacious and has fewer side effects.

Other Vaccines

Some travelers, including missionaries, physicians, and anthropologists, need special consideration. These individuals live for prolonged periods in developing countries or are at special risk for contracting certain highly contagious diseases. Consideration should be given to immunization with hepatitis B, Japanese B encephalitis, plague, and rabies vaccines. In general, such consultations should be referred to a qualified travelers' clinic.

Malaria Prophylaxis

Malaria prophylaxis is a major problem for international travelers because of the high and increasing prevalence of drug resistance by the parasite. The need for, as well as the type of, prophylaxis is dependent upon the exact itinerary within a given country, since transmission risk is quite regional. For example, malaria transmission does not occur in most urban centers in Southeast Asia (e.g., Bangkok), but highly drug-resistant strains of *Plasmodium falciparum* may be encountered in the countryside. Recommended chemoprophylactic regimens have changed frequently within the past few years. Detailed information on malaria risk must be updated frequently. In general, travelers to areas where chloroquine-sensitive *P. falciparum* strains are exclusively found (Central America, the Caribbean, North Africa, and the Middle East) should take chloroquine phosphate (300 mg base or 500 mg salt) weekly starting 2 weeks before, during, and for 6 weeks after leaving areas in which malaria is endemic. Travelers to areas where chloroquine-resistant *P. falciparum* is common should take mefloquine (Larium), 250 mg a week starting a week before travel, during travel, and for 4 weeks after. These areas currently include Southeast Asia, sub-Saharan Africa, South America, and South Asia. Alternative regimens include weekly chloroquine with back-up treatment for presumptive breakthrough malaria with 3 tablets of pyrimethamine-sulfadoxine (Fansidar). Daily doxycycline (100 mg) is another reasonable alternative. No antimalarial regimen is completely effective in Burma, rural Thailand, or some parts of East Africa, where mefloquine resistance is a growing problem. Because of these facts, emphasis must be given to the use of netting, screens, and insect repellants as well as to the prompt diagnosis and treatment of any febrile episodes (temperature > 102°F [39°C]) overseas.

Traveler's Diarrhea

Between 20 and 50% of individuals traveling to developing countries will develop diarrhea during or shortly after their trip. The risk is highest when traveling to India, Latin America, Africa, the Middle East, and South Asia. The average duration of an episode of traveler's diarrhea is 3 to 6 days. About 10% of episodes last longer than 1 week. The diarrhea may be accompanied by abdominal cramping, nausea, headache, low-grade fever, vomiting, or bloating. Fewer than 5% of persons have fever greater than 101°F (38°C), bloody stools, or both. Travelers with these symptoms may not have simple traveler's diarrhea and should see a physician at once (see Chapter 103).

Diarrheal illness (including cholera) can be avoided through care with food and water. All water should be presumed to be unsafe. Salads are often contaminated by protozoal cysts and, along with street vendor foods, are the most dangerous foods encountered by most travelers. Food should be well cooked, including meat, seafood, and vegetables. Milk is often unpasteurized; therefore, dairy products should be avoided.

Bismuth subsalicylate (Pepto-Bismol) can be used as a prophylactic measure (2 tablets 4 times a day) or used to treat acute bouts of diarrhea (1 oz every 30 minutes for 8 doses). Diphenoxylate (Lomotil) and loperamide (Imodium) may give some symptomatic relief of diarrhea but should be avoided if the diarrhea is severe, fever exists, or blood is present in the stool. Trimethoprim-sulfamethoxazole (Bactrim), doxycycline (Vibramycin), or one of the newer quinolones with or without concomitant use of loperamide can be taken orally for 3 to 5 days to treat episodes of diarrhea. These regimens reduce the duration of symptoms and are effective against a wide variety of bacterial pathogens, including most *Shigella* and *Salmonella* species. Prophylactic antibiotics are not generally recommended except for very short trips because of the emergence of resistant strains and the development of photosensitivity or other reactions to prophylactic medications.

General Health Information

Other potentially dangerous activities overseas include exposure to dogs and cats (rabies), swimming in fresh water (schistosomiasis or leptosporosis), walking barefoot (hookworm or strongyloidiasis), and insect bites. In addition to malaria, many diseases, including dengue, sleeping sickness, and yellow fever, are transmitted by biting insects.

Special Problems

Pregnant Women

Live virus vaccines are contraindicated in pregnant women and greatly complicate pretravel preparations. Chloroquine probably can be used safely. Travel to areas of chloroquine-resistant malaria is of great risk and should be strongly discouraged. No drug regimen to prevent or treat chloroquine-resistant malaria is safe in pregnancy, and malaria in a pregnant woman is a medical emergency for both the mother and her fetus.

Acquired Immunodeficiency Syndrome (AIDS)

Travelers and host countries are increasingly concerned about AIDS. Many countries, including the United States, now bar entry to AIDS patients. Several countries require HIV serologic testing for all travelers applying for more than a 3-month visa, which requires official documentation well in advance of travel. Patients with HIV infection need special preparation prior to travel to developing countries because of their increased susceptibility to certain illnesses (e.g., pneumococcal infection and tuberculosis).

Most international travelers are concerned about the risk of acquiring AIDS while abroad. AIDS is acquired by the same activities associated with transmission in the United States. Most legitimate concerns center on untested blood or nonsterile needles, which might be used in an emergency. In general, a few hospitals in almost all countries frequented by tourists now have sterile needles and screen their blood supply.

THE RETURNING TRAVELER

With the exception of skin testing for tuberculosis, asymptomatic returning travelers generally do not need screening tests. The clinical problems that most often arise in travelers soon after return are fever and diarrhea, whereas eosinophilia is the most common cause for later referral. Of the three, fever is most important, since delay in the diagnosis of *P. falciparum* malaria can be fatal. Fever should always prompt consideration of malaria until proved otherwise in travelers returning from countries where malaria is endemic, even if they are still taking prophylactic drugs. It is important to speciate the malaria with a thin and thick blood film, since this affects therapy. Chloroquine-sensitive *P. falciparum* is treated with 1 gm of chloroquine given orally, followed by 500 mg at 6, 24, and 48 hours. For *Plasmodium vivax* and *Plasmodium ovale* (also generally chloroquine-sensitive), this regimen is followed by primaquine daily for 14 days to eradicate hepatic forms. Resistant *P. falciparum* is treated with quinine sulfate, 650 mg given orally every 8 hours for 3 days, and tetracycline, 250 mg given orally every 6 hours for 10 days. All patients with suspected resistant infection should be hospitalized. In smear-negative cases in which clinical suspicion remains high, repeated smears every 8 to 12 hours should be obtained. If fever is not due to malaria, then tuberculosis, typhoid fever, hepatitis, enteric infections, and amebic liver abscess should be considered.

Traveler's diarrhea unresponsive to empirical antibiotics and persistent until the traveler returns home often represents giardiasis. Three stool specimens for ova and parasites, one stool examination for red blood cells and white blood cells, and a stool culture are usually warranted. Unfortunately, *Giardia lamblia* may be missed in up to one third of cases even after this work-up. If clinical suspicion is high, an empirical course of metronidazole (500 mg po tid × 7 days) is usually justified. Antibiotic-resistant bacteria, amebiasis, temporary lactose intolerance, bacterial overgrowth, and tropical sprue should also be considered.

Eosinophilia in a returning traveler is less common and usually manifests weeks or months after travel. It is usually caused by any one of a variety of helminth infections. A stool specimen for ova and parasites is indicated but may be negative during the tissue-migrating phase of many intestinal worms or in tissue nematode infections, such as filariasis or onchocerciasis. Management of the more common parasitic infections encountered in travelers is included in the next section. Finally, it should be remembered that some diseases acquired abroad can take several years to manifest symptoms. When presenting with an unknown illness, all travelers should be advised to remind their doctor of past international travel.

PROTOZOAL AND HELMINTHIC INFECTIONS

Protozoal Infections in the United States
(Table 110–1)

Worldwide, the incidence of parasitic infections is increasing. This is due in part to the emergence of antimicrobial resistance (e.g., malaria) and an increasing number of susceptible hosts, especially those with HIV infection. Protozoal infections in the United States occur more frequently in selected patient populations and may be particularly severe in immunocompromised hosts. For example, giardiasis and amebiasis are common causes of diarrhea in homosexual men. Babesiosis is very severe in asplenic individuals, and *Toxoplasma* encephalitis primarily affects patients with AIDS.

Amebiasis and Giardiasis

Giardiasis is a common cause of persistent, nonbloody diarrhea in returning travelers. Although *G. lamblia* is prevalent throughout much of the developing world, travelers from St. Petersburg, Russia, have had consistently high attack rates, sometimes exceeding 50% for large tour groups. Homosexual males also have a high prevalence of infection because of specific sexual practices. The diagnosis is generally made by identification of ova or trophozoites on stool examination (at least three stool specimens

TABLE 110–1	Protozoal Infections				
Protozoan	**Setting**	**Vectors**	**Diagnosis**	**Special Considerations**	**Treatment**
Endemic in US					
Babesia microti	New England	Ixodid ticks, transfusions	Thick or thin blood smear	Severe disease in asplenic persons	Quinine and clindamycin
Giardia lamblia	Mountain states	Humans, ? small mammals	Microscopic exam or stool or duodenal fluid exam	Common in homosexual men, travelers, children in day care	Quinacrine or metronidazole
Toxoplasma gondii	Ubiquitous	Domestic cats, raw meat	Clinical; serologic confirmation	Pregnant women, immunosuppressed host (AIDS)	Pyrimethamine and sulfadiazine
Entamoeba histolytica	Southeast	Human	Microscopic exam of stool or "touch prep" from ulcer	Common in homosexual men, travelers, institutionalized persons	Metronidazole
Cryptosporidium sp.	Ubiquitous	Human	Acid-fast stain of stool	Severe in immunosuppressed hosts (AIDS)	None
Trichomonas vaginalis	Ubiquitous	Human	"Wet prep" of genital secretions	Common cause of vaginitis	Metronidazole
Primarily Seen in Travelers and Immigrants					
Plasmodium sp.	Africa, Asia, South America	*Anopheles* mosquito	Thick and thin blood smear	Consider in returning travelers with fever	Dependent upon regional resistance pattern (see text)
Leishmania donovani	Middle East	Sandfly	Tissue biopsy	Consider in immigrants with fever and splenomegaly	Pentostam
Trypanosoma sp.	Africa, South America	Reduvid bugs, transfusion	Direct exam of blood or CSF	Very rare in travelers, transfusion associated	Supportive

AIDS = Acquired immunodeficiency syndrome; CSF = cerebrospinal fluid.

should be examined). The drug of choice for adults is metronidazole, 500 to 750 mg 3 times a day for 7 days.

Like *Giardia, Entamoeba histolytica* is transmitted via the fecal-oral route; the vast majority of infected individuals are asymptomatic. In contrast to *Giardia*, invasive extraintestinal illness can occur, and thus it is important to treat even asymptomatic individuals. When *E. histolytica* causes acute illness, it is generally manifested by bloody diarrhea. In the United States, amebic dysentery is occasionally misdiagnosed as ulcerative colitis or Crohn's disease and the administration of corticosteroids may cause significant worsening and toxic megacolon. Stool examination for ova and parasites is generally diagnostic, but sigmoidoscopy may be required with either a touch preparation of the punctate ulcers or a biopsy. Serology is useful to rule out this diagnosis. This is especially important in individuals from industrialized countries, since the background serologic positivity is quite low in this population. Extraintestinal amebiasis generally presents as hepatic liver abscess (see Chapter 102).

Protozoal Infections Common in Travelers and Immigrants (see Table 110–1)

Malaria

Management of this parasitic infection is discussed under "The Returning Traveler."

Leishmaniasis

Cutaneous and mucocutaneous leishmaniasis should be considered in any traveler returning from the Middle East or endemic areas of Latin America who has a persistent skin or mucous membrane lesion. Diagnosis is made by tissue biopsy. Visceral leishmaniasis should be suspected in immigrants with fever and splenomegaly. Diagnosis is made by bone marrow biopsy and culture. Cutaneous leishmaniasis is generally self-limited. Other types are treated with Pentostam (sodium stibogluconate), 20 mg/kg/day for up to 20 days.

African Trypanosomiasis

In Africa, this protozoal infection causes sleeping sickness. Although only rarely imported into developed countries, it should be suspected in systemically ill patients from Africa presenting with fever, headache, and confusion. Many patients will remember a painful chancre at the site of an insect bite. Diagnosis is made by direct examination of the blood, lymph aspirate, or cerebrospinal fluid. Treatment is not uniformly effective and should be supervised by an expert in the field.

Chagas' Disease (American Trypanosomiasis)

Trypanosoma cruzi is the most common cause of heart failure in South America, particularly Brazil. Transmission is through contact with feces from infected reduvid bugs (kissing bugs). Most cases are asymptomatic for decades and then manifest with cardiomegaly, megaesophagus, or megacolon. Diagnosis of acute disease is made by direct examination of the blood. Early diagnosis is critical, as patients may respond to nitrofuran or nitroimidazole derivatives. Chronic cases are suspected on the basis of serology, but background seropositivity is high in many endemic countries. Treatment of chronic Chagas' disease is largely supportive.

Helminthic Infections Common in the United States (Table 110–2)

Pinworm

Enterobiasis is common in the United States, particularly among children. Perianal pruritus is the major clinical presentation. Infection is maintained by fecal-oral contamination. Diagnosis is made by the application of cellophane tape to the anus and subsequent direct examination for ova. Treatment is with mebendazole, 100 mg given once. It is advisable to treat all family members, and repeated doses may be necessary.

TABLE 110–2	Helminthic Infections				
Helminth	**Setting**	**Vectors**	**Diagnosis**	**Treatment**
Endemic in US				
Pinworm (enterobiasis)	Ubiquitous	Human	Direct exam for ova	Mebendazole, albendazole
Ascaris lumbricoides	Southeast	Human	Stool exam for ova	Mebendazole, albendazole
Trichuris trichiura	Southeast	Human	Stool exam for ova	Mebendazole, albendazole
Hookworm	Southeast	Human	Stool exam for ova	Mebendazole, albendazole
Common in Travelers and Immigrants				
Strongyloides stercoralis	Developing world	Human	Stool exam for larvae	Thiabendazole, ivermectin
Schistosoma sp.	Developing world	Snails	Stool exam for ova	Praziquantel
Wuchereria sp.	Asia	Mosquitos	Nocturnal blood exam	Ivermectin
Onchocerca volvulus	Africa, South and Central America	Blackfly	Biopsy	Ivermectin
Loa loa	Africa	Mosquitos	Blood exam, clinical setting	Ivermectin

Other Intestinal Nematodes

Ascaris (giant roundworm), *Ancylostoma duodenale* and *Necator americanus* (hookworm), and *Trichuris* (whipworms), still endemic in the United States, are extremely common in immigrants and are ubiquitous in the developing world. Most individuals are asymptomatic. Ascariasis and hookworm may cause transient pulmonary infiltrates with eosinophilia during the tissue migratory phase of infection. Heavy *Ascaris* infection may cause intestinal, biliary, or pancreatic obstruction, but generally the patient is alerted to infection by the passage of a 6- to 8-inch-long dead adult worm. Hookworm infection can be associated with iron deficiency. Diagnosis is made on the basis of stool examination for ova and parasites. Each of these worms can be eradicated with appropriate antihelminthic therapy.

Helminth Infections Common in Travelers and Immigrants (see Table 110–2)

Strongyloidosis

Strongyloides stercoralis is a common cause of eosinophilia in immigrants, particularly those from Southeast Asia. Infection can persist for years; many men who served in the Pacific theater during World War II or in Vietnam still harbor active infections. Although usually asymptomatic, infection can cause diarrhea, abdominal pain, and malabsorption. This helminth can cause life-threatening disseminated infection in individuals immunosuppressed by cancer chemotherapy, steroids, or HIV infection. Diagnosis may be made by stool examination, but this is not a very sensitive technique. Treatment with thiabendazole twice daily for 2 days is curative in more than 90% of immunocompetent hosts.

Schistosomiasis

Schistosoma mansoni (Africa, South America, and the Caribbean), *Schistosoma japonicum* (Philippines, China, and Indonesia), and *Schistosoma mekongi* (Cambodia, Laos, and Vietnam) are the most common causes of hepatosplenic enlargement in the world. Chronic infection can lead to an unusual form of periportal hepatic fibrosis, obstruction of portal blood flow, and bleeding esophageal varices. Unsuspected cases in the United States are often misdiagnosed as hepatitis B or alcohol-induced liver disease. A clue to the correct diagnosis is that the liver is enlarged, in contrast to the small, shrunken liver of alcoholic cirrhosis. *S. japonicum* can also cause seizures, which result from aberrant central nervous system migration of adult worms. *Schistosoma haematobium* (Africa) commonly causes hematuria and leads to urinary obstruction. Diagnosis is made by examination of stool or urine for ova and parasites.

Lymphatic Filariasis

Wuchereria bancrofti and *Brugia malayi* cause elephantiasis throughout the tropics. Patients may present with acute lymphadenitis or asymptomatic eosinophilia. Occasional patients have pulmonary symptoms, infiltrates, and marked eosinophilia (tropical pulmonary eosinophilia). The diagnosis is made by finding microfilariae in blood specimens obtained at midnight. Treatment currently consists of a single oral dose of ivermectin, but this does not kill the adult worms.

Loa Loa

Eyeworm is endemic in West and Central Africa. Patients present with transient pruritic subcutaneous swellings. Eosinophilia is universal. In the United States, cases are often misdiagnosed for years as chronic urticaria. In rare patients, the adult worm can be visualized as it crosses the anterior chamber of the eye, giving this worm its common name. Diagnosis is generally suspected on clinical grounds and is confirmed by biopsy.

River Blindness

Infection with *Onchocerca volvulus* occurs in West and Central Africa as well as South and Central America. Although the most severe manifestations occur in the eye, the most common clinical presentation in the United States is recurrent pruritic dermatitis. The diagnosis can be made by direct examination of skin snips for microfilariae; a specific serologic test is also available. Ivermectin is the treatment of choice.

Clonorchiasis

The Chinese liver fluke, *Clonorchis sinensis*, is important to diagnose in Asian immigrants. Symptoms may be confused with those of biliary tract disease. If untreated, infection can lead to cholangiocarcinoma. Praziquantel is curative.

Cysticercosis

The invasive larval form of pork tapeworm is the most common cause of seizures throughout the world, as well as in young adults in Los Angeles, chiefly immigrants from Mexico. Typically, patients present with new onset of seizures or severe headache. A single ring-enhancing lesion is the characteristic finding on computed tomographic (CT) scan. The diagnosis may be confirmed by an immunoblot assay using peripheral blood. Praziquantel is curative but may precipitate focal cerebral edema and seizures by killing other cysticercariae within the cerebrospinal fluid. An expert should be consulted prior to treatment.

Intestinal Tapeworms

Three intestinal tapeworms commonly infect humans: *Taenia saginata* from raw beef, *Taenia solium* from raw pork, and *Diphyllobothrium latum* from raw fish. Most individuals are asymptomatic, but *T. solium* can cause invasive disease (cysticercosis) if ova of the adult worm are ingested by humans. *D. latum* is associated with vitamin B$_{12}$ deficiency. All three are treated with praziquantel.

Hydatid Disease

This disease commonly manifests as a cystic liver mass in emigrants from sheep-raising parts of the world. Diagnosis is important, since rupture of the cyst can lead to dissemination. Diagnosis is often suspected owing to the appearance of the cyst (calcified wall and dependent hydatid "sand") on abdominal CT scan. Serology can be helpful but is occasionally negative if the cyst has not leaked. Currently, primary therapy is the surgical removal of the cyst without spillage of its contents.

REFERENCES

Gardner P (ed.): Health issues of international travelers. Infect Dis Clin North Am 1992;6:275–510.

Mahmoud AAF: Tropical medicine: Current problems and possible solutions. Infect Dis Clin North Am 1995;9:265–274.

US Public Health Service, Department of Health and Human Services: Centers for Disease Control and Prevention: Health Information for International Travel, 1995. Washington, DC, Government Printing Office. Updated on a weekly basis with the blue summary sheet.

Neurologic Disease

Section XIV

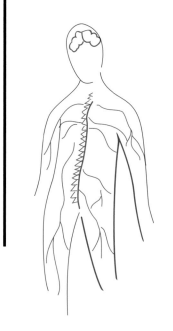

111

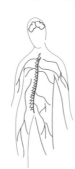

Neurologic Evaluation of the Patient

Neurologic disorders can be divided clinically into three principal diagnostic categories. First, distressing symptoms that often exist without associated clinical or laboratory evidence of tissue abnormalities (Table 111–1). These tend to be the most frequent complaints that bring patients to general physicians and, often, the most difficult to diagnose definitively and manage successfully. Second, intrinsic neuromuscular or neurologic disorders that affect either peripheral nerve and muscle or the central nervous system or both as a result of intrinsically abnormal genetic, developmental, autoimmune, neoplastic, or degenerative processes (Table 111–2). Third, disorders that derive from abnormalities in other body systems or the environment to damage the central nervous or neuromuscular system (see Table 111–2). The essence of clinical diagnosis lies in the physician's being able to identify with a high degree of probability which of these three categories most likely caused the patient's symptoms and signs. The progressive questions listed in Table 111–3 greatly ease this task and usually can be answered at least tentatively by obtaining a careful history and clinical neurological examination. Properly obtained laboratory tests can then be called upon to confirm or specifically identify the accurate diagnosis.

To minimize error and maximize the chance of early, effective treatment the physician must systematically approach patients with potentially neurologic complaints and answer four fundamental questions, as outlined in Table 111–4.

THE NEUROLOGIC HISTORY

The neurologic history in most respects is similar to the general medical history. Many neurologic diseases, however, are not accompanied by either abnormal physical or laboratory findings, so that the history often supplies a greater proportion of the diagnostically relevant information than does a medical history. Furthermore, because neurologic abnormalities affect such important functions as thinking, moving, and feeling, most patients will perceive that something is awry even before physical signs appear. Physical findings not previously recognized by the patient or family may often be irrelevant or even misleading. By contrast, recent symptoms, such as mild weakness or alterations of sensation, often reflect disease even if the

process is still too subtle to be detected by physical examination. Because neurologic symptoms are so keenly sensed, a careful history often allows the examiner to localize the disease anatomically and to understand its pathophysiology even before he or she begins the physical examination.

Certain guidelines aid in taking complete and accurate histories:

Require Precision

Do not accept jargon or diagnoses from the patient. For example, a patient who complains of dizziness may mean vertigo (a vestibular symptom), lightheadedness (potentially caused by anxiety or, less often, cardiovascular disease), syncope, ataxia, diplopia, or psychogenic dissociation—all of which have very different implications.

Both Listen and Ask

Elicit the history in the patient's own words and, whenever possible, without interruption. However, the physician must ask direct questions to encourage relevance, achieve precision, and place each symptom in its correct context. If the information is not volunteered, ask about the temporal profile of the complaint: Was the onset abrupt or gradual? Has the symptom(s) ever appeared previously? Is it static, progressive, waxing and waning, or improving? Inquire into the intensity and frequency of the symptoms: Has anything relieved them? Have there been precipitating factors?

Form Hypotheses

One must sift and distill the information in order to focus on what is relevant and weed out the irrelevant. Concurrently, one must form anatomic and/or pathophysiologic hypotheses about the nature of the symptoms and gradually refine them into etiologic terms as the history develops.

Hypotheses should favor illnesses that are *probable* (i.e., common diseases are more likely than rare diseases), *serious* (e.g., brain tumors should be excluded before di-

TABLE 111–1	Common Neurologic Symptoms Often Unaccompanied By Structural or Laboratory-Detectable Abnormalities

Headache
Backache
Dizziness
Insomnia
Chronic fatigue
Anxiety or panic
Hysteria or simulation
Manic-depressive symptoms
Schizophrenic symptoms

TABLE 111–3	Crucial Questions in Neurologic Diagnosis

1. Does the patient have a nervous system disorder? Do psychological mechanisms play an important role in the genesis of symptoms?
2. What part(s) of the nervous system are affected? Is the lesion peripheral (muscle; neuromuscular junction; peripheral nerve or roots) or central (i.e., above or below the foramen magnum)? If above, above or below the tentorium? Either way, are there one or several lesions, left or right, symmetrical or asymmetrical? What specific tests may give useful answers?
3. What are the mechanisms (structural or physiologic, vascular, neoplastic, inflammatory)?
4. What is the cause (etiology)?

agnosing tension headache), *treatable* (e.g., combined systems disease and spinal cord meningioma should be ruled out before making a diagnosis of multiple sclerosis), and *novel* (some patients do have rare diseases, and these should not be forgotten).

Always Cover the Main Points of a Complete History

However justified the chief complaint appears to be, ensure that other physical or psychological disabilities are not playing a role. In particular, inquire about the patient's mood (e.g., is he/she depressed or suicidal?), his/her usual daily activities and whether the illness interferes with them, sexual function, and his/her own view of the illness and what effects it produces. Always ask about alcohol and drug intake, both prescription and recreational.

End by Summarizing

Summarize the history for the patient, asking if the summary is correct and if anything has been missed. Such a summary tends to reassure patients and offers a chance to supply information and to correct misunderstandings.

Obtain Further History from the Family and Friends

If the history appears incomplete, and especially when the history suggests changes in mental state or consciousness, the family, friends, and colleagues should be asked to supply missing elements.

Gear the Neurologic Examination to Hypotheses Generated by the History

The hypotheses generated during the course of the history determine which of the nonroutine neurologic maneuvers the physician will carry out during the examination.

THE NEUROLOGIC EXAMINATION

A screening neurologic examination, as outlined in Table 111–3, takes only a few minutes. More time may be

TABLE 111–2	Etiologic Categories of Neurologic Diseases

Intrinsic Causes
Genetic or metabolic
Developmental
Autoimmune
Neoplastic
Degenerative

Extrinsic Causes
Extraneural organ failure
Toxic or nutritional
Vascular
Infectious
Traumatic
Psychogenic

TABLE 111–4	Important Elements of the Neurologic Examination

Level of arousal
Mental status
  Orientation, mood, language, memory, intellect, thought
Station and gait
Cranial nerves
Motor system
  Strength, tone, muscle bulk, adventitious movements, coordinated activity
Peripheral sensory system
  Pin, temperature, vibration, proprioception, object identification
Reflexes
  Deep tendon
  Abdominals
  Plantar
  Anal wink
Autonomic system
  Blood pressure
  Sphincter
Vascular system
  Carotid pulse and bruits; distal arteries

required to evaluate areas that the history suggests may be disordered. Note the *level of arousal:* awake and alert, drowsy and lethargic, responsive only when externally stimulated (stuporous), or behaviorally unarousable, even to vigorous external stimulation (comatose)? Examine the *mental state* as you take the history. Persons who give articulate and comprehensive histories with accurate attention to detail and dating of complaints rarely suffer mental impairment. Nevertheless, when any doubt exists, check (1) orientation, particularly for place and date; (2) short-term memory (the most vulnerable memory function) by asking the patient to repeat three unrelated words 5 minutes after he/she has heard them; and (3) the capacity to abstract, by interpreting proverbs and by recognizing similarities and differences (boy-dwarf, apple-pear). Because anxiety can interfere with cognitive functions, one must be patient and reassuring. A formal quantitative screening examination such as the "mini mental status" examination (Table 111–5) can rapidly and usefully define suspected cognitive dysfunction.

Observe the patient's *stance* and *walk*. A patient who can turn briskly, walk on heels and toes, do a deep-knee bend, and tandem walk has no substantial disability of motor or coordinative functions of the lower extremities.

Examine the *cranial nerves:* test visual acuity and visual fields in all patients and scrutinize the optic fundi for abnormalities of the blood vessels, retina, or optic disc. Quickly test pupillary activity, ocular movements, corneal reflexes, jaw movement, facial movement, hearing, swallowing, speaking, and breathing. Postural tests of labyrinthine function need not be administered in the absence of a history of dizziness or vertigo.

Assess *upper extremity* form, strength, and proprioception by having the patient extend the arms forward in a supinated position and spread the fingers. Any of the following suggest an abnormality: a tremor affects the arm or index finger in the finger-nose test, eyes opened or closed; an outstretched arm drifts when the eyes are closed; arm jerks or muscle twitching appears. If the patient complains of weakness or sensory loss, the arms should be tested individually.

Any significant sensory loss of the extremities will almost certainly have been described by the sentient patient during the history. Accuracy demands careful sensory testing of each dermatome and peripheral nerve in the area of complaint. Screen *deep tendon reflexes* by testing at biceps, triceps, brachioradialis, knees, and ankles. Test the plantar responses, recalling that equivocal Babinski signs usually are not abnormal. *Autonomic activity* and *sphincter functions* usually can be estimated from the history. Careful assessment of sphincter tone, voluntary sphincter contraction, the anal wink reflex, and perianal sensation are essential if complaints of urinary-fecal incontinence or recent impotence exist. Always test for postural hypotension when evaluating autonomic impairment or dizziness. Palpate and, if appropriate, auscultate the carotid arteries, aorta, and peripheral pulses for evidence of vascular disease.

Do not be misled by equivocal neurologic signs. In office practice, many anxious patients hyperdiscriminate and interpret mild changes in pin prick or vibratory perception as important. When persons complain of sensory disturbance, ask them to map its distribution before examining them.

DIAGNOSTIC TESTS: SCOPE AND LIMITATIONS

Technology has remarkably increased the accuracy of neurologic diagnosis but, if overused, needlessly raises the cost of medical care. Before ordering, the judicious physician must consider the precise advantages conferred by each positive or negative test.

Tissue Analysis

Lumbar Puncture (LP)

Performed with proper indications, this safe and simple technique indirectly assesses biochemical abnormalities in the extracellular fluid of the central nervous system (CNS). Because headache and backache can follow an LP, the procedure should be reserved for specific indications (Table 111–6). The test is mandatory and usually diagnostic for leptomeningeal infection or cancer. The test also establishes the diagnosis (in the presence of a normal computed tomographic [CT] scan) of pseudotumor cerebri or idiopathic intracranial hypotension. The total protein concentration gives nonspecific information about the presence of nervous system disease and assists in the diagnosis of polyneuropathies. Protein electrophoresis may assist in the diagnosis of multiple sclerosis, paraprotein abnormalities, and other inflammatory diseases of the nervous system. Patients should not receive anticoagulants for a presumed stroke unless an LP or a brain image has ruled out intracranial hemorrhage. LP should not be performed in patients with suspected intracranial mass le-

TABLE 111–5	Mini Mental Status Examination*

Test	Score
What is the year, season, date, day, month?	5
Where are you: state, county, town, place, floor?	5
Name three objects: State slowly and have patient repeat (repeat until patient learns all three).	3
Do reverse serial 7s (five steps) or spell "world" backwards.	5
Ask for three unrelated objects above.	3
Name from inspection a pencil, a watch.	2
Have patient repeat "No if's, and's, or but's."	1
Follow a three-stage command (1 pt each). (Take a paper in your hand, fold it, and put it on the floor.)	3
Read and obey the command "Close your eyes."	1
Write a simple sentence.	1
Copy intersecting pentagons.	1

* Of a possible total score of 30, most patients with advanced dementia score below 15, whereas those with uncomplicated depression score above 25. Mixed or transient cognitive impairments produce scores that fall between normals and those with irreversible dementia.

TABLE 111-6	Considerations for Performing a Lumbar Puncture (LP)

Indications for Test

Absolute (before brain imaging)
  Suspicion of acute CNS infection unaccompanied by primary neurologic signs and symptoms
  Before anticoagulant therapy for cerebrovascular disease (only if no image available)
Relative (following brain imaging)
  Increased intracranial pressure suspected, CT or MRI normal
  Suspicion of cryptic nervous system disease
  Intrathecal therapy for meningeal leukemia or fungal meningitis
  Symptomatic treatment of severe headache from subarachnoid hemorrhage or pseudotumor cerebri

Contraindications to Test

Absolute: Tissue infection in region of puncture site
Relative
  Intracranial or infraspinal mass lesion known or probable
  Bleeding tendency (anticoagulant or thrombocytopenia)
  Increased intracranial pressure due to mass lesions

Diagnostic Evaluation of CSF

Routine: Cell count and differential, protein content, glucose level, Gram's stain, bacterial cultures, xanthochromia
Special studies: Malignant cytology, oligoclonal bands, paraproteins, selected studies for Lyme disease, tuberculosis, syphilis, viral antibodies, and so on

Complications of Test

Common Headache, backache
Rare: Transtentorial or foramen magnum herniation; worsening of spinal tumor symptoms; spinal epidural hematoma (in patients with bleeding tendency); herniated or infected disc; reaction to anesthetic agent; meningitis (contaminated needle)

CSF = Cerebrospinal fluid; CNS = central nervous system; CT = computed tomography; MRI = magnetic resonance imaging.

sions until after a brain scan has been obtained and diagnostic uncertainty remains. The tests in Table 111–4 are most commonly ordered. Small needles and technically smooth punctures are the best ways to reduce the risk of post-LP headache.

Tissue Biopsy

Diagnostic biopsies of muscle, peripheral nerve, or brain are largely confined to major specialty centers. When indicated, they sometimes can provide answers achievable in no other way.

Imaging Techniques (Fig. 111–1)

Computed Tomography (CT) and Magnetic Resonance Imaging (MRI). Modern techniques of imaging and computed tomography (CT) and magnetic resonance imaging (MRI) identify most structural diseases of the brain and spinal cord. A negative test often reassures the patient (and his physician) that no serious structural disease is present. However, the tests are expensive, seldom diagnose metabolic or inflammatory disorders, and should not substitute for clinical judgment.

Magnetic resonance imaging is available in many centers and its technical advantages make it superior to CT scanning except in patients with cardiac pacemakers or intracranial metal clips (Table 111–7). MRI is unaffected by bone and usually does not require the injection of contrast material. Furthermore, images can be produced in any plane, whereas CT images are limited to horizontal and coronal planes. MRI frequently reveals lesions, including tumors, arteriovenous anomalies, and areas of demyelination, that CT scanning fails to detect. No irradiation is involved. New MRI technology has the capacity to study functional brain activity as well as to monitor brain changes during illnesses such as acute stroke or trauma.

Positron Emission Tomography (PET)

PET is an isotopic CT method for imaging focal cerebral blood flow and metabolism. Although resolution is poorer than with MRI, the technique's ability to measure metabolic rate (e.g., by increased focal oxygen or glucose consumption) helps differentiate low-grade from high-grade brain tumors and may distinguish radiation damage from recurrent brain tumors in treated patients.

Single Photon-Emitting Computed Tomography (SPECT)

Single photon-emitting computed tomography also can identify functional patterns, but less exactly than either MRI or PET. SPECT uses a gamma camera placed over the scalp to detect I-131 emitted from a lipid-soluble molecule that, after intravenous injection or inhalation, almost immediately enters the brain in proportion to the organ's regional blood flow. The result provides a semiquantitative, static map of regional cerebral function as deduced from the geography of its energy-supplying blood flow.

Myelography

MRI has largely replaced plain radiographs and myelograms in diagnosing problems involving the spine and spinal cord. Occasionally, to obtain finer definition of spinal root lesions, myelography is conjoined with CT scanning. The test is particularly valuable for identifying herniated discs as well as compression of the spinal cord, cauda equina, or nerve roots.

Angiography

The blood vessels of the brain and spinal cord can be visualized either by injection of contrast material directly into an artery or by the injection of a larger amount of contrast material intravenously, with the images enhanced by computerized subtraction techniques. These approaches generally are reserved for specialized radiologic centers.

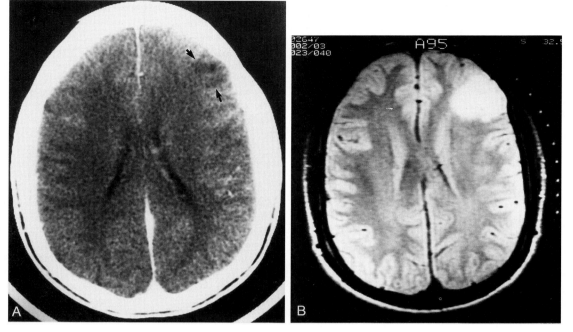

Figure 111-1

Comparison of imaging techniques in a patient suffering from a low-grade glioma of the left frontal lobe. The computed tomography (CT) scan (*A*) was taken after an injection of double the standard dose of contrast material. It shows only a vague area of hypodensity in the frontal lobe (*arrows*). Magnetic resonance scan (*B*) taken at the same level within a few days of the CT scan reveals a large area of hyperdensity caused by the altered proton density of the low-grade tumor. A biopsy revealed a low-grade glioma. The patient had suffered a single generalized convulsion and had no other neurologic signs or symptoms.

New computer programs are likely to enable MRI to replace arteriography for many diagnostic indications.

Electrodiagnostic Studies (Table 111–8)

Electrodiagnostic tests can be extremely useful in the differential diagnosis of neurologic disease, but they do not substitute for a clinical formulation derived from a careful history and neurologic examination. Individually, such tests are expensive and are best reserved for evaluating patients with uncertain diagnoses or to answer specific questions concerning the history and examination. They should be interpreted only in light of the history and neurologic findings.

TABLE 111–7	MRI Versus CT in Neurologic Diagnosis

Advantages of MRI

  No bone artifact on images
  Gadolinium contrast agent safer than iodine
  Resolution (1–2 mm) and tissue discrimination generally better
  Parasagittal planes of section available

Disadvantages of MRI

  Contraindicated with cardiac pacemakers or metal intracranial clips
  Difficult for critically ill patients
  Engenders claustrophobia

CT = Computed tomography; MRI = magnetic resonance imaging.

Electroencephalography (EEG)

EEG records the electrical activity of the cerebral cortex. The test is particularly helpful in the differential diagnosis of seizures, especially if an attack occurs spontaneously or can be evoked during the recording process. It also helps differentiate seizures from metabolic encephalopathy, and it aids in distinguishing between organic and psychogenic causes of unresponsiveness. The absence of EEG activity, properly recorded, supports the diagnosis of brain death.

Nerve Conduction Studies

Nerve conduction studies (see Table 111–8), electromyography and neuromuscular transmission studies are discussed in Chapter 122.

Evoked Potentials

External stimuli evoke changes in the electrical activity of the brain. Using signal-averaging techniques, scalp recordings can often identify these stimuli. Clinically useful tests include visual evoked potentials (VEPs), brain stem auditory evoked potentials (BAEPs), and somatosensory evoked potentials (SEPs). VEPs can identify abnormalities of central response time in one or both eyes even when visual acuity is normal. They are particularly useful

TABLE 111–8	Noninvasive Electrical Studies of the Nervous System		
Test	**Some Indications**	**Comments**
Electroencephalogram (EEG)	Any brain dysfunction, especially epilepsy	Sensitive but not specific; relatively inexpensive
Visual evoked potentials (VER)	Tests integrity of optic nerve and cerebral visual pathway	Sensitive for asymptomatic optic neuritis (e.g., multiple sclerosis); not usually required clinically
Brain stem auditory evoked potentials (BAER)	Tests integrity of auditory pathways	Sensitive for acoustic nerve tumors and brain stem disease
Somatosensory evoked potentials (SEP)	Tests integrity of central sensory pathways	Sensitive for spinal cord and lower brain stem disease
Nerve conduction velocity	Tests rate of conduction in peripheral nerve	Distinguishes demyelination from axonal disease; sometimes establishes site of nerve compression
Neuromuscular transmission studies	Myasthenia gravis, Lambert-Eaton syndrome, botulism	Noninvasive but unpleasant
Electromyogram (EMG)	Identifies denervated areas of muscle, detects reduced muscle action, identifies myopathic changes	Helps identify lower motor neuron disorders, nerve root compression; helps distinguish neurogenic from myopathic disorders

for identifying optic nerve and brain abnormalities in patients with clinical signs of brain stem and spinal cord disease such as multiple sclerosis. BAEPs, elicited by brief clicks presented to one ear, identify abnormalities of the acoustic nerve and its brain stem pathways. Abnor-malities are associated with lesions in the cerebellopontine angle and the brain stem. This test is particularly useful in identifying hearing abnormalities in infants. SEPs are used to identify compressive, demyelinating, or metabolic disturbances affecting central sensory pathways, particularly in the spinal cord. A new technique of magnetically stimulating the brain and recording evoked motor potentials in the extremities may have future clinical value.

Genetic Identification

Of an approximately 100,000 genes that create and maintain the normal development and life of human beings, approximately 60,000 are thought to contribute to neurologic or muscular functions. Several thousand genes appear to act exclusively in the development and maintenance of the brain and its direct connections. At this writing, the specific genetic underpinnings have been identified for more than 100 neurologic abnormalities, with more and more added each month. Presently, gene analysis is expensive and seldom provides an important tool in clinical neurologic diagnosis. As gene expressions and their post-translational functions become better understood, however, gene therapy almost certainly will depend upon accurate, routine diagnostic testing to obtain successful results.

REFERENCES

Aminoff MS, Greenberg DA, Simon RP: Clinical Neurology. 3rd ed. Stanford, CT, Appleton & Lange, 1996.
Bradley WG, Daroff RB, Fenichel GM, Marsden CD: Neurology in Clinical Practice. 2nd ed. 2 vols. Boston, Butterworth-Heinemann, 1995.
Neurology. Part 14. *In* Bennett JC, Plum F (eds.): Cecil Textbook of Medicine. 20th ed. Philadelphia, WB Saunders, 1996, pp 1957–2171.
Patten J: Neurological Differential Diagnosis. 2nd ed. Berlin, Heidelberg, and New York, Springer-Verlag, 1995.
Rowland LP (ed.): Merrit's Textbook of Neurology. 9th ed. Baltimore, Williams & Wilkins, 1995.

112

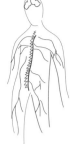

Disorders of Consciousness and Higher Brain Function

The human conscious state expresses the interaction of two major neurologic functions: arousal and cognition. The recurrent, circadian cycling of wakefulness and sleep is a phylogenetically primitive behavioral activity that is regulated predominantly by nuclear structures contained within the rostral brain stem, the ventromedian hypothalamus, and the basal forebrain. Mental content and learned behavior, by contrast, express the workings of more complicated neural mechanisms that depend on millions of interacting nerve and supporting cells located in the gray matter of the cerebral hemispheres and their directly related subcortical nuclei, the thalamus and basal ganglia.

This chapter discusses abnormalities of consciousness from several aspects. It first addresses problems related to normal and abnormal sleep and then describes a variety of pathologic alterations of the overall conscious state that pose serious threats to the brain and the integrity of the individual.

A. Sleep and Its Disorders

PHYSIOLOGY

Normal sleep-wake cycles are regulated chronologically by the small suprachiasmatic nucleus of the hypothalamus. Within the hypothalamus itself, posterior areas stimulate arousal, whereas anterior neuronal populations actively stimulate sleep. Cholinergic nuclei located in the anterior pontine tegmentum send fibers to both the hypothalamus and the basal forebrain. The action of this ascending system contributes critically to arousal and sleep states and may influence cerebral cognitive activity as well. Rapid eye movement (REM) sleep, for example, depends on the integrity of these pontine structures.

Normal sleep, as monitored by electroencephalogram (EEG) studies, proceeds in four deepening stages, plus REM. Stage 1 is transitional and may account for brief, drowsy episodes during wakefulness or the entry into sleep's later stages. Deep, satisfying sleep in stages 3 or 4 affects children and young adults but gradually disappears

after about the age of 50 years, so that elderly persons normally awaken several times during the night. REM sleep activity remains throughout life. Its biologic value is unknown although most recallable dreams appear to occur during REM periods.

Individual needs for sleep among healthy persons normally vary widely from as little as 4 to 5 hours per day to as much as 9 or 10. Moderate exercise reduces the latent period to fall asleep and may predispose to deeper, longer sleep periods. Anxiety, preoccupation, depression, drugs such as caffeine, and somatic conditions such as fever, pain, and cardiopulmonary disease all contribute to subjective difficulties in sleeping. Distressing insomnia or hyposomnia can have several aspects. Older persons generally sleep with less satisfaction than do younger ones. Some insomniacs complain of an increased latent period before sleep occurs, whereas others report middle-of-the-night or early-morning awakenings. Although subjectively distressing, such common variations produce little or no physiologic harm. Sleep studies of patients with "insomnia" find that periods of sleep almost always are longer than the subject believes. What the subject remembers is the awakenings. Severe insomnia, a reduction of total sleep to 3 to 4 hours or less per day, whatever the cause, appears to reduce mental efficiency.

COMMON SLEEP DISORDERS

Insomnia of recent origin is best handled by reassurance, with efforts directed toward correcting underlying medical or psychological problems and, if necessary, the parsimonious prescribing of mild sedatives. Such a cautious approach may fail to please all patients, but most chronic insomnia is extremely difficult to treat effectively because all successful soporifics sooner or later induce tolerance when taken in nonaddicting amounts. Acute insomnia due to intercurrent illness, acute physical or emotional pain, jet lag, and the like is best treated in otherwise healthy persons with small doses of the short-acting benzodiazepines, zolpidem, 10 mg, or triazolam, 0.125 mg at bedtime. Milder agents such as benadryl, chloral hydrate, or flurazepam may be preferable for elderly patients or those with fever or systemic illness. With any of these agents, half the manufacturer's recommended dose usually suffices for nonhabituated elderly persons. Tricyclic antidepressants, with the entire dose taken at bedtime, help in the management of the insomnia of depression. Alcohol, although widely employed, is a poor choice of sedative; it shortens the sleep latency interval but tends to shorten the duration of sleep and to produce unpleasant hangovers. Tolerance often occurs, resulting in patients taking increasing doses to achieve an effect.

Hypersomnia, defined arbitrarily as a sustained 20 to 30% increase over the norm for any given person, can reflect overwhelming fatigue, psychological depression, or serious neurologic disease. Chronic or recurrent hypersomnia is a symptom most often of narcolepsy or of one of the sleep apnea syndromes.

Narcolepsy is a chronic disorder of unknown cause characterized by recurrent brief episodes of uncontrollable drowsiness. It usually starts in the late teens or early 20s, accompanied by one or more of the following experiences: (1) *sleep attacks* consisting of sudden, uncontrollable, and inappropriately timed episodes of rapid eye movement sleep that interrupt normally scheduled wakefulness; (2) *cataplexy,* a phenomenon of abrupt muscular hypotonia precipitated by surprise or emotion; (3) *hypnagogic hallucinations,* intense dreamlike experiences accompanying the twilight zone between sleep and wakefulness; (4) *sleep paralysis,* an overwhelming sense that one cannot move, occurring during the moments of awakening from sleep. All these features may be experienced to some degree by normal persons, but in narcolepsy the symptoms intensify to the point of disrupting social and vocational occupations or producing dangerous situations such as drowsy driving. The predisposition to narcolepsy appears to be inherited as an autosomal dominant trait, with most narcoleptics possessing the specific DQB1 0602 haplotype. The clinical expression of the narcoleptic syndrome varies considerably, and its underlying cause is unknown. Medications are of limited value, although therapy with methylphenidate helps some sufferers. In intractable cases, symptomatic treatment with other amphetamine congeners or monoamine oxidase inhibitors occasionally brings relief.

Sleep disturbances that can occur in otherwise normal persons include enuresis (bedwetting), night terrors, nightmares, sleep walking, and sleep talking. All of these conditions predominantly affect children. Although tension, anxiety, or other psychological problems may accentuate the tendencies, they are probably not the cause. Imipramine, 25 to 50 mg at bedtime, helps some cases of enuresis. Several of the other disorders improve with the taking of short-acting benzodiazepines at bedtime. Most of the conditions subside during late adolescence or adulthood.

Restless legs or intermittent general bodily restlessness is either a presleep phenomenon or interrupts sleep, particularly in elderly persons. No specific treatment exists, but avoiding rich dinners and alcohol sometimes helps.

References

Aldrich MS: The neurobiology of narcolepsy-cataplexy. Prog Neurobiol 1993;41:533–541.

Kryger MH, Roth T, Dement WC: Principles and Practice of Sleep Medicine. 2nd ed. Philadelphia; WB Saunders, 1994.

B. Pathologic Alterations of Consciousness

SUSTAINED IMPAIRMENTS OF CONSCIOUSNESS

By definition, sustained impairments of consciousness can last for a matter of hours to indefinitely (Tables 112–1 and 112–2). Primary disturbances of arousal include *stupor* and *coma.* Organically caused, acutely occurring, sustained, but reversible abnormalities of the content of consciousness are termed *delirium* or *metabolic encephalopathy;* impaired arousal and attention usually accompany the latter states. Sustained disturbances of consciousness may be caused by either pathologic

TABLE 112–1	Consciousness and Its Alterations: Definitions

Consciousness. The awake state of awareness of self and environment.

Coma. An eyes-closed state of unarousable, sleeplike behavior in which patients lack any recognizable evidence of awareness of inner thoughts or outer events.

Stupor. A state of psychological unresponsiveness that can be interrupted only by vigorous and sustained external stimulation.

Hypersomnia. Sleep behavior that consistently exceeds the subject's norm by 25 to 30% or more.

Delirium, also known as confusional state. An acute or subacute state characterized by a transient reduction in the clarity of awareness of the environment. Symptoms include impaired memory, at least partial disorientation, misperceptions, poor judgment, and delusions. Prolonged confusional states may be difficult to distinguish from the early stages of chronic dementia. Agitated or severe forms of delirium most often accompany toxic or infectious illnesses. Affected patients become boisterous and restless; many suffer hallucinations, usually of a visual nature. A dreamlike state characterized by a loss of self-recognition can occur, as can reversals of sleep-wake cycles, accompanied by episodic insomnia or hypersomnia.

Vegetative state. A condition reflecting severe brain damage characterized by retained sleep-wake cycles and absent cognitive activity. Relatively normal autonomic thermal control, chewing, swallowing, breathing, and circulatory regulation often remain. Behavioral responses consist of no more than primitive motor reflexes or instinctive emotional patterns of agitation or crying.

Locked-in state. An uncommon condition in which severe damage to central or peripheral motor pathways prevents all communication. Affected patients remain conscious but cannot express it because communication is paralyzed. Either bilateral interruption of the corticospinal tracts in the brain stem or severe motor polyneuropathy can cause the condition. Comparable but less prolonged experiences affect conscious patients who are intubated for life-support ventilation.

Brain death. The permanent loss of all essential brain functions, despite the continued activity of artificially supported heart, lungs, and other viscera. Brain death has been accepted as representing death of the person in most of the United States as well as Western Europe. Table 112–2 provides diagnostic criteria.

interruptions of the upper brain stem–hypothalamic arousal mechanisms or global-diffuse organic impairments of cerebral regions that regulate mental and behavioral functions. Restricted, focal psychological impairments such as aphasia, selective perceptual loss, or specific learning deficits are described in a later part of the chapter, as are the permanent declines in cognitive function called dementia.

Mechanisms and Diagnosis of Comatose States

Mechanisms

Disorders that can damage the brain so extensively or strategically as to interrupt consciousness fall into three general categories (Table 112–3): (1) supratentorial mass lesions such as neoplasms or hemorrhages that either (a) directly invade or destroy the posterior ventromedial diencephalon or (b) enlarge so as to compress these basal diencephalic areas or herniate them through the tentorial notch; (2) structural subtentorial lesions that bilaterally damage or destroy the midbrain–upper pontine activating-arousal systems; and (3) diffuse metabolic or multifocal structural abnormalities that simultaneously or in close succession cause widespread, severe cerebral hemispheric dysfunction. These latter conditions can depress arousal mechanisms either directly or by abruptly removing their normal feedback stimulation from the cerebral cortex. Many of these diffuse or multifocal conditions have chemical rather than structural causes. Such nonstructural illnesses may produce no abnormalities on brain imaging and create a challenge in diagnosis and management.

TABLE 112–2	Criteria for Diagnosis of Brain Death

1. Nature and duration of coma must be known
    a. Known structural disease or irreversible systemic metabolic cause
    b. No chance of drug intoxication or hypothermia below 32°C; no paralyzing or sedative drugs recently given for treatment
    c. Six-hour observation of no brain function is sufficient in cases of known structural cause when no drug or alcohol is involved in cause or treatment; otherwise, 12 to 24 hr plus a negative drug screen is required
2. Absence of cerebral and brain stem function
    a. No behavioral or reflex response to noxious stimuli above foramen magnum level
    b. Fixed pupils
    c. No oculovestibular responses to 50-ml ice water calorics
    d. Apneic off ventilator with oxygenation for 10 min (many centers require a rise in $PaCO_2 \geqq 20$ mmHg during apnea)
    e. Systemic circulation may be intact
    f. Purely spinal reflexes may be retained
3. Supplementary (optional) criteria* (any one acceptable)
    a. EEG isoelectric for 30 min at maximal gain
    b. No circulation present on cerebral blood flow examination

*May be useful if medicolegal issues are in question or when taking organs for transplantation, especially within <6 hours of the time that diagnosis is first reached.
EEG = Electroencephalogram.

TABLE 112–3	Common Causes of Stupor and Coma

I. Supratentorial lesions
   A. Compressing or herniating the diencephalon against the upper brain stem (common): cerebral hemorrhage, large cerebral infarction, subdural hematoma, epidural hematoma, brain tumor, brain abscess (rare)
   B. Directly invading or destroying the posterior ventromedial diencephalon (less common): neoplasms, infarcts, encephalitis
II. Subtentorial lesions (compressing or damaging the upper pontine midbrain reticular formation): pontine or cerebellar hemorrhage, midbrain–upper pontine infarction, tumor, cerebellar abscess, acute demyelination (rare)
III. Metabolic and diffuse lesions
   A. Exogenous psychoactive drugs or poisons
   B. Anoxia or ischemia
   C. Mixed encephalopathies: pathologic aging, postoperative state, systemic infection, therapeutic drugs in various combinations
   D. Hepatic, renal, pulmonary, pancreatic insufficiency
   E. Hypoglycemia
   F. Infections: meningitis, encephalitis
   G. Multifocal small structural lesions, e.g., metastases, emboli, thrombi
   H. Concussion and postictal states
   I. Ionic and electrolyte disorders
   J. Nutritional deficiency
IV. Psychogenic unresponsiveness

Approach to the Unconscious Patient

Once the history is obtained, physical and laboratory tests provide crucial clues. An evaluation of motor and neuro-ophthalmologic signs plus an appraisal of the initial breathing pattern often yields the most useful clinical information in reaching a provisional diagnosis. Brain imaging abets clinical localization and reveals most coma-producing mass or destructive lesions if they exist. Systematic studies of blood, urine, cerebrospinal fluid (CSF), and other tissues offer specific indications of the causes of many of the metabolic encephalopathies. The following paragraphs amplify these principles.

Supratentorial Mass Lesions (Fig. 112–1). The most frequent supratentorial causes of acutely or subacutely altered consciousness consist of expanding hemispheric masses that can press the surrounding cerebrum, shifting it either downward to displace the diencephalon against the midbrain or down and laterally to compress the temporal lobe against the thalamus and midbrain.

According to their anatomic locations in the cerebrum, most supratentorial masses cause signs of focal cerebral dysfunction before they produce discernible changes in consciousness (Table 112–4). The initial clinical signs may be behavioral-psychological or can consist of sensorimotor abnormalities on the opposite side of the body. As such cerebral masses grow in size, they displace the thalamus and hypothalamus, reducing arousal and causing bilateral abnormal motor signs. Brain stem–controlled pupillary reflexes, conjugate eye movements, and oculovestibular responses remain largely or completely spared in early supratentorial coma. Unless the progressive diencephalic compression is halted, however, the process proceeds to transtentorial herniation.

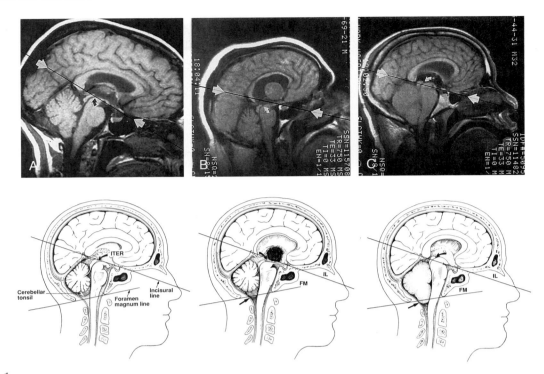

Figure 112–1

Midsagittal diagrams and magnetic resonance images (MRI) of a normal adult brain compared with downward and upward transtentorial herniation as well as foramen magnum herniation. *A,* Normal 45-year-old male brain. The incisural line (IL) defines the plane of the tentorial opening, which extends from the junction between the vein of Galen and the cerebral venous straight sinus posteriorly to the anterior clinoid process. The iter, the rostral opening of the aqueduct of Sylvius *(black curved arrow),* lies on or within 2 mm of the IL. The cerebellar tonsils remain well above the foramen magnum (FM). *B,* Downward transtentorial herniation due to a chronic colloid cyst lying in the third ventricle (dark round shadow on diagram). The *curved white arrow* on the MR scan points to the aqueduct, posterior thalamus, and mesencephalon, which are displaced 8 mm caudally of the IL. The cerebellar tonsils are visible at the level of the foramen magnum. *C,* Upward tentorial plus foramen magnum herniation has occurred secondary to a cerebellar lymphoma in a 32-year-old man with HIV-1 infection. The cerebellum is enlarged. The iter *(black curved arrow)* and the rostral mesencephalon have herniated 6 mm above the IL, and the brain stem is flattened against the base of the skull. The cerebellar tonsils have herniated into the foramen magnum. (From Plum F: Sustained impairments of consciousness. *In* Bennett JC, Plum F [eds.]: Cecil Textbook of Medicine. 20th ed. Philadelphia, WB Saunders, 1996, p 1971.)

Primary destructive or invasive lesions of the posterior paramedian thalamus/hypothalamus are well-established but relatively unusual supratentorial causes of stupor and coma. The area can be selectively damaged by stroke secondary to rostral basilar artery occlusion; by neoplasms, particularly primary lymphomas; by granulomas such as those of sarcoid; or by acute encephalitis. With any of these conditions the chief clinical manifesta-tion usually consists of gradually or acutely progressing hypersomnia, sometimes blending into unarousable sleep lasting most of the 24-hour day. Specific diagnosis depends on other signs of thalamic or brain stem dysfunc-tion plus information gained from imaging studies and, less often, CSF analysis.

HERNIATION SYNDROMES (see Fig. 112–1). Transtentorial

TABLE 112–4	Characteristics of Structural Supratentorial Lesions Leading to Coma

Initiating symptoms usually cerebral-focal: aphasia; focal seizures; contralateral hemiparesis, sensory changes, or neglect; frontal lobe behavioral
changes; headache
Dysfunction moves rostral to caudal in the brain: e.g., focal motor →
bilateral motor → altered level of arousal
Abnormal signs usually confined to a single or adjacent anatomic level
(not diffuse)
Brain stem functions spared unless herniation develops

TABLE 112–5	Signs of Central and Uncal Transtentorial Herniation

	Central	Uncal
Arousal	Declines early	Declines late
Pupils	Small, equal, reactive	Ipsilateral dilation
Oculocephalics	Full, conjugate	Unilateral third nerve palsy
Motor	Decerebrate early	Decerebrate late
Breathing	Sighs, yawns, periodic	Central hyperventilation, late

herniation can occur in either a downward or an upward direction. Downward herniation can take two forms (Table 112–5). *Central compression-herniation* squeezes and eventually displaces the midline diencephalon caudally toward and through the tentorial notch against the midbrain. As this occurs, the level of arousal declines, bilateral upper motor neuron signs tend to replace early focal cerebral signs, and signs of hypothalamic dysfunction ensue, including small, light-reactive, equal pupils. Evidence of brain stem dysfunction (e.g., eye movement changes) appears as the midbrain becomes severely compressed by the downward shift. *Uncal (lateral) herniation* results when a lesion occupying the temporal fossa expands and pushes the ipsilateral uncus over the edge of the ipsilateral tentorium, thereby compressing the third nerve and midbrain (see Fig. 120–1). Reduced consciousness and bilateral motor signs appear relatively late, the earliest evidence of serious trouble usually being incipient dilation of the pupil. Either form of herniation warns of impending upper brain stem compression and calls for quick and effective action to prevent irreversible neurologic damage.

SUBTENTORIAL LESIONS. Subtentorial lesions cause coma by damaging or compressing the activating systems located in the tegmentum of the upper pons and midbrain. Because the reticular formation surrounds or lies adjacent to oculomotor pathways and upper brain stem cranial nerve nuclei, the onset of stupor or coma caused by subtentorial lesions always is accompanied by signs of damage to upper cranial nerves. Also, most subtentorial lesions causing coma have a structural nature that magnetic resonance imaging (MRI) can identify. Table 112–3 lists their most common causes and Table 112–6 gives their characteristic signs and symptoms.

METABOLIC, DIFFUSE, AND MULTIFOCAL DISORDERS PRODUCING DELIRIUM OR UNCONSCIOUSNESS. Table 112–3 lists major examples. They tend to affect the brain diffusely and characteristically produce symptoms and signs of both widespread cerebral and concurrent brain stem dysfunction. Depending on the particular illness, its severity, and its rate of appearance, symptoms in metabolic multifocal encephalopathy can include cognitive changes, a reduction in arousal, or both. Acute self-induced drug overdose or sudden, severe hypoglycemia, for example, can precipitate acute coma with few prodromal symptoms. By contrast, mild drug intoxication or a moderate reduction in blood sugar is more likely to be reflected by sustained confused or bizarre behavior.

Signs and Symptoms (Table 112–7). Characteristic in the early stages is an acute or subacute confusional state accompanied by restlessness and reduced alertness. Mental status examination (Table 111–5) reveals impaired recall, poor concentration, and often disorientation. Confabulation, obtundation, and stupor follow in varying degrees and combinations. Fluctuations in behavior are common; some patients may alternate widely between stupor and agitation. Symptoms of delirium tend to be accentuated by nightfall and unfamiliar surroundings.

Characteristic motor changes include tremor, asterixis, and multifocal myoclonus. The tremor of delirium tends to be coarse, irregular, rapid at 8 to 10 Hz, and intensified by movement. Bilateral asterixis or multifocal myoclonus arising acutely or subacutely and accompanying a recent impairment of consciousness is pathognomonic of metabolic encephalopathy. Seizures, hyperactive stretch reflexes, and even focal signs sometimes accompany several of the metabolic encephalopathies such as drug withdrawal, global cerebral anoxia, hypoglycemia, hyperosmolar coma, and fulminating hepatic encephalopathy. Such focal signs usually are transient and accompanied by other neurologic changes that reflect diffuse or multifocal brain disease.

Pupillary light reflexes usually are preserved in metabolic coma. Exceptions include the following: poisoning with hyoscine, strong narcotics, or glutethimide; deliberate or accidental contact with mydriatics; and irreversible anoxia-asphyxia. Except in cases of severe sedative overdose, spontaneous conjugate eye movements or conjugate oculovestibular reflexes are preserved until the terminal phases of most metabolic comas.

Breathing alterations are common: vigorous hyperpnea (Kussmaul breathing) accompanies the metabolic acidosis of diabetes, uremia, lactic acidosis, and organic alcohol ingestion, whereas less prominent overbreathing reflects the alkaloses of hepatic disease, septic shock, and early salicylism. Hypoventilation is prominent in carbon dioxide encephalopathy, whether due to pulmonary disease or medullary respiratory depression caused by drugs or hypoglycemia.

TABLE 112–7 | **Characteristics of Metabolic Encephalopathy**

Often associated with aging, multiple medications, change in environment, and acute systemic illness
Confusion, lethargy, delirium often precede or replace coma
Motor signs, if present, are usually symmetric
Bilateral asterixis, myoclonus appear
Pupillary reactions usually preserved; tonic calorie-induced eye movements are often present
Sensory abnormalities are usually absent
Moderate hypothermia is common
Abnormal signs reflect incomplete brain dysfunction simultaneously affecting multiple anatomic levels

---

TABLE 112–6 | **Characteristics of Subtentorial Lesions Causing Coma**

Onset of coma often sudden
Symptoms of brain stem dysfunction may precede coma
Localizing brain stem signs always present
  Caloric responses disconjugate or absent
  Pupil(s) abnormal: pinpoint (pons), fixed (midbrain), irregular and/or unequal (midbrain-pontine)
  Often bizarre signs: ocular bobbing, ataxic breathing, etc.
  Often signs of cerebellar or bilateral motor dysfunction

TABLE 112–8	Signs of Psychogenic Pseudocoma

Lids close actively and often resist examiner's attempt to open them
Breathing: eupnea or acute hyperventilation
Pupils responsive or dilated (self-administered cycloplegics)
Oculocephalic responses unpredictable; caloric tests produce quick nystagmus
Motor responses unpredictable and often asymmetric or bizarre
No pathologic reflexes; EEG normal awake

EEG = Electroencephalogram.

Psychogenic Unresponsiveness

This can accompany several psychiatric disorders, including the catatonia of schizophrenia or severe depression as well as hysteria or malingering. Sometimes, the clinical picture may superficially resemble metabolic coma. Certain signs differentiate, however (Table 112–8). Careful examination reveals a normal general physical and somatic neurologic condition. Psychogenically unresponsive patients may resist answers during attempts to appraise mental status, but only hysterics or malingerers provide false ones. Those with closed eyes resist passive opening of the lids, and when the lids are passively raised, they shut abruptly when released; neither is true in organic coma. Pupils are briskly reactive unless mydriatics have been self-instilled, ice water calorics give normal responses, and the electroencephalogram (EEG) is normal. One must always remember, however, that much hysteria arises in the setting of organic disease, presumably due to excess anxiety.

Emergency Diagnosis and Management of Coma

Only a few disorders cause sudden, acute coma (Table 112–9). When related events or a history is unavailable, one proceeds to stabilize the condition immediately with the steps outlined in Table 112–10. The examiner then carefully but rapidly evaluates signs and, if possible, past events as indicated in Tables 112–11 and 112–12. The preliminary stabilization and examination should require no more than a few minutes. Except when infection seems likely, brain images should be obtained as soon as possible to determine whether a surgical procedure is in-

TABLE 112–9	Common Causes of Sudden Acute Coma

Brain trauma (see Chapter 117)
Acute intracranial hemorrhage
  Subarachnoid (see Chapter 116)
  Extradural (see Chapter 117)
  Intracerebral, intrapontine (see Chapter 116)
Drug poisoning (see Table 112–22)
Epileptic attacks (see Chapter 118)
Acute ischemic pontine–mesencephalic stroke
Hypoglycemia
Acute infection: meningitis

TABLE 112–10	Emergency Management of Coma

1. Assure airway and oxygenation.
2. Maintain adequate systemic circulation.
3. Give thiamine, 50–100 mg intravenously.
4. Give glucose after first obtaining blood for analysis.
5. Stop generalized seizures.
6. Restore blood acid-base and osmolar balance but do not change serum sodium by more than 15 mOsm/day.
7. Treat infection specifically.
8. Ameliorate extreme body temperature (>41° or <35°C).
9. Consider naloxone.
10. Control agitation-tremulousness with lorazepam or haloperidol.

dicated. In the absence of signs of acute meningitis, lumbar puncture is best withheld until an MRI or computed tomography (CT) scan excludes an acute intracranial mass. EEG is helpful only when serial seizures (status epilepticus) due to petit mal or partial complex seizures produce an acute confusional state.

Most cases of acute coma of unknown cause result from self-induced drug poisoning, and patients lacking definite alternative diagnoses must be managed for this possibility until another cause is established. Among older persons, especially those with chronic illness or receiving multiple medications, metabolic encephalopathies also are common. These occur especially in the hospital setting where confusion, obtundation, or delirium due to a mixture of adverse causes can complicate the course of many acute medical or surgical illnesses. Standard blood chemistries plus a search for offending medications frequently reveal the cause of such conditions.

BRIEF AND EPISODIC ALTERATIONS OF CONSCIOUSNESS

Table 112–13 lists disorders that produce recurrent, short-lived, relatively stereotyped alterations in perceptions, psychological feeling states, somatic functions, or global consciousness. Although each of these conditions produces fairly characteristic symptoms and signs, only hypoglycemia, seizure disorders, or certain forms of syncope (e.g., with cardiac arrhythmia) are associated with diagnostic laboratory findings and then only during the episodes. Accordingly, the cause of most episodes of brief loss of consciousness must be inferred from retro-

TABLE 112–11	Keys to Clinical Diagnosis of Coma

Pursue history diligently and provide immediate lifesupport (see Table 112–10).
How do signs of dysfunction evolve?
  Rostral-caudal? (Supratentorial)
  Focal brain stem from onset? (Subtentorial)
  Multifocal diffuse? (Metabolic-diffuse)
  Do they represent nonphysiologic abnormalities? (Psychogenic)
Obtain emergency brain scan.
Move to specific tests or treatment.

TABLE 112–12	Helpful Clues in Early Diagnosis of Coma
Fever	Meningitis, encephalitis, postictal state, acute bacterial endocarditis, scopolamine poisoning
Hypothermia	Myxedema, hypoglycemia, drug poisoning, brain stem infarct
Signs of trauma	Cerebral contusion; extradural, subdural, or parenchymal hematoma
Severe hypertension	Cerebral or subarachnoid hemorrhage; hypertensive encephalopathy
Hypotension	Occult (usually gastrointestinal) bleeding, septic shock, hypovolemia, poor cardiac output, depressant drug poisoning
	Tachycardia >180/min, bradycardia <40/min; poor cardiac output
Arrhythmias	Tricyclic antidepressant overdose, myocardial infarction
Hyperventilation	Diabetic ketosis; uremia; organic alcohol poisoning; lactic acidosis, hepatic coma; salicylate poisoning
Hypoventilation	Pulmonary insufficiency, depressant drug or opiate poisoning, low brain stem infarct or hemorrhage
Petechiae	Meningococcemia, thrombocytopenic and non-thrombocytopenic purpura, bacterial endocarditis
Pink skin	Carbon monoxide poisoning
Stiff neck	Acute meningitis, subarachnoid hemorrhage

spective evidence. In such instances, the patient's age, the medical history, and, especially, an accurate recounting of symptoms or reports of direct observers provide the greatest help in diagnosis.

Syncope describes brief loss of consciousness due to a global reduction in cerebral blood flow. The disorder almost always is due to an abrupt or semiabrupt reduction of cardiac output, most frequently secondary to acutely impaired right heart output (cardiac rhythm maintained) or severe left heart output (asystole or severe arrhythmia) (see Table 8–8).

Syncope due to reduced right heart filling usually results from pooling of blood in capacitance veins of the

TABLE 112–13	Brief, Often Recurrent Disorders of Global Neurologic Function

Brief Loss of Consciousness

Traumatic concussion (see Chapter 118)
Syncope (see Tables 9–9 and 119–7)
Hypoglycemia (see Chapter 72)
Seizures (see Chapter 119)

Recurrent Psychological Disturbances

Hyperventilation attacks
Panic attacks
Fugue states

Episodic Neurologic Dysfunction Without Impaired Arousal

Transient global amnesia
Cerebral transient ischemic attacks
Drop spells
Migraine

lower extremities or trunk. Most often, this comes from the triggering of vasodepressor reflexes (vasodepressor syncope, sometimes called neurocardiogenic syncope). Other causes include orthostatic hypotension secondary to depleted blood volume, hypotensive drugs, and peripheral neurologic disease. Mechanical increases in pulmonary resistance such as those that may accompany severe coughing or acute pulmonary infarction are less frequent mechanisms. Cardiac tamponade interferes with both right and left heart filling and output.

Vasodepressor syncope (simple fainting) exceeds in frequency all other causes of acute brief unconsciousness combined. Simple fainting tends to be a recurrent problem in some individuals; a few give a family history of the disorder. No associated neurologic or cardiac abnormality can be found in most cases. Attacks are engendered by emotional crises, acute painful visceral stimuli, hyperventilation, micturition, recent ascent to high altitude, and, in susceptible persons, various combinations of alcohol, hunger, and drugs. Often, one can identify no precipitating cause. Attacks begin in some persons with a brief prodrome of anxiety, giddiness, diaphoresis, and nausea before collapse. Others precipitously sink to the floor as heart rate and blood pressure fall and cardiac output declines. Except with prolonged asystole, syncope always occurs in the erect or sitting position, never when a person is supine. Patients with vasodepressor syncope are pale and sweaty and may have one or two generalized clonic twitches as a result of a profound faint (convulsive syncope). Incontinence is unusual, but vomiting, micturition, and diarrhea commonly follow the attack. In young persons with a negative physical examination and characteristic history, physiologic or structural disease almost never is present and laboratory studies need not be extensive. Tilt-table test results are not reliable in predicting future recurrences. Electrophysiologic testing of cardiac rhythms is best limited to patients with known or probable heart disease. Hysteria and drug-alcohol intoxication are the chief resemblers. Table 119–7 outlines the differences from minor seizures. Simple fainting can affect persons older than 50 years, but a first episode in that age group deserves evaluation to rule out serious cardiac disorders. Cerebral transient ischemic attacks rarely simulate syncope. Occasionally, vasodepressor syncope accompanies attacks of severe migraine in adolescents and young adults.

Syncope resolves too quickly to treat except posturally by placing the subject supine and elevating the lower extremities; there are no effective preventive measures except when severe cardiac disorders are found and corrected. For benign vasodepressor syncope, avoiding offending foods as well as eliminating bouts of alcohol ingestion without accompanying food may help.

Other causes of briefly altered unconsciousness are uncommon or discussed elsewhere (see Table 112–12). Hyperventilation attacks more closely resemble the syndrome of panic than syncope. Affected patients may complain of feeling unreal, floating, or dizzy, but they do not lose contact with the environment. Perioral paresthesias, a sense of suffocating dyspnea, and carpopedal spasm are diagnostic. Propranolol, up to 40 mg 3 times daily, or amitriptyline in doses up to 50 mg daily, may reduce the frequency of panic attacks. Propranolol is especially helpful in warding off stage fright.

REFERENCES

Kapoor WN: Evaluation and management of syncope JAMA 1992; 268: 2553.
The Multi-society Task Force on PVS: Medical aspects of the persistent vegetative state. N Engl J Med 1994;330:1499–1508, 1572–1579.
Plum F, Posner JB: Diagnosis of Stupor and Coma. 3rd ed. Philadelphia, FA Davis, 1982.
Taylor D, Lewis S: Delirium. J Neurol Neurosurg Psychiatr 1993;56: 1742–1751.

C. Focal Disturbances of Higher Brain Function

REGIONAL SYNDROMES

The two cerebral hemispheres supplement each other functionally in a variety of cognitive and sensorimotor tasks (Fig. 112–2). Certain abstract functions, however, are more or less strongly lateralized in the adult human brain. Language and manual functions, for example, are strongly lateralized to the left, so-called dominant hemisphere, in most brains. Structures mediating spatial recognition, especially that dealing with the perceived relationship of the person to his/her external environment, are more commonly lateralized to the right, nondominant hemisphere. Several less prominent motor or sensory skills are less strongly lateralized; their qualities lie beyond the scope of this text but are briefly summarized in Tables 112–14 and 112–15.

LANGUAGE AND APHASIA

The critical areas for language processing include Wernicke's area, which extends posteriorly along the superior temporal gyrus from the primary auditory cortex to the angular gyrus and adjacent inferior parietal lobe cortex. From that area, a stout fiber bundle, the arcuate fasciculus, interconnects Wernicke's area with Broca's area of the inferolateral frontal cortex (Fig. 112–3).

Language function is generated entirely or predominantly from the left hemisphere in roughly 95% of the population. Dominance for handedness is less exclusive: about 15% of persons are left-handed or ambidextrous, but only a third of left-handers possess a right hemisphere that is dominant for language. Most left-handers tend to have some language function in both hemispheres, so that they seldom become completely and permanently aphasic from unilateral injuries or surgical resections from either hemisphere.

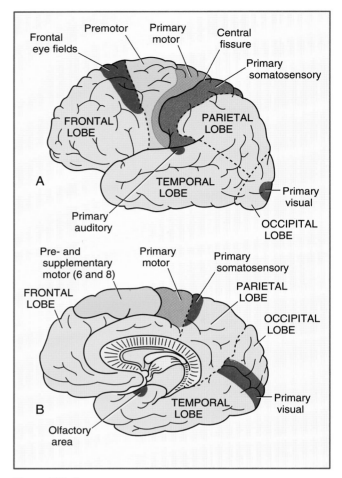

Figure 112–2
Major anatomic and functional areas of the cerebral hemispheres. *A,* Lateral surface. *B,* Medial surface.

Aphasia or *dysphasia* consists of a loss or impairment of language function as a result of damage or dysfunction in the specific language areas of the dominant hemisphere (Table 112–16). *Dysarthria,* by contrast, consists of a disturbance in the articulation of speech.

Broca's aphasia is characterized by severe disturbances in expressing either spontaneous or commanded speech and writing. Comprehension is relatively better but

TABLE 112–14	Syndromes of Frontal Lobe Injury
Unilateral Motor-Premotor Damage	**Large Prefrontal-Premotor or Bilateral Damage**
Contralateral spastic weakness, more distal than proximal	Emotional outbursts
Contralateral seizures: focal hand, face, foot (rare); adversive body or eyes	Lack of or indifference to insight
Broca's aphasia (dominant hemisphere)	Antisocial behavior
Impaired conceptualization and planning, either hemisphere	Reduced attention
Mutism ± apathy	

TABLE 112–15	Syndromes of Parietal Lobe Damage

Postcentral cortex
  Homunculus-patterned contralateral impairment of somesthetic abstraction: Stereoanesthesia-astereognosis
Inferior parietal lobe
  Dominant (left): Aphasia, apraxia, acalculia, right-left disorientation
  Nondominant (right): Spatial disorientation; perceptual neglect, especially contralaterally; inappropriate affect, sometimes delirium
  Large lesions: Anosognosia

incompletely preserved, with things spoken being better understood than things read. Many patients with Broca's aphasia also have an associated right hemiparesis or hemiplegia, the result of an adjacent vascular lesion affecting the internal capsule.

Wernicke's aphasia consists of an incapacity to recognize the nature or meaning of symbolic sensory stimuli, including language, or to connect learned words with either inner thoughts or stored memories. Affected patients cannot recognize spoken, written, or symbolized language or gestures. They tend to articulate a fluent nonsense with a natural, meaningless rhythm. Insight is minimal and prognosis is poor.

Many aphasic patients show mixtures of the preceding categories. As a rule, however, expressive defects correlate with frontal lobe injury, whereas receptive and word-finding deficits are associated with temporoparietal abnormalities. *Conduction aphasia* is characterized by a fluent, Wernicke-like pattern coupled with the ability of the patient to repeat after the examiner phrases and often long sentences. The responsible lesions lie near but not within the primary speech areas.

Global aphasia describes the combined severe loss of all major aspects of language function due to frontotemporal damage in the dominant hemisphere.

Mutism, the inability to speak or make sounds, can accompany acute left pre–Broca area lesions, bilateral frontal lobe damage, the locked-in state (see Table 112–1), or hysteria. All but the last-mentioned produce associated signs of organic brain disease.

Dysarthria consists of the inability to articulate speech clearly because of abnormal innervation or mechanical disease of the vocal apparatus. Most affected patients can at least make sounds. Causes include severe

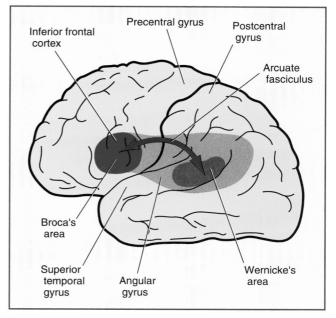

Figure 112–3
Primary language areas in the dominant cerebral hemisphere. Damage to Broca's area or Wernicke's area produces characteristic language abnormalities (see Table 112–15). Injury to the surrounding stippled areas causes less classic language impairments, including conduction aphasia. The arcuate fasciculus interconnects the two areas.

bulbar or pseudobulbar paralysis as well as vocal dystonia.

Apraxia refers to a disturbance of the ability to perform learned motor acts despite the retention of sufficient sensory and language function to understand the command and enough crude motor capacity to carry it out (praxis). The condition most commonly accompanies deep lesions of one or both parietal lobes.

Agnosia is the inability to recognize a complex sensory stimulus or body part despite the preservation of elemental perceptions and language. The phenomenon accompanies certain large parieto-occipital–posterior temporal lobe lesions. It most often is caused by a large stroke or one of the degenerative dementias.

Anosognosia defines a striking neuropsychological abnormality in which an individual can neither recognize

TABLE 112–16	Principal Aphasia Types			
	Locus of Lesion	**Speech**	**Comprehension**	**Associated Signs**
Broca's area	Inferior posterior frontal lobe	Halting; reduced; nonfluent	Good	Often right hemiparesis; self-aware; frustrated
Wernicke's area	Superior-lateral posterior temporal lobe	Abundant, fluent, semantic nonsense	Poor to absent	Often none
Conduction	Supramarginal gyrus; primary auditory cortex or insular region	Fluent but some expressive defects	Poor to absent	Often none
Global	Large frontotemporal lesions	Dense, expressive, nonfluent language loss; brief expletives may remain	Poor	Usually right hemiparesis or hemiplegia

a common percept nor recall that such recognition ever existed.

MEMORY

An accurate memory is an indispensable function of the normal adult brain. The content of memory can be large or small, as can the ability to learn. Severe loss of memory or an inability to learn represent handicaps that characterize mental retardation (not discussed in this text) or varying degrees of disability, of which the greatest is dementia. Table 112–17 lists various patterns of memory that can be impaired in brain diseases.

Memory Mechanisms

Storage of both perceived events and motor skills is distributed widely in the brain, especially in the parietal-temporal areas for perceptual-verbal memories or prefrontal regions for motor skills. The agnosias described earlier reflect damage to such distributed areas. Memory formation and retrieval of perceptions, by contrast, appear to require the integrity of the hippocampal areas of the temporal lobe and the thalamus. The considerable redundancy of memory-processing functions means that clinically severe memory impairment usually requires extensive unilateral or bilateral injury. Illustrating this, bilateral damage to or surgical removal of the hippocampus results in profound and usually permanent deficits in intermediate memory affecting especially the verbal-visual-spatial spheres. Similarly, bilateral damage to several paramedian areas of the thalamus and probably the mammillary bodies results in a profound memory disturbance, the most severe form of which produces a Korsakoff syndrome.

The development and retrieval of long-term memories relate in incompletely understood ways to cholinergic and other autonomic projections that link the subcortical basal forebrain with the hippocampus and areas of the association cortex. Degeneration of these projections is a prominent accompaniment of Alzheimer's and certain other dementias.

TABLE 112–18	Most Common Memory Disorders

Benign forgetfulness of aging
Severe amnesia of dementia
Severe head trauma
Transient global amnesia
Thiamine deficiency (Korsakoff's)
Episodic asystole or hypoglycemia (acute brain anoxia)
Encephalitis, stroke(s), brain tumor
Psychogenic amnesia

Clinical Memory Disorders (Table 112–18)

Many middled-aged and elderly persons experience an increasing, relatively isolated difficulty in recalling proper names and recent events of minor importance. This benign forgetfulness bears no consistent relationship to the progressive dementias and is best treated with prompt and vigorous reassurance.

Even modest head trauma temporarily interrupts memory-mediating neural connections. Concussive injuries frequently produce an initially severe retrograde and lesser anterograde amnesia; usually the memory loss disappears with time.

Transient global amnesia (TGA) largely affects persons older than 65 years. The condition consists of an acute onset of amnesia for time, place, and past memory, usually lasting for 3 to 12 hours. Affected persons can identify themselves but are severely distressed about the experience. Most TGA attacks reflect temporary vascular insufficiency affecting the hippocampal memory areas or their thalamic connections. Temporal lobe seizures or hysterical fugue states are the principal conditions to be distinguished from this disorder, but most TGA attacks are readily diagnosed clinically. Most episodes neither leave residual limitations nor carry a strong risk of recurrence.

TABLE 112–17	Patterns of Memory

Anterograde: New memories laid down after a particular time or event
Retrograde: Memories extending back from a particular event (e.g., brain trauma)
Short-term or "working": Holding in the mind the memory of an image or event for ±30 to 60 seconds
Long-term: Memory processed into storage after 30 to 60 seconds (recent long-term memories tend to disappear before remote ones)
Explicit: Recall of autobiographic experiences, facts, thoughts; explicit memory is often lost in dementia
Implicit: Sometimes called procedural; includes learning motor skills and many automatic reactions; implicit memories often spared in dementia
Instinctive: Genetically transmitted memories, largely affecting automatic motor acts, mood or behavioral patterns, visceral sensations

TABLE 112–19	Organic and Psychogenic Amnesia Compared	
	Organic	**Psychogenic**
Time frame	Recent worse than remote	Unpredictable mixture of recent and remote, often for circumscribed events
Pattern	Anterograde amnesia as bad as retrograde	No anterograde amnesia except in total fugues ("who am I?")
	Emotionally important events recalled better	Such events often "forgotten"
Self-recognition	Intact except with severe delirium or seizures	May be denied
Behavior	Questions about illness asked repeatedly	Often no questions asked

Psychogenic memory impairment can affect either recent or remote recall, usually in clinically recognizable patterns. Table 112–19 compares the principal features of organic and psychogenic amnesia. In general, with organic disturbances in memory, emotionally reinforced material is recalled better than neutral events. Also, with organic memory loss, disorientation is worst for time, less for place and persons, and never for self; remote events are recalled better than recent ones, and cues often improve recall. By contrast, psychogenic amnesia tends to be greatest for emotionally important events, may delete from the patient's memory well-defined blocks of past events while leaving intact the recall of preceding or following material, and may affect remote memories equally with recent ones.

Treatment

Many patients with acute post-traumatic amnesia recover spontaneously. Patients with other forms of organic amnesia do less well unless the memory loss was caused by drugs or intercurrent illness. Neither medications nor diets have proved useful in treatment.

REFERENCE

Heilman KM, Valenstein E: Clinical Neuropsychology. 3rd ed. New York, Oxford University Press, 1993.

D. Dementia

GENERAL CONSIDERATIONS

Dementia describes a sustained or permanent, multidimensional decline of intellectual function that interferes seriously with the individual's social or economic adjust-

TABLE 112–20 Major Causes of Progressive Dementia

1. Senile dementia—Alzheimer-type	50%
2. Multi-infarct (arteriosclerotic)	10%
3. Combination of 1 and 2	15%
4. Communicating hydrocephalus	
5. Alcoholic or post-traumatic	15%
6. Huntington's disease	
7. Intracranial mass lesions	
8. Uncommon or mixed with above:	10%
Chronic drug use; Creutzfeldt-Jakob; metabolic (thyroid, liver, nutritional); degenerative (spinocerebellar, amyotrophic lateral sclerosis, parkinsonism, multiple sclerosis, Pick's, Wilson's, epilepsy); AIDS dementia; static postanoxic dementia	

AIDS = Acquired immunodeficiency syndrome.

ment. Table 112–20 lists causes of dementia and their approximate frequency. Several, such as Huntington's disease, Creutzfeldt-Jakob disease, and acquired immunodeficiency syndrome (AIDS), are discussed elsewhere in this book.

Static dementia follows acute brain injury and once a few days or weeks have elapsed, remains either fixed or improves only modestly. Severe head injury, global brain ischemia from cardiac arrest, large intracranial neoplasms or hemorrhages with their surgical removal, or infections such as severe encephalitis or meningitis are typical causes. *Progressive dementias* may begin either suddenly or insidiously but, by definition, worsen with the passage of time, often ending in total incapacity or death.

Early Clinical Manifestations

Acute, static dementia seldom provides a problem in diagnosis. Most often the issue becomes not whether a mental decline has occurred but to what degree and how the patient can restructure his or her world to new, possibly permanent limitations.

Early diagnosis in the progressive dementias may be difficult because both families and patients may attribute cognitive deterioration to ordinary personality variations. Initial symptoms involve deterioration in mood, personality, recent memory, judgment, and the capacity to form abstractions. Families or work associates usually detect a change before the patient does, and persons who live by intellectual efforts may display limitations relatively earlier than do those with routine or manual jobs. Some patients become so apathetic as to seem depressed. Furthermore, late-life depression often takes its roots in a dementing illness. In other instances, great anxiety, increased irritability, or paranoia can disrupt a once pleasant personality. Loss of recent memory is universal. Appointments are missed, plans forgotten, and stories of recent events become narrated repeatedly with little insight. Eventually, orientation fails, first for days, then years, then months, and finally for place. Interest lags. Debts may be accumulated silently, property unwisely sold, accounts lost, and meals cooked twice over or served half-done. Mental capacities can fluctuate without apparent relationship to external events. In Alzheimer's disease and some of the other progressive primary dementias, social amenities tend to be retained until late in the course. By contrast, incontinence, vulgarity, soup on the shirt, and a disheveled appearance characterize the mental deterioration that accompanies frontal lobe disease, intracranial mass lesions, or chronic drug-alcohol abuse.

Diagnosis

All patients with symptoms of subacute or chronic brain disease should receive a brief evaluation of mental function such as represented by the Mini Mental Status (see

TABLE 112–21	Potentially Treatable Dementias

Chronic medication; drug or alcohol exposure
Intracranial mass lesions
Communicating hydrocephalus
Deficiency of vitamin B_1, B_6, or B_{12}
Chronic hepatic encephalopathy
Wilson's disease
Syphilis
Granulomatous meningitis

TABLE 112–22	Therapeutic Drugs Potentially Causing Confusion or Delirium

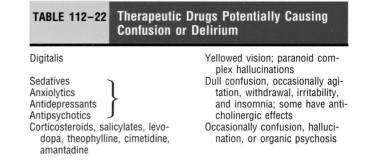

Digitalis	Yellowed vision; paranoid complex hallucinations
Sedatives Anxiolytics Antidepressants Antipsychotics	Dull confusion, occasionally agitation, withdrawal, irritability, and insomnia; some have anticholinergic effects
Corticosteroids, salicylates, levodopa, theophylline, cimetidine, amantadine	Occasionally confusion, hallucination, or organic psychosis

Table 111–5). For further quantitation, the assistance of a trained psychologist may be helpful. In mild to moderate dementia, early learned verbal capacities remain but everyday memories and performance deteriorate.

In addition to a pertinent history and physical examination, baseline initial evaluation for all demented patients should include a complete blood count (CBC), standard chemistry screen, Venereal Disease Research Laboratory (VDRL) test, serum free thyroxine (T_4) index, thyroid-stimulating hormone (TSH) level, and cobalamin level. A CT or MRI head-brain scan should be obtained whenever clinical findings leave diagnosis in doubt. A few causes of dementia are potentially treatable, including those listed in Table 112–21. Most of these can be suspected at the time of the patient's initial evaluation. Special tests for the others need be applied only when specific clinical indications exist.

Pseudodementia is a term applied to reversible states in which chronic drug intoxication, depressive illness, or psychogenic fugue states seemingly impair memory (see Table 112–17) or cognition. Aging persons are especially susceptible to the first two. Among drugs, the barbiturates, benzodiazepines, butyrophenones, tricyclic antidepressants, monoamine oxidase (MAO) inhibitors, anticholinergics, corticosteroids, and digitalis are frequently responsible (Table 112–22).

THE MOST FREQUENT DEMENTIAS
(Table 112–23)

Alzheimer's Presenile and Senile Dementia (ASD)

This devastating increasingly frequent disorder occasionally affects persons younger than 50 years but becomes prevalent in later years, affecting about 5% of all persons older than 70 years and as many as 20% over age 80. Classic neuropathology includes abnormal intraneuronal filaments, *tangles,* combined with collections of amyloid protein, *plaques,* that engulf the detritus of degenerated neurons. The changes most frequently and heavily involve the hippocampus and amygdala as well as the association cortical areas of the parietal, temporal, and frontal lobes. Prominent neuronal losses affect the same areas. Neurochemical abnormalities remain poorly understood, but ascending cholinergic and norepinephrine regulatory pathways are prominently damaged. Risk factors include age over 70 years, a family history of Alzheimer's disease or Down syndrome, severe past head trauma, or the inheritance of the apolipoprotein E-e4 allele.

Recent years have seen major advances in the genetics of Alzheimer's disease. Aside from the apoE-e4 allele, which provides an important susceptibility factor for late-

TABLE 112–23	Characteristics of the Most Common Dementias			
Type	**Incidence and Risks**	**Major Features**	**Laboratory Findings**
Alzheimer's dementia (AD)	5–10% <80 yr; >20% >80 yr. Rarely autosomal dominant; 25% have affected relatives.	Neat appearance; social amenities preserved until late; event and spatial memory loss produce disorientation. Patients have little insight; many display nocturnal restlessness-agitation. Sensorimotor abnormalities are absent.	None relevant. Brain images are normal or show mild atrophy.
Multi-infarct dementia	>60 yr. Hypertension, smoking, diabetes, and hyperlipidemia increase the risk.	Successive strokes, large and small. Rarely, gradually progressive. Upper motor neuron abnormalities common on examination.	MRI shows multiple strokes or diffuse, T2-weighted "bright spots" in hemispheric white matter.
Hydrocephalic dementia	60 yr. Can follow head trauma (accidents, boxing, surgery, meningeal infection or bleeding). Often no antecedents are identified.	Mild to moderate slowness of thinking, global dementia; broad-based, stiff, shuffling gait; incontinence. Mild bilateral upper motor neuron dysfunction, legs > arms.	CT or MRI shows dilated cerebral ventricles, effaced hemispheric sulci. CSF pressure normal in most.
Parkinson's disease (PD)	Dementia coexists in 20–50% over age 65.	Cognitive loss accompanies advanced PD, often with associated depression. Clinically resembles AD.	None relevant.

CSF = Cerebrospinal fluid; CT = computed tomography; MRI = magnetic resonance imaging.

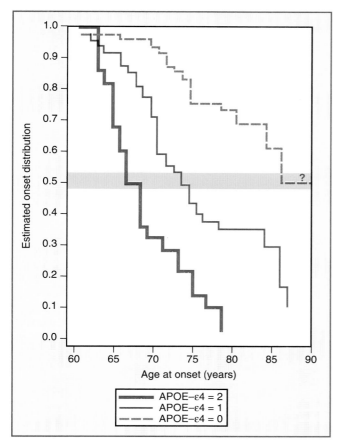

Figure 112–4
The influence on age of onset of Alzheimer's dementia (AD) among individuals possessing two, one, or zero APOE-ε4 alleles. Subjects belonged to 42 families known to be susceptible to late-onset AD. As diagrammed, 50% of carriers of a double ε4 allele developed AD at approximately 65 to 68 years. Fifty percent of those with a single allele developed the disease at 73 to 74 years, whereas surviving persons having no ε4 alleles had about a 50% risk at an age older than 85 years. (Adapted from Corder EH, Saunders AM, Strittmatter WJ, et al.: Gene dose of apolipoprotein E type 4 allele and the risk of Alzheimer's disease in late-onset families. Science 1993;261:921–924. Copyright 1993 American Association for the Advancement of Science.)

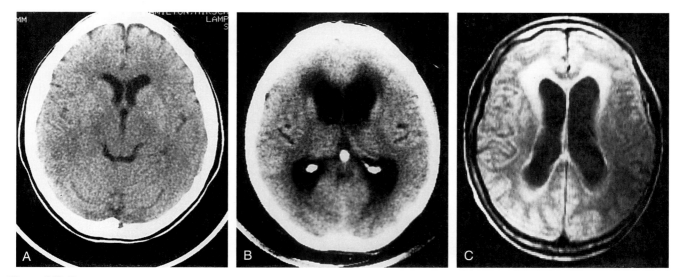

Figure 112–5
Communicating hydrocephalus. A 61-year-old woman 7 years following uncomplicated removal of carcinoma of the lung developed symptoms of headache and depression of mood. Neurologic examination and computed tomographic (CT) evaluation (*A*) were considered unremarkable. Over the next 4 months she became increasingly withdrawn, occasionally incontinent, and finally disoriented. She developed a broad-based ataxic gait, and CT scan showed ventricular dilatation (*B*). Magnetic resonance imaging (MRI) confirmed the ventricular enlargement and showed periventricular increased signals typical of edema (*C*). Spinal fluid contained increased protein, glucose 25 mg/dl, and malignant cells. Cerebrospinal fluid (CSF) pressure was 180 mm in the lateral recumbent position. Her alertness and gait temporarily improved following spinal drainage.

life Alzheimer's (Fig. 112–4), three gene abnormalities have been identified as responsible for early-onset familial clusters of the disease. Abnormalities on chromosome location 21q21 predispose to an abnormal amyloid protein expressed as an autosomal dominant form of the illness as well as to early Alzheimer changes superimposed on Down syndrome. Two somewhat similar abnormalities in neural membrane proteins derive from abnormal chromosome 14q24.3 and on chromosome 1; both mutations are uncommon and produce autosomal dominant, early-onset Alzheimer's in small, geographically remote, or widely scattered family clusters.

Clinically, ASD usually begins insidiously with memory impairment, personality alterations, and affective shallowness giving way at varying rates to severe amnesia for past events and for spatial relationships. Language errors later develop. Social amenities are preserved until late in the disease. Focal neurologic abnormalities or convulsions are not a feature. Specific diagnostic laboratory markers are lacking except in early-onset (below age 40 years) cases, which may result from identifiable gene abnormalities. Clinical diagnosis in typical cases, however, reaches about an 85% concordance with postmortem findings. The duration of ASD varies widely between extremes of 3 to 20 years, with patients declining slowly toward a terminal near-vegetative state. Death comes from pneumonia or intercurrent illness. Alzheimer variants have been described in association with the late stages of parkinsonism and occasionally with motor neuron disease. No effective treatment has been established, but haloperidol in small amounts often is useful in calming excessive agitation in the late stages.

Multi-Infarct Dementia

This occurs as a result of successive large and small strokes, affecting the cerebral hemispheres and their deep subcortical nuclei. Hypertension, diabetes mellitus, or hyperlipidemia most often underlie the vascular changes. The usual clinical picture is of successive, cumulative episodes of focal neurologic worsening, resulting in a disheveled appearance, accompanied commonly by aphasia, focal neurologic deficits, and CT or MRI that show multiple lucencies reflecting past infarctions. Occasionally, successive small strokes in hypertensive patients result in a less obviously episodic decline but a progressive amnesia.

Progressive Hydrocephalic Dementia

The condition is caused by chronic interference with the CSF absorption pathways that lie over the surface of the hemispheres. Ultimate causes include acutely or remotely occurring inflammatory or neoplastic meningitis, subarachnoid hemorrhage, and traumatic head injury; in many instances the initiating mechanism escapes detection. Principal diagnostic features include age greater than 55 years; moderate, diffuse cognitive decline; fatigue on exercise; urinary urgency-incontinence; and a broad-based, moderately spastic ataxic gait, usually accompanied by extensor plantar responses. Brain images show abnormal cerebral ventricular dilatation accompanied by reduced vertical sulcus markings, usually coupled with evidence of periventricular edema (Fig. 112–5). Some patients improve following surgical ventricular shunting.

REFERENCES

Arnold SE, Kumar A: Reversible dementias. Med Clin North Am 1993; 77:215–230.

Beal MF: Aging, energy and oxidative stress in neurodegenerative disease Ann Neurol 1995;38:357–368.

Corder EH, Saunders AM, Strittmatter WJ et al: Gene dose of apolipoprotein E type 4 allele and the risk of Alzheimer's disease in late-onset families. Science 1993;261:921–923.

Selkoe DJ: Aging brain, aging mind. Sci Am 1992;267: Sept. 135–142.

113

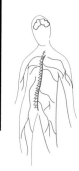

Disorders of Mood and Behavior

A. Psychiatric Disorders

Table 113–1 lists the most common types of mood and behavior disorders. This text treats these disorders only briefly, devoting attention to conditions that may enter the differential diagnosis of common medical problems. It is likely that future discoveries will bring greater knowledge of the mechanisms of psychiatric disorders and a clearer understanding of the interface between so-called organic and psychogenic illnesses. In the meantime, however, one must sift out for most patients with chronic medical problems the relative degrees of both psychological and physical distress and give due weight to each in devising treatment. The Diagnostic and Statistical Manual of Mental Disorders IV (DSM IV) of the American Psychiatric Association (1994) provides objective diagnostic criteria for psychiatric disorders that, if rigorously applied, will help to minimize diagnostic errors.

SCHIZOPHRENIC DISORDERS

The term schizophrenia describes a group of symptomatic psychological disorders, possibly of different origins, that are characterized by disturbances of mind and personality, including hallucinations, delusions, and altered behavior toward others. The common thread consists of a disturbance in the form and content of thought and a deterioration in psychosocial functioning, which often causes downward social mobility. The disorder, which affects about 1% of the population, sometimes can be mimicked by structural or physiologic-pharmacologic diseases involving the brain's limbic system, and the diagnosis requires that such structural disease be absent. The symptoms of schizophrenia usually begin during adolescence or early adulthood. Thought blocking and a lack of emotional warmth are frequent early symptoms. Many patients suffer from auditory hallucinations in which they either hear their own thoughts aloud or hear voices derogating their behavior. Others experience delusions that their actions or thoughts are controlled by outside forces that command them to carry out unwanted acts. Schizophrenic persons often appear vague, unresponsive, and unemotional, with awkward, slowed thinking and ideas poorly related to one another. The affect is often flat or inappropriate. Some schizophrenic patients show facial grimaces or tics that can resemble chorea or other extrapyramidal disorders. Others become immobile (catatonia), their apathy and indifference resembling frontal lobe disturbances.

The cause or causes of schizophrenia are unknown, although recent studies employing brain imaging techniques describe abnormalities in the structure and function of the left temporal lobe. Along the same lines, studies of identical twins have shown a strong genetic basis for the disorder. Early claims for a chromosomal locus for the disease have not been confirmed.

Diagnosis rests on recognizing the distinctive symptoms and ruling out other potential causes for the emotional and personality disorders. Schizophrenic patients, if their cooperation can be assured, are oriented and show no abnormality of cognitive functions. Sometimes it is difficult to distinguish schizophrenia from an affective psychosis. The distinction is important because treatment differs and prognosis is considerably better in the affective psychoses.

The treatment of schizophrenia requires considerable expertise. Neuroleptic drugs including phenothiazine, butyrophenones, and thioxanthenes have been the past mainstays. Difficulties in patient compliance and side effects however, make pharmacotherapy best left to experts. Long-term use of phenothiazines predisposes more than 10% of patients to *tardive dyskinesias* in the form of either continuous orolingual facial movements or, less commonly, dystonic movements of the trunk or extremities. Because tardive dyskinesia may persist even when neuroleptics are discontinued, one should attempt to control psychotic symptoms with the smallest possible dose. With early, appropriate treatment, the condition remits in about one third to one half of patients, and another 30% are able to live in the community.

Recently, atypical antipsychotics such as clozapine and resperidone have been developed. Both act on serotonergic as well as dopaminergic receptors. Neither precipitates extrapyramidal complications. Approximately 30% of patients who have not responded to traditional antipsychotics improve with clozapine. A 1% incidence of agranulocytosis makes monitoring imperative.

TABLE 113–1	Psychiatric Disorders of Mood and Behavior

Major psychoses
    Schizophrenic disorders
    Affective disorders
Major neuroses
    Anxiety disorders
    Somatoform disorders
    Dissociative disorders
    Factitious disorders
    Not attributable to a mental disorder, e.g., malingering

AFFECTIVE DISORDERS

The category includes a group of disorders characterized by an excessive disturbance of mood, whether elation or depression. The major patterns include recurrent episodes of either manic or depressive behavior or both (bipolar disorders), with attacks recurring repeatedly but usually clearing after weeks or months with or without treatment. The pathogenesis is unknown, although monozygotic twin studies suggest a major genetic component. Between episodes most patients behave relatively normally.

Depression

The most common affective disorder is depression (Table 113–2). Depression is a feeling of sadness and misery, usually accompanied by lowered self-esteem ranging from feelings of inadequacy and incompetence to a full-blown delusion that the patient is evil and responsible for many of the world's ills. The delusions distinguish *psychotic* from *situational* depressions (i.e., excessive sadness related to a true environmental event).

The diagnosis of depression may be difficult. At first contact, depressed patients with severe psychomotor retardation may be considered mistakenly to suffer from an organic dementia. Features listed in Table 113–3 help to distinguish between these conditions. The second challenge lies in distinguishing severe depression from physical illness. Many patients complaining of somatic symptoms have lost weight and may look so ill that the physician searches for a disease such as cancer without considering depression as the primary process. Early morning awakening, loss of appetite, and, particularly, recent-onset headache unaccompanied by structural disease should suggest depression; direct questioning about mood is essential. Patients should be asked if they feel blue or hopeless. If so, one should ask them gently and supportively if they have considered suicide as an option. An affirmative answer greatly strengthens the diagnosis and suggests a need for psychiatric consultation.

An additional diagnostic task is to identify depression in the setting of established physical illness or environmental stress. Such reactions can too easily be regarded as appropriate to the situation. Profound depression, even in terminally ill patients, is not the rule but its

TABLE 113–2	Common Manifestations of Depression

Feelings of sadness and low self-esteem
Delusions of self-evil, often bizarre
Insomnia (most) or hypersomnia
Relative anorexia, weight loss, apathy
Ill-founded aches and pains, especially headache and backache
Complaints of mental loss despite normal cognitive tests

presence adds great misery. The physician should consider it an added illness meriting specific treatment.

Finally, one also must distinguish structural disease of the brain from psychogenic apathetic depression. In doubtful instances obtaining a brain scan or appropriate laboratory test provides accurate differentiation.

Most depression responds to appropriate treatment with antidepressant drugs. Until recently the tricyclic antidepressant drugs such as amitriptyline, given in appropriate doses, were the drugs of choice. When used, they should be started in low doses and gradually increased. This gradual approach is particularly important in the elderly to avoid excessive sedation and hallucinations. If a tricyclic is given as a single dose at night, it promotes sleep, frequently relieving almost immediately one of the most disturbing symptoms in the depressed patient. The full psychological benefit usually takes 2 to 4 weeks. Other antidepressant drugs include monoamine oxidase inhibitors, tetracyclic antidepressants, and trazodone. Recently developed serotonin-reuptake inhibitors such as fluoxetine, paroxetine, and sertraline have come into wide usage. All are effective and free of anticholinergic side effects. The *Physicians' Desk Reference* should be consulted for dosage. Benzodiazepines are not useful and may exacerbate depression. If antidepressant drug therapy fails, electroshock therapy is often efficacious, particularly in patients with psychotic depression.

Mania

Manic signs and symptoms are the antithesis of depression, producing elation, grandiosity, and constant restless

TABLE 113–3	Features Distinguishing Depression from Dementia	
	Depression	**Dementia**
Duration of symptoms	Weeks to months	Months to years
Insight	Hypochondriacal	Often minimal
Prominent personalities and events	Recalled	Forgotten
Speech	Sparse to mute	Mute to excessive
Vegetative signs: insomnia, constipation, anorexia	Prominent	Minimal
Nocturnal behavior	Better	Worse
Sensorimotor changes	Absent	Often present
Brain images or EEG	Normal	Often abnormal

EEG = electroencephalogram.

activity. Alternating episodes of manic "highs" with depressive "lows" are termed *bipolar disease.* In the earliest stages of mania, patients actually may become more productive. As time passes, however, many deteriorate. Manic persons are easily distracted, show flight of ideas, and some become so grandiose and implausible as to be recognized easily as "crazy." Patients with intense mania may go for days without sleep and yet deny fatigue. The mood can suddenly change to anger and violence with little or no provocation.

The diagnosis of mania is usually easy because of the typical symptoms. Sometimes thyrotoxicosis, structural disease of the limbic system, or corticosteroid drug intoxication can mimic mania. Alternately, it may be difficult to distinguish a manic episode from schizophrenic agitation, but the extreme self-confidence that accompanies mania or a history of bipolar swings usually confirms the diagnosis.

The treatment of mania is difficult, in part because patients feel well and see no need for medicine. Phenothiazines or butyrophenones often control agitated behavior. Lithium is the mainstay. The drug is usually given in doses ranging from 900 to 1800 mg/day. Higher doses should be left to expert psychopharmocologists. Plasma levels should be kept below 2 mEq/L; excessive levels lead to confusion, disorientation, tremor, anorexia, and, sometimes, seizures with permanent neurologic damage. Maintenance lithium in patients with a history of manic psychosis or bipolar disease often prevents further episodes.

Anxiety Disorders (Table 113–4)

Abnormal anxiety is an unpleasant mood of tension and apprehension related to fear but not focused on an immediately stressful situation or object of danger. Anxiety is generally accompanied by autonomic symptoms including tachycardia, perspiration, dry mouth, and sometimes hyperventilation. In predisposed individuals, perception of autonomic changes, particularly palpitations (tachycardia) and lightheadedness (hyperventilation), increases the anxiety, thereby intensifying the autonomic symptoms.

The cause of the primary anxiety disorders is unknown. The condition is common, with a prevalence rate

TABLE 113–4	The Primary Anxiety Disorders

Phobic disorders
    Agoraphobia with panic attacks
    Agoraphobia without panic attacks
    Social phobia
    Simple phobia
Anxiety states
    Panic disorder
    Generalized anxiety disorder
    Obsessive-compulsive disorder
Post-traumatic stress disorder
    Acute
    Chronic or delayed
Atypical anxiety disorder

TABLE 113–5	Diagnostic Criteria for Panic Disorder Without Agoraphobia

A. Both (1) and (2):
  (1) recurrent unexpected panic attacks
  (2) at least one of the attacks has been followed by 1 month (or more) of one (or more) of the following:
    (a) persistent concern about having additional attacks
    (b) worry about the implications of the attack or its consequences (e.g., losing control, having a heart attack, "going crazy")
    (c) a significant change in behavior related to the attacks
B. Absence of agoraphobia
C. The panic attacks are not due to the direct physiological effects of a substance (e.g., a drug of abuse, a medication) or a general medical condition (e.g., hyperthyroidism).
D. The panic attacks are not better accounted for by another mental disorder, such as social phobia (e.g., occurring on exposure to feared social situations), specific phobia (e.g., on exposure to a specific phobic situation), obsessive-compulsive disorder (e.g., on exposure to dirt in someone with an obsession about contamination), posttraumatic stress disorder (e.g., in response to stimuli associated with a severe stressor), or separation anxiety disorder (e.g., in response to being away from home or close relatives).

With Agoraphobia

A. Both (1) and (2):
  (1) recurrent unexpected panic attacks
  (2) at least one of the attacks has been followed by 1 month (or more) of one (or more) of the following:
    (a) persistent concern about having additional attacks
    (b) worry about the implications of the attack or its consequences (e.g., losing control, having a heart attack, "going crazy")
    (c) a significant change in behavior related to the attacks
B. The presence of agoraphobia
C. The panic attacks are not due to the direct physiological effects of a substance (e.g., a drug of abuse, a medication) or a general medical condition (e.g., hyperthyroidism).
D. The panic attacks are not better accounted for by another mental disorder, such as social phobia (e.g., occurring on exposure to feared social situations), specific phobia (e.g., on exposure to a specific phobic situation), obsessive-compulsive disorder (e.g., on exposure to dirt in someone with an obsession about contamination), post traumatic stress disorder (e.g., in response to stimuli associated with a severe stressor), or separation anxiety disorder (e.g., in response to being away from home or close relatives).

of about 1% and a higher incidence in women. Genetic as well as behavioral-developmental factors undoubtedly play a role. Anxiety disorders have a higher concordance in monozygotic than in dizygotic twins, generally run in families, and are often associated with alcoholism. A disproportionate number of patients have mitral valve prolapse.

Clinically, anxiety states include (1) *phobias,* which can vary from simple phobic fears of particular objects, to agoraphobia, fear of being either alone or in public places, (2) panic attacks marked by fear, apprehension, and feelings of impending doom without underlying cause (Table 113–5), and (3) a generalized and constant feeling of fear and apprehension.

The diagnosis usually is easy: no organic disease produces such a litany of sensory experiences. Having such patients hyperventilate often reproduces their symptoms and distinguishes the disorder from a primary cardiac or neurologic abnormality. Only rarely can structural disease be responsible for attacks of autonomic dysfunction that appear to have their origin in panic. Some temporal lobe seizures can produce an aura of intense fear or anxiety associated with abnormalities of pulse and respiration, in early stages indistinguishable from panic attacks. Such seizures, however, culminate in a recognizable psychomotor attack or a generalized convulsion. Sudden changes in cardiovascular function, such as arrhythmias or acute hypertension (as from a pheochromocytoma), can mimic panic or anxiety attacks. The strongest clinical clue to such organically generated episodes is their recent onset.

Behavioral therapy and pharmacologic agents may ameliorate recurrent panic attacks. Behavior modification has been useful in the treatment of phobias. Useful drugs for generalized anxiety disorders and panic attacks include monoamine oxidase inhibitors, tricyclic antidepressants, and modest doses of anxiolytic agents such as the benzodiazepines. Beta blockers such as propranolol sometimes help patients with major autonomic symptoms, especially those who have mitral valve prolapse as well.

Somatoform, Dissociative, and Factitious Disorders

The essential feature is physical symptoms unexplained by either demonstrable organic findings or known physiologic mechanisms, accompanied by evidence of severe psychologic instability. Somatoform or dissociative disorders putatively differ from factitious disorders or malingering in that the symptoms are believed not to be under conscious control. Somatoform disorders are often grouped together under the rubrics of "hysteria" or conversion reaction.

Somatoform disorders can produce almost any of the symptoms of physical illness (Table 113–6). Most *conversion symptoms* involve the nervous system and consist of abnormalities of consciousness or gait, paralysis, sensory loss, blindness, hearing loss, speech loss, or seizures. (Many patients with pseudoseizures also have true epilepsy.) Non-neurologic somatic complaints such as nausea, multiple aches and pains, excessive fatigue, and weakness are common conversion symptoms that often lead to excessively repeated medical studies until their nonsomatic origins are realized.

Conversion symptoms occur in a variety of forms, some more elaborate than others. Most often, they arise in patients with severe repressed or expressed anxiety who displace their inner symptoms onto a fixed idea of disease located in a specific organ or member. Less often, such symptoms are superimposed on those of an actual organic disease, presumably as an attention-getting device or an unconscious displacement of vaguely sensed ill health onto a less emotionally threatening sensory or motor infirmity.

A third variety, called *Munchausen's syndrome,* involves persons who actively simulate organic disease, ei-

TABLE 113–6	Diagnostic Criteria for Somatization Disorder

A. A history of many physical complaints beginning before age 30 years that occur over a period of several years and result in treatment being sought or significant impairment in social, occupational, or other important areas of functioning.

B. Each of the following criteria must have been met, with individual symptoms occurring at any time during the course of the disturbance:
  (1) *four pain symptoms:* a history of pain related to at least four different sites or functions (e.g., head, abdomen, back, joints, extremities, chest, rectum, during menstruation, during sexual intercourse, or during urination)
  (2) *two gastrointestinal symptoms:* a history of at least two gastrointestinal symptoms other than pain (e.g., nausea, bloating, vomiting other than during pregnancy, diarrhea, or intolerance of several different foods)
  (3) *one sexual symptom:* a history of at least one sexual or reproductive symptom other than pain (e.g., sexual indifference, erectile or ejaculatory dysfunction, irregular menses, excessive menstrual bleeding, vomiting throughout pregnancy)
  (4) *one pseudoneurological symptom:* a history of at least one symptom or deficit suggesting a neurological condition not limited to pain (conversion symptoms such as impaired coordination or balance, paralysis or localized weakness, difficulty swallowing or lump on throat, aphonia, urinary retention, hallucinations, loss of touch or pain sensation, double vision, blindness, deafness, seizures; dissociative symptoms such as amnesia; or loss of consciousness other than fainting)

C. Either (1) or (2):
  (1) after appropriate investigation, each of the symptoms in Criterion B cannot be fully explained by a known general medical condition or the direct effects of a substance (e.g., a drug of abuse, a medication)
  (2) when there is a related general medical condition, the physical complaints or resulting social or occupational impairment are in excess of what would be expected from the history, physical examination, or laboratory findings

D. The symptoms are not intentionally produced or feigned (as in factitious disorder or malingering)

Reprinted with permission from the Diagnostic and Statistical Manual of Mental Disorders, Fourth Edition. Copyright 1994 American Psychiatric Association. From American Psychiatric Association: Diagnostic and Statistical Manual of Mental Disorders, Fourth Edition. Washington DC, American Psychiatric Association, 1994.

ther by symptoms alone or by self-medication or self-mutilation in order to deceive medical personnel. Many such persons either have been health care workers or have had close association with health professionals. Typical examples are individuals who induce "idiopathic" hypokalemia by ingesting surreptitiously obtained diuretics or nondiabetics who self-inject insulin to simulate disease-produced hypoglycemia. Some memorize the details of medical textbooks in order to present a credible story of a severe disease such as acute intermittent porphyria. Others have been known to ingest anticoagulants in an effort to imitate a cryptic blood dyscrasia. Munchausen's syndrome is a serious disease with a high incidence of self-invited invasive medical procedures and operations. Women predominate in its incidence. Characteristically, as the cause of their symptoms begins to be recognized, patients travel from hospital to hospital until the nature of their illness becomes apparent. Most refuse psychiatric assistance and continue to insist that their medical complaints have an organic origin. Many eventually commit suicide.

Malingering, that is, conscious simulation of nonexistent sensations or motor loss, is more common in men, especially when the illness is work-related or influences retirement benefits. The diagnosis can be difficult to prove but should be suspected when signs and symptoms are physiologically absurd and good evidence of potential secondary gain of either a psychological or financial nature can be identified.

Dissociative disorders consist of sudden, temporary alterations in self-aware consciousness not caused by structural or physiologic disease of the nervous system. Such disturbances include the following:

1. *Factitious amnesia* for either a circumscribed event or all past life events, not associated with recent memory impairment as tested by routine instruments (see also Table 112–19).
2. *Fugue states,* episodes in which individuals disappear from their ordinary location, travel elsewhere, and assume a new identity, denying knowledge of their previous existence.
3. *Multiple personalities,* conditions in which individuals claim several exclusively different inner selves, each one freed of responsibility for the knowledge or acts of the absent self-persona.
4. *Depersonalization disorders,* in which persons claim a change in their self-perception so that they lose or alter their sense of reality. Fleeting feelings of depersonalization are fairly widespread among normal individuals, especially children and adolescents. Similar experiences lasting for seconds or a few minutes in duration occur with temporal lobe epilepsy. Long periods of depersonalization almost always reflect psychological rather than physiologic abnormalities of the brain.

Diagnosis of the above disorders often is far from easy and depends heavily on the physician's experience and level of suspicion. Whether the symptoms follow a neurologic, systemic, or psychiatric pattern, the key to their understanding lies in the fact that they are inexplicable on a physiologic basis.

All of these conditions are difficult to treat. Physical, particularly neurologic, symptoms in their early stages can often be relieved by a matter-of-fact approach in which the physician reassures the patient but avoids initiating a long discussion of the symptom's pathogenesis. Firmness and personal support often restore strength to a hemiplegic hysteric and sight to a blind one. At the same time, psychological support should be given to relieve anxiety and to ameliorate the environmental stresses that produced the symptoms in the first place. Many such patients, however, are intractable to treatment. This is especially true of those with Munchausen's syndrome, dissociative states, and malingering.

REFERENCES

Kaplan H, Saddock B (eds.): Comprehensive Textbook of Psychiatry. 6th ed. Baltimore, Williams & Wilkins, 1995.

Kaplan H, Saddock B (eds.): Pocket Handbook of Psychiatric Drug Treatment. Baltimore, Williams & Wilkins, 1993.

Marsden CD: Hysteria–A neurologist's view. Psychol Med 1986; 16: 277–288.

Ross CA, Pearlson GD: Schizophrenia, the heteromodal association neocortex and development; potential for a neurogenetic approach. Trends Neurosci 1996; 19:171–176.

B. Drug and Alcohol Abuse

Drug abuse is a huge medical-social problem worldwide. Almost any drug as well as many household substances, including some common plants, can produce toxic changes if ingested in large amounts. Most abused drugs, as well as those taken for suicidal purposes, exert their primary effects on opiate receptors in the brain. Drugs, including alcohol, that affect higher brain function generally possess in varying combinations and severity the addiction-promoting potentials of *psychological dependence* leading to craving, *tolerance-habituation* leading to the ingestion of increasing amounts of drugs to achieve a constant effect, and *physical dependence* leading to neurogenic withdrawal phenomena unless the drug is taken continuously. Individual susceptibility to these changes varies widely and is influenced by both environmental and inherited qualities. Whatever these contributions may be, however, the physician's level of suspicion and his or her courage in facing the patient with the evidence provide the key to obtaining proper treatment.

THERAPEUTIC DRUG OVERDOSE

This condition is frequent, especially among the elderly, whose susceptibility is enhanced both by poor memories for what they have taken and their involutionally weakened neurologic and metabolic reserves. The chief offenders are listed in Table 113–7. Several of these agents, such as digitalis and corticosteroids, can cause confusion and hallucinations in standard therapeutic doses, especially in patients over age 70.

TABLE 113–7	Therapeutic Drugs Potentially Causing Confusion or Delirium
Drug	**Side Effects**
Digitalis	Yellowed vision; paranoid complex hallucinations
Sedatives, Anxiolytics, Antidepressants, Antipsychotics	Dull confusion, occasionally agitation, withdrawal, irritability, and insomina. Some have anticholinergic effects
Corticosteroids, salicylates, levodopa, theophyllilne, cimetidine, amantadine	Occasionally confusion, hallucination, or organic psychosis

TABLE 113–8	Common Drug Poisonings Affecting Arousal and/or Behavior

Drug	Signs and Symptoms Mild	Signs and Symptoms Severe	Diagnostic Test	Treatment
Opiates				
Heroin Morphine Meperidine Methadone Hydromorphone Oxycodone Levorphanol	"Nodding" drowsiness, small pupils, urinary retention, slow and shallow breathing; skin scars and subcutaneous abscesses; duration 4–6 hours; with methadone, duration to 24 hours	Coma; pinpoint pupils, slow irregular respiration or apnea, hypotension, hypothermia, pulmonary edema	Response to naloxone Urine	Naloxone, 0.4 mg intravenously or intramuscularly; repeat at 15-minute intervals if patient responds and gradually increase intervals; repeat in 3 hours if necessary; if no response by second dose, suspect another cause; treat shock; find and detect infection
Sedatives–Hypnotics				
Alcohol Barbituates Chloral hydrate Glutethimide (Doriden) Meprobamate (Equanil)	Confusion, rousable drowsiness, delirium, ataxia, nystagmus, dysarthria, analgesia to stimuli	Stupor to coma; pupils reactive, usually constricted; oculovestibular response absent; motor tonus initially briefly hyperactive, then flaccid; respiration and blood pressure depressed; hypothermia.	Blood, urine, breath Blood Blood Blood	Intubate, ventilate, lavage; drainage position; antimicrobials; keep mean blood pressure >90 mm Hg and urine output >300 ml per hour; avoid analeptics; hemodialyze severe phenobarbital poisoning
Benzodiazepines (Librium, Valium, Tranxene, Atavan, Dalmane, etc.)	Usually taken with another sedative if poisoning is attempted	Coma seldom severe if drug taken alone	Blood	As above; diuresis of little help
Toxic Hyperactives				
Amphetamines Methylphenidate	Euphoria, sometimes paranoid, repetitive behavior; dilated pupils, tremor, hyperactive reflexes; hyperthermia, tachycardia, arrhythmia	Agitated, assaultive and paranoid excitement; occasionally convulsions; hyperthermia; circulatory collapse	Blood	Chlorpromazine
Cocaine	Similar but less prominent than above; less paranoid, often euphoric	Twitching; irregular breathing, tachycardia, arrhythmia, occasionally convulsions; myocardial infarction; acute stroke; vasculitis; chronic paranoid psychosis or depression	Blood, urine	Diazepam plus labetalol for cardiovascular crisis
Monoanine oxidase inhibitors (Parnate, Nardil, Eutonyl, etc.)	Hypertensive crises; agitation, drowsiness; ataxia	Hypotension; headache; chest pain; agitation; coma, seizures and shock	Clinical	Symptomatic; gastric lavage
Neuroleptics (phenothiazines, butyrophenones, etc.)	Acute dystonia, somnolence, hypotension	Coma; convulsions (rare); arrhythmias; hypotension	Blood	Anticholinergics; diphenhydramine; symptomatic; gastric lavage
Psychedelics (lysergic acid diethylamide, mescaline, psilocybin, phencyclidine)	Confused, disorientation, perceptual distortions, distractability withdrawn or eruptive, leading to accidents or violence; wide-eyed, dilated pupils; restless, hyperreflexic; less often, hypertension or tachycardia	Panic		Reassure; diazepam satisfactory; avoid phenothiazines
Scopolamine-Atropine (knockout drops, Transderm delirium)	Agitation or confusion, visual hallucinations, dilated pupils, flushed and dry skin	Florid toxic disoriented delirium, visual hallucinations; later, amnesia, fever, dilated fixed pupils, hot flushed dry skin, urinary retention		Reassure; sedate lightly; avoid phenothiazines; do not leave alone

Continued

TABLE 113–8	Common Drug Poisonings Affecting Arousal and/or Behavior *Continued*			
	Signs and Symptoms			
Drug	**Mild**	**Severe**	**Diagnostic Test**	**Treatment**
Antidepressants				
Tricyclics (Tofranil, Elavil, Desipramine, etc.)	Restlessness, drowsiness; tachycardia; ataxia; sweating	Agitation; vomiting; hyperpyrexia, sweating; muscle dystonia, convulsions; tachycardia or arrhythmia	Blood	Symptomatic; gastric lavage; for severe cases, intensive care, anticonvulsants, and antiarrhythmics
Lithium	Mild lethargy	Sustention-intention tremor, lethargy; muteness with appearance of distraction; coma; multifocal seizures; slow or fluctuating course	Blood	Hydrate if mild; hemodialyze for delirium, coma, or convulsions
Acid-Forming Intoxicants				
Methanol (formic); ethylene glycol (oxalic and hippuric); other organic alcohols	Inebriation with hyperpnea	Progressive hyperventilation; drunkenness, stupor; eventually convulsions and death; early blindness with methanol	Blood shows increasingly severe anion gap acidosis	Inhibit hepatic alcohol dehydrogenase by giving alcohol until acidosis controlled treat acidosis vigorously
Salicylates				
Aspirin	Tinnitus, dyspnea	Older persons: confusional state or toxic delirium leading to stupor, convulsions, coma	Blood salicylate >60 mg/dl	Alkaline diuresis

Reproduced with permission from Bennett JC, Plum F (eds.): Cecil Textbook of Medicine, 20th ed. Philadelphia, WB Saunders, 1996, p. 1975.

RECREATIONAL-SEDATIVE DRUG ABUSE AND POISONING (Table 113–8)

Marijuana

This widely used, predominantly inhaled agent, depends primarily on metabolites of delta-9-tetrahydrocannabinol for its pharmacologic action. Autonomic effects include conjunctival congestion, tachycardia, flushing, orthostatic hypotension, dry mouth, and sometimes vomiting. Psychic reactions depend considerably on the user and the setting in which the drug is inhaled. Users report perceptual enhancement, euphoria, a sense of timelessness, infectious joviality, and drowsiness. Coordination and reaction time are impaired. Mild tolerance and physical dependence usually develop, but most persons suffer only moderately adverse effects. Physiologic effects include respiratory tract irritation, tachycardia, decreased sperm formation, and, possibly, reduced fertility. Enduring psychic changes are uncertain. Acutely, depression, panic, paranoia, and toxic psychosis have been reported. Some chronic heavy users become unable to undertake goal-directed efforts, but whether the trait precedes or follows cannabis use is uncertain.

Central Nervous System (CNS) Depressants

Those most frequently abused include benzodiazepines, short-acting barbiturates, and other sedatives, especially methaqualone (Quaalude) and methyprylon (Noludar). The agents are mostly ingested orally and are widely used to counteract insomnia and anxiety. Most self-medicators develop mild habituation. Severe addiction can develop among secret sedative users, much as it does among closet alcoholics. Street use of all the CNS depressants is usually combined with marijuana, alcohol, or cocaine.

Withdrawal symptoms commonly follow the removal of any of these drugs after heavy usage, usually beginning 2 to 6 days after cessation. Symptoms consist of heightened insomnia, anxiety, and apprehension, together with tremulousness and mild autonomic changes. Withdrawal from chronic heavy barbiturate use is particularly distressing and causes symptoms and signs similar to those of the alcohol abstinence syndrome. Treatment is similar to that of alcohol withdrawal syndromes and consists of reintroducing the drug, then tapering it gradually to avoid symptoms. Overprescribing by physicians commonly underlies addiction to these drugs. Barbiturates probably should be avoided except for the treatment of epilepsy. All CNS depressant drugs tend to intensify preexisting feelings of psychological depression, contraindicating their use for treating such symptoms.

Cocaine

This powerfully addicting agent is predominantly insufflated but also can be taken by mouth, vein, or absorption through mucous membranes. Its use has increasingly spread among adolescents and young adults, especially in the free-based form termed "crack." Mortality climbs apace. Physiologic effects include local anesthesia, fever, tachycardia, hypertension, pupillary dilation, peripheral vasoconstriction, tachypnea, and anorexia. Psychologically, users report feelings of increased energy, alertness, and psychic power, often coupled with irritability and some anxiety. Reportedly, intravenous use or the smoking of crack induces an intense, euphoric "rush" followed by a craving to repeat the experience. Complications include social dissolution associated with craving, ulceration of the nasal septum, intracranial stroke-causing angiitis, occasionally convulsions and, with high doses, coma and death. Amphetamine abuse can cause somewhat similar experiences and complications. Treatment of cocaine abuse consists of withdrawal in a protective environment plus giving benzodiazepines or phenothiazines to control severe agitation. Psychological dependence is strong, leading to repetitive or continuous use, with a "crash" of debilitated disorganization and deep sleep at the end. Postwithdrawal craving reportedly is intense and protracted, leading to frequent recidivism even after weeks or months of abstinence.

Opiates

Heroin, morphine, methadone, and meperidine are the chief offenders, in that order. Two principal medical problems arise with their acute use: accidental or intentional overdose and the development of complications resulting from idiosyncratic reactions, infections, and immunologic abnormalities. Efforts by amateur chemists to produce psychedelic congeners have sometimes generated molecular variants with disastrous results, as exemplified by a recent miniepidemic of chemically induced severe parkinsonism.

Acute overdose with opiates produces stupor or coma, pupillary miosis, and slow, irregular, shallow breathing. Body temperature and blood pressure fall, seizures can occur, and some patients develop acute pulmonary edema. Treatment of acute overdose consists of immediately giving naloxone, a powerful opiate antagonist, intravenously or, if no veins can be found, intramuscularly. If no immediate response occurs, the injection should be repeated. Because the effects of naloxone wear off within 2 to 3 hours and the depressant effects of the opiates can last much longer, the antagonist should be repeated at 2- to 3-hour intervals until all evidence of a response disappears. Stuporous or hypoventilating patients who do not respond immediately should be treated according to the general program for care of the patient in coma (see Table 113–9).

Chronic opiate addicts can develop severe withdrawal symptoms consisting of yawning, anxiety, restlessness, rhinorrhea, lacrimation, and influenzal symptoms within minutes after receiving naloxone. The symptoms can be reduced by clonidine or ameliorated by small doses of narcotics. Naloxone should be confined to overdose situations and not employed in a nonemergency setting either as a diagnostic measure or to induce withdrawal.

Complications of illicit narcotic use include arrhythmias, pulmonary edema, and convulsions due to adulterants. Opiate users suffer a high incidence of bacteriologic infections of skin, veins, blood, heart, and lung. Many develop viral hepatitis and AIDS (see Chapter 109). Serious neurologic complications consist of neuropathy, myelopathy, optic neuritis, and myriad infections, including tetanus and brain abscess.

Tricyclic Antidepressants

These agents possess potentially serious cardiovascular effects, oral doses of more than 2 gm often being lethal. Because behavioral changes can take some hours to develop and blood levels may not be easily available, patients reporting acute self-overdose should have an immediate electrocardiogram (ECG). The presence of a widened QRS to greater than 100 msec indicates serious toxicity and a need for intensive supervision and cardiac monitoring. A more common presentation consists of a state of stupor or coma, combined with anticholinergic signs reminiscent of atropine poisoning and the presence of cardiac arrhythmias on the ECG. Treatment in alert patients consists of ipecac-induced vomiting and in stuporous ones of gastric lavage followed by activated charcoal instillation. Convulsions and arrhythmias are treated by appropriate standard measures. Otherwise, management follows that outlined in Table 113–9. Most tricyclics have metabolic half-lives of many days, so that monitoring and intensive treatment can be required for as long as a week in severe cases.

Salicylate Poisoning

Salicylate intoxication can occur in older adults as an accident of overzealous attempts to relieve pain and in adolescents and young adults as intentional overdose. Salicylates in high doses uncouple oxidative phosphorylation, and aspirin adds acid radicals. The resulting acid-base disturbance in adults is almost diagnostic: tissue glycolysis produces intracellular lactacidosis, which produces an acid urine and stimulates the brain stem respiratory centers. The result is a mixed respiratory alkalosis-metabolic acidosis with an elevated blood pH, a low Pa_{CO_2}, and low serum bicarbonate. Early symptoms include tinnitus, deafness, disequilibrium, drowsiness, and moderate delirium. With blood levels greater than 60 mg/

TABLE 113–9	Emergency Management of Coma

1. Assure airway and oxygenation.
2. Maintain adequate systemic circulation.
3. Give thiamine, 50 to 100 mg intravenously.
4. Give glucose after first obtaining blood for analysis.
5. Stop generalized seizures.
6. Restore blood acid-base and osmolar balance but do not change serum sodium by more than 15 mOsm/day.
7. Treat infection specifically.
8. Ameliorate extreme body temperature ($>40°$ or $<35°C$).
9. Consider naloxone.
10. Control agitation-tremulousness with lorazepam or haloperidol.

dl, stupor, coma, and potentially fatal convulsions can ensue. Treatment consists of gastric lavage and intravenous or oral bicarbonate solutions, using alkaline diuresis as an end point.

Phencyclidine (PCP)

PCP is currently the most widely abused of the psychedelic-hallucinogenic group of drugs that include, among numerous others, lysergic acid diethylamide (LSD), amphetamines, and scopolamine. Most users describe a state of altered perception in which dreams and heightened reality become indistinguishable. Excess inhalation or ingestion of PCP can induce ataxia, confusion, aggressive violence, prolonged psychotic states, coma, or convulsions. Treatment is symptomatic, but the "bad trip" may be shortened by acidifying the urine with ammonium chloride and applying continuous gastric suction to accelerate excretion of the drug.

Nonethyl Alcohols

Most cases of poisoning from these agents occur in alcoholics or drug abusers unaware of the toxic nature of the substance. Methanol and ethylene glycol both produce potentially fatal metabolic acidosis through their metabolic products. The hepatic enzyme alcohol dehydrogenase acts on both substrates to produce acid products. Inhibiting alcohol dehydrogenase by giving 4-methylpyrazol or 5 to 10 gm of ethyl alcohol per hour by mouth or vein effectively halts this highly toxic step and is the treatment of choice. Severe poisoning requires maintaining ethanol blood levels of 100 to 150 mg/dl for at least 48 to 72 hours while stabilizing blood acid-base levels with bicarbonate buffer. Ethylene glycol may cause subsequent renal damage from oxylate and hippurate crystalluria.

ALCOHOL ABUSE AND ITS COMPLICATIONS

Ethyl alcohol is the oldest and still most widely taken psychotropic drug. Used by more than half of all Americans and abused by 1 in 20, the agent creates a huge medical and sociologic problem.

Pharmacology

Ethanol is usually ingested as a fraction of some vehicle of distinctive taste such as beer (5%), wine (12%), or various stronger agents containing 20 to 50% alcohol (40 to 100 proof). Ethanol enters the blood within minutes from the stomach and intestine and quickly penetrates all aqueous body compartments, including the brain and alveolar air. Ethanol is excreted through the lungs by physical diffusion and detoxified by hepatic dehydrogenase at a rate that approximates 8 ml/hour, clearing about 15 mg/dl/hour from the blood.

TABLE 113–10	Blood-Alcohol Levels and Symptoms	
Level (mg/dl)	**Sporadic Drinkers**	**Chronic Drinkers**
50 (party level)	Congenial euphoria	No observable effect
75	Gregarious or garrulous	Often no effect
100	Incoordinated; legally intoxicated	Minimal signs
125–150	Unrestrained behavior Episodic dyscontrol	Pleasurable euphoria or beginning incoordination
200–250	Alertness lost → lethargic	Effort required to maintain emotional and motor control
300–350	Stupor or coma	Drowsy and slow
>500	Some die	Coma

Blood levels of alcohol correlate directly with clinical signs and symptoms, with chronic alcoholics showing great tolerance compared with novices (Table 113–10). In less than near-fatal amounts, aside from producing vasodilation and gastric irritation, alcohol exerts almost all its acute effects on the central nervous system, acting entirely as a depressant. The earlier euphoriant-excitatory stage reflects a removal of higher inhibitory effects from limbic system restraints, and larger doses increasingly depress first forebrain and then brain stem functions. Death from acute intoxication usually results from central respiratory depression followed by circulatory failure.

Clinical Features

Acute Intoxication

The behavioral effects of acute intoxication vary with the user, ranging among social drinkers from pleasant conviviality to angry argumentativeness. A small number of younger male drinkers develop pathologically severe, aggressive, violent behavior—*dyscontrol*—for which they later claim no memory. The syndrome has potentially dangerous consequences, and its diagnosis calls for total abstinence and immediate psychiatric referral. *Alcoholic blackouts,* periods of amnesia lasting for several hours or more during or at the end of a heavy drinking bout, are a sign of serious intoxication bordering on anesthesia. When recurrent, they signify impending or already existing alcoholic addiction.

Treatment of acute alcoholic attacks depends upon the degree of intoxication and the associated blood levels. Mild drunkenness requires no treatment. More severe intoxication producing heavy drowsiness or stupor deserves attention, especially if one does not know whether or not additional drugs have been ingested. The level of CNS depression can increase rapidly as alcohol is absorbed, and stuporous drunks need close attention to vital functions. Alcoholic deep stupor or coma requires hospital monitoring until symptoms subside. Patients with associated severe trauma or fever need especially close evaluation for potentially masked neurologic injury, blood loss, or infection.

Withdrawal Syndromes

Headache, giddiness, difficulty in concentrating, nausea, and mild tremulousness characterize the well-known *hangover*. Classic but unproved remedies or preventives include forcing nonalcoholic fluids while still intoxicated, avoiding the ingestion of agents such as red wines or brandies, and taking antacids. When hangover appears, another alcoholic drink aborts most of the symptoms but represents an early step toward the development of chronic alcoholism.

The serious withdrawal states of chronic alcoholism consist of prominent tremulousness, rum fits, and delirium tremens (DTs). They usually are preceded by years of problem drinking and precipitated by continuous alcoholic ingestion lasting many days or weeks.

Tremulousness, insomnia, and agitation, although much more common, symptomatically blend into DTs, discussed below. Each reflects a state of central adrenergic hyperexcitation that emerges as alcohol's inhibitory influence dissipates. *Withdrawal convulsions* (rum fits) consist of single or short runs of generalized seizures, usually with no focal features. Their necessary stimulus consists of no more than a falling blood alcohol level and, in contrast to the more delayed appearance of DTs, they can occur during the course of a prolonged spree within hours of the last drink. About one third are followed by the DTs if abstinence continues. Treatment is symptomatic, using diazepam to stop the seizures and dampen the often associated tremulousness. Interictal laboratory tests, including computed tomography (CT) scans and electroencephalograms (EEGs), show no specific abnormality, but if focal seizures occur a brain scan should be done to rule out a localized lesion such as subdural hematoma. Prophylactic anticonvulsants confer no protection.

Delirium tremens represents the most serious, occasionally fatal withdrawal complication of alcohol, usually appearing only after a decade or more of fairly continuous, heavy drinking. The course is worsened when complicated by systemic infection, hepatic insufficiency, or head trauma. A somewhat similar although less florid condition affects patients withdrawing from chronic heavy barbiturate use, and the treatment described below applies equally well to that syndrome. Either alcoholic or *barbiturate withdrawal* DTs can arise unexpectedly in patients abruptly withdrawn from these drugs in association with admission to hospital for conditions such as trauma or emergency surgery.

Characteristically, DTs most often emerge 3 to 5 days after complete alcohol or drug withdrawal. First symptoms consist of tremulousness, disorientation, visual hallucinations, and agitation. Prominent signs of beta-adrenergic autonomic hyperactivity include fear, sweating, tachycardia, hypertension, tachypnea, and incontinence. Many affected patients are malnourished and display associated signs of hepatic insufficiency, gastritis, dehydration, infection, polyneuropathy, myopathy, or Wernicke's syndrome. Treatment consists of sedation with a drug cross-tolerant for alcohol, diazepam being most useful (Table 113–11). Huge amounts of the drug may be required: authorities report that as much as a total of 215

TABLE 113–11	Treatment of Severe Tremulousness or Delirium Tremens

1. Attempt control by reassurance and observation.
2. Treat systemic problems promptly.
3. Give thiamine first; continuously supply and balance electrolytes and other vitamins.
4. Treat uncontrollable agitation: Control with diazepam, 10 mg intravenously (IV) given slowly followed by 5–10 mg IV slowly every 5 minutes, to induce calmness. Once calm, maintain with diazepam, 5–10 mg IV or more every 1–4 hours.

mg given in successive smaller doses may be necessary to control agitation initially. Some patients may need as much as 1200 mg given intravenously during the first 60 hours in order to remain calm.

Chronic Alcoholism

This condition is widespread and requires the physician's constant vigilance to detect it sufficiently early to modify its course. Psychological dependence, closet drinking, increasing social lapses, frequent hangovers, and an increasing number of nights out with "old friends" are danger signals. Blackouts, absenteeism, drunken driving, occupational downgrading, or any medical complications including repeated physical injury imply serious trouble.

Even to get a potential alcoholic to consider that he or she has a psychological-medical problem can be a thankless and often unsuccessful task. Nevertheless, the doctor must try. Success usually requires sustained and effective psychotherapy by an experienced therapist plus participation in a reinforcement group such as Alcoholics Anonymous. Several industries and large universities recently have established such groups, reporting successes as high as 70% or more once persons come to realize that their jobs are on the line and their employer is genuinely interested. Disulfiram (Antabuse) produces conditioned avoidance to alcohol by introducing a violently adverse reaction to its ingestion. Its use is best supervised by experienced therapists.

Complications of Alcohol Abuse

Drunkenness contributes to a large fraction of deaths and severe injuries from traffic accidents, trauma, murder, suicide, and the inadvertent overdose of other drugs. Chronic complications can affect many body organs (Table 113–12). Some of these may be due to a direct, but tenuously established, toxic effect. Nutritional deprivation, however, causes the majority. Alcohol contains 7 calories per gram, but most of its vehicles include negligible amounts of vitamins, trace metals, or other nutrients, including protein. Alcoholics, supplying their immediate energy needs by carbohydrates, can wear the mask of nutritional good health for years while their brains, nerves, livers, and hearts degenerate to a degree that, sooner or later shortens their mental capacity and lives.

TABLE 113–12	Major Non-Neurologic Complications of Alcoholism

Heart

Cardiomyopathy
Arrhythmia
Hyperlipidemia

Gastrointestinal

Gastritis
Hepatitis-cirrhosis
Pancreatitis
Head, neck, and esophageal cancer
Malabsorption

Blood

Iron or folate deficiency
Anemia
Thrombocytopenia
Prothrombin deficiency

Endocrine

Male sexual impairment
Increased fetal risk

Immune System

Increased susceptibility to infection and impaired healing

Electrolyte Disturbances

Hypocalcemia
Hypomagnesemia
Hypophosphatemia
Acute water intoxication
Alcoholic hyperosmolality
Alcoholic ketosis

TOXIC AND DEFICIENCY NEUROLOGIC DISORDERS RELATED TO ALCOHOLISM AND NUTRITIONAL DEPRIVATION (Table 113–13)

In addition to chronic alcoholism, severe nutritional insufficiencies can accompany any debilitating, energy-consuming illness, such as metastatic cancer, disseminated infection, thyrotoxicosis, advanced connective tissue disease, impaired intestinal absorption, and chronic behavioral disorders. Nutritional insufficiency with these illnesses only occasionally is confined to a single vitamin or nutrient although thiamine lack is perhaps most prevalent. Signs that suggest nutritional failure include apathetic listlessness, darkening of the skin, a sore red tongue, fissuring at the corners of the mouth, burning feet, progressive unexplained weight loss, and unexplained anemia. This section focuses on the most common neurologic compli-

TABLE 113–13	Major Neurologic Complications of Severe Alcoholism

Amblyopia and optic atrophy
Progressive cerebral degeneration and dementia
Peripheral neuropathy
Myopathy
Wernicke-Korsakoff disease
Parenchymatous cerebellar degeneration

cations, all of which occur more with alcoholism than any other single disorder in the United States.

Chronic severe alcoholics suffer an increased incidence of middle-life–onset *optic neuropathy,* a condition marked by reduced visual acuity, central or paracentral scotomas, and normal optic fundi. Dietary and vitamin therapies sometimes bring improvement. Advanced problem drinkers can develop CT-imaged *cerebral atrophy* and signs of dementia as early as the fourth decade. Abstinence sometimes reverses the severity of these changes.

Alcoholic-nutritional peripheral neuropathy usually occurs only in company with advanced, mixed nutritional deprivation and improves only with total replacement and weight gain. The disorder produces axonal degeneration affecting predominantly the small pain- and temperature-mediating fibers in the distal lower extremities. Because nerve conduction velocity depends on the integrity of the larger, touch-mediating peripheral fibers, that test can remain normal in the early stages of the neuropathy. Distal motor loss occurs relatively early. Spontaneous, often burning, pain and autonomic neuropathy commonly affect advanced cases. Deep tendon reflexes disappear in a distal-to-proximal pattern. Recovery, often incomplete, requires months or years of renourishment.

Alcoholic myopathy is confined to chronic, severe alcoholics and can have either an acute or a chronic onset. The acute form consists of sudden transient rhabdomyolysis, often following a cluster of rum fits or possibly other trauma. It includes muscle pain, tenderness, cramping, weakness, and an elevated serum creatine kinase. Severe cases can develop myoglobinuria with associated renal complications. Chronic myopathy consists of diffuse proximal muscle wasting and weakness disproportional to any existing neuritic impairment. It improves gradually with nutritional replacement.

Wernicke-Korsakoff disease reflects the acute and chronic CNS effects of severe, sustained thiamine depletion in the face of a continued caloric intake. In the United States, severe alcoholism most often causes the disorder, but other impoverished diets, such as nonsupplemented hospital glucose infusions, hemodialysis, various food faddisms, and hyperemesis gravidarum, can lead to the same condition. The brain pathologic changes include axonal demyelination, neuronal loss, glial proliferation, endothelial thickening, and petechial pericapillary hemorrhages. The oculomotor, vestibular, and medullary autonomic nuclei as well as the brain stem reticular formation suffer the greatest damage. At higher levels the mammillary bodies, the mediodorsal thalamic nuclei, and scattered cortical regions including the hippocampus suffer most.

Clinically, patients with acute Wernicke's disease are confused, often drowsy or semistuporous, ataxic, and dysarthric. Partial or complete external ophthalmoplegia and nystagmus are cardinal features. Further examination often discloses tachycardia, orthostatic hypotension, hypothermia, and a diffuse analgesia. The pupils seldom are affected, but almost any motor cranial nerve can be partially paralyzed. Most patients have at least mild signs of peripheral neuropathy. Treatment consists of giving thiamine, 100 mg parenterally, upon suspicion of the diagnosis, followed by replenishment of blood volume and electrolytes. Glucose administration should not precede thiamine treatment, as its metabolic processing can precipitate acute worsening. Evidence of severe anemia, hepatic insufficiency, or infection should be corrected and the patient watched closely for evidence of impending seizures or DTs. General good nourishment and efforts to halt the destructive slide of chronic alcoholism necessarily follow.

Wernicke's disease is readily diagnosed clinically, provided that one has enough history to suspect thiamine deficiency. The eye signs provide a critical clue: only acute idiopathic polyneuropathy, myasthenia gravis, botulism, and intoxication with phenytoin are likely to cause a similarly acute symmetric or asymmetric bilateral external ophthalmoplegia with preserved arousal. Of these, only Wernicke's disease and, rarely, phenytoin intoxication produce mental changes. The response to thiamine injection is usually diagnostic: the ophthalmoplegia usually begins to improve within a matter of hours to a day or so, a response produced with no other disorder.

Korsakoff's amnestic syndrome usually emerges as the acute confusional delirium of Wernicke's disease subsides. Affected patients show a profound, relatively isolated loss of recent memory for events. This, coupled with a placid lack of insight, often leads to total disorientation mixed with absurd conversations or answers to questions (confabulation). Arousal, language functions, and remote memories are spared. Korsakoff's arises only after either several preceding attacks of Wernicke's encephalopathy or an unusually severe one. Treatment is as for Wernicke's. About half the patients treated for the first time improve to the point of regaining independence.

Acute cerebellar degeneration occurs most often in alcoholics as a complication of an acute superimposed, severe binge. Its pathogenesis remains unclear but may reflect acute alcoholic damage to chemically vulnerable regional neurons. The symptoms reflect acute neuronal degeneration in the anterior and superior cerebellar vermis, leading to a gradually or suddenly appearing broad-based, stiff-legged ataxia unaccompanied by incoordination in the upper extremities or nystagmus. Many patients have an associated nutritional peripheral neuropathy.

Central pontine myelinolysis (CPM), sometimes termed *osmotic demyelination syndrome,* occurs as a complication of severe, relative hyponatremia or its treatment, usually following the correction of serum sodium levels at or below 110 mEq/L. Such severe hyponatremia can be a complication of prolonged alcoholism but more often arises in association with severe systemic illness. The disorder consists of the development of a symmetric zone of demyelination affecting the basis pontis of the brain stem, leading to lethargy or stupor, a quiet confused delirium, and more or less severe quadriparesis. Other symmetric brain areas may also demyelinate. Best evidence suggests that the abnormality most often follows the overly rapid correction of severe hyponatremia. Most authorities recommend raising the serum sodium in patients with profound hyponatremia by no more than about 0.5 mEq/hr. Most examples of CPM become visible on MRI or CT brain images within a week or so after onset. Many patients treated symptomatically recover in a matter of weeks. Some, however, never become normal.

REFERENCES

Arky R, et al: Physicians' Desk Reference. Montvale, NJ, Medical Economics Co, 1996.

Meyer RE: The disease called addiction: emerging evidence in a 200-year debate. Lancet 1996; 347:162–166.

O'Brien CP: Drug abuse and dependence. *In* Wyngaarden JB, Smith LH Jr, Bennett JC (eds.): Cecil Textbook of Medicine. 19th ed. Philadelphia, WB Saunders Co, 1992, pp 47–55.

Olson KR, et al.: Poisoning and Drug Overdose. Norwalk, Appleton and Lange, 1994.

114

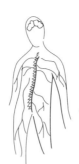

Disorders of Autonomic Function

The autonomic nervous system contains three major components. One links the brain to the pituitary gland via the hypothalamus to regulate the peripherally located endocrine organs (see Chapter 65). The second diffusely projects to higher brain centers cholinergic, noradrenergic, and serotoninergic pathways that originate, respectively, in ventral basal forebrain nuclei, the pontine locus ceruleus, and the raphe nuclei of the midbrain and pons. These ascending systems, along with others originating in the posterior hypothalamus, modulate arousal as well as cognitive and emotional expression. The third component consists of descending and peripheral autonomic sympathetic and parasympathetic pathways that originate in the hypothalamus and other brain stem centers and connect via sympathetic and parasympathetic ganglia with the viscera and the extremities to regulate internal homeostasis.

HYPOTHALAMUS (HT)

Direct damage to the HT can impair normal arousal mechanisms; interfere with trophic regulation of the pituitary gland; blunt learning, memory, and emotion; and disrupt mechanisms that regulate body temperature, visceral functions, water balance, and feeding behavior. Table 114–1 lists the principal disorders that result from dysfunction of the system.

Disturbances of Temperature Regulation

Sustained relative *hypothermia* or *poikilothermia*, with body temperatures varying with the environment and falling below 35°C, can follow destructive lesions of the posterior hypothalamus or adjacent midbrain. Hypothermia also accompanies several metabolic comas as well as depressant drug poisoning. In addition, impaired autonomic responses to dehydration and ambient cooling frequently affect alcoholics and elderly persons, increasing their susceptibility to cold exposure and intensifying fluid loss and hypothermia. Small epidemics of exposure-induced hypothermia have been reported among residents of insufficiently heated nursing homes. Body temperatures below 33 to 34°C usually induce severe apathy or stupor, a reduction in amplitude of vital signs, and palpably cold skin. Treatment of core temperatures between 31° and 35°C consists of gradual rewarming by blankets in a warmed environment. Heating blankets set at 38°C, tub immersions at 40° to 42°C, or warmed peritoneal dialysis can be employed for persons with colder core temperatures. Fluids and auxiliary treatment are guided by specific cardiac or infectious complications.

Episodic hypothermia is an uncommon disorder, probably representing a form of diencephalic epilepsy; body temperature episodically drops to 32°C or less, associated with reduced alertness, mental slowness or confusion, and, usually, cardiorespiratory irregularities. Some affected patients respond to antiepileptic therapy.

Hyperthermia accompanies several disorders, including hypothalamic damage as well as heat exhaustion, heat stroke, and malignant hyperthermia. *Neurogenic hyperthermia* occurs as an acute phenomenon in association with several disorders affecting the hypothalamic region. Fever can rise to potentially fatal levels of 42°C or higher. If standard antipyretic measures fail, adding small doses of opiates sometimes ameliorates the elevated temperature. Other measures are discussed under heat stroke. Subacute or chronic fever almost never results from primary hypothalamic disorders.

Heat Exhaustion and Heat Stroke (Table 114–2)

These conditions result from combinations of high environmental temperature, increased generation of body heat, and decreased bodily adaptive functions. Muscular heat cramps commonly follow exhausting exercise in hot weather. They respond quickly to fluid and salt ingestion. *Heat exhaustion* results from continued heat generation in the presence of a gradual net loss of water or salt and water. Muscle cramps progress to impairment of cardiovascular mechanisms manifested by feelings of giddiness, dizziness, and syncope. With more protracted and severe exposures, fever and delirium follow. Sweating continues until the late stages. Treatment consists of cool spongings or tubs plus generous salt and water replacement.

Heat stroke, a potentially fatal disorder, characteristically affects its victims during the summer's first severe heat wave or upon the sudden movement of vigorously active young persons from a cool to a hot climate, such as occurs with troops during warfare. As with heat exhaustion, risk factors include a lack of acclimatization,

TABLE 114-1	Principal Nonendocrine Disorders of Autonomic Regulation

Central (mainly hypothalamic)
  Emotional disorders
    Panic; panic disorder; psychosomatic illnesses; cardiac arrhythmias
  Thermoregulatory disorders
    Hyperthermia (rare)
      Acute trauma, local diencephalic region surgery, encephalitis, heat stroke, malignant hyperthermia, malignant neuroleptic syndrome
    Hypothermia-poikilothermia
      Episodic hypothermia (primary, developmental); destructive HT damage; metabolic (sedative drugs, hypoglycemia); senility or nutritional impairment plus exposure
  Water balance
    ADH dysregulation: SIADH; essential hypernatremia (i.e., disconnection between HT osmoreceptor and ADH regulation); episodic hyperdipsia with hyponatremia (some is behavioral, some centrally induced)
  Feeding behavior
    Hyperphagia-obesity (medial HT)
    Anorexia-inanition (rare, lateral HT)
  Arousal-sleep disorders
Peripheral-central autonomic insufficiencies or dysregulation
  Idiopathic autonomic insufficiency (Shy-Drager syndrome)
  Visceral organ dysregulation: cardiovascular, gastrointestinal, genitourinary
  Tetanus (autonomic components)
  Inherited dysautonomia (e.g., Riley-Day)
Peripheral autonomic disorders
  Polyneuropathy: generalized inflammatory-demyelinating, selective acute autonomic neuropathy, diabetes, syphilis (tabes), acute intermittent porphyria, amyloidosis, leprosy, geriatric
  Reflex sympathetic dystrophies

HT = Hypothalamus; ADH = antidiuretic hormone; SIADH = syndrome of inappropriate antidiuretic hormone.

old age and infirmity, alcoholic excess and, especially, the ingestion of anticholinergic or antipsychotic drugs. Heat stroke results when high ambient temperatures and humidity combine to generate heat and prevent its loss while, at the same time, age, neurologic disease, or drugs impair central autonomic mechanisms. Clinical signs include hyperpyrexia greater than 41°C; hot, dry skin; and increasing prostration, confusion, stupor and, finally, coma accompanied by signs of brain stem dysfunction. Associated abnormalities can include tachycardia, ST and T wave abnormalities on the electrocardiogram (ECG), hypotension, consumption coagulopathy, signs of dehydration, potassium and sodium depletion, and hepatic damage. Treatment is aimed at bringing core temperature below 39°C in an ice tub bath and meeting systemic problems, including high-output heart failure, as they arise. Mortality and permanent neurologic disability relate directly to the duration of hyperthermia and the prompt effectiveness of its treatment.

Malignant Hyperthermia and Neuroleptic Malignant Syndrome

Malignant hyperthermia is a rare autosomal dominant disorder that results from a point mutation in the ryanodine receptor of skeletal muscle. The error leads to excessive calcium release from muscle sarcoplasm during anesthetic induction. Immediately after a preoperative administration of succinylcholine followed by an inhalation anesthetic, diffuse, severe skeletal muscle contraction takes place, producing generalized rigidity, increased heat production, and potentially fatal fevers of 39 to 42°C or greater. Treatment consists of quick interruption of anesthesia, intravenous administration of dantrolene, and vigorous efforts to counteract fever and systemic lactacidosis. Blood relatives of those who show the disorder should be pretested for potential susceptibility before receiving general anesthesia. The *neuroleptic malignant syndrome,* a less frequent idiosyncratic response, follows a similar clinical pattern, with hyperthermia, muscle rigidity, autonomic instability, and reduced consciousness following administration of one or more of the drugs cited in Table 114–3. The pathogenesis is poorly understood. Treatment consists of neuroleptic withdrawal, cooling measures, and bromocriptine or another dopamine agonist.

Disorders of Water Balance

1. Hypoplasia or direct damage to the supraoptic or paraventricular nuclei or their major connections to the posterior pituitary gland leads to antidiuretic hormone (ADH) deficiency and the disorder *diabetes insipidus.*
2. Neurogenic imbalance or biologically erroneous signals from peripheral receptors or their central nervous system (CNS) connections can lead to *inappropriately increased ADH* secretion, producing excessive hemodilution and hyponatremia.
3. HT-engendered failure of thirst associated with reduced ADH secretion causes the rare condition of *essential hypernatremia,* in which appetite for water is lacking despite pathologically elevated serum sodium levels.

TABLE 114-2	Heat Exhaustion and Heat Stroke Compared	
	Heat Exhaustion	**Heat Stroke**
Time of occurrence	Any hot weather	First sustained heat wave
Principally affected	Elderly hypodipsics, young heavy laborers, strenuous athletes	Elderly; infirm; obese; alcoholics; psychotics
Principal pathogenesis	Salt or water loss	Failure of heat loss
Contributing factors	Prolonged exercise	Antiperspirants; anticholinergics, phenothiazines, diuretics, neuroleptics; old age; dehydration
Body temperature	37–38.5°C	39–43°C
Sweating	Usually present	Absent
Treatment	Fluids and adjusted electrolytes	Prompt body cooling (ice water immersion)

TABLE 114-3	Chief Drug Groups Associated with the Neuroleptic Malignant Syndrome

Phenothiazines
Butyrophenones
Thioxanthines
Other antipsychotic agents
Sudden discontinuation of anti-Parkinson drugs
Dopamine-depleting agents

Changes in serum sodium that exceed 30 mEq/L in either direction accompanying any of these disorders should be treated with deliberate slowness to avoid producing *acute osmotic encephalopathy.* (See also Chapter 112, page 793.) Optimal management should restrict serum sodium changes to less than 20 mEq/L per 24 hours.

CENTRAL AND PERIPHERAL AUTONOMIC INSUFFICIENCIES

Generalized systemic *autonomic insufficiency* (pandysautonomia) can occur on either a central or a peripheral basis. Diffuse, moderate sympathetic-parasympathetic dysfunction accompanies occasional cases of parkinsonism and several of the late-life cerebellar degenerations. *Multiple system disorder* is an uncommon midlife, slowly progressive, degenerative condition that affects central and, to a lesser degree, peripheral autonomic pathways, accompanied by variable abnormalities in cerebellar, extrapyramidal and, occasionally, corticospinal motor systems. Cardinal symptoms and signs include male impotence, anhidrosis, orthostatic hypotension, absent autonomic cardiovascular reflexes, impaired pupillary control, gastrointestinal hypomotility, urinary retention or incontinence, hoarseness, and signs of parkinsonism or cerebellar dysfunction. Affected patients develop refractory bradycardia, orthostatic hypotension, and symptoms of lightheadedness or syncope when assuming the erect or even the sitting position. Treatment is symptomatic and consists of counteracting the hypotension with elastic stockings, increasing fluid intake, and giving mineralocorticoids to assist in blood volume expansion.

Central-peripheral autonomic dysfunction of a more benign but protracted type is responsible for a variety of psychosomatically engendered functional abnormalities involving the heart, gastrointestinal tract, and urogenital system.

Autonomic abnormalities including severe hypotension also can accompany a number of peripheral neuropathies as noted in Table 114-1. The association is particularly frequent with diabetic neuropathy. Moderate autonomic dysfunction consisting of persistent tachycardia, impaired volume reflexes, and mild orthostatic insufficiency accompanies most examples of *acute inflammatory neuropathy* of the Guillain-Barre type. Pandysautonomia or peripheral autonomic insufficiency contributes importantly to the major symptoms of *idiopathic orthostatic hypotension.* Similarly, tachycardia, neurogenic ECG changes, fluctuating hypertension, and abnormal sweating patterns mark the course of acute tetanus, porphyria, and inherited amyloidosis.

The elderly are particularly susceptible to autonomic dysfunction as a result of gradual degeneration of central-peripheral adaptation pathways plus an increasing susceptibility to the autonomic side effects of commonly used medications. Reflex and spontaneous shivering or sweating declines and impairs adaptation to extremes of environmental temperature in the elderly. Baroceptors, vasculotonic reflex controls, gastrointestinal reflexes, and urogenital controls gradually deteriorate as well. As a result, postural hypotension, reduced exercise tolerance, abnormal bradycardia, dyspepsia and constipation, male impotence, and urinary incontinence frequently plague life's later years. A host of cardiotropic, antidepressant, and psychotropic drugs can intensify these susceptibilities. Treatment of these common geriatric problems requires both patience and resourcefulness. Anecdotal evidence suggests that continued exercise and close attention to diet and blood volume may ameliorate many of these difficulties; it may be, however, that only the still healthy are capable of such self-regulation. Otherwise one treats symptomatically, minimizing both prescription and other drug use, checking on the autonomic effects of necessary medications, and treating bowel and bladder problems with the mildest possible remedies that may help. The references that follow discuss these problems in greater detail.

REFERENCES

Loewy AD, Spyer KM: Central Regulation of Autonomic Functions. New York, Oxford Press, 1990.

McLeod JG, Tuck RR: Disorders of the autonomic nervous system. Part 1: Pathophysiology and clinical features. Ann Neurol 1987; 21:419; Part 2. Investigation and treatment. Ann Neurol 1987; 21:519.

Saper C: Autonomic disorders and their management. *In* Bennett JC, Plum F (eds.): Cecil Textbook of Medicine. 20th ed. Philadelphia, WB Saunders Co, 1996, pp 2007–2014.

115

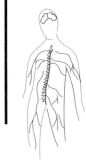

Disorders of Sensory Function

A. Pain and Painful Syndromes

PAIN AS A SIGNAL OF DAMAGE

Pain (Table 115–1) is the most common symptom for which patients seek medical assistance. Additionally, chronic pain is probably the most vexing problem that physicians face. Pain has two aspects: the first is an emotionally neutral perception of a stimulus that is usually sufficiently strong to produce tissue damage; the second is an affective response to the perception of that stimulus. Pain implies damage to the organism, either physical or psychological, and chronic pain, if untreated, itself damages the organism. Figure 115–1 schematizes the central pathways carrying different modalities of sensation, including pain.

DIAGNOSIS OF PAINFUL DISORDERS

Pain can be either acute or chronic; pain of more than 3 months' duration is usually considered chronic. Several clinical features differentiate acute from chronic pain. Patients suffering from severe acute pain usually give a clear description of its location, character, and timing.

TABLE 115–1	Aspects of Pain

Definition

An unpleasant sensory and emotional experience associated with either actual or potential tissue damage, or described in terms of such damage (International Association for Study of Pain)

Temporal Characteristics

Acute (less than 3 months)
Chronic (more than 3 months)

Physiology

Somatic
Visceral
Neuropathic

Pathogenesis

Structural
Psychophysiologic
Delusional

Signs of autonomic nervous system hyperactivity with tachycardia, hypertension, diaphoresis, mydriasis, and pallor are often present. Acute pain usually responds well to analgesic agents, and psychological factors often play only a minor role in pathogenesis. By contrast, patients suffering from chronic pain describe less precisely the localization, character, and timing of the pain, and, because the autonomic nervous system adapts, signs of autonomic hyperactivity disappear. Furthermore, chronic pain usually responds less well to analgesic agents, and psychological colorings are usually more pertinent than with acute pain. All of these factors may lead the physician to believe that the patient exaggerates his complaints. Because there are no reliable objective tests to assess chronic pain, the physician is advised to accept the patient's report, taking into consideration age, cultural background, environment, and psychological factors known to alter reaction to pain.

Chronic pain can be divided into three somewhat overlapping categories in decreasing order of frequency:

1. Chronic pain associated with *structural disease*, such as occurs with rheumatoid arthritis, metastatic cancer, or sickle cell anemia, may be characterized by episodes of pain alternating with pain-free intervals or by unremitting pain waxing and waning in severity. Psychological factors may play an important role in exacerbating or relieving pain, but treatment of the pain by analgesics or correcting the underlying disease is usually most helpful.
2. *Psychophysiologic disorders.* Structural disease, such as a herniated disc or torn ligaments, may once have been present, but whether or not structural disease was ever present, psychological factors may have altered central synaptic mechanisms so as to engender pain perceptions long after the underlying deficit has healed. Affected patients tend to respond poorly to analgesic drugs, but often respond well to combination therapy directed at the end-organ (i.e., injection of trigger points, behavioral therapy in muscles) and discussing disturbing psychological factors.
3. *Somatic delusions.* Pain caused by neither structural nor physiologic disorders occurs in patients with severe psychiatric disturbances such as psychotic depres-

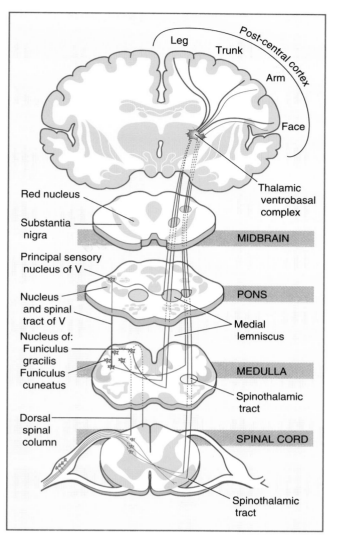

Figure 115-1

Simplified schematic anatomy of central ascending sensory pathways. Somatosensory fibers mediating predominantly touch and proprioceptive sensations either directly or, less often, after a synapse in the dorsal horn, pass rostrally up the ipsilateral dorsal spinal column to reach the gracile and cuneate relay nuclei in the medulla oblongata. At that point, the fibers decussate to form the contralateral medial lemniscus, which projects directly to the ventroposterolateral component of the thalamic ventrobasal complex (TVC). Fibers mediating pain and temperature information synapse in the substantia gelatinosa of the ipsilateral spinal dorsal horn, then traverse the cord over the immediate and next rostral segment to form the contralateral ascending spinothalamic tract, which projects predominantly to the TVC and other nuclei (not shown). Note the nucleus and spinal tract that extends along the brain stem from the trigeminal nucleus in the pons to the substantia gelatinosa of second cervical segments. Secondary fibers emanating from the nucleus carry pain afferents from the face, mouth, and pharyngolaryngeal structures. Most of these fibers decussate at the cervicomedullary level to join the opposite spinothalamic tract and accompany it to the thalamobasal complex. The practical neurologic aspect of this anatomic arrangement is that the nucleus tractus spinal V in the lower brain stem lies close to the spinothalamic tract serving the opposite side of the body. As a result, intrinsic lesions of the lower brain stem may sometimes produce a reduction or loss of ipsilateral facial pain sensation along with a total hemisensory loss of pain from face to toes on the opposite side of the body.

sion or schizophrenia. Such pains are described in sufficiently vague and bizarre terms and distributions as to indicate the diagnosis. Effective treatment depends on psychiatric treatment.

Pain associated with either structural or psychophysiologic disorders can arise from somatic, visceral, or neural structures. *Somatic pain* results from activation of peripheral receptors and somatic efferent nerves, without injury to the nerves themselves. The pain can be either sharp or dull but is typically well localized and intermittent. *Visceral pain* results from activation of visceral nociceptive receptors and visceral efferent nerves and is characterized as a deep aching, cramping sensation, often referred to cutaneous sites. *Neuropathic pain* results from injury to peripheral receptors, nerves, or the central nervous system. It is typically burning and dysesthetic and often occurs in an area of sensory loss (e.g., postherpetic neuralgia). The autonomic nervous system plays a significant modulatory role in all three types of pain, most prominently in visceral and deafferentation pain. Somatic and visceral pain are readily managed with a wide variety

of nonopioid and opioid analgesics, anesthetic blocks, and neurosurgical approaches. In contrast, neuropathic pain may respond poorly to either analgesics or anesthetic and neurosurgical procedures.

Referred pain is perceived at a site remote from the source of the noxious disturbance. It is evoked by disease of deep structures that are usually innervated by the same dermatome. Referred pain may be associated with cutaneous hyperalgesia and even relieved by procaine injection into the area of referral. When pain is referred to the same dermatome or myotome that includes the diseased structure (e.g., pain down the medial aspect of the arm [T1–T2] produced by myocardial infarction or angina pectoris, or diaphragmatic irritation causing shoulder pain [C4]), it is often helpful in diagnosis. However, pain is sometimes referred at a great distance from the primary site to segments not similarly innervated, in which case the mechanism is perplexing (e.g., anginal pain referred to the jaw, gallbladder pain felt in the chest or shoulder). Various theories have been suggested to account for referred pain. Such theories as division of the same nerve into deep (visceral) and superficial branches, release of chemical mediators in the nervous system, and convergence of cutaneous and visceral nerves into common synaptic pools at the spinal cord all might explain the dermatomal referral of pain but fail to explain pain at remote sites.

HEADACHE AND OTHER HEAD PAIN

Head pain can result from distortion, stretching, inflammation, or destruction of pain-sensitive nerve endings as a result of either intra- or extracranial disease in the distribution of any of the cranial and upper cervical nerves. Most head pain, however, arises from extracerebral structures and carries a benign prognosis. Table 115–2 classifies the common causes of headache.

Because headache is so common and so rarely due to structural disease, excessive application of expensive and highly technical laboratory procedures to its diagnosis and management substantially increases unnecessary medical costs. Nevertheless, in some instances a timely brain image by computed tomography (CT) scan or magnetic resonance imaging (MRI) or a lumbar puncture can give life-saving information about an otherwise undiagnosable problem. The following principles may help to manage the individual patient:

1. A complete history, with special attention to the location and character of the pain; associated symptoms (e.g., nausea, paresthesias); precipitating, exacerbating, and relieving factors; and previous history of headache can usually establish the diagnosis. The physical and laboratory examinations are rarely helpful unless the history suggests structural disease. (Examples include:

	Migraine	Tension
TABLE 115–3	**Differential Diagnosis of Migraine and Tension Headache**	
Intensity	Moderate to severe	Mild to moderate
Duration	4–48 hr	Minutes to weeks
Location	Unilateral (parieto-temporal)	Bilateral (variable)
Precipitating factors	Food, alcohol, menstruation, bright lights, exercise	Fatigue, anxiety
Age	Children, adolescents, and young adults	Any
Sex	Females more than males	Either
Associated symptoms	Nausea, vomiting, photophobia, phonophobia, malaise	Tight, tender muscles
Treatment	Dark room, sleep; analgesics; sumatriptan; ergot; prophylactic drugs	Analgesics and/or antidepressants
Diurnal pattern	Morning, often interrupts sleep	Anytime, usually afternoon or evening, rarely interrupts sleep

headaches of recent origin have a consistently focal distribution that follow trauma or that begin after the age of 30 years or have a first, explosive onset.) Most patients with headache, however, suffer from either vascular headache of the migraine type or tension-type headaches (Table 115–3).
2. Electroencephalographs (EEGs) and skull radiographs are not useful in the diagnosis of headache. When an imaging test is required, MRI is the preferred choice.
3. Diagnostic lumbar puncture should be performed with any acute headache that (a) is accompanied by fever or (b) is explosive or the most severe, sudden headache ever suffered (a history typical of acute subarachnoid hemorrhage). In an emergency setting, lumbar puncture should be deferred until after CT scanning with other acute headaches not suggestive of infectious meningitis.

TABLE 115–2	**Pathophysiologic Classification of Headache**

Vascular Headache

Migraine headache
  Classic migraine
  Common migraine
  Complicated migraine
  Variant migraine
Cluster headache
  Episodic cluster
  "Chronic" cluster
  Chronic paroxysmal hemicrania
Miscellaneous vascular headache
  Carotodynia
  Hypertension
  Orgasmic, exertional, and cough headache
  Hangover
  Toxins and drugs
  Occlusive vascular disease

Cranial Neuralgias

Tension-Type Headache

Common tension headache
Depressive equivalent
Conversion reaction
Temporomandibular joint dysfunction
Atypical facial pain

Traction-Inflammation Headache

Cranial arteritis
Increased or decreased intracranial pressure
Extracranial structural lesions
Pituitary tumors

Extracranial Structural Lesions

Paranasal sinusitis and tumors
Dental infections
Otitis
Ocular lesions
Pituitary tumors
Cervical osteoarthritis

From Posner JB: Headache and other head pain. *In* Bennett JC, Plum F (eds.): Cecil Textbook of Medicine. 20th ed. Philadelphia, WB Saunders Co, 1996, pp 2031–2036.

Migraine and Other Vascular Headaches

The term *vascular headache* applies to a group of clinical syndromes of unknown etiology in which the final step in pathogenesis of the pain appears to be dilation or irritation of one or more branches of the carotid artery (particularly the superficial temporal artery), leading to stimulation of nerve endings supplying that artery. The pain threshold of these nerve endings is lowered by release of neurotransmitters or other substances from nerve endings in the vessel wall.

Migraine is characterized by recurrent headaches, often severe, frequently beginning unilaterally, and usually associated with malaise, nausea and/or vomiting, and photophobia (see Table 115–3). The disorder often begins in childhood, affects women more often than men, and runs in families. The disorder may be preceded by an aura (migraine) or may not (common migraine).

In *classic migraine* (about 15 to 20% of migraine patients), brief (up to 30 minutes) neurologic dysfunction precedes or, less often, accompanies headache. The neurologic symptoms are usually visual, consisting of bright flashing lights (scintillation or fortification scotomas) beginning in the center of a homonymous visual half-field and radiating outward toward the periphery over 10 to 30 minutes. Other neurologic disturbances can include unilateral paresthesias of the hand and perioral area, aphasia, hemiparesis, and hemisensory defects. Neurologic symptoms usually disappear before the headache begins. If the neurologic symptoms are unilateral, the headache almost always affects the other side. *Migraine equivalent* (e.g., recurrent attacks of neurologic dysfunction that mimic the migraine alone but do not culminate in headache) may be confused with transient ischemic attacks or focal seizures. If the neurologic dysfunction continues into or outlasts the duration of the headache, the disorder is called *complicated migraine*. In rare instances, permanent cerebral infarction may occur.

A recent survey suggests that 11 million Americans suffer from migraine headaches with moderate to severe disability. Other vascular headache syndromes are less common, but each has distinctive clinical findings. Most acute vascular headaches last only several hours and are best treated by rest in a quiet, dark room accompanied by a mild analgesic agent such as aspirin, acetaminophen as a nonsteroidal analgesic (Table 115–4). Occasionally, and when severe nausea is present, more potent analgesics such as codeine or Demerol may be required. Such drugs should generally be avoided, however, partly because they add to nausea and because of their potential for abuse. Patients with prolonged or severe migraines may be considered for one or another of the agents listed in Table 115–4.

Cluster headaches (Table 115–5) are short-lived attacks of extremely severe, unilateral head pain that occur in clusters, often occurring several times daily and lasting several weeks, only to disappear for months or years before recurring. The diagnosis is established by the characteristic history. Because the headaches frequently recur at known times, the ingestion of ergotamine tartrate prophylactically an hour or two before the expected headache may abort the headache. Sumatriptan as well as the serotonin inhibitor methysergide also is often successful in preventing cluster headaches.

Tension-Type Headache (Table 115–6)

So-called tension-type headaches are characterized by a steady, nonpulsatile, unilateral or bilateral aching pain, usually beginning in the occipital region but often involving frontal or temporal regions as well. They are frequently accompanied by tender posterior cervical, temporalis, and masseter muscles. Unique among headaches, the pain may be constantly present for days, weeks, or months. Tension-type headaches are more frequent in

TABLE 115–4	Pharmacotherapy of Migraine Headaches	
	Drug	**Adverse Effects or Comments**
Mild cases	Metoclopramide (antinauseant); aspirin; acetaminophen; non-steroidal anti-inflammatory drugs (NSAIDs)	Few
Moderate to Severe	Ergotamine tablet; dihydroergotamine (available in US only for intramuscularly injection)	Ergotamine poisoning
Severe	Ergotamine or sumatriptan, orally or intramuscularly	Ergotamine poisoning; helps 80% of patients but 25–50% relapse and require another injection or dose within 1–24 hr; rarely induces angina or myocardial infarction in patients with cardiac history or heavy smokers
Prophylaxis	Ergotamine-caffeine tablets or suppositories; ergotamine tartrate (sublingual), dihydroergotamine; chronic beta-blockers (e.g., propranolol); amitriptylene and other tricyclics; methysergide; valproate; NSAIDS	Methysergide is valuable, but continuous use can induce retroperitoneal fibrosis. 1 month holidays every 5th month recommended

women, in individuals who are tense and anxious, and in those whose work or posture requires sustained contraction of posterior cervical, frontal, or temporal muscles. Similar headaches often reflect a serious depression or other psychologic abnormalities. Some authorities believe that the pain syndrome represents dysregulations of central sensory systems rather than originating in peripheral pain receptors. The symptoms of common migraine and

TABLE 115–5	Characteristics of Cluster Headache

1. Severe unilateral orbital, supraorbital, and/or temporal pain lasting 15–180 min, often at the same time each day
2. Headache associated with at least one of the following signs on the side of pain:
   a. Conjunctival injection
   b. Lacrimation
   c. Nasal congestion
   d. Rhinorrhea
   e. Forehead and facial sweating
   f. Miosis
   g. Ptosis
   h. Eyelid edema
3. Frequency of attacks: from 1 every other day to 8 per day
4. Occur in cluster of 3–6 wk; rarely chronic

TABLE 115–6	Classification of Tension-Type Headaches

Common tension headache
Depressive equivalent
Conversion reaction
Post-traumatic headache
Temporomandibular joint dysfunction
Atypical facial pain

tension-type headaches overlap and many patients suffer from both.

Tension headache variants include the so-called temporomandibular joint (TMJ) syndrome with unilateral or bilateral head pain, usually in the temporal region and in the jaw, often radiating into the ear. *Post-traumatic headaches* are dull, generalized, aching head pains that follow head injury. The disorder can blend into *depressive headache,* a chronic generalized headache, usually vaguely described, sometimes associated with dizziness and unsteadiness.

Atypical facial pain or atypical facial neuralgia describes a syndrome characterized by steady aching face pain, usually unilateral, localized to the lower part of the orbit, maxillary area, and sometimes the jaw. The pain begins without a known precipitating episode and may last for hours or indefinitely. It may spread to involve the head or neck, and the muscles of the jaw and neck often become tender. The disorder almost exclusively affects tense, anxious, and often chronically depressed women, often in early middle age. Early accurate diagnosis can minimize expensive laboratory tests and avoid addicting drugs or mutilating surgical or dental procedures.

Headache from Intracranial Disorders

Most of the intracranial disorders that cause headache (Table 115–7) are discussed under their respective headings.

In *acute and subacute meningitis* the headache is usually generalized, throbbing, and severe. It may be rapid or gradual in onset, and by the time it is fully developed is associated with nuchal rigidity. The diagnosis is established by lumbar puncture. In *subarachnoid hemorrhage,* the initial sudden headache is caused by an abrupt alteration of intracranial pressure. This immediate pain is succeeded by a chronic persistent headache, often accompanied by increasing nuchal rigidity that results from a chemical meningitis caused by the blood.

Intracranial hypotension, usually from loss of spinal fluid from lumbar puncture or a dural tear, decreases the buoyancy of the brain so that the organ descends when the upright position is assumed, exerting traction on structures at its apex and compression on structures at its base. Occasionally, the small bridging veins that enter the sagittal sinus may rupture and cause subdural hematomas. *Intracranial hypertension* causes headaches when vascular and neural structures over the apex or at the base of the brain are unevenly stretched or inflamed by tumor or

TABLE 115–7	Headache from Intracranial Disorders

Increased Intracranial Pressure
Benign intracranial hypertension
High-pressure hydrocephalus

Increased Venous Pressure
Septic or aseptic intracranial thrombophlebitis
Extracranial venous occlusion

Decreased Intracranial Pressure
Cerebrospinal fluid leakage
Post-lumbar puncture headache

Infection
Meningitis
Encephalitis
Subdural abscess
Empyema

Vascular Disorders
Subarachnoid hemorrhage
Intracranial hematoma

Tumors
Brain
Pituitary

edematous brain. The most common cause is brain tumor. Another cause of increased intracranial pressure headache is *pseudotumor cerebri* (benign intracranial hypertension).

Pituitary tumors can produce headache by stretching and distorting pain-sensitive structures at the base of the skull, particularly the diaphragma sellae. Pain is generally referred to the frontal or temporal regions bilaterally and may on occasion be referred to the vertex or occipital regions. Acute headache occurring with *pituitary apoplexy* usually results from infarction of or hemorrhage into the tumor. Sudden expansion may compromise the overlying optic chiasm, leading to visual loss, or invade the laterally lying cavernous sinus, producing ocular palsies. Pituitary apoplexy often is best treated surgically by emergency drainage of the hemorrhagic or infarcted material.

Extracranial Structural Headache (Table 115–8)

Nasal and Sinus Headache

Most so-called sinus headache is in reality migraine or tension-type headache. True sinus headache results from acute inflammation of the paranasal sinuses, which produces pain localized over the involved sinus and is asso-

TABLE 115–8	Headache from Intracranial Disorders

Paranasal sinusitis and tumors
Dental infections
Otitis
Ocular lesions
Cervical osteoarthritis
Cranial arteritis

ciated with the stigmata of acute infection. Sinus radiographs and a physical examination are diagnostic.

Dental Pain

Severe dental pain can be extremely difficult to localize because pain may spread to other teeth or distant tissues that may exhibit surface hyperalgesia, tenderness, and vasomotor reactions. Patiently tapping each tooth for tenderness, using a blunt object or rod, often gives a localizing clue. Dental radiographs usually are diagnostic.

Aural Pain

Pain in the vicinity of the ear can be caused by disease of the teeth, tonsils, larynx and nasopharynx, TMJ, or cervical spine and its soft tissues. Pain in the ear can be associated with vascular headaches, atypical facial pain, and herpes zoster of the fifth and seventh cranial nerves as well as, rarely, the glossopharyngeal nerve. Primary ear disease is relatively infrequent—but important—as a source of headache, because it almost always indicates inflammatory or destructive disease.

Eye Pain and Headache

Errors of refraction (hypermetropia, astigmatism, anomalies of accommodation), ocular muscle imbalance (strabismus), glaucoma, and iritis are universally described as causing headache. For most, the headache is mild in degree and usually starts around and over the eyes and subsequently radiates to the occiput and back of the head. The pain of glaucoma or iritis begins in the eye, can become severe, and then later extends to include a periorbital distribution.

Temporal Arteritis

Sometimes known as giant cell arteritis, this disorder of late life affects predominantly white women. The most prominent symptom usually consists of a new, severe, sustained, steady or throbbing headache most often located in the temporal region of the scalp and accompanied by a tender, nodular, or incompressible artery in the area. Head pain also may affect the masseter or sternocleidomastoid muscles, occasionally as the chief symptom. Associated symptoms may include malaise, fatigue, weight loss, low-grade fever, and proximal myalgia affecting the pectoral or pelvic girdle areas (*polymyalgia rheumatica*). The erythrocyte sedimentation rate (ESR) usually rises to 60 mm/hr or more. Pathological examination of the offending temporal artery usually shows an inflammatory response, often with partial or complete occlusion of the lumen. Autoimmune processes presumably provide the cause.

Temporal arteritis represents a medical emergency, since delaying proper treatment increases the risk of retinal artery occlusion, thereby producing partial or complete functional loss of vision in the affected eye. High-dose corticosteroid treatment should be started immediately in the presence of a probable clinical diagnosis. Firm diagnosis can be established by temporal artery biopsy performed immediately before or after starting therapy. A remarkable resolution of symptoms within 12 to 18 hours following steroid therapy is almost as reliable. Long-term management is directed at maintaining a normal ESR and gradually reducing or ceasing steroids as soon as possible. Bimonthly follow-ups of symptoms and ESR are desirable to detect relapses.

Cranial Neuralgias

Several distinctive, extremely severe, paroxysmal head pains can result from sudden episodic, intrinsic, and excessive discharges from a cranial nerve. The most common are trigeminal or glossopharyngeal neuralgia.

Trigeminal Neuralgia

Trigeminal neuralgia is characterized by sudden, lightning-like paroxysms of pain in the distribution of one or more divisions of the trigeminal nerve. Age groups are important: onset after 50 years usually reflects a vascular compression by a tortuous artery at the base of the brain. Onset in younger persons more often results from a gasserian ganglion tumor or multiple sclerosis. Some can follow a brain stem stroke.

The history is diagnostic. The pain occurs as brief, lightning-like stabs frequently precipitated by touching a trigger zone around the lips or the buccal cavity. At times, talking, eating, or brushing the teeth serves as a trigger. The pains rarely last longer than seconds, and each burst is followed by a refractory period of several seconds to a minute during which no pain can be precipitated. The pain is limited to the distribution of the trigeminal nerve, usually involving the second or third division or both. Spontaneous remissions are common. Between paroxysms of pain, the patient is asymptomatic. The pain rarely occurs at night. Ordinarily, the neurologic examination is entirely normal. Sensory changes in the distribution of the trigeminal nerve should prompt a careful search for structural disease such as tumor.

Carbamazepine is the initial treatment of choice for trigeminal neuralgia; phenytoin and baclofen are occasionally effective. The drugs are not analgesics and are effective only for specific kinds of pain such as trigeminal neuralgia, glossopharyngeal neuralgia, and the lightning pains of tabes dorsalis. If medical treatment fails, either radiofrequency lesions of the gasserian ganglion (to block sensory conduction) or surgical relief of vascular pressure on the nerve is indicated.

Glossopharyngeal Neuralgia

Glossopharyngeal neuralgia is characterized by pain similar to that of trigeminal neuralgia but originating in the posterolateral pharynx and ipsilateral ear in the distribu-

TABLE 115–9	Miscellaneous Causes of Headache

Headache Associated with Substances or Their Withdrawal

Ergotamine abuse and withdrawal
Analgesic abuse and withdrawal
Alcohol abuse and withdrawal (hangover)
Caffeine withdrawal
Nitrates/nitrites (hot dog headache)
Monosodium glutamate (Chinese restaurant syndrome)
Carbon monoxide

Headache Associated with Systemic Infection or Fever

Headache Associated with Metabolic Abnormality

Hypoxia and ischemia
Dialysis

TABLE 115–10	Pain-Sensitive Structures in and Around the Spine

Sensitive	Insensitive
Ligaments	Ligaments
Anterior and posterior longitudinal ligaments	Intraspinous and ligamentum flavum
Facets	Vertebral body
Articular cartilage	Intervertebral disc
Capsule	
Nerve roots	
Paraspinal muscles	

tion of the glossopharyngeal and vagus nerves. Occasionally patients suffer cardiac slowing or brief arrest (syncope) during attacks of pain as a result of the intense afferent discharge over the glossopharyngeal nerve. Carbamazepine is often effective, but, if drugs fail, glossopharyngeal nerve roots can be sectioned in the posterior fossa. Symptomatic glossopharyngeal neuralgia is occasionally the presenting complaint in a patient with a tonsillar tumor. Careful examination of the pharynx and tonsillar fossa for mass lesions must be carried out.

Table 115–9 lists less frequent causes of headache.

NECK AND BACK PAIN

About 80% of individuals suffer significant low back pain at least once, and the annual incidence is 5%. Next to alcoholism, back pain is the leading cause of time lost from work. Most neck and back pain, although incapacitating, is transient and neither life-threatening nor associated with obvious pathologic abnormalities. By and large, symptoms outweigh findings on physical examination or imaging studies. Furthermore, a pathophysiologic diagnosis is elusive, making rational therapy impossible beyond giving simple analgesics. Fortunately for all concerned, most patients suffering from back pain recover within a few weeks regardless of treatment. Only 4% are disabled longer than 6 months.

Pain in the neck or back may arise from one or more of several pain-sensitive structures (Table 115–10). Table 115–11 lists common causes of neck or back pain. Most acute neck or back pain (the classic "crick") is probably caused by muscle strain and spasm due to unaccustomed exercise, stretching or perhaps viral infection. Such pains are transient and not life-threatening (see also myofascial pain, below). The pain usually disappears within days or a few weeks no matter what the treatment. Most chronic neck or back pain is either myofascial in origin or associated with vertebral arthritis or intervertebral disc disease, the former causing pain by compression of small nerve twigs supplying the facet joints and the periosteum of the vertebral bodies, the latter causing pain by compression of the nerve root. More rarely, tumors and inflammatory or degenerative arthritic lesions of the spine may be responsible. Specific findings resulting from

intervertebral disc disease are discussed in Chapter 122. Spinal cord tumors or congenital abnormalities are described in Chapter 116.

Evaluation of neck or back pain begins with a history. Most benign pain is of acute or subacute onset and frequently follows some unaccustomed physical activity by minutes to hours, particularly lifting or bending. With other forms, patients awaken in the morning feeling stiff and sore after unusual exercise. Sometimes low back pain begins acutely, frequently on arising in the morning, without any obvious precipitating event. Most neck pain begins as a stiff neck, often on awakening, without a previous history of unusual activity. Similar short-term pain experiences may occur episodically over many years. Most benign neck or back pain is dull or aching in quality, exacerbated by movement, and relieved by rest. Affected patients are comfortable when recumbent and immobile or at least are able to find one position that relieves the pain. Pain that is present when the patient is immobile and that cannot be relieved by postural manipulation should lead to a search for a serious disorder.

TABLE 115–11	Common Causes of Neck and/or Back Pain

Trauma

Muscle strain or spasm
Subluxed facet joints
Compression fractures (osteoporosis)

Psychophysiologic

Muscle tension and spasm
Fibromyalgia

Degenerative Disorders

Herniated disc
Spondylosis
Spinal stenosis
Osteoarthritis

Neoplasm

Extradural (usually malignant)
Intradural extramedullary (usually benign)
Intramedullary (either benign or malignant)

Inflammation

Arthritis
Osteomyelitis of vertebral body
Disc infection

Likewise, pain that radiates in a clear dermatomal distribution is probably a result of nerve root compression, especially if there are paresthesias or loss of sensation. By contrast, radiating pain in a nondermatomal distribution often accompanies neck and back muscle spasms; it usually does not portend serious neurogenic disease.

The physical and neurologic examinations may reveal a cause for the pain. Systemic disease such as cancer, urinary tract infection, pelvic disease, or abdominal aneurysm may cause back pain because a lesion impinges on the vertebral body or paravertebral structures. Evidence for neurologic disease such as weakness, sensory loss, or reflex abnormalities suggests spinal cord or nerve root dysfunction. Evaluation of such dysfunction is discussed in Chapters 116 and 122.

In the absence of a clear abnormality on physical examination, conservative treatment of back pain with immobility, heat, analgesics, and sometimes physical therapy ameliorates symptoms in a short period of time without the necessity of substantial laboratory evaluation. Even in the absence of neurologic signs, however, if pain persists after conservative treatment, radiographic and laboratory evaluation become mandatory.

MYOFASCIAL PAIN

A major part of head, back, and neck pain arises from skeletal muscle, particularly from the paravertebral muscles. Unaccustomed exercise causes soreness and tenderness in the involved muscles but is rarely a source of patient complaint. Prolonged tonic contraction of skeletal muscles, however, has a pathogenesis that originates in psychological tension, resentment, and anxiety and may produce pain, the cause of which is not immediately apparent to the patient. Examples are chest pain from contraction of the pectoralis majors, posterior thoracic or lumbar pain from paraspinous muscle contraction, and abdominal pain from rectus muscle contraction. The pain is initially localized over the area of muscle contraction but may spread widely in a distribution characteristic for the muscles involved. The affected muscles are usually tender to palpation, and one often finds a particularly tender area somewhere in the muscle, called a *trigger zone,* which, when palpated, reproduces the distribution of the spontaneous pain. One common variant of myofascial pain is the *fibrositis/fibromyalgia syndrome,* a disorder of middle-aged women characterized by generalized musculoskeletal pain, morning stiffness, disturbed sleep and fatigue (nonrestorative sleep), and at times vague complaints of digital swelling or paresthesias. Symptoms often overlap those of somatoform disorders and chronic fatigue syndrome. Headache and "irritable bowel" symptoms are common, and most patients are concurrently anxious or depressed. Tender points can be found on examination in most or all of the 14 sites illustrated in Figure 115–2. It is likely that other myofascial and referred pain syndromes are fragments of the fibromyalgia syndrome.

The pathophysiology of myofascial pain is poorly understood, and the treatment is often frustratingly difficult. In some patients mild analgesic drugs (aspirin), heat,

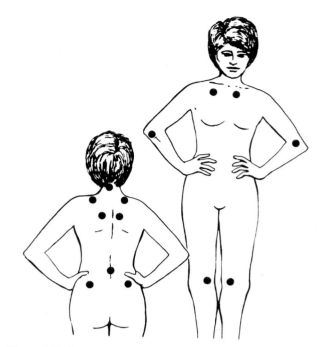

Figure 115–2

Tender point map: 14 sites of local tenderness. The unilateral sites are at the intertransverse and/or interspinous ligaments of C4 to C6 and the interspinous ligament at L4 to L5 and the bilateral sites at the upper borders of the trapezius, the supraspinatus origins at the medial border of the scapula, the upper outer quadrants of the buttocks, the second costochondral junctions, the lateral epicondyles, and the medial fat pads of the knees. (From Wolfe F: The clinical syndrome of fibrositis. *In* The fibrositis-fibromyalgia syndrome. Am J Med 1986; 81[Suppl 3A]; with permission.)

and massage yield temporary or long-term relief. In other patients, massage or even injection of trigger points with local anesthetics gives relief. Biofeedback with the patient trying consciously to relax contracted muscles recorded by surface electromyography (EMG) has been reported to be useful. Antidepressants are modestly effective and produce at least a short-term remission in about 20% of patients. For most patients, a combination of the above physical methods with investigation and treatment of the underlying psychological disorder is necessary if long-term relief is to be achieved.

CAUSALGIA AND REFLEX SYMPATHETIC DYSTROPHY

The terms apply to severe pain, usually burning in quality and associated with autonomic changes including swelling, vasomotor instability, and abnormalities of sweating. If the injury has involved a peripheral nerve, particularly the sciatic or median nerve, the syndrome is called *causalgia.* If there has been no trauma, or if the syndrome follows a visceral illness (e.g., myocardial infarction), the term applied is *reflex sympathetic dystrophy.* The exact pathophysiology of the disorder is unknown, but abnormal activity of the sympathetic nervous system contributes importantly to both the pain and the autonomic symptoms.

Severe burning pain, is usually the first symptom after the injury. The pain is continuous, worsened by emotional stress, and sometimes so severe that moving or touching the limb is intolerable. At first the pain is localized to the site of injury or the distribution of the nerve injured, but it often spreads to involve the entire extremity. Vasomotor changes develop early, first with vasodilation (warm and dry skin) and later vasoconstriction (edema, cyanosis, and cool skin). Other abnormalities include hyper- or hypohidrosis, atrophy of the skin and subcutaneous tissues, and osteoporosis. The entire symptom complex is rarely present in any one patient, and one sign or symptom usually predominates. Untreated, the disorder eventually can lead to muscle atrophy, fixation of joints, and a useless extremity. The mechanism is poorly understood.

Treatment is sometimes effective, particularly if begun early. Repeated local anesthetic infiltration of the painful site with lidocaine sometimes leads to relief. If local measures fail, most patients are relieved by sympathetic ganglion block, which, if repeated, may give permanent relief. A short course of corticosteroids has been reported to be effective.

Phantom limb sensations or pain describe sensory illusions of the continued existence of a proximally or distally amputated portion of an extremity. The illusions can consist of explicitly sensing that the lost part presently occupies a particular position in space or, worse, can simulate distressing causalgia-like paresthesias or pains emanating from the now-absent member.

The mechanisms generating these bizarre phenomena remain unexplained although some findings suggest that they may reflect plastic changes in nerve connections in the sensory thalamus.

REFERENCES

Campbell JK, Caselli RJ: Headache and other craniofacial pain. *In* Bradley WG, Darott RB, Fenichel GM, Marsden CD: Neurology in Clinical Practice: 2nd ed. Boston, Butterworth-Heinemann, 1996, pp 1683–1720.

Dotson RM: Causalgia-reflex sympathetic dystrophy-sympathetically maintained pain. Myth and reality. Muscle Nerve 1993; 16:1049–1055.

Olesen J, Tfeit-Hansen P, Welch KMA: The Headaches. New York, Raven, 1993.

Wall PD, Melzack R (eds.): Textbook of Pain. London, Churchill Livingstone, 1994.

Weinstein JN (ed.): Clinical Efficacy in The Diagnosis and Treatment of Low Back Pain. New York, Raven, 1992.

B. The Special Senses

The special senses, by definition, process the exteroceptive systems of the brain including smell, taste, vision, audition, and the experience of equilibrium as it relates to gravity and position in real or perceived space. With the

possible exception of smell, impairments of these systems become immediately apparent to patients and often provide a primary complaint. Nevertheless, even in asymptomatic persons a brief screening examination sometimes may reveal an important deficiency of which the patient remains unaware.

ABNORMALITIES OF SMELL AND TASTE

Smell

Table 115–12 lists common causes of anosmia. Most acquired disturbances of smell result from transient or sustained diseases of the nasal mucous membranes that obstruct access to or dry out or deaden the receptor areas. Such disorders seldom are complete and they commonly respond to local treatment. No satisfactory treatment has been found for neurogenic anosmias. Affected patients must be warned explicitly to avoid gas heating and to install smoke alarms to compensate for the life-threatening hazards of the defect. *Dysosmia* is a distortion of olfactory perception (normal odors perceived as a foul smell) that may occur without prior anosmia or during the recovery phase from anosmia. The cause most often lies in paranasal infections or, sometimes, in psychiatric illness. Hallucinations of smell, usually of a foul quality, occur with epileptogenic lesions affecting the region of the amygdala and are termed uncinate fits.

Taste

Much of what is perceived as taste derives indirectly from olfaction, which should be checked in any patient complaining of taste loss. Disorders that directly cause taste abnormalities are listed in Table 115–12. Epileptic discharges occasionally cause gustatory hallucinations.

TABLE 115–12	Common Causes of Sustained Loss of Taste and Smell	
	Taste	**Smell**
Local	Radiation therapy	Allergic rhinitis, sinusitis, nasal polyposis, bronchial asthma
Systemic	Cancer, renal failure, hepatic failure, nutritional deficiency (B_{12}, zinc), Cushing's syndrome, hypothyroidism, diabetes mellitus, infection (influenza), drugs (antirheumatic and antiproliferative)	Renal failure, hepatic failure, nutritional deficiency (B_{12}), Cushing's syndrome, hypothyroidism, diabetes mellitus, infection (viral hepatitis, influenza), drugs (nasal sprays, antibiotics)
Neurologic	Bell's palsy, familial dysautonomia, multiple sclerosis	Head trauma, multiple sclerosis, Parkinson's disease, frontal brain tumor

From Baloh RW: Smell and taste. *In* Bennett JC, Plum F (eds.): Cecil Textbook of Medicine. 20th ed. Philadelphia, WB Saunders, 1996, p 2014.

Psychologically depressed or paranoid patients often complain of a foul taste, but taste perception is usually normal.

DISORDERS OF VISION AND OCULAR MOVEMENT

Vision

Introduction and Definitions

A knowledge of the anatomy of visual pathways is important in clinical diagnosis, because lesions damaging or interrupting the visual sensory system can usually be discretely localized by history and visual field examination (Fig. 115–3). As Figure 115–3 indicates, partial or complete visual loss in one eye, sparing the other, implies damage to the retina or optic nerve anterior to the chiasm, whereas a visual field abnormality affecting both eyes originates at or posterior to the chiasm; the more congruent the visual fields, the more posterior lies the lesion. *Scotomas* are areas of relative or complete visual loss (see Fig. 115–3, point 8). *Central scotomas* severely decrease vision because the macular fibers are damaged, whereas scotomas away from the macula may hardly be noticed by the patient. Visual field abnormalities impairing half or nearly half of the field are termed hemianoptic. A *homonymous hemianopia* implies a postchiasmal lesion; a *bitemporal hemianopia* a chiasmal lesion; and an *altitudinal hemianopia*, whether unilateral or bilateral, vascular damage to retinal structures. Smaller defects involving only a quarter of the visual field are called *quadrantanopia*. Homonymous *superior quadrantanopia* implies temporal lobe damage, whereas homonymous *inferior quadrantanopia* implies parietal lobe damage. *Scintillating scotomas* refer to hallucinations of flashing lights. When bilateral, such abnormalities imply an abnormal discharge of the postgeniculate visual system. The disorder is common in migraine and also in seizures originating from the occipital lobe.

Diseases Causing Visual Impairment

Test visual acuity in each eye with the patient wearing glasses or, if untreated myopia is suspected, by the addition of a pinhole held against the lens. Corrected vision in either eye of less than 20/40 suggests an associated cataract, retinal, or neurologic disorder, and further workup is indicated. Most patients are immediately aware of unilateral central visual loss but some patients may fail to notice such amaurosis, particularly in the nondominant eye, until they inadvertently close the other one. Color sensation in each eye should be tested. Acquired diminution of color vision strongly suggests a lesion of the optic nerve; even when visual acuity is normal the patient may note that colors appear "washed out" in the involved eye. *Visual fields* in all four visual quadrants should be tested, comparing the patient's field with the examiner's. Many patients, particularly with cerebral lesions, may be un-

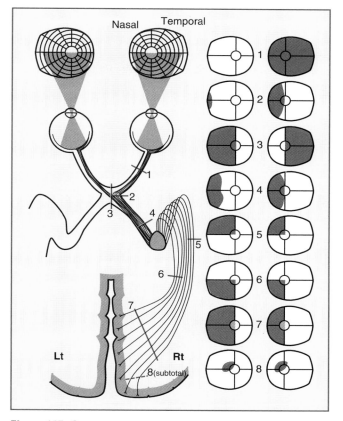

Figure 115–3

Visual fields that accompany damage to the visual pathways: 1, Optic nerve: unilateral amaurosis. 2, Lateral optic chiasm: grossly incongruous, incomplete (contralateral) homonymous hemianopia. 3, Central optic chiasm: bitemporal hemianopia. 4, Optic tract: incongruous, incomplete homonymous hemianopia. 5, Temporal (Meyer's) loop of optic radiation: congruous partial or complete (contralateral) homonymous superior quadrantanopia. 6, Parietal (superior) projection of the optic radiation: congruous partial or complete homonymous inferior quadrantanopia. 7, Complete parieto-occipital interruption of optic radiation. Complete congruous homonymous hemianopia with psychophysical shift of foveal point often sparing central vision, giving "macular sparing." 8, Incomplete damage to visual cortex: congruous homonymous scotomas, usually encroaching at least acutely on central vision. (From Baloh RW: Neuro-ophthalmology. *In* Bennett JC, Plum F [eds.]: Cecil Textbook of Medicine. 20th ed. Philadelphia, WB Saunders, 1996, p 2015.)

aware of a visual field defect although the astute patient may report that he or she bumps into things or recently has had an automobile accident on the "blind side." The field should be tested with first unilaterally and then bilaterally presented objects. In particular, bitemporal defects should be sought, as they may be the only sign of an asymptomatic pituitary tumor. Normal visual fields with unilateral testing but an abnormal field (in particular a left-field defect) when the two fields are tested bilaterally (extinction) suggests a cerebral defect. Suspicious findings on bedside confrontation or a positive history warrants formal perimetry by a specialist.

Corneal, lenticular, or vitreous diseases that are severe enough to produce visual symptoms can usually be detected by funduscopic inspection. *Glaucoma* with high intraocular pressure causes either slow or rapid visual loss associated with ring or annular scotomas and a deeply cupped optic disc. Visual loss may be preceded by halos seen around illuminated lights and pain in the affected eye. Diagnosis must be confirmed by tonometry. *Retinal detachment* gives rise to unilateral distortions of visual images that may be mistaken for monocular scintillating scotomas. Detachment can usually be identified by irregularities seen in the retina on funduscopic examination.

UNILATERAL VISUAL LOSS. Serious visual loss from optic nerve lesions can affect either one or both eyes asymmetrically, leading to nonhomonymous visual defects; the pupillary light reflex is diminished to the same degree as is vision. Most acute or subacute optic nerve disease is due to demyelinating disease (optic neuritis), vascular disorders (retinal or optic nerve ischemia from arterial embolism or occlusion), or neoplastic lesions. The history is important; if the visual loss is abrupt, whether transient or permanent, the cause is usually vascular. A slower onset over hours or days suggests demyelination; progressive visual loss over weeks or months implies a compressive lesion (e.g., tumor). If the disorder is at the nerve head, it produces papilledema, but if more posteriorly the same disease process can cause a central scotoma or even blindness with no immediately visible change in the optic nerve. *Demyelinating optic neuritis* is usually initially unilateral. It may be a symptom of multiple sclerosis, but many patients with optic neuritis recover and some avoid later neurologic dysfunction. Demyelinating optic neuritis has a particular predilection for the myelinated fibers that supply the macula, thus leading to central scotomas. Peripheral vision may remain intact. *Ischemic optic neuropathy* may be a symptom of temporal arteritis or more often occurs in late middle-aged patients as a result of arterial embolism. In patients with ischemic optic neuropathy, the second eye also tends to become involved, but no treatment can prevent it. *Tumors* can usually be identified by either funduscopic examination, brain imaging, or both. Acute and *transient monocular blindness* are usually a result of embolization of the central retinal artery or one of its branches. The emboli may originate from an athero-sclerotic plaque in the carotid or ophthalmic artery or from thrombotic material in the left heart or on cardiac valves such as may complicate rheumatic heart disease and mitral valve prolapse.

BILATERAL VISUAL LOSS. Gradually developing bilateral retinal or optic nerve disease occurs with heredodegenerative conditions, vascular diseases such as diabetes, or idiopathic (senile) macular degeneration. Leber's optic atrophy affects predominantly young men in early adulthood, creating bilateral functional blindness within a matter of months to a few years. Transmission is sex-linked autosomal and due to abnormal maternal mitochondrial gene activity. These conditions can be diagnosed by funduscopic or slit lamp examination. Acute *transient bilateral blindness* (bilateral visual obscuration) is usually a symptom of increased intracranial pressure; it is almost always associated with severe papilledema and can occur with either brain tumors or pseudotumor cerebri.

Acute or subacute bilateral optic neuritis may reflect a demyelinating process, but most examples are due to toxic-nutritional problems or inherited optic atrophy rather than multiple sclerosis. Most chiasmal lesions in the adult result from tumors compressing that structure; the most common are pituitary adenomas, but also include craniopharyngiomas, meningiomas, and large aneurysms of the carotid artery. In small children, optic gliomas are a major cause of chiasmal visual loss. Lesions of the optic tract producing incongruous homonymous field defects are usually caused by infarcts or, less commonly, tumors. Disorders posterior to the optic tract produce congruent field defects that usually involve macular fibers. When the lesion is occipital, sparing the occipital pole (which often has a bilateral supply from both the middle and the posterior cerebral artery), macular fibers may be spared. The phenomenon can be identified by careful visual field testing. Most postchiasmal visual loss is caused by cerebral vascular disease or tumor.

Bilateral damage to the visual radiation or occipital cortex produces *cortical blindness*. Such blindness is characterized by a normal funduscopic examination, normal pupillary light reflexes, and often unawareness of the blindness on the part of the patient. Most transient cortical blindness is a symptom of basilar artery insufficiency, hypertensive encephalopathy, or more rarely of migraine. The condition may also occur transiently following a generalized seizure. Why the cerebral cortex is so vulnerable to these diffuse cerebral disorders is not clear. Cortical blindness, because of the preservation of pupillary reflexes, may at first be confused with a conversion reaction (hysteria). An examination of visual evoked responses will establish the diagnosis.

Any complaint of visual loss, particularly unilateral and transient, is an emergency. Lesions that involve one eye often can soon involve the second, and transient or incomplete lesions can become permanent or complete. Many disorders of the visual system are caused by vascular disease, inflammation, or tumors and are potentially treatable. Accordingly, a rapid and meticulous examination is necessary: first to localize the site of the lesion by funduscopic and visual field examination and then to identify its pathogenesis (usually by a CT or MRI scan). These steps may lead to treatment that preserves vision. Examples of sight-saving procedures include reduction of pressure in acute glaucoma, the early use of corticosteroids for the treatment of cranial arteritis, anticoagulation for crescendo carotid or basilar insufficiency, and prompt surgical decompression for the appropriate treatment of tumors.

Pupils

Inspect the *pupils* in both dim and bright light (significant anisocoria may be present in only one). Pupillary inequalities of 1 mm or less are rarely important (15% of normal individuals have some anisocoria). Note the size of the palpebral fissure. Ptosis with a small pupil suggests a

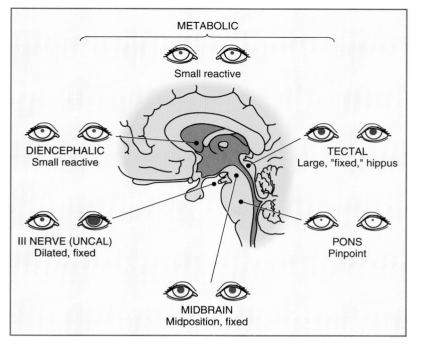

Figure 115-4
Pupillary responses in comatose patients. The schematic shows abnormalities resulting from damage to various points along the central pupillary pathways. In patients with metabolic encephalopathy, pupils are small and reactive, as are pupils resulting from diencephalic damage, such as occurs with early herniation. Lesions of the upper brain stem usually produce unilaterally or bilaterally large or midposition fixed pupils, whereas pontine lesions result in pinpoint pupils. (From Plum F, Posner JB: Diagnosis of Stupor and Coma. 3rd ed. Philadelphia, FA Davis, 1980; with permission.)

Horner's syndrome; ptosis with a large pupil, a partial third nerve palsy. Pupillary reactions should be tested using a bright light in a relatively dim room. The reaction should be brisk and symmetric. The bright light is moved quickly from one eye to the other. If there is dilation of one pupil as the light is moved to it from the other side, one should suspect an abnormality of the optic nerve in that eye. The accommodative pupillary response can be tested by asking the patient first to look into the distance and then at the examiner's finger held a foot from his nose. The pupils should constrict symmetrically and rapidly. A balance between sympathetic and parasympathetic (oculomotor nerve) fibers (Fig. 115-4) determines the size of the pupil. The pupillary light reaction is determined on the afferent side by visual sensory fibers originating in the retina and traveling through the optic nerve, chiasm, and tract to the midbrain and on the efferent side by parasympathetic fibers that arise in the oculomotor nucleus of the midbrain (Table 115-13).

When *sympathetic fibers* are damaged, the pupil narrows (the light reaction is still normal) and the palpebral fissure becomes smaller as the upper lid descends and the lower lid elevates (Horner's syndrome). The eye, however, does not close as it does with oculomotor nerve lesions. Sweat fibers may be involved as well, leading to anhidrosis on the entire half of the body if the damage is central, on the ipsilateral face and neck if the damage is between the spinal cord and the superior cervical ganglion, or on the medial side of the forehead only if the damage is above the superior cervical ganglion.

Horner's syndrome may be caused by vascular damage to the hypothalamus or brain stem, but lesions in those loci produce other neurologic signs that locate the disorder. An isolated Horner's syndrome may be the first sign of a lung cancer of the superior sulcus or may occur with tumors or other diseases involving the carotid artery. In some instances the cause of the disorder is not found. Horner's syndrome is valuable as a localizing diagnostic sign but in and of itself does not require treatment in that it impairs neither vision nor ocular motor function.

Parasympathetic disorders occur unilaterally with any lesion of the oculomotor nerve, particularly those that compress the nerve, such as tumors or aneurysms. Cerebral herniation leads to pupillary dilation if it directly compresses the third nerve or to bilaterally midpositioned and fixed pupils if it affects the midbrain.

The pupils are not always equal in size. Essential

TABLE 115-13 Frequent Causes of Pupillary Abnormalities

Small pupils	Large Pupils	Reaction to Light
Sympathetic paralysis	Parasympathetic paralysis	Reduced or absent
Argyll Robertson pupil	Holmes-Adie pupil	Nonreactive
Pontine hemorrhage	Post-traumatic iridoplegia	
Opiates	Mydriatic drops	
Pilocarpine drops	Glutethimide overdose	
	Cerebral death	
	Atropine or scopolamine poisoning	
	Amphetamine or cocaine poisoning	
Old age	Childhood	Reactive
Horner's syndrome	Anxiety	
	Physiologic anisocoria	

Modified from Patten J: Neurological Differential Diagnosis. 2nd ed. London, New York, Springer, 1995.

anisocoria (lifelong difference in the sizes of the pupils with a normal light reaction) occurs in about 15% of normal people. Tonic (Adie's) pupil is a somewhat larger than normal pupil that constricts little or not at all to light and shrinks slowly on accommodation. It constricts more than normal when dilute pilocarpine is instilled, suggesting that the pupil is parasympathetically denervated (denervation hypersensitivity). The disorder may be unilateral or bilateral and when symptomatic is characterized by a long delay in focusing when the patient attempts to move from far to near vision. There may be pain or a dazzling sensation when affected patients exit from a dark to a light room. In some persons the disorder is associated with absent deep tendon reflexes *(Adie's syndrome),* but neither the pupillary nor the reflex disorder causes serious disability.

Argyll Robertson pupils are small (1 to 2 mm), unequal, irregular, and fixed to light. They constrict briskly on accommodation. Their principal causes are neurosyphilis and diabetic and certain other autonomic neuropathies. Unexplained unilaterally or bilaterally dilated pupils with visual blurring can result from accidental or intentional instillation of mydriatics such as scopolamine or atropine. Such an abnormality is typified by failure of the pupil to constrict promptly with 1% pilocarpine.

Damage to visual fibers (the afferent arc of the pupillary light reflex) leads to the "paradoxical pupillary response," in which the direct reaction to light is impaired (because the afferent information is not carried to the oculomotor nerve), but the consensual reaction to light directed in the other eye is normal because the efferent information reaches both oculomotor nerves. The response is best seen when a bright light is rapidly moved from a normal to a visually impaired eye; the consensually constricted pupil in the impaired eye then dilates.

Ocular Movement

Examination and Definitions

Examine *eye movements* first by asking a patient to voluntarily move his or her eyes laterally and up and down and then to track a flashlight in the same directions. Failure of voluntary movement with normal following movements suggests a supranuclear brain disorder (e.g., a progressive supranuclear palsy). Failure of conjugate movement, either voluntarily or on tracking, also suggests a supranuclear disorder. Disconjugate movements suggest a brain stem or peripheral disorder. Inquire about double vision and look for nystagmus on forward, lateral, and upward gaze. Unsustained nystagmus on extremes of gaze is usually physiologic. Sustained nystagmus unassociated with vertigo is probably due to a central lesion.

Patients with ocular paralyses complain either of blurred vision ("like a ghost on a television set") or frank diplopia. Horizontal diplopia implies either lateral rectus (abducens nerve) or medial rectus (oculomotor nerve) dysfunction. Vertical or oblique diplopia must involve other muscles. The patient should be closely questioned about the onset of the diplopia (progressive worsening after onset suggests compressive lesions; sudden onset,

vascular lesions). Inquire about diurnal pattern (most diplopia worsens with fatigue but diplopia absent in the morning and present later in the day suggests myasthenia gravis). Ask about relationship to other neurologic symptoms. In a patient complaining of diplopia, try to determine by examination the position in which the diplopia is most marked. This defines the ocular muscle (or muscles) involved. Deviations of ocular muscles too subtle to be observed by the examiner may be perceived as diplopia to the patient. Red glass testing should be left to experts. In the hands of a nonspecialist it more often misleads than helps. Intermittent diplopia suggests myasthenia gravis, and one should attempt to fatigue the muscles by sustained repetitive action to produce the abnormality. All patients complaining of diplopia in whom an immediate cause is not apparent should have a Tensilon test. Frank abnormalities of ocular movements on examination without diplopia suggest a slowly developing, long-standing lesion such as ocular myopathy with the patient suppressing the experience of diplopia. Monocular diplopia is usually caused by disease of lens or retina and only rarely by psychogenic or cerebral disease.

Abnormal disjunctive eye movements can result from disturbances at several levels of the neuraxis. These include abnormalities in the action of individual muscles (ocular myopathies), the myoneural junction (myasthenia gravis), the oculomotor nerve, the three paired nuclei in the brain stem, or the internuclear medial longitudinal fasciculus that yokes the eyes in parallel movement. The term *strabismus* refers to an involuntary deviation of the eyes from normal physiologic position. Nonparalytic strabismus is due to an intrinsic imbalance of the ocular muscle tone and is usually congenital. Paralytic strabismus results from defects in ocular muscle innervation and implies a neuromuscular disorder. A congenital strabismus may be compensated during life only to become manifest with aging, fatigue, or systemic disease. Patients with strabismus often suppress vision in one eye in order to prevent diplopia. If this occurs in early infancy, the suppressed eye develops permanent reduction of vision *(amblyopia ex anopsia).* This does not occur if strabismus develops later in life.

Defects in ocular movement resulting from faulty action of the eye muscles or their peripheral innervation (such as the third, fourth, and sixth cranial nerves) are called ocular paralyses. Abnormalities of conjugate gaze are called gaze paralyses and result from disease of supranuclear structures.

Ocular Paralyses

The *abducens* (sixth cranial) nerve subserves the lateral rectus muscle. Selective involvement of the nerve anywhere along its pathway, leads to isolated weakness of abduction of the affected eye. If the nucleus itself is involved, there is also a gaze paresis to the ipsilateral side as a result of damage to supranuclear structures in the same area. The *trochlear* (fourth cranial) nerve subserves the superior oblique muscle, which intorts the eye and moves it down when it is medially deviated. All other muscles, including the pupilloconstrictor and the levator of the upper lid, are controlled by the *oculomotor* (third cranial) nerve. Abnormalities of the cranial nerves in the brain stem are almost always associated with other neurologic signs and are usually caused by vascular disturbances, tumors, or demyelinating disease. The peripheral nerves may be involved individually or together by lesions lying anywhere from their site of exit in the brain stem to where they enter the muscle. The nerves are most widely separated in the posterior fossa and run closest to each other in the cavernous sinus and superior orbital fissure. Accordingly, compressive lesions in the cavernous sinus usually cause multiple unilateral ocular palsies, whereas those in the posterior fossa may cause single (sometimes bilateral) nerve dysfunction. Intrinsic lesions of the third nerve (e.g., diabetic neuropathy) often spare the pupil, whereas compressive lesions (tumors and aneurysms) involve the pupil early. Table 115–14 lists the major causes of acute ophthalmoplegia.

Conjugate Paralysis

Conjugate movement of the eyes is regulated by supranuclear pathways that descend from the forebrain to reach the medial longitudinal fasciculus in the brain stem. Unilateral cerebral hemispheric disease resulting from hemorrhage, infarct, or tumor acutely paralyzes conjugate gaze to the contralateral side and often causes deviation of the eyes to the ipsilateral side. Sometimes, particularly in deep-lying hemispheral hemorrhages involving the thalamus, the eyes deviate in the opposite direction. The eye deviation can usually be overcome by vestibular stimulation and is generally transient. Lesions of brain stem pathways cause more permanent conjugate paralysis to the ipsilateral side, with the eyes at rest deviating slightly to the contralateral side. This abnormality usually cannot be overcome by vestibular stimulation.

Lesions of the medial longitudinal fasciculus (MLF), which connects the third and sixth nerves in the brain stem, lead to *internuclear ophthalmoplegia,* in which the eyes at rest may either be parallel or show a mild skew deviation but move disjunctively on lateral gaze. (Skew deviation results from any of a number of lesions involving the brain stem and has little localizing value.) A characteristic of internuclear ophthalmoplegia is that during lateral gaze toward the side of the MLF lesion, the ipsilateral eye abducts and shows nystagmus, whereas the contralateral, adducting eye partially or completely fails to move nasally because of the absence of ascending impulses to reach the opposite third nerve nucleus. Internuclear ophthalmoplegia may be caused by an infarct from small vessel disease (e.g., systemic lupus erythematosus, hypertension) or by demyelinating disease. Bilateral internuclear ophthalmoplegia almost always results from multiple sclerosis.

HEARING AND ITS IMPAIRMENTS

Symptoms of Auditory Dysfunction

Test hearing clinically by having the patient listen to a softly ticking watch or by rubbing one's fingers a few inches from the ear. The examiner can use his or her own hearing as a standard. If hearing is diminished, the Weber test should be carried out. Lateralization to the poorly hearing side suggests conductive loss. Lateralization to the normally hearing side suggests a sensorineural abnormality. More thorough evaluation of hearing requires audiometry.

Two symptoms reflect disease of the auditory system: the first is hearing impairment, sometimes associated with pitch distortion (diplacusis) as well as a decrease in the intensity of sound. The second is tinnitus, a sound heard in the ear or head not arising from the external environment. Hearing loss is termed conductive (external and middle ear), sensorineural (cochlea and auditory nerve), or central (brain stem and cerebral hemispheres). Figure 115–5 provides an algorithm for diagnosing nonobvious causes of hearing loss.

Conductive hearing loss is characterized by equal loss of hearing at all frequencies and by well-preserved speech discrimination once the threshold for hearing is exceeded. The ear often feels full, as if blocked. Bone conduction exceeds air conduction and, if unilateral, the Weber test (tuning fork in the center of the head) is referred to the deaf ear. Persons with *sensorineural hearing loss,* typically hear low tones better than high-frequency ones. They often find it difficult to hear speech mixed with background noise; small increases in the intensity of sound may cause discomfort (recruitment). Air conduction exceeds bone conduction and the Weber test refers to the hearing ear. With hearing loss resulting from cochlear disease (usually due to selective destruction of hair cells), diplacusis and recruitment are common. *Central hearing loss* is rare and requires bilateral lesions of such areas as the inferior colliculus, medial geniculate bodies, or temporal lobe. When the primary receiving areas (Heschl's gyrus) are destroyed, hearing is diminished or absent even for pure tone. Damage to association

TABLE 115–14	Major Causes of Acute (< 48 Hr) Ophthalmoplegia
Condition	**Diagnostic Features**
Bilateral	
Botulism	Contaminated food; high-altitude cooking; pupils involved
Myasthenia gravis	Fluctuating degree of paralysis; responds to edrophonium chloride (Tensilon) IV
Wernicke's encephalopathy	Nutritional deficiency; responds to thiamine IV
Acute cranial polyneuropathy	Antecedent respiratory infection; elevated CSF protein
Brain stem stroke	Other brain stem signs
Unilateral	
Carotid-posterior	Third cranial nerve, pupil involved communicating aneurysm
Diabetic-idiopathic	Third or sixth cranial nerve, pupil spared
Myasthenia gravis	As above
Brain stem stroke	As above

IV = Intravenous; CSF = cerebrospinal fluid.

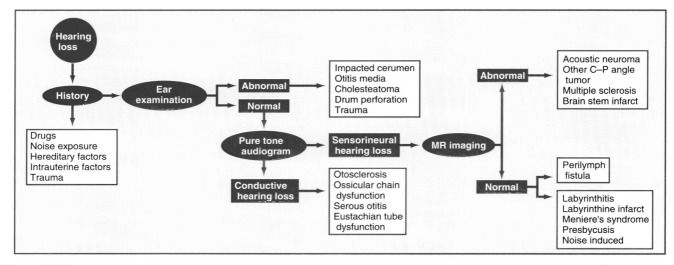

Figure 115-5

Evaluation of deafness (unilateral and bilateral). MR = Magnetic resonance. (Modified from Baloh RW: Hearing and equilibrium. *In* Bennett JC, Plum F [eds.]: Cecil Textbook of Medicine. 20th ed. Philadelphia, WB Saunders, 1996, p 2022.)

areas in the superior temporal gyrus may leave an ability to hear sounds without comprehending their meaning.

Causes of Hearing Loss

Conductive hearing loss arises from abnormalities of the external or middle ear and can raise hearing threshold no more than 60 dB, because bone conduction is intact. Otoscopic examination may reveal obstruction in the external auditory meatus by *impacted cerumen*, canal infection, or similar causes. A *fluid-filled middle ear*, a result of middle ear infection (otitis media), reduces movement of the ossicles against the oval window. If the otoscopic examination is negative, *otosclerosis*, a process in which the annular ligament that attaches the stapes to the oval window overgrows and calcifies, is a likely diagnosis. Chronic tinnitus sometimes marks the early stages of this process, which reduces ossicular transmission via the window to the cochlear basement membrane.

Sensorineural hearing loss from genetically determined deafness may be present at birth or develop in adulthood. The diagnosis of *hereditary deafness* rests on the finding of a positive family history.

Acute unilateral deafness usually has a cochlear basis. Bacterial or viral infections of the labyrinth, head trauma with fracture or hemorrhage into the cochlea, or vascular occlusion of a terminal branch of the anterior inferior cerebellar artery can damage the cochlea and its hair cells. An acute, idiopathic, occasionally reversible, unilateral hearing loss strikes young adults and is presumed to reflect either a viral infection or a vascular disorder of the cochlea. Sudden unilateral hearing loss, often associated with vertigo and tinnitus, can result from a perilymphatic fistula. Such fistulas may be congenital, follow stapes surgery, or result from severe or mild trauma to the inner ear.

Drugs can cause sudden bilateral hearing impairment. Salicylates, furosemide, and ethacrynic acid can cause intense tinnitus and transient deafness when taken in high doses. Aminoglycoside antibiotics can destroy cochlear hair cells in direct relation to the height of their serum concentrations, causing permanent hearing loss. Some anticancer chemotherapeutic agents, particularly cisplatin, can produce similar effects. Subacute, relapsing cochlear deafness occurs with *Meniere's syndrome*, a condition associated with fluctuating hearing loss and tinnitus, recurrent episodes of abrupt and often severe vertigo, and a sensation of fullness or pressure in the ear. Recurrent endolymphatic hypertension (hydrops) is believed to cause the episodes. Pathologically, the endolymphatic sac is dilated and contains atrophic hair cells. The resulting deafness is subtle and reversible in the early stages but subsequently becomes permanent. What hearing remains is characterized by *diplacusis* (a different pitch heard in the affected ear) and loudness recruitment (quiet sounds are not heard but loud sounds are heard as loud as or louder than in the good ear). The disorder is usually unilateral. When bilateral (<20% of cases), it begins in one ear before the other.

Gradually progressive hearing loss with age (*presbycusis*) reflects deterioration in the cochlear receptor system with degeneration of the hair cells, especially at the base. As a result, higher tones are lost early, a change similar to that which follows the recurrent trauma of noise-induced hearing loss from exposure to loud military or industrial noises or blaring music. Unilateral hearing loss that begins and progresses insidiously is characteristic of a benign neoplasm of the cerebellopontine angle (e.g., acoustic neurinoma); an MRI scan usually establishes the diagnosis.

Treatment of Hearing Loss

The best treatment is prevention. Early detection of noise- or drug-induced hearing loss and removal of the offending agent often preserves hearing. Otosclerosis can often be corrected by surgery; closure of a perilymph fistula may improve hearing. Hearing aids help patients with conductive hearing loss, and some newer hearing aids may help patients with cochlear or other sensorineural abnormalities.

Tinnitus

Tinnitus is the term applied generally to extraneous noises heard in one or both ears. Most tinnitus is chronic, of no pathologic importance, and can be overcome by the physician's reassurance and the patient's withdrawing attention from the symptom. Table 115–15 lists possible causes of tinnitus of recent onset. Tinnitus is either *objective,* i.e., the patient hears a real sound, one that can usually be heard by the examiner with a stethoscope, or *subjective,* i.e., the sound arises from an abnormal discharge of the auditory system and cannot be heard by the observer. Most objective tinnitus has a benign cause, but the finding may also be an early sign of increased intracranial pressure. Such tinnitus, which can be obliterated by pressure over the jugular vein, probably arises from turbulent flow in compressed venous structures at the base of the brain.

Subjective tinnitus can arise from anywhere in the auditory system. A faint, moderately high-pitched metallic ring can be observed by almost everyone if he/she concentrates attention on auditory events in a quiet room. Sustained, louder tinnitus accompanied by audiometric evidence of deafness occurs in association with either conductive or sensorineural disease. Tinnitus observed with otosclerosis tends to have a roaring or hissing quality. That associated with Meniere's syndrome often produces sounds that vary widely in intensity with time and quality, sometimes including roarings or clangings. Tinnitus with other cochlear or auditory nerve lesions tends to be higher pitched and ringing in quality.

Treatment

If the underlying disorder causing objective tinnitus can be corrected, tinnitus may disappear. Masking noises placed into the ear occasionally make patients more comfortable and better able to function.

TABLE 115–15	Principal Causes of Sustained Tinnitus	
Objective	**Subjective**
Normal joint or muscle sounds	Most are normal
Patent eustachian tube (synchronizes with breathing)	Drugs: quinine, quinidine, salicylates, indomethacin, rarely others.
Pulse-related: vascular malformations (very rarely, intracranial tumor or elevated pressure)	Meniere's: often intense, can include loud roarings or clangings
Continuous: venous hum	Otosclerosis: roaring, hissing

DIZZINESS AND VERTIGO

Symptoms and Signs

Dizziness

The symptom of "dizziness" expresses any of a number of internal experiences, of which labyrinthine-vestibular vertigo is perhaps the easiest to describe but far from the most common patient complaints (Table 115–16). The experience of true vertigo is usually explicit: a sensation that either the self or the surroundings are vigorously whirling in a continuous direction that can last for seconds or, in lesser intensity, several minutes or more. By contrast, most dizziness is not vestibular in origin and reflects feelings of lightheadedness or "spaciness," a brief sensation of dysequilibrium on sudden standing from a sitting or supine position, a sense of presyncope, or feelings of unsteadiness when walking. Dizziness with these qualities often emerges as a somatoform response to mild cases of influenza, excessively long hours at the work place, looking out over the void from the retaining rails of high buildings, episodes of recognized anxiety, and epochs of emotional depression. Hyperventilation episodes sometimes accompany the attacks in anxious persons. Patients with somatoform disorders and chronic fatigue syndrome often complain of chronic dizziness that remains refractory to either medications or urgings to change lifestyles. Mild doses of benzodiazepines or serotonin uptake inhibitors such as fluoxetine are widely consumed by such persons but unpredictable in their beneficial effects. Many patients improve with reassurance and one of the above drugs, but management often is difficult in chronic, nonvertiginous cases.

Pathogenesis of Vertigo

The vestibular system consists of the finely tuned bilateral semicircular canals and otolithic apparatus of the inner ear as well as their central connections. Any imbalance in input-output between the paired vestibular end-organs or their primary receiving areas in the vestibular nuclei that is not caused by a true movement of the head or body produces a mismatch between vestibular stimulation and

TABLE 115–16	Differential Diagnosis of Dizziness in Approximate Order of Frequency

1. Anxiety-hyperventilation
2. Lightheadedness or presyncope
3. Transient fatigue or intercurrent illness
4. Vertigo
   Benign positional
   Pathologic (disease of labyrinth, VIII nerve, brain stem)
5. Diplopia or other primary visual abnormalities
6. Ataxia
   Cerebellar dysfunction
   Proprioceptive loss
7. Dissociative episodes
8. Partial complex seizures

that going to other sense organs (especially the eyes and proprioceptive organs). The result is the illusory sensation of movement in space called vertigo. Vertigo is the only direct symptom of a vestibular abnormality, but because the vestibular system influences other neural systems, vertigo may be accompanied by autonomic symptoms (nausea, vomiting, diaphoresis), motor symptoms (ataxia, past pointing, falling), or ocular symptoms (oscillopsia—a visual sensation that the environment is moving). The clinical sign of a vestibular abnormality is *nystagmus,* a rhythmic to-and-fro movement of the eyes. Patients suffering from vertigo and nystagmus have an abnormality, either physiologic or pathologic, of the labyrinthine-vestibular system. As already noted, many patients are unable to distinguish vertigo from lightheadedness or other dizziness, and the physician must first determine whether the patient is truly vertiginous.

Nystagmus reflects an imbalance in the complex neural network that involves the visual pathways, the labyrinthine proprioceptive influences from neck muscles, the vestibular and cerebellar nuclei, the reticular formation of the pontine brain stem, and the oculomotor nuclei (Table 115–17). It can be of two types *jerk nystagmus* consists of a slow phase away from the visual object followed by a quick saccade back toward the target. The quick eye movement describes the direction of (compensatory) jerk nystagmus. Benign jerk nystagmus, at the extremes of lateral gaze, is a common finding without pathologic significance. When bidirectional gaze-evoked nystagmus is prominent or involves vertical as well as horizontal movements to an equal degree, excessive sedative or anticonvulsant drug ingestion is most often the cause. Sustained gaze-evoked nystagmus with combined horizontal and torsional components inhibited by fixation suggests a peripheral lesion, whereas vertical nystagmus, particularly that which is not inhibited by fixation, suggests a central lesion. *Pendular nystagmus* is slow and coarse and equal in rate in both directions. It is usually congenital in origin or develops after birth as a result of severe visual impairment but can occasionally be a symptom of cerebellar or brain stem disease.

Several unusual forms of nystagmus have neurologic localizing qualities: *Dissociated nystagmus* (unequal in the two eyes) implies a brain stem lesion. *Periodic alternating nystagmus* consists of a horizontal jerk nystagmus that changes its direction periodically. It has been associated with a variety of posterior fossa abnormalities, especially those involving the region of the craniocervical junction. *Downbeat nystagmus* produces downward jerks with the eyes in the primary gaze position; it often reflects a craniocervical abnormality such as the Arnold-Chiari malformation but can occur with parenchymal lesions such as multiple sclerosis. Some normal persons have the capacity to induce *voluntary nystagmus,* which is extremely rapid, occurs in short bursts of 10 to 15 seconds or so, is present on the extremes of gaze, and may be unequal in the two eyes.

Other abnormalities of conjugate eye movements include *ocular flutter,* consisting of brief, intermittent horizontal oscillations arising from the primary gaze position. *Ocular myoclonus* consists of continuous, rhythmic, pendular oscillations, most often vertical, with a rate of 2 to 5 beats per second. Often it accompanies palatal myoclonus and has a similar pathogenesis. *Opsoclonus* is a pattern of rapid, chaotic, conjugate, repetitive saccadic eye movements ("dancing eyes"). These disorders reflect cerebellar or brain stem dysfunction and also can emerge as a remote effect of systemic neoplasm, especially neuroblastoma in children. *Ocular dysmetria* consists of saccadic overshoots or undershoots of conjugate eye movement during rapid saccadic shifts of visual fixation. The phenomenon reflects cerebellar dysfunction.

Laboratory Tests of Vestibular Function

Bedside *caloric tests* induce vertigo. With the patient lying supine and the head elevated approximately 30 degrees, water 7°C above or below body temperature is douched against the tympanic membrane. In the normal situation, cold water produces nystagmus away from the side of stimulation (because of inhibition of the horizontal semicircular canal) and warm water nystagmus to the side of stimulation (because of stimulation of the semicircular canal). An astute patient suffering from labyrinthine vertigo can often tell which stimulation reproduces the symptoms, thus assisting in the localization of the lesion. Absence of the caloric response on one side suggests ipsilateral labyrinthine failure. Because most peripheral nystagmus is partially inhibited by the visual fixation of the open eyes, accurate quantitative evaluation may require *electronystagmography,* electrical recording of the eye movement with the eyes closed.

Causes of Vertigo

Vertigo can be either physiologic or pathologic. *Physiologic vertigo* occurs when there is a mismatch among the vestibular, visual, and somatosensory systems induced by an external stimulus. Common examples of physiologic vertigo include motion sickness, height vertigo (the sensation that occurs when one looks down from a great height), and visual vertigo (the sensation sometimes felt when one views a motion picture of a roller coaster or other violent movement). In almost all instances, the diagnosis is clear from the history. One exception may be head extension vertigo, a sensation of vertigo or postural

---

TABLE 115–17	Frequent Patterns of Nystagmus and Their Significance

Jerk nystagmus (slow drift away from target, quick jerk back).
Equal, prominent, bidirectional horizontal or vertical jerk nystagmus: sedative or anticonvulsant medication.
Sustained horizontal or torsional nystagmus inhibited by fixation: peripheral abnormality.
Vertical, non-inhibited vertical nystagmus: brain stem lesion.
Dissociated nystagmus between two eyes: brain stem lesion.
Downbeat jerk nystagmus: low ponto-medullary dysfunction (Arnold-Chiari malformation, cerebellar tumor, multiple sclerosis).
Ocular bobbing (coarse rapid conjugate down-jerks with slow return to horizontal): severe pontine lesion or anoxic encephalopathy.

imbalance induced with the head maximally extended while standing (ceiling painter's vertigo) or, in elderly persons, with the head vigorously extended during head washing. The symptoms are probably mainly due to strong proprioceptive stimulation of the vestibular nuclei by neck muscles but vestibular artery insufficiency may play a part. *Motion sickness,* which occurs when a person is a passenger in a moving vehicle, is often exacerbated by sitting in a closed space or reading, thereby giving the visual system the miscue that the environment is stationary. The symptom may be relieved by looking at the environment and watching it move. *Height vertigo* caused by a mismatch between sensation of normal body sway and lack of its visual detection can often be relieved by the patient either sitting or visually fixing on a nearby stationary object.

Pathologic vertigo usually arises from an abnormality of the vestibular system but less commonly can be produced by visual or somatic sensory disorders. Vestibular vertigo can be caused by disease of either the peripheral or central vestibular apparatus (Table 115–18). In general, peripheral vertigo is more intense, more likely to be associated with hearing loss and tinnitus, and often leads to nausea and vomiting. Nystagmus associated with peripheral vertigo is frequently inhibited by visual fixation. Central vertigo is generally less severe, more sustained, and often associated with other signs of CNS disease. The nystagmus of central vertigo is not inhibited by visual fixation and frequently is disproportionately prominent to the degree of vertigo. Figure 115–6 illustrates the diagnostic approach to the vertiginous patient.

Benign positional vertigo is a common disorder of middle and old age that accounts for the symptoms of at least half of such patients with true vertigo. Typically, the patient first experiences severe whirling vertigo immediately after turning over, first lying down in bed at night, arising in the morning or, occasionally, during sleep. Less commonly, the patient may experience similar symptoms when he or she turns suddenly while standing or walking. Usually the symptoms are greatest when the patient lies on the side with the affected ear undermost. The vertigo is delayed for several seconds following the motion, is sudden in onset, is severe and often frightening, and may be accompanied by nausea or vomiting. The patient usually reports that the vertigo ceases when he or she moves out of the position that causes it, but in fact if he or she remains in that position, it rarely lasts more than a minute. The pathophysiology of the disorder is not established. Some authorities have postulated that debris from otoliths (cuprolithiasis) may enter the posterior semicircular canal to artificially stimulate it in the dependent position. The diagnosis is made by the characteristic history. The symptoms and nystagmus sometimes can be reproduced by seating patients erect on an examining table, then quickly moving them to the supine position. The illness usually lasts several weeks and then resolves, but may recur. If the patient has the classic history and physical findings, no further evaluation is necessary. If the history or findings are atypical, the condition must be distinguished from other causes of vertigo and nystagmus, such as tumor or infarct of the posterior fossa. Typical benign positional vertigo is rarely associated with such conditions. The preventive treatment for most patients lies in reassurance plus a series of conditioning exercises in which patients are taught to repetitively reproduce the sudden head movements 10 to 20 times each morning and evening.

Peripheral Vestibulopathy

This disorder, also called *acute labyrinthitis* or *vestibular neuronitis,* may occur as a single bout or may recur repeatedly over months or years. The vertigo is acute, and sometimes so severe that patients are unable to sit or stand without vomiting and ataxia. They prefer to lie absolutely still in bed with the involved ear uppermost. Attacks sometimes follow a respiratory infection. Nystagmus is invariably present, usually horizontal or rotatory, and directed away from the involved labyrinth. The severe symptoms usually improve substantially within 48 to 72 hours, allowing the patient to be up and about. Many patients however report that for weeks or months following the episode sudden movements of the head produce mild vertigo or nausea. Although the disorder is called *acute labyrinthitis,* suggesting a viral infection of the labyrinth, EMG evoked potential studies suggest that in many patients there are accompanying eighth nerve or brain stem abnormalities. The disorder induces considerable discomfort but disappears spontaneously in a matter of days to a week or so.

Labyrinthine fistulas have been reported to produce episodic vertigo. Fistula testing by a skilled otolaryngologist should establish that diagnosis. Some have suggested that acute vertigo can result from compression of the vestibular nerve by blood vessels of the posterior fossa in a manner analogous to trigeminal neuralgia. Other peripheral causes of vertigo include Meniere's syndrome and the taking of vestibulotoxic drugs, most of which are also ototoxic. Vertigo may be an additional symptom in patients suffering from *sudden hearing loss.* The pathogenesis of the disorder is unknown but may be vascular in

TABLE 115–18	Causes of Vestibular Vertigo or Dysequilibrium
Peripheral Causes	**Central Causes**
Peripheral vestibulopathy	Brain stem ischemia
Labyrinthitis and/or vestibular neuronitis*	Cerebellopontine angle tumors
	Demyelinating disease
Acute and recurrent peripheral vestibulopathy	Cranial neuropathy
	Seizure disorders (rare)
Benign positional vertigo*	Heredofamilial ataxia
Meniere's syndrome*	Spinocerebellar degeneration
Vestibulotoxic drugs	Friedreich's ataxia
Focal labryrinthine-third cranial nerve	Olivopontocerebellar atrophy
disease	Other central causes
Trauma	Brain stem tumors
Cancer	Cerebellar degenerations
Infection	Paraneoplastic syndromes
Otosclerosis	
Perilymph fistula	

* Common causes of acute severe vertigo.

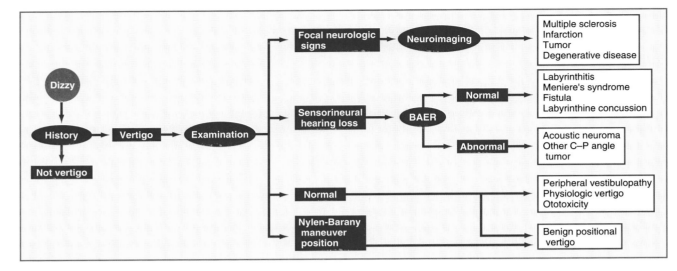

Figure 115–6

Evaluation of vertigo. BAER = Brain stem auditory evoked response. (Modified from Baloh RW: Hearing and equilibrium. *In* Bennett JC, Plum F [eds.]: Cecil Textbook of Medicine. 20th ed. Philadelphia, WB Saunders, 1996, p 2025.)

some, viral infections in others. Bacterial infection of the labyrinth or occasionally otitis media causes vertigo. Degenerative and genetic abnormalities of the labyrinthine system can cause vertigo. *Cervical vertigo* is the term given to the feelings of dysequilibrium associated with head movement described by some patients with cervical osteoarthritis or spondylosis. The disorder probably is caused by unbalanced input from cervical muscles to the vestibular apparatus. Acute neck strain may be occasionally associated with vertigo. Local anesthetics injected into one side of the neck can produce vertigo and ataxia by a similar lack of balanced input. No nystagmus accompanies these disorders.

Central Vertigo

Central causes of vertigo, less common than peripheral causes, produce less severe vertigo than that resulting from peripheral lesions, no hearing loss or tinnitus, and associated neurologic signs of brain stem or cerebellar dysfunction.

Cerebrovascular Disease

If ischemia, infarction, or hemorrhage affects the brain stem or cerebellum, vertigo accompanied by nausea and vomiting is a relatively common symptom. Occipital headache as well as nystagmus and other neurologic signs suggesting brain stem or cerebellar dysfunction usually accompany vertigo. Rarely, vertigo (nonpositional) is the sole symptom of *transient ischemic attacks* of the brain stem, but most patients suffering such attacks during a stroke report headache, diplopia, facial or body numbness, and ataxia as well.

Cerebellopontine Angle Tumors

Most tumors growing in the cerebellopontine angle (e.g., acoustic neuroma, meningioma) grow slowly, allowing the vestibular system to accommodate. Thus they usually produce vague sensations of dysequilibrium rather than acute vertigo. Frequently such neoplasms produce complaints of tinnitus, hearing loss, and a sensation that the person is being pulled or pushed to one side when he or she walks. Occasionally episodic vertigo or positional vertigo heralds the presence of a cerebellopontine angle tumor. Virtually all affected patients have retrocochlear hearing loss and decreased or absent caloric responses on the involved side. CT or MRI scans through the temporal bone and posterior fossa usually reveal the tumor.

Demyelinating Disease

Acute vertigo may be the first symptom of *multiple sclerosis,* although only a small percentage of young patients with acute vertigo eventually develop multiple sclerosis. Vertigo may also be a symptom of *parainfectious encephalomyelitis* or, rarely, *parainfectious cranial polyneuritis* of the Guillain-Barré type. In these instances, the accompanying neurologic signs establish the diagnosis.

Cranial Neuropathy

A variety of acute or subacute illnesses affecting the eighth cranial nerve can produce vertigo as an early or sole symptom, the most common being *herpes zoster.* The *Ramsay Hunt syndrome (geniculate ganglion herpes)* is characterized by vertigo and hearing loss, variably associated with facial paralysis and sometimes pain in the ear. The typical lesions of herpes vesicles, which may follow the appearance of neurologic signs, are found in the external auditory canal and sometimes over the palate. Whether herpes zoster is ever responsible for vertigo in the absence of the full-blown syndrome is not certain. *Granulomatous meningitis* or *leptomeningeal metastases* and cerebral or systemic *vasculitis* may involve the eighth nerve, producing vertigo as an early symptom. In these disorders, cerebrospinal fluid (CSF) analysis usually suggests the diagnosis.

Seizure Disorders

Patients suffering from temporal lobe epilepsy occasionally suffer vertigo as the aura. Vertigo in the absence of other neurologic signs or symptoms, however, is never caused by epilepsy or other diseases of the cerebral hemispheres.

Other Central Causes

Many structural lesions of the brain stem or cerebellum, particularly if rapid in onset, may cause vertigo. In a few instances, vertigo may initiate the symptoms of *paraneoplastic brain stem degeneration*. As with *brain stem tumors, cerebellar degenerative diseases* and other structural disease of the brain stem and posterior fossa, there are usually other neurologic symptoms, almost always including signs of brain stem or cerebellar dysfunction, in addition to the vertigo and nystagmus.

Treatment

The best treatment of symptomatic vertigo is to cure the underlying disease. In many instances, however, that is not possible and one must resort to symptomatic treatment. In acute vertigo, such as occurs with labyrinthitis, most patients insist on bedrest. Vestibulosedative drugs such as meclizine or diazepam may be helpful. Prochlorperazine suppositories can be used to circumvent vomiting. Vestibulosuppressive drugs such as meclizine also sometimes help more chronic vertiginous disorders. Scopolamine, 0.4 to 0.8 mg, together with methylphenidate, 5 mg orally, may give relief of vertigo, particularly motion sickness. Transdermal scopolamine paste-on units placed behind the ear have been reported to be effective in preventing motion sickness for up to 72 hours. If head or neck movement precipitates vertigo, a cervical collar sometimes relieves the symptoms.

REFERENCES

Baloh RW, Honrubia V: Clinical Neurophysiology of the Vestibular System. 2nd ed. Philadelphia, FA Davis Co, 1990.

Leigh RH, Zee DS: The Neurology of Eye Movement. 2nd ed. Philadelphia, FA Davis Co, 1991.

Sullivan M, Clark MR, Fische M, et al: Psychiatric and otologic diagnoses in patients complaining of dizziness. Arch Intern Med 1993; 153: 1479–1484.

116

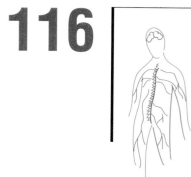

Disorders of the Motor System

A. Mechanisms of Normal and Abnormal Motor Function

The normal human voluntary motor system originates in the premotor areas of the frontal lobe cortex and sends its messages caudally, via the corticospinal tract after the basal ganglia and cerebellum have added their postural, reinforcing, and coordinating influences (Fig. 116–1). Additional descending influences from the red nuclei, vestibular nuclei, and brain stem reticular formation converge with descending corticospinal pathways on bulbospinal motor neurons to activate integrated, functionally automatic motor programs. At every level afferent feedback impulses from muscle, nerve, spinal segment, brain stem, cerebellum, basal ganglia, and cortex guide the efferently directed action so as to assure its healthy success. Figures 116–2 and 116–3 indicate the corticobasal ganglia and corticocerebellar loops that unconsciously precede every voluntary and most involuntary movements that we humans make.

Disease potentially can affect selectively every level of the motor system from muscle to brain. Table 116–1 briefly lists most common anatomic locations of diseases affecting the motor system. Later sections of this chapter discuss most of them in greater detail. The first step in recognizing any of these categories lies in evaluating symptoms and signs, giving specific attention to deciding whether the origin of the complaints lies in the peripheral (muscles, nerves, roots) or the central nervous system (CNS). Once the latter decision is reached, it becomes easier to ferret out exactly which level or which component of motor control is most likely to be the offender. Because many diseases of the human motor system are unaccompanied by specific neurodiagnostic laboratory abnormalities, the carefulness of the clinical examination and the examiner's ingenuity often provide the most reliable guide to the nature of the patient's illness. Laboratory tests for examining neuromuscular disease are described in Chapter 111.

SIGNS AND SYMPTOMS OF MOTOR DYSFUNCTION

Fatigue and Weakness

Fatigue refers to a perception of intellectual or manual physical exhaustion that may follow or even precede concerted mental and/or physical effort. Normal degrees of activity-related fatigue require little more than a common sense appraisal. Pronounced fatigue after the act can have either an organic or a psychological pathogenesis. Localized muscular fatigability most often reflects a regional disorder, deconditioning or aging of the nerves or muscles; when accompanied by detectable, exercise-induced local reductions in muscle strength, the symptom is characteristic of myasthenia gravis. Chronic, generalized fatigability can accompany a number of specifically diagnosable systemic illnesses, such as chronic liver disease, chronic well-characterized immune disorders, or widespread malignancy. Neurologic disorders that characteristically produce fatigue include myasthenia gravis, progressive muscular dystrophy, motor neuron disease, Parkinson's disease, stroke, severe trauma, and multiple sclerosis. All of these conditions produce other clinical abnormalities that identify their specific cause. More difficult to understand and classify are states of long-lasting, generalized weakness coupled with feelings of pre-effort fatigue for which no objectively verifiable cause can be found. Variously called over the years neurasthenia, effort syndrome, and, at present, chronic fatigue syndrome, the condition is widespread in Western industrial nations. Infectious disease specialists have searched vigorously but thus far fruitlessly for a cause of chronic fatigue syndrome.

Chronic fatigue syndrome affects two principal cate-

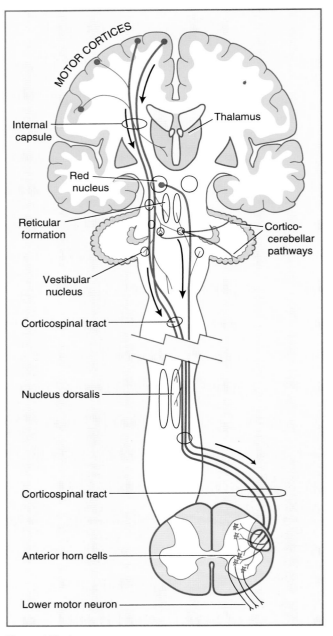

Figure 116-1
Normal human voluntary motor system.

Far more common than epidemic chronic fatigue are sporadic cases. Indeed, chronic fatigue is the seventh most common complaint presented to primary care physicians. In addition to feeling chronically tired, with or without undertaking physical activity, many affected patients complain of multiple functional symptoms including abdominal pain, bizarre pain patterns affecting other body parts, menstrual complaints, sleep disorders, headaches, vague myalgias, and postexercise fatigue. Many of the complaints overlap those found in the equally poorly understood disorder *fibromyalgia* (see Chapters 85 and 90). Others are consistent with patterns seen in somatoform disorders (Ch 112). In keeping with science news reports, which recurrently report new organic causes for the syndrome, most affected patients believe strongly or unshakably that they suffer from a chronic virus infection or other externally generated disorder. Careful psychiatric and past history evaluation, however, characteristically discloses chronic somatoform illness long preceding the putatively recent onset of fatigue. Fully three quarters of chronic fatigue patients fulfill criteria for having at least one psychiatric disorder in their lifetime, and several studies have found evidence for major depressive episodes in as many as 50%, past or present. A consistent feature in all studies has been that patients with chronic fatigue syndrome avoid expressing psychiatric symptoms unless specifically asked and they tend to dissociate their somatic complaints from their mood disorder.

Although it is possible that chronic fatigue syndrome may have both somatic and psychosomatic causes, one should not ignore the latter because several studies report that antidepressives coupled with cognitive behavioral group therapy can bring relief to as many as half such patients. Experience suggests that repeated efforts to find organic causes for the symptoms not only fail to improve symptoms but also block other, psychologically based efforts at treatment. Among other steps, in addition to strong psychological counseling efforts, chronically fatigued patients should be urged to undertake full physical and mental activity.

Weakness, a more specific symptom than fatigue, refers to an impaired capacity to conduct a voluntary motor act due to a loss of muscular power. The term *paresis* is synonymous. *Paralysis* designates more complete loss of motor function. Most weakness or paralysis results from disease or dysfunction of the central or peripheral nervous system or the muscles. Sometimes, however, muscle guarding and immobility that surround injured or inflamed areas of the trunk or extremities can cause the false appearance of weakness when motion accentuates the pain. The qualities of hysterical weakness are described below.

The history is of major importance in recognizing the nature and significance of weakness. Most persons promptly recognize a recently developing or rapidly progressing muscle motor loss but tend to ignore insidiously developing, painless weakness until it produces substantial functional disability (e.g., inability to climb stairs). Families or physicians may sometimes detect such gradually evolving limitations (e.g., limping or dragging a leg) before the patient does. Conversely, although most patients with motor system disorders complain of "weak-

gories of patients. One is represented by a small fraction of persons who, by all past records, were healthy and energetic until struck by an ill-defined, generalized, flu-like illness. Following the latter, prostrating, isolated fatigue limits their normal physical and mental activity for periods lasting many weeks, months, or even indefinitely. Some examples of this ordinarily self-limited disorder have erupted in mini-epidemics among primary caregivers. Many efforts have been made to establish an infectious nature for the condition. Only one, however, which suggested a chronic immunologic reaction to human herpes virus type 6, has provided strong evidence that the epidemic disorder may have an organic cause.

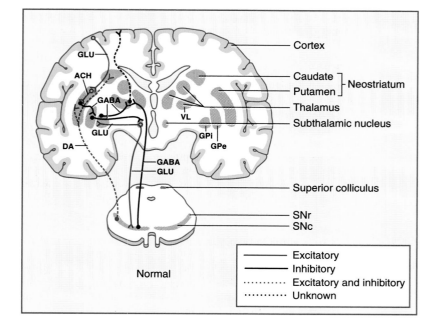

Figure 116–2
Anatomy of the basal ganglia and their connections. ACh = Acetylcholine; GABA = γ-aminobutyric acid; GLU = glutamate; GP = globus pallidum (e = external, i = internal); DA = dopamine; SN = substantia nigra (c = compacta, r = reticulate); VL = ventrolateral. Note the feedback loop that proceeds from cerebral prefrontal areas to the basal ganglia and eventually back from basal ganglia to thalamus to motor cortex. This ultimately regulates the descending corticospinal motor system. (From Jancovic J: The extrapyramidal disorders. *In* Wyngaarden JB, Smith LH Jr, Bennett JC [eds]: Cecil Textbook of Medicine. 19th ed. Philadelphia, WB Saunders, 1992, p. 2129.)

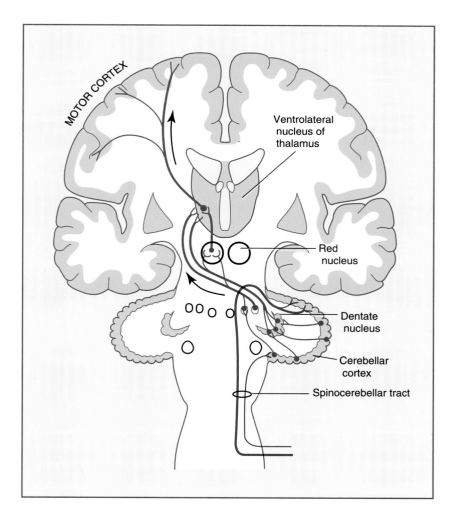

Figure 116–3
Corticocerebral loop.

TABLE 116–1	Principal Disorders of the Motor System from Distal to Proximal

Muscular
    Dystrophies, metabolic myopathies, inflammatory
       myopathies (myositis)
Myoneural junction
    Myasthenia, Lambert-Eaton syndrome, botulism
Peripheral nerve disorders
    Polyneuropathy
    Mono- or focal neuropathy
Radiculopathies and lower motor neuron diseases
Spinal cord diseases
Cerebellar ataxias
Extrapyramidal movement disorders
Corticospinal diseases (disorders of the upper motor neuron)

ness," an occasional patient may use the term *numbness* to indicate why objects drop from the weak hand. In other instances, patients use the term *weakness to* mean fatigability, asthenia, or even incoordination. Patients should be pressed to be specific about the terms they use and, if they are truly weak, to describe which motor acts are limited. In the legs, for example, proximal muscle weakness is usually characterized by difficulty getting out of low chairs, arising from the toilet seat, or climbing stairs, whereas distal motor weakness is characterized by tripping because of failure to dorsiflex the foot while walking on irregular ground or when climbing stairs or curbs. Shoulder girdle weakness is characterized by difficulty using a hair dryer or lifting heavy objects to a high shelf, whereas distal extremity weakness is noted in manipulative tasks such as turning keys, opening door knobs, or unscrewing jar tops.

Patterns of Neurologic and Muscular Weakness

Corticospinal tract dysfunction weakness can be divided into respective patterns of upper motor neuron and lower motor neuron disability (Table 116–2). *Upper motor neuron lesions* arising at the cerebral level typically produce regional weakness predominating in the hand and arm, the lower face, or the foot and leg, in that order of

TABLE 116–2	Clinical Signs of Upper and Lower Motor Neuron Lesions

	Upper	Lower
Paralysis	Mostly distal, distributed in major body part	Proximal or distal: distributed by nerve, plexus, root or anterior horn cell anatomy
Atrophy	Minimal, late, disuse	Prominent, early, neurotropic
Fasciculations	Absent	Often present
Spasticity	Present	Absent
Deep tendon reflexes	Increased	Decreased or absent
Babinski's sign	Present	Absent

frequency. A hemiparesis (face, arm, and leg) can originate from the cerebrum, as can face-hand-arm weakness. Face-leg weakness, sparing the arm, implies two anatomically distinct lesions, whereas arm-leg weakness sparing the face can originate anywhere along the corticospinal pathway between the internal capsule and the upper cervical cord. Upper motor neuron weakness typically affects skilled movement, with paresis being more marked distally than proximally in the limbs. Various components of *spasticity* emerge, including increased muscular resistance to passive stretch with lengthening and shortening reactions, increased deep tendon reflexes, and abnormal postural responses to stimulation including decorticate, decerebrate, and spinal flexor responses and the classic Babinski's sign (extensor plantar response). Upper motor neuron lesions seldom severely paralyze the face and never completely so. As a result, the brow and orbicularis oculi, like other bodily midline muscle groups, are relatively spared. Atrophy of the limbs, if it occurs at all, is mild and due to disuse. The electromyogram (EMG) usually shows no abnormality beyond a reduction or loss of voluntary contraction activity.

Disease of the lower motor neuron, including the anterior horn cells, the motor nerve root, or the motor nerve, causes a classic syndrome (see Table 116–2). Weakness is focally distributed according to areas of denervation, so that a major clue to anatomic diagnosis lies in distinguishing among the respective paralytic patterns produced by damage to spinal cord, ventral motor root, plexus, or peripheral nerve. Characteristic sensory defects accompany many of these causes. With severe denervation-weakness, visible muscle atrophy begins within days. Motor resistance is subnormal, deep tendon reflexes diminish or disappear, and, with proximally originating denervation, fasciculations may become visible through the skin. Electric signs of denervation, including first fibrillation and later fasciculation, begin within 3 to 4 weeks of injury.

Among *basal ganglia diseases,* asthenia is prominent in parkinsonism and chorea. Some patients in the early stages of parkinsonism complain of a hemiparetic weakness that can misleadingly suggest corticospinal tract dysfunction. Most persons with Parkinson's disease, however, suffer only mild to moderate weakness but report disproportionately prominent difficulty in initiating and continuing movements, "as if starting through molasses." Their limbs show rigidity rather than spasticity, their deep tendon reflexes are at most only moderately increased, and they lack Babinski's sign or other evidence of pathologic reflex spasticity.

Cerebellar diseases, especially those of the hemisphere and dentate nuclei, cause ipsilateral asthenia and weakness. Ataxia and incoordination are prominent. Muscle resistance to passive stretch is, if anything, reduced, but deep tendon reflexes may be moderately hyperactive, and impaired cerebellar regulation of the stretch reflex can cause pendular swinging of the knee jerk. Pathologic reflexes and muscle atrophy are lacking.

Nerve-muscle junctional disease is of two kinds. The more frequent, myasthenia gravis (MG), consists of an autoimmune blockage of the acetylcholine receptor in the muscle. The other, the Lambert-Eaton myasthenic syndrome involves immunologic blockage of presynaptic calcium channels that reduces release of neurotransmitter from the nerve terminals. Weakness in MG affects most often the oculomotor, bulbar, and proximal limb muscles, which rapidly fatigue with quick successive action. Weakness in the less common Lambert-Eaton syndrome, by contrast, affects mainly the distal limbs, is maximal with first effort, and lessens with repeated tries. Atrophy occurs in neither disorder except when severe chronic MG induces muscle disuse. Muscle tone is normal, deep tendon reflexes are usually preserved or reduced, and sensation is unaffected. Properly performed EMGs are diagnostic.

Myopathies, diseases intrinsic to muscle, produce insidiously beginning weakness that symmetrically affects anatomic groups in patterns characteristic of the particular variant of degenerative (dystrophic), metabolic (e.g., thyrotoxic), or inflammatory (myositis) disease. Weakness occasionally remains constant (congenital myopathy) but usually progresses either slowly (dystrophy), rapidly (metabolic or inflammatory myopathy), or episodically (periodic paralysis). Resistance to passive stretch is normal, but the muscles may be tender (myositis), show myotonia (congenital myotonia, myotonic dystrophy), be abnormally soft (thyrotoxicosis), look abnormally large (pseudohypertrophy), or feel unduly firm (connective tissue infiltration). Deep tendon reflexes are preserved until late in the course except in hypokalemic myopathy. Serum enzymes often are abnormal in muscular dystrophy, and EMGs in many instances are characteristic. Sensation remains intact.

Major Abnormal Movements

Table 116–3 lists the major conditions causing nonparoxysmal, focal, or generalized abnormal gross skeletal muscle movements. Several of the focal movements can be confused with epileptic attacks (see Chapter 119). Categories overlap, especially those of dystonia, chorea, athetosis, and dyskinesia.

Myotonia comprises a prolonged (seconds) involuntary contraction of a group of adjacent muscle fibers following a self-limited, voluntary effort or an abrupt local percussion as with a reflex hammer. A genetically caused abnormality of the postsynaptic muscle membrane produces self-repetitive muscle membrane depolarizations and afterdischarges that lead to sustained fiber shortening.

Cramps describe a sudden, painful, abrupt shortening of muscles. Motor units during cramps fire at about 300 per second, much faster than the most vigorous voluntary contraction. The high rate of discharge causes a sustained, strong muscular contraction and secondarily induces pain. Both aspects can be relieved by stretching the affected muscle or by massage. Central mechanisms may also be involved, because certain conditions are associated with a propensity to cramps: partial denervation (especially amyotrophic lateral sclerosis), pregnancy, and electrolyte disorders (especially water intoxication and hyponatremia). Cramps attributed to hypo-osmolarity are seen in some patients treated by maintenance hemodialysis. They respond to treatment with hypertonic solutions of glucose or sodium.

Cramps occur commonly in otherwise normal individuals, especially the elderly. Some people with or without a family history of cramps are more susceptible than others for unknown reasons. Cramps that occur only at night or after sustained exercise can sometimes be prevented by quinine sulfate, 0.3 gm taken orally. Others can occur frequently during the day, occasionally so often that the individual is effectively crippled. Phenytoin, 0.3 to 0.6 gm daily, may be helpful in these patients, but some are resistant to this as well as to other drugs that may be tried, including diazepam, carbamazepine, and diphenhydramine. Patients with benign fasciculations (lacking weakness, wasting, or other signs of motor neuron disease) seem especially prone to frequent cramps.

Tetany is a special form of cramp, identified by its predilection for flexor muscles of the hand and extensors of the fingers, its association with laryngospasm, and its relationship to hypocalcemia. Tetany can be painful. It differs from other cramps electromyographically in a characteristic rhythmic grouping of discharging potentials. Hyperventilation-induced tetany is sometimes overlooked as a cause of cramps or laryngospasm.

Muscle fibrillation consists of continuously recurrent spontaneous contractions of single muscle fibers, largely invisible and due usually to denervation but sometimes to dystrophic degeneration of single fiber membranes. The phenomenon reflects hypersensitivity of the muscle membrane and contractile system to circulating or locally diffusing acetylcholine (ACh). *Fasciculations* represent spontaneous, synchronous, recurrent depolarization-contractions of the fibers of a single motor unit or of a group of partially denervated motor units that have been reinnervated by fibers from adjacent, still-conducting motor axons. The pathogenesis reflects denervation hypersensitivity to ACh of the damaged motor axon. Fasciculations of larger motor units and grouped motor units are visible through the skin.

Myokymia has been used to describe a variety of apparently different disorders characterized by cramps in association with continuous spontaneous rippling of muscle. The EMGs in some cases show prolonged trains of

TABLE 116–3	Major Movement Disorders

Tremor
    Parkinson's
    Cerebellar
    Familial—senile
Chorea
    Huntington's
    Sydenham's
    Lupus- or pregnancy-related
Ballism
Dystonia
Athetosis (congenital)
Dyskinesia
    Hemifacial spasm
    Levodopa-associated
    Tardive
Myoclonus
Tics

spontaneous potentials, whereas in others grouping of potentials is found. Some patients have difficulty in relaxing grip, a phenomenon called *neuromyotonia* because, unlike myotonia, the muscular activity is abolished by neuromuscular blocking agents, indicating a neural rather than a muscular origin. At least some affected persons possess antibodies reacting with voltage-gated potassium channels in the neural membrane.

In patients with severe myokymia, continuous shortening of muscle leads to abnormal postures and abnormally increased resistance to passive movement. Such abnormalities are often due to central neurologic disorders and are thought to result from poorly understood genetically related autoimmune disorders. Some affected patients suffer fluctuating rigidity of axial and limb muscles and continuous EMG activity despite vigorous attempts to relax. The resulting disorder has been labeled *stiff-man syndrome*. Ordinary cramps may be superimposed upon the persistent stiffness. Phenytoin, carbamazepine, diazepam, or mexiletine in therapeutic doses may bring dramatic relief. The condition may have several causes; in several cases antibodies have been demonstrated against central gamma-amino-butyric acid (GABA) receptors.

Tremor (Table 116–4). *Essential tremor* or *benign familial tremor* is an accentuation of a physiologic, 8- to 12-Hz rhythmic oscillation that can affect the distal arms, the

TABLE 116–4   Characteristics of Common Tremors

	Associated Disorder	Position	Frequency, Character
Essential	Normal or anxiety-accentuated	Sustained posture	8–12 Hz Oscillating, distal extremities
Familial	Autosomal pattern of inheritance; linked to essential tremor	Sustained posture Intention	8–12 Hz Oscillating head-neck, distal extremities
Parkinson's	Basal ganglia disease Wilson's disease	Resting or postural Not intention	4–7 Hz Reciprocally alternating Tongue, facial muscles, distal extremities
Cerebellar	Vermis, anterior cerebellar	Action-intention tremor. Rhythmic regular titubation of trunk, lower extremities	Coarse, 3–6 Hz Oscillating
	Spinobulbar cerebellar input	Distal lower extremity	Coarse, somewhat irregular ataxia
	Neocerebellar dentate outflow	Distal upper extremity	Often irregular. Increases as target is approached
Asterixis	Metabolic encephalopathy, particularly hepatic	Outstretched tongue or, more often, hands. Flaplike appearance	Coarse 1–3 Hz Rapid twitches with variable intervals between

head, or, less often, the vocal apparatus. Coarse in its pattern but absent at complete rest, the tremor begins with the maintenance of posture and is accentuated by voluntary, intentional movement, sometimes to an incapacitating degree. The abnormality depends on cerebellar mechanisms as well as basal ganglia dysfunction and can be blocked by lesions placed in the ventrolateral nucleus of the thalamus. Essential tremor varies widely in intensity and can appear at any age but becomes more common and prominent in elderly life *(senile tremor)*. It is not accompanied by rigidity, akinesia, ataxia, or weakness, and its predisposition is transmitted as an autosomal dominant trait. Alcohol in small amounts and, less often, anxiolytic agents suppress the movement. The beta-blocker propranolol reduces the intensity of the tremor in about 25% of affected persons. Primidone and baclofen are useful for some patients.

Resting or *parkinsonian tremor,* a 4- to 7-Hz oscillation, reflects the alternating contractions of agonist-antagonist muscles, most often of the distal extremities, especially the hand ("pill rolling"). Less frequently the lower facial muscles, the tongue, or the lower extremities are involved. The tremor worsens with anxiety or fatigue and tends to quiet down or briefly disappear with relaxation or periods of intense manual concentration. As with all abnormal movements of basal ganglia origin, parkinsonian tremor disappears during sleep. Its genesis is believed to reflect excess cholinergic activity in the striatum, leading to an abnormally high GABA output from the putamen to the pallidum. The tremor can be abolished by lesions of the thalamic ventrolateral nucleus and is improved by antiparkinsonian drugs, as discussed below.

Intention (cerebellar) tremor can take any of three patterns. One relates to damage of the vermis and anterior lobe and results in an oscillating, rhythmic ataxia of the trunk and lower limbs during attempts to walk (titubation). A second, associated with lesions of the afferent spinocerebellar input, produces a more irregular, high-steppage, shaking ataxia of the lower extremities, which can blend into titubation. The third, resulting from damage to the dentate outflow pathway of the superior peduncle, produces the classic hand or foot intention tremor, consisting of an irregular, coarse 3- to 6-Hz distal oscillation that increases in amplitude and irregularity as the voluntarily moving extremity approaches its object. In all instances, cerebellar tremor reflects a disruption in the balance between afferent impulses to the roof nuclei of the cerebellum and the immediately following inhibitory loop that normally feeds back on these roof nuclei from the Purkinje cells. Cerebellar intention tremor so far has resisted efforts at pharmacologic control.

Asterixis is an irregular, flaplike tremor, distributed more distally than proximally, that involves the extremities, less often the tongue, with a frequency varying from less than 1 to as high as 3 Hz. It is most often observed to accompany the metabolic encephalopathies and usually is accompanied by an accentuated physiologic tremor. Its mechanism reflects a brief loss of muscle contraction in muscles controlling extension of the involved member, followed by a rapid myoclonic-like flexor movement during recovery.

Chorea describes involuntary, nonrhythmic, irregularly distributed, coarse, quick twitching movements affecting the face, tongue, and proximal and distal extremities. Slower athetoid twistings sometimes intersperse themselves concurrently. Mild cases may resemble little more than anxiety-provoked fidgets, whereas the appearance of severe forms blends into a generalized dystonia. Efforts at sustained muscular contraction accentuate the disorder, which possesses features of both basal ganglia and cerebellar dysfunction. Pharmacologically, the phenomenon most closely resembles the effects of central dopamine hyperactivity. *Ballism* consists of irregular, abrupt, repetitive, wide-amplitude flinging movements of the limbs initiated predominantly by proximal girdle muscles. Less prominent distal choreiform movements often accompany the condition, which involves body parts opposite to an infarcted or, rarely, otherwise damaged subthalamic nucleus. Usually unilateral in distribution (hemiballismus), the condition is ameliorated by haloperidol or reserpine. Ordinarily it subsides spontaneously within a few weeks after onset.

Dystonia can accompany several basal ganglia disorders and is the major sign of a primary movement disorder of late childhood, adolescence, or adult life. The abnormality is characterized by bizarre sustained or spasmodic twisting or turning motions, most but not all of which affect more distal body parts. The distinctive feature of the movements is that they involve the simultaneous tonic co-contraction of agonist and antagonist muscle groups. Brief dystonia usually lasts for a second or more, a rate somewhat faster than in *athetosis,* a slow, proximally distributed twisting observed most commonly in children who have suffered perinatal or infantile basal ganglia-thalamic damage. Most dystonic movements also tend to recur in longer spasms, sometimes lasting minutes to hours at a time. Dystonia can be generalized or restricted, inherited or acquired. It can arise as a distinct, idiopathic disorder or as an accompaniment to several basal ganglia diseases, including Huntington's chorea and Wilson's disease. The pathophysiology and pharmacologic basis of dystonic movements are poorly understood. Several phenothiazine derivatives, however, can induce acute dystonia as an idiosyncratic response in susceptible hosts. Structural lesions involving the basal ganglia–thalamic motor pathways sometimes cause a contralateral hemidystonia. The anticholinergic, antihistamine drug diphenhydramine hydrochloride blocks acute drug-induced dystonia but not the naturally occurring form.

Motor tics are sudden, quick, irregular, stereotyped movements of variable complexity that repetitively involve similar but not identical groups of muscles. They can come on at any age, most often in adolescence or young adulthood, and most frequently involve the face, eyes, or mouth but seldom the extremities. Some mild forms represent psychologically generated habit patterns. More severe examples, often combined with bizarre barkings or the shouting of scatologic and other obscenities, comprise *Gilles de la Tourette's syndrome.*

Myoclonus consists of sudden, abrupt contractions of single muscles or restricted groups of muscles, most frequently affecting the limbs, less often the trunk. The phenomenon has many causes and can arise from abnormally excitable gray matter at any level of the nervous system. Single generalized myoclonic jerks occur normally as startle responses or when drifting off to sleep. Myoclonic seizures generated from the cerebrum usually occur in distal muscles, whereas myoclonus generated in the lower brain stem or spinal gray matter usually has a proximal distribution that affects the pectoral girdle, trunk, or pelvic girdle. Myoclonic jerks accompany several forms of epilepsy. They also occur in a multifocal pattern in association with several metabolic encephalopathies, especially those associated with uremia or penicillin intoxication. They can complicate severe cerebral anoxia or accompany prion (Creutzfeldt-Jakob) disease.

Palatal myoclonus relates more to a form of continuous tremor than to true myoclonus. The condition consists of rhythmic, regular, 2- to 3-Hz contractions of the soft palate and, less commonly, the adjacent pharynx. It arises in association with infarction or degeneration of the pathway that links together the dentate, red nucleus, and inferior olive. Unlike the tremors of basal ganglia or cerebellar origin, palatal myoclonus persists during sleep. The serotonin precursor 5-hydroxytryptamine sometimes ameliorates the contractions, which have been attributed to denervation hypersensitivity of medullary olivary neurons.

Hemifacial spasm can affect the motor distribution of either facial nerve, producing rapidly recurring, painless, nonstereotyped fragmentary twitching of any of the facial muscles. The condition persists into sleep and has been attributed to ephaptic cross-conduction of fibers within the facial nerve secondary to damage caused by long-standing intracranial compression from an overlying branch of the basilar artery. Surgical decompression sometimes relieves the condition, which is disfiguring but neither painful nor dangerous.

REFERENCES

Dawson DM, Sabin TD: Chronic Fatigue Syndrome. Boston, Little, Brown & Co., 1993.

Lane TJ, Manu P, Mathews DA: Depression and somatization in the chronic fatigue syndrome. Am J Med 1991; 91:335–344.

B. Movement Disorders

The term *movement disorders* refers to a group of neurologic conditions generated by abnormalities that arise in the brain and affect resting skeletal muscles in a nonparoxysmal manner so as to produce gross, functionally inappropriate activity in the face, limbs, or trunk. All appear only during the waking state and all are believed to represent dysfunction or damage initially related primarily to the basal ganglia and its subcortical connections with the thalamus. Included anatomically are the symmetrically placed deep cerebral nuclei of the caudate nucleus and putamen (together known as the striatum), the globus pallidus or pallidum, the subthalamic nucleus, and the substantia nigra of the midbrain (see Fig. 116–2). The functions of the basal ganglia are best deduced from their diseases. The ganglia especially influence the control of trunk and proximal appendicular movement by feeding information forward to the frontal cortex before that region sends its final signals to the craniospinal motor neurons via the corticospinal tract. In fact, secondary interruption of the corticospinal pathway ameliorates or interrupts pre-existing signs of basal ganglia dysfunction. This observation has led to diseases of the basal ganglia being termed *extrapyramidal disorders*. The basal ganglia exert a major influence on the planning of movement and in establishing the postural "set" or "platform" upon which corticospinal influences superimpose learned motor activity.

The basal ganglia contain a distinct neurotransmitter anatomy. Corticostriatal and thalamostriatal afferents are both excitatory in their action, probably employing glutamate as a transmitter (see Fig. 116–2). The well-known nigrostriatal input employs dopamine. Dopaminergic synapses probably exist on all neuronal types within the striatum, although the functionally most important receptors appear to lie on the axon terminals of incoming corticostriate fibers. The striatum also contains many cholinergic interneurons believed functionally to counterbalance the dopaminergic input. This latter action may help to explain why anticholinergic drugs sometimes improve the symptoms of parkinsonism. Most of the outputs of the basal ganglia to their known projection areas employ the inhibitory transmitter GABA. A number of neuropeptides also have been identified in the nuclei, but their functional significance remains uncertain.

PARKINSONISM

Parkinsonism is a syndrome consisting, in variable combinations, of slowness in the initiation and execution of movement (bradykinesia), increased muscle tonus (rigidity), tremor, and impaired postural reflexes. The underlying pathogenesis is primarily a defect in the dopaminergic pathway that connects the substantia nigra to the striatum. In idiopathic or postencephalitic parkinsonism, the deficiency results from degeneration of the pigmented dopamine-secreting neurons in the substantia nigra, whereas most drug-induced parkinsonism reflects a blocking of dopamine receptors in striatal neurons. Several rare diseases that cause degeneration of striatal receptor neurons also produce clinical parkinsonism but fail to improve with the use of levodopa or its congeners. Similar therapeutic limitations apply to the parkinsonian manifestations that sometimes accompany advanced vascular diseases, neoplasms, and certain degenerative disorders, such as progressive supranuclear palsy, the Shy-Drager form of generalized idiopathic autonomic insufficiency, and some of the progressive cerebellar degenerations. In most of these conditions treatment with dopamine agonists confers few, if any, benefits.

Parkinson's Disease

This idiopathic disorder of adults has its highest incidence in men over 40 years. The cause is unknown. Epidemio-logic studies have traced some examples to long-preceding influenza epidemics, and a few others to the illegally synthesized opiate MPTP. The occurrence of the latter effect hints that other exogenous agents may also contribute to the cause. Most patients, however, relate no hint of a specific cause or a family predisposition. The early motor deficits can be traced to incipient degeneration of nigral dopamine-transmitting cells. Later, refractory motor, autonomic, and mental abnormalities develop in many cases, implying degeneration of striatal receptor mechanisms plus, sometimes, degeneration of the locus ceruleus and the basal nucleus of Meynert.

Symptoms and Signs (Table 116–5)

Most cases of idiopathic parkinsonism begin with weakness, tremor, or both. Early in the disease, most patients describe motor slowness, stiffness, or easy fatigability in a single limb or hemiparetic distribution. The typical 4- to 7-Hz resting tremor affects approximately 70% but may not exist at all in some patients, especially those affected by prominent rigidity.

Patients with parkinsonism often have a diagnostically typical appearance. The body stoops stiffly forward, bent at the knees, hips, and neck, with arms held close to the sides and flexed at the elbows. Steps are small or shuffling, turns are taken slowly, and patients with advanced cases tend to accelerate their gait uncontrollably (festination) or, less often, to suffer from retropulsion. The outstretched, often trembling hands are extended at the wrist and thumb and flexed at the metacarpophalangeal joints (pill rolling posture). The face becomes masklike, unblinking, and often greasy. Speech becomes slurred, monotonous, and sometimes barely understandable. Handwriting becomes cramped and small in size. Deep tendon reflexes can be of average, slightly increased, or decreased amplitude. Percussion of the eyebrow brings out Myerson's sign, the failure of the blink reflex to adapt to repeated gentle taps. Other abnormal motor reflexes are absent early, but Babinski's sign sometimes emerges as a late change, reflecting the development of corticospinal tract dysfunction. The limbs of most patients display a nonspastic, steadily increasing resistance to movement, often interrupted by an 8-Hz tremor, conferring the classic "cogwheel" rigidity. Behavioral disorders are common. Many if not most patients become depressed in the early stages, and as many as half develop dementia by 7 or more years after onset.

Drug-induced parkinsonism can follow the taking of several antipsychotic agents given chronically in high doses. Chief present offenders are the phenothiazines and

TABLE 116–5	Major Features of Parkinson's Disease
Mental	Slowed thinking, mild dementia, depression, insomnia, drug effects (usually late changes)
Autonomic	Sexual difficulties, sweats, seborrhea, constipation, fatigue
Postural	Stooped, bent stance, festination; shuffling gait
Motor	Asthenia, tremor, hypokinesia, rigidity

butyrophenones, both of which pharmacologically block dopamine receptors in the striatum and may interfere with the dopamine output of nigral cells as well. Other toxic syndromes in addition to typical parkinsonism can occur with these agents, including a diffuse motor restlessness; acute dystonic reactions that dissipate with anticholinergic, antihistamine, or diazepam therapy; and oculogyric crises, which reflect an oculomotor dystonia. Drug-induced parkinsonism may somewhat benefit from anticholinergic agents but fails to subside with levodopa. The late complication of tardive dyskinesia is discussed below.

Treatment

Three major lines of treatment offer help to victims of Parkinson's disease (Table 116–6). First, the physician must understand and respond to the fear that the disease engenders, the high incidence of depression it causes, and the mild to moderate intellectual decline that sooner or later affects most cases. Second, a consistent plan for pharmacotherapy must be developed. Third, surgical procedures are increasingly considered to treat patients with refractory cases. Present approaches include thalamic stimulation, thalamotomy to relieve tremor, pallidotomy, and transplants of fetal nigral cells or tissue into the striatum. Thus far, all lie in the realm of investigative procedures and should be confined to use in major medical centers.

Most authorities in the United States currently try to defer treatment with dopaminergic drugs as long as possible in an effort to delay proportionately the late, toxic stages of levodopa therapy. (No well-established evidence supports this view.) Ordinarily, selegiline, the antioxidant drug that prevents MPTP-induced parkinsonism in animals, is initiated, usually at 5 mg twice a day. On theoretical grounds, many authorities recommend concurrent administration of vitamin E capsules. After an interval to allow any undesirable side effects of selegiline to develop (they are uncommon), a trial of amantadine, 100 mg twice a day, may be added. Unless clinically beneficial effects appear within 1 month, the latter drug should be discontinued and replaced by the anticholinergic trihexyphenidyl in small doses of 2 mg 3 times a day. The dose can be advanced slowly according to tolerance and symptom relief. Ultimately, these agents become insufficient to control symptoms of parkinsonism and either levodopa-carbidopa or pergolide (a dopamine agonist) must be used to attempt symptom control. When this stage is reached, it is wise to seek consultative assistance in further management, as several options exist to maximize long-term benefits.

Given over a long period of time or in high doses, both levodopa and the anticholinergic drugs can produce limiting side effects. Full benefits of levodopa seldom last more than 5 to 7 years, and large doses or long usage eventually produce uncontrollable abnormal movements of the trunk and extremities, termed dyskinesias. Furthermore, with time, the dose acts more briefly and is followed by intermittent, unpredictable periods of immobility (the "off" effect). Anticholinergic drugs are prone to cause dry mouth, visual blurring, and, occasionally, urinary retention; nightmares or daytime delirium can be a distressing consequence in the elderly.

Many patients become depressed during the course of Parkinson's disease, some suicidally so. Current antidepressant drugs, namely, the serotonin uptake inhibitors, may ameliorate these symptoms.

Progressive Supranuclear Palsy

This is an uncommon disorder of middle-aged or older persons marked by insidiously developing and progressive degenerative changes in the basal ganglia, basal nuclei, and cerebellum. Clinical features include a Parkinson-like rigidity and loss of postural reflexes combined with rigidity of the body and a postural dystonia marked by extension of the head. A progressive external ophthalmoplegia, consisting of paralysis first, of voluntary conjugate vertical gaze, and later of lateral gaze, is diagnostic. Full-range tonic abnormal oculocephalic reflex responses during arousal emerge concurrently and are easily elicited by bedside examination. A moderate dementia usually accompanies the motor changes. Dopamine-agonist drugs occasionally bring symptomatic improvement but progression is relentless.

Huntington's Disease

Huntington's disease is an uncommon inherited disorder transmitted as an autosomal dominant trait with complete penetrance. Recent research has succeeded in placing the Huntington gene, at chromosome 4p16.3. The annual gene product has been identified and labeled *huntington*. The abnormal gene itself contains an abnormal excess of the trinucleotide cytosine-adenine-guanine which both determines the 100% penetrance of the disease and serves as an accurate diagnostic measurement for gene carriers.

Huntington's disease affects striatal neurons, especially the small GABA-transmitting cells and scattered nerve cells in the frontal lobe cortex, claustrum, subthalamus, and cerebellar Purkinje and dentate systems. Gliosis is prominent. Neurochemically, GABA, acetylcholine, and angiotensin II decline in the striatum, with less severe

TABLE 116–6	Treatment of Parkinson's Disease (PD)
General measures	Maintain full physical and social activities.
Emotional	Outline cognitive and emotional encouragements and reassurances. If necessary, provide pharmacologic antidepressants.
Pharmacologic	Start with selegiline. Test effects of amantadine and anticholinergics; continue if tolerated *and* helpful. Add levodopa-carbidopa to selegiline if signs of PD remain prominent. If or when levodopa side effects develop, try slow-release preparations or dopa agonists.
Surgical	Last resort, still experimental and for experts only: stereotaxic thalamotomy or pallidotomy, transplants of dopamine-generating fetal cells or tissue.

reductions affecting substance P, cholecystokinin, and enkephalin. Somatostatin-containing neurons are selectively preserved.

The principal clinical changes include dyskinesia, altered behavior, and dementia. Most cases begin between ages 30 and 50. Early motor symptoms often include dystonic posturing and rigidity, but these changes give way to prominent choreiform activity in most affected adults. Signs of corticospinal tract dysfunction or sensory changes are lacking. Eccentricity, inappropriateness, a loss of social amenities, excess irritability, and sexual hyperactivity can mark the early stages. Occasionally, a schizophreniform illness precedes the motor abnormality by several years. Depression is common and suicide occurs frequently, in part because the progressing dementia often fails to blunt insight.

Diagnosis comes from recognizing the characteristic progressive generalized choreiform activity accompanied by behavioral or personality changes, especially in a person with a tell-tale family history. Spontaneous mutations are uncommon, but some affected persons inevitably lack knowledge of their true antecedents. Computed tomography (CT) or magnetic resonance imaging (MRI) scans in fully developed cases show cerebral atrophy, especially of the caudate and putamen, to a degree that is almost specific to the disease. Symptomatic treatment is aimed at minimizing the distressing movements, with reserpine or baclofen. Psychological symptoms may require major antipsychotic drugs for their control. Current genetic knowledge allows for accurate genetic counseling for family members of known cases, but in the absence of preventive measures many such persons decline the opportunity. The principal disorders to be considered in differential diagnosis are as follows: *Gilles de la Tourette's syndrome* most often is transmitted in an autosomal dominant pattern, but such patients have an earlier onset, show motor tics rather than chorea, and lack the behavioral-mental changes. *Senile chorea* is a rare disorder beginning in persons older than 60 years. Many but not all such cases have the Huntington gene. The abnormal movements usually are less prominent than in Huntington's, and the degree of dementia is less. *Hemiballismus* is a disorder of older persons. A reversible adult chorea also can develop in association with lupus erythematosus or thyrotoxicosis. It has an abrupt onset and gradually disappears within weeks or months.

Sydenham's Chorea

This now uncommon, self-limited disorder usually lasts 2 to 6 months and is considered an autoimmune disorder related to rheumatic fever. It occurs most often in children under the age of 15 years but can sometimes affect pregnant women or persons with systemic lupus erythematosus. Choreiform activity in Sydenham's chorea takes a fidgety, fragmented form, sometimes difficult to separate from habit tics. Affected children are clumsy and often dysarthric and walk unsteadily. An inability to sustain tonic movement, such as steadily protruding the tongue or sustaining an uninterrupted grasp of the examiner's fingers, is common to all the choreas.

Treatment is symptomatic. Recurrent attacks occur in as many as one third of affected children.

DYSTONIA

Dystonia can appear either as part of a primary basal ganglia disease or as a symptom secondary to a number of other conditions affecting those structures (Table 116–7). The chronic dystonias include a group of uncommon disorders of inherited or sporadic origin. A number of families have now been identified with a genetic marker at the 32–q34 region of chromosome 9. Also, a dopa-responsive dystonia has been linked to an abnormality located on chromosome 9. The specific cause and pathophysiology are unknown for any of these conditions, and no neuropathologic changes have been found consistently in the brain. An imbalance of neurotransmitter function in the basal ganglia has been postulated, but specific neurochemical candidates remain elusive, inasmuch as both dopamine excess and presumed dopamine receptor blockade can induce acute transient dystonic movement.

Severe generalized dystonia, sometimes called *dystonia musculorum deformans,* begins predominantly in young children and adolescents, most often beginning with an equinovarus posturing of the foot or a tonically flexed hand, then spreading to involve the neck, face, and trunk in nearly continuous, recurrent, intense, involuntary, asymmetric contractions. The movements, which characteristically lead to prolonged spasms, eventually produce bizarre contortions with severe musculotendinous contractures. Ensuing bone deformities can produce scoliosis,

TABLE 116–7	The Major Dystonias

Primary Dystonia		
Conditions	**Inheritance**	**Age of Onset**
Generalized dystonia	Autosomal recessive Autosomal dominant Sporadic	Childhood Adolescence or adulthood
Focal dystonia Foot-leg or hand-arm	Inherited or sporadic	Mostly adulthood, occasionally late
Blepharospasm	Sporadic	Late adulthood
Facial mandibular (Meige's syndrome)	Sporadic	Late adulthood
Spasmodic torticollis	Mostly sporadic, occasionally autosomal recessive	Adulthood Middle adulthood
Occupational dystonia Writer's cramp Musician's cramp	Sporadic	Early-middle adulthood

Secondary Dystonia	
Chronic	**Acute**
Wilson's disease Huntington's disease Postencephalitic Severe cerebral anoxia-ischemia Manganese poisoning	Head trauma Phenothiazines Butyrophenones Levodopa

chest deformities, and a foreshortening of natural height. Lesser degrees of the illness can arise during adulthood and tend to produce restricted impairments of the lower or upper extremities.

Spasmodic torticollis is the most common of the focal dystonias. It affects predominantly the muscles of the neck and shoulders, which bilaterally and simultaneously contract to produce recurrent unilateral head turning or head extension. Elevations of the shoulder and, often, platysmal contractions may accompany the movements of the head and neck. In mild cases the movement can be restrained by the subject's placing gentle antagonistic pressure against the chin or occiput. More severe examples can spread to produce spastic dysphoma and hand-arm dystonia. Discussion of other forms of focal dystonia can be found in the references.

Treatment of the dystonias is unsatisfactory. High doses of the anticholinergic drug trihexyphenidyl somewhat relieve a few patients. The use of carbamazepine or diazepam occasionally has been reported favorably in others. Stereotaxic surgical attacks on the thalamus benefit some children with severe generalized dystonia but carry a high risk of complications and must be regarded as desperation measures. Recently, investigators have reported success with judiciously repeated fractional injection of botulinum toxin into the periocular muscles of patients with incapacitating blepharospasm.

DYSKINESIA

The dopamine-induced dyskinesia of chronic treated parkinsonism has been described above. *Tardive dyskinesia* follows the chronic ingestion and, often, withdrawal of antidopaminergic antipsychotic drugs. The activity consists of abnormal, semirhythmic involuntary movements affecting the mouth (lingual-oral-buccal), trunk, or extremities. Once it starts, the condition almost always remains permanently. A few cases are known to have appeared within a few days of phenothiazine medication, but in most instances, the complication follows prolonged drug use. Its appearance can be delayed until weeks, months, or even years after stopping the drugs. The facial movements most often consist of chewing, tongue darting, and grimacing. Other forms include repeated flexion and extension of the trunk, piano playing–like successive contraction of the fingers and toes, and repetitive steppings of the feet while standing erect. Supersensitivity of the dopamine receptors of the basal ganglia is believed to be the cause. Reserpine or, in the presence of continued psychosis, a higher dose of antidopaminergic antipsychotics sometimes bring partial relief. Tardive dyskinesia is a disfiguring, seriously disturbing, and frequent complication. The potential for producing it should discourage the use of phenothiazine drugs for any but serious medical-psychiatric problems. *Meige's syndrome,* a dystonia involving the jaw and lower face, somewhat resembles tardive dyskinesia but produces slower, more twisting movements. There is no necessary history of antipsychotic medication. Baclofen or valproate has been reported to improve selective cases.

REFERENCES

Fahn S, Bressman SB, Brin MF, Greene P, Duroisin RC, Burke RE: Movement disorders. *In* Rowland LP (ed.): Merritt's Textbook of Neurology. 9th ed. Baltimore, Williams & Wilkins, 1996, pp 695–736.
Jankovic J: The extrapyramidal disorders. *In* Bennett JC, Plum F (eds.): Cecil Textbook of Medicine. 20th ed. Philadelphia, WB Saunders, 1996, pp 2042–2049.

C. The Major Cerebellar Ataxias

The cerebellum receives afferent information from the limbs and trunk, from the vestibular-cochlear apparatus, and from pontine relays derived from the descending corticospinal tract. It divides its output among the vestibular nuclei, structures involved with axial and distal extremity motor control, and, in large measure, the premotor-motor cortex via the red nucleus and thalamus (see Fig. 116–3). Evidence indicates that the cerebellum influences both the planning and smooth regulation of voluntary movement by its projections to cerebral cortical motor areas.

SIGNS AND MECHANISMS OF CEREBELLAR DYSFUNCTION

Disorders of the cerebellum or its principal connections produce characteristic *symptoms* and *signs,* including easy fatigability; *ataxia* of gait; an inability to control the range of movement, producing under- or over-shoot; impairment of rapidly alternating movements; an inability to synergize motion around two or more joints; *postural* or *intention tremor; dysarthria;* and, possibly, *nystagmus* with the fast component toward the side of the cerebellar lesion.

Ataxias linked to the cerebellum and its major afferent and efferent connections fall into three major anatomic-symptomatic groups (Table 116–8). These include (1) diseases affecting predominantly the afferent spinocerebellar and associated spinal pathways, (2) diseases or disorders involving the cerebellum proper and its immediate outflow tracts, and (3) diseases in which cerebellar involvement comprises only part of a widespread degeneration of central nervous system (CNS) structures. Clinically, the signs and symptoms of the three categories sometimes overlap, but distinction usually is possible. Mass lesions or demyelinating disorders affecting the cerebellar system usually can be identified by computed tomography (CT) or magnetic resonance imaging (MRI). The following paragraphs describe the principal degenerative disorders affecting the system.

Spinocerebellar disease produces a wide-based, lurching sensory ataxia due to impairment of ascending proprioceptive and spinocerebellar pathways. At their worst, patients stagger from side to side, stepping with high, irregularly placed feet that often pound the floor as

TABLE 116–8	Principal Syndromes of the Cerebellum and its Connections

I. Primarily Spinocerebellar Signs and Symptoms
  A. Inherited spinocerebellar ataxias (childhood or adolescent onset, chronic course, few positive sensory symptoms)
    1. Molecular genetic defect uncertain: Friedreich's ataxia (chromosoma 9) and its variants;
    2. Genetic defect known: phytanic acid α-hydroxylase deficiency (Refsum); deficiency of α-tocopherol transfer protein and abetalipoproteinemia
  B. Acquired spinal sensory ataxia (acute, subacute, or insidious onset): polyneuropathy; sensory polyradiculopathy (tabes dorsalis); vitamin B_{12} deficiency; spinal cord damage (e.g., multiple sclerosis, neoplasm)

II. Primarily Cerebellar Symptoms
  A. Inherited autosomal dominant and sporadic adult degenerations: restricted olivopontocerebellar atrophy (young to mid-adulthood); ataxia-telangiectasia (childhood onset)
  B. Developmental abnormalities (onset of signs varies, progressive): basilar impression; Arnold-Chiari malformation
  C. Nutritional-immunologic (mostly adult onset, acute or subacute course)
    1. Acute, reversible parainfectious cerebellar ataxia of children
    2. Alcoholic-nutritional cerebellar degeneration
    3. Paraneoplastic cerebellar–brain stem degeneration
  D. Structural cerebellar lesions (acute or subacute course): trauma, neoplasms, hemorrhage, anoxia-ischemia, severe hyperthermia
  E. Intoxication (acute or subacute or chronic): alcohol; sedatives; anxiolytics; phenytoin; anticancer agents

III. Cerebellar-Plus Symptoms
  A. Autosomal inherited or sporadic system degenerations (mid-adulthood onset, gradual progression)
    1. Olivopontocerebellar atrophy (OPCA) plus, variably, spasticity, parkinsonism, sensory changes, optic atrophy, retinitis pigmentosa, ophthalmoplegia, dementia
    2. Shy-Drager syndrome of autonomic insufficiency plus parkinsonism plus ataxia (multiple system atrophy)
  B. Acquired disseminated disorders affecting cerebellar and other systems (e.g., cancer, abscess)

they walk. Large afferent fibers carrying position and vibratory sense from the lower extremities degenerate, leading to rombergism and an accompanying loss of deep tendon reflexes. Sometimes, involvement of descending corticospinal pathways results in pathologic reflexes, whereas direct cerebellar involvement can impair coordination of oculomotor as well as upper extremity muscles.

Within the cerebellum itself, damage or degeneration of the posterior midline *floccular nodular area* produces a narrow-based ataxia with a tendency to fall backwards plus nystagmus on lateral and, sometimes, downward gaze. Dysfunction of the more anterior midline *vermis* and *anterior lobe* is more common and accompanies especially deep midline cerebellar tumors, alcohol-nutritional deficiencies or paraneoplastic degeneration. A broad-based, stiff-legged ataxia often is accompanied in severe cases by an oscillating, rhythmic sustention tremor of the trunk and lower extremities (titubation). Deep tendon reflexes tend to be accentuated, but nystagmus is uncommon unless Wernicke's disease (see Chapter 113) disease concurrently affects the vestibular nuclei.

Lateral hemispheric lesions characteristically produce subtle signs consisting of mild ipsilateral incoordination and perhaps hypotonia. If they directly involve the cerebellar roof nuclei or outflow pathways, they cause in the upper extremities the classic signs of cerebellar incoordination and tremor as described in the first paragraph of this section. Lesions that expand the cerebellum to compress the adjacent brain stem or infiltrate it produce the additional symptoms and signs of headache, nausea, vomiting, cranial nerve abnormalities, or long tract dysfunction.

PRIMARY CEREBELLAR DEGENERATIONS

Many forms of injury, deficiency, or trauma can injure cerebellar function, but those deriving from genetically related forces provide the greatest challenge (Table 116–9). The primary degenerations include a heterogeneous, uncommon group of system degenerations in which neuroaxonal death variously affects afferent pathways to the cerebellum, the cerebellum itself, and, often, trans-synaptically connected CNS structures. The group often is designated as *olivopontocerebellar atrophy (OPCA)*. The abnormal chromosome has been found in most variants, with the specific gene and sometimes abnormal gene product identified in many. Although one can identify more or less distinct syndromes of spinocerebellar and primary cerebellar degeneration, different diseases may overlap considerably in their neuropathology; phenotypes can differ clinically in single kindreds. Related conditions include peroneal muscular atrophy, other degenerative neuropathies, hereditary spastic paraplegia, motor neuron disease, atypical forms of parkinsonism, and the Shy-Drager form of progressive autonomic insufficiency. Such combinations sometimes are referred to as multiple systems atrophy. Most of the CNS system degenerations are uncommon, but their specific molecular abnormalities are rapidly being discovered. Three of the autosomal types, although possessing genes located on different chromosomes, demonstrate abnormally long cy-

TABLE 116–9	Principal Causes of Spinocerebellar and Cerebellar Ataxias in Late Adolescents and Adults

I. *Non-inherited*
  A. Infections
    1. Parainfections in children (reversible) associated with viral infection (measles)
    2. Paraneoplastic cerebellar degeneration (anti-Yo antibody)
    3. Early in Creutzfeld-Jakob (prion) disease
  B. Metabolic
    1. Systemic: hepatic encephalopathy, hyperammonemia, hypothyroidism
    2. Mitochondrial disease (Ramsay-Hunt; Kearns Sayre syndrome; MERRF [myoclonic epilepsy with ragged red fibers])
    3. Defective DNA repair; ataxia telangiectasia, Cocayne's syndrome
    4. Cerebellar infarction or hemorrhage
    5. Alcoholic thiamine deficiency
    6. Demyelinating and deficiency (B_{12}) disease
    7. Severe anoxia and hyperthermia
II. *Inherited*
  A. Autosomal recessive ataxias: Friedreich's (mostly children-adolescents)
  B. Late-onset autosomal dominant ataxias: olivopontocerebellar atrophy (OPCA) and its variants

tosine-adenosine-guanine (CAG) repeats on the abnormal gene. The following section describes the most frequent types; the references contain more extensive discussions as well as descriptions of the rarer entities.

Friedreich's Ataxia

Friedreich's ataxia, the prototypic spinocerebellar degeneration, affects children and young adults. The syndrome can be produced by more than one defect but the gene responsible for the most commonly identified phenotype locates to chromosome 9. It can be transmitted in autosomal dominant or autosomal recessive patterns, but sporadic cases are common. Neuronal loss involves the dorsal root ganglia and the spinal cells of origin of the spinocerebellar tracts, with degeneration beginning caudally and progressing rostrally. Axonal loss and demyelination affect the spinal nerves, the dorsal column, and the spinocerebellar tracts as well as the descending corticospinal tract. Some cases show cell loss in the cerebellum and occasionally in brain stem nuclei as well.

Friedreich's ataxia typically begins insidiously, usually before age 10 years, and progresses steadily. Most patients become unable to walk unassisted during their third decade. Position and vibratory sense are lost initially in the lower extremities, and this plus the corticospinal defect leads to an increasing sensorimotor staggering ataxia accompanied by atrophic, hypotonic lower limbs with areflexia and extensor plantar responses. By their late teens or 20s, most patients develop dysarthria and many have nystagmus. Orthopedic changes include a characteristic pes cavus deformity (which can affect some family members as the sole mark of the abnormal trait) as well as a mild to moderate scoliosis and, sometimes, a high arched palate. Low intelligence affects some victims from the start, whereas a few appear to decline mentally as they proceed through their 20's. Associated, less common, abnormalities include optic atrophy, retinal degeneration, deafness, and anterior horn cell degeneration. Many victims develop cardiac enlargement and most show conduction defects on the electrocardiogram (ECG). Some develop heart failure; few survive beyond 40 years. Diagnosis usually is apparent from the patient's appearance and physical findings. Among laboratory tests, none is specific except in the specific deficiency syndromes, most of which appear sufficiently distinctive clinically to prompt appropriate biochemical study. Visual evoked potentials are abnormally slow in most cases of either spinocerebellar or primary cerebellar ataxia, and somatosensory evoked potentials tend to be particularly slowed in Friedreich's ataxia but not in olivopontocerebellar atrophy. The spinal fluid is normal.

Roussy-Lévy ataxia closely resembles Friedreich's ataxia except that the condition runs a much slower course, often with little progression into adulthood. Deep tendon reflexes along with position and vibration sensations are spared, and extensor plantar responses fail to develop. Other family members may show evidence of the more common peroneal muscular atrophy or hereditary spastic paraplegia.

Olivopontocerebellar Degeneration (OPCD)

This loose category includes a group of uncommon, progressive degenerative disorders of adult life that produce cerebellar dysfunction with or without signs of degeneration in other motor-sensory systems, including the spinal cord, cerebellar outflow pathways, basal ganglia, autonomic nervous system, optic nerves, and even cerebral cortex.

Pathologically, the most frequent denominator of the OPCD group is degeneration of the inferior olive and the pontine-cerebellar relay nuclei, with degeneration and demyelination of their respective climbing axons into the cerebellum. Trans-synaptic death occurs in the target cells of the cerebellar cortex. Less consistent abnormalities affect neurons and their axons in the more remote neurologic structures mentioned above. Degeneration of the basal ganglia and central autonomic neurons usually is prominent in the Shy-Drager variant.

OPCD can affect either sex, as early as age 20 but most often begins between the ages of 40 and 60 years. Transmission is largely autosomal dominant but sporadic cases are far from rare. Furthermore, identical genotypes often result is dissimilar phenotypes. Currently gene loci associated with autosomal dominant ataxia include 6p22–p23, 12p12–ter, 12q23–24.1, 16q24–ter, 14q24–q32 and, 14q24.3–qter. Three of these contain the CAG triple repeat abnormality. Progression is relatively rapid, and most patients become totally dependent within 6 years of onset. Initial symptoms and signs include a relatively wide-based ataxia accompanied by incoordination of the upper extremities and dysarthria. Dysmetria usually remains worse in the lower than the upper extremities. The limbs become hypotonic but deep tendon reflexes are preserved except when spinal degeneration occurs. Most patients develop nystagmus. Among those with basal ganglia involvement, parkinsonian signs emerge during the moderately advanced stages of the illness. Babinski signs and other manifestations of corticospinal tract dysfunction occur late if at all. Some patients develop palatal myoclonus. Functional dementia accompanies the late stages of approximately one third of cases.

No specific test is diagnostic of OPCD. Brain stem auditory evoked potentials are abnormal in a majority. Differential diagnosis requires ruling out the conditions listed in sections II and III of Table 115–8. MRI usually discloses cerebellar and pontine atrophy and rules out other structural lesions. Nutritional disease and possible drug intoxication can be identified by the history. Paraneoplastic syndromes are discussed in Chapter 120.

The cause being unknown, only symptomatic treatment can be offered.

Ataxia-Telangiectasia

This disorder affects spinal cord, cerebellum, and basal ganglia functions. The illness begins in early childhood, inherited as an autosomal recessive trait with the gene mapping to chromosome 11q. Progressive ataxia of gait, incoordinated upper extremities, facial and appendicular choreoathetosis, and opsoclonus are characteristic. Most affected children become wheelchair-bound and begin to show mental retardation by the second decade. Prominent telangiectases stud the conjunctivae, the ears, the nose, and the cheek areas. The disease includes thymic hypoplasia with a severe deficiency of IgA. Patients suffer a high incidence of endocrine abnormalities, respiratory infections, chromosomal aberrations, and neoplasms. Most die before age 20 years.

REFERENCES

Harding AE: Cerebellar and spinocerebellar disorders. In Bradley WG, Daroff RB, Fenichel GM, Marsden CD (eds.): Neurology in Clinical Practice. 2nd ed. Boston, Butterworth-Heinemann, 1996, pp 1773–1792.

Rosenberg RN: Autosomal dominant cerebellar phenotypes: The genotype has settled the issue. Neurology 1995; 45:1–5.

D. Mechanical Lesions of the Spine and Spinal Cord

The spinal cord interconnects the brain with the neurologic structures serving the extremities and trunk. It carries sensory fibers from the periphery to the brain and motor instructions, including those that control autonomic function (e.g., bladder and bowel), from the brain to the periphery. Fibers subserving different sensory modalities (e.g., pain, temperature, vibration, position) are sorted into different pathways in the spinal cord (see Fig. 122–1). Moreover, the different modalities cross to the contralateral side at different levels. Descending motor fibers that lie contralateral to their target nuclei in the brain become ipsilateral in the spinal cord (see Fig. 116–1). As a result, dissociated sensory and motor abnormalities (Table 116–10) mark syndromes of the spinal cord and help the examiner to identify the site of the lesion in both the cephalocaudal direction (e.g., arm weakness implies a cervical cord lesion, paraplegia a thoracic or lumbar lesion) and also in the transverse plane. Such localization may also suggest a diagnosis. For example, Brown-Séquard syndrome is a common presenting finding in extradural tumors and radiation myelopathy, whereas a central cord or anterior commissure lesion suggests trauma or syringomyelia.

SPINAL CORD NEOPLASMS

Neoplastic growths that cause nerve root or spinal cord disorders can begin in the paravertebral, extradural, intradural, or intramedullary compartments. Most neoplasms that cause spinal cord compression are extradural and metastatic. Most extradural neoplasms originate in the vertebral body and compress spinal roots or cord without invading them. Most intradural neoplasms also cause

TABLE 116–10	**Clinical Signs of Spinal Cord Lesions**	
Anatomic Site	**Neurologic Findings**	**Pathologic Example(s)**
Transverse myelopathy	Paraplegia or quadriplegia with sensory and autonomic loss	Trauma Cord compression by tumor
Brown-Séquard syndrome (hemicord section)	Ipsilateral spastic hemiparesis or leg-only paresis with position and vibration loss; and contralateral pin and temperature sensation loss	Radiation myelopathy
Posterolateral column syndrome	Spastic paraparesis with position and vibration loss but preserved pin and temperature sensation	Multiple sclerosis AIDS myelopathy
Anterior cord syndrome	Spastic quadriparesis or paraparesis with pin and temperature sensation loss but preserved position and vibration sensation	Anterior spinal artery occlusion
Central cord syndrome (cervical)	Flaccid weakness of arms with normal legs ± pin and temperature sensation loss	Trauma (hematomyelia)
Anterior commissure syndrome	Bilateral loss of pin and temperature sensation with or without flaccid weakness; sometimes sacral segments spared	Syringomyelia

AIDS = Acquired immunodeficiency syndrome.

symptoms by compressing spinal roots or cord without invading, but unlike extradural neoplasms, the majority are benign and slow-growing. Intramedullary neoplasms cause symptoms by both invading and compressing spinal structures; the tumors may be either benign or malignant.

Paravertebral Tumors

Neoplastic lesions that begin in or metastasize to the extraspinal paravertebral space often cause serious and perplexing neurologic problems. The tumor may extend longitudinally within the paravertebral space, progressively compressing nerve roots as it grows. At times, the tumor may grow through an intervertebral foramen and compress not only the nerve root but also the spinal cord. Rarely, spinal cord symptoms may be caused by ischemia from compression of radicular arteries that supply the spinal cord. If the tumor lies lateral to the immediate paravertebral space, it may compress the brachial, lumbar, or sacral plexus, causing symptoms similar to root compression but with a different pattern of sensory and motor loss.

The symptoms of extravertebral tumors begin insidiously with severe, unrelenting pain, often with a burning quality. The pain is localized just lateral to the spine and radiates, bandlike, in the distribution of the involved dermatome or dermatomes (see Fig. 122–2). If the lesion involves abdominal or thoracic roots, objective motor and sensory changes often are minimal, but autonomic changes may be prominent or the only neurologic sign. *Hyperhidrosis* occurring in a band coinciding with the site of the pain strongly suggests the diagnosis. When the tumor involves cervical or lumbar roots, the pain may be soon followed by numbness in the fingertips or toes with accompanying weakness and reflex diminution, depending on the roots involved. Autonomic changes, including anhidrosis or hyperhidrosis, can affect the arm or leg, whereas Horner's syndrome and/or diaphragmatic paralysis often accompany cervical or upper thoracic paravertebral tumors. The diagnosis of paravertebral tumors is best established by MRI scan at the level suggested by the clinical findings. The MRI also can determine whether the lesion has grown through the intervertebral foramen or has eroded vertebral bodies.

The differential diagnosis of paravertebral tumor includes several disorders that can cause paravertebral pain with or without compression of nerve roots. *Psychophysiologic muscle tension* syndromes often cause paravertebral low back or neck pain. In some instances, there may be radiation of the pain, but usually in a nondermatomal distribution. Examination often reveals marked tenderness of muscle, which sometimes can be relieved by injecting the trigger point with saline solution or a local anesthetic. Temporary improvement of pain after such injections does not imply that structural disease is absent, because trigger points can equally well be a reaction to spinal or nerve root disease. In muscle tension syndrome, autonomic, sensory, or motor changes are not present. Disease of the kidneys and other viscera lying in the retroperitoneal space may cause pain similar to that of paravertebral tumors, but the pain usually does not radiate and is not associated with autonomic, motor, or sensory changes. Percussion of the involved viscera reproduces the pain that is usually described as a dull ache rather than a neurogenic burning pain. Entrapment neuropathies occasionally mimic the symptoms of paravertebral tumor.

The management of paravertebral masses depends on the diagnosis. In patients known to have cancer, particularly lymphomas or carcinomas of the breast or lung, the tumor can be assumed to be metastatic and should be treated with radiation therapy and, if available, chemotherapy. If the patient has no known primary lesion, resection may be attempted, both to establish a diagnosis and to decompress the nerve roots. Once biopsy establishes diagnosis, further therapy such as radiation or chemotherapy can be chosen.

Extradural Tumors

Extradural neoplasms can compress spinal roots and cord in one of two ways. Either they arise in vertebrae surrounding the spinal cord and grow into the epidural space, or they arise in the paravertebral space and grow through the intervertebral foramen so as to compress the cord without involving either vertebral or paravertebral structures. Most extradural neoplasms are metastatic from carcinomas of the breast, lung, prostate, or kidney or from malignant melanoma. Some extradural neoplasms arise de novo in the vertebral bodies (e.g., chordoma, osteogenic sarcoma, myeloma, chondrosarcoma). A minority of extradural neoplasms are benign (e.g., chordoma, osteoma, osteoid osteoma, angioma). Pain, the first symptom, may precede other symptoms of spinal cord compression by weeks or months, depending on the rate of growth of the tumor. Rarely, extradural neoplasms may be painless, with the first symptoms being those of spinal cord dysfunction. The first spinal cord symptoms other than pain usually consist of corticospinal tract dysfunction with weakness, spasticity, and hyperreflexia, followed by paresthesias with loss of vibration and position sense. Unless the lesion compresses the conus medullaris or the cauda equina, bladder and bowel dysfunction are late signs. As with other causes of spinal cord compression, extradural neoplasms cause symptoms first distally and later proximally. Thus, even thoracic and cervical neoplasms generally cause weakness and numbness in the legs before trunk and upper extremity muscles are involved. The diagnosis of extradural spinal cord compression must be suspected by the history of pain followed by signs and symptoms of spinal cord dysfunction and confirmed by imaging studies. In about 85% of patients suffering from extradural spinal cord compression, plain radiographs reveal bone lesions at the site of compression. In the few remaining patients, radionuclide bone scan or CT or MRI scan may demonstrate a bone lesion. The diagnosis of extradural spinal cord compression and its localization can be made by either MRI or myelography. The differential diagnosis of extradural neoplasms includes inflammatory disease of bone and epidural abscess (e.g., vertebral tuberculosis, bacterial osteomyelitis), acute or subacute epidural hematomas, herniated intervertebral discs, spondylosis, and, very rarely, extreme extramedullary hematopoiesis (in patients with severe and chronic anemias) or epidural lipomatosis (in patients on chronic steroid therapy). A definitive diagnosis can be made by biopsy of the lesion during the course of a decompressive operation or by percutaneous needle biopsy of the involved vertebral body.

The treatment of extradural neoplasms depends on the cause. Most neoplasms that cause extradural spinal cord compression are malignant and progress rapidly. Thus, the early diagnosis and vigorous emergency treatment of extradural spinal cord compression is mandatory (Table 116–11). The treatment includes corticosteroids (dexamethasone, 16 to 100 mg daily) to decrease spinal cord edema. In patients not known to be suffering from a primary cancer, metastatic disease remains the most common cause of extradural spinal cord compression, but a definitive diagnosis can be made only by biopsy. Such patients should begin corticosteroid therapy followed by surgery with removal of as much tumor as possible for both diagnostic and therapeutic purposes. When a primary cancer already has been diagnosed, treatment consists of radiation therapy and chemotherapy (if an effective agent

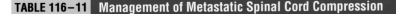

| TABLE 116-11 | Management of Metastatic Spinal Cord Compression |

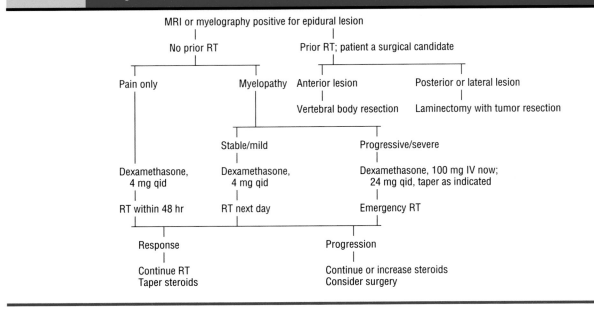

IV = Intravenous; MRI = magnetic resonance imaging; RT = radiation therapy.

is available). Benign extradural tumors require surgery and usually can be completely removed.

Intradural Extramedullary Tumors

Most intradural tumors are benign. Meningiomas and neurofibromas are the two most common types. Teratomas, arachnoid cysts, and lipomas are less common causes. *Meningiomas* occur especially in middle-aged and elderly women, predominantly in the thoracic spinal cord. Another common site is the foramen magnum. Meningiomas grow slowly. Pain is the first symptom in most patients, but in about 25% the growth is painless. Because meningiomas are often located on the posterior aspect of the cord, paresthesias and sensory changes beginning distally in the lower extremities are a frequent early symptom and are often mistaken for peripheral neuropathy. As the disease progresses, however, the development of corticospinal tract signs indicates the spinal origin of the symptoms. Even when spinal cord signs and symptoms are obvious, the occasional lack of pain may lead one to suspect a degenerative or demyelinating disease such as multiple sclerosis rather than a neoplasm. In patients with meningiomas, the lumbar puncture reveals an elevated cerebrospinal fluid (CSF) protein content well above that found in degenerative or demyelinating diseases. MRI with contrast enhancement usually establishes the diagnosis. The treatment of spinal cord compression from meningiomas is surgical removal. Because the tumor grows slowly and the cord can adapt to compression, even patients with severe neurologic disability often recover fully.

The second most common cause of intradural spinal cord compression is *neurofibroma*. Because these tumors usually arise from the dorsal root, radicular pain is often the first symptom, preceding spinal cord compression by months or years. When spinal cord compression develops, it progresses slowly. Some patients with spinal neurofibromas suffer from neurofibromatosis (see Chapter 122). As neurofibromas grow through the intervertebral foramen, they enlarge it, a finding appreciated by an appropriately positioned radiograph. The CSF protein is almost always elevated. The diagnosis is established by MRI scan. Surgical extirpation of the lesion usually leads to recovery.

Occasionally, metastatic tumors involving the leptomeninges produce intradural but extramedullary mass lesions. Pain is almost always a prominent early symptom, and spinal cord compression develops more rapidly than it does with the more benign intradural tumors. In addition, malignant cells are usually found on CSF examination. The glucose concentration may be low and the protein concentration elevated. The treatment of intradural malignant neoplasms is radiation therapy and chemotherapy. Complete surgical extirpation is almost always impossible.

Intramedullary Tumors

The most common intramedullary spinal tumors are astrocytomas (usually benign) and ependymomas. Other tumors that occasionally cause intramedullary spinal lesions are hemangioblastomas, lipomas, and metastases (Fig. 116-4). Pain is an early symptom of most intramedullary tumors, and signs of spinal cord dysfunction progress rapidly or slowly depending on the growth characteristics of the tumor. Intramedullary tumors are often associated with syringomyelia, the syrinx sometimes lying at a dis-

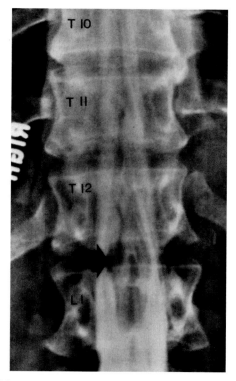

Figure 116-4

An intramedullary metastasis. A man with oat cell carcinoma of lung, in remission, complained of progressive weakness of the lower extremities and loss of bladder, bowel, and sexual function. A metrizamide myelogram revealed an area of enlargement at the conus medullaris *(arrow)*, indicating a hematogenous metastasis to the spinal cord.

tance from the primary tumor and producing its own symptoms of spinal dysfunction. The diagnosis is established by MRI. In some patients with long-standing benign intramedullary lesions, plain radiographs of the spine may show widening of the spinal canal and erosion of the pedicles. The differential diagnosis includes intramedullary abscesses and syringomyelia without tumor. A definitive diagnosis is established by biopsy. Successful surgical removal of intramedullary tumors is possible, particularly with ependymomas and hemangioblastomas but sometimes with gliomas as well. A highly skilled and experienced surgeon, is necessary for tumors to be removed without increasing neurologic disability. If the tumor cannot be totally excised, postoperative radiation may delay recurrence.

VASCULAR DISORDERS OF THE SPINAL CANAL

Extradural, intradural, and intramedullary vascular disorders all can cause spinal cord compression. The most common and serious extradural vascular disease is *spinal epidural hematoma.* Hemorrhage into the spinal epidural space may occur spontaneously or be associated with trauma, a bleeding diathesis, or a vascular malformation. The condition occurs particularly among patients being treated with anticoagulants. It may occasionally follow

lumbar puncture, particularly in patients with bleeding abnormalities or those receiving anticoagulants. The hemorrhage usually arises from the epidural venous plexus and tends to collect over the dorsum of the spinal cord, covering several segments. The clinical picture is characterized by the sudden or rapid onset of severe localized back pain and spinal cord dysfunction, often leading to complete paraplegia or cauda equina symptoms in several hours. If the patient has a known bleeding disorder, the clinical diagnosis is easily established. In patients without known bleeding or clotting disorders, the differential diagnosis includes acute epidural abscess and acute transverse myelopathy. Most patients showing spinal cord compression require emergency surgical evacuation. The longer the delay in decompression, the less likely is recovery.

Spinal arteriovenous malformations may cause symptoms by hemorrhage (Fig. 116-5), compression, or ischemia. Spinal subarachnoid hemorrhage is characterized by the sudden onset of back pain, often with a radicular component, with or without the development of signs of spinal cord compression. A lumbar puncture reveals evidence of subarachnoid hemorrhage with red cells, xanthochromic spinal fluid, and usually an elevated protein concentration. The diagnosis of spinal subarachnoid hemorrhage often can be suspected clinically because symptoms begin with back pain rather than with headache as in intracranial hemorrhage.

Vascular malformations within the substance of the spinal cord may give rise to intramedullary hemorrhage (hematomyelia) as well as subarachnoid hemorrhage. The sudden development of partial or complete transverse myelopathy is the most common onset.

Spinal arteriovenous malformations may gradually compress the spinal cord or produce episodes of spinal ischemia. In such cases, patients present with slowly progressive or episodically worsening symptoms. Transient

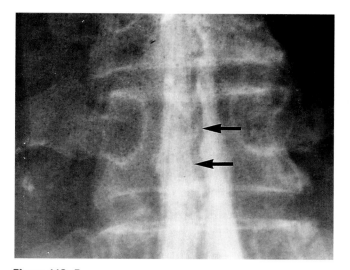

Figure 116-5

Spinal arteriovenous malformation. A metrizamide myelogram demonstrates a tangle of abnormal vessels *(arrows)* on the surface of the cord.

exacerbation of symptoms may occur in association with menstrual periods or pregnancy.

Complete or partial recovery of function can follow episodes of spinal cord ischemia or even small hemorrhages. The unchanging localization of the attacks and the prominence of pain help differentiate symptoms caused by arteriovenous malformations from other recurrent neurologic disorders such as multiple sclerosis. MRI usually identifies an arteriovenous malformation. Advances in microsurgery and invasive neuroradiology have increased considerably the chances for satisfactory removal or obliteration.

INHERITED AND DEVELOPMENTAL SPINAL STRUCTURAL DISORDERS

Congenital anomalies of the spine are common and are often encountered on radiographs of patients with or without associated neck or low back pain. Some congenital anomalies such as *spina bifida occulta* are so common as to be considered variants of normal and are probably never responsible in and of themselves for low back pain. Other congenital anomalies that are usually asymptomatic but are possible causes of neck or back pain include *facet tropism* (misalignment of the facets on the two sides of the corresponding vertebral body; several authorities believe that this increases rotational stress on the facet joints and may cause back pain); *transitional vertebrae* (e.g., sacralization of a lumbar vertebra or lumbarization of a sacral vertebra), altering spinal mechanics, resulting in instability and mechanical stress and sometimes producing back pain; and *spondylolisthesis* (forward slipping of one vertebral body onto another, caused by a defect between the articular facets).

A third group of congenital anomalies of the spine are likely to cause not only neck or back pain but also neurologic disability. These include basilar impression, which is often associated with Arnold-Chiari malformation. Severe spinal scoliosis or kyphosis, congenital stenosis of the lumbar or cervical spinal canal, anterior and lateral spinal meningoceles, and diastematomyelia are other causes of back pain and neurologic disability.

Abnormalities of the Craniocervical Junction

Basilar impression consists of invagination of the odontoid process into the foramen magnum. Occasionally the condition arises from occipital bone softening due to Paget's disease, fibrous dysplasia, or cancer. More often basilar impression occurs as a congenital defect, often associated with anomalies of the foramen magnum, the Arnold-Chiari malformation, or syringomyelia. Symptoms of congenital basilar impression may be delayed until the third or fourth decade of life and reflect the presence of either vertebral artery compression-ischemia or direct medullopontine compression-displacement. Occipital headache, vertigo, nystagmus, dysarthria, dysphagia, ataxia, abnormalities of central respiratory control, and

long tract signs begin insidiously and progress gradually. Many patients develop a secondary obstructive hydrocephalus. Diagnosis is suggested by the clinical findings plus an abnormally short neck. MRI reveals not only the protrusion of the odontoid process above the foramen magnum but also can identify the presence of an Arnold-Chiari malformation.

The *Arnold-Chiari malformation* is a developmental displacement of the cerebellar tonsils through the foramen magnum, with (type II) or without (type I) elongation of the medulla and lower end of the fourth ventricle into the cervical canal. Symptoms can resemble those described for basilar impression, can be due entirely to obstructive hydrocephalus, or can reflect a progressive cerebellar ataxia. Rarely, intermittent headache and/or syncope may be the only symptom(s). MRI is diagnostic (Fig. 116–6). Treatment of either basilar impression or the Arnold-Chiari malformation causing progressive neurologic deficits consists of surgical decompression of the foramen magnum or, when appropriate, ventricular shunting to relieve hydrocephalus.

Syringomyelia refers to a cavity within the central spinal cord, arising most often at the cervical level and proceeding caudally (see Fig. 116–6). Syringomyelia can arise either as a congenital abnormality or in association with spinal canal/cord mass lesions. In the congenital form spinal syringes may be associated with independent cavities in the medulla (syringobulbia) or can penetrate caudally into the thoracic and lumbosacral regions.

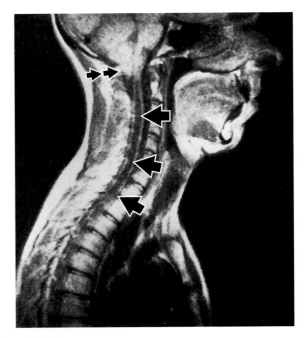

Figure 116–6

Midsagittal magnetic resonance image of Arnold-Chiari malformation *(small black arrows)* and syringomyelia *(three white-black arrows)* in a 33-year-old man. Note the cerebellar tonsils extending below the posterior rim of the foramen magnum *(dark structure immediately above the black arrow)*. The syrinx extends from the medulla well into the thoracic cord.

Pathologically, syringomyelic cavities are anatomically located in the center of the cord. As life advances, the syrinx progressively replaces the centrally located gray matter of the posterior and anterior horns of the spinal cord and interrupts the decussating spinothalamic pain-carrying fibers in the anterior commissure. Most spinal syringes are associated with other congenital malformations, including the Arnold-Chiari malformation (see Fig. 116–6), fusion of the cervical vertebrae, or malformations at the lumbosacral region, including spina bifida and associated meningomyelocele. About one third develop in the presence of intraspinal tumors or extend from the scanned proximal end of traumatically caused spinal cord transections.

Clinical manifestations of congenital syringomyelia most often begin in the second or third decade, frequently affecting the hands or upper trunk with a typically dissociated impairment of pain and temperature sensation coupled with preservation of the senses of touch, vibration, and joint position. Progressive muscular atrophy usually develops in the involved segments, especially in the upper extremities, and commonly leads to kyphoscoliosis. The analgesia results in painless ulcers, burns, and traumatic arthropathy. As a rule, areflexia marks the upper extremities, whereas upper motor neuron signs eventually develop in the legs, accompanied in those members by reduced vibratory and position sensations. In most affected patients the disease process progresses slowly but relentlessly.

In patients with syringobulbia, dissociated impairment of pain and temperature develops over the face, along with nystagmus, pharyngeal and vocal cord paralysis, and lingual atrophy.

Clinical diagnosis is usually not difficult once considered. Leprosy, other rare and acquired peripheral neuropathies, and intramedullary destructive or neoplastic lesions of the spinal cord and brain stem are the only insidiously developing conditions that cause widespread dissociated loss of pain and temperature sensation. Leprosy can be dismissed if the subject has not been raised in an endemic area, and neither it nor other peripheral neuropathies produce signs or direct images of spinal cord dysfunction. The important consideration is whether or not an associated spinal neoplasm exists. MRI definitively outlines most syrinxes and neoplasms if present. Treatment generally is unsatisfactory although foramen magnum decompression has halted the progression of some patients with an associated Arnold-Chiari malformation.

REFERENCES

Braakman R: Management of cervical spondylitic myelopathy and radiculopathy. J Neurol Neurosurg Psychiatry 1994; 57:257–263.

Kanner RM: Low back pain. Semin Neurol 1994; 14:272–278.

Oldfield EH, Muraszko K, Shawker TH, et al.: Pathophysiology of syringomyelia associated with Chiari I malformation of the cerebellar tonsils. Implications for diagnosis and treatment. J Neurosurg 1994; 80:3–15.

Posner JB: Mechanical lesions of nerve roots and spinal cord. *In* Bennett JC, Plum F (eds.): Cecil Textbook of Medicine. 20th ed. Philadelphia, WB Saunders, 1996; pp 2141–49.

117

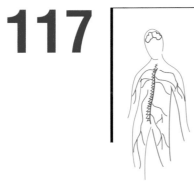

Cerebrovascular Disease

Cerebrovascular diseases include disorders of the arterial or venous circulatory systems or their contents that produce or threaten to produce injury to the central nervous system (CNS). The general term stroke describes the functional neurologic injury. The cause of stroke can be either *anoxic-ischemic,* the result of arterial insufficiency with failure to supply sufficient oxygen and substrate to the tissue, or *hemorrhagic,* the result of abnormal bleeding into or around CNS structures. *Arteriovenous malformations* of the brain or spinal cord can produce neurologic abnormalities by bleeding, producing ischemic damage, or acting as space-occupying lesions.

ANATOMY AND PATHOPHYSIOLOGY OF THE CEREBRAL CIRCULATION

Anatomy

The cerebral arterial circulation derives from four major extracerebral (neck) arteries, the paired vertebral arteries (VA) and the internal carotids (ICA) (Fig. 117–1). Acute, complete occlusion of these extracranial arteries can result at any age from atherosclerosis, embolization, inflammation, intrinsic arterial disease, or trauma. Age and the effectiveness of the intracranial arterial anastomotic pattern determine whether ischemic brain damage ensues.

THE POSTERIOR INTRACRANIAL CIRCULATION. Inside the skull the two VAs first give off the two posterior cerebellar arteries (PICA), then fuse to form the basilar artery (BA) at the ventral pontine-medullary junction. The BA, in turn, divides at its apex into the two posterior cerebral arteries (PCA), having, along its course, generated the bilateral anterior inferior cerebellar (AICA) and superior cerebellar arteries (SCA). The VA, BA, PCA, and their tributaries supply the entire brain stem, most of the thalamus, and the posteromedial aspects of the cerebral hemispheres.

THE ANTERIOR INTRACRANIAL CIRCULATION. Each ICA gives off the retinal artery from the carotid siphon and then, soon after it enters the skull, divides into an ipsilateral anterior (ACA) and middle cerebral artery (MCA) and posterior communicating artery. The ACAs supply the medial surfaces of the hemispheres as far back as the

parietal lobe. The MCAs irrigate the hemispheres' lateral surfaces as well as the basal ganglia and the central core of hemispheric white matter of each side.

The Circle of Willis

In most persons, the circle of Willis is a potentially effective intracranial anastomotic pathway that compensates for sudden focal reductions in blood flow at the base of the brain. Congenital asymmetry of the VAs and narrowing or absence of its anterior or posterior communicating segments are relatively common and may reduce the circle's anastomotic effectiveness. Beyond the circle, the major intracranial arterial beds anastomose over the surface of the brain through tiny interconnecting pial arterioles, most of which are too small to compensate for major arterial occlusions. The drainage fields of the penetrating arteries, descending from the pial surface into the deep white matter or subcortical nuclei, enjoy little anastomotic protection.

Physiology

Cerebral arteries contain less muscle, no elastic tissue, and less adventitia than systemic arteries. The reduced musculature especially affects the junctions where major branches diverge from the large arteries at the base of the brain, creating vulnerable points from which most intracranial aneurysms arise.

The Blood-Brain Barrier

This barrier insulates the brain and its extracellular fluid, including the cerebrospinal fluid (CSF), from many of the body's blood-borne chemical perturbations, such as circulating drugs, immunogenic antigens, and electrolyte changes. The anatomic barrier lies in the intracranial endothelium, where tight intercellular junctions weld the entire inner vascular surface into a continuous membranous sheet. As a result, only nonpolar materials that have a small molecular size, are lipid soluble, or are transported across the membrane by specific carrier systems or pumps transgress the endothelium with any rapidity.

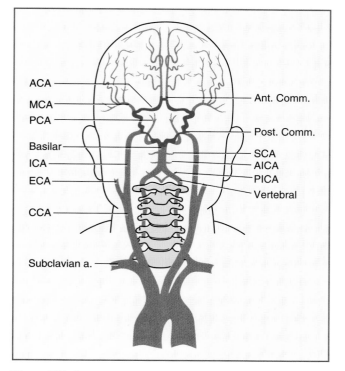

Figure 117–1
Coronal view of the extracranial and intracranial arterial supply to brain. Vessels forming the circle of Willis are highlighted. ACA = Anterior cerebral artery; AICA = anterior inferior cerebellar artery; Ant. Comm. = anterior communicating artery; CCA = common carotid artery; ECA = external carotid artery; ICA = internal carotid artery; MCA = middle cerebral artery; PCA = posterior cerebral artery; PICA = posterior inferior cerebellar artery; Post. Comm. = posterior communicating artery; SCA = superior cerebellar artery. (Modified from Lord R: Surgery of Occlusive Cerebrovascular Disease. St. Louis, CV Mosby, 1986; with permission.)

Transient breaches of the barrier occur under a variety of circumstances but have little ill effect on brain function. Sustained, partial barrier alteration occurs in areas of cerebral neoplasms, inflammation, trauma, or necrosis and contributes to the formation of edema associated with such conditions. Severe damage to barrier transport mechanisms can intensify brain infarction during ischemia.

Autoregulation

The brain's resistance arterioles adjust their degree of constriction according to the metabolic requirements of the tissue and the systemic blood pressure (BP). Normally, the arterioles automatically and locally dilate in response to increases in local brain functional activity, and constrict as functional requirements decline. Similarly, they dilate as systemic blood pressure falls and intrinsically constrict as it rises. Although the two responses are independently regulated, they synergize to fulfill the brain's metabolic need. The normal limits of cerebral autoregulation to intra-arterial pressure extend between approximately 60 and 160 mm Hg of systemic mean pressure. Impaired autoregulation to pressure

changes can contribute to brain injury in several circumstances, including brain trauma, acute mass lesions, and large strokes. At such times widespread abnormal vasodilatation allows the intracranial pressure (ICP) to rise, sometimes to levels that approach the arterial blood pressure. Impaired arterial autoregulation also can accompany severe hypertension (mean BP greater than 160 torr), in which case intense elevations of intrinsic systemic blood pressure can produce both vascular and brain tissue injury.

EPIDEMIOLOGY AND RISK FACTORS

Stroke takes a worldwide toll, affecting especially persons 55 years and older. Although the incidence has declined somewhat in recent years, only heart disease and cancer exceed stroke as causes of death and disability in developed countries.

Table 117–1 lists the major immediate causes of stroke. In addition, a number of systemic conditions and social habits predispose to the arterial and hematologic changes that cause stroke (Table 117–2). *Hypertension* adversely affects the heart and induces progressive narrowing of the cerebral arterioles; it creates the greatest risk factor but smoking lies close behind. The increasingly successful treatment of hypertension and the reduction in smoking habits have been major factors reducing stroke incidence in the United States. Population studies show an especially strong association among dietary salt intake, hypertension, and cerebral hemorrhage.

Alcoholic excess increases stroke risk, with several studies reporting an increase of severe strokes immediately following bouts of heavy intoxication. Modest alcohol ingestion on the order of one to two glasses of wine

TABLE 117–1	Causes of Acute Cerebral Ischemia

Mainly Focal

Arterial disease, thrombotic or embolic
Cardiac emboli
Functional arterial spasm or constriction
a. Migraine
b. Subarachnoid hemorrhage
c. Acute or subacute bacterial meningitis
Intracranial venous sinus of venous thrombosis

Mainly Global

Absolute or functional (ventricular fibrillation) asystole >30 sec in duration
Severe decline in cardiac output
   Shock
      Bradycardia <30–40 beats/min
      Cardiac tamponade
      Severe heart failure
Three- or four-vessel stenosis of cervical arteries plus TIA
Profound anemia: HCT usually <20
Profound hypoxemia: Pa_{O_2} <35–40 mm Hg
Carbon monoxide poisoning
Prolonged status epilepticus
Disseminated intravascular coagulation
Fat embolization

HCT = Hematocrit; TIA = transient ischemic attacks.

TABLE 117–2	Most Frequent Risk Factors in Stroke

Hypertension
Smoking
Excess salt intake
Myocardial infarction
Auricular fibrillation
Diabetes mellitus
Alcohol abuse
Homocysteinemia
Obesity
Severe carotid stenosis
Parental stroke

per day may actually reduce stroke risk. Elevated serum homocysteine levels are common in European and American adult men and can be corrected by folic acids, 200–400 μg daily. The stroke risk associated with current oral contraceptives is uncertain.

ISCHEMIC STROKE

Etiology and Mechanisms

Focal ischemic stroke is caused by either embolic or thrombotic occlusion of a major artery in the neck or head. *Global ischemic stroke* results in total failure of blood supply, such as follows cardiac arrest or, rarely, severe impairments of the oxygen supply to the brain.

Vascular Factors

These can be either primarily thrombotic or embolic, as listed in Table 117–3. In either case, the critical event is reduction of blood flow to the brain.

Hematogenous Factors

Table 117–3 lists the major causes. Except for anesthetic or industrial accidents that result in severe reductions in inhaled oxygen, or carbon monoxide poisoning, which blocks oxyhemoglobin formation, uncomplicated hypoxemia and anemia are uncommon causes of ischemic stroke since arterial oxygen supplies must be reduced to about 40% of normal before cerebral insufficiency develop. This level of anoxemia is likely to produce cardiac as well as cerebral difficulties. In the absence of severe hypotension, acute hemorrhage, or anatomic abnormalities in the cervicocranial circulation, isolated hemoglobin levels greater than 7 to 8 gm/dl or Pa_{O_2}, values greater than 40 to 45 mm Hg seldom can be incriminated as primary causes of stroke. Indeed, because of blood flow adjustments or chronic exposure, even lower hemoglobin values may cause no symptoms.

Among the coagulopathies causing stroke, *physiologic platelet aggregation* deserves specific attention. Vascular changes producing partial or complete ischemia in the brain stimulate an immediate increase in platelet aggregation in the abnormal areas. Similarly, ulcerated arteriosclerotic plaques attract fibrin-platelet aggregations to their surface as part of the healing process. The ensuing detritus provides a potential source for the extension of a thrombosis or the formation of artery-to-artery emboli.

Blood Flow and Tissue Factor

The brain and spinal cord metabolize at the highest basal rate of any large organ, consuming approximately 20% of the body's resting oxygen requirement. The brain contains practically no reserves of oxygen and only tiny stores of glucose, its normal substrate. As a result, any severe reduction of blood supply threatens the organ's vitality. In most instances, cerebral autoregulation and increased tissue oxygen extraction can support normal or nearly nor-

TABLE 117–3	Vascular and Hematologic Factors Contributing to Stroke

Mural Abnormalities

A. Extracranial-intracranial atherosclerosis
  1. Thrombotic narrowing or occlusion of cervical vessels
  2. Ulcerated aortocervical plaques generating platelet-fibrin or cholesterol emboli
  3. Thrombotic occlusion of intracranial vessels
B. Inflammatory-immunologic vascular occlusions
  1. Extracranial only (cranial arteritis)
  2. Extracranial and intracranial
    a. Generalized polyarteritis
    b. Septic emboli (bacterial endocarditis)
  3. Intracranial only
    a. Bacterial or granulomatous arteritis
    b. Amphetamine or cocaine-like drugs
    c. Idiopathic
C. Invasion or compression of arterial or venous vascular walls by trauma, neoplasms

Embolic Disorders

A. Artery-to-artery: platelet or cholesterol emboli from aortocervical atherosclerotic plaques
B. Cardiogenic
  1. Mural (post–myocardial infarction)
  2. Atrial
  3. Valvular
    a. Septic (endocarditis)
    b. Nonseptic (rheumatic, atherosclerotic, mitral prolapse, nonbacterial endocarditis)
  4. Neoplastic (arterial myxoma)
C. Latent atrial septal defect with right-to-left emboli from deep vein thrombosis
D. Fat embolism
E. Air embolism
F. Clamp dislodgement of aortic plaques during bypass surgery
G. Hematologic abnormalities
  1. Hematocrit >55
  2. White blood cell count >500,000
  3. Thrombocytosis >600,000
  4. Platelet hyperaggregability
  5. Elevated homocysteine levels
H. Hemoglobinopathies and autoimmunopathies
  1. Sickle cell disease
  2. Paraproteinemia
  3. Lupus anticoagulant
  4. Cardiolipin antibody

mal brain function despite blood flow reductions down to about 40% of normal. Below this threshold, though, a small additional decline can cause membrane failure and brain cell death. Partial or complete vascular occlusion (focal ischemia) and profound hypotension (global ischemia) represent the most common causes of such catastrophes. Any significant degree of anemia, hypoxemia, or hypercoagulability accentuates the hazards.

How long severe anoxia or ischemia must last to cause irreversible brain damage is uncertain. Humans faint by about the eighth second of asystole, but much evidence suggests that some brain tissues can recover from severe partial ischemia lasting as long as an hour or more.

Heart and systemic vascular diseases are the most important associated factors causing clinical stroke (Table 117–4). Most focal stroke results from emboli lodging in the intracranial arteries, with about 40% coming from the heart and the remainder from artery-to-artery emboli, most of which are presumed to originate from the aortic arch or carotid-vertebral arteries. Cardiac arrhythmias account for most instances of embolism or global cerebral ischemia among older persons. Furthermore, the statistical risk of future myocardial infarction in stroke patients is as great as or greater than the risk of a repeated cerebral event. Mitral valve prolapse, which can cause valvular or subvalvular thrombi, is found 6 times more frequently than normal among persons below age 45 with acute stroke. Similarly, a greatly increased incidence of focal stroke is associated with atrial fibrillation of whatever cause. Anterior wall myocardial infarction (MI) produces a high incidence of left ventricular thrombi; if not treated prophylactically with anticoagulants, as many as 40% of such patients suffer stroke during convalescence from the MI. Table 117–4 lists common causes and manifestations of acute embolic stroke.

Neuropathology of Ischemic Brain Damage

The process of *cerebral infarction* damages or destroys all tissue elements, including neurons, glial cells, and blood vessels. Within a matter of hours, osmotic gradients drag water into the necrotic tissue and inflammatory-immune reactions add to the mass effect. Tissue factors including excess excitatory stimulation of ischemic recep-

TABLE 117–4	Findings Suggesting Cardiac-Embolic Origin for Focal Stroke

Persons <45 yr with no evident systemic risk factors but mitral prolapse
Known heart disease: rheumatic aortic or mitral valve; atrial fibrillation; recent anterior wall infarction; murmur plus unexplained fever (subacute bacterial endocarditis [SBE]); chronic cardiomyopathy; mitral annular calcification
Multiple cerebral arteries involved
Emboli in other organs
Hemorrhagic infarct
Demonstrated internal carotid artery narrowing >70%
Changing cardiac murmurs (SBE or nonbacterial thrombotic endocarditis [NBTE])

tors, tissue lactic acidosis, and free radical formation may enlarge and extend the damage. Infarction characteristically follows prolonged anoxia-ischemia such as occurs with vascular occlusion and can be focal or multifocal in nature depending on the pattern of affected vessels. Large infarcts involve the vascular territory of the major intracranial arteries. Small infarcts, 5 to 8 mm or so in diameter, sometimes called *lacunes*, result from occlusion of arteriolar branches. Lacunes especially result from occlusion of the terminal branches supplied by the middle cerebral and basilar arteries.

Hemorrhagic infarcts are marked by scattered areas of escaped red cells in the ischemic tissue, occurring most often at the periphery of an infarcted area. The mechanism is thought to represent reperfusion of damaged arterial endothelium, allowing diapedetic bleeding to occur.

Selective neuronal necrosis describes damage restricted to specifically located nerve cells, sparing glial and vascular elements. When caused by anoxia, the process affects selectively vulnerable neurons located in the hippocampus, the deeper level of the cerebral cortex (laminar necrosis), and the cerebellar Purkinje cells. Characteristically selective neuronal death follows brief periods of acute cardiac arrest, prolonged status epilepticus, and profound hypoglycemia and has been attributed to a transient excess of excitatory neurotransmitter activity in the vulnerable area. Subsequent severe hippocampal damage produces the most frequent cause of memory loss following cardiac arrest, whereas Purkinje cell damage is a major factor in causing the distressing condition of postanoxic myoclonus.

Clinical Definitions of Stroke (Table 117–5)

Transient ischemic attacks (TIAs) are defined as periods of focal, acute neurologic insufficiency lasting from a few minutes to an hour or so, followed by complete functional recovery. Presumably, emboli composed of fibrin, platelets or, rarely, cholesterol crystals that arise in the heart or large cervical arteries are responsible for most TIAs. Less frequent sources include tiny fragments of cardiac valvular vegetations or hematogenous abnormalities within the affected vessels. Severe narrowing of greater than 75% of a common or internal carotid artery in the neck may account for some cases on a hemodynamic basis. Magnetic resonance imaging (MRI) discloses the presence of small areas of brain infarction in about half the cases.

Completed stroke refers to a sustained ischemic event sufficient to produce neuronal necrosis or infarction in at least part of the territory of an affected cerebral artery. The ensuing neurologic defect can last days, weeks, or permanently. Even after maximal recovery, at least minimal neurologic difficulties often remain. The clinical severity of completed strokes depends upon the particular arterial bed, the size of the associated infarct, and the functional neuroanatomy of the area affected by the lesion. Completed *minor strokes* involving only distal branches of the middle cerebral or basilar artery, for example, produce only restricted neurologic damage compared to *major strokes* that involve the main areas sup-

TABLE 117–5 Principal Patterns of Acute Stroke

Transient Ischemic Attacks
Brief episodes of focal neurologic deficits lasting 2–3 min to at most a few hours; no residual defects. May affect the distal distribution of the retinal, internal carotid, middle cerebral, or basilar artery.

Completed Stroke
Acute, sustained functional neurologic loss lasting from days to permanently in the distribution of one or more branches of the intracranial arteries.
Minor strokes
Limited functional deficits and small size, detected by brain imaging.
Major strokes
Severe sensorimotor or cognitive impairments. Brain images typically show either a large lesion or one involving the paramedian distribution of the vertebrobasilar system.
Evolving stroke
An unusual condition in which a restricted neurologic insufficiency, usually motor, starts focally but spreads relentlessly over a matter of hours to involve adjacent functional areas supplied by the parent intracranial artery.

plied by the middle cerebral or basilar arteries. A clinically important point is that minor strokes causing limited neurologic impairment in a vascular territory sometimes warn of impending thrombosis of the larger parent artery. Accordingly, in the early hours following onset of neurologic damage it may be difficult or impossible to distinguish minor completed strokes from reversible ischemic neurologic deficits or even the beginnings of a more serious stroke in evolution.

Stroke in evolution refers to a condition wherein ischemic neurologic deficits begin in a focal or restricted distribution but spread gradually in a pattern reflecting involvement of more and more of the anatomic territory supplied by a middle cerebral or basilar artery. These early hours represent a critical time period to attempt therapy. Occasionally, stroke can evolve for longer periods, up to a week or so, but such a pattern more often reflects the presence of ischemia or bleeding related to a neoplasm or arteriovenous malformation. The pathogenesis of most evolving strokes probably consists of the extension of thrombus from an initial clot along the affected artery. Some may reflect hemodynamic instability with insufficiency spreading into the penumbral margin of ischemic zones at the edge of the initially hypoperfused area. Evolving stroke must be differentiated from the less specific and temporary neurologic worsening that sometimes results when cerebral edema complicates large, completed strokes as described below.

Major Stroke Syndromes (Table 117–6)

Ischemia of the Internal Carotid Artery (Anterior Circulation) System

Both thromboses and emboli can occlude the anterior cerebral circulatory system. Emboli are especially common because of the large size of the system and the fact

that so many emboli from the heart find their first escape up the large common carotid arteries.

Transient Ischemic Attacks Affecting the Internal Carotid Artery (ICA) Distribution

About one third of these events are associated with *stenosis-ulceration* or severe stenosis (> 75%) in the ipsilateral common or internal carotid artery, usually at its bifurcation. Thrombi from the heart or the proximal aorta cause most of the rest. A few carotid TIAs may be caused by hematogenous abnormalities producing small, spontaneously arising endovascular clots.

Anterior circulation TIAs almost entirely affect either the retinal artery or MCA circulation, with the two involved concurrently about 10% of the time. Isolated ophthalmic artery TIAs have the least serious prognosis.

TABLE 117–6 Major Stroke Syndromes

I. Anterior Circulation (ICA and tributaries)
A. TIAs
1. Retinal artery. Brief (10–30 sec), often repeated, unilateral graying-out of vision reflecting ophthalmic arterial insufficiency, ipsilateral to propagating ICA. Pupil sluggish, retina pale, vessels underfilled, cholesterol emboli sometimes visible.
2. MCA, Intermediate length (2–50 min) usually stereotyped, producing contralateral upper motor neuron (UMN) face-hand or hemiparetic weakness, sometimes aphasia or dysarthria. Sensory symptoms or seizures uncommon. Images show small lesions in approximately 50%.
B. Completed stroke
1. ICA-MCA distribution. Onset usually abrupt, a few evolve for 24 hr. Residua last days to indefinitely. Neurologic changes can include contralateral face, face-hand, hemiplegic, or sensorimotor weakness, attention-neglect, or aphasia if large lesion arises in dominant hemisphere, neglect if lesion in nondominant hemisphere. Seizures affect 5%; brain edema plus large strokes can lead to stupor. Brain images rule out hemorrhages and almost always reveal infarction by 24 hr.
2. ACA distribution. Incidence uncommon, some asymptomatic, others cause contralateral sensory–upper motor neuron weakness of leg-foot, occasionally Broca's aphasia.

II. Posterior Circulation (VA, BA, PCA)
A. TIAs
1. Duration 5–55 min. Attacks often complex and symptoms may vary in different patients as well as in the same patient during different attacks. Table 117–7 lists typical symptoms.
B. Completed stroke
1. VA, PICA syndrome: ipsilateral headache, ataxia, paralysis of swallowing and tongue; pain loss, ipsilateral face and contralateral body; Horner's syndrome, ipsilatera; vomiting.
2. PICA, AICA, and SCA occlusions each can result in acute cerebellar infarction. The text describes complete syndromes.
3. BA trunk:
Lower (vertebrobasilar junction). Lower extremity paraplegia or tetraplegia, bizarre eye movements, small pupils, breathing irregularities, often coma.
Rostral (basilar apex–PCA junction). Variable: hemiplegia or diplegia; pupillary and oculomotor paralysis; stupor or coma; visual field defects; amnesia.
4. PCA:
Distal branches: Quadratic or hemianopic visual field loss.
Proximal branches to thalamus: memory loss, sensorimotor hemiplegias.

Symptoms consist of a rapidly developing (10 seconds or so) unilateral graying-out of vision of one eye (amaurosis fugax). The episodes usually last for seconds, rarely for more than a few minutes, after which normal vision nearly always returns. Retinal examination during the attack may disclose conspicuous narrowing of both arteries and veins, sometimes with blood flow being so slow that venous filling appears segmented. Yellow, refractile, residual retinal arterial spots represent cholesterol crystals. Their presence implies cholesterol detached from an upstream arterial plaque and a greater potential risk for future irreversible embolic ischemia.

Symptoms of TIAs affecting the MCA distribution depend upon the functional neuroanatomy of the ischemic field. Peripheral branch occlusions characteristically cause transient, restricted hand-arm or face-hand-arm paresis with or without accompanying somesthetic sensory loss. Occlusions distal to the point where the lenticulostriate artery branches from the MCA in the dominant hemisphere can cause transient aphasia. More proximal occlusions produce transient motor hemiparesis with or without associated language defects. Neither altered consciousness nor confusion ordinarily accompanies ICA-MCA TIAs, most of which last less than 10 to 20 minutes. Seizures are rare.

INTERNAL CAROTID ARTERY OCCLUSION. *Acute* occlusion of the previously fully patent vessel can result from atherosclerosis, immunologic-inflammatory disease, traumatic arterial dissection, massive embolism, or surgical ligation performed in an effort to halt traumatic bleeding or entrap an intracranial aneurysm. Most spontaneous ICA occlusions develop at the site of a previously severe stenosis, either at the carotid bifurcation or, less frequently, in the intracranial siphon.

The neurologic effects of either severe stenosis or total ICA occlusion depend on the patient's age, the rate at which closure occurs, the presence or absence of ulcerated endothelial plaques, and the degree of intracranial anastomotic compensation. Stenoses of less than 85% usually cause little or no reduction in blood flow and few symptoms unless thrombi form on ulcerated plaques and break off as emboli. Plaques containing calcification are especially dangerous. Autopsy and arteriographic studies suggest that many ICA occlusions that evolve gradually cause neither symptoms nor structural brain damage. Neurologic injury with the remainder ranges from small, deep focal cerebral infarctions to massive strokes that involve the entire distribution of the ipsilateral middle and, sometimes, anterior cerebral arteries.

Small completed strokes or TIAs precede symptoms of major acute stroke due to ICA occlusion in as many as 20% of cases, usually reflecting progressive stenosis or plaque formation. If a major hemispheric lesion does occur, neurologic symptoms and signs affecting the MCA distribution characteristically develop rapidly, with their intensity depending on the size of the subsequent brain lesion. Ipsilateral or bitemporal headache may accompany the onset of occlusion. Focal motor or generalized seizures accompany the acute stage of about 5% of large ICA-MCA distribution infarcts.

Although diagnosis of an ICA-MCA distribution stroke usually is easily made on clinical grounds, a confirming computed tomographic (CT) of MRI image is useful to rule out hemorrhage or other unexpected causes. Clinical diagnosis of internal carotid artery/narrowing or occlusion is not reliable and in most cases requires imaging studies by noninvasive methods (ultrasound or Doppler flow estimates or arterial MRI).

External palpation of the neck is an unreliable sign in diagnosis of ICA occlusion, because internal and external carotid arteries cannot reliably be distinguished from one another. A total absence of cervical arterial pulsations in the region of the angle of the jaw or over the facial arteries suggests the uncommon event of common carotid or combined internal-external carotid artery occlusion. Bruits heard predominantly or entirely over the carotid bifurcation area immediately below the angle of the jaw suggest an underlying stenosis of either the ICA or external carotid artery (ECA) or both. Generally, the harsher the bruit, the more likely that it reflects severe stenosis, especially if accompanied by a palpable thrill. Only bruits that disappear as auscultation moves down the neck toward the clavicle can be regarded confidently as emanating from the carotid bifurcation.

MIDDLE CEREBRAL ARTERY (MCA) OCCLUSION. Embolism represents the most frequent cause of MCA occlusion. Other mechanisms include extension of clot from an occluded internal carotid artery, intrinsic atherosclerosis, and endovascular thrombosis. The onset of symptoms and signs usually is rapid, taking seconds or minutes to evolve, and commonly silent, producing no more than a sense of paralysis or "deadness" in contralateral body parts. Affected patients, if asleep at onset, may notice no difficulty until they attempt to arise after awakening. The immediate neurologic deficit, as with carotid occlusion or ICA-MCA TIAs, depends upon where along the MCA the occlusion rests. Major MCA strokes in either hemisphere tend to produce contralateral hemiplegia. Those affecting the dominant hemisphere tend to cause aphasia, whereas those lying in the nondominant right hemisphere tend to produce confusional states, spatial disorientation, and various degrees of sensory and emotional neglect. Severe inattentiveness, stupor, or coma with unilateral cerebral stroke is limited to patients in whom acute, large, dominant-hemisphere lesions produce global aphasia or those who develop severe secondary, brain, edema and diencephalic compression-herniation.

ANTERIOR CEREBRAL ARTERY (ACA) OCCLUSION. The anterior cerebral artery has two major parts: (1) the basal portion, extending from the ICA to join the anterior communicating artery, and (2) the interhemispheric portion, supplying the ipsilateral medial frontal lobe as far posteriorly as the sensorimotor foot area. Occlusion of the interhemispheric branch produces an acute focal sensorimotor defect in the contralateral foot and distal leg. Proximal ACA occlusion may cause no neurologic deficits if a patent anterior communicating artery carries blood from the opposite carotid supply. Lacking such a collateral, ischemia may affect deep frontal lobe nuclei to cause (in the dominant hemisphere) Broca's or anterior conduction aphasia. TIAs rarely affect the ACA distribution; recurrent paresthesias or weakness involving a single foot-leg is more consistent with cerebral seizures or, less often, recurrent ischemia in the vertebral-basilar system.

Ischemia of the Vertebral-Basilar (Posterior Circulation) System

The BA and two intracranial VAs are supplied rostrally by the posterior communicating arteries and caudally from the cervical VAs, which originate from the subclavians. Variation in the patency of these sources has several possible effects. With both ends of the double supply open, narrowing or even occlusion of a VA or even the BA sometimes can occur without causing symptoms. Emboli are less frequent in the posterior than the anterior circulation, whereas primary atherosclerotic occlusion affects the BA and VAs more frequently than the carotid systems.

VERTEBRAL-BASILAR TIA. The nature of the complex and variable symptoms and signs depends on the anatomic distribution of ischemia (Table 117–7). Often the neurologic changes vary from attack to attack in the same person. This variability contrasts with carotid TIAs, in which recurrent episodes in the same patient tend to remain stereotyped.

OCCLUSION OF VA OR BA. Occlusion of these arteries and their main branches, the PICA, AICA, and SCA, can cause several different syndromes depending on the rostral-caudal brain level of the arterial stoppage, the point of occlusion along the length of the vessel, and whether the involvement includes the paramedian vessels, circumferential arteries, or both (see Table 117–6).

PCA OCCLUSIONS. Atherosclerosis located at the basilar take-off or emboli that lodge more peripherally most often account for these occlusions. Distal obstructions result in homonymous or quadrantic hemianopias, whereas more proximal stoppage produces infarction of the sensory thalamus and sometimes the lateral midbrain as well.

The effects of BA occlusion at the apex depend upon whether the obstruction includes the posterior cerebral arteries, the arteries supplying the overlying diencephalon, the vessels feeding the midbrain, or some combination thereof. Loss or reduction of consciousness is common and is often associated with a variety of paralyses affecting pupillary, gaze, and oculomotor functions. If the cerebral peduncles are affected, decorticate or decerebrate motor posturing and paralysis ensue. Residua may include inattention, dementia, memory loss, visual field defects, gaze palsy, and sensory or motor impairments. More caudally placed occlusions of the BA, if they selectively affect paramedian vessels, impair consciousness and produce disconjugate eye movements, unequal pupils, and signs of bilateral upper motor neuron dysfunction. Bizarre irregularities in breathing patterns often emerge.

Complete basilar occlusion affecting both paramedian and circumferential vessels usually produces incomplete ischemic transection of the brain stem. Affected patients are comatose and show pinpoint, irregular, or unequal pupils, bilateral conjugate gaze paralysis, or internuclear ophthalmoplegia and tetraplegia. Few survive more than a few days.

UNILATERAL VA OCCLUSION. Unilateral VA occlusion is asymptomatic in about 50% of cases. When symptoms do occur, they produce the syndrome of the posterior inferior cerebellar artery. Signs of mild ipsilateral cerebellar dysfunction are accompanied by ipsilateral lower motor neuron paralysis of cranial nerves IX, X, and XII, coupled with pain and temperature loss contralaterally on the body and ipsilaterally on the face. An ipsilateral Horner's syndrome usually is present.

ACUTE CEREBELLAR INFARCTION. Infarction can occur when occlusion strikes any of the three main cerebellar arteries, principally the inferior branch. If the cerebellum swells from ischemic edema sufficiently to distort the brain stem and obstruct the normal CSF outflow, serious complications may occur. Symptoms initially include ipsilateral occipital headache and signs of mild cerebellar dysfunction followed by increasing occipital head pain, often vomiting, and the development of ipsilateral cranial nerve defects. Progression, if it occurs, usually develops within 12 to 36 hours and is marked by more severe headache and drowsiness or stupor. CT scans in such instances show an enlarged, hypodense cerebellar hemisphere; with fourth ventricle obstruction and lateral ventricle enlargement. Lateral ventricular drainage can prevent further damage or death.

Spinal Stroke

Ischemic infarction due to atherosclerotic arterial occlusion rarely affects the spinal cord. More common is anoxic-ischemic injury associated with prolonged hypotension (shock) or compression by intraspinal mass lesions. Arterial lesions, when they occur, almost always involve the anterior spinal artery, atherosclerotic obstruction striking most often at the level of the cervical radicular artery or one or two segments below. Inflammatory and immune arteritides are, if anything, more frequent than atherosclerotic obstructions, especially in younger persons, and tend to occur at the T4 level. In both instances, neurologic damage develops acutely or rapidly, usually reach-

TABLE 117–7	**Most Common Symptoms of Vertebral-Basilar TIAs**
Paramedian Arteries (midline of BA)	**Circumferential Arteries (PICA, AICA, SCA, PCA)**
Transient global amnesia	Nonpositional vertigo
Diplopia	Unilateral face or body paresthesias
Episodic, paroxysmal drowsiness	
Paraparesis or tetraparesis	Episodic hemianopia or scintillations
Ataxia	
Dysarthria	Unilateral posterior headache

ing a maximum within 24 hours of onset, and produces a transverse myelopathy affecting the anterior half of the cord. Lower motor neuron abnormalities sometimes can be detected at the level of the lesion combined with asymmetric, bilateral impairment of pain and temperature sensations beginning one or two dermatomes below. Injury to corticospinal pathways results in upper motor neuron dysfunction caudal to the level of occlusion. Dysfunction of bowel, bladder, and male sexual activities usually accompanies these abnormalities.

Cerebral Venous Thrombosis

Obstruction of the cerebral venous sinuses or their main tributaries has several potential causes (Table 117–8) with puerperal factors being the most common. Sagittal sinus occlusions pose the greatest risk, causing in many instances bilateral hemorrhagic infarctions in parasagittal frontal-parietal areas leading to potentially fatal brain edema. Symptoms include headache, lethargy, bilateral weakness of the legs and, to a lesser degree, arms, and seizures. Often, the clinical picture resembles a progressive encephalopathy or even viral encephalitis. CT or MRI scans can be highly suggestive by showing one or more bilateral hemorrhagic infarctions in parasagittal cerebral areas. Diagnosis rests on imaging the occluded sinus by sagittal MRI or, definitively, by invasive cerebral arteriography aimed at delineating cerebral venous architecture.

Untreated, evolving symptomatic cerebral venous thrombosis carries a 25 to 40% mortality rate. Early treatment with intravenous heparin can reduce morbidity/mortality by half or more if applied within a few hours or days of onset.

Hypertensive Encephalopathy (HE)

HE is an abnormal, dangerous state of multifocal cerebral ischemia induced by a severely, acutely, or subacutely elevated blood pressure (Table 117–9). The condition has become uncommon thanks to the widespread use of effective antihypertensive drugs.

The pathogenesis of HE relates to the effect of high systemic intravascular pressure on the brain's arterioles. If elevated tension exceeds the upper limits of normal cerebral autoregulation, a combination of multifocal arteriolar

TABLE 117–8	Major Causes of Cerebral Venous and Sinus Thrombosis in Approximately Declining Order of Frequency

Late pregnancy and postpartum state
Coagulant factors associated with malignancy, disseminated intravascular coagulation, thrombotic purpura
Idiopathic
Severe dehydration or intrinsic hyperviscosity
Neoplastic invasion of anterior sagittal sinus
Septic extension from face, sinus, mastoid, brain abscess

TABLE 117–9	Hypertensive Encephalopathy
Immediate cause	Acute, severe hypertension; erythropoietin treatment for renal cancer
Associated illnesses	Renal disease, eclampsia, abrupt withdrawal of antihypertensive drugs, pheochromocytoma
Manifestations	Acute headache, nausea, vomiting, confusion or stupor, cortical blindness, convulsions, transient motor changes
Findings	BP usually >200/130; retinal hemorrhages or papilledema; relatively normal renal function (BUN <100); MRI shows disseminated small or confluent areas of acute leukoencephalopathy
Treatment	Reduce mean BP by 30–40 mm Hg/hr, avoiding abrupt major declines (controlled nitroprusside drip most reliable); treat seizures with diazepam IV

BP = Blood pressure; BUN = blood urea nitrogen; IV = intravenous; MRI = magnetic resonance imaging.

vasodilatation and vasoconstriction occurs, producing diffusely distributed small zones of microhemorrhages and ischemia.

Differential diagnosis of HE includes acute uremia (blood urea nitrogen > 100 mg/dl), encephalitis (fever, no severe hypertension, usually slower course), cerebral venous sinus thrombosis, acute lead encephalopathy, disseminated intravascular coagulation, and acute bacterial endocarditis.

HE requires urgent treatment using intravenously regulated sodium nitroprusside to lower blood pressure promptly to levels within the upper range of autoregulation (mean 130 ± 10 mm Hg). Later, within 12 hours or so, systemic pressures can be reduced more gradually so as to allow arterioles to adapt and reduce the risk of inducing focal cerebral hypoperfusion. Long-term control of the underlying hypertension must be pursued vigorously.

Diagnosis and Differential Diagnosis in Ischemic Stroke

Clinical understanding plus judiciously chosen confirmatory laboratory tests give accurate diagnosis in nearly all instances. Age, mode of onset, the presence or absence of known risk factors or previous vascular events, and whether or not the neurologic deficit fits a known vascular distribution provide the chief clues. The first minutes or hours of observation show whether a stroke is a TIA, is progressing, or, for the moment, has completed its ravages. The general history and physical examination often disclose the presence or absence of stroke-causing systemic diseases (see Table 117–1), especially those of the heart or great vessels. These steps, combined with routine laboratory studies (urinalysis, complete blood count and smear, standard chemical and electrolyte screening, electrocardiogram [ECG] chest radiography) provide accurate diagnosis most of the time. A CT or MRI head scan should be obtained for any first completed or progressive stroke, because about 4% of such patients have other disorders such as a neoplasm, hematoma, vascular malformation, or abscess. CT or, if unavailable, lumbar puncture should be done before anticoagulants are administered. One should recall, however, that even large cerebral infarcts may not produce abnormalities on the CT scan until as late as 24 to 48 hours after onset.

Ischemic stroke seldom affects persons less than age 50 except in association with specific risk factors or identifiable toxic or systemic causes. Patients lacking such apparent antecedents deserve especially careful appraisal.

Differentiation among TIAs, progressive stroke, minor completed stroke, and severe completed stroke is implicit in their presentations. Several conditions, however, can be mistaken for stroke and vice versa (Table 117–10). Seizures usually are not difficult to distinguish from TIAs because the latter rarely cause positive motor signs, are less long-lasting, and produce no postictal effects. Postictal paralysis usually can be distinguished from stroke by its association. Glaucoma or other local diseases of the eye, cranial arteritis, and migraine represent alternate potential causes of unilateral visual loss. Complicated migraine can produce symptoms suggesting acute stroke or vertebral-basilar TIA. The patient's age and past history usually are distinguishing. Benign positional vertigo differs from basilar TIAs by its strict link to positional stimuli and its lack of associated symptoms of brain stem dysfunction. Similar specific associations identify acute labyrinthitis or Meniere's disease as well as the nonspecific dizzy feelings experienced by many elderly persons. Cardiac arrhythmias rarely cause symptoms resembling TIAs, just as TIAs rarely cause syncope. Subdural hematomas or large, unruptured intracranial aneurysms sometimes produce brief attacks that are indistinguishable from carotid TIAs and that may have a similar embolic pathogenesis. Stroke almost always can be distinguished from deep cerebral hemorrhage or brain tumor by CT imaging. Afebrile brain abscesses or granulomas can similarly be identified. Cervical-cerebral angiography has little usefulness in evaluating acute stroke. Its place in managing aftercare is described below.

Etiologic diagnosis guides both acute and chronic management (see Tables 117–1 to 117–4). Echocardiography and cardiac wall motion studies can identify potential sources of emboli in patients with mitral prolapse, valvular stenosis, or anterior wall infarctions and detect the rare atrial myxoma. Electroencephalograms and other clinical neurophysiologic studies seldom provide useful information. Noninvasive investigations, such as ultrasonic or Doppler flow studies, applied to the carotid systems are more useful in planning preventive care than acute management. Generally speaking, the more restricted and reversible the initial neurologic injury, the more assiduously one searches for specific causes for which treatment might reduce the risk of future brain damage.

Management of Acute Stroke

Many pharmacologic agents have been tested unsuccessfully as treatments for acute stroke, including glutamate-receptor blockers, calcium-channel blockers, antioxidants, and others. Thrombolytic agents including streptokinase and tissue plasminogen factors have similarly been tested but thus far the dangerous tendency of streptokinase to induce fatal cerebral hemorrhage has limited its usefulness. In a recent single-trial testing, tissue plasminogen factor (tPA) has been found to improve outcome in acute strokes by 30% if administered 180 minutes or less after the onset of symptoms. Stringent criteria, outlined in Figure 117–2, govern the use of tPA to minimize complications. Whether new agents from drug families already tested unsuccessfully will bring future success remains to be seen.

General management of acute stroke consists of providing general medical and nursing care, reducing hypertension or hyperviscosity if present, and taking steps to prevent acute or future worsening of the neurologic deficit. Acutely, one attempts to halt progressing stroke, to prevent recurring cerebral emboli, and to stabilize patients with fluctuating neurologic changes with the least possible deficit. The development of ischemic brain edema may require therapeutic attention after 24 to 48 hours.

The Use and Choice of Anticoagulants

Aspirin therapy has been sufficiently protective against recurrent thromboembolism that it can be recommended as immediate therapy in acute stroke. Anticoagulants have known value in protecting against certain well-documented risk factors in stroke. Table 117–11 outlines widely accepted guidelines for using these agents in acute and chronic stroke. One must be cautious when employing anticoagulants since the treatment can cause dangerous bleeding of about 1 to 2% per year, even in experienced hands. Heparin therapy is initiated at the time of admission to hospital: in patients describing repetitive, closely spaced TIAs; in those with progression of stroke signs during the immediately preceding hours or minutes; in those observed to have increasing neurologic deficits superimposed acutely on what at first appear to be minor strokes; and in patients demonstrating fluctuating signs and symptoms of vertebral-basilar or carotid ischemia. In all such instances other than TIAs, either a CT scan or, when imaging is unavailable, a lumbar puncture must be performed to rule out hemorrhage. Heparin should be delayed for at least 2 hours after the lumbar puncture to reduce the risk of spinal epidural bleeding. Anticoagula-

TABLE 117–10	Conditions Misdiagnosed as Stroke	
Mistaken for Stroke	**Mistakenly Diagnosed as Stroke**
Focal seizures called TIAs	Complicated migraine
Glaucoma attributed to retinal artery occlusion	Subdural hematoma
Benign vertigo or Meniere's disease considered vertebral-basilar TIA	Occasional large aneurysms causing TIAs
Vasodepressor syncope regarded as minor stroke	Hemorrhage or infarction in neoplasms

TIA = transient ischemic attack.

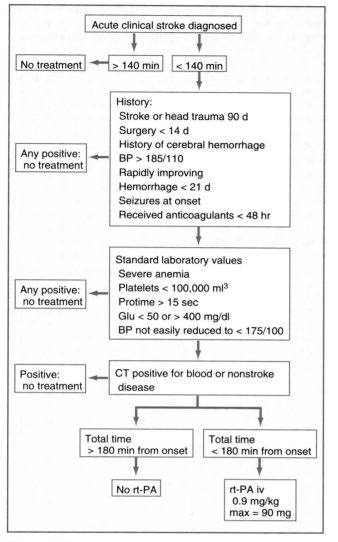

Figure 117–2

Evaluating acute stroke for safe rtPA therapy. (From National Institute of Neurological Disorders and Stroke rt-PA Stroke Study Group: Tissue plasminogen activator for acute ischemic stroke. N Engl J Med 1996; 333:1581–1587.)

tion is contraindicated in the presence of factors listed in Table 117–11.

Anticoagulation is stopped in most patients, except those with atrial fibrillation (AF), after 2 to 4 weeks. Anticoagulants have no demonstrated benefit for patients with completed acute stroke of more than 2 to 4 hours' duration. Such patients immediately should proceed to the preventive measures listed in Table 117–12.

Ischemic Cerebral Edema

At least some degree of edema surrounds all cerebral infarcts. Ischemic edema generally becomes detectable within 12 to 24 hours following infarction and continues to increase for as long as 72 hours thereafter. Large, edematous hemispheric infarcts can produce sufficient

brain swelling to cause transtentorial herniation. Similar enlargement in the cerebellum may compress the brain stem or obstruct CSF outflow pathways. Either can be fatal.

Cerebral edema produces hypodense areas detectable by brain imaging surrounding a more or less distinct region of recent infarction. Such changes usually cannot be imaged by CT until at least 48 hours after the ictus.

Unless postischemic edema produces serious shifts of the brain within the skull, the process produces few or no symptoms. Treatment of major degrees of swelling requires correcting or treating systemic medical complications and, if herniation threatens, giving intravenously a dehydrating agent such as mannitol in an effort to shrink the brain. Passive, sustained hyperventilation briefly reduces the intracranial volume by inducing arterial vasoconstriction lasting 1 to 2 hours. Diuretic drugs produce minimal benefit. The induction of anesthetic coma has no therapeutic value. Corticosteroid drugs are contraindicated in the treatment of stroke; they do not benefit necrotic edema and may accentuate neurologic damage.

Medical Management of Stroke Patients and Risk Factors

Once past the acute phase of stroke, treatment consists of whatever rehabilitation is necessary, plus the initiation of

TABLE 117–11	**Use of Anticoagulants in Stroke**

I. Acute Therapy
  A. Indications
     Repetitive TIAs clustered closely together within a single day or a few days. Acutely progressive weakness in stroke.
  B. Procedure
     Initiate with heparin. Start warfarin concurrently and discontinue heparin when prothrombin time reaches 1.5 × normal. Continue warfarin 3–4 wk except in atrial fibrillation (AF). With acute completed stroke, start aspirin (ASA) therapy only.
  C. Contraindications
     Hypertension, either systolic >170 mm Hg or diastolic >100 mm Hg; uremia; bleeding diathesis; intracranial bleeding (by CT or LP); LP within past 2 hr.
II. Prophylactic or Chronic Therapy
  A. Indications
     Acute anterior wall myocardial infarction with mural thrombus formation. Procedure: high-dose heparin continuing with warfarin until thrombi dissolve.
     Chronic atrial fibrillation with any or all of the following risk factors:
       1. Congestive heart failure within 3 mo
       2. History of hypertension
       3. Previous thromboembolism
       4. Left ventricular dysfunction and/or enlarged left atrium measured by echocardiography
       5. Chronic cardiac valvular disease
     Atrial fibrillation with none of these risk factors is more safely treated with chronic ASA.
  B. Procedure: Initiate and maintain warfarin to maintain prothrombin time 1.5 × normal chronically.
  C. Contraindications:
     Same as in I.C. above.

CT = Computed tomography; LP = lumbar puncture; TIA = transient ischemic attack.

measures designed to reduce the risk of future stroke, myocardial infarction, or other vascular complications (see Table 117–12).

Aspirin and ticlopidine enjoy proven success in preventing recurrent stroke and myocardial infarction. Both drugs inhibit platelet aggregation but by different biochemical steps. Current evidence indicates that ticlopidine may be somewhat more effective than aspirin overall but is more expensive and produces severe neutropenia in about 1% of those exposed. Neither dipyridamole nor sulfinpyrazone has proven value in stroke prophylaxis. Patients with atrial fibrillation who are less than 60 years of age and suffer none of the specific risk factors mentioned in Table 117–12 can safely and effectively be treated with aspirin rather than warfarin.

Surgical Treatment

Table 117–13 lists indications and contraindications for carotid endarterectomy as a preventive measure. In North American and British studies, only patients who had both arteriographically confirmed ICA stenosis of greater than 70% and a history of an ipsilateral TIA or actual stroke within the preceding 3 months showed a highly significant longevity and freedom from stroke when compared with nonsurgical controls 18 months postoperatively. Rates for severe stroke or death were cut approximately in half. No benefit from surgery was demonstrated in either study for patients with less than 70% carotid stenosis, in those who had not suffered recent preoperative events, or those with complete carotid occlusion. Evidence indicates that high surgical morbidity-mortality rates contraindicate carotid endarterectomy in patients with evolving strokes. Other contraindications include recent major strokes, myocardial infarction, uncontrolled hypertension, and severe systemic metabolic problems.

TABLE 117–12	Treatment Risk Factors in Stroke

Proven Benefits

Stop smoking
Reduce systolic hypertension >160 mm Hg by at least 20 mm Hg, if possible to below 150 mm Hg; reduce diastolic pressure >90 mm Hg by at least 10 mm Hg, if possible to 85 mm Hg or below
Take daily aspirin, 0.6 gm, or ticlopidine, 0.5 gm/day as platelet antiaggregant
Treat selected symptomatic patients surgically for carotid stenosis of >70%
If obese, lose weight

Possible Benefits

Exercise
Lower cholesterol
Surgical carotid endarterectomy in asymptomatic patients with >70% stenosis
Use alcohol modestly
Control diabetes

TABLE 117–13	Carotid Endarterectomy and Stroke Prevention*

Indications	Contraindications or Uncertainties
Good general health	Severe medical problems
If hypertensive, treated	No history of recent ipsilateral TIA or stroke
Internal carotid stenosis 70–90%	Inexperienced or unskilled surgeon
Ipsilateral stroke or TIA within 3–6 mo	Internal carotid artery either completely or <70% occluded
Surgeon available with morbidity-mortality record <2%	

TIA = Transient ischemic attack.

Prognosis in Stroke

About one fourth of patients with acute completed stroke die during hospitalization. Advanced age, severe brain stem dysfunction, coma, and serious associated heart disease all worsen the outlook. Among survivors, about 40% of all patients with acute stroke make a good functional recovery. The degree and rate depend on the initial severity, the amount of improvement within the first 2 weeks, age, and how much language or cognitive difficulty persists. Few patients with pronounced Wernicke's aphasia or functional dementia regain full independence. Motor flaccidity or dense hemisensory defects persisting past the first weeks similarly reduce the probability of future independence.

Prognosis for patients with TIAs depends on the presence or absence of associated risk factors, especially cardiac. A variety of studies indicate a combined risk of about 12% per year for either stroke, myocardial infarction, or death (from either) following the onset of these minor cerebrovascular events. The annual risk of such consequences climbs to about 20% among patients with major strokes.

SPONTANEOUS PARENCHYMAL CEREBRAL HEMORRHAGE

Spontaneous (nontraumatic) cerebral hemorrhage may occur primarily into the substance of the brain (intracerebral or parenchymal) or over its surface (subarachnoid). Table 117–14 lists the major causes. Cerebral hemorrhage totals about 15% of all clinically detectable strokes but assumes greater medical importance because of its serious consequences. Table 117–15 lists the most characteristic manifestations.

Hypertensive-Atherosclerotic (H-A) Cerebral Hemorrhage

Roughly 80% of spontaneous parenchymal cerebral hemorrhages fall into this category. Long-standing hypertension antedates the bleed in about two thirds of cases, with

TABLE 117–14	Nontraumatic Causes of Intracranial Hemorrhage

I. Intracerebral Hemorrhage
  A. "Hypertensive" atherosclerotic hemorrhage: large; occurs mainly in basal ganglia, thalamus, cerebellum, pons. Often clinically catastrophic. Derives directly from degenerative-atherosclerotic vascular injury. Only 60% occur in hypertensives.
  B. Lobar hemorrhages: smaller; arise in polar regions of frontal, temporal, or occipital-parietal lobes. More common in elderly and in association with amyloid angiopathy or small vascular malformation. Some are asymptomatic.
  C. Hemorrhage from vascular malformations: large and small; many are cryptic lobar.
  D. Uncommon: bleeding into brain tumors; accompanying blood dyscrasias or anticoagulants; from inflammatory vasculopathies; secondary to venous infarction.

II. Subarachnoid Hemorrhage
  A. 85% arise from congenital berry aneurysms; 10–15% penetrate brain parenchyma.
  B. 15% cause not found.

the incidence of bleeding generally paralleling the intensity and duration of that disorder. With or without hypertension, rupture reflects an area of weakening leading to hemorrhage from penetrating arterioles of approximately 100 to 150 μm in diameter. Spontaneous bleeding can affect almost any part of the brain, although the most common sites for H-A hemorrhages are into the deep cerebral regions of the internal capsule, basal ganglia, and thalamus, as well as into the central pons and the deep nuclear regions of the cerebellum (Figs. 117–3 and 117–4).

In contrast to ischemic stroke, which commonly occurs during sleep, most H-A cerebral hemorrhage begins during wakefulness, often associated with exertion. Sudden severe headache, "the worst in my life," often announces the onset, followed within minutes to hours by neurologic signs whose nature and severity reflect the site and extent of the bleeding. Characteristically, systemic examination discloses hypertension, sometimes to a temporarily severe degree, and, commonly, cardiac enlargement as well as hypertensive or atherosclerotic changes in the retinal arteries.

Basal Ganglia–Internal Capsular Hemorrhage

The onset headache commonly arises ipsilateral to the bleed and is followed shortly by a progressive contralateral hemiparesis, often accompanied by the eyes deviating toward the side of the lesion owing to damage to the adjacent frontal eye fields. Convulsions are common and can take either a generalized grand mal pattern or a focal one that involves the body contralateral to the bleeding. In the latter case, the eyes often deviate away from the lesion during the seizure. Rupture into the lateral ventricle is frequent and precipitates autonomic symptoms of shivering, nausea, and vomiting. Large hemorrhages greater than 2.5 to 3 cm in diameter frequently cause coma within a few hours, and many such cases go on to severe disability or death. Smaller hematomas cause less neurologic damage, and ultimate improvement may be considerable.

Thalamic Hemorrhage

Although serious, these often are smaller and less devastating. Contralateral sensory loss, hemianopia, and hemiparesis or hemiplegia are characteristic. Compression of the tectum-midbrain commonly induces drowsiness, which only occasionally proceeds to coma. Gaze palsies are common and include defects in upward gaze. Eyes cast down and laterally at rest provide an almost pathognomonic sign of bleeding in this area. Midbrain compression may transiently cause pupillary inequality or fixation.

Pontine Hemorrhage

The events are defined in Table 117–15. Most patients die. Those who survive usually are left quadriplegic and totally dependent.

Cerebellar Hemorrhage

Unilateral occipital headache often announces the onset followed by ipsilateral incoordination-ataxia of the ex-

TABLE 117–15	Characteristics of Acute, Spontaneous, Severe Cerebral Hemorrhage			
	Headache	Motor-Sensory Signs	Gaze-Preference	Consciousness
Basal ganglia–internal capsule	Ipsilateral to bleed generalized severe	Contralateral hemiplegia, convulsions	Eyes deviate toward lesion	Coma frequent
Thalamic	Either or both sides, moderate	Contralateral hemiparesis, hemianopia; often hemisensory defect	Eyes deviate down and contralateral to lesion	Drowsy to coma with large lesions
Pontine	Cataclysmic global	Stertorous breathing, bilateral posturing	Pupils pinpoint, bilateral lateral gaze paralysis, ocular bobbing	Coma within seconds to minutes
Cerebellar	Ipsilateral to bleed, occipital	Ipsilateral incoordination, dysarthria, facial weakness	Weakness, paralysis of ipsilateral conjugate gaze	Late stupor or coma implies brain stem compression

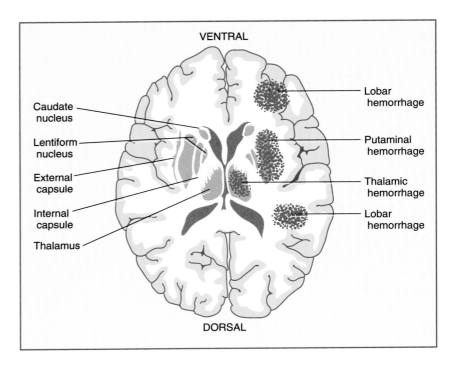

Figure 117–3
Horizontal section through the cerebral hemispheres illustrating frequent sites of thalamic, putaminal, and lobar hemorrhages.

tremities, slurred speech, and sometimes nausea and vomiting. Disequilibrium, ipsilateral facial weakness, and diplopia with ipsilateral conjugate gaze paralysis often follow within a matter of hours and may reflect either dissection of the hematoma into the lateral pons or only compression of that structure. The development of a reduced level of consciousness or of signs of upper motor neuron dysfunction affecting the extremities suggests the development of brain stem compression.

Lobar Hemorrhage

These occur in peripheral distribution in the white matter of the cerebral or cerebellar hemispheres. They usually are smaller and produce fewer acute or permanent neurologic abnormalities than the deep hypertensive-atherosclerotic hematomas described above. Among younger persons, many arise from image-detectable arteriovenous malformations or as complications of sympathomimetic

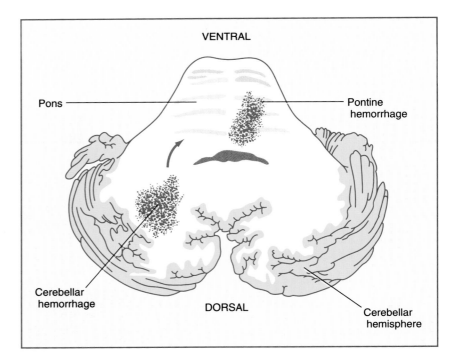

Figure 117–4
Horizontal section through pons and adjacent cerebellum showing common hemorrhage sites. The *arrow* shows a frequent line along which cerebellar hemorrhage can dissect into the pons.

drug abuse. Cerebral amyloid angiopathy is the leading cause in the elderly and commonly manifests with Alzheimer's disease.

Diagnosis

Hemorrhage into brain tumors occasionally may be indistinguishable from acute stroke, but large bleeds cause far more severe symptoms. Headache, severe hypertension, acute prostration, nausea and vomiting, convulsions, autonomic signs, and loss of consciousness are all more characteristic of deep cerebral hemorrhage than of ischemia. If blood reaches the subarachnoid space or if downward or upward herniation threatens, the neck stiffens. CT scan is diagnostic for hemorrhage but not for the cause of bleeding. Patients who are not hypertensive, who are young, or who have less than devastating neurologic deficits deserve arteriography to seek a potentially treatable vascular anomaly. Lumbar puncture can precipitate fatal intracranial herniation and should be avoided unless brain imaging is unavailable and acute bacterial meningitis seems a strong possibility.

Treatment

Treatment consists of bringing the blood pressure to nearly normotensive levels and applying supportive measures. When clinical signs and CT examination suggest that a cerebellar hemorrhage is compressing the brain stem or causing acute hydrocephalus, lateral ventricular decompression, clot removal, or posterior fossa decompression may be life-saving. Efforts to drain acute cerebral hemorrhages surgically are seldom successful. Lives may be saved but outcomes often are devastating.

Few patients in coma from cerebral hemorrhage survive, and those with extensive brain stem damage remain neurologically devastated. Considerable spontaneous neurologic recovery, however, often follows even moderately large hemorrhages in the peripheral parts of the cerebral or cerebellar hemispheres, because the blood dissects between much of the tissue rather than totally destroying it.

INTRACRANIAL ANEURYSMS

Intracranial aneurysms occur in three characteristic forms: fusiform, mycotic, and congenital berry aneurysms.

Fusiform aneurysms represent ectatic dilatations of the basilar or intracranial portion of the carotid artery. They develop a sausage-like or irregular bulbous shape, sometimes reaching a size of 5 to 10 cm in diameter. Usually they produce no symptoms, but sometimes their large size compresses adjacent tissues or cranial nerves to cause local neurologic dysfunction. Basilar artery fusiform aneurysms characteristically cause multiple bilateral asymmetric cranial nerve dysfunction extending anywhere from the third to the tenth nerve. Similarly large aneurisms of the intracranial carotid artery may cause ipsilateral visual loss or contralateral hemiparesis. Such aneurysms seldom rupture, and they resist successful surgical therapy.

Mycotic aneurysms arise in the course of bacterial endocarditis when septic emboli lodge in a peripheral cerebral vessel, producing endothelial ischemia at the embolic site. Infecting bacteria subsequently invade the arterial wall, and the resulting weakening invites aneurysmal blowout. Mycotic aneurysms are often multiple and characteristically arise peripherally on the cerebral arterial tree. Some resolve with antibiotic treatment, but those that remain after sterilizing the cardiosystemic infection should be treated surgically.

Congenital berry aneurysms arise at bifurcation points along the circle of Willis at the base of the brain (Fig. 117–5). In the anterior circulation they form especially at the junctions between the anterior cerebral and anterior communicating arteries and between the middle cerebral and either the posterior communicating or carotid arteries. Similar aneurysms can balloon out at one of the several major tributary points along the basilar-vertebral axis. Berry aneurysms vary considerably in size from a few millimeters to 1 to 2 cm or more in diameter. Those larger than 1.5 to 2 cm in diameter are commonly termed "giant" and carry a particular risk of rupture.

Berry aneurysms are thought to result from a congenital defect that affects adventitial tissue and muscle at arterial branch points along the base of the brain. The weak point allows aneurysmal formation and eventual rupture. Similar aneurysms also occur in association with certain brain tumors, presumably owing to the release of an as yet undetected angiotrophic factor. Congenital aneurysms are more common in persons with long-standing hypertension, especially those suffering from coarctation of the aorta and polycystic kidney disease. Some persons have multiple intracranial aneurysms. Heredity creates a low but definite predisposition.

Clinical Manifestations of Aneurysmal Rupture and Subarachnoid Hemorrhage (SAH)

These can be divided into five phases: onset, the first week of acute symptoms, the risk of secondary ischemic infarction, the development of communicating hydrocephalus, and the indications for and outcome of surgery.

The usual first symptom is sudden excruciating headache, sometimes followed by brief syncope, the latter resulting either from a neurogenically induced cardiac arrhythmia or from the brief concussion that accompanies the sudden rise in intracranial pressure. Subsequent effects depend on the locus and extent of the bleeding. Small warning leaks sometimes occur, causing a severe headache (sentinel headache) that then subsides over the following few days. Larger bleeds confined to the subarachnoid space produce more severe and sustained head pain, followed in 12 to 24 hours by signs of meningeal inflammation as red blood cells lyse and release irritating pigments into the CSF.

Stiff neck at onset implies a large hemorrhage either arising in the posterior fossa or producing acutely elevated intracranial pressure with descent of the cerebellar tonsils. Retinal hemorrhages can appear within minutes of the onset of subarachnoid bleeding. Either focal neuro-

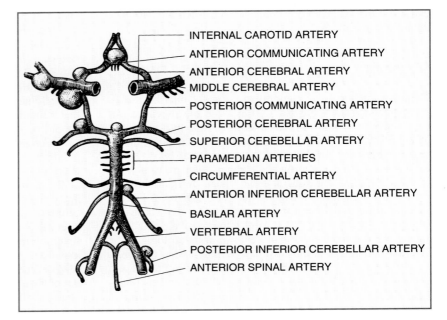

Figure 117–5
The more common sites of berry aneurysm. The diagrammatic size of the aneurysm at the various sites is directly proportional to its frequency at that locus.

INTERNAL CAROTID ARTERY
ANTERIOR COMMUNICATING ARTERY
ANTERIOR CEREBRAL ARTERY
MIDDLE CEREBRAL ARTERY
POSTERIOR COMMUNICATING ARTERY
POSTERIOR CEREBRAL ARTERY
SUPERIOR CEREBELLAR ARTERY
PARAMEDIAN ARTERIES
CIRCUMFERENTIAL ARTERY
ANTERIOR INFERIOR CEREBELLAR ARTERY
BASILAR ARTERY
VERTEBRAL ARTERY
POSTERIOR INFERIOR CEREBELLAR ARTERY
ANTERIOR SPINAL ARTERY

logic signs or a reduced state of consciousness at onset imply that blood has dissected into the brain. Severe bleeds can immediately produce coma because bleeding dissects into the brain or ruptures into the ventricular system. Persistent coma implies a poor prognosis. After the first day, the development of new focal motor or neurologic abnormalities reflects either rebleeding or cerebral infarction caused by secondary arterial vasoconstriction induced by the subarachnoid blood.

By a few hours after the onset of bleeding, a variety of systemic and secondary changes may complicate the picture. The initial bleed may stimulate the release of systemic catecholamines, which produce diffuse myocardial micronecrosis and abnormalities in the ECG. Acutely, systemic hyperglycemia, leukocytosis, and fever have a similar adrenergic pathogenesis. Subsequently, fever, leukocytosis, and delirium can last a week or more owing to a continuing blood-induced chemical meningitis. Most severely ill patients with acute SAH secrete inappropriately high levels of antidiuretic hormone, predisposing to hyponatremia. Late symptoms of lethargy, continued delirium, stupor, or diffuse, mild upper motor neuron abnormalities may reflect the development of communicating hydrocephalus secondary to blockage of CSF absorption pathways.

Diagnosis

The first principle is to respect the development of sudden severe headache in a previously well adult. Although many such "thunderclap headaches" turn out to be benign, when serious doubt exists, one should obtain a CT scan, which detects most subarachnoid hemorrhages, or a lumbar puncture, taking care to identify intrinsic bleeding by centrifuging bloody fluid and looking for a discolored supernatant.

For more obviously acutely ill patients with typical symptoms, CT scan is the laboratory procedure of choice; if no blood is visualized, lumbar puncture can then be done to identify other potentially serious causes of sudden acute headache. CT scans also show the presence of large clots in the subarachnoid space or brain and provide a baseline for future comparison in the event of subsequent unexplained worsenings. Contrast CT scans or MRI obtained with contemporary instruments often outline aneurysms of greater than 5 mm in diameter as well as arteriovenous abnormalities that may have caused the hemorrhage.

Acute subarachnoid hemorrhage is a life-threatening illness that should be dealt with by specialized personnel. Once the condition is diagnosed, patients should be referred immediately to experienced neurosurgeons in a tertiary medical center. Arteriography is indispensable for identifying the presence and location of aneurysms and should be performed by skilled neuroradiologists as soon as possible. In poor-risk patients or when it is anticipated that surgery will be done elsewhere, no value is gained by adding the hazards of arteriography to the already precarious state.

Management and Prognosis

Optimal treatment for aneurysmal subarachnoid hemorrhage consists of surgical clipping of the leaking vessel as soon as possible after onset. Good-risk patients operated on within a day of acute bleeding enjoy the highest survival and the fewest neurologic complications. Prognosis is substantially worse in patients whose early course is complicated by reduced arousal, confusion, or severe somatic neurologic deficits. Of all SAH patients, two thirds die within 1 month (many without reaching a hospital), with about one fourth of the survivors being severely disabled. The first 2 weeks after onset carry the greatest risk of rebleeding, amounting to about 30%. Among patients whose aneurysms cannot be treated successfully, rebleeding with a two thirds risk of mortality continues at a rate of about 3% per year.

Medical therapy for acute SAH consists of bed rest, mild sedation, and nonopiate pain relief. The calcium channel–blocker nimodipine lowers by one third the incidence of cerebral infarction after SAH and should be started immediately, employing oral doses of 60 mg every 4 hours for 21 days.

Surgery should be deferred or avoided in patients who are neurologically unstable, in those with major neurologic deficits, and in those who are stuporous or comatose. Similarly, most authorities avoid immediate surgery for patients whose arteriograms show arterial vasospasm. Continued obtundation not explained by focal damage but associated with CT evidence of progressive hydrocephalus sometimes can be relieved by ventricular shunting. It is not established whether operating on intracranial aneurysms more than 30 days following the bleed has any advantage over the natural history of the disease.

ARTERIOVENOUS MALFORMATIONS (AVMs)

Four types of vascular malformations can affect the brain including: (1) capillary telangiectases, seldom a cause of clinical abnormalities; (2) venous angiomas. One form constitutes the Sturge-Weber syndrome; larger ones occasionally may rupture or, when in the spinal cord, can produce tissue compression. (3) Small-vessel *cavernous angiomas*, which sometimes provide an occult source of intracerebral hemorrhage. (4) Arteriovenous malformations (AVMs) consisting of snakelike vascular tangles in which arteries connect directly with veins. AVMs can affect any part of the brain or spinal cord and can range in diameter from a few millimeters to 10 cm or more. Most arise from congenital abnormalities of the arterial wall at points where two or more major intracranial arteries conjoin, such as in the deep frontoparietal area where the distal branches of anterior, middle, and poste-

rior cerebral arteries converge. Most AVMs gradually increase in size and characteristically produce their symptoms in persons over age 30 years.

AVMs can cause three kinds of neurologic disability: (1) as many as half leak intermittently, producing parenchymal or subarachnoid hemorrhages that usually are smaller and less dangerous than those resulting from hypertensive hemorrhage or ruptured berry aneurysms; (2) some cause focal epileptic seizures; and (3) others slowly enlarge, producing progressive neurologic deficits. A small percentage of AVMs are associated with unilateral headaches resembling classic migraines; among all migraines, however, this is a rare cause.

Surgical treatment of AVMs, although often successful, is technically difficult. Invasive neuroradiologic techniques often have better success. Moderate-sized AVMs discovered incidentally by CT scan or arteriography and causing no symptoms are best left alone. Similarly, patients with seizures as their only manifestation often are best treated with anticonvulsants alone. AVMs smaller than 3 cm in diameter often can be coagulated by proton beam or focused gamma ray radiation. The risk of neurologic damage or fatal bleeding in intracranial AVMs is relatively low, and cases should be judged individually in experienced neurologic centers.

REFERENCES

Adams HP, Biller J: Ischemic cerebrovascular disease. *In* Bradley WG, Daroff RB, Fenichel GM, Marsden CD (eds.): Neurology in Clinical Practice. 2nd ed. Vascular Diseases of the Nervous System. Boston, Batterworth-Heinemann, 1996; pp 993–1047.

Bronner LL, Kanter DS, Manson JE: Primary prevention of stroke. New Engl J Med, 1995; 333:1392–1400.

Case CS: Intracerebral hemorrhage. *In* Bradley WG, Daroff RB, Fenichel GM, Marsden CD (eds.): Neurology in Clinical Practice. 2nd ed. Vascular Diseases of the Nervous System. Boston, Butterworth-Heinemann, 1996.

National Institute of Neurological Disorders and Stroke rt-PA Stroke Study Group: Tissue plasminogen activator for acute ischemic stroke. New Engl J Med 1996; 333:1581–1587.

Pulsinelli WA, Levy DE: Cerebrovascular diseases. In Bennett JC, Plum F (eds.): Cecil Textbook of Medicine. 20th ed. Philadelphia, WB Saunders, 1996, pp 2057–2080.

118

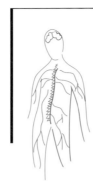

Trauma to the Head and Spine

HEAD/BRAIN INJURY

Pathophysiology

An average of 52,000 persons in the United States die each year from traumatic brain injury; since 1900, more than half of these resulted from firearms. Meanwhile, motor vehicle deaths declined by 22% reflecting the success of preventive measures in this area.

Open, *focal brain injuries* caused by crush or penetrating objects affect specific regions, usually of the cerebrum. *High-velocity penetrating missiles* can emit shock waves that injure more remote areas of the hemispheres and brain stem. Most focal injuries produce relatively restricted problems requiring largely acute surgical treatment. The consequences of *closed head injury* are different and depend upon the intensity of impact, the direction of the resulting movement of the cranium, and whether or not complications arise. Heavy alcohol intake or illicit drug intoxication increases the incidence and worsens its effects. Complicating systemic illnesses adversely influence management and outcome.

Most of the brain damage that comes from closed head injury results from impact-caused acceleration-deceleration forces. Inertia carries the gelatinous brain forward against the suddenly immobile skull, injuring structures both under the point of injury and 180 degrees away (contrecoup) (Fig. 118–1). Concurrent torsional injuries to the head literally shear white matter fibers away from their origins and/or destiny, thereby devastating normal cerebral connectivity. In such circumstances, the presence or absence of a fracture is relatively irrelevant; it is the brain that suffers most.

The care of severe head injuries falls largely into the provinces of neurosurgeons or emergency medicine personnel. General physicians are more concerned with acute, roadside first aid and, especially, the chronic effects of mild head injury that does not require acute hospital admission.

Severe Head Injury

Whether or not consciousness has been lost, the presence or absence of associated neurologic abnormalities involving neuro-ophthalmologic, motor, and breathing functions provides the best index of severity. Later on, severity can be judged by the duration of coma and how long anterograde or retrograde amnesia lasts. Table 118–1 provides an algorithm.

Mild injuries are those in which persons report feeling only dazed or semisyncopal and have normal neurologic findings. Neither hospitalization nor laboratory testing is needed so long as the patient can be depended upon to report potential complications and there are no abnormal neurologic signs. If doubt exists, discretion recommends obtaining a computed tomographic (CT) scan to rule out incipient extradural or parenchymal hematoma. When CT scan is available, skull radiographs are useless.

Concussion defines brief loss of consciousness or global memory loss with no immediate or delayed neurologic residua detectable by clinical or radiographic study. The boxer's knockout epitomizes the abnormality: for a few seconds awareness disappears, the pupils dilate and fix, breathing stops, the heart slows, and muscles become flaccid. Anterograde amnesia can last as long as an hour or so, but observable recovery begins within seconds to minutes and completes itself within hours. Psychosensory symptoms such as giddiness, anxiety, and apprehension may remain for days or longer. Brain imaging studies show no abnormality, and no treatment is indicated other reassurance and, sometimes, anxiolytics.

Intermediate diffuse brain injuries extend the length of unconsciousness to as much as an hour or so and are followed by a proportionately greater injury and slower recovery of orientation and behavior. Associated drunkenness can make appraisal difficult, but in the earliest stages cautious evaluation requires that one attribute any neurologic changes directly to the trauma. Many patients are transiently disoriented, and others show mild or moderate focal neurologic abnormalities. Patients with intermediate-level injuries require hospitalization to guard against complications and to control possible agitated behavior. More active treatment seldom is necessary. Most patients younger than about age 40 years recover completely within days to weeks. Loss of consciousness for as little as 24 to 36 hours in older persons may be followed by permanent psychological and intellectual limitations.

Severe diffuse injury is judged by the patient's clinical response rather than the nature of the trauma. Serious neurologic damage usually is apparent from the start, al-

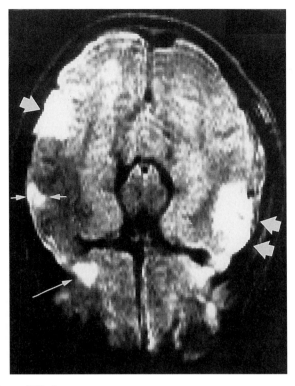

Figure 118–1
Magnetic resonance image of closed head injury showing cerebral edema–contusion at point of impact *(two large arrows)* and 180 degrees opposite *(one large arrow)* in a 22-year-old woman. An extradural hematoma had been removed at the impact site 6 days earlier. Small arrows indicate additional contusions. The patient recovered completely.

TABLE 118–1	An Algorithm for Managing Acute, Severe Head Injury

Patient Awake

Focal signs or severe headache:
  Absent: watch 1–2 hr; give phone number to call if symptoms arise.
  Present: watch but get brain image; observe until stable. If image
    negative, follow above.

Patient Unconscious, Obtunded, or Confused

At accident:
  Place supine on flat carrying surface.
  Evaluate and clear airway.
  Seek and staunch hemorrhage.
    Await paramedics, who have antishock agents and transporting
      equipment.
  Give no opiates.
In emergency room (if possible a trauma center):
  Intubate and deliver 30–50% oxygen.
  Assist ventilation as needed.
  Start intravenous line with large-gauge needle.
  Treat shock; avoid hyponatremia.
  Stop seizures; avoid steroids and opiates; give antibiotics as indicated.
  Obtain neurosurgical consultation; if delayed, complete systemic and
    neurologic examinations and obtain brain computed tomography
    scan.
  Assign to critical care experts decisions about whether to treat sys-
    temic or neurologic injuries first.

though exceptions exist. For example, following seemingly mild head trauma, an occasional child or adolescent can develop within minutes to an hour or so massive and sometimes fatal brain edema. More commonly, severe, unanticipated brain edema or infarction can be delayed for several hours to a day or more in adults. Even hemorrhages can postpone their appearance for a matter of days to a week or so. Patients who undergo these delayed responses account for as many as 20% of fatal head injuries.

Management of Acute Head Trauma and Its Complications

Emergency Management

Whether at the accident scene or hospital emergency room, proper immediate steps may save both lives and brains. The algorithm given in Table 118–1 outlines the general approach.

Hospital Management

Patients with severe trauma should be treated in an intensive care setting, where standard critical care measures are the mainstay. Potential complications (Table 118–2) include the early onset of severe brain edema and/or hemorrhage, the development of extradural hematomas, the presence of depressed skull fractures with intracranial infection, and the development of carotid sinus fistulae. The references provide details of these acute management problems. The general physician's role in head injury becomes most important during later convalescent periods.

Post-Traumatic Problems

These conditions fall into the province of general physicians and neurologists and often produce difficult management problems (Table 118–3).

TABLE 118–2	Late Complications of Acute Brain Trauma

Self-Limited

Postconcussion syndrome
Benign, delayed post-traumatic encephalopathy

Serious

Intellectual, personality, and motor decline
Post-traumatic epilepsy
Chronic subdural hematoma
Dementia pugilistica (boxers)

TABLE 118–3	Problems Faced by General Physicians/ Neurologists Managing Head Injury

Acute
Delayed post-traumatic encephalopathy
Subacute-Chronic
Post-traumatic epilepsy
Subdural hematoma
Late post-traumatic dementia or dementia pugilistica
Postconcussion syndrome

Acute Briefly Delayed Post-Traumatic Encephalopathy

This is an unusual syndrome that principally affects children or adolescents. Approximately 15 minutes to 2 hours or so following a minor head injury, such as falling from a low swing, the young person becomes obtunded or stuporous, often with nausea or vomiting. Despite these potentially alarming early symptoms, most patients recover uneventfully, but focal neurologic deficits including cortical blindness sometimes can last for several hours or, very rarely, permanently. The cause is not known, although the visual loss may be secondary to posterior cerebral artery compression during transient edema-induced transtentorial herniation. Similarly unexplained are rare instances of parenchymal cerebral hemorrhage that can arise from hours to a matter of a week or more following relatively mild, initially uncomplicated cerebral trauma.

Post-Traumatic Epilepsy

This condition, mainly associated with convulsive attacks, ranges in incidence from 50% after penetrating brain injuries down to about 5% following unconsciousness-producing closed head injury. In an effort to protect against such convulsive attacks, most authorities treat asymptomatic patients with penetrating brain injuries prophylactically with phenytoin or carbamazepine for up to 2 years following severe injury.

Whether such treatment protects against post-traumatic epilepsy remains uncertain. If seizures do occur, the drugs mentioned represent the treatment of choice.

Chronic Subdural Hematomas

These represent significant complications after head injury. The onset of symptoms can be weeks to months after injuries that are usually mild and sometimes so trivial as to have been forgotten. Age over 50, alcoholism, and the anticoagulated state are important predisposing factors. A sustained, new headache and fluctuating mental dullness are the most common symptoms, often associated with hypersomnia and sometimes with hemiparesis. The varying symptoms presumably reflect small rebleedings or the development of transient intracranial pressure

elevations associated with impaired cerebral arterial autoregulation. Accurate diagnosis requires brain imaging, which in symptomatic cases shows brain shift or, with bilateral hematomas, smaller than normal ventricles and few sulci at the vertex. Magnetic resonance imaging (MRI) is diagnostically superior because CT films obtained within a matter of a few weeks after injury may not distinguish the hematoma from the surrounding brain (Fig. 118–2). Small or moderate hematomas can be treated by observation with or without administering corticosteroids to reduce potential brain swelling. Larger clots, particularly those causing abnormal neurologic signs or symptoms, are best treated surgically.

Delayed Dementia Following Brain Trauma and the apoE ε4 Allele

This can affect two cohorts, each representing a different kind of injury but both disproportionately including persons carrying the apolipoprotein apoE ε4 allele. It has been known for some time that acute brain trauma results in beta-amyloid deposition in brain. More recent evidence shows that persons with a history of head injury associated with an hour or more of unconsciousness and possessing the apoE ε4 allele have a 10-fold increased risk of developing late-life Alzheimer's disease. Controls of similar age possessing the apoE ε4 allele but having no head injury suffer only a 2-fold risk over the non-allele population.

Dementia pugilistica, the "punch drunk" syndrome, clinically affects former boxers older than age 55 years, although psychological tests may show a less serious degree of intellectual deterioration even before age 40. Victims develop progressive motor slowness, clumsiness, dysarthria, ataxia, memory loss, and incontinence. The syndrome relates directly to the number of former fights, with an incidence of about 20% among those who box professionally 6 to 9 years or more. Brain images show cerebral atrophy and ventricular dilatation. Postmortem brain analyses reveal prominent neurofibrillary degeneration, diffuse deposition of beta-amyloid protein in apoE ε4 carriers and, in a subset of such carriers, cerebral amyloid angiopathy potentially leading to later life cerebral hemorrhage.

Postconcussion Syndrome (PCS)

Sometimes called *mild traumatic brain injury* or *post-traumatic stress disorder,* this syndrome characteristically follows mild head injuries. Similar symptoms may ensue after other forms of acute psychologically threatening trauma such as "whiplash" injury. To be considered postconcussive, the initial head trauma must have induced unconsciousness lasting no more than seconds to minutes, precipitated no evident focal neurologic abnormalities, and induced a period of anterograde amnesia lasting for minutes to hours. Brain imaging is uninformative.

Headache, giddy sensations, irritability, difficulty in concentration, and vague apprehension of impending ca-

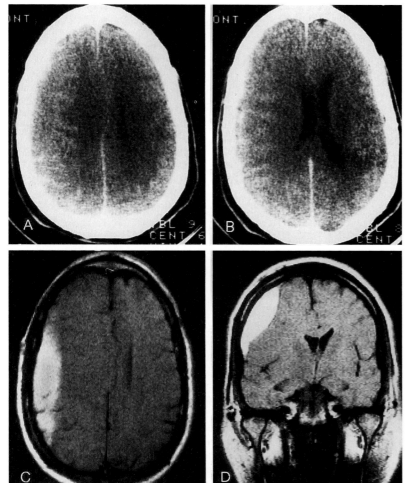

Figure 118–2

An isodense subdural hematoma invisible on computed tomographic scan (*A* and *B*) is readily disclosed by a concurrently obtained magnetic resonance imaging (*C* and *D*). The patient had suffered from headache, loss of mental acuity, fatigue, and disequilibrium for 4 months. He was unable to tandem walk, but examination otherwise was unremarkable. He recovered completely following drainage of the hematoma.

tastrophe constitute the major symptoms of PCS. Physical and laboratory signs of biologically significant neurologic or systemic dysfunction usually are lacking, and the condition gradually passes with time, medication having no specific effect. No cause is known. Contrary to common opinion, compensation or previous psychological problems appear to have little influence on the incidence or duration of the disorder. Antidepressants have shown little benefit. Management consists of reassurance plus symptomatic treatment for headache, neck pain, or dizziness. Whatever the treatment, half to two thirds of sufferers will lose their major symptoms in 6 months and all but about 5 to 10% will have returned to full activity within a year, albeit with some residual sense of intellectual quickness. The presence of a supportive physician provides the most important therapy.

SPINAL CORD INJURY

Severe spinal cord injury is relatively uncommon but often is both devastating and prolonged in its consequences. Most affected persons are younger than 30 years of age. The intraspinal contents can be concussed, contused, lac-

erated, macerated, or sheared, depending upon the nature of the initiating injury.

The principal mechanisms of spinal injury are dislocation with or without fracture at the atlas-axis junction, fracture-dislocations with or without bony fragmentation at other spinal levels, and penetrating missile or stab wounds. Less frequent causes derive from severe hyperflexion or hyperextension of the cervical spine in persons who suffer from an abnormally narrow spinal canal.

Patterns of Spinal Cord Injury and Their Resulting Disabilities

Complete Versus Partial Cord Injury

This can usually be discerned almost immediately following injury. Neurologic findings in complete injury reflect functional cord transection. Flaccid motor paralysis develops below the level of damage accompanied by total anesthesia in the same distribution. Bladder and bowel functions are lost, and prognosis for neurologic recovery is poor, irrespective of treatment.

Partial spinal injury is more common with cervical

than thoracic cord trauma and can take several forms. Any discernible voluntary movement or sensory perception found distal to the injury at the time of accident means that the injured cord or nerve roots possess a capacity for recovery that only time will define.

Spinal Concussion

The most common cause is high-velocity missile wounds that pass close to the spinal canal but fail to damage the cord severely. Distal neurologic loss never is complete, and recovery occurs within hours to days.

Central Cord Damage

Usually due to trauma, central cord damage affects primarily the lower cervical segments, usually with patchy hemorrhage centered along or adjacent to the spinal central canal (hematomyelia). Severe external blows or local fractures without serious canal displacement are the most common causes. The upper extremities become more paralyzed and insensate than the lower; sensory changes at and immediately below the cervical level affect pain and temperature more than touch; bladder and male sexual paralysis are common.

Cervical Hyperextension and Hyperflexion Injury

Mild or inconsequential paraparesis affecting legs more than arms is typical in cervical hyperextension, coupled with painful paresthesias in the arms and hyposensitivity to position and vibratory testing below the lesion. *Hyperflexion injury* may produce tetraparesis or tetraplegia accompanied by bilateral pain and temperature impairment below the lesion. Urinary retention often ensues. Both hyperextension (posterior cord) and hyperflexion (anterior cord) injuries can vary widely in severity, and many patients regain considerable function. Mixed or unilateral injuries produce variants of the *Brown-Séquard syndrome* of hemicord damage.

Intraspinal damage at or distal to the first lumbar spinal level injures the *conus medullaris* or *cauda equina*. The result may produce various mixtures of flaccid paralysis, distal mixed sensory loss, and autonomic-sexual paralysis affecting the pelvic girdle and lower extremities.

Whiplash Injury

A collection of painful symptoms can follow acute hyperextension-flexion of the neck without symptoms or signs of traumatic nerve root or cord dysfunction. The nature of the injury is an acute sprain; symptoms similar to those incurred in mild postconcussion disorders commonly arise and usually are not related to either potential compensation or intrinsically neurotic personalities. Symptoms last less than 6 months in over half the victims and remain permanent only in about 4%. Standard early treatment includes adequate analgesia plus strong reassurance by the physician. Soft collars and professional physical therapy contribute importantly.

Treatment

Management at the scene of the accident consists of maintaining ventilation, protecting against shock, and immobilizing the neck and spine to prevent further damage. Recent controlled studies show that methylprednisolone given intravenously in doses of 30 mg/kg of body weight within 8 hours after the onset of trauma and followed by 5.4 mg/kg infused hourly for 23 hours reduces the amount of eventual neurologic dysfunction. Persons with severe spinal injuries are best cared for in experienced centers. Open surgical treatment confers little benefit and only adds another trauma. Acute and postacute management for quadriplegics or paraplegics requires treatment in specialized centers.

REFERENCES

Alexander MP: Mild traumatic brain injury: Pathophysiology, natural history, and clinical management. Neurology 1995; 45:1253–1260.

Chiles BW, Cooper PR: Acute spinal injury. New Engl J Med 1996; 334:514–520.

Pearce JMS: Polemics of chronic whiplash injury. Neurology 1994; 44: 1993–1997.

Radanov BP, Sturzenegger M, Di Stefano G: Long-term outcome after whiplash injury. Medicine 1995; 74: 281–297.

119

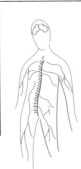

Epilepsy

An *epileptic seizure* consists of an episode of uncontrollable, abnormal motor, sensory, or psychological behavior caused by repetitive, hypersynchronous, abnormal electrochemical activity originating in the cerebrum. *Epilepsy* is a chronic disorder characterized by recurrent seizures in which the attacks themselves become the target for specific therapy. Many seizures occur sporadically in conditions that are not part of the disease of epilepsy. These can result from a variety of causes such as electroconvulsive therapy, profound syncope, the ingestion or withdrawal of certain drugs or toxins, or any of several kinds of infections or acute injuries of the brain.

Seizure disorders fall into two general etiologic groups: (1) *primary or idiopathic epilepsy,* which predominantly reflects genetic predisposition but the cellular-molecular cause remains largely or entirely unknown; and (2) *secondary or symptomatic epilepsy,* in which seizures result from a known structural or metabolic disease of the brain.

INCIDENCE AND GENERAL ETIOLOGY

Seizures can begin at any time of life (Table 119–1). Population studies in several developed countries worldwide indicate that 2 to 4% of all persons suffer from recurrent seizures at some time during their lives. Third World countries as well as First World inner-city areas show incidence rates almost twice as high.

PATHOPHYSIOLOGY

Focal seizures produce abnormal unilateral movements or sensations as well as stereotyped behavioral patterns that express the pathologic excitation of specific parts of the cerebral hemispheres. Most often, they originate in association with anatomically restricted lesions of gray matter such as scars, tumors, arteriovenous malformations, or focal areas of inflammation. *Generalized seizures,* by contrast, express themselves with bilateral motor abnormalities, usually accompanied by at least a brief loss of consciousness. They reflect either a diffuse hyperexcitable propensity of brain cells or the presence of a deeply lying, cryptic epileptogenic abnormality that involves centrally located subcortical activating mechanisms. Focally

originating ictal discharges can become generalized when they project bilaterally to widespread cerebral areas. Certain anatomic areas of the cerebrum are especially disposed to producing seizures. These include the frontal lobes, the medial temporal lobes (limbic system), the diencephalic reticular formation, and, to a lesser degree, the occipital lobes.

Genetic factors influence susceptibility to both generalized and focal epilepsy. Generalized epilepsies, such as petit mal absences and febrile convulsions, are usually transmitted as an autosomal dominant trait with variable penetration. The blood relatives of patients with chronic focal seizures originating in the temporal lobe also show an above-normal incidence of seizure disorders.

The specific brain mechanisms that cause seizure discharges to start, spread, or stop are poorly understood. Abnormalities that have been suggested include: (1) intrinsic neuronal receptor and molecular channel changes that could induce abnormal ionic conductance across synapses, (2) abnormal neurotransmitter synthesis leading to deficiencies of inhibitory or excesses in excitatory neurotransmitters, and (3) deficiencies in genetically regulated intracellular enzymes that normally affect the capacity of the neurons or glial cells to pump ions and repolarize.

CLINICAL SEIZURE PATTERNS (Table 119–2)

Individual epileptic attacks can last from a few seconds to several minutes in duration, with the pattern of the symptoms often reflecting the functional anatomy of the seizure focus. Seizures and their effects can be divided into several stages. The *aura,* the first self-experienced symptom, usually reflects the anatomic focus where the seizure begins. The *attack* itself follows and subsequently gives way to the *postictal period,* during which headache, drowsiness, or focal neurologic abnormalities can remain, often for minutes, occasionally for hours or even days.

Partial Seizures

Partial seizures consist of repetitive attacks of uncontrollable, focal neurologic dysfunction. The attacks are described as *simple* if only a restricted form of behavior or experience is expressed (equivalent to the aura) and con-

TABLE 119-1	Principal Causes of Seizures by Age of Onset
Neonatal	Developmental insufficiency or brain injury
Infantile	Congenital malformations, perinatal injury, metabolic disorders
Children and adolescents	Mainly genetic
Adults over 20	Some genetic; otherwise, cerebral neoplasms; drug-alcohol withdrawal; brain injury by trauma, stroke, infection, or surgery

sciousness remains intact. Attacks are called *complex* if the pattern of neurologic symptoms and signs evolves or if consciousness is impaired or lost. The initiating signs and symptoms offer the best clinical localizing evidence for the brain area that contains the epileptogenic lesion.

Partial motor seizures can arise from epileptogenic foci in the primary motor, premotor, supplementary motor, or prefrontal areas of either frontal lobe. Lateral prefrontal, supplementary motor, and premotor foci all cause adversive seizures. Motor components in partial motor seizures can begin and remain as simple aversion of the head and eyes away from the side of the focus, can include extension or raising of the contralateral arm and turning of the trunk, and occasionally can include crude vocalizations or, if arising in the dominant hemisphere, speech arrest. Because of abundant anatomic transcortical and thalamic interconnections, frontal seizure discharges can either produce contralateral motor activity or rapidly precipitate generalized convulsions. With lesions lying far anterior in the frontal lobes, consciousness may be lost concurrently with or even before any focal movements begin. By contrast, most patients with focal seizures aris-

TABLE 119-2	Classification of Epileptic Seizure Patterns

I. **Partial seizures** originate from a focal, usually structural lesion in the brain and may express either a single symptom without altered consciousness (simple) or changing symptoms associated with altered consciousness (complex).
  A. Motor (includes monomyoclonic)
  B. Sensory
  C. Psychological
  D. Partial complex: behavioral seizures with altered consciousness, usually of limbic-temporal lobe origin
II. **Generalized seizures** cause at least momentary loss of consciousness except some myoclonic attacks.
  A. Nonconvulsive
    1. Absence (petit mal)
    2. Atypical absence
    3. Atonic
    4. Myoclonic
  B. Convulsive
    1. Tonic-clonic (grand mal)
    2. Tonic only
    3. Clonic only
III. **Atypical or unclassified seizures** usually do not impair consciousness.
  A. Paroxysmal tonic spasms
  B. Spinal myoclonus

ing from supplementary or premotor areas remain aware for at least the beginning of the attack.

Primary motor (rolandic) seizures produce the classic *jacksonian* epileptic attack, John Hughlings Jackson being the English neurologist who first deduced the significance of the pattern. Rhythmic, clonic twitching begins in the contralateral thumb or corner of the mouth and most often spreads gradually to produce adjacent movements from thumb to hand to arm to face. Occasionally, the spread goes from face to hand. Either way, spread to a generalized convulsion is common. Many jacksonian seizures are followed by transient or sustained postictal *Todd's paralysis* of the limb.

Partial sensory seizures produce the classic epileptic aura: a sensory presentiment that represents the time and place of the seizure onset. Most common are epigastric rising sensations that emanate from discharges affecting the frontal lobe insular cortex, followed in frequency by somatosensory tingling or numbness (postcentral gyrus), simple visual phenomena (mostly occipital), vertigo (superior temporal gyrus), or vague cephalic or generalized body sensations (no localizing value). Lesions in and around the temporal uncus cause foul-smelling hallucinations that often blend into other temporal lobe symptoms.

Partial complex seizures of temporal lobe–limbic cortex origin represent the most frequent form of chronic epilepsy, amounting to about 40% of total cases. About half begin before age 25 years, and most are associated with discernible structural lesions in the temporal limbic area. Frequent causes include developmental anomalies, residua of early-life brain infection or severe febrile convulsions, head trauma, neoplasms, and, in later life, stroke or focal atrophy. Most partial complex seizures begin in foci that lie along the medial portion of the temporal lobe or the adjacent inferior frontal limbic area from which they spread posteriorly along the temporal lobe limbic cortex. They often project transcallosally to the opposite medial temporal area. Attacks also can spread into deep diencephalic structures to produce generalized convulsions. Consciousness and memory usually are severely dulled or lost during the evolution of the attack.

The aura of partial complex seizures is the first symptom of the attack (Table 119–3). It commonly identifies the seizure's anatomic origin and sometimes comprises the entire episode. More often, early, consciously perceived symptoms spread into stereotyped automatic movements that can take several forms (Table 119–4). Partial complex seizures usually last 1 to 2 minutes, seldom as long as 5, and are followed by slow reorientation accompanied by headache and drowsiness. Most affected patients show temporal lobe spikes or slow foci in interictal electroencephalograms (EEGs), provided that records during sleep are obtained. Sometimes, however, deep limbic discharges may go undetected altogether by skull surface electrodes.

Many patients suffering from temporal epilepsy display abnormal interictal behavior, including ruminative obsessiveness, religiosity, circumstantiality, hypersensitivity, and self-absorption, as well as hypergraphia.

Differential diagnosis of partial complex seizures includes mainly petit mal absences and psychiatric fugue states. Petit mal absence attacks are abrupt in onset and

TABLE 119–3	Frequent Early Symptoms of Limbic-Temporal Lobe Seizures

Symptom	Locus of Origin
Foul odor, "uncinate fit"	Temporal uncus-amygdaloid area
Micropsia or macropsia	Middle-inferior temporal gyrus
Déjà vu (intense familiarity)	Parahippocampal-hippocampal area
Jamais vu (environmental unfamiliarity)	
Fragments of voices, phrases, songs	Auditory association cortex
Lip smacking, abdominal pain, borborygmi, epigastric rising, cardiac arrhythmia	Insular, temporal-polar limbic cortex
Dreamy feelings, fear, pleasure, anger	Parahippocampal and septal areas

offset, last only a few seconds, usually are unaccompanied by subjective self-awareness, do not produce auras or automatisms, and are associated with a diagnostic EEG abnormality. Psychiatric fugues can be more difficult to distinguish, especially from true psychomotor attacks in patients who have normal EEGs. Psychiatric states, however, include a past history of sustained psychiatric or behavioral aberration and last longer than seizures. Also, they lack the characteristic evolution from aura to attack to a drowsy and confused postictal state. Often, they have a self-rewarding relationship to life situations that is lacking in true epilepsy. Partial complex seizures do not offer a satisfactory explanation for unprovoked violence or planned crime.

Generalized Epilepsies

Secondary Generalization

As noted earlier, many partial seizures can evolve rapidly into generalized convulsions before the epileptic discharge burns itself out. Occasionally the generalized seizure explodes before any focal behavioral sign exposes itself. In such instances meticulous electroencephalographic study, brain imaging, or restricted postictal weakness may indicate the focus and its causative lesion.

TABLE 119–4	Common Ictal Manifestations of Limbic Partial Complex Seizures

Autonomic:	Flushing, pallor, tachypnea, nausea, eructation-borborygmi, sweating, cardiac arrhythmia
Cognitive:	Intense déjà vu (familiarity), jamais vu (spatial amnesia), forced thinking, dreamlike states, depersonalization
Affective:	Laughing, fear, rage, depression, elation
Sensory:	Olfactory hallucinations, macropsia, micropsia, familiar voice fragments, visualized objects or scenes, emotional experiences (dreamy states)
Motor:	Staring with lip smacking, chewing, semipurposeful rubbing; confused, bizarre behavior; walking or, occasionally, running; postictal confusion or drowsiness

Primary Generalized Epilepsies

These can take several forms depending upon the patient's age at onset and the extent and nature of any associated structural or metabolic disease of the brain. The generalized epilepsies can be divided conveniently according to whether or not they produce major convulsions.

NONCONVULSIVE GENERALIZED EPILEPSY (Table 119–5). *Absence seizures (petit mal)* usually begin between ages 2 and 12 years, almost always before age 20. No structural or metabolic disease has as yet been identified as the cause, although genetic studies show an approximately 40% incidence of EEG abnormalities among first-degree relatives. Neither intelligence nor other neurologic functions are impaired.

Simple absence attacks last no more than 1 to 2 seconds and are characterized by a blank stare, often accompanied by mild 3- to 4-Hz blinking of the eyelids. The child's head droops, the lids and sometimes the arms jerk rhythmically, and there may be brief motor automatisms and enuresis. In severely affected children, dozens to 100 or more such episodes can occur in a single day. More protracted, *complex absence attacks* can last for 15 to 30 seconds, rarely as long as a minute.

Both the clinical pattern and the EEG are typical (Fig. 119–1). The EEG contains repeated bursts and runs of symmetric 3.5-Hz activity. Overbreathing for 60 to 180 seconds often induces both the electrical abnormality and the seizures. Atypical seizures or EEG patterns that differ from the aforementioned suggest one of the less benign generalized childhood epilepsies. About half the children with petit mal seizures develop generalized tonic-clonic convulsions before the age of 20. Status epilepticus with petit mal seizures is described in a later section.

Myoclonus defines a brief, unexpected, and uncontrollable jerk of the entire body or a focal portion of the trunk or one of the extremities. The phenomenon often

TABLE 119–5	Types of Nonconvulsive, Generalized Epilepsy

Absence seizures (petit mal): Common childhood condition with high genetic influence and no structural brain abnormalities. Diagnostic EEG. Good cognitive prognosis.
Adult petit mal status: A rare middle-life disorder producing sustained dulled behavior; EEG resembles petit mal. Only some patients respond to standard anticonvulsants. Some deteriorate intellectually.
Myoclonus: Benign (juvenile) epileptic myoclonus. Fairly common. Begins in late childhood or adolescence. Autosomal dominant abnormality of chromosome 6. Clinically mild. EEG relates to petit mal.
Secondary myoclonic epilepsy: Several severe degenerative diseases of children and adults cause generalized or multifocal myoclonic attacks. Acquired causes include anoxia, encephalitis, severe trauma, and Creutzfeldt-Jakob disease.
Atonic-akinetic epilepsy and infantile spasms reflect developmental delay: Severe myoclonic, atonic, or spasmogenic illnesses of infancy and young childhood. Can result in injuries.
Palatal myoclonus: Is not myoclonus but a rhythmic 120 beats/min tremor of the soft palate associated with brain stem–cerebellar disease.

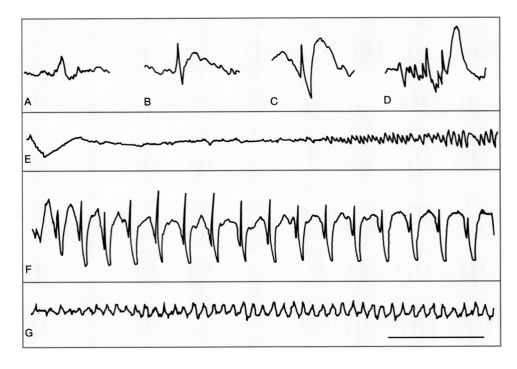

Figure 119–1
Electroencephalographic patterns in seizure disorders. *A,* Interictal sharp wave. *B, C,* Interictal spike-and-wave complexes. *D,* Interictal poly-spike-and-wave complex. *E,* Recruiting rhythm typical of the onset of a generalized convulsion. *F,* Repetitive spike-and-wave discharges typical of absence seizures. *G,* Rhythmic pattern seen with temporal lobe seizures. *Line* at the bottom right of the figure represents 1 second. (From Engel J: The epilepsies. *In* Wyngaarden JB, Smith LH, Bennett JC [eds.]: Cecil Textbook of Medicine. 19th ed. Philadelphia, WB Saunders, 1992, p 2208.)

occurs normally during presleep drowsiness. Diffuse, multifocal, or repetitive myoclonus, however, is abnormal and occurs in several degenerative toxic and infectious neurologic disorders as well as in several of the severe childhood epilepsies (see Table 119–5).

Bilateral benign (juvenile) epileptic myoclonus consists of bilateral repetitive mild myoclonic jerks affecting girls more than boys and arms more than legs. The disease usually begins during early adolescence, and the symmetric jerks especially involve the shoulders and arms. Often, the EEG contains bifrontal 3.5- to 4-Hz sharp and slow activity similar to that found in absence seizures. The disorder pathogenically and genetically lies close to petit mal and carries a similar modest risk of future tonic-clonic seizures. It responds to similar medication, especially sodium valproate, but may be so mild as to require no treatment. Table 119–5 describes other, less common forms of myoclonic attacks.

GENERALIZED CONVULSIVE EPILEPSY. Generalized convulsive epilepsy can take either the tonic-clonic or tonic form.

Tonic-clonic (grand mal) seizures can begin at any age. Most produce loss of consciousness at onset, although patients occasionally report a brief rising epigastric sensation as the attack begins. Any focal manifestations in the evolution of the attack or in the postictal period suggest a localized structural cause rather than a generalized basis for the seizure. Prodromal warnings (not auras) sometimes precede the attacks by several hours and can include a change in mood, a sense of apprehension, insomnia, or loss of appetite. Sometimes clusters of repetitive myoclonus anticipate a convulsion. As the convulsion begins, patients may cry out unconsciously. They

stiffen tonically in extension, usually with muscles contracted so tightly as to arrest breathing. Deep cyanosis follows before relaxation and a first post-tonic breath ensue. Such vigorously tonic phases seldom last as much as a minute but may be repeated several times over. Gradually, hyperextension gives way to a series of rapid successive clonic jerks of neck, trunk, and extremities. Finally, flaccid relaxation ensues, accompanied by stertorous breathing, pallor, and profuse salivation. Hypertension, tachycardia, and heavy perspiration accompany the motor changes. The pupils may be briefly fixed and moderately dilated during the tonic convulsions. Absent oculocephalic reflexes, hyperactive deep tendon reflexes, and extensor plantar responses can outlast the seizure for several minutes, but these changes usually disappear as the patient awakens 2 to 3 minutes after the relaxation phase begins. Many patients bite their tongues or lose sphincter control during attacks. Sometimes the tonic contractions are so strong that they compress dorsal or upper lumbar vertebrae. Other serious injuries are uncommon. Fatigue, muscle weakness and soreness, generalized headache, and drowsiness follow grand mal attacks. Occasionally, confusion can last for several hours. Most patients sleep postictally and awaken several hours later with only muscle soreness to remind them that a convulsion has occurred.

During the convulsive movements of generalized seizures, EEG recordings disclose rapidly repeating spike discharges followed by sharp-slow activity as clonic contractions supervene. Postictally the record becomes abnormally slow, sometimes for several hours. The interictal EEG can be normal in about 20% of instances but usually contains spike-slow complexes, bursts of abnormally slow activity, or mixtures of spike and slow activity in bursts or in short, 10- to 20-second runs appearing symmetrically over the scalp (see Fig. 119–1).

Unusual Seizures and Other Conditions That Respond to Antiepileptic Medication

In predisposed persons, a variety of sensory stimuli can precipitate *reflex epilepsy*. Photogenic seizures can be triggered by stroboscopic lights, driving past a stand of trees that filters the sun, looking at video games, or waving the hand in front of eyes fixed upon bright illumination. The ensuing generalized seizure can take the form of myoclonus, an absence attack, or a tonic-clonic convulsion. Closely related are seizures elicited by looking at certain geometric patterns or, rarely, by reading. Polarized glasses may reduce the stimulus intensity of photosensitive attacks; valproic acid is the most effective anticonvulsant.

Familial paroxysmal choreoathetosis is a rare disorder inherited as an autosomal dominant or recessive trait and characterized by paroxysms of choreiform, dystonic, and athetoid body torsions occurring during full consciousness. Stress or sudden movement can precipitate the episodes. Phenytoin or carbamazepine relieves most cases.

Recurrent torsion spasms consist of episodic dystonic spasms affecting the face, trunk, and extremities in patients with multiple sclerosis. Body movement or startling stimuli can precipitate the attacks, which do not interfere with consciousness. The EEG remains normal, but phenytoin or carbamazepine treatment prevents the episodes.

Anticonvulsants also can favorably affect other disorders that result from an excess of central or peripheral excitation. Included are myokymia and *lightning pains*—episodic, severe, flashlike pains affecting the extremities, associated most often with neurosyphilis or diabetic neuropathy. Carbamazepine sometimes reduces the pain of herpes zoster, as well as trigeminal or glossopharyngeal neuralgia.

Diagnosis

Given evidence that a seizure, automatism, or other brief episode of altered brain function has occurred, the major questions are whether it is epileptic and, if so, of what type and cause. The patient's description of the experience or a witness's accurate observation of an attack usually provides the most rewarding information. The setting of the attack often suggests acute causes such as drug withdrawal, central nervous system (CNS) infection, trauma, or stroke; a history of recent-onset seizures in an adult suggests an intracranial mass lesion and a more chronically sustained or remote history of attacks suggests chronic epilepsy. Any focal feature reported either as an aura or during or following the seizure suggests a structural brain lesion demanding appropriate investigation. The pattern of an attack as well as the patient's age immediately delimits the possible types and causes (Table 119–6).

Physical and neurologic examinations should identify any evidence of either systemic illness or structural neurologic disease. Laboratory studies should include lumbar puncture in any child or adult with new-onset seizures or

TABLE 119–6	Major Clinical Features of Postinfantile Epilepsy	
Age	**Major Cause**	**Types of Seizures**
Children <15 yr	Idiopathic and genetic epilepsy	Generalized (grand mal) Febrile convulsions Petit mal absence Adolescent myoclonus Partial complex attacks (uncommon)
	Developmental defects; birth trauma; inherited biochemical disorders; acute central nervous system (CNS) infection-inflammation; post-traumatic or postinfectious	Generalized grand mal Partial motor, sensory, or psychological attacks, simple or complex Disseminated or multifocal myoclonus Partial or generalized
Adults 15–25+ yr	Idiopathic and genetic epilepsy	Generalized (grand mal) convulsions Polymyoclonus Partial complex seizures
	Acute CNS infection-inflammation; traumatic–post-traumatic; drug intoxication or withdrawal; brain tumor or arteriovenous malformation	Generalized or partial seizures
Adults >25 yr	Brain tumor; CNS infection-inflammation; traumatic–post-traumatic; withdrawal; acute or poststroke	Generalized or partial seizures

suspected of developing CNS infection. Single seizures seldom affect the cerebrospinal fluid (CSF) content, but major motor status epilepticus temporarily can raise the protein concentration and generate up to 100 white cells per mm^3. If, in children, the history, findings, or EEG suggests a focal abnormality, or in any adult, a contrast-enhanced MRI or CT scan is indicated.

The EEG is critical in diagnosing the type of epilepsy and its best therapy. The normal EEG contains fairly rhythmic, bilaterally symmetric potentials, with amplitudes ranging from about 20 to 200 mV (see Fig. 119–1). The typical EEG frequencies recorded in healthy adults are 8.5 to 13 Hz, called alpha; 13 to 30 Hz, called beta; 4 to 7 Hz, called theta; and 0.5 to 4 Hz, called delta. Wakeful persons at rest typically show a dominant alpha rhythm, which accelerates into less rhythmic, faster frequencies during concentrated attention and after ingesting certain drugs. Frequencies of 8 Hz and slower occur normally during drowsiness or sleep; such slowing during wakefulness commonly reflects an abnormality of brain function. Regionally localized or asymmetric bursts of slowing, sharp waves, or spikelike waves characteristically reflect focal disturbances in brain function, whereas, paroxysmal and symmetric slow, sharp, or sharp-slow activity is typical of primary epilepsy. EEG findings, however, must be interpreted with caution because 20% of patients with clinically typical epilepsy can have normal records, whereas 2 to 5% of persons who never have a seizure can express occasional epileptic-like sharp waves or sharp-slow activity in the EEG. Most laboratories routinely employ hyperventilation and stroboscopic stimulation to activate potential EEG abnormalities. Atypical electrode placements, sleep studies, and telemetry are diagnostic tools utilized by specialists. Chief to be considered in the differential diagnosis at all ages are syncope, pseudoseizures and other factitious attacks among adolescents and younger adults, and cerebral transient ischemic attacks in older patients.

Syncope provides the biggest problem, because one seldom can observe the attack and retrospective histories incline toward ambiguity. Furthermore, syncope often recurs in children and adolescents and, when severe, may terminate in a brief, nonepileptic convulsion. Syncope always occurs when sitting or standing except when associated with episodic cardiac arrest (Table 119–7). Attacks of syncope last a shorter time than seizures, produce characteristic changes in appearance and motor behavior, cause no postictal confusion or headache, and often are linked to emotional or visceral stimulation. Persons with syncope characteristically lack EEG abnormalities, and neither anticonvulsants nor other medications reliably improve the condition.

Factitious pseudoseizures provide a diagnostic challenge because they often occur in persons who suffer from organic epilepsy as well. Most hysterical seizures occur in emotionally stressful settings or to achieve secondary gain. Certain features suggest pseudoseizures: rapidly rolling the head or body from side to side, an alternating thrashing of the extremities, or pelvic thrusting. Few hysterics soil or injure themselves during attacks, whereas many epileptics do. Nevertheless, hysterics or malingerers can be good actors and their attacks can fool even experienced observers. A dependable but expensive way to differentiate organic from hysterical major motor seizures is to obtain a serum prolactin level immediately postictally: the level rises with true convulsions but not with hysteria. Accurate diagnosis in puzzling cases is best achieved by epilepsy centers equipped to monitor behavioral and EEG activity in 24-hour epochs.

Episodic psychogenic fugue states or attacks of behavioral dyscontrol sometimes become confused with partial complex seizures. Most such episodes bear little resemblance to the stereotyped automatisms of temporal lobe epilepsy. As with major convulsion-like attacks, a strongly abnormal EEG inclines one toward a diagnosis of epilepsy. In difficult cases, telemetric monitoring of behavior concurrently with EEG recording can assist diagnosis.

Cerebral transient ischemic attacks (TIAs) rarely produce symptoms resembling epilepsy, because their principal effects consist of ischemic hypofunction rather than epileptic hyperfunction. Occasionally, however, aphasic speech arrest can occur with TIAs, and a few TIA patients develop contralateral or generalized trembling of the extremities which may resemble epileptic phenomena. The recent development of symptoms, the vascular distribution of the changes, the lack of an epileptogenic lesion on clinical evaluation or brain imaging, and the presence of other signs of systemic or cerebral vascular disease almost always lead to the correct diagnosis.

Several other kinds of episodic events may briefly suggest seizures but can be dismissed by obtaining a careful history or description of the attack. These include rapid breath-holding attacks in young children; migraine, which in children sometimes causes ataxia, vomiting, visual hallucinations or delirium, and stupor; narcolepsy-cataplexy; hyperventilation spells; and drop attacks in older adults. Nonepileptic causes of recurrent seizures include hypocalcemia, occurring spontaneously in children and following parathyroidectomy in adults, hypoglycemia at any age, and recurrent alcohol or depressant drug withdrawal.

MANAGEMENT

The goal is to halt the attacks completely. With symptomatic epilepsy this is followed by efforts to eradicate the cause, whereas in idiopathic seizure disorders antiepileptic therapy must be supplemented by efforts to help the patient adjust to a disease that brings fear to most and shame to many.

Control of Seizures

The ultimate goal is to achieve complete seizure control with minimal or absent antiepileptic drug toxicity. At present, medication suppresses seizures completely in about 60% of patients with chronic epilepsy, and substantially improves another 15 to 20%. Many of the uncontrollable patients suffer from a serious underlying disease of the brain, whereas others resist compliance with therapeutic instructions. Certain principles, however, may enhance success with pharmacologic regimens.

TABLE 119–7	Major Distinctions of Syncope From Seizures	
Sign	**Syncope**	**Seizures**
Prodromes	Usually nausea, "swimming" sensation, faintness; sometimes none	Aura or epigastric rise Often none
Onset	Sitting or erect	Any position
Awareness of attack	Always present	Sometimes absent (petit mal absences)
Motor activity	Usually none, occasionally brief clonic-tonic spasms. Convulsions may follow cardiac arrests	Focal, tonic, clonic, sustained
Duration	Seconds	0.5–2 min
Cardiovascular	Pulse slow, weak	Pulse fast, strong
Appearance	Pale, sweating	Flushed, salivating
Postictal	Oriented, sweaty, nauseated; sometimes vomiting, diarrhea	Confused, headache, drowsy
Electroencephalogram	Normal	Abnormal

1. Many persons have a single seizure with no recurrence. Accordingly, one should start long-term treatment on patients after a single, first attack only when a defined cause can be found that is likely to generate recurrences. Special social or vocational circumstances may override this rule. The principle of avoiding chronic treatment for only a single event also applies to uncomplicated febrile convulsions.
2. If repeated seizures occur, diagnose the probable type and give the single preferred medication in full recommended therapeutic dose.
3. If a single drug does not control the seizures, even at toxic levels, try another. Similarly, if the first anticonvulsant causes serious side effects, withdraw it but immediately initiate the next most effective agent. If efforts at single drug therapy fail, most patients are best referred to a specialized center for consultation, because combined therapy is often difficult to regulate without producing toxicity. Always adjust medications gradually so as to accomplish maximal seizure control with minimal side effects.
4. Never stop anticonvulsant medications for generalized seizures abruptly. Status epilepticus may result.

Choice of Anticonvulsants

Table 119–8 lists an arbitrary order of preference for effective anticonvulsants for various types of chronic epilepsy. Table 119–9 summarizes some of the major toxicities of these agents. As with any potent medication, physicians and patients should read package inserts before prescribing. Notwithstanding these precautions, one must remember that recurrent seizures constitute a physically dangerous, emotionally devastating, and intelligence-threatening risk. By comparison, the incidence of potential complications of antiepileptic therapy is almost trivial.

Use of Drug Levels in Management

The determination of blood levels can be a valuable adjunct to treatment. "Therapeutic" blood levels reflect empirically established values at which most patients acquire seizure control without toxic side effects. Many patients become well-controlled (or occasionally toxic) below the maximal therapeutic level, whereas others show no ill effects despite blood values above this point. In all instances the clinical response, not the blood level, defines the goal of the treatment.

Drug level determinations are especially useful within 2 to 3 weeks after beginning therapy so as to determine the patient's compliance, judge metabolic response to the medication, and compare the pharmacologic and clinical effects. They also can be helpful when drug dosage is changed: individual detoxification mechanisms can be saturated when antiepileptic drugs are increased or can overact to cause subtherapeutic ranges when the dose is reduced. Blood levels should be rechecked when patients are placed on an additional anticonvulsant or receive other medications that may influence hepatic enzyme systems.

TABLE 119–8	**Current Best Drugs for Epilepsy**		
Type of Seizure and Drug	Usual Total Adult Dose (gm)	Daily Doses	Therapeutic Blood Levels (μ/ml)
Generalized tonic-clonic			
Carbamazepine	0.8–1.2	3–4	8–12
Valproate	1–4	4	50–100
Phenytoin	0.3–0.5	2	10–20
Phenobarbital	0.1–0.25	1	15–40
Absence seizures			
Ethosuximide	0.75–2.0	2	40–100
Valproate		Same as above	
Clonazepam	0.002–0.008	3	0.01–0.05
Partial epilepsies			
Carbamazepine		Same as above	
Phenytoin		Same as above	
Valproate		Same as above	
Phenobarbital		Same as above	
Clonazepam		Same as above	
Gabapentin	2.4	3	
Lamotrigine	0.3–0.4	2	

An occasional blood level determination obtained during the course of chronic, effective therapy helps patients to understand the need for continued compliance. When seizures are well controlled, blood levels need be checked no more than annually.

TABLE 119–9	**Toxicity of Common Antiepileptic Drugs**

Carbamazepine

Dose-related: mental slowing, nausea, drowsiness, ataxia, nystagmus
Idiosyncratic: exanthema, inappropriate antidiuretic hormone secretion, leukopenia, aplastic anemia (rare), hepatic toxicity (rare)

Phenytoin

Dose excess: tremor, vertigo, nystagmus, ataxia, drowsiness
Hypersensitivity: gingival hyperplasia, hirsutism, coarse features, exanthema

Valproate

Dose-related: increased appetite, hair loss, tremor, ataxia, drowsiness
Idiosyncratic: toxic hyperammonemia, hepatic toxicity

Phenobarbital

Dose excess: drowsiness, mental slowing, dysarthria, ataxia, nystagmus
Idiosyncratic: exanthema

Primidone

Same as phenobarbital (seldom used)

Ethosuximide

Dose-related: dyspepsia, hiccup, headache, insomnia
Idiosyncratic: psychotic behavior, aplastic anemia (rare)

Clonazepam

Dose-related (in up to 50%): sedation, muscular hypotonia, ataxia, oral and tracheobronchial hypersecretion

Gabapentin

Dose-related: sedation

Lamotrigine

Idiosyncratic: rash (10%), particularly in combination with valproate

Special Management Problems

Status Epilepticus

In this condition seizures follow one another so rapidly that new attacks begin before the previous one has ceased. Attacks that follow in close succession but with brief periods of reawakening between are designated *serial seizures*. Either condition can occur with partial or generalized epilepsy. Status epilepticus is of special concern because the successive or continuous epileptic activity sometimes can damage the brain permanently. If, however, an accurate witness is unavailable, one must wait to be sure that epileptic attacks are continuing before initiating the treatment outlined in Table 119–10.

Partial motor status, an uncommon condition sometimes known as partial continuous epilepsy, occurs in several forms and can last for hours, days, or even as long as a year or more. The seizure frequency can range from as little as one every 3 seconds to as many as several per second. The motor attacks can consist of as little as a highly focal, myoclonic, repetitively localized twitch to jerks that involve most of the limb or even half the body, not always affecting precisely the same muscles. In general, cerebral lesions cause partial motor seizures in the face or distal upper extremity, whereas brain stem or spinal lesions tend to cause proximal myoclonic activity. Large strokes cause about half the cases, whereas trauma, neoplasms, or encephalitis produces the rest. Sometimes the cause never becomes clear. Partial continuous epilepsy often resists all efforts at treatment.

Partial complex status produces a sustained state of confusion associated with stereotyped motor and autonomic automatisms. Some attacks produce a suddenly beginning schizophreniform or stuporous state, whereas others are marked by bizarre, detached activity. Patients may resist assistance in their fuguelike state, which can last for hours and sometimes days. The EEG usually shows continuous slow and spike activity predominating over one or both temporal areas, commonly asymmetrically. Occasionally, surface recordings may be only mildly abnormal, but epileptiform activity can be detected by nasopharyngeal leads or from electrodes placed deep in the brain. Treatment should be initiated promptly, as the effects of prolonged seizures can permanently impair memory and intellect.

Absence status (petit mal status) occurs in two forms. The more common resembles partial complex status and consists of semiconfused automatic behavior accompanied by closely spaced or continuous runs of 3- to 4-Hz spike and wave activity on the EEG. The condition occurs in patients with known petit mal and usually is confined to adolescents or occasionally young adults. Most episodes last less than 30 minutes. Similar behavioral attacks of prolonged (days to months) automatisms associated with confusion, EEG abnormality, and sometimes gradual interictal mental deterioration can occur in older persons with no history of epilepsy. Most such attacks can be halted with intravenous diazepam.

Major generalized motor status epilepticus creates a life-threatening medical emergency. Repetitive convulsions lasting an hour or so commonly produce residual brain damage. The most frequent cause is abrupt withdrawal of anticonvulsant medications from a known epileptic. Other precipitants include withdrawal of alcohol or drugs in a habitual user, cerebral infection, trauma, hemorrhage, or neoplasm. Treatment of the convulsions and protection of the brain are of immediate concern and should take the form outlined in Table 119–10. Identification of the cause of the attacks must be undertaken as soon as possible after seizures stop.

Febrile Convulsions

Convulsions caused by fever occur mainly in neurologically healthy children between the ages of 6 months and 5 years who recurrently develop single generalized seizures when affected by an acute, fever-producing illness. Factors that increase the chance of having a future chronic epileptic disorder include age less than 1 year at onset, convulsions lasting longer than 15 minutes or coming in clusters, any pre- or postictal sign of neurologic abnormality, or a family history of epilepsy. Present practice is to do everything possible to limit the course of the single convulsion but to place only children who have high risk factors on medication.

Menstruation, Genetic Counseling, and Pregnancy

A number of women with epilepsy suffer an increase in seizures during the days immediately preceding and following the onset of menses. Acetazolamide, 250 to 500 mg daily, taken prophylactically or a modest increase in medication during the susceptible days often counteracts the problem.

TABLE 119–10	**Treatment of Adult Status Epilepticus or Serial Seizures**

Convulsive tonic-clonic or complex partial status

1. Assure the airway, give O_2, check blood pressure (BP) and pulse. Intubate if needed. Assess oxygenation regularly. Establish a venous line and draw blood for glucose, calcium, hyper or hypo-osmolar indicants. If indicated, measure pH, Pao_2, $Paco_2$.
2. Promptly start infusion and give 50 ml of 50% glucose. Give thiamine 100 mg IV.
3. Infuse diazepam intravenously 5 mg/min until seizures stop or to total 20 mg. Also start phenytoin 50 mg/min to total 18 mg/kg. Monitor electrocardiogram and BP.
4. If convulsions persist, give *either* (1) phenobarbital 100 mg/min or as loading dose to 20 mg/kg, *or* (2) 100 mg diazepam in 500 ml dextrose 5% run in at 40 ml/hr. Monitor ventilation closely and assist if necessary.
5. If convulsions persist, start anesthesia with pentobarbital, intubation, and, if seizures persist, neuromuscular blockade. Monitor the electroencephalogram continuously.

Serial tonic-clonic or partial motor status

1. Steps 3 and 4 above but do not induce coma.

Petit mal status

1. Diazepam as in step 3 followed by oral ethosuximide, valproic acid, or both.

Persons with seizure disorders should be advised about the hereditary risks to the fetus. Best evidence suggests that 4 to 10% of the offspring of patients with generalized primary epilepsy will suffer one or more seizures. This compares to a risk of about 1.5% in the general population. Rates in the partial epilepsies differ less clearly from the norm.

Chronic anticonvulsant medication often requires adjustment during pregnancy because blood volume increases and drug pharmacokinetics change. Blood level monitoring during the latter half of pregnancy can be useful in managing the difficult-to-control woman. During pregnancy, it is advisable to give vitamins and supplements, including calcium. Some authorities recommend that all woman of childbearing age take 1 mg folic acid daily to protect against developmental defects. Vitamin K, 5 mg twice weekly, should be given orally during the final 6 weeks, with a parenteral supplement administered to the mother and infant at the time of delivery. Breast feeding is not contraindicated in women taking antiepileptics.

Teratogenic Effects

Children of mothers or fathers taking antiepileptic medication have a birth defect risk 2 to 3 times that of the general population. Seizures, however, offer a greater risk to the mother and fetus than does the generally low rate of birth defects associated with antiepileptic drugs. Two agents, trimethadione and valproate, have been incriminated with especially high teratogenicity in experimental studies. Phenytoin, phenobarbital, and carbamazepine use during pregnancy all have been associated with neurodevelopmental difficulties. Given all factors, phenobarbital probably has the least teratogenic effect.

Surgical Therapy

In addition to attempting to remove specific mass or destructive brain lesions that include seizures among their symptoms, several forms of surgical treatment may halt or ameliorate medically intractable, chronic seizure disorders. Procedures include, for particular indications, local resection of seizure foci, anterior temporal lobe resections, section of the corpus callosum, and, rarely, subtotal hemispherectomy. Such approaches are best conducted in large medical centers sponsoring specialized programs for the treatment of epilepsy.

Psychosocial Management

The presence of incompletely controlled epilepsy and its frequent association with other neurologic limitations often create large emotional problems for the patient. In addition, disorders that cause partial complex seizures may result in aberrant personality traits that intensify isolation. Outbreaks of frustration, depression, and suicide are more frequent among patients with epilepsy than in the general population. A reduced libido and hyposexuality have been noted in males with partial complex seizures. By contrast, in the absence of associated brain damage, most persons with epilepsy score in the normal range on intelligence tests. Many persons with controlled epilepsy have performed superbly at every level of professional, governmental, artistic, and business life.

Patients with seizure disorders are helped most by bringing the attacks under control, but reassurance, sensitivity, and optimistic social guidance aid immeasurably. Once seizures are under control, affected persons should be encouraged to live a normal life using common sense as their guide. Body-contact and high-risk sports are best avoided unless seizures have been completely controlled for well over a year; high diving, deep water or underwater swimming, high alpine climbing, boxing, and head-contact football are ill advised. Most states grant automobile driver's licenses to patients with epilepsy provided that no seizures have occurred for at least a year. Life and health insurance policies are available under special circumstances. The Epilepsy Foundation of America can assist patients with these and other social-vocational considerations.

Discontinuation of Medication

One considers stopping antiepileptic medication either (1) because seizures continue and all concerned believe the drugs are ineffective or (2) because seizures have been completely controlled for a long time. The first condition is uncommon and must be approached cautiously because of the dangers of precipitating status epilepticus. The latter decision can be considered between patient and doctor when absence seizures have been fully suppressed for 2 or 3 years and other types of seizures for 3 to 5 years. The patient's value system, economic and social factors, and knowledge of risks all should contribute to the decision. Between 20 and 50% of those who discontinue treatment experience recurrent seizures, which may be more difficult to control than the original attacks. Particularly likely to relapse are persons whose initial seizures lasted longer than 6 months, were difficult to control, or were associated with any specific neurologic abnormality. A moderate or severely abnormal EEG represents an additional risk of recurrence if treatment stops. In general, most socioeconomically stable, well-controlled adult epileptics should stop anticonvulsant medication only if they show drug toxicity. For most, the cost of relapse is just too high.

REFERENCES

Brodie MJ, Dichter MA: Antiepileptic drugs. New Engl J Med 1996; 334:168–175.

Delgado-Escueta AV, Janz D: Consensus guidelines: Preconception counseling, management, and care of the pregnant woman with epilepsy. Neurology 1992; 42(suppl. 5):149.

Dodson WE, De Lorenzo RJ, Pedley TA, et al: Treatment of convulsive status epilepticus: Recommendations of the Epilepsy Foundation of America's working group on status epilepticus. JAMA 1993; 270:854.

Pedley TA: The epilepsies. *In* Bennett JC, Plum F (eds.): Cecil Textbook of Medicine. 20th ed. Philadelphia, WB Saunders, 1996, pp 2113–2125.

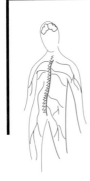

120

Intracranial Neoplasms, CNS Complications of Cancer, and States of Altered Intracranial Pressure

INTRACRANIAL NEOPLASMS

Introduction and Definitions

Intracranial tumors can arise from any structure within the intracranial cavity. Most begin in the brain, but the pituitary, pineal region, cranial nerves, and leptomeninges are also sites of neoplastic degeneration. Furthermore, any of these structures may be the site of metastatic spread from tumors that arise outside the nervous system. Intracranial tumors are not rare; they are the second most common cancer in children, and in adults malignant brain tumors are more common than Hodgkin's disease. Brain lymphoma and malignant glioma appear to be increasing in incidence. Also, the incidence appears to be increasing as the population ages. Symptomatic metastatic intracranial tumors are equal to or greater in number than primary neoplasms (Table 120–1).

Intracranial tumors can be classified both by site of origin and by histologic type. Most arise from neuroectodermal elements (the precursor of both neurons and glia). The terms *benign* and *malignant* applied to brain tumors reflect histologic criteria that reflect local growth rate rather than propensity to metastasize. Even highly malignant primary brain tumors rarely metastasize, although they may spread locally from the parenchyma to seed the leptomeninges and spinal cord. Also, many "benign" brain tumors recur despite treatment and eventually lead to the demise of the patient. Others may undergo "malignant degeneration" that alters their biologic potential.

Classification

Neuroectodermal Tumors

The most common neuroectodermal tumor is the *astrocytoma*. Astrocytomas can arise anywhere in the brain or spinal cord and infiltrate surrounding normal structures. Small nests of tumor cells often can be found several centimeters from the main bulk. In some instances, astrocytomas may have a multicentric origin or, more rarely, infiltrate the entire neuraxis (gliomatosis cerebri). Some, particularly cerebellar astrocytomas of childhood, may lie quiescent for decades after only partial resection. About half of astrocytomas grow slowly. The others consist of rapidly growing tumors that include the anaplastic astrocytoma and the glioblastoma multiforme. In adults, benign astrocytomas have a prognosis of 4 to 7 years, anaplastic astrocytomas 1.5 to 2.5 years, and glioblastoma usually 1 year or less. *Oligodendrogliomas* usually grow more slowly than astrocytomas and tend to calcify. Glial tumors are often mixed, so that elements of oligodendroglioma may be found within a tumor that is primarily astrocytic in origin, and areas of benign astrocytoma may be found within a malignant glioblastoma. Because of the heterogeneity of such tumors, small biopsies may give misleading diagnostic and prognostic information. Primary *lymphomas* of the nervous system are increasing in frequency in both immunosuppressed and immunocompetent individuals. They are often multifocal in the brain and seed the leptomeninges. Common sites of *ependymoma* growth include the fourth ventricle in children and the spinal cord in children and adults. Malignant ependymomas of the fourth ventricle often spread to involve the leptomeninges. *Medulloblastomas* arise from a primitive neuroectodermal cell, usually in the cerebellum, and likewise may seed throughout the cerebrospinal fluid (CSF). They are predominantly tumors of childhood and are highly malignant, but 60% of children treated by surgery and radiation therapy now survive more than 5 years. In children, astrocytomas represent half of all cerebellar tumors, medulloblastomas and ependymomas making up the rest.

TABLE 120-1	Common Intracranial Tumors in Adults		

| | Primary (50%) | | |
Metastatic (50%)	Brain Tumor (70%)		Other Intracranial Tumor (30%)
Lung 40%	Glioblastoma	40%	Meningioma 80%
Breast 20%	Anaplastic astro-	20%	Acoustic neuroma 10%
Melanoma 20%	cytoma		Pituitary adenoma 5%
Miscellaneous 20%	Astrocytoma	15%	Miscellaneous 5%
	Lymphoma	10%	
	Oligodendroglioma	5%	
	Miscellaneous	10%	

Mesodermal Tumors

The most common mesodermal tumor is *meningioma.* Meningiomas are usually benign and arise in certain favored sites: along the dorsal surface of the brain, the base of the skull, the falx cerebri, the sphenoid ridge, or within the lateral ventricles. Although these tumors are benign, they often reach a large size before they are discovered and may be difficult to remove. Furthermore, they may recur even after apparently complete surgical extirpation. The most common cranial nerve tumor is the *acoustic schwannoma* (neurilemoma, acoustic neuroma). Early discovery of such tumors has been possible in recent years because of the development of refined auditory tests and magnetic resonance imaging (MRI), thereby enabling these tumors to be removed frequently via a translabyrinthine approach or treated by radiosurgery. *Pituitary adenomas* may begin as intrasellar masses and extend into extrasellar locations, causing visual loss. *Microadenomas,* asymptomatic except for their hormone secretion, can now be identified by high-resolution computed tomographic (CT) scan or MRI of the pituitary. *Craniopharyngiomas* are developmental tumors derived from Rathke's pouch and may be intrasellar or suprasellar in location; they are frequently calcified and often cystic. *Pineal region* tumors occur primarily in children. They rarely originate from the pineal gland itself but instead are germinomas, often curable by chemotherapy and radiation. The benign *colloid cyst* usually grows in the anterior third ventricle. Vascular tumors include *arteriovenous malformations,* which are not truly neoplastic, and the *hemangioblastomas,* which are. The latter tumors, when located in the brain stem or cerebellum, may be part of the von Hippel–Lindau syndrome that includes hemangioblastomas elsewhere in the body. Congenital tumors include the craniopharyngiomas, *chordomas* (which arise at the base of the brain or the lumbosacral area from the primitive notochord), *dermoids,* and *teratomas.* Granulomas and parasitic cysts come from tuberculomas, cryptococcosis (toruloma), sarcoidosis, and cysticercosis.

Metastatic Tumors

These can spread to any part of the intracranial cavity and tend to exhibit growth characteristics similar to their parent neoplasm. Metastatic tumors, unlike primary tumors, tend to be well-circumscribed rather than infiltrative and are easier to remove in toto than are primary neoplasms.

Symptoms and Signs

Because they arise within the closed box of the skull, intracranial tumors tend to cause symptoms and signs

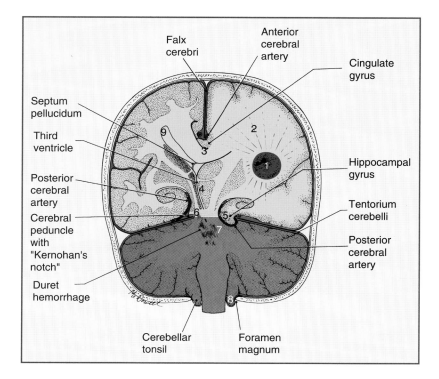

Figure 120-1
Schematic representation of the pathophysiology of clinical symptoms caused by a brain tumor. A mass lesion *(black sphere)* and surrounding edema *(dashed lines)* enlarge the hemisphere, obliterating normal sulci and shifting normal structures caudally and across the midline. The tumor and surrounding edema destroy and displace normal tissue in the hemisphere, producing contralateral neurologic signs (e.g., weakness and sensory loss). Obliteration of subarachnoid spaces by the mass lesion raises intracranial pressure, producing generalized signs (e.g., headache and papilledema). Shifts of normal brain cause symptoms at a distance and may lead to cerebral herniation (see Chapter 112). (Adapted from Cairncross JG, Posner JB: *In* Yarbro JW, Bornstein RS [eds.]: Oncologic Emergencies. New York, Grune and Stratton, 1981, with permission; from Posner JB: Neurologic Complications of Cancer. Philadelphia, FA Davis, 1995, p 9.)

while still relatively small. Symptoms may be caused by any of the four following factors (Fig. 120–1). (1) The tumor invades, irritates, or replaces normal tissue. This probably accounts for only a minority of symptoms in brain tumors but is particularly characteristic of low-grade infiltrating gliomas. (2) The tumor growth compresses normal tissues. As intracranial tumors grow, they compress surrounding tissues and cause shifts of normal brain structures. Blood vessels are compressed as well, leading to ischemia of the surrounding tissue. (3) New vessels formed in the growing brain tumor do not possess a blood-brain barrier (the anatomic-physiologic structure that excludes proteins, ionized substances, and many water-soluble chemotherapeutic agents from the normal central nervous system [CNS]). The blood-brain barrier also breaks down in compressed tissue surrounding a brain tumor. As a result, edema forms both within and around the tumor, which adds to the mass in the brain. Furthermore, because the brain has no lymphatics, removal of edema is slow. That edema produces many of the symptoms of intracranial tumors is attested to by the dramatic response that most brain tumor symptoms show to corticosteroids. These drugs, which decrease brain edema by restoring the integrity of the blood-brain barrier, substantially ameliorate symptoms for most patients with brain tumors without having a biologically significant effect on the growth of the tumor. (4) Large or small strategically located tumors (third ventricular and fourth ventricular tumors, leptomeningeal tumors) obstruct CSF pathways, leading to hydrocephalus. The resulting inability of normally formed CSF to escape from the ventricular system or the subarachnoid space further adds unwanted mass and raises intracranial pressure.

The mass of a brain tumor plus the attendant edema and hydrocephalus all may lead to herniation of normal cerebral structures under the falx cerebri, through the tentorium or foramen magnum (see Chapter 112).

The symptoms and signs caused by brain tumors depend on the location of the tumor and its histopathology (rapidity of growth). Sudden changes in tumor size resulting from hemorrhage, necrosis, or obstruction of CSF pathways can cause additional symptoms. Symptoms and signs may be divided into three major categories: (1) *generalized,* largely due to increased intracranial pressure; (2) *focal,* a result of ischemia and/or compression of normal brain at the site of the tumor; and (3) *false localizing,* a result of shifts of cerebral structures, causing neurologic abnormalities at a distance from the tumor.

Generalized Symptoms and Signs

The most common symptoms of increased intracranial pressure is *headache.* The head pain may be felt at the site of the tumor but more commonly is diffuse. In its early stages, the typical brain tumor headache is mild, tends to occur early in the morning when the patient first awakens, and disappears as the patient assumes an upright posture and breathes more deeply, thus lowering intracranial pressure. As the tumor enlarges, headaches become more constant and severe and are often exacerbated by coughing, bending, or sudden movement of the head.

Later, headaches may awaken the patient at night. Headaches are common symptoms only occasionally caused by brain tumors, but their onset in a patient not previously prone to headache or a recent change in headache pattern should alert the physician to the possibility of increased intracranial pressure. *Papilledema* occurs in about one tenth of patients with an intracranial neoplasm, probably as a result of obstruction of CSF pathways. Papilledema is much more common in children and young adults than it is in the elderly. *Vomiting,* with or without preceding nausea, is a common symptom of intracranial hypertension in children but less so in adults. Vomiting usually occurs early in the morning before breakfast. It is often, but not always, accompanied by headache. Vomiting is more common in posterior fossa tumors but can occur with any tumor that raises intracranial pressure. *Mental changes* are also common. Patients first become irritable and then later quiet and apathetic. They retire to bed early, arise later (unless the early morning is accompanied by headache), and nap during the day. They are forgetful, seem preoccupied, and often appear psychologically depressed. Psychiatric consultation is frequently procured before the diagnosis of brain tumor is suspected. In patients with mass lesions and intracranial pressure, *plateau waves* are a common phenomenon. Plateau waves are increased in intracranial pressure that last between 5 and 20 minutes. They are caused by failure of normal cerebral vascular autoregulation so that an abrupt increase in cerebral blood volume occurs, causing the intracranial pressure to rise. Such pressure waves can increase an already high intracranial pressure by as much as 60 to 100 mm Hg. The wave may be asymptomatic but more commonly is accompanied by neurologic symptoms including headache, brief visual loss, altered consciousness, and sometimes weakness of the extremities. These episodic changes in neurologic function usually last only a few minutes and may be precipitated by a sudden rise from a lying position; by alterations in intracranial pressure associated with coughing, sneezing, or straining; or even by tracheal suctioning.

Focal Symptoms and Signs

The location of a brain tumor determines not only whether the growth is more likely to produce generalized or focal signs but also the type of focal signs it produces. Tumors arising in relatively silent areas of the brain (such as the frontal pole) may grow to large size, raise intracranial pressure, and cause severe signs of generalized brain dysfunction before focal signs are evident. Similarly, tumors obstructing the ventricular system, particularly at the outflow of the third and fourth ventricles, also produce generalized signs before focal signs become evident. On the other hand, tumors arising in primary rather than association cortex are more likely at their onset to produce focal symptoms and signs. Tumors of the visual system cause visual loss or visual field deficits before generalized signs develop. Tumors of the sensorimotor cortex cause weakness and sensory change. In addition, because certain areas of the frontal lobe, temporal lobe, and sensorimotor cortex have a relatively low threshold for epileptic discharges, seizures are often an early symptom. If the tumor is in the sensorimotor cortex, the seizures take a focal sensory or motor pattern. Tumors arising in more silent areas can cause unrecognized focal epileptogenic discharges, which generalize to produce a grand mal seizure. Seizures are the most common presenting symptom of meningiomas and of low-grade infiltrating astrocytomas and oligodendrogliomas.

Cranial nerve tumors include trigeminal and acoustic schwannomas or meningiomas. Fifth nerve tumors are characterized by pain and sensory loss in the face, the pain sometimes resembling that of trigeminal neuralgia. Eighth nerve tumors are characterized by slowly progressive hearing loss with or without loss of balance. Both can be treated surgically.

A number of different tumors growing in the *pituitary fossa* and/or the *suprasellar* cistern lead to a combination of neurologic and endocrinologic abnormalities. The most common sellar tumor is the pituitary adenoma, a benign growth that often secretes excessive amounts of the hormone made by its parent cell. The tumors often remain very small, the only symptoms produced being those of hypersecretion of prolactin (amenorrhea-galactorrhea syndrome in women), growth hormone (acromegaly), or adrenocorticotropic hormone (Cushing disease). Other adenomas, however, can grow to a large size, compressing and destroying the normal pituitary gland and leading to hypopituitarism and diabetes insipidus. As such tumors grow superiorly, they compress the diaphragma sella, a pain-sensitive structure, and cause headache. Immediately above the diaphragma sella lies the optic chiasm, compression of which leads to bitemporal hemianopsia. If the tumor grows laterally, it encounters the oculomotor nerves in the cavernous sinus, producing ocular palsies. Some pituitary tumors outgrow their blood supply. In this instance, patients suffer sudden hemorrhage or necrosis into the tumor, producing the syndrome of *pituitary apoplexy.* A previously asymptomatic patient presents to the physician with acute headache plus visual changes (bitemporal hemianopsia or blindness) and sometimes oculomotor palsies. The patient is often febrile, with a stiff neck from spillage of blood and necrotic tissue into the subarachnoid space. A CT scan usually reveals a pituitary mass, often hemorrhagic. Emergency treatment with hormonal replacement and, often, decompression usually leads to a good outcome. Tumors arising in the *parasellar area* may cause visual loss simultaneous with or even before pituitary failure. The first sign of pituitary failure in these instances is usually diabetes insipidus; in children, failure of sexual development and obesity are common problems, probably resulting from compression of the hypothalamus. Craniopharyngiomas, optic gliomas, meningiomas, and sometimes large carotid aneurysms cause masses in this area, as do germinomas (ectopic pinealoma).

Most tumors arising in the *pineal area* are germinomas, teratomas, or other embryonal growths. These tumors are common in children, boys more than girls. They produce their symptoms by compression of the sylvian aqueduct, leading to hydrocephalus. Compression of fibers in the upper brain stem early on leads to loss of upward gaze and sometimes pupillary fixation. Occasion-

ally compression of the inferior colliculus causes deafness. A definitive diagnosis of pineal region tumor is important because the germinomas are usually curable, whereas most of the others are not. *Leptomeningeal* tumors usually result from spread of a primary brain or systemic tumor to the leptomeninges; occasionally lymphomas or melanomas arise in the leptomeninges. Metastatic leptomeningeal invasion is common from lymphomas, leukemias, or solid tumors such as carcinomas of the breast and malignant melanomas. Primary tumors of the nervous system that commonly seed the meninges include medulloblastomas, malignant ependymomas of the fourth ventricle, and germinomas. Symptoms of leptomeningeal involvement may occur before the primary tumor has declared itself. The first symptoms are often those of increased intracranial pressure from hydrocephalus (see Fig. 113–4). Additional symptoms include seizures from invasion of the cortex, cranial nerve palsies from infiltration of nerves passing through the subarachnoid space, and spinal root dysfunction, often involving the lower extremities and the bladder as a result of infiltration of the cauda equina. The diagnosis is suspected by the presence of diffuse or multifocal signs of CNS dysfunction and usually can be established by the identification of malignant cells in the CSF.

False Localizing Symptoms and Signs

Growing tumors mold the surrounding normal brain and displace adjacent and remote structures from their normal positions. When these structures are shifted, they may be compressed by nearby dura, by bone at the base of the skull, or by the bony foramina through which the cranial nerves pass. Compression of normal structures at a distance from the growing tumor leads to focal neurologic signs that may incorrectly localize the tumor. These false localizing signs usually occur with slow-growing tumors arising in relatively silent areas. Examples of well-recognized false localizing signs include diplopia as a result of displacement compression of the sixth nerve at the base of the brain, hemianopsia caused by tentorial herniation that compresses the posterior cerebral artery and produces ischemia to the occipital lobe, and tinnitus, vertigo, or hearing loss from compression of the eighth nerves as they pass through the internal auditory canal. False localizing signs rarely produce a diagnostic problem nowadays because of the availability of accurate imaging techniques. False localizing signs can also occur with pseudotumor cerebri or intracranial hypotension, in which their recognition is particularly important if one is to avoid unnecessarily exhaustive laboratory evaluation or inappropriate surgery.

Diagnostic Tests

In any patient clinically suspected of harboring an intracranial neoplasm, MRI is the test of choice (Fig. 120–2). It can identify tumors sometimes missed by CT scan (low-grade gliomas and small posterior fossa lesions) and often helps differentiate tumor from arteriovenous malfor-

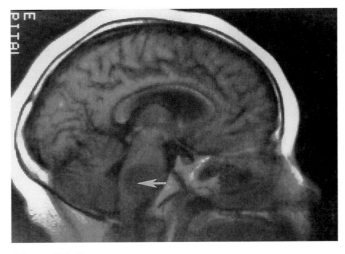

Figure 120–2
Magnetic resonance imaging (MRI) scan of an 18-year-old man with progressive cranial nerve symptoms suggesting a brain stem tumor. The computed tomographic (CT) scan was normal. Sagittal MRI reveals a mass *(arrow)* in the pons.

mations better than does CT. Meningiomas are often difficult to distinguish from normal structures by MRI, unless the scan is enhanced by intravenous gadolinium. Radionuclide brain scan, skull radiographs, and electroencephalograms (EEGs) add nothing to the diagnosis. If a leptomeningeal tumor is suspected by the presence of unexplained hydrocephalus or a diffuse encephalopathy without focal abnormalities on a brain image, lumbar puncture should be performed to look for the typical changes of pleocytosis, malignant cells in the CSF, elevated protein, and hypoglycorrhachia (low glucose con-

tent). At times, contrast-enhanced MRI or myelography identifies small tumors on the nerve roots.

Imaging techniques reveal the presence but not the exact nature of a lesion. Thus, neither CT nor MRI can definitively distinguish between the histologic types of tumors, nor can they reliably differentiate between neoplasms and other tumors such as abscesses or granulomas. Angiography is useful primarily to assist the surgeon in defining the proximity of the tumor to nearby arteries and veins. If a lesion is present and cannot clearly be identified on clinical grounds, biopsy is necessary before treatment is undertaken. When the lesion is accessible, surgical excision not only establishes the diagnosis but also provides the first step in the treatment of the patient. If the lesion is not accessible, CT- or MRI-directed stereotactic needle biopsy often can establish the diagnosis definitively.

Treatment

The treatment of intracranial neoplasms varies depending on the nature of the neoplasm, its location, and the general condition of the patient, but certain general principles apply. When there is a single lesion and it is surgically accessible, it should be removed to whatever degree possible. Although some patients undergoing surgery of intracranial neoplasms suffer increased neurologic dysfunction, the majority improve because the surgery relieves compression of brain structures. The advantages of surgery are that it cures some patients (pituitary adenoma, most meningiomas, cerebellar astrocytomas), it ameliorates symptoms in the majority of patients, and the debulking of a large malignant lesion allows time for other slower-acting therapeutic modalities to be effective. It

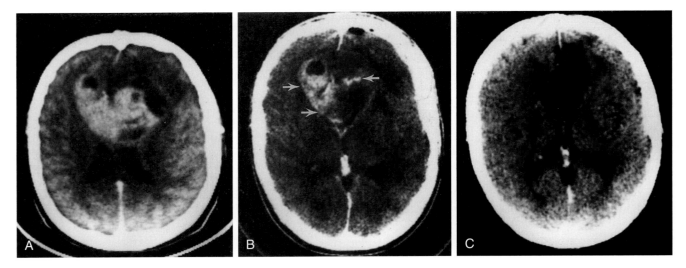

Figure 120–3
Results of treatment of glioblastoma multiforme. A 32-year-old man presented with headaches, seizures, and papilledema. A large contrast-enhancing bifrontal mass was partially extirpated and then treated with radiation therapy and chemotherapy. *A,* The mass prior to therapy. *B,* The mass shortly postoperatively, indicating that there had been a major but incomplete resection. A residual tumor is indicated by the arrows. *C,* CT scan 2.5 years later. The site of surgical extirpation is indicated by the lucent area. There is no evidence of contrast enhancement, suggesting that the residual tumor has been eradicated. The patient became asymptomatic.

also definitively establishes the diagnosis. An exception is the primary brain lymphoma, the diagnosis of which should be established by stereotactic needle biopsy only. Treatment of that disorder is chemotherapy with or sometimes without radiation.

Most intracranial neoplasms cannot be cured surgically (Fig. 120–3). For them, the second line of treatment is radiation therapy (RT). RT is delivered either to the site of the tumor only (e.g., gliomas), to the entire neuraxis (e.g., medulloblastomas), or to the whole brain (e.g., multiple metastases). RT improves both survival and quality of life in most patients with malignant tumors. It probably also favorably affects the course of more benign tumors such as astrocytomas and recurrent meningiomas.

Chemotherapy, when added to RT, enhances both survival and quality of life of some patients with lymphoma and malignant astrocytomas, but its role in other intracranial neoplasms is not yet well established.

SPINAL NEOPLASMS

Spinal tumors originate from the same cell types as do intracranial tumors, and the same principles of diagnosis and treatment apply to them as to intracranial tumors. They are discussed in detail in Chapter 116.

PARANEOPLASTIC SYNDROMES

When patients with systemic cancer (i.e., cancer that arises outside the CNS) develop nervous system dysfunction, metastasis is usually the cause. However, cancer also exerts deleterious effects on the nervous system in the absence of direct metastatic involvement (paraneoplastic syndromes). Recognition of these nonmetastatic neurologic complications can prevent inappropriate and perhaps harmful therapy directed at a nonexistent metastasis. Because at times the neurologic symptoms precede the discovery of the cancer, nervous system symptoms can lead the physician to the diagnosis of an otherwise occult neoplasm. An almost bewildering variety of neurologic disorders have been ascribed to effects of systemic cancer (Table 120–2). However, most patients with nervous system dysfunction not caused by metastases are eventually found to be suffering from systemic infections, from vascular or metabolic disorders that affect the nervous system secondarily, or from unwanted side effects of cancer therapy.

Remote Effects

Remote effects of cancer on the nervous system describes nervous system dysfunction of unknown cause occurring either exclusively or with greater frequency in patients with cancer.

Remote effects are not common, probably affecting less than 1% of patients with cancer. Circulating antibodies against the target nervous system organ can be found in some patients suffering from remote effects (Table

| TABLE 120–2 | Nervous System Paraneoplastic Syndromes |

I. Remote Effects
  A. Brain and cranial nerves
    1. Dementia
    2. Bulbar encephalitis
    3. Subacute cerebellar degeneration (opsoclonus)*
    4. Optic neuritis (retinal degeneration)
  B. Spinal cord
    1. Gray matter myelopathy
      a. Subacute motor neuropathy
      b. "Autonomic insufficiency"
    2. Subacute necrotic myelopathy
  C. Peripheral nerves and roots
    1. Subacute sensory neuronopathy (dorsal root ganglionitis)*
    2. Sensorimotor peripheral neuropathy
    3. Acute polyneuropathy, Guillain-Barré type
    4. Autonomic neuropathy
  D. Neuromuscular junction and muscle
    1. Polymyositis and dermatomyositis (dermatomyositis in older men)*
    2. Lambert-Eaton myasthenic syndrome
    3. Myasthenia gravis (thymoma)
    4. Neuromyotonia
II. Metabolic, Hormonal, and Nutritional Abnormalities
  E. Metabolic encephalopathy
    1. Destruction of vital organs
      a. Liver (hepatic coma)
      b. Lung (pulmonary encephalopathy)
      c. Kidney (uremia)
      d. Bone (hypercalcemia)
    2. Elaboration of hormonal substances by tumor
      a. "Parathormone" (hypercalcemia)
      b. "Corticotropin" (Cushing's syndrome)
      c. Antidiuretic hormone (water intoxication)
    3. Competition between tumor and brain for essential substrates
      a. Hypoglycemia (large retroperitoneal tumors)
      b. Tryptophan (carcinoid)
    4. Malnutrition

---

* Neurologic disorders that may precede diagnosis of cancer and strongly suggest its presence.

120–3). In a few instances, injection of the antibody or extracts of tumor into experimental animals has reproduced portions of the clinical syndrome, suggesting an autoimmune mechanism with the antigen originating in the tumor. Not all patients harbor such antibodies, and other suggestions for the cause of remote effects have included viral infections, toxins secreted by the tumor, and nutritional deprivation.

A few neurologic syndromes are highly characteristic of remote effects. These include subacute cerebellar degeneration, subacute sensory neuronopathy, and the myasthenic syndrome.

Subacute cerebellar degeneration caused by cancer has a clinical picture sufficiently characteristic to suggest strongly that cancer is present even if the neurologic symptoms predate the appearance of the tumor. There is usually a subacute onset of bilateral and symmetric cerebellar dysfunction, the patient being equally ataxic in arms and legs. Severe dysarthria is usually present; vertigo, diplopia, and nystagmus are common. The CSF may have as many as 40 lymphocytes/mm³ and an elevated protein and IgG concentration. The disease, which may

TABLE 120–3	Antineuronal Antibodies Associated with Remote Effects of Cancer on the Nervous System				
Antibody	**Neuronal Reactivity**	**Neuronal Antigens**	**Cloned Genes**	**Tumor**	**Paraneoplastic Symptoms**
Anti-Hu (also ANNA-1)	Nucleus > cytoplasm (all neurons)	35–40 kD	HuD, HuC, Hel-N1	SCLC,* neuroblastoma, sarcoma, prostate	PEM, PSN, PCD autonomic dysfunction
Anti-Yo (also PCAb)	Cytoplasm Purkinje cells	34, 62 kD	CDR34, CDR62	Ovary,* breast,* lung	PCD
Anti-Ri (also ANNA-II)	Nucleus > cytoplasm (CNS neurons)	55, 80	Nova	Breast,* gynecological,* lung, bladder	Ataxia, opsoclonus
Anti-Tr	Cytoplasm Purkinje cells	?	—	Hodgkin's	PCD
Anti-VGCC	Presynaptic NMJ	VGCC ? 64 kD 37 kD	MysB Synaptotagmin	SCLC*	LEMS
Anti-retinal	Photoreceptor Ganglion cells	23, 65, 140, 205 kD	Recoverin	SCLC,* melanoma gynecological	CAR
Anti-amphyphisin	Presynaptic	128 kD	Amphyphisin	Breast, SCLC	Stiff-man, PEM

* The most frequently associated cancers.
CAR = cancer-associated retinopathy; CNS = central nervous system; LEMS = Lambert-Eaton myasthenic syndrome; NMJ = neuromuscular junction; PCD = paraneoplastic cerebellar degeneration; PEM = paraneoplastic encephalomyelitis; PSN = paraneoplastic sensory neuronopathy; SCLC = small cell lung cancer.

be associated with any cancer, precedes the discovery of the neoplasm by a few weeks to 3 years in more than half the patients, and it tends to run a progressive course over weeks to months, rendering the patient severely disabled. Cerebellar atrophy may be seen on MRI, particularly if done late in the course of the illness. Characteristic pathologic changes consist of diffuse or patchy loss of Purkinje cells in all areas of the cerebellum. There may be lymphocytic cuffs around blood vessels, particularly in the deep nuclei. This illness can be distinguished from cerebellar metastases by the symmetry of its signs and the absence of increased intracranial pressure. It differs from alcoholic-nutritional cerebellar degeneration because dysarthria and ataxia in the upper extremities are prominent in the paraneoplastic cerebellar degenerations but are usually mild or absent in the alcoholic variety. The hereditary cerebellar degenerations rarely run so rapid a course. At times the disorder stabilizes or improves with successful treatment of the tumor. Antibodies to cerebellar Purkinje cells have been found in the serum of some patients.

Another, less common cerebellar syndrome is that of *opsoclonus* (spontaneous, conjugate, chaotic eye movements most severe when voluntary eye movements are attempted). Opsoclonus is frequently associated with cerebellar ataxia and myoclonus of the trunk and extremities. It is most common in children as a remote effect of neuroblastoma. In children, the neurologic symptoms respond to adrenocorticosteroid therapy and to treatment of the tumor.

Subacute sensory neuronopathy is marked by loss of sensation with relative preservation of motor power. The illness usually precedes the appearance of the carcinoma and progresses over a few months, leaving the patient with a moderate or severe disability. Pathologically, there is destruction of posterior root ganglia with perivascular lymphocytic cuffing and wallerian degeneration of sensory nerves. Many of the patients have inflammatory and degenerative changes in brain and spinal cord as well. The entity is rare and there is no treatment. Some patients harbor an antibody that reacts with an antigen found in the nuclei of neurons throughout the peripheral and central nervous systems.

The *myasthenic syndrome* (Lambert-Eaton syndrome) is associated with small cell lung cancer (or rarely other cancers) in about two thirds of patients; the other one third do not have cancer (see also Chapter 123).

Injury from Therapeutic Radiation

When parts of the nervous system are included within an ionizing irradiation portal, adverse effects may result (Table 120–4). The likelihood of adverse effects is related to the total dose of radiation, the size of each fraction, the total duration over which the dose is received, and the volume of nervous system tissue irradiated. Other factors such as underlying nervous system disease (e.g., brain tumor, cerebral edema), previous surgery, concomitant use of chemotherapeutic agents, and individual susceptibility make it impossible to define precisely a safe dose for any given individual. However, certain guidelines allow the radiation therapist to calculate generally safe nervous system doses. Adverse effects may involve any portion of the central or peripheral nervous system and may occur acutely or be delayed weeks to years following irradiation.

TABLE 120–4	Radiation Injury to the Nervous System	
Time After Radiation Therapy	**Organ Affected**	**Clinical Findings**
Primary Injury		
Immediate (min to hr)	Brain	Acute encephalopathy
Early delayed (6–16 wk)	Brain	Somnolence, focal signs
	Spinal cord	Lhermitte's sign
Late delayed (mo to yr)	Brain	Dementia, focal signs
	Spinal cord	Transverse myelopathy
	Peripheral nerves	Paralysis, sensory loss
Secondary Injury (yr)	Several	Brain, cranial, and/or peripheral nerve sheath tumors
	Arteries (atherosclerosis)	Cerebral infarction
	Endocrine organs	Metabolic encephalopathy

Clinical Manifestations

Acute encephalopathy may follow large radiation doses to patients with increased intracranial pressure, particularly in the absence of corticosteroid prophylaxis. Immediately following treatment, susceptible patients develop headache, nausea and vomiting, somnolence, fever, and occasionally worsening of neurologic signs, rarely culminating in cerebral herniation and death. Acute encephalopathy usually follows the first radiation fraction and becomes progressively *less* severe with each ensuing fraction. This disorder is believed to result from increased intracranial pressure and/or brain edema from radiation-induced alteration of the blood-brain barrier. It responds to corticosteroids. Acute worsening of neurologic symptoms does not occur after spinal cord irradiation.

Early delayed encephalopathy or *myelopathy* appears 6 to 16 weeks after therapy and persists for days to weeks. In children, the encephalopathy commonly follows prophylactic irradiation of the brain for leukemia and is called the *radiation somnolence syndrome*. The disorder is characterized by somnolence, often associated with headache, nausea, vomiting, and sometimes fever. The EEG may be slow, but there are no focal signs. In adults, the syndrome usually follows irradiation for brain tumors and is characterized by lethargy and worsening of focal neurologic signs. Both disorders usually respond to steroids, but if untreated they resolve spontaneously. In adults with brain tumor, the MRI may transiently worsen, leading one to suspect growing tumor. In children, lumbar puncture rules out the potential diagnosis of meningeal leukemia. *Early delayed myelopathy* follows radiation therapy to the neck or upper thorax and is characterized by Lhermitte's sign (an electric shock–like sensation radiating into various parts of the body when the neck is flexed). The symptoms resolve spontaneously. Early delayed radiation syndromes are believed to result from demyelination, possibly due to radiation-induced, transient damage to oligodendroglia.

Late delayed radiation injury appears months to years following radiation and may affect any part of the nervous system. In the brain, there are two clinical syndromes. Diffuse injury may follow whole-brain irradiation either to patients without brain tumors (prophylactic irradiation for oat cell carcinoma) or to some patients with primary and metastatic brain tumors. The disorder is characterized by dementia without focal signs. MRI reveals cerebral atrophy and pathologic changes are nonspecific; there is no treatment. Focal radiation damage affects patients who receive either focal brain irradiation during therapy of extracranial neoplasms or whole-brain irradiation for intracranial neoplasms. Neurologic signs suggest a mass and include headache, focal or generalized seizures, and hemiparesis. Brain MRI show a hypodense mass, sometimes with contrast enhancement. Neuropathologic features include coagulative necrosis of white matter, telangiectasia, fibrinoid necrosis and thrombus formation, and glial proliferation and bizarre multinucleated astrocytes. The clinical and MRI findings cannot be distinguished from those of brain tumor, and the diagnosis can be made only by biopsy. A hypometabolic positron emission tomographic scan (PET scan) suggests radiation necrosis rather than recurrent tumor. Corticosteroids sometime ameliorate symptoms. The treatment, if the disorder is focal, is surgical removal. *Late delayed myelopathy* is characterized by progressive paralysis, sensory changes, and sometimes pain. A Brown-Séquard syndrome (weakness and loss of proprioception in the extremities of one side with loss of pain and temperature sensation on the other) is often present at onset. Patients occasionally respond transiently to steroids, and the disorder may stop progressing, but generally patients become paraplegic or quadriplegic. Pathologic changes include necrosis of the spinal cord. *Late delayed neuropathy* may affect any cranial or peripheral nerve. Common disorders are blindness from optic neuropathy and paralysis of an upper extremity from brachial plexopathy after therapy for lung or breast cancer. The pathogenesis is probably fibrosis and ischemia of the plexus. There is no treatment.

Radiation-induced tumors, including meningiomas, sarcomas or, less commonly, gliomas, may appear years to decades after cranial irradiation and may follow even low-dose radiation therapy. Malignant or atypical nerve sheath tumors may follow irradiation of the brachial, cervical, and lumbar plexuses. The CNS may also be damaged when radiation alters extraneural structures. Radiation therapy accelerates *atherosclerosis,* and cerebral infarction associated with carotid artery occlusion in the neck may occur many years after neck irradiation. Endocrine (pituitary, thyroid, parathyroid) dysfunction from radiation may be associated with neurologic signs. Hypothyroidism from radiation may also cause an encephalopathy.

NON-NEOPLASTIC ALTERATIONS OF INTRACRANIAL PRESSURE

Introduction and Definitions

Intracranial pressure is determined by rates of CSF formation and absorption and by cerebral venous pressure, the last a reflection of systemic venous pressure. Lumbar puncture pressure in the lateral decubitus position accurately reflects intracranial pressure in most instances. Depending on the patient's degree of relaxation, the normal CSF pressure ranges between 65 and 195 mm of CSF (5 to 15 mm Hg), although pressures as high as 250 mm of CSF have been reported in apparently normal individuals. Nevertheless, pressures above 170 are suspect, and pressures above 200 should be considered abnormal until proven otherwise. CSF pressure is not affected by obesity. Elevated CSF pressure measured at lumbar puncture does not necessarily reflect neurologic disease; elevation of the head of the bed can raise the lumbar CSF pressure, although it lowers intracranial pressure. Elevation of systemic venous pressure, such as occurs acutely with coughing, abdominal straining, or crying and chronically with congestive heart failure or venous obstruction of the superior vena cava or jugular veins, raises intracranial pressure. Hypercapnia (e.g., pulmonary disease, excessive sedation) increases the cerebral blood volume and thus CSF pressure. Conversely, if the patient is positioned with the head down, lumbar puncture pressure is lower, although intracranial pressure becomes higher. The loss of CSF around the needle hole between the time the needle enters the subarachnoid space and the manometer is placed also lowers intracranial pressure. When all of these artifactual causes of altered intracranial pressure are eliminated, the most common cause of intracranial hypertension is intracranial tumor and the most common cause of intracranial hypotension is a CSF leak following lumbar puncture or myelogram.

Intracranial Hypertension

Pseudotumor Cerebri

As the name suggests, this disorder is characterized by increased intracranial pressure in the absence of a tumor or obvious obstruction of CSF pathways. The cause is usually not established, although a number of CNS or systemic illnesses appear to play a role. Pseudotumor can follow head trauma, middle ear disease, internal jugular vein ligation, oral contraceptive use, pregnancy, and polycythemia vera, all conditions that suggest possible cerebral venous occlusion. In a few such patients, MRI or angiograms show sagittal or lateral sinus occlusion. The disorder has also been reported in patients on prolonged corticosteroid therapy, after steroid withdrawal, with Addison's disease or hypoparathyroidism, and with ingestion of drugs such as vitamin A, nalidixic acid, and tetracycline. Most cases, however, are idiopathic.

The disorder usually affects young (ages 20 to 30), obese females, is characterized by headache, papilledema, and at times visual obscurations (sudden momentary, usually bilateral visual loss). It has a benign prognosis.

Most patients with pseudotumor present to the physician with headache and papilledema. In a few, headaches are absent and the disorder is discovered because of either brief visual losses (obscurations) or papilledema found on routine ophthalmologic examination. Sometimes there is no papilledema or only unilateral papilledema

even though intracranial pressure is grossly elevated. Visual obscurations do not portend visual loss. However, whether or not they occur, 10 to 15% of patients lose some vision during the course of the disease, varying from small scotomata to, rarely, total blindness. Other clinical symptoms that are less common but that may concern the physician include vomiting, diplopia, vertigo, tinnitus, neck pain and stiffness, orbital pain, drowsiness, and dysesthetic sensation. These false localizing signs probably result from minor shifts of normal structures engendered by the intracranial hypertension. The disorder usually runs a benign course, with the headache and papilledema resolving in several weeks to several months, although in many patients intracranial pressure as measured at lumbar puncture remains elevated for months to years.

The diagnosis of pseudotumor is suspected clinically and established by the presence of elevated intracranial pressure in a patient with a normal MRI or CT scan. The CSF pressure is usually above 300 mm and its composition is normal, although some patients may have a relatively low protein count (below 15 mg/dl). Venous occlusions can usually be detected by MRI. A few errors in diagnosis occur in patients with an anomalous elevation of the optic discs (pseudopapilledema) or, very rarely, in patients with diffuse infiltrating gliomas of the brain (gliomatosis cerebri). The first can be ruled out by appropriate ophthalmologic tests, including fluorescein angiography, and the second usually by MRI and time.

Treatment is symptomatic. Weight loss helps. Repeated lumbar punctures sometimes relieve the headaches, and some physicians believe that corticosteroids are helpful. Only if there is evidence of progressive visual loss is therapeutic intervention mandatory. In that instance, the best treatment appears to be fenestration of the optic nerve sheath; sometimes shunting the CSF from the lumbar sac into the peritoneum is required.

Hydrocephalus

An increase in the amount of ventricular fluid enlarges the cerebral ventricular system. *Obstructive hydrocephalus* can result from either stenosis or occlusion of CSF pathways within the ventricular system (noncommunicating) or from stenosis or occlusion of subarachnoid pathways outside the ventricular system (communicating). *Nonobstructive hydrocephalus* results from passive enlargement of the ventricular system because of atrophy of brain substance (hydrocephalus ex vacuo). Obstructive hydrocephalus is often but not always associated with intracranial hypertension and, when acute, may be rapidly fatal. The more chronic the hydrocephalus, the more likely the intracranial hypertension is to be either mild or undetectable (normal pressure hydrocephalus) and the more likely are the symptoms to be indolent.

Acute hydrocephalus, such as occurs with sudden obstruction of the ventricular system (e.g., colloid cyst of the third ventricle, subarachnoid or cerebellar hemorrhage), is characterized by sudden severe headache, vomiting, lethargy, and sometimes coma. If the ventricular system is not decompressed, herniation and death can occur. *Subacute* (subarachnoid hemorrhage, meningitis, leptomeningeal neoplasia) or *chronic hydrocephalus* (congenital aqueductal stenosis, spinal cord tumors, idiopathic normal pressure hydrocephalus) is usually characterized by progressive lethargy, apathy, and dementia, often associated with an unsteady gait and urinary urgency or incontinence. There may be bilateral corticospinal tract signs, particularly in the lower extremities, with hyperactive knee and ankle jerks and extensor plantar responses. If the pressure is grossly elevated, patients may develop headache and papilledema, but these are uncommon.

The presence of enlarged ventricles is detected easily by MRI or CT scan. Unfortunately, it is not always easy to distinguish on the scan between obstructive hydrocephalus and hydrocephalus ex vacuo unless the cause (e.g., tumor) can be identified. A lumbar puncture revealing an elevated intracranial pressure assists in the diagnosis, but because some patients with obstructive hydrocephalus have a relatively normal intracranial pressure, that test likewise may not give a definitive diagnosis. In patients with classic symptoms of chronic hydrocephalus (i.e., dementia, gait unsteadiness, and incontinence), removal of CSF at lumbar puncture sometimes relieves symptoms, indicating both that CSF obstruction is producing the symptoms and that ventricular shunting will be therapeutic.

Intracranial Hypotension

Intracranial hypotension usually follows lumbar puncture but occasionally results from spontaneous or traumatically induced tears of the dura, leading to leakage of subarachnoid fluid. The resulting low CSF pressure is characterized by headache beginning occipitally and radiating frontally when the patient assumes the erect posture. The headache is sometimes associated with nausea, vomiting, photophobia, and a stiff neck. Some patients develop diplopia from abducens nerve paralysis. Auditory symptoms such as tinnitus and vestibular dizziness also can occur. The symptoms probably result because the brain, unsupported by CSF, shifts downward when the erect posture is assumed. The diagnosis is easily made on clinical grounds if the patient has undergone a lumbar puncture or myelogram a few days previously, but can be established only by performing a lumbar puncture and noting the low CSF pressure if no such history is present. In some patients the MRI scan reveals contrast enhancement of the cranial meninges. Symptoms usually resolve spontaneously but in a few instances may persist, in which case a search for the site of the leak should be made. Some investigators have recommended epidural injection of a few milliliters of the patient's blood to patch a dural leak following lumbar puncture. In a few instances of spontaneous or traumatic dural tears, surgical repair of the leak has been necessary.

REFERENCES

Posner JB: Neurologic Complications of Cancer. Philadelphia, FA Davis, 1995.
Wen PY, Black PML (eds.): Brain tumors in adults. Neurol Clin 1995; 13:701–974.

121

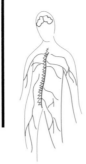

Infectious and Inflammatory Disorders of the Nervous System

The central nervous system (CNS) is subject to attack by many of the same infectious agents and antigen-antibody reactions that affect the remainder of the body. As is true with systemic infections, bacterial, fungal, and parasitic diseases of the nervous system are particularly likely to occur when the body's resistive mechanisms have been breached. Viral infections of the nervous system are also common, especially in immunosuppressed hosts. Except for so-called slow viruses, discussed in this section, viral diseases of the nervous system are described in Chapter 97. Chapter 92 discusses factors that predispose to infections of the nervous system.

BACTERIAL INFECTIONS OF THE BRAIN

Bacterial infections of the CNS may be parenchymal, meningeal, or parameningeal. Parenchymal lesions include brain abscesses as well as some of the complications of bacterial endocarditis and venous thrombosis. The most common meningeal infection, acute bacterial meningitis, is discussed in Chapter 97 and in the references for this chapter. Less common *parameningeal infections* include brain and spinal epidural or subdural abscesses (subdural empyema).

Bacteria most often reach the nervous system from a prior site of infection in a systemic organ, except when abnormal pathways connect the CNS and the surface of the body. Examples of such connections may follow CNS trauma, surgical procedures, or the development of spontaneous cerebrospinal fluid (CSF) fistulas. Such pathways should be sought in patients with repeated CNS bacterial infections. The offending organism is often *Streptococcus pneumoniae*.

Intracranial Abscesses

Intracranial abscesses consist of areas of acute bacterial inflammation (early in the course) or pus localized to one of the intracranial compartments (i.e., the epidural space, the subdural space, or the brain itself).

Epidural Abscess

Epidural abscesses usually arise by direct extension from adjacent osteomyelitis, mastoiditis, or infection of the paranasal sinuses. In the early stages, signs and symptoms amplify those of infection of the extracranial site from which they arose; for example, head pain, local swelling, and redness commonly overlie epidural abscesses originating from frontal sinuses. Fever usually is present accompanied by leukocytosis with a preponderance of polymorphonuclear leukocytes. Focal neurologic signs are uncommon, and increased intracranial pressure is usually absent. In the early stages, the CSF usually contains at most a few lymphocytes with a slightly elevated protein; often the fluid remains normal. If the initial disorder is untreated, the infection may breach the dura to produce a subdural empyema, bacterial meningitis, or brain abscess. Alternately, if the epidural inflammation lies close to a large venous sinus, thrombophlebitis with sinus occlusion often may complicate the infection. The extent of an epidural abscess is usually easily defined by brain images as a mass occupying the epidural space and compressing the underlying brain. Whether cranial or spinal, such abscesses in their early stages often can be treated successfully with appropriate antibiotics alone (the organism having been identified by culture of purulent material obtained from the ear or sinuses). In some instances, particularly when the abscess is large or when it fails to shrink rapidly with antibiotic therapy, surgical drainage is required.

Subdural Abscess

Most subdural abscesses (subdural empyemas) arise from infection of paranasal sinuses or the middle ear (otitis media). Organisms from the primary infection follow cranial venous channels, often producing thrombophlebitis as they go through the dura into the subdural space. Occasionally, traumatically induced subdural hematomas become secondarily infected to form subdural empyemas. The site of the empyema depends on the site of the primary infection. Those of the paranasal sinuses usually extend over the frontal lobe, whereas those from ear infections penetrate the skull posteriorly both above and below the tentorium. The inflammatory reaction excited by the organism may form a membrane that completely walls off the collection of pus.

Most patients with subdural empyema suffer the signs and symptoms of sinusitis or otitis prior to the onset of the empyema. As the intracranial abscess develops, the initial pain usually worsens and spreads more widely. Fever, if not already present, usually develops, the white blood cell count rises, and patients often become drowsy and may vomit. Secondary thrombophlebitis of the brain may ensue and cause the focal neurologic signs of seizures or hemiparesis. Eventually the intracranial pressure rises, and a fulminant course may produce death within a few days if no treatment is undertaken. The diagnosis is suggested by a history of pre-existing infection combined with local physical abnormalities. Brain imaging defines both the site of primary infection and the subdural collection of pus. The CSF is usually under increased pressure and may contain several hundred cells with an elevated protein but normal glucose concentration. Lumbar puncture, however, is ill-advised in patients suspected of subdural empyema because no organisms will be recovered and the rapidly increasing intracranial pressure threatens to produce cerebral herniation.

Subdural empyema almost always requires surgical drainage. If combined with appropriate antibiotic therapy, this step usually relieves the symptoms and cures the patient if the disease is detected in its earliest stages. Unfortunately, diagnosis is often delayed, resulting in a mortality of about 25%. Most deaths result from venous sinus thrombosis with secondary cerebral infarction or meningitis. Heparin anticoagulant therapy may reduce the neurologic damage from such thromboses.

Brain Abscess

Brain abscess is the most common intracranial abscess. Like those of the epidural and subdural spaces, parenchymal abscesses of the brain can arise by direct extension along venous channels from infections in the paranasal sinuses or the ear. Currently, however, most arise by hematogenous spread from infections elsewhere in the body. Metastatic abscess probably originates from a transient bacteremia with organisms lodging in capillary vessels of the brain. The process begins as a focal inflammatory encephalitis, followed in days or weeks by encapsulation of pus to form a true abscess. Unlike the typically identifiable primary site of infection in epidural or subdural abscesses, the systemic infection in brain abscesses may already have resolved without having produced symptoms. Some patients with brain abscess give a history of dental manipulation or mild urinary tract infection several weeks earlier; others have had lung infections. Congenital cyanotic heart disease and arteriovenous shunts in the lungs increase the risk of brain abscess because the lungs normally filter out circulating bacteria. Immunosuppressed patients often develop multiple rather than the single brain abscesses that most often affect patients with normal immunity.

The primary site of the infection determines the offending organism. Common agents include an aerobic or microaerophilic *Streptococcus* as well as enteric bacteria. In traumatic brain abscesses, staphylococci are common; *Clostridium* occasionally is present. Many of the infections are mixed, Rarer causes of abscesses include *Actinomyces* and *Nocardia*. Tuberculous abscesses are uncommon in the United States but frequent in less-developed countries.

The site of a brain abscess depends partly on its source. Those that originate in the middle ear generally invade the temporal lobe or cerebellum, those in the paranasal sinus penetrate the frontal lobe, and those from penetrating injuries involve the wound site. Hematogenous abscesses can affect any part of the brain, although most distribute themselves along the territory of the middle cerebral artery.

Most abscesses produce symptoms similar to but more rapidly progressive than those of a brain tumor. It is uncommon for patients to suffer from fever, substantial tenderness of the skull, or an elevated white blood cell count. Instead, patients present with headache, signs of increased intracranial pressure, and focal signs that depend on the site of the lesion. Focal or generalized seizures are common. Occasionally, the onset is strokelike.

DIFFERENTIAL DIAGNOSIS. This includes brain tumor and less often cerebral infarct. Abscess should be suspected if a patient suffers one of the predisposing causes (e.g., immune suppression, cyanotic heart disease, arteriovenous shunting in the lungs) or if a systemic bacterial infection has occurred in the recent past. A history of a draining ear or evidence of otitis media, particularly when clinical symptoms and signs point to a lesion in the temporal lobe or cerebellum, strengthens the likelihood of brain abscess, as does a history of purulent sinusitis. If fever exists or the white blood cell count is elevated (neither usually is the case), the diagnosis favors abscess. Lumbar puncture should not be performed because of the risk of cerebral herniation. Brain images are helpful but not always specifically diagnostic. Characteristically they show a hypodense lesion surrounded by a contrast-enhancing ring. Similar rings also can rim primary and metastatic brain tumors as well as recent cerebral infarcts. A thin, smooth-walled ring suggests an abscess, whereas a thick, irregular ring is more common with brain tumor (Fig. 121–1). In some instances surgical exploration is required to make the diagnosis.

THERAPY. Brain imaging has revolutionized the diagnosis and treatment of brain abscess because early diagnosis often permits starting antibiotics before extensive pus formation and mass effect have occurred. For abscesses 3 cm or smaller, antibiotics alone usually suffice, the choice depending on the suspected causal organism. If the organism is not known, a combination of penicillin and metronidazole in high doses for a period of about 6 weeks is usually effective. Serial imaging helps greatly in judging the effectiveness of antibiotic therapy and deciding when, if ever, surgical extirpation is necessary. Even after full

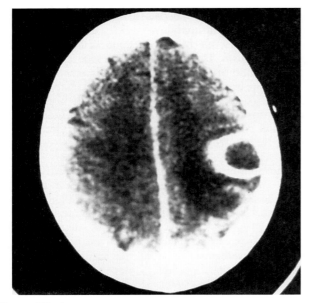

Figure 121–1

Computed tomographic (CT) scan showing a brain abscess. A woman presented to physicians after a focal seizure followed by headache and weakness of the arm. Dental work had been performed several weeks before. CT scan revealed a contrast-enhanced, ringlike mass surrounded by edema. It is not possible on this scan to differentiate tumor from abscess. At surgery a well-encapsulated abscess was encountered.

recovery the contrast-enhancing ring may persist for many weeks and does not imply that the abscess is still active. Large abscesses, failure of antibiotic therapy to either shrink the lesion or improve the clinical course, or the presence of a doubtful diagnosis all mandate surgical removal or, for surgically inaccessible lesions, stereotactic needle biopsy and drainage. With early detection and vigorous antimicrobial treatment, most patients do not need surgery and recover with few sequelae other than a tendency to seizures, which can be controlled by anticonvulsants. This approach has reduced the mortality from brain abscesses in some series to about 5%.

Cortical and Venous Sinus Thrombophlebitis

Bacterial infections of the CNS may cause cerebral thrombophlebitis with secondary occlusion of the large dural sinuses. The most common sites of infective sinus occlusion are the lateral sinus (a complication of acute or chronic otitis media), cavernous sinus (a complication of orbital or nasal sinus infection), and the superior sagittal sinus, usually occluded by direct extension of infected clot from the first two. Cortical veins may be involved either by direct contact with an infection in the epidural or subdural space or by the extension of infective clot from the sinuses.

The symptoms of *lateral sinus occlusion* depend on the rapidity of the occlusion and the importance of that sinus in draining the brain's blood. Because the two lateral sinuses are often of different sizes, slowly developing occlusion of the smaller one usually causes no symptoms at all. Occlusion of the dominant lateral sinus is often heralded by headache and papilledema. Focal signs are absent unless the occlusion spreads to involve the jugular vein, in which case pain, swelling, and a palpable cord in the neck may develop. If the occlusion spreads to the inferior petrosal sinus, abducens and trigeminal nerve involvement (Gradenigo's syndrome) can occur and, if the jugular bulb is involved, dysarthria, dysphagia, and neck weakness (jugular foramen syndrome) ensue.

Cavernous sinus occlusion causes a florid picture, often resulting from staphylococcal infection of the face or sinus. Symptoms begin with fever, headache, nausea, vomiting, and seizures. Proptosis affects the ipsilateral eye with chemosis and ophthalmoplegia, to which sensory loss in the distribution of the first division of the trigeminal nerve sometimes is added (all result from the third, fourth, fifth, and sixth nerves passing through the cavernous sinus). Papilledema is a late event.

Sagittal sinus occlusion is characterized by headache and, often, papilledema. If acute in onset and involving the posterior distribution of the sinus, bilateral hemorrhagic infarction of the brain develops, sometimes producing bilateral hemiparesis more marked in the leg and proximal arm than in the hand and face.

The diagnosis of sinus occlusion or corticothrombophlebitis should be suspected in a patient with a head or neck infection who develops signs of increased intracranial pressure with or without focal neurologic signs. The diagnosis of sinus occlusion can easily be made by magnetic resonance imaging (MRI), which distinguishes clot from flowing blood in vessels, or by digital intravenous angiogram (Fig. 121–2); the tests do not distinguish between infective and noninfective thromboses.

Infective sinus thrombosis is usually successfully treated with appropriate antibiotics; sometimes despite treatment the clot propagates to cause severe cerebral infarction and even death. Recent evidence indicates that prompt diagnosis of sinus thrombosis, followed by heparin-warfarin therapy, substantially reduces mortality and prevents or reverses neurologic damage.

Bacterial Endocarditis

The disseminated emboli of subacute bacterial endocarditis affect the nervous system of a quarter to a third of patients with that disease (Table 121–1). The most common symptom is that of an embolic stroke characterized by the acute onset of focal motor weakness. Multiple small emboli may cause confusion, hallucinations, and lethargy with or without fleeting focal signs. Infected emboli lodged in cerebral blood vessels sometimes induce aneurysm formation (mycotic aneurysm), typically located in the distal portion of cerebral arteries. The distribution differs from that of congenital aneurysms, which locate themselves more proximally. *Mycotic aneurysms* often rupture to cause severe cerebral or subarachnoid hemorrhage. Resolution of the aneurysms after antibiotic therapy has been reported, but the danger of rupture is so

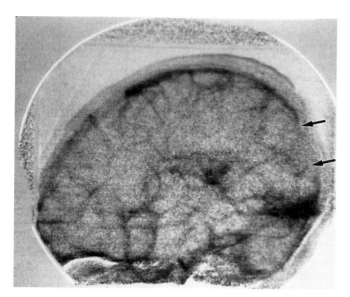

Figure 121-2

Digital venous angiogram, lateral view, patient facing left, in a patient with sagittal sinus occlusion. The procedure is generally more effective in demonstrating the cerebral venous system than is an arteriogram, because the cerebral hemispheres are filled with contrast material simultaneously. The patient had a bland occlusion of the posterior sagittal sinus *(arrows)*. Inflammatory sinus occlusions have a similar appearance.

great that, once they are found, surgical clipping usually is performed. As in other disorders causing sepsis, brain abscesses can result from either acute or subacute bacterial endocarditis.

Spinal Infections

The spinal leptomeninges are bathed by the same CSF and suffer from the same kinds of meningeal infections and inflammatory processes that affect the brain. Subdural and epidural collections of pus, however, can be localized to the spinal canal. Their clinical pictures differ from their counterparts in the intracranial cavity. Spinal cord parenchymal abscesses are exceedingly rare. They usually

TABLE 121-1	Major Neurologic Complications of Bacterial Endocarditis*

Cerebral infarction
Multiple microemboli (diffuse encephalopathy)
Meningeal signs and symptoms
Seizures
Microscopic brain abscesses
Visual disturbances
Cranial or peripheral neuropathy
Mycotic aneurysm
Subarachnoid hemorrhage (with or without identifiable mycotic aneurysm)

---

* Cerebral infarction or embolic encephalopathy affects as many as one third of cases, in many producing the first symptoms.

reach the spinal cord, as they do the brain, by hematogenous spread.

Spinal Abscess

Most *spinal epidural abscesses* arise at the cervical or lumbar levels and extend from an infected focus in an adjacent vertebral body (osteomyelitis) or soft tissues. *Staphylococcus aureus* is the most common organism. Other abscesses arise either by hematogenous invasion or by direct extension from a paravertebral infected focus. Depending on the virulence of the organism, clinical signs may develop either rapidly or slowly. In either case, neck or back pain is the most prominent symptom. The pain is usually severe and, in its early stages, well-localized. Tenderness of the spine surrounds the site of the infection. As the illness develops, pain may spread in a dermatomal distribution as nerve roots are irritated by the inflammatory process. Unless effective treatment is started at this stage, progressive weakness and sensory loss (myelopathy) develop below the site of the lesion and may lead to paraplegia in hours to days. Most patients with acute epidural abscesses are febrile and toxic, with an elevated white blood cell count. These findings may be less prominent with more chronic processes but the erythrocyte sedimentation rate is usually elevated. Radiographs of the vertebral body may not become abnormal for several weeks following the onset of symptoms. MRI of the spine, however, can detect the epidural lesion and are the diagnostic measure of choice. If MRI is unavailable, computed tomographic (CT) scans are almost as useful. Percutaneous tapping of the abscess may enable bacteriologic diagnosis. If spinal imaging is unavailable, a myelogram can outline the epidural mass. CSF obtained at the time of myelography is characterized by pleocytosis (up to several hundred white cells), elevated protein, and a normal glucose concentration; organisms are rarely cultured. In more chronic processes the pleocytosis may be absent.

Spinal subdural empyemas, usually caused by *S. aureus,* are more likely to be associated with meningitis and spinal cord infarction than are epidural abscesses but otherwise present with similar clinical changes. The diagnostic and therapeutic approaches are similar to those for epidural abscess.

With spinal epidural or subdural abscesses antibiotic therapy should be started as soon as one suspects the diagnosis. In the past, surgical drainage was considered imperative in acute abscesses. Recently, some of these lesions detected by imaging in their early stages have been cured with antibiotics alone. If signs of myelopathy or nerve root involvement develop, however, the patient should be surgically decompressed. The outcome is usually satisfactory in patients who are not already paralyzed when treatment is started.

DIFFERENTIAL DIAGNOSIS. Acute or subacute spinal abscesses must be differentiated from *acute or subacute transverse myelitis* and from *spinal epidural or subdural hematomas* (usually a disorder of patients with abnormal coagulation). Chronic spinal abscesses must be distinguished from *tumor.* In the acute disorder, fever, toxicity, and a history of prior infection support the diagnosis of abscess, and a carefully done myelogram or CT scan reveals the lesion to be extradural. Acute transverse myelopathy is associated either with a normal myelogram or with swelling of the spinal cord itself. With chronic abscesses, differentiation between tumor and infection may be more difficult. Both conditions can produce radiographic changes in the vertebral bodies. Inflammation is more likely to affect two contiguous vertebral bodies across an intravertebral disc, whereas tumors are usually restricted to individual vertebral bodies. If the diagnosis is in doubt, biopsy of the vertebral body or decompression of the epidural space is necessary to make the differentiation.

Neurosyphilis and *tuberculosis* of the nervous system are discussed in Chapter 97.

SLOW VIRUS INFECTIONS OF THE NERVOUS SYSTEM

The term *slow virus infection* designates a group of transmissible disorders in which a long latent period separates the time between first inoculation and subsequent development of disease. Several such infections, not all attributable to true viruses, can selectively attack the human nervous system (Table 121–2). Two retroviruses, the human immunodeficiency virus type 1 (HIV-1) and the human T cell lymphotrophic virus type 1 (HTLV-1), invade the nervous system of apparently healthy persons and require months to as much as several years to express their serious effects. Discussion of HIV-1 and its impact can be found in Chapter 108. HTLV-1 recently has been identified as the cause of *tropical spastic paralysis* as well as a myelopathy occurring in the Kyushu district of Japan and termed HTLV-1/HAM. The virus has also been

implicated in acute T-cell lymphoma/leukemia. The neurologic disorder is prevalent in tropical and semitropical belts worldwide and is encountered in the United States principally among Caribbean immigrants and Southeastern blacks. HTLV-1 can be transmitted sexually, by breast-feeding, and by transfusion. Usual age of onset is between 35 and 45 years, with an insidious onset and slow progression of spastic paraparesis followed by loss of bladder and bowel control. Peripheral or cranial nerves are sometimes affected. Diagnosis is made by detection of the virus as well as identification of high-level antibody synthesis and oligoclonal bands in the CSF. Treatment consists of immunosuppression or apheresis but at best brings modest improvements.

Subacute sclerosing panencephalitis, caused by measles virus, and a somewhat similar progressive panencephalitis, caused by rubella viruses, are severely damaging brain disorders attributable to persistent defective viral replication. Both affect children fatally, usually beginning many months to several years after the initial viral infection and pursuing a slow course. Widespread measles and rubella vaccination have all but erased the diseases in the United States.

Progressive multifocal leukoencephalopathy (PML) results from the invasion of the papovavirus, JC virus, into the brain. Rare in its incidence, PML affects patients with autoimmune deficiency syndrome (AIDS) or other disorders impairing T lymphocytes or macrophage-mediated immune responses. Gradually beginning but insidiously progressive cerebral demyelination produces signs of major sensory impairment coupled with characteristic white matter abnormalities on MRI. Occasionally the disease remits spontaneously but so far no useful treatment has been found.

Creutzfeldt-Jakob disease (CJD) is a rare form of mid-life, rapidly progressive transmissible dementia affecting patients worldwide with intellectual loss, signs of upper motor neuron impairment, ataxia, and myoclonus. The disease closely resembles or is identical with *kuru,* a disorder discovered among members of a cannabalistic New Guinea tribe 40 years ago and found to be transmissible into the brains of animals with several years delay in appearance. CJD has been transmitted to animals as well as between humans by the successive use of intracerebral electrodes, by cornea transplants, and by at least one batch of human-derived pituitary gland growth hormone given to children for replacement therapy. An essentially identical clinical and pathologic condition exists as an autosomal dominant hereditary disease called *Gerstmann-Straussler-Scheinker syndrome (GSS)* or hereditary Creutzfeldt-Jakob disease. Both the hereditary and the sporadic disease are marked by the conversion from normal to abnormal of a naturally occurring *prion* protein, genetically coded on chromosome 20. Presumably, the transmitted human agent, which is identical to the one that causes animal transmission in scrapie, a sheep disease, and in cattle (mad cow disease) in some way denatures the recipient's normal prion protein. The novel agent replicates in amounts that eventually become fatal to CNS cells. Several alleles of the prion protein have been found in the hereditary GSS syndrome. There is no

TABLE 121–2	Slow Virus Infections of the Nervous Systems	
Disorder	**Virus/Agent**	**Classification**
AIDS (see Ch. 108)	Human immunodeficiency virus 1 (HIV-1)	Retrovirus (RNA)
HTLV-1 associated myelopathy (HAM); tropical spastic paraparesis	Human T-cell lymphotrophic virus Type 1 (HTLV-1)	Retrovirus (RNA)
Progressive multifocal leukoencephalopathy	JC virus	Papovavirus (DNA)
Subacute sclerosing panencephalitis	Measles virus	Paramyxovirus (RNA)
Progressive rubella panencephalitis	Rubella virus	Togavirus (RNA)
Creutzfeldt-Jakob disease, kuru, Gerstmann-Straussler-Scheinker syndrome	Denatured normal body protein	Hereditary, infectious, and sporadic transmission

AIDS = Acquired immunodeficiency syndrome.

treatment for CJD, and almost all affected victims die within 6 to 18 months after symptoms first appear. Risks to healthcare workers have been extremely small or absent.

DEMYELINATING AND OTHER CNS INFLAMMATORY DISORDERS OF PROBABLE IMMUNE CAUSE

Demyelinating Disorders

Disorders with a relative predilection for damaging CNS myelin are listed in Table 121–3. Those that have an immune basis are discussed here. Others, if they affect primarily adults, are described elsewhere in the text under appropriate headings.

Several disorders are believed to result from abnormal immune mechanisms that cause CNS dysfunction by damaging the myelin sheaths covering axons. The conditions appear to have their primary effect on the oligodendroglial cells, which are responsible for the production and maintenance of the myelin sheaths. The acute lesions of these demyelinating disorders usually contain lymphocytes and macrophages. Production of IgG within the CNS is characterized by an elevated CSF-to-serum IgG ratio. In their severe forms, the disorders also can damage other structures in demyelinated areas, including axons and astrocytic cells.

Multiple Sclerosis (MS)

This is by far the most common of the presumed immune demyelinating disorders of the CNS. It is more common in women and usually causes its first symptoms between the ages of about 20 and 40 years. Classically it is characterized by remissions and exacerbations of neurologic

TABLE 121–3	Demyelinating Disorders

A. Unknown cause
1. Multiple sclerosis
2. Devic's disease
3. Optic neuritis
4. Acute transverse myelopathy

B. Parainfectious disorders
1. Acute disseminated encephalomyelitis
2. Acute hemorrhagic leukoencephalopathy

C. Viral infections
1. HTLV-1 associated myelopathy
2. Progressive multifocal leukoencephalopathy
3. Subacute sclerosing panencephalitis

D. Nutritional disorders
1. Combined systems disease (vitamin B_{12} deficiency)
2. Demyelination of the corpus callosum (Marchiafava-Bignami disease)
3. Central pontine myelinolysis

E. Anoxic-ischemic sequelae
1. Delayed postanoxic cerebral demyelination
2. Progressive subcortical ischemic encephalopathy

TABLE 121–4	Symptoms and Signs of Multiple Sclerosis Listed in Declining Order of Frequency

Symptoms
Unilateral visual impairment
Diploplia
Paresthesias
Ataxia or unsteadiness
Vertigo
Fatigue
Muscle weakness
Ocular disturbance, especially internuclear ophthalmoplegia
Urinary disturbance
Dysarthria or scanning speech
Mental disturbance

Signs
Optic neuritis
Internuclear ophthalmoplegia
Nystagmus
Spasticity or hyperreflexia
Babinski's sign
Absent abdominal reflexes
Dysmetria or intention tremor
Impairment of central sensory pathways
Labile or changed mood

dysfunction affecting several different sites in the CNS over many years (lesions disseminated in space and time). Typically, at onset an otherwise healthy person suffers an acute or subacute attack of unilateral loss of vision, true vertigo, ataxia, paresthesias, incontinence, diplopia, dysarthria, or paralysis (Table 121–4). The symptoms result from a focus of inflammatory demyelination (which later scars to form a plaque) in the white matter of the brain (most frequently periventricular), brain stem, or spinal cord. The demyelination acts to slow or block conduction of nerve impulses, thereby producing neurologic dysfunction. The symptoms are usually painless, remain for several days to weeks, and most often partially or completely resolve. After a period of relative freedom, new symptoms appear. Although individual frequencies vary widely, the average rate of exacerbations is about one every other year. In some patients, however, the clinical course consists of progressive neurologic dysfunction; this usually takes the form of a slowly progressive myelopathy characterized by spasticity and ataxia, predominantly of the lower extremities. In other instances, one or two attacks may be the sole clinical expression of the disease for an entire lifetime. On average, about 60% of MS patients remain fully functional 10 years after the first attack, and 25 to 30% continue this way for 30 or more years after the onset. Statistically, the disorder does not greatly decrease life expectancy, although some middle-aged patients become severely disabled and die prematurely of complications.

ETIOLOGY. The etiology of MS is unknown, although most clues indicate immunologic and genetic factors. The disease is far more common in the northern and southern temperate latitudes than in more equatorial regions. Young children who move from a tropical to a temperate area increase their likelihood of contracting multiple sclerosis, and vice versa. The findings suggest an infective agent acquired early in life (a slow or retrovirus, or exposure to a childhood infection). An immune disorder is suggested not only by the inflammatory infiltrates sometimes seen in the perivascular areas of the demyelinated plaques but also by the fact that a decrease in suppressor lymphocytes in the serum usually precedes acute attacks. A relapsing encephalomyelitis resembling MS has been produced by injection of myelin antigens into experimental animals. Genetic predisposition is suggested by the fact that haplotype DW2 is found in about 65% of MS patients, compared with 15% of control subjects, and there is a high coincidence in monozygotic twins. In addition, the disorder is uncommon in Asians and African blacks, including those who are born in the United States.

DIAGNOSIS. The diagnosis depends upon identifying in persons of appropriate age clinical evidence of lesions that have affected different areas of CNS white matter at intervals separated in time by at least 2 months (Table 121–5). When doubt exists, laboratory evidence of CNS immune dysfunction or of imaged white matter lesions should be sought. Clinically, however, otherwise healthy persons who suffer relapsing and remitting neurologic dysfunction over a long period of time (e.g., diplopia in year one, sensory loss in an arm in year three, urgency incontinence in year five) almost certainly have MS. Furthermore, evidence of more than one widely spaced lesion in the nervous system (e.g., optic neuritis plus internuclear ophthalmoplegia) strongly suggests disseminated sclerosis in a younger person who lacks evidence of other disease.

Certain symptoms strongly suggest the diagnosis of MS. These include bilateral internuclear ophthalmoplegia, Lhermitte's sign (electric shock–like sensation radiating to the extremities initiated by neck flexion), and an exacerbation of neurologic symptoms associated with acute febrile illness.

The laboratory examination is helpful but not definitive. Most patients have an elevated CSF gamma globulin level as well as discrete (oligoclonal) bands found in the gamma region on agarose or polyacrylamide gel electrophoresis. Multiple CSF oligoclonal bands (more than two)

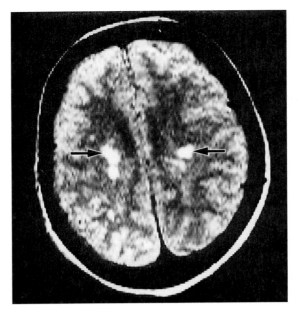

Figure 121–3

A magnetic resonance image from a patient with multiple sclerosis (MS). Multiple lesions of the white matter *(arrows)* with a predilection for periventricular areas strongly support the diagnosis of MS in a patient with an appropriate history and physical findings.

strongly support a diagnosis of MS in clinically appropriate cases, although other inflammatory diseases of the nervous system also can produce oligoclonal bands. Spinal, auditory, or visual evoked responses can reveal additional subclinical lesions in doubtful cases. Most helpful from a laboratory standpoint is MRI, which usually reveals characteristic white matter lesions scattered through brain and/or spinal cord (Fig. 121–3). CT scanning provides less sensitive detection.

Early diagnosis can be difficult in some cases, particularly in the absence of the typical remitting and exacerbating history, and when neither CSF nor MRI findings are as yet characteristic. Often, early symptoms are primarily sensory and sometimes appear to take bizarre, nonanatomic distributions, leading the physician to worry about a conversion reaction. Occasionally signs in MS may be severe and apparently unifocal, at first suggesting a brain or spinal cord tumor or vascular disease. Conversely, difficulty can arise with small brain stem structural abnormalities. Such lesions can give rise to a potentially misleading collection of cranial nerve, sensory, cerebellar, and motor signs that at first suggest demyelination. To prove a disseminated disorder in a patient with prominent brain stem signs requires evidence of dysfunction of structures not represented in the brain stem (e.g., optic neuritis, visual field deficit) or spinal cord. Visually evoked responses often help because MS-related optic nerve involvement is common and often causes abnormalities of conduction in the nerve without clinical symptoms. A difficult differential diagnosis in patients with prominent recurrent symptoms and signs of lower brain stem dysfunction lies between MS with remitting and exacerbating symptoms and small arteriovenous anomalies

TABLE 121–5	Criteria for the Diagnosis of Multiple Sclerosis

Clinical definite multiple sclerosis*: Evidence by history, neurologic examination, or both of at least two distinct attacks separated in time and producing objective evidence of neurologic dysfunction involving separate areas of central white matter. A related laboratory abnormality such as abnormal visual evoked responses, magnetic resonance imaging of white matter lesions, or cerebrospinal fluid oligoclonal banding can be taken as one objective sign.

Clinically probable multiple sclerosis: Two distinct, verified clinical neurologic attacks involving different areas of the nervous system plus existing clinical evidence of one relevant area of neurologic dysfunction or one of the laboratory abnormalities cited above.

* Reprinted from Neurology V13, page 227, 1983 by permission of Little, Brown and Company (Inc).

of the medulla or pons, which can produce recurrent symptoms by repetitive small hemorrhages. MRI usually solves the problem.

THERAPY. One can treat the symptoms of MS, but so far not the disease. Many physicians believe that acute bouts of neurologic dysfunction resolve more quickly when treated with short-term administration of corticosteroids. No evidence indicates that such treatment brings long-term benefit. The immunomodulatory cytokine interferon-beta has shown favorable results in reducing the frequency of clinical attacks of MS. The agent also reduces the rate of appearance of cerebral demyelinating lesions as detected by MRI. Other immunosuppressive agents also have been used chronically for treatment, but with either therapy long-term improvement has been difficult to prove. The illness understandably frightens patients, and sympathetic reassurance and follow-up supervision provide considerable support. Patients severely disabled by late symptoms, which generally include spasticity and bladder and bowel dysfunction (see Table 121–4), often are best treated in multidisciplinary clinics or centers where physical therapy, psychological support, family counseling, and supportive medical therapy are all available.

Acute Disseminated Encephalomyelitis (ADE)

This monophasic demyelinating inflammatory disorder can appear after viral infections or as a complication of vaccination. The condition usually produces multifocal brain and spinal cord symptoms but may be restricted to one area, particularly the optic nerve (acute optic neuropathy) or spinal cord (acute transverse myelopathy). When related to an antecedent viral infection, ADE usually occurs 6 to 10 days after the appearance of the other systemic symptoms. When it follows vaccination, it usually begins 10 days to 3 weeks after the injections. At times a similar syndrome can appear in the absence of any identifiable exposure. The pathogenesis is believed to comprise an antigen-antibody response, the antigen being either the injected vaccination protein or the infecting virus. Clinically ADE typically produces acute headache, fever, and multifocal neurologic signs. The most severely affected patients develop delirium, stupor, or coma. Seizures are relatively common. The CSF is characterized by pleocytosis (20 to 200 lymphocytes per mm^3) and usually an elevated gamma globulin. Protein concentration may be a little elevated, but glucose concentration is usually normal. Myelin basic protein can be identified in the CSF of some patients. The electroencephalogram (EEG) is usually diffusely abnormal, with widespread slowing, but does not have the characteristic focal slow and sharp wave activity of herpes simplex encephalitis.

ADE produces clinical and CSF manifestations similar to those of acute viral encephalitis and cannot be distinguished from that disorder by clinical findings. Since neither ADE nor acute viral encephalitis, save for herpes simplex, can be treated definitively, such a differentiation is not crucial. Despite its presumed immune

mechanism, neither corticosteroids nor other immunosuppressive agents have been effective in treatment.

Acute hemorrhagic leukoencephalitis is a fatal, rare variant of acute encephalomyelitis. The illness usually occurs after an upper respiratory infection and is characterized by sudden headache, seizures, and rapid progression to coma. Patients often die within a few days. CSF often shows more polymorphonuclear leukocytes than lymphocytes. The brain at autopsy is swollen, with bilateral and asymmetric hemorrhages scattered throughout the white matter. There is no known treatment.

Acute Transverse Myelopathy (Myelitis)

Acute transverse myelopathy is a clinical syndrome characterized by the rapid onset of ascending or transverse spinal cord dysfunction, usually involving primarily the midthoracic or high thoracic–low cervical cord. The disorder usually begins with abrupt, severe back pain and sometimes fever and malaise. In a matter of 12 to 24 hours, weakness and paresthesias appear in the lower extremities, sometimes with radicular pain at the level of the uppermost involved cord segments. Occasionally the disease is painless. In its severest form, complete paralysis and loss of sensation and autonomic function develop below the highest level of the lesion. In less severe forms there may be patchy loss of sensation with bilateral corticospinal tract signs predominating or a Brown-Séquard syndrome. In a few patients, the spinal cord signs ascend for hours to a week or two and reach a stable level, usually in the upper thoracic cord. Late recurrences occasionally develop.

About half the patients give a preceding history of banal infection, usually upper respiratory, or of a vaccination. The myelopathy is presumably a delayed immune response. Rarely, the illness is associated with an occult neoplasm.

The CSF usually contains 50 to 100 white cells and a slightly elevated protein concentration. The diagnostic problem is to distinguish acute transverse myelopathy from parameningeal infection with secondary involvement of the cord. The history and findings in transverse myelopathy may mimic those of epidural or subdural infections. Arteriovenous malformations of the spinal cord can engender similar symptoms. Accurate diagnosis can be established by MRI. If MRI is not available, myelography may be undertaken to rule out infection or hemorrhage. Sometimes, the spinal cord of patients with acute transverse myelopathy may be misleadingly swollen, producing a complete block to myelographic dye. Care must be taken to distinguish the swollen cord from an epidural or subdural block.

There is no effective treatment for the disorder. About one third of patients recover spontaneously.

Other Demyelinating Disease

Devic's disease (neuromyelitis optica) is a clinical syndrome characterized by transverse myelopathy and optic neuropathy, usually bilateral. The two symptoms usually occur within days or weeks of each other. The disease is generally thought to be a variant of MS, but in many instances the spinal cord necrosis is considerably more intense than one finds in the demyelinating plaques of most cases of MS.

Acute optic neuritis can either occur as a symptom of MS or arise in independent isolation.

Reye's Syndrome

Reye's syndrome is a parainfectious encephalopathy that usually follows influenza type A or B or varicella viral infections. The disease affects children far more frequently than adults. It is thought that heavy aspirin ingestion may be a cofactor risk. Attacks damage several mitochondrial enzyme activities in liver and brain, producing serum hyperammonemia, lactic acidosis, and elevation of free fatty acids. The onset of Reye's syndrome usually occurs as signs of the initial flu-like disorder begin to subside and includes headache, intractable vomiting, and lethargy or stupor. Patients may rapidly become comatose. The diagnosis is confirmed by evidence of marked elevation of hepatic enzymes in the serum but without hyperbilirubinemia, and an elevated arterial ammonia level. In children, hypoglycemia may occur. The CSF, is unremarkable. Mortality is high in comatose patients, with mitochondrial abnormalities found in both liver and brain at autopsy. Careful control of increased intracranial pressure using hyperosmolar agents, as well as correction of hypoglycemia and electrolyte abnormalities, allows some persons to recover.

REFERENCES

Autel JP: Multiple sclerosis. Neurolog Clin 1995; 13:1–23.

Del-Curling O Jr, Gower DJ, McWhorter JM: Changing concepts in spinal epidural abscess. A report of 29 cases. Neurosurgery 1990; 27:185.

Leys D, Christians JL, Derambure PL, Hladley JP, Lesoin F, Rosseaux M, Jomin N, Petit H: Management of focal intracranial infections. Is medical treatment better than surgery? J Neurol Neurosurg Psychiatry 1990; 53:472.

Newsom-Davis J: The Highlings Jackson Lecture: Autoimmunity and the nervous system. J Roy Soc Med 1995; 88:639–643.

Prusiner SB, Hsiao KK: Human prion diseases. Ann Neurol 1994; 35:385–395.

Tunkel AR, Scheld WM: Acute bacterial meningitis. Lancet 1995; 13:1675–1680.

122

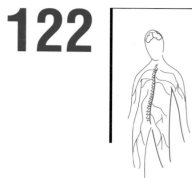

Motor Nerve, Nerve Root, Peripheral Nerve, and Neurocutaneous Disorders

PERIPHERAL NERVE DISORDERS

Gross Structural Relations

These are most simply described as they relate to the spinal cord. Somewhat more complex principles apply to the cranial motor neurons and somatic afferent peripheral pathways.

Figure 122–1 diagrams the structures that link the peripheral and central nervous system at approximately spinal level C5. The large lower motor neurons lie in the anterior (ventral) horn of the spinal cord and send their large and small fibers directly via the motor root and subsequent motor nerves to skeletal muscle receptors. (Smaller nerve fibers innervate the intramuscular muscle spindles that set the sensitivity of the stretch reflex.) Sensory roots enter the dorsal horn of the cord having been relayed by large and small neuron bodies located in the dorsal root ganglia. Distal to the ganglion, peripheral motor and sensory fibers fuse into a single peripheral nerve as they leave or approach the intervertebral foramen (not illustrated). Dorsal and ventral rami emanating from the proximal nerve root split to innervate the back with dorsal branches and the body and limbs with ventral rami. These latter further subdivide into brachial and lumbar plexuses to serve the upper and lower extremities.

The ultimate peripheral nerve patterns of the body then emerge either from these last mentioned complexes or, along the back and trunk, from the dorsal or ventral rami, respectively. Figure 122–2 outlines the usual distribution of the ultimate cutaneous fields of the major peripheral nerves and dermatomes on the body. By and large, peripheral nerve abnormalities arise distal to the region of the emergent ventral spinal rami and their plexuses whereas dermatomal sensory or motor abnormalities reflect impairments of dorsal sensory or ventral motor roots adjacent to or near the spinal outlet.

Anatomic Involvement of the Peripheral Nervous System

Anatomically, disorders of the peripheral nervous system can affect a single or several spinal nerve roots (radiculopathy), brachial or lumbar plexuses (plexopathies), and single or multiple nerves (Table 122–1).

MICROSCOPIC INVOLVEMENT. Diseases of the peripheral nervous system may affect one or more of three structures: (1) the cell body (neuronopathy), (2) the axon (axonopathy), or (3) the Schwann cells and/or their metabolic product, the myelin sheath (demyelinating neuropathy). Any of these processes may be focal, leading to mononeuropathy (involvement of a single nerve) or multiple mononeuropathy (involvement of several different single nerves), or diffuse, causing polyneuropathy. Polyneuropathies usually are symmetrical and most often involve the distal nerves of the extremities (see Table 122–1). The distal nature of most polyneuropathies reflects the fact that the longest nerves are the most metabolically active and thereby vulnerable. Although each of the anatomic and pathologic disorders listed in Table 122–1 can have distinctive clinical symptoms, there is considerable overlap. Furthermore, individual etiologic agents, such as diabetes or cancer, may cause more than one type of neuropathy.

In *demyelinating neuropathy*, segments of myelin degenerate, usually from immunologic or infectious causes. Clinically, demyelinating neuropathy is characterized by functional failure of large myelinated fibers, leading to decreased light touch, position, and vibration sensation, as well as to weakness and reduction or absence of deep tendon reflexes. A relative sparing of lightly myelinated or unmyelinated fibers partially preserves temperature and pain sensation, although these modalities become involved in severe cases. The onset of demyelinating neuropathy may be rapid, and with Schwann cell proliferation and remyelination, recovery may be equally rapid.

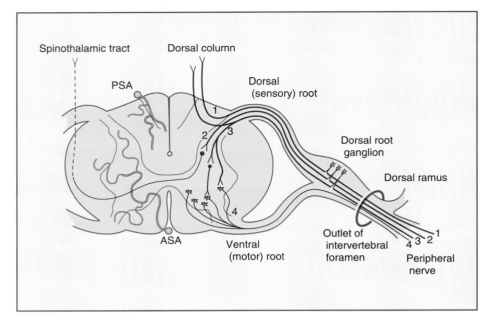

Figure 122-1

Simplified representation showing the relation between the C5 spinal cord level and its peripheral nerve structures. ASA = Anterior spinal artery; PSA = posterior spinal artery. Numbers on peripheral nerve represent the following: 1, Pacinian corpuscle (touch); 2, free nerve ending (pain); 3, muscle spindle afferent; 4, motor nerve efferent. (Modified from Waxman SG, de Groot J: Correlative Neuroanatomy. 22nd ed. Norwalk, CT, Appleton & Lange, 1995.)

Because the myelin sheath can be involved anywhere throughout its peripheral course, demyelinating neuropathy, although usually symmetric, sometimes affects both proximal and distal fibers to a similar degree. Cranial nerves are often involved, as well as peripheral nerves. The cerebrospinal fluid (CSF) protein is elevated in diffuse demyelinating neuropathies because of damage to spinal roots. Electrical studies of demyelinated nerves reveal that conduction velocity is slowed, often to 20 or 25% of normal values, and the amplitude of the action potential is small because it is dispersed over a longer duration.

Axonal neuropathy is characterized by degeneration of the distal ends of long axons, with secondary loss and degeneration of the myelin sheath. The disorder usually causes an equal loss of all sensory modalities, although in some instances small axons carrying pain and temperature suffer disproportionately. The first symptoms are usually sensory, with paresthesias or sensory loss of the tips of the fingers and toes. Only later, as the sensory loss spreads more proximally, does motor involvement occur in a typical "stocking and glove" distribution. Unlike demyelinating neuropathy, recovery is usually slow because of the slow rate of regeneration of the damaged axons. Spinal roots usually are not involved and the CSF protein remains normal. Electrically, axonal neuropathies are characterized by normal or only slightly (10 to 15%) slowed conduction velocity and by small sensory action potentials.

Neuronopathies affect the cell body of sensory or motor nerves, causing either acute or gradual onset of sensory and/or motor loss, often with little or no prospect of recovery.

Diagnostic Measures

The gross configuration of abnormalities affecting the spinal column, spinal cord, and peripheral branches can be visualized readily by advanced magnetic resonance imaging (MRI) and computed tomographic (CT) imaging. These instruments are less helpful in diagnosing disease in peripheral nerves or neuromuscular structures. For these areas, electrophysiologic tests and, sometimes, nerve or muscle biopsy may be essential to making an accurate diagnosis.

Electrophysiologic Studies of Nerve and Muscle

NERVE CONDUCTION STUDIES. Percutaneous electrical stimulation of a peripheral nerve generates an action potential. For motor nerves, electrodes are placed over a muscle to record the evoked muscle action potential. One stimulates the nerve innervating that muscle at various points along its length; the conduction velocity is the time required for the impulse to travel from each site of stimulation to the onset of the evoked muscle response. For sensory nerves, cutaneous nerve branches are stimulated distally with recording electrodes placed over the nerve at various proximal sites. These peripheral nerve and muscle electrophysiologic studies assist in determining whether disease involves nerve, muscle, or both and in determining the distribution of the abnormality. They facilitate the differentiation of demyelinating neuropathy from axonal neuropathy, neuropathy from radiculopathy, and primary muscle disease from disease of the motor unit. Demyelinating neuropathies affect mainly large fibers and slow the conduction velocity. When disease damages axons in addition to myelin, the decrease in the number of axons that can be electrically activated results in a diminution in the size of the compound action potential.

ELECTROMYOGRAPHY (EMG). EMG is performed by inserting a needle electrode into a muscle to record the structure's electrical activity. Normal muscle is silent at rest, but denervated or diseased muscle membranes become

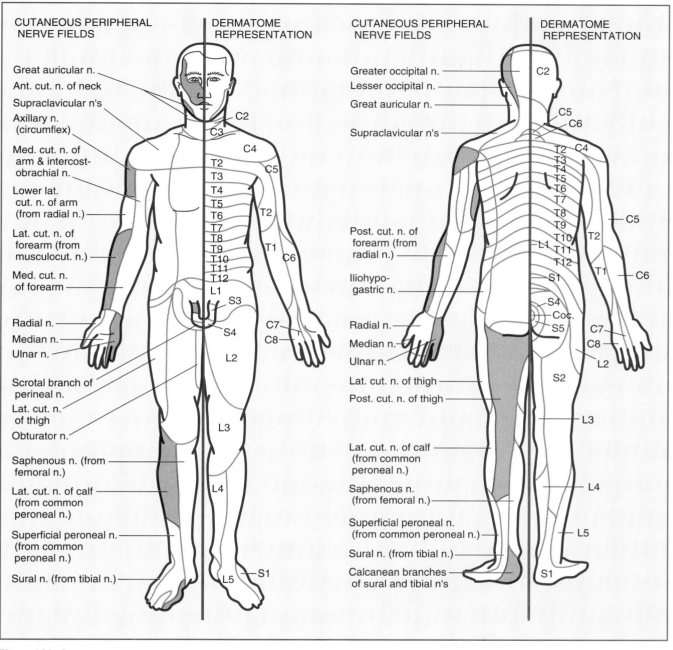

Figure 122-2

The cutaneous fields of the major peripheral nerves and dermatomes seen on the anterior (*left*) and posterior (*right*) surfaces of the body. (Redrawn from Haymaker W, Woodhall B: Peripheral Nerve Injuries. Philadelphia, WB Saunders Co., 1953.)

spontaneously excitable, generating fibrillation potentials of small amplitude. When the nerve or motor neuron is diseased, entire motor units may become spontaneously active. The resulting fasciculations are often visible and can be detected by the electrode. Furthermore, when damaged axons cease to innervate muscle fibers, the remaining axons gradually sprout collaterals that reinnervate the denervated fibers; as a result, during voluntary contraction the few remaining muscle units show a decrease in their

number and an increase in the size of their electrical potentials. When the patient voluntarily contracts the muscle being examined, action potentials appear and with full voluntary contraction cannot be distinguished from one other (interference pattern). With neurogenic weakness, the interference pattern is reduced or disappears because of the paucity of voluntary action potentials. By contrast, in primary disease of muscle, the size of motor units decreases as muscle fibers degenerate because each

TABLE 122-1	Anatomic Distributions and Causes of Peripheral Nerve and Root Disorders

Lesion	Clinical Examples
Radiculopathy	Herniated cervical or lumbar disc, spondylosis, malignancy
Plexopathy	
Brachial	Acute autoimmune plexopathy, traction-trauma, metastases, Pancoast lung cancer
Lumbar	Proximal femoral or sciatic "neuropathy": diabetic, retroperitoneal hemorrhage, paraspinal infection, malignancy, obstetric-gynecologic problems
Mononeuropathy	
Single	Compression entrapment
Multiple	Diabetic, periarteritis, autoimmune connective tissue disorders
Diffuse (polyneuropathies)	
Axonopathy	Nutritional deficiency Toxic exposure, diabetes, uremia, rare inherited
Myelinopathy	Inflammatory-immune (Guillain-Barré and its variants)
Neuropathies, axonal or myelin	Lower motor neuron disorders (ALS), paraneoplastic sensory neuronopathies, hereditary

nerve now innervates fewer fibers. During voluntary contraction the number of activated units remains normal, but their amplitude declines; the interference pattern remains normal. In primary myopathies, the distribution abnormality helps in characterizing the myopathy itself. Table 122–2 provides a guide to the usefulness of and pertinent changes in electrophysiologic tests in various neuromuscular disorders. The EMG must be interpreted in light of

TABLE 122-2	Typical Electrophysiologic Features of Neuropathies and Myopathies

	Nerve Conduction Velocity	Electromyography
Inflammatory myopathy or dystrophy	Normal	Fibrillations; positive sharp waves; small motor units
Metabolic myopathy	Normal	Small motor units
Axonal neuropathy	Normal	Fibrillations; positive sharp waves; fasciculations; large motor units with distal predominance
Demyelinating neuropathy	Slowed diffusely	Normal motor units
Radiculopathy	Normal	Fibrillations; positive sharp waves; fasciculations; large motor units if chronic
Motor neuron disease	Normal	Fibrillations; positive sharp waves; fasciculations; large motor units diffusely

the clinical findings, because occasional fibrillation potentials may be found in healthy individuals. Also, myopathies and neuropathies sometimes produce confusingly similar changes.

NEUROMUSCULAR TRANSMISSION STUDIES. Diseases of the neuromuscular junction are characterized by normal nerve conduction velocity and a usually normal EMG. Repetitive electrical activation of the neuromuscular junction, however, produces either an abnormal diminution (myasthenia gravis) or an abnormal facilitation (Lambert-Eaton myasthenic syndrome, botulism) of the successively evoked muscle action potential.

MONO- AND POLYNEUROPATHIES AFFECTING SOMATIC CRANIAL NERVE FUNCTIONS
(Table 122–3)

Several disorders cause acute or chronic dysfunction of one or more cranial nerves. *Acute cranial nerve mononeuropathies* include optic neuropathy. Ocular motor mononeuropathies (i.e., sudden, selective dysfunction of cranial nerves III, IV, or VI) usually have a vascular basis. An example is *diabetic ophthalmoplegia*, which generally occurs in mildly affected diabetics, sometimes before the diagnosis of diabetes is made. It is characterized by the painful onset of paralysis in a single cranial nerve (most commonly the oculomotor, sparing the pupil). The pain resolves in a few days and the paralysis subsides over a few months. Similar disorders affecting nondiabetics are called acute ocular neuropathy, which likewise has a benign prognosis. The differential diagnosis includes compression lesions (i.e., orbital or intracranial tumor or intracranial aneurysm) and inflammatory lesions (meningitis).

Aside from *trigeminal neuralgia*, the trigeminal nerve suffers rarely from a bilateral form of sensory neuropathy associated with connective tissue autoimmune disease (Sjögren's syndrome) or malignancy. Loss of sensation in a single peripheral branch of the nerve (V1, 2, or 3) usually reflects underlying malignancy. Selective weakness rarely affects the motor fibers of the nerve, and then, mostly by malignant invasion. Involvement of any kind of the descending trigeminal nucleus and tract in the lower pons and medulla can impair pain sensation to the ipsilateral face in a more-or-less "onion peel" manner, spreading out from perioral areas.

Acute facial palsy is usually of unknown cause and has a benign prognosis (Bell's palsy). The disorder may follow a banal infection or exposure to a draft and usually begins with mild pain behind the ear, followed within several hours by paralysis of the muscles supplied by the facial nerve. Unilateral loss of taste is common (chorda tympani). Recovery usually begins within 2 months, and within 9 months to 1 year 80% of patients report virtually normal function. The pathogenesis of the disorder is believed to be an infectious-inflammatory swelling of the facial nerve in the facial canal of the middle ear, leading in severe cases to an acute compression neuropathy. Recent evidence suggests that herpes simplex invasion may trigger the process. Differential diagnosis includes herpes

TABLE 122–3	Cranial Nerves: Functions and Principal Impairments	
Nerve	**Normal Function**	**Disorders**
I. Olfactory	Smell/taste	See text
II. Optic	Carries visual exteroceptors	See text
III, IV, VI. Oculomotor, trochlear, abducens	Regulate direction of gaze	See text
V. Trigeminal	Sensory branches: carry somatic receptor impulses serving upper brow/face (V1); middle face and upper gums/teeth (V2); and lower face/gums (V3). Motor branches: travel with V3 to innervate jaw muscles	Sensory impairment of touch, topical recognition, pain in all three roots Pain pathways are relayed by descending spinal trigeminal nucleus-tract before crossing to contralateral spinothalamic tract in lower brain stem
VII. Facial	Innervates facial muscles. Chordotympani branch supplies taste fibers to anterior tongue	
VIII. Acoustic-vestibular	Carries auditory and vestibular information to pontine brain stem	See text
IX. Glossopharyngeal	Overlaps vagus in function	
X. Vagus	Carries both autonomic (parasympathetic) fibers innervating viscera as well as somatic efferent and afferent fibers. Somatic fibers innervate pharyngeal-laryngeal muscles; afferent fibers include pharyngeal-vocal receptor systems as well as tracheal, pulmonary, and gastrointestinal receptors	Ipsilateral paralysis and anesthesia of soft palate, pharynx, larynx
XI. Accessory	Carries motor fibers emanating from lower nucleus ambiguus to join vagus efferents. Spinal components emanate from C2–C6 segments to innervate sternocleidomastoid and upper trapezius muscles	Involvement can result from cancers involving meningeal or jugular foramenal areas of skull. More frequent causes are trauma or acute brachial neuropathy
XII. Hypoglossal	Innervates ipsilateral tongue muscles. Paralyzed tongue points towards side of weakness	Lower motor neuron involvement can occur mechanically from regional cancers or innately from myasthenia gravis, cranial neuropathies, or, most frequently, amyotrophic lateral sclerosis

zoster as well as tumors and basal meningitis (e.g., Lyme disease, sarcoid). Bilateral facial weakness of sudden onset suggests either inflammatory-immune neuropathy or Lyme disease. Gradual development of facial diplegia suggests sarcoid or meningeal cancer.

The most important aspect of management in severe facial palsies is to protect the cornea. Patients with acute, severe peripheral facial paralysis cannot close the eye, and the cornea should be protected with a lens when out of doors and the eye should probably be patched at night. Although the evidence of efficacy is weak, many physicians who encounter a patient with Bell's palsy during the first 46 to 72 hours of paralysis treat the disorder with a short course of corticosteroids (60 mg of prednisone daily for 1 week, with gradual tapering over the next week) when not otherwise contraindicated.

Facial hemispasm is characterized by unilateral, recurring, rapid, locally migrating twitches of bundles of facial muscles most often occurring around the eye or mouth. The disorder usually begins in middle to elderly life and is initially intermittent in bursts of minutes to an hour or so but often becomes nearly continuous. Sensory changes are lacking and most examples reflect the compression of the facial nerve at the base of the brain by an adjacent artery. Surgical separation of the two usually halts the problem. *Facial synkinesias* are late consequences of Bell's palsy and consist of spontaneous contractions of unrelated facial muscles in association with intended movement such as eye blinking. *Facial myokymia* consists of spontaneous, continuous, vermicular waves of small facial muscle contractions usually caused

by a structural brain stem lesion adjacent to the facial nucleus.

The glossopharyngeal and vagal nerves act in close concert. Injury to different sensory fibers from the lateral pharynx and ear canal can produce *glossopharyngeal neuralgia*. Swallowing and vocal function can be paralyzed by damage to the nucleus ambiguus in the brain stem from stroke or locally placed neoplasms, or to the emerging vagus nerve fibers that exit the skull via the jugular foramen to reach the striated musculature of the pharynx or vocal cords. Gradual unilateral involvement may induce only moderate dysfunction, but sudden central unilateral destruction of the nuclei (e.g., acute stroke) can cause transient but relatively severe swallowing dysfunction and hoarseness. Bilateral injury, such as may occur with cranial polyneuropathy, poliomyelitis, meningeal cancer, or a pseudobulbar palsy, can halt swallowing or the capacity to clear the pharynx. Endotracheal intubation or tracheostomy is usually necessary to prevent choking. Progressive lower motor neuron degeneration of pharayngeal fibers due to amyotrophic lateral sclerosis produces similar problems.

Multiple cranial nerve neuropathies are uncommon except as they complicate tumors at the base of the skull (e.g., nasopharyngeal carcinoma), leptomeningeal metastases, or meningitis (e.g., tuberculosis, sarcoid, Lyme disease). Idiopathic multiple cranial neuropathies typically begin with pain in the eye or face; paralysis develops acutely, often responds to treatment with corticosteroids, and may be recurrent. The most common and well-defined condition is the Tolosa-Hunt syndrome, characterized by unilateral paralysis of muscles supplied by oculomotor, trochlear, and abducent nerves, sometimes accompanied by sensory loss in the first division of the trigeminal nerve. The disorder is thought to result from granulomatous inflammation of the superior orbital fissure or cavernous sinus. Similar syndromes can involve lower cranial nerves or a combination of oculomotor and lower cranial nerves. When the disorder is painless and symmetric it may represent a restricted form or initial manifestation of the Guillain-Barré syndrome (GBS).

Pseudobulbar palsy describes spastic, bilateral weakness due to damage of supranuclear motor pathways affecting cranially innervated striated muscles extending from the trigeminal down to the hypoglossal nerves. At its maximal degree, the result is a slow, grinding, effortful dysarthria coupled with difficulties in chewing and swallowing meaty foods and, sometimes, choking on fluids. Hyperactive jaw, facial, and pharyngeal reflexes often accompany the weaknesses. Muscle atrophy is absent and excessive involuntary limbic expressions of crying or, less often, laughing may accompany the motor problems.

Other immune polyneuropathies not related to GBS are those associated with *multiple myeloma*, particularly of the osteoblastic variety, and *benign monoclonal gammopathies*. The neuropathy in these instances slowly progresses and has a sensorimotor distribution with no distinct systemic signs other than the alterations of serum proteins. The pathogenesis is thought to have an immune basis in which gamma globulin produced in excess by the primary disorder binds to the nerves to react with a myelin-associated glycoprotein and cause demyelination. In the case of multiple myeloma, treatment of the primary disease sometimes leads to amelioration of the neuropathy.

Metabolic Neuropathies

Several metabolic or nutritional diseases are associated with polyneuropathy (Table 122–4). Diabetic neuropathy is especially common and can take several forms (see Chapter 71).

These subacute or chronic sensorimotor neuropathies have few individually characteristic signs, and the diagnosis is usually suggested by identifying the underlying systemic disease. For example, most patients with the peripheral neuropathy of acute intermittent porphyria have mental changes and/or abdominal pain preceding the onset of the neuropathy. Likewise the characteristic slow reflexes of hypothyroidism are usually present in addition to the sensorimotor polyneuropathy. In any patient suffering from a chronic progressive sensorimotor polyneuropathy, a careful search for metabolic disorders is essential to establish the diagnosis.

Toxic Neuropathies

Table 122–5 lists some of the toxins known or believed to cause polyneuropathies. In general, polyneuropathies produced by toxins are sensorimotor in pattern, although a few, such as those caused by acrylamide and pyridoxine

TABLE 122–4 Metabolic and Nutritional Diseases of Peripheral Nerves

Endocrine

Diabetes (polyneuropathy)
Hypothyroidism
Acromegaly (usually entrapment neuropathies)

Nutritional

Vitamin deficiency
    Thiamine (beriberi, Wernicke's disease)
    Pyrodoxine (isoniazid toxicity)
    Vitamin B_{12} (pernicious anemia, gastrectomy)
Multiple factors (alcohol)
Malnutrition (Vitamins B_6 and E)

Renal (uremia)

Hepatic

Porphyria
Chronic liver failure

toxicity, produce predominantly sensory changes. In every instance of obscure polyneuropathy, a careful occupational history and search for intoxicants, either knowingly or unknowingly ingested, is warranted.

Hereditary Neuropathies

Table 122–6 lists the most often encountered types, among which the *Charcot-Marie-Tooth* groups have by far the largest prevalence. Three principal genotypes exist with several different genetic patterns; nevertheless, the phenotype remains relatively similar among the group, albeit with somewhat different ages of onset. Early symptoms usually include a weakness-deformity of the feet that impairs walking and running. Distal, symmetric mus-

TABLE 122–5 Some Causes of Toxic Neuropathies

Pharmaceutical Agents	Other Agents
Antiretrovirals	Acrylamide (truncal ataxia)
Chloramphenicol	Arsenic (sensory, brown skin, Mees' lines)
Cisplatin	Carbon disulfide
Clioquinols	Cyanide
Ethambutol	Dichlorophenoxyacetic acid
Gold	Biologic toxin in diphtheritic neuropathy
Isoniazid†	Ethylene oxide
Nitrofurantoin*	*n*-Hexane (glue fumes)
Nitrous oxide	Lead (wrist drop, abdominal colic)
Perhexiline	Mercury
Pyridoxine†	Methyl bromide
Stilbamidine	Organophosphates (cholinergic symptoms, delayed onset of neuropathy)
Suramin	
Taxol	Thallium (pain, alopecia, Mees' lines)
Thalidomide	Trichloroethylene (facial numbness)
Vincristine	

* Predominantly motor.
† Predominantly sensory.
Modified from Schaumburg HH: Toxic neuropathies. *In* Wyngaarden JB, Smith LH Jr, Bennett JC (eds.): Cecil Textbook of Medicine. 19th ed. Philadelphia, WB Saunders, 1992, pp 2246–2247.

TABLE 122-6	Hereditary Neuropathies of Adulthood

Charcot-Marie-Tooth Disease

Type 1. Autosomal Dominant, Gene Location:

1A = C17p11.2, hypertrophic
1B = C1q22, nonhypertrophic, often mild
1C = gene not located, phenotype similar

Type 2. C1 p

Type 3. Dejerine-Sottas Gene C17p11.2, Hypertrophic

Neuropathy, severe disability

Familial Amyloid Polyneuropathies (Four Subtypes)

Porphyric Neuropathy

Rare Neuropathies Sometimes Affecting Adults:

Fabry's disease; leukodystrophies; Refsum's disease; Tangier disease; abetalipoproteinemia (vitamin E deficiency due to mutation in microsomal transfer protein); mitochondrial neuropathies; hereditary sensory and autonomic neuropathies (rare except in infants-neonates)

cle atrophy develops, creating a "stork-leg" clinical image. Sensory impairment usually affects peroneal nerve distribution. In many cases, the distal upper extremities become atrophied as well but usually undergo no sensory impairment. As noted, some forms are due to recurrent demyelination and repair of the nerves produces a palpable hypertrophic neuropathy. Despite their genetic etiology, clinical severity ranges widely from case to case, even within families. The ultimate degree of weakness varies widely from patient to patient but only rarely becomes completely incapacitating. Treatment consists of supportive efforts to counter progressive weakness.

Inherited amyloid neuropathy is due to an autosomal dominant defect of the transthyretin (prealbumin) gene. Neurologic disability usually appears during early adulthood and affects predominantly small neural fibers mediating pain and autonomic functions. The course is invariably progressive and most victims die before age 50 years.

Critical Illness Polyneuropathy

A significant number of patients with sepsis and multiorgan failure who are intubated and admitted to intensive care units develop weakness, hyporeflexia, and electrophysiologic signs of motor and sensory axonal dysfunction. Most patients who develop such "critical illness" or "intensive care unit" polyneuropathy have been critically ill for 2 weeks to 1 month. The disorder is often first suspected when the patient cannot be weaned from a respirator. Most patients who survive the underlying illness recover over several months. The exact pathogenesis of the axonal neuropathy is not known.

NEUROCUTANEOUS SYNDROMES

The category includes a relatively large number of mainly inherited disorders that concurrently involve the nervous system and the skin. The most common disorders that

extend into or begin in adult life all express an autosomal dominant trait and include neurofibromatosis, types 1 and 2; tuberous scelerosis; and von Hippel–Lindau disease. Sturge-Weber syndrome, a sporadic congenital malformation of the cephalic venous microvasculature, commonly impairs mental development and often is complicated by seizures. Most affected children reach adulthood.

Diagnostic Measures

The gross configuration of abnormalities affecting the spinal column, spinal cord, and peripheral branches can be visualized readily by advanced MRI and CT imaging devices. These instruments are less helpful in diagnosing disease in peripheral neural or neuromuscular structures. For these areas, electrophysiologic tests and, sometimes, nerve or muscle biopsy may be essential to making an accurate diagnosis.

THE MOTOR NEURON DISEASES

The term *motor neuron disease* refers to a group of chronic neurologic disorders affecting the anterior horn cells of the spinal cord and lower brain stem plus, in many instances, the large motor neurons of the cerebral

TABLE 122-7	Principal Motor Neuron Diseases

Hereditary Progressive Spinal Muscular Atrophy (SMA)

Autosomal, related to 5q11.2–11.3
Infantile SMA (type 1)—Werdnig-Hoffmann
Perinatal (most die before 2 yr)
Kugelberg-Welander SMA type 3 (see text)

Hexosaminidase Deficiency

Onset childhood or adolescent

Kennedy Disease

Xq21.3–22. Rare. Bulbar-spinal atrophy, beginning after 40 yr with dysarthria, dysphagia, and slow course

Nonhereditary Progressive Spinal Muscular Atrophy (Adult Form)

Rare
Insidious onset, 35–50 yr
Distal > proximal weakness; no spasticity
Cranial symptoms minimal or absent
Survive normally

Primary Lateral Sclerosis

Rare
Age of onset 50 ± 10 yr
Progression slow but continuous
Mean survival about 20 years
No laboratory markers
Asymmetric progressive spastic weakness involves lower > upper limbs but eventually bulbar functions
Premature death, 7–20+ yr from onset
No lower motor neuron or sensory changes

Amyotrophic Lateral Sclerosis (2nd Variants)

Sporadic/familial (rare)
Bulbar-spinal, spinal-bulbar, pure spinal variants. Glutamate toxicity postulated. Familial group analysis shows mutation on Cr21q 22.1–22.2 resulting in superoxide dismutase deficiency

cortex that give rise to the corticospinal tract (Table 122–7). Sensory changes and cerebellar dysfunction are absent. If both upper and lower motor neuron abnormalities are found, the disorder is called *amyotrophic lateral sclerosis* (ALS). *Progressive bulbar palsy* is a variant of ALS that causes relatively rapidly advancing upper and lower motor neuron involvement of the muscles of the jaw, pharynx, and tongue. A small number of adults develop only a slow, progressive muscle atrophy and weakness accompanied by fasciculations but no spasticity. A few will have a family history of the disorder, but most cases are sporadic examples of progressive muscular atrophy (PMA) type 2. The rarest form of pure motor neuron disease begins as bilateral upper motor neuron disease affecting the extremities *(progressive lateral sclerosis),* the bulbar muscles *(pseudobulbar palsy),* or both (see Table 122–7). Lower motor neurons are spared in such cases. Amyotrophic lateral sclerosis may be associated with a form of late-life dementia characterized by prominent signs of frontal lobe dysfunction.

Motor neuron disease may first affect bulbar muscles, one or both of the extremities on one side of the body, the lower or upper extremities symmetrically, or all four limbs simultaneously. The disorder's incidence increases with advancing age and progresses over 2 to 7 years until death. A subacute developing but reversible motor neuron disease, difficult to distinguish from ALS, also has been reported in a few patients in the United States. The bulbar form has the shortest course, PMA the longest (often more than 10 years), and ALS intermediate. The disease rarely takes an autosomal dominant form. Recent group analyses of this disorder have revealed evidence of a mutation on chromosome (Cr) 21 involving the toxic formation of zinc-copper superoxide dismutase. Other experimental leads suggest that the disease may be related to excess glutamate activity or free radical formation leading to cellular auto-oxidants. Endemic outbreaks in the Mariana Islands have also been identified, but whether the risk factors are environmental or genetic remains undiscovered.

The typical patient with ALS develops progressive limb weakness affecting distal more than proximal areas, and especially affecting the small muscles of the hand. Early atrophy and fasciculations are prominent. Some patients may have muscle cramps, but sensory symptoms are rare. The deep tendon reflexes are usually preserved in the early phase of the disease, at least in the upper extremities. Signs of upper motor neuron involvement may develop at any time but almost always appear by the time muscle involvement has lasted a year. Characteristically bladder and bowel functions remain unaffected. ALS spares the extraocular muscles but in the late stages can interfere with supranuclear oculomotor control. Some patients show signs of emotional lability. Intellectual functions deteriorate in approximately 5%. The CSF is normal. Electrodiagnostic testing is helpful. The motor nerve conduction velocities remain normal even in the presence of severe atrophy, a finding that separates this disorder from the peripheral motor neuropathies, in which conduction velocities are reduced.

In its classic form, ALS, with painless weakness and atrophy of the hands, fasciculations in the entire upper

TABLE 122–8	Differential Diagnosis of Amyotrophic Lateral Sclerosis (ALS)	
Disease	**Distinguishing Features**
Benign fasciculations	No weakness, atrophy, or EMG abnormality
Motor neuron diseases	
Lead or mercury toxicity*	Increased lead or mercury levels
Benign focal amyotrophy	Onset in young; strictly focal; no upper motor neuron signs
Postpolio progressive muscular atrophy	Little true evidence of progressive muscular degeneration; slow course; no upper motor neuron signs; mechanical problems usually present
Subacute motor neuronopathy in lymphoma	Plateau in few months, later improvement
ALS in lung cancer or B cell dyscrasia*	Improves on treatment of tumor
Adult spinal muscular atrophy	Symmetric, slow course; no upper motor neuron signs; rare
Thyrotoxic myopathy with fasciculations*	Myopathic EMG
Compressive myelopathy due to cervical spondylosis or extra-medullary tumor*	Sensory symptoms; no lower motor neuron signs in legs; cord compression on MRI or myelography
Immune-mediated multifocal motor neuropathy*	Multifocal nerve conduction block; high antiganglioside antibody titers

* Treatable conditions.
EMG = Electromyography; MRI = magnetic resonance imaging.

extremities, and spasticity and reflex hyperactivity of the legs with extensor plantar responses can hardly be mistaken for any other disease. Less classic findings, however, may make it more difficult to differentiate on clinical grounds alone (Table 122–8).

Similar problems may be encountered in the rare condition of *multifocal motor neuropathy.* This progressive bulbar palsy must be distinguished from myasthenia gravis, myopathies, and in particular polymyositis. Upper motor neuron signs such as a hyperactive jaw jerk and emotional lability and spastic speech establish the presence of motor neuron disease. Marked atrophy and fasciculations of the tongue likewise establish that diagnosis. If these findings are absent, an edrophonium test and EMG of bulbar muscles may be necessary to make the distinction. Early in its course, if motor neuron disease affects only a few contiguous muscles, it must be distinguished from nerve root plexus disease or intramedullary neoplasms or syrinxes. Along with the absence of sensory changes, the finding of widespread electromyographic abnormalities plus the recognition of typical clinical abnormalities usually establishes the diagnosis of motor neuron disease.

Wohlfart-Kugelberg-Welander disease (PMA type 3) is a form of progressive muscular atrophy that begins during late childhood, adolescence, or early adulthood with symptoms that include proximal muscle atrophy, weakness, and fasciculations. Genetically, the illness relates to Cr5q11–q13. Reasons for its lesser severity have not been determined. It progresses slowly and is usually compatible with a lifespan into the third or fourth decade. The onset in the first and second decade of life of proximal weakness and atrophy with fasciculations but a very slow progression without evidence of upper motor neuron involvement distinguishes the disorder from ALS. If fasciculations are not prominent, EMG findings (denervation with the insertional irritability of polymyositis) and the results of muscle biopsy distinguish the neurogenic disease from acquired or inherited myopathies. The cause of the disorder is unknown. Specific therapy is not available. Similar syndromes, sporadically appearing, have not been related to the Cr5q11−q13 gene locus.

OTHER ANTERIOR HORN CELL DISEASES. *Monomyelic* (benign focal) *amyotrophy* is an uncommon disorder in which lower motor neurons supplying one extremity (usually an arm) are affected. The disease mostly involves young men. It begins in the second or third decade and progresses over a period of 2 to 4 years and then stops. The patient is left with a variable degree of weakness in the involved extremity, but the disease does not generalize and is usually not disabling. *Poliomyelitis* is an acute, viral inflammatory disease affecting anterior horn cells that once was a major cause of paralysis in the industrial world before the development of an effective polio vaccine. A similar but much less severe weakness can occasionally be caused by other neurotropic viruses. The *post-polio syndrome* is characterized by overall weakness developing years after recovery from acute paralytic poliomyelitis. The disorder appears to be a "wear and tear" problem, resulting in increasing mechanical difficulties in moving body parts with permanently overburdened surviving muscles.

FOCAL RADICULOPATHY AND NEUROPATHY

Most focal neuropathies result from vascular disease, compression, or trauma. Clinically, the mononeuropathies are characterized by sensory and/or motor loss (usually both) in the anatomic distribution of all or part of a nerve root, nerve plexus, or peripheral nerve. One can determine the site of the injury clinically by observing the anatomic distribution of dysfunction (e.g., an injury to the radial nerve at the humerus causes weakness of the brachioradialis muscle and extensors of the wrist and fingers; it spares the triceps muscle because radial nerve fibers in the triceps depart from the nerve more proximally in the upper arm).

Trauma and Compression

Most monoradiculopathies and mononeuropathies are caused by trauma and result from compression, transection, or stretching of the nerve root or the nerve itself. The most frequent disabling disorder is entrapment of a cervical or lumbar nerve root by a herniated intervertebral disc as the root passes through the intervertebral foramen. Mild injury to a nerve may leave the nerve structurally intact but cause a conduction block first by ischemia and subsequently by demyelination. Acute ischemic lesions recover rapidly when pressure is released; if demyelination ensues, the nerve recovers more slowly. A more severe injury interrupts the axons but leaves the connective tissue sheaths intact. Such lesions are common in closed crush injuries. Depending on the degree of damage, recovery may be partial or complete, but it proceeds slowly. The most severe injury is transection of both axons and connective tissue sheaths, such as occurs with severe stretch injuries or penetrating wounds. Recovery does not occur unless the nerve is surgically repaired, and even then the prognosis is poor.

Acute Trauma

Any portion of the peripheral nervous system can be damaged by trauma. In wartime, penetrating wounds of peripheral nerves and nerve plexuses are major causes of disability. In peacetime, traumatic peripheral nerve lesions usually result from closed crush or traction injuries. The *brachial plexus* is a major site of traction injuries, commonly resulting from motorcycle accidents or compression injury when the arm is hyperabducted, as under anesthesia. The former injuries are usually permanent, the latter transient. Other acute compression injuries sometimes follow general anesthesia for surgery. Still others that are induced by alcohol or sedatives include radial nerve palsy from compression of the nerve in the radial groove of the humerus (Saturday night palsy). Others include peroneal nerve palsy from compression between the surface and the head of the fibula (crossed-leg palsies), ulnar palsy (often from compression by an intravenous board in the ulnar groove at the elbow), and sciatic palsies from compression of the buttocks or ill-placed injections into that site.

Chronic Compression Radiculopathies and Myelopathies

HERNIATED INTERVERTEBRAL DISC. When disc material herniates into the lateral vertebral canal, it may compress spinal roots as they enter the intervertebral foramen. (See Fig. 122−2.) Occasionally, the disc herniates more centrally, compressing either the spinal cord in the cervical or thoracic area or the cauda equina in the lumbar area. The specific signs and symptoms of herniated discs depend partly on whether the predominant compression affects the spinal cord or nerve root, and partly on the level at which the neural structures are compressed (Table 122−9). Thoracic disc herniations are rare, but may compress the spinal cord as well as the emerging root.

The most common symptom of herniated disc is pain. Local pain is felt as a dull aching in the neck or back, with an associated stiffness of those structures, frequently occurring episodically in response to minor current or remote trauma. Muscle spasm often splints the neck or back. Radicular (i.e., dermatomal, Fig. 122−3) pain may occasionally be the first sign of disc disease but more often follows repetitive bouts of local pain. Both local and radicular pain have the characteristics of being exacerbated by activity and relieved by rest.

Raising the intraspinal pressure by coughing, sneez-

TABLE 122–9	Signs and Symptoms of Herniated Disc					
Site of disc herniation	C4–C5	C5–C6	C6–C7	L3–L4	L4–L5	L5–S1
Involved root	C5	C6	C7	L4	L5	S1
Pain	Medial scapula, lateral border of arm	Lateral forearm, thumb, and index finger	Posterior arm, lateral hand, mid-forearm, and medial scapula	Down to medial malleolus	Back of thigh, lateral calf, dorsum of foot	Back of thigh, back of calf, lateral foot
Sensory loss	Lateral border of upper arm	Lateral forearm, including thumb	Mid-forearm and middle finger	Medial leg to malleolus	Dorsum of foot	Behind lateral
Reflex loss	Biceps	Supinator	Triceps	Knee jerk	None	Ankle jerk
Motor deficit	Deltoid, supraspinatus, infraspinatus, rhomboids	Biceps, brachioradialis, brachialis (pronators and supinators of forearm)	Latissimus dorsi, pectoralis major, triceps, wrist flexors	Inversion of foot	Dorsiflexion of toes and foot (latter L4 also)	Plantar flexion and eversion of foot

ing, or straining increases the pain sharply. Directly stretching the compressed root also aggravates the pain. In the upper extremities, extending the arm and laterally flexing the neck away from the extended arm often reproduces radicular pain. In the lower extremities, raising the extended leg with the patient in the recumbent position frequently reproduces the pain of an L5 or S1 radiculopathy. If pain is felt on the opposite side as well (crossed straight-leg raising), the sign suggests herniated disc disease.

If an intervertebral disc herniates medially, rather than laterally, the symptoms may mimic a spinal tumor except that with disc disease there may be little or no

pain. The diagnosis of herniated disc is deduced from the characteristic clinical symptoms and findings. Both CT and especially MRI are effective in identifying most disc disease and in most cases are sufficient for preoperative localization of the site of herniation.

No consensus exists about the preferred management of herniated discs. Most physicians believe that the first step is bed rest. Surgery is indicated when (1) bed rest fails, and the patient is incapacitated by severe, intractable pain; (2) a centrally placed lumbar disc compresses the cauda equina, producing urinary dysfunction; or (3) there is motor weakness caused by compression of the spinal cord. Some believe that peripheral motor weakness caused by root compression is also an indication for immediate surgery, but such weaknesses often disappear spontaneously with time. Several microsurgical approaches have been found to relieve the compression with minimal morbidity.

SPONDYLOSIS. Spondylosis is a term applied to chronic degenerative disease of intervertebral discs associated with reactive changes in the adjacent vertebral bodies. Most spondylosis causes no symptoms, except when the reactive tissue compresses a nerve root or the spinal cord. When this occurs, the signs and symptoms resemble those of a herniated disc, but the onset is less abrupt and the treatment often is more difficult. In both the cervical and lumbar areas, spondylosis is more likely to produce spinal cord or cauda equina symptoms if the sagittal diameter of the spinal canal is further impinged upon by osteophytes (canal stenosis). The signs and symptoms of *cervical spondylosis* result from compression either of the spinal cord or its emerging roots and are thus similar to those of a herniated disc (see Table 122–9). Most patients suffer either radiculopathy or myelopathy but not both. The classic picture of *cervical spondylotic myelopathy* is one of little or no pain but slowly developing weakness, atrophy, and fasciculations in the upper extremities, particularly the small muscles of the hand, or an insidiously developing spastic paraparesis with decreased proprioception in the legs. At first the findings may suggest a diagnosis of amyotrophic lateral sclerosis. However, cervical spondylosis usually produces sensory changes, particularly vibration loss in the lower extremities, whereas in amyotrophic lateral sclerosis fasciculations arise from areas

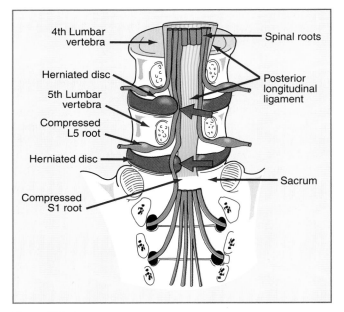

Figure 122–3

Schematic view of nerve root compression by a lumbar herniated disc. Note that the posterior longitudinal ligament tapers as it travels caudally, leaving vulnerable lateral areas into which the disc can herniate and compress the nerve root destined for the next lower exit foramen. Note also that a more laterally placed herniation of the L4–5 interspace would entrap the L4 root in the intervertebral canal (not shown). (Reprinted with permission from Posner JB: Back pain and epidural spinal cord compression. Med Clin North Am 1987; 71:185.)

wider than single motor roots. The differential diagnosis includes other compressive lesions of root and spinal cord.

When neurologic signs suggest that cervical spondylosis is causing a myelopathy, MRI is the examination of choice, often making more invasive myelography unnecessary (Fig. 122–4).

Having established the diagnosis, many physicians prefer to begin conservative treatment with cervical traction and stabilization of the neck with a soft collar. If the patient develops progressive neurologic signs, especially weakness and atrophy or spasticity, surgical therapy may be indicated.

The aforementioned considerations also apply to *lumbar spondylosis.* The symptoms resemble those of herniated disc, often occurring at multiple levels. Often patients with spinal stenosis from either spondylosis or congenital narrowing of the lumbar spine develop pseudoclaudication of the lower extremities. Typically, walking evokes or accentuates symptoms and signs of pain, paresthesias, and weakness. All of the symptoms may disappear when the exercise stops, even though the person remains standing. At times similar symptoms may be exacerbated by prolonged standing and relieved only by sitting or lying down. Pseudoclaudication of the cauda equina may be distinguished from intermittent vascular claudication in several ways (Table 122–10). With severe

TABLE 122–10	Distinguishing Features of Neurogenic Pseudoclaudication and Vascular Claudication in the Lower Extremities	
Function	**Neurogenic**	**Vascular**
Vascular pulses during exercise	Remain	Predictably and stereotypically disappear
Deep tendon reflexes	Often remain at rest	Absent at rest
Skin temperature	Warm	Cool
MRI or CT myelogram of lumbar spine	Severe canal narrowing or obstruction	Usually normal for age
Vascular Doppler signals	Intact	Reduced or near absent
Treatment	Spinal surgery	Angioplasty

CT = Computed tomography; MRI = magnetic resonance imaging.

lumbar stenosis, conservative treatment usually fails and decompressive laminectomy becomes the treatment of choice.

Acute-Subacute Plexopathies

BRACHIAL PLEXOPATHY. The brachial plexus is constructed by mixed nerve roots from C5–T1 which fuse into upper, middle, and lower trunks above the level of the clavicle and redistribute into lateral, posterior, and medial cords below that landmark. Symptoms include several patterns of weakness, pain, and sensory loss in structures about the pectoral girdle. Table 122–11 lists frequent causes.

ACUTE AUTOIMMUNE BRACHIAL NEURITIS. This condition is characterized by the abrupt onset of severe pain, usually in the distribution of the axillary nerve (over the lateral shoulder) but at times extending into the entire arm. Males of young age predominate. The acute pain generally subsides after a few days to a week. Usually coincident with the subsidence of the pain, weakness of the proximal arm becomes apparent. The serratus anterior is the most commonly paralyzed muscle, but other muscles of the shoulder girdle, including the deltoid and muscles of the upper arm, may be paralyzed as well. Rarely, most of the arm and even the ipsilateral diaphragm are paralyzed. Sensory loss is usually restricted to the distribution of the axillary nerve. Weakness may last weeks to months and be accompanied by severe atrophy of the shoulder girdle. Total recovery occurs in most patients within several months to 2 or 3 years. The disorder has been reported to follow upper respiratory infection or an immunization, but often there is no antecedent illness.

LUMBOSACRAL PLEXOPATHY. The lumbosacral plexus is constructed by mixed spinal roots from T12–S3. Predominant contributions go to femoral, sciatic, and obturator nerves. Clinical expression includes proximal pain and weakness in anterior thigh muscles (femoral) or posterior thigh and buttocks. Table 122–11 lists frequent causes.

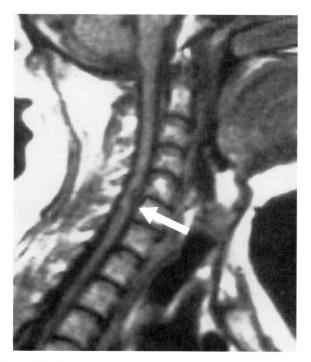

Figure 122–4
Cervical disc herniation causing myelopathy. Magnetic resonance imaging (MRI) from a middle-aged patient with a 1-year history of numbness in the right arm and progressive spastic weakness of both legs. There was no pain. Although MRI does not image bone, the bone marrow in the vertebral bodies is clearly visible. The herniated disc impinging on the cervical cord between C5 and C6 can be easily seen *(arrow).*

TABLE 122–11	Principal Causes of Nerve Plexopathy

Brachial

Traumatic stretching—avulsion
Backpack pressure plexopathy
Thoracic outlet syndrome (rare)
Clavicle and/or rib fracture
Cancer: pulmonary apex, brachial metastases
Radiation injury
Malplaced nerve blocks
Autoimmune brachial neuropathy

Lumbar

Pregnancy
Hemorrhage due to blood dyscrasias, anticoagulants
Pelvic cancer and/or radiation
Pelvic and/or spinal fracture
Paraspinal abscesses
Metabolic-inflammatory: diabetic; vasculitic

Chronic Compression Neuropathies

In order to reach their peripheral targets, many nerves must pass through narrow channels where they can become chronically compressed in fibrosseous tunnels, angulated and stretched over arthritic joints or bony structures, or recurrently compressed by repeated trauma. Table 122–12 lists the major compression neuropathies.

CERVICAL RIB AND THORACIC OUTLET SYNDROME. The brachial plexus as it passes through the thoracic outlet can be compressed by a cervical rib or by normal bone, muscles, and fibrous tissue. The compression usually occurs when the arm is abducted and may involve the subclavian artery as well as the plexus. Symptoms include paresthesias of ulnar fingers and rarely weakness and wasting of the small hand muscles. The sensory abnormalities usually respond to avoiding the abducted position. Surgical removal of the first rib and fibrous band sometimes is performed as treatment, but its indications and benefits are controversial.

CARPAL TUNNEL SYNDROME. The increasing use of typewriters and computers by the blue-collar work force has catapulted this syndrome into a major disability claim, sometimes on limited physical evidence. In classic in-

TABLE 122–12	Common Sites of Nerve Entrapment

Median nerve
  Carpal tunnel—wrist
  Pronator muscle—elbow
Ulnar nerve
  Elbow
  Wrist
Radial nerve—humeral groove
Brachial plexus—thoracic outlet
Sciatic nerve—buttock (sciatic notch)
Peroneal nerve—behind knee
Lateral femoral cutaneous nerve—inguinal ligament
Cervical and lumbar root—intervertebral canal

stances the median nerve is pathologically compressed at the wrist as it passes deep to the flexor retinaculum. Symptoms include numbness, tingling, and burning sensations in one or both palms and in the fingers supplied by the median nerve, including the thumb, index, middle, and lateral half of the ring finger. Some patients complain that all fingers become numb, but this is difficult to confirm objectively. Pain and paresthesias are most prominent at night and often interrupt sleep. The pain is prominent at the wrist but may radiate to the forearm, rarely to the shoulder. Both pain and paresthesias are relieved by loose shaking of the hands. In some patients, symptoms may persist for years without objective signs of median nerve damage. In others, sensory loss may appear over the tips of the fingers and/or weakness can develop in the median nerve–innervated thumb muscles in association with atrophy of the lateral aspect of the thenar eminence.

Additional predisposing factors include gardening, house painting, meat wrapping, or typing. Other causes include pregnancy, myxedema, acromegaly, rheumatoid arthritis, and primary amyloidosis.

The diagnosis is based on clinical symptoms, and the demonstration of a conduction block at the wrist by motor nerve velocity studies. If rest and splinting fail, treatment is section of the transverse carpal ligament, decompressing the nerve.

ULNAR PALSY. The ulnar nerve may be entrapped at the elbow (cubital tunnel) or at the wrist. Injury may also occur years after a malunited supracondylar fracture of the humerus with bony overgrowth (tardive ulnar palsy). Contrary to the findings in the carpal tunnel syndrome, muscle weakness and atrophy characteristically predominate over sensory symptoms and signs. Patients notice atrophy of the first dorsal interosseous muscle and difficulty performing fine manipulations of the fingers. There may be numbness of the small finger, the contiguous half of the ring finger, and the ulnar border of the hand.

MERALGIA PARESTHETICA. This is the most common pure sensory mononeuropathy. It results from compression of the lateral cutaneous nerve of the thigh as it passes under the inguinal ligament. Numbness or burning sensations occur over the lateral thigh; sometimes prolonged standing or walking provokes the symptoms. Weight reduction may help, but in many cases the condition subsides spontaneously. A similar sensory syndrome can affect the dorsal aspect of the thumb when a tight watchband compresses a cutaneous branch of the radial nerve.

Infectious Focal Neuropathies

Cranial nerves and nerves of the cauda equina may be damaged by acute bacterial meningitis, subacute meningitis (e.g., tuberculosis), or less commonly, chronic meningitis (e.g., fungal meningitis). Common infections of the peripheral nervous system include herpes zoster, leprosy, Lyme disease, and acquired immunodeficiency syndrome (AIDS).

Vascular Neuropathies

Several diseases that affect small or medium-sized vessels may lead to ischemia or infarction of isolated peripheral nerves. The most common disorder is a mononeuropathy that complicates *diabetes*. Mononeuropathy or multiple mononeuropathies commonly arise as early complications or first symptoms of *periarteritis nodosa*. Less commonly, rheumatoid arthritis, systemic lupus erythematosus, hypersensitivity angiitis, Sjögren's syndrome, or Wegener's granulomatosis may cause a similar peripheral neuropathy. Vascular neuropathies are characterized by the acute onset of motor and sensory loss in the distribution of one or more single peripheral nerves. With the passage of time, other nerves become involved. Depending on the intensity of the vasculitis, the neurologic deficit may resolve after weeks or months, only to affect another nerve at a distant place. Severe cases can involve so many nerves that the condition resembles a polyneuropathy rather than a mononeuritis multiplex. Usually a careful history distinguishes the focal onset of the latter.

POLYNEUROPATHY

Inflammatory/Immune Polyneuropathies

GUILLAIN-BARRÉ SYNDROME. Several acute and chronic polyneuropathies derive from a known or probable immune basis (Table 122–13). The mechanism of neurologic dysfunction is usually demyelination initiated by an antimyelin-antiganglioside antibody. The most frequent of these disorders is the Guillain-Barré syndrome (GBS, or acute postinfectious polyneuropathy). GBS has a peak incidence in young or middle-aged persons and can affect all races and both sexes. The disorder is characterized by a rapidly progressive, predominantly motor neuropathy that may paralyze all voluntary muscles, including those controlling respiration and/or cranial motor nerve functions. Sensory changes are usually milder than motor abnormalities and may include no more than tingling paresthesias in the hands and feet. Only rarely does sensory loss predominate. *Acute cranial polyneuropathy,* either with or without prominent peripheral nerve involvement, often reflects the presence of a slightly different antiganglioside antibody. Pain is common in GBS, as is some

---

TABLE 122–13 | Autoimmune Peripheral Neuropathies

Acute Inflammatory Neuropathy (Guillain-Barré Syndrome)
  Demyelinating
  Axonal
  Cranial (Miller Fisher variant)
Chronic Inflammatory Demyelinating Neuropathy
  Subacute sensory neuropathy (paraneoplastic)
  Paraproteinemic neuropathies
  Acute brachial plexopathy
  Sensorimotor
  Pure motor

---

degree of autonomic dysfunction. Many patients suffer from hypertension or cardiac arrhythmias, the latter being the usual cause of the 5% death rate.

Characteristically, patients developing GBS report having had a mild respiratory or gastrointestinal infection in the preceding 2 or 3 weeks. Other predisposing factors are surgical procedures and Hodgkin's disease. Predominant symptoms include weakness evolving from feet to hands, with about 10 to 15% of patients describing paresthesias in those members. Fever is absent. Typical is a steady progression of increasing loss of strength ascending the limbs over a matter of hours or days. As many as 10% of patients develop swallowing difficulties and about 1 in 20 develop respiratory insufficiency. Abnormal laboratory findings include a CSF lymphocytosis of up to 20 lymphocytes per mm^3 and within a few days an elevated CSF protein level above 100 mg/dl, usually without an accompanying pleocytosis. In most instances, strength approaches normal over several weeks to months. Patients who require respiratory support and cardiovascular monitoring improve more slowly and some retain partial weakness indefinitely. These considerations often lengthen hospital stay. Prompt, accurate diagnosis is imperative for acute GBS since plasmapheresis or infused human immunoglobulin given soon after onset usually can halt the disease's progression and accelerate its recovery. Steroids provide no help and sometimes worsen progression.

GBS VARIANTS. Two other acute, immune polyneuropathies resemble GBS in their relatively rapid onset, their relationship to antecedent minor illnesses, their symmetry of involvement, and their reversibility by apheresis or human immunoglobulin. *Ataxic-ophthalmoplegic neuropathy* predominantly affects oculomotor nerves, other cranial nerves, and proprioceptive sensory nerves arising from the lower limbs. The other, much more dangerous variant causes an acute, *noninflammatory axonal neuropathy*. The pattern of onset and progression of the diseases resembles that of classic GBS. Prompt immune therapy appears to halt the process but once severe paralysis occurs it often remains for long periods and, sometimes, permanently. Epidemiologic studies have found a close linkage to preceding campylobacter infection. The highest prevalence of the illness has been found among Chinese provincial children.

MULTIFOCAL MOTOR NEUROPATHY. This uncommon condition affects predominantly young men, with an insidiously beginning, distal and asymmetric weakness coupled with mild muscle atrophy and fasciculations, but no sensory changes. It presumably has an autoimmune pathogenesis. Strength loss characteristically exceeds muscle atrophy, deep tendon reflexes are reduced or absent, and spasticity is absent. Diagnosis can be suspected by the gradual nature of symptoms plus electrodiagnostic studies showing slowed motor nerve conduction time. Anti-immune therapy provides inconsistent results.

NEUROFIBROMATOSIS. The disorder(s) express a trait with a high spontaneous mutation rate (40 to 60% of cases are clinically sporadic). There are two forms of the disorder.

Neurofibromatosis 1 (von Recklinghausen's disease) is caused by an abnormality in neurofibromin, expressed normally at the gene locus 17q11.2. Characteristic stigma include pigmented skin lesions (café au lait spots), multiple tumors of spinal or cranial nerves (neurofibromas composed of proliferating fibroblasts or neurilemmal sheath cells), skin tumors, and frequently, intracranial meningiomas. There is an increased association with pheochromocytomas, cystic lung disease, renal vascular lesions causing hypertension, fibrous dysplasia of bone, and medullary thyroid carcinoma, as well as other tumors of endocrine glands. The tumors can overlap in the region of the brachial or sacral plexus to produce large plexiform neuromas that can evolve into malignant sarcomas. Intracranial astrocytomas and glioblastomas occur with a greater than normal frequency. Stenosis of the aqueduct with noncommunicating hydrocephalus is sometimes observed.

Neurofibromatosis 2 reflects a defect in the protein merlin, genetically expressed at 22q11.21–13.1. Less common than neurofibromatosis 1, the disorder is characterized by bilateral acoustic neuromas. Cutaneous manifestations may be absent, but meningiomas and spinal neurofibromas occur with increased frequency.

TUBEROUS SCLEROSIS. This neurocutaneous disorder is inherited as an autosomal dominant trait. Its triad of findings, all present by late childhood, including facial nevi (adenoma sebaceum), epilepsy, and mental retardation, result from a defect in the protein tuberin, generated at 16p13.3. Subtle cases occasionally produce problems in the differential diagnosis of early or late adolescent epilepsy, and funduscopic examination can disclose nodules or phakomas of the retina that look neoplastic but in fact are stable and similar in structure to the adenoma sebaceum. Some patients develop intracranial or optic gliomas. Rhabdomyomas of the heart as well as renal tumors and neoplasms of the endocrine organs can be observed.

STURGE-WEBER DISEASE. This disease reflects a sporadic congenital malformation of the cephalic venous microvasculature. The port wine–colored capillary hemangiomas involve specific trigeminal dermatomes on the face, accompanied by a similar malformation of the underlying meninges and cerebral cortex. Diagnosis is made by observing the disfiguring stain. General or focal motor seizures may occur with or without associated mental retardation and require antiepileptic medication. The disfiguring stain deserves cosmetic repair if possible.

VON HIPPEL–LINDAU DISEASE. This condition is inherited in a simple autosomal dominant pattern and is characterized by hemangioblastomas of the cerebellar hemispheres with associated angiomas of the retina and cystic changes in the kidney and pancreas. Recent evidence maps the abnormal gene to chromosome 3p25 in the region associated with renal carcinoma. Hemangioblastomas can sometimes arise in the brain or spinal cord. An association with pheochromocytomas, polycythemia, and several forms of cancer has been noted.

REFERENCES

Bradley WG, Daroff RB, Fenichel GM, Marsden CD (eds.): Neurology in Clinical Practice. 2nd ed. Chapters 79–82. Boston, Butterworth-Heinemann, 1995.

Brown RH: Amyotrophic lateral sclerosis: Recent insights from genetics and transgenic mice. Cell 1995; 80:687–692.

Brown RH: Superoxide dismutase and familial amyotrophic lateral sclerosis: New insights into mechanisms and treatment. Ann Neurol 1996; 39:145–146.

Dyck PJ, Thomas PK, Griffin JW, Low PA, Podulsio JF (eds.): Peripheral Neuropathy. 3rd ed. Philadelphia, WB Saunders, 1993.

Gomez MR: Neurocutaneous diseases. *In* Bradley WG, Daroff RB, Fenichel GM, Marsden CD (eds.): Neurology in Clinical Practice. Boston, Butterworth-Heinemann, 1995, pp 1561–1582.

Schaumberg HH, Berger AR, Thomas PK (eds.): Disorders of Peripheral Nerves. 2nd ed. Philadelphia, FA Davis, 1992.

123

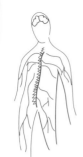

Disorders of Myoneural Junction and Skeletal Muscle

A. Disorders of Myoneural Junction

Three kinds of abnormalities can cause dysfunction or disease of the myoneural junction:

1. Impaired postjunction receptor mechanisms cause myasthenia gravis.
2. Deficiency of acetylcholine release characterizes the Lambert-Eaton myasthenic syndrome as well as the toxicity of botulism and the adverse effect of certain chemical poisons.
3. Depolarizing or nonpolarizing blockage of the action of acetylcholine at the muscle receptor mechanism can be caused by several drugs and poisons, the most notorious being curare.

Neuromuscular junction disorders are characterized by weakness and often by fatigability of muscle, so that repetitive use of the muscle often leads to increased weakness. In some, but not all, of the diseases, cranial and respiratory muscles are peculiarly susceptible. Drugs may cause or exacerbate pre-existing neuromuscular junction disorders. They are particularly likely to cause postoperative respiratory depression. The major disorders are listed in Table 123–1.

MYASTHENIA GRAVIS

Myasthenia gravis is an autoimmune disease caused by circulating antibodies that damage acetylcholine receptors lying within the postsynaptic muscle membrane. The condition may occur in isolation or be associated with other autoimmune disorders, such as systemic lupus erythematosus and hyperthyroidism. It is usually associated with an abnormality of the thymus gland, either hyperplasia (65%) or a thymoma (10 to 15%). Myasthenia gravis is accompanied by accumulation of lymphocytes in muscle and other organs, an increased frequency of nonspecific antibodies against nuclear antigens, and the presence of antithyroid antibodies. Two facts confirm that a circulating substance plays a major role in production of the weakness: (1) transplacental passage of a substance oc-

curs, so that infants born to myasthenic women suffer transient myasthenia-type bulbar weakness. Symptoms subside as the antibody supplied to the infant by the mother disappears, usually within a week to a month. (2) Plasmapheresis relieves symptoms in patients with the disease.

Myasthenia gravis may begin at any time, including the newborn, but in young adulthood the incidence is about 3 times more common in women than men whereas in older persons, men and women are equally affected. Most cases are sporadic.

The disease is characterized by weakness and fatigability. Weakness usually begins in the extraocular muscles, with ptosis and diplopia. The symptoms may be localized to the ocular muscles or generalized, mild or severe (Table 123–2). Symptoms tend to become more prominent toward the end of the day, following fatiguing activity, or with continuous use of extraocular muscles, such as in driving or reading. Closing the eyes or relaxing the muscles for a few minutes makes the symptoms subside. Other bulbar muscles may also be affected, with difficulty in swallowing, chewing, or speaking, becoming more noticeable after sustained activity of the involved muscles or when the patient is otherwise fatigued. If limb weakness develops, it more often affects proximal than distal muscles. Respiratory weakness alone or in combination with swallowing paralysis is the most feared complication. Patients who are otherwise not severely affected may unexpectedly develop acute breathing failure during a respiratory infection.

The history commonly suggests the condition and the physical examination usually confirms it. The key maneuver lies in bringing out weakness that develops with repetitive movements in extraocular or other muscles. For example, if one directs an affected patient to look fixedly at an object on the ceiling, after 30 or 40 seconds, the lids begin to droop and the eyes may diverge. In a symptomatic patient, an intravenous injection of *edrophonium chloride* (Tensilon), an anticholinesterase agent, leads to rapid amelioration of clinical symptoms

TABLE 123–1 | **Disorders of Neuromuscular Transmission**

Autoimmune
    Myasthenia gravis
    Lambert-Eaton myasthenic syndrome

Toxic
    Botulism
    Tick paralysis
    Drug-induced
    Pesticide (organophosphate) poisoning

Congenital
    Familial infantile myasthenia*
    End-plate acetycholinesterase deficiency*
    Slow-channel syndrome†
    End-plate AChR deficiency*
    High-conductance fast-channel syndrome*
    Paucity of synaptic vesicles and reduced quantal release‡
    Putative abnormality of ACh-AChR interaction‡

*Autosomal recessive inheritance.
†Autosomal or X-linked recessive inheritance.
‡Autosomal-recessive inheritance suspected.

and improved or normal muscle function for a few minutes, until the drug effects wear off. Positive results in a symptomatic patient are so dramatic that they establish the diagnosis. False-positive results can occur with increased muscular effort by the patient during the test and often can be identified by similar responses to a placebo. Occasionally, very weak muscles may be refractory to edrophonium, giving rise to false-negative results. Additional confirmatory evidence is provided by electromyographic (EMG) response to nerve stimulation. Repetitive stimulation of the nerve induces a rapid decline in the muscle action potential, the electrical counterpart of muscle fatigability. Other electrophysiologic tests are described in the references. Eighty to ninety per cent of patients with myasthenia gravis harbor antibodies against the acetylcholine receptor. False-positive tests are extremely uncommon, although patients in remission may continue to have elevated levels of antibodies.

The diagnosis of myasthenia gravis must be distinguished from *neurasthenia,* a subjective feeling of weakness and fatigability caused by psychological disorders, as well as by other myopathies and neuropathies. Attention to the effects of pharmacologic agents and electrical tests of muscle almost always establishes the diagnosis.

The treatment of myasthenia has several goals. (1) Increase the effectiveness of acetylcholine released at the myoneural junction by the anticholinesterase drugs neostigmine and pyridostigmine. Excessive treatment can cause weakness because cholinesterase inhibitors may produce a depolarizing block at the neuromuscular junction. In addition, the augmented release of acetylcholine may cause distressing abdominal cramping. Because the autonomic acetylcholine receptors of the gut are muscarinic, they can be blocked by oral atropine-like agents without affecting the nicotinic neuromuscular receptors. (2) Remove the circulating antibody. Plasmapheresis has proved to be a safe and beneficial but short-lasting treatment for most patients with myasthenia. It sometimes is used to improve severely weak patients and may keep them free of symptoms for days to weeks. (3) Thymectomy is a well-established treatment that improves about 85% of patients by reducing production of the antibody. All patients with generalized myasthenia should be considered for thymectomy. Another method of suppressing production of the antibody is to use immunosuppressive drugs, either corticosteroids or azathioprine. Corticosteroids in high doses often exacerbate myasthenia symptoms. That risk is minimized by starting the drug at low doses and advancing slowly. After a few days or a week patients begin to improve. Azathioprine can also be used to suppress antibody formation.

Patients with myasthenia are prone to develop sudden worsening of symptoms, particularly associated with respiratory infections. Such patients are best treated in intensive care units with respiratory support. Plasmapheresis may hasten resolution of such *myasthenic crises.*

THE LAMBERT-EATON MYASTHENIC SYNDROME

The *Lambert-Eaton myasthenic syndrome* is an uncommon autoimmune disorder in which antibodies reduce the voltage-dependent calcium channel at the neuromuscular junction. Repetitive stimulation of the nerve leads to a facilitation of the muscle action potential rather than a diminution. In about two thirds of instances, the disorder represents a paraneoplastic phenomenon associated with small cell lung cancer; the remaining one third occur without an underlying illness. Patients complain of proximal weakness of limb muscles, particularly in the lower extremities, and increased fatigability. They also suffer paresthesias in the thighs, a dry mouth and, in men, impotence. Examination reveals proximal weakness, but strength may increase as the patient attempts to sustain the contraction (the clinical counterpart of the electrical facilitation). Deep tendon reflexes are hypoactive or absent, particularly at the knees and ankles. Mild ptosis is common, but other cranial nerve abnormalities are not. Diagnosis is confirmed by the typical history and examination plus an EMG. Overt lung cancer, if it develops at all, may follow the neuromuscular symptoms by months to years. As in myasthenia gravis, plasmapheresis often relieves the symptoms.

TABLE 123–2 | **Classification of Myasthenia Gravis**

  I. Ocular myasthenia
 IIA. Mild generalized myasthenia with slow progression; no crisis; drug-responsive
 IIB. Moderate generalized myasthenia; severe skeletal and bulbar involvement, but no crisis; drug response less satisfactory
 III. Acute fulminating myasthenia; rapid progression of severe symptoms with respiratory crisis and poor drug response; high incidence of thymoma; high mortality
 IV. Late severe myasthenia; same as III, but takes 2 yr to progress from Classes I or II; crisis; high mortality

OTHER JUNCTIONAL DISORDERS

The *slow channel syndrome* results from a rare autosomal dominant disorder that slows closure of the acetylcholine receptor ion channel. It may present in adult life with weakness, fatigability, and atrophy of cervical, shoulder girdle, and forearm muscles. Other muscles, including those innervated by cranial nerves, may be involved as well. This clinical picture can resemble refractory myasthenia gravis, especially because the EMG declines as in myasthenia gravis; the disorder responds poorly to anticholinesterases.

Botulism is caused by the exotoxin of *Clostridium botulinum* and occurs following the ingestion of bacterially contaminated, improperly canned food. The toxin interferes with acetylcholine release at the neuromuscular junction. Symptoms usually begin within a few days of ingestion with blurring of vision, diplopia, and difficulty in swallowing and chewing. Gastrointestinal symptoms may precede the neurologic symptoms, and the weakness spreads rapidly to cause paralysis of cranial and respiratory muscles and lesser paralysis of arms and legs. The pupilloconstrictor fibers are affected early in the disorder, producing loss of visual accommodation. If electrical neuromuscular transmission studies are performed early, the findings may resemble the myasthenic syndrome. The disease may produce death from respiratory paralysis unless artificial respiration is started promptly. The history, its explosive onset and progression, and its normal spinal fluid protein distinguish botulism from the ophthalmoplegic form of the Guillain-Barré syndrome, which it can resemble closely. If appropriate critical care is provided, full recovery usually occurs.

Tick paralysis is a disorder caused by a tick neurotoxin that blocks transmission at the neuromuscular junction. Most cases occur in children, particularly girls, in whom the tick embeds in the skin near the hairline and goes unnoticed. After 5 or 6 days, paresthesias and progressive weakness develop, which may progress to flaccid paralysis of cranial and respiratory muscles and the extremities. Cerebrospinal fluid (CSF) protein is normal and the paralysis subsides promptly following removal of the parasite.

Aminoglycoside antibiotics rarely interfere with neuromuscular transmission. The most common manifestation is postoperative apnea without other evidence of paralysis, particularly in the presence of renal failure, leading to high antimicrobial drug levels. Some patients may have a flaccid quadriplegia that responds to administration of calcium and quinidine. Other drugs that can cause or exacerbate myasthenic syndromes include tetracycline, antiarrhythmic agents (procainamide, quinidine), beta-adrenergic blockers (propranolol, timolol), phenothiazines, lithium, trimethaphan, methoxyflurane, and magnesium given parenterally or in cathartics.

Organophosphate pesticides containing long-acting anticholinesterases cause weakness from acetylcholine receptor desensitization and may also cause delirium. Atropine and pralidoxime reverse the symptoms.

Several rare congenital or hereditary disorders of function of the neuromuscular junction can cause weakness in infants and newborns.

REFERENCE

Engel AG, Franzini-Armstrong C (eds.): Myology, Basic and Clinical. 2nd ed. New York, McGraw-Hill, 1994, pp 1769–1835.

B. Disorders of Skeletal Muscle

Muscle, the largest organ in the body, can be directly affected by several diseases primary to the structure itself or by the secondary effects of a number of systemic illnesses. Most myopathies are characterized by muscle weakness (usually of proximal but sometimes distal muscles) and atrophy (sometimes pseudohypertrophy). Myopathies can usually be distinguished from neuropathies by clinical examination, serum enzyme measurement, and EMG (Table 123–3).

To distinguish among the myopathies often requires a muscle biopsy, which may have to be studied biochemically and by electron microscopy. Recent genetic discoveries promise to allow genetic identification of carriers and prenatal diagnosis of most muscular dystrophies.

Table 123–4 classifies the myopathies. This text places its emphasis on disorders that are common or that have characteristic clinical findings. A more extensive discussion of the myopathies as well as the identification of the more than 25 abnormal genes that cause muscle disease can be found in A.G. Engel's chapter in the Cecil Textbook of Medicine, 20th edition.

MUSCULAR DYSTROPHIES

Muscular dystrophies (Table 123–5) are inherited myopathies characterized by progressive weakness usually beginning early in life.

Duchenne dystrophy is an X-linked recessive disor-

TABLE 123–3	Clinical Clues Differentiating Muscle from Nerve Disease	
	Myopathy	**Neuropathy-Neuronopathy**
Distribution	Mainly proximal and symmetric	Distal if symmetric; nerve or root distribution if mono- or multifocal
Atrophy	Late and mild	Early and prominent
Onset	Usually gradual	Often rapid
Fasciculations	Absent	Sometimes present
Reflexes	Lost late	Lost early
Tenderness	Diffuse in myositis	Focal in nerve or root disease
Cramps	Rare	Common
Sensory loss	Absent	Often present
Muscle enzymes	Usually elevated	Usually not or slightly elevated

From Engel AG: General approach to muscle diseases. *In* Bennett JC, Plum F (eds.): Cecil Textbook of Medicine. 20th ed. Philadelphia, WB Saunders, 1996, p 2160.

TABLE 123-4	Myopathies

Muscular dystrophy (see Table 123–5)
Myotonias (see Table 123–6)
Inflammatory myopathies
   Infections (e.g., toxoplasmosis, trichinosis, viral)
   Immune processes: polymyositis, dermatomyositis, inclusion body myositis, sarcoidosis, polymyalgia rheumatica, eosinophilic syndromes
Endocrine myopathies (see Section X)
   Hyperthyroidism and hypothyroidism
   Hyperparathyroidism
   Hyperadrenalism (glucocorticoids)
   Hyperpituitarism
Periodic paralysis (see Table 123–7)
Metabolic myopathies
   Glycogen storage diseases
   Lipid storage diseases
   Mitochondrial diseases
Congenital muscle disorders
Drugs and toxins

der of boys (rarely girls) characterized by painless weakness that is maximal in the pelvic girdle and thighs, less prominent about the shoulders, and least prominent in the distal extremities. The abnormal gene positioned on band Xp21 fails to produce *dystrophin,* a 400-kd protein whose absence allows calcium and complement components to enter and destroy muscle fibers. The disorder reveals itself with increasing clumsiness when the child begins to walk (beyond 18 months). Affected boys run awkwardly and rise from the floor by placing hands on knees and

TABLE 123-5	Principal Muscular Dystrophies and the Location of Their Abnormal Genes*

Dystrophy	Location
X-Linked Recessive Dystrophies	
Duchenne/Becker dystrophy	Xp21
Emery-Dreifuss dystrophy with joint contractures and atrial paralysis	Xq28
Autosomal Recessive Dystrophies	
Severe childhood (limb-girdle) muscular dystrophy	13q12
Scapulohumeral (limb-girdle) muscular dystrophy	15q
Autosomal-recessive distal muscular dystrophies	Several genes
Congenital muscular dystrophies	Several genes
Autosomal Dominant Dystrophies	
Myotonic dystrophy	19q13
Facioscapulohumeral dystrophy	4q35
Autosomal dominant scapuloperoneal dystrophy	
Dominantly inherited adult-onset limb-girdle dystrophy	5q
Oculopharyngeal dystrophy	
Autosomal dominant distal dystrophies	Several genes

*For a more comprehensive review, see Engel AG: Muscular dystrophies. *In* Bennett JC, Plum F (eds.): Cecil Textbook of Medicine. 20th ed. Philadelphia, WB Saunders, 1996.

using the hands to walk up the thighs (Gowers' sign). With time the calf muscles appear abnormally enlarged (pseudohypertrophy). Gradually the weakness becomes more severe, and adolescents are usually wheelchair-bound. Genetically incurred reduced intelligence is common, and many boys develop brain atrophy during their teens. Death occurs in early adulthood. The presymptomatic diagnosis can be made early by finding an elevated serum creatine kinase. The mutation rate is high, and in about two thirds of individuals no other family member is affected. Efforts to provide substitution therapy have thus far been ineffective. Duchenne must be distinguished from two similar dystrophies: *Becker's dystrophy* reflects the presence of an abnormality in dystrophin rather than its absence. The disease also is X-linked but has its onset later in childhood or adolescence and has a slower or more variable tempo (some patients function well into adult life). *Emery-Dreifuss dystrophy* also begins later and is more benign than Duchenne dystropy; pseudohypertrophy is lacking and serum enzymes remain normal or only slightly increased. Associated cardiac arrhythmias can lead to sudden death.

Limb-girdle dystrophies describe a group of disorders affecting muscles of the pelvic and shoulder girdle, usually beginning late in childhood or adolescence. They affect girls as often as boys, and progress at variable rates. Pseudohypertrophy is uncommon. Muscle biopsy and EMG may be necessary to distinguish this disorder from a similar proximal neurogenic disorder—the Wohlfart-Kugelberg-Welander syndrome (see Table 122–7).

Facioscapulohumeral dystrophy appears during late childhood or adulthood and is characterized by prominent weakness in the perioral muscles of the face and eventually weakness of eye closure. Latissimus dorsi degeneration leads to scapular winging, with the sternal head of the pectoral muscle being affected more than the clavicular. The shoulder and pelvic girdle muscles are also affected. Weakness of the trunk muscles may cause severe scoliosis. The disorder is transmitted as an autosomal dominant trait with variable but usually extremely slow progression.

Ocular muscular dystrophy is a slowly progressive disorder characterized by ptosis and progressive external ocular paralysis. The pupils are spared, and both eyes are usually affected symmetrically, so that diplopia is uncommon. Involvement of head, neck, and limb musculature varies from family to family. Because each oculomotor nerve fiber supplies only a few muscle fibers, it can be difficult to distinguish neuropathies from myopathies by either EMG or histologic examination of the eye muscles. Accordingly, the distinction between ocular myopathies and neuropathies rests on findings in other skeletal muscles. In some ocular myopathies, the skeletal muscles of the neck or limbs contain abnormally large mitochondria in increased numbers, producing a characteristic "ragged red fiber" appearance on trichrome stains.

Distal myopathy, unlike most muscular dystrophies, affects distal leg and hand muscles first. It is rare and can be identified only by characteristic signs of myopathy on EMG and muscle biopsy. *Scapuloperoneal dystrophy,* with its distal weakness in the legs, resembles neurogenic peroneal atrophy, but there is no sensory loss and proximal weakness often affects the shoulder girdle. The disorder is transmitted as an autosomal dominant trait with relatively slow progression.

Treatment of Inherited Dystrophy

No specific treatment exists. Physical therapy along with splints and braces may keep many patients walking who would otherwise be confined to a wheelchair. Corticosteroids have been reported to slow the progression of Duchenne dystrophy.

OTHER INHERITED MYOPATHIES

Several rare congenital or inherited biochemical defects can cause lifelong muscle weakness. Among these are congenital myopathies, glycogen storage diseases, lipid storage diseases, and mitochondrial myopathies.

Congenital myopathies are a group of disorders characterized by mild weakness that generally persists unchanged throughout life. The cause is not known; a few are familial and many are sporadic. The disorders are present at birth, and their chief importance lies in distinguishing them from the more severe progressive muscular dystrophies and neonatal anterior horn cell disorders. A number of glycogen storage diseases cause muscle symptoms. *McArdle's disease,* type 5 glycogen storage disease, results from an absence of muscle phosphorylase, so that patients are unable to break down glycogen during anaerobic exercise. They are usually asymptomatic until early adolescence or early adulthood, when they develop painful muscle cramps (actually contractures) after exercise. Myoglobinuria and renal failure may ensue, and patients may eventually become weak. A similar deficit results from phosphofructokinase deficiency. The diagnosis of both is established by the failure of venous lactate to rise during ischemic exercise. Biochemical study of biopsied muscle defines the exact enzyme deficiency. *Lipid storage* and *mitochondrial myopathies* usually become symptomatic in childhood and can be responsible for neurologic symptoms in addition to muscle weakness. The references provide sources that discuss these conditions more extensively.

MYOTONIAS

Table 123–6 classifies muscle diseases associated with myotonia. Myotonia results from an abnormality of the muscle membrane leading to delayed relaxation. The diagnosis is easily made clinically by asking a patient to grip one's fingers and then quickly let go. Its characteristic EMG displays repetitive action potentials that may wax or wane over many seconds when the needle is inserted or after the patient attempts to relax from a voluntary contraction. The most common myotonic abnormality is *myotonic dystrophy,* with a population incidence of 1 in 7500 births. The autosomal dominant disorder

TABLE 123–6	Myotonias and Their Genetic Associations		
Conditions		**Genetic Locus**	**Abnormality**
Myotonic muscular dystrophy		19q13.3	Myosin kinase
Myotonia congenita		7q35	Chloride channel
Paramyotonia congenita		17q23.1–25.3	Sodium channel
Hyperkalemic periodic paralysis		17q23.1–25.3	Sodium channel

causes progressive, primarily distal muscle weakness, myotonia, cranial muscle weakness, and endocrine abnormalities. The gene lies on chromosome 19 with linkage to the gene encoding complement C3. The disorder may begin early in life or be delayed into adulthood. Affected persons have facial weakness with ptosis, difficulty puckering the lips, and dysarthria. Additional wasting involves the temporalis and masseter muscles. Selective weakness and wasting affect the sternocleidomastoid muscles, giving the neck a long, swan-like appearance.

Extremity muscles are affected distally. Myotonia occurs primarily in the hands, usually as the first symptom. It becomes less severe as weakness develops and may not be easy to identify in the late stages. Almost all patients eventually develop cataracts, and men experience early frontal baldness and testicular atrophy. Conduction defects in the heart may lead to cardiac arrhythmias, and cardiomyopathy may cause congestive heart failure. General functional disability usually appears by the fourth decade. There is no effective treatment.

Myotonia congenita is rarer and occurs in both autosomal dominant and recessive forms. The disease begins in infancy and is characterized by diffuse myotonia, which makes the child stiff when initiating exercise but looser as activity continues. Affected persons move clumsily and have a stiff and wooden appearance. Cold generally worsens the symptoms. The disorder is annoying more than disabling. Drugs such as phenytoin and quinine may relieve symptoms.

Paramyotonia congenita is a rare disorder of autosomal dominant inheritance that clinically resembles myotonia congenita but with periodic paralyses. A genetic defect exists at the skeletal muscle sodium channel. Facial, forearm, and hand muscles are predominantly involved; cold exposure can either worsen or singularly precipitate the myotonia. Similar myotonias sometimes occur in hyperkalemic paralysis, and paramyotonia may simply be a manifestation of the more common periodic paralysis.

DRUG, NUTRITIONAL, AND TOXIC MYOPATHIES

With the exception of corticosteroids, drug-induced myopathy is rare. *Steroid myopathy* complicates the course of almost every patient treated for more than a few weeks with pharmacologic doses of corticosteroids and can even occur after a long period of doses that are considered close to replacement. Patients receiving every-other-day steroid therapy seem to have less myopathy. Muscle enzymes and EMG are usually normal. Other drugs that can cause myopathy include vincristine, chloroquine, bretylium, emetine, ipecac, carbenoxolone, guanethidine, epsilon-aminocaproic acid, penicillamine, colchicine, amiodarone, lovastatin, isoretinoic acid, cocaine, zidovudine, and clofibrate. Thiazide diuretics, the repeated use of laxatives, or the ingestion of other drugs that cause potassium loss may lead to chronic hypokalemia and a proximal myopathy that may be acute at onset, with elevated serum enzymes and even necrosis on muscle biopsy. For severe weakness to occur, the serum potassium concentration must fall below 2 mEq/L. Chronic alcoholism and malnutrition can lead to severe proximal muscle weakness.

PERIODIC PARALYSES

Periodic paralyses (PP) by definition are characterized by recurrent attacks of flaccid weakness, often accompanied with modest changes in serum potassium. The hereditary forms (Table 123–7) are transmitted as an autosomal dominant trait although seemingly sporadic clinical examples are relatively frequent. Pathophysiologically, they are characterized as *channelopathies*, reflecting their impairment of ion channels in skeletal muscle fibers.

Hypokalemic PP reflects an abnormality in the dihydropyridine receptor gene that functions as a voltage-gated calcium channel. The disorder is characterized by sudden attacks of flaccid weakness, usually beginning in late childhood or adolescence and frequently occurring at night after a large carbohydrate meal. The attacks may totally paralyze the extremities and trunk, sparing the respiratory, bulbar, and cranial muscles, and may last a day or more before spontaneously resolving. During the course of the attack, the serum potassium is usually low (e.g., 2.5 to 3 mEq/L), and the patient may respond to oral or intravenous potassium. Repeated attacks can lead to permanent weakness. Muscle biopsy shows vacuoles within muscle fibers. The *hyperkalemic* variety links to a mutational defect on the sodium-channel protein. The disorder begins in early childhood with attacks that occur more frequently than the hypokalemic variety, are usually milder, and generally last only minutes to hours rather than days. Typically, the hyperkalemic attack begins while the patient is resting after vigorous exercise. Lid lag and Chvostek's sign may be present along with prominent myalgias. During attacks, the serum potassium usually rises to between 5 and 7 mEq/L, and some patients develop myotonia, often limited to percussion myotonia of the tongue. Although the serum potassium levels and the clinical symptoms separate typical examples of the hypo- and hyperkalemic disorders, the conditions overlap, and many patients suffer periodic paralyses without alteration of the serum potassium.

The diagnosis of periodic paralysis is made by the typical history and confirmed by finding an abnormal serum potassium level during an acute attack. If an acute attack is not observed, one may be precipitated (in the hypokalemic form by glucose and insulin or in the hyperkalemic form by potassium), but this should be done only in a hospital setting where one is prepared to deal with complications. Thyroid function should be assessed in all patients suffering hypokalemic periodic paralysis; diuretic ingestion or other secondary courses (see Table 123–7) should be suspected if the serum potassium falls below 2.5 mEq/L.

MYOGLOBINURIA

Myoglobinuria results when major injuries to muscles lead to *rhabdomyolysis* and release of myoglobin into the serum and urine, giving the urine a brown-rust color. Myoglobinuria occasionally occurs as a hereditary disease but more often relates to sporadic muscle injuries. Affected muscles may be in the extremities or trunk; cranial and respiratory muscles seldom are affected. Crush injury is a common cause, as is pressure injury to muscles, resulting from a patient's lying immobile after poisoning from sedatives or carbon monoxide. Prolonged unconsciousness in the snow likewise can lead to myoglobinuria, as can arterial occlusion by tourniquet or embolism. Snake bites and binge alcohol ingestion also can cause myoglobinuria, as can malignant hyperthermia. Even normal people may develop some degree of myoglobinuria after vigorous exercise. Strenuous exercise among army recruits, during ritual hazing, or in marathon runners leads to myoglobinuria in a small percentage of individuals. In addition to the discoloration of the urine, the clinical syndrome is characterized by muscle aches and swelling as well as some weakness. Symptoms may persist for several days, even though the pigment in the urine rarely lasts more than 4 hours. The major potential complication is kidney injury due to myoglobin plugging the renal tubules. The disorder should be considered as a possible cause of acute renal failure of uncertain etiology. Myoglobin can be identified spectrophotometrically in the urine.

TABLE 123–7	Hereditary and Secondary Periodic Paralyses
Hereditary	**Gene Locus**
Hypokalemic	1q31
Hyperkalemic	17q23.1–25.3
Without myotonia	
With myotonia	
With paramyotonia	
Paramyotonia congenita	17q23.1–25.3
Secondary	
Hypokalemic	
Thyrotoxic	
Urinary potassium wastage	
Gastrointestinal potassium wastage	
Barium intoxication	
Hyperkalemic	
Renal insufficiency	
Adrenal insufficiency	

REFERENCES

Engel AG: Diseases of muscle (myopathies) and neuromuscular junction. *In* Bennett HC, Plum F (eds.): Cecil Textbook of Medicine. 20th ed. Philadelphia, WB Saunders, 1996, pp 2158–2173.

Griggs RC, Mendell JR, Miller RG: Evaluation and Treatment of Myopathies. Philadelphia, FA Davis, 1995.

Hoffman EP: Voltage-gated ion channelopathies: Inherited disorders caused by abnormal sodium, chloride, and calcium regulation in skeletal muscle. Annu Rev Med 1995; 46:431–441.

The Aging Patient

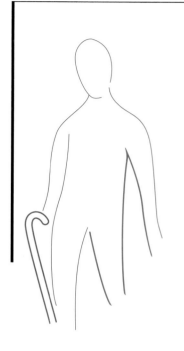

Section XV

124

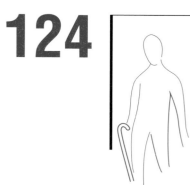

The Biology of Aging

A precise definition of normal physiologic aging remains elusive. Although probably regulated by intrinsic cellular mechanisms, the process of aging is modulated by a number of environmental influences. Because the lifetime experiences of each individual are unique and the combined effects of all environmental stimuli are impossible to calculate, it is frequently difficult to differentiate whether a measured alteration noted in older persons represents an inevitable consequence of the aging process or a potentially preventable disease. This issue has significant clinical implications. It would be important to know, for example, how much of the physiologic decline seen with advancing age could be prevented by utilizing reasonable prophylactic measures.

The response of the whole organism to the aging process varies by organ system (Fig. 124–1, Table 124–1). Certain organs, such as the kidneys, lungs, and immune system, develop age-related declines in basal physiologic function. Many other organs, such as the heart, bone marrow, and liver, maintain a level of basal physiologic function comparable to that of the younger individual. However, the process of aging in most organ systems is characterized by a reduction in reserve capacity manifested by a blunted and more variable response to increased stimulation. This diminished reserve capacity renders older persons less able to maintain homeostasis when subjected to physiologic stress. As a consequence of these age-related changes, the elderly are more susceptible to disease and slower to recover from an injury or disease complication than is a younger person. For example, compared with younger individuals, the elderly are more susceptible to and less able to survive many infectious diseases because of an age-associated decline in their host defense mechanisms, particularly their cell-mediated immunity. These same alterations in immune function are also thought to contribute to the higher incidence of cancer seen in the elderly.

The intrinsic cellular mechanisms that cause aging have yet to be identified with certainty. However, a number of theories have been postulated. The *programmed aging theory* states that aging is programmed by genetic mechanisms. The resulting age-related alterations in cellular function become manifest as a decline in immunologic and neuroendocrine function that eventually contributes to susceptibility to disease and eventual death. An alternate theory states that aging is the consequence of an *accumu-lation of random genetic errors* that over time results in impaired protein synthesis and a deterioration in cellular function. Cells normally produce free radicals such as hydrogen peroxide and superoxide as byproducts of metabolism. According to the *free radical theory,* aging is characterized by a progressive decline in the ability of cells to neutralize these metabolites rapidly, and this eventually results in irreversible cellular damage. A progressive decline in the *DNA repair capability* of cells has also been theorized to be the cause of aging. According to this theory, the decreased ability to repair damage to DNA results in errors in RNA and protein synthesis that eventually have an adverse effect on cellular function.

THE DEMOGRAPHICS OF AGING AND IMPLICATIONS FOR HEALTH CARE

As has been the case since the turn of the century, America is continuing to grow older. Between 1900 and 1980, the proportion of the population over the age of 65 grew from 4% to approximately 12%. By the year 2030, when most of the postwar baby boom generation will be over the age of 65, the elderly will constitute more than 20% of the population. The largest percentage of increase will occur in subjects over the age of 85 (Fig. 124–2). This phenomenal aging of society is the consequence of improved life expectancy and a gradually falling birth rate. Because of differences in life expectancy, by the age of 75 there are twice as many females as males.

Advancing age is associated with a higher prevalence of both acute and chronic disease and an increasing risk of becoming functionally dependent. Roughly 5.3% of adults between the ages of 65 and 75 require assistance with *basic activities of daily living* (bathing, dressing, walking, use of the toilet, and transferring from bed to chair). Slightly fewer than 6% require assistance with *instrumental activities of daily living* (cooking, shopping, use of the telephone, household chores, and handling household financial matters). By the age of 85, these figures increase dramatically to 35% and 40%, respectively (Fig. 124–3). Functional dependence greatly increases the need for both acute and chronic health care and amplifies the risk of institutionalization.

The dramatic growth in the proportion of the popula-

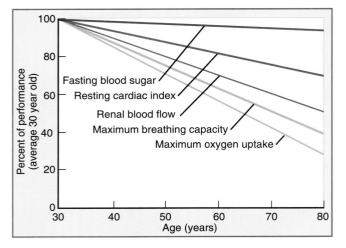

Figure 124–1
Percentage of decline, between ages 30 and 80 yr, in a number of physiologic functions.

TABLE 124–1	Age-Related Decline in Physiologic Functions

Organ System	Age-Related Decline in Function
Special senses	Presbyopia
	Lens opacification
	Decreased hearing
	Decreased taste, smell
Cardiovascular	Impaired intrinsic contractile function
	Decreased conductivity
	Decreased ventricular filling
	Increased systolic blood pressure
	Impaired baroreceptor function
Respiratory	Decreased lung elasticity
	Decreased maximal breathing capacity
	Decreased mucus clearance
	Decreased arterial Po_2
	Impaired chemoreceptor regulation of respiration
	Increased risk of secondary infection
Immune	Decreased cell-mediated immunity
	Decreased T cell number
	Increased T suppressor cells
	Decreased T helper cells
	Loss of memory cells
	Decline in antibody titers to known antigens
	Increased autoimmunity
Endocrine	Decreased hormonal responses to stimulation
	Impaired glucose tolerance
	Decreased androgens and estrogens
	Impaired norepinephrine responses
Autonomic nervous system	Impaired response to fluid deprivation
	Decline in baroreceptor reflex
	Increased susceptibility to hypothermia
	Impaired gastrointestinal motility

tion that is elderly has important economic consequences for the health care system and the nation. Because of the increasing need for health care with advancing age, the elderly are heavy consumers of health care resources. Although representing only 12% of the population, the elderly account for 33% of all hospital admissions, 44% of all hospital days, and the vast majority of visits to physicians. Approximately 36% of all health care dollars are spent on the elderly. A large proportion of these expenditures are incurred in the last year of life. Hospitalization accounts for 40% of older persons' health care costs, with visits to physicians and nursing home care each contributing 20%. Medicare is the major provider of health care for the elderly ($70 billion), with Medicaid contributing $20 billion and third-party payers $10 billion.

Although high-technology acute care is readily available to most older persons, gross deficiencies exist in the delivery of primary and preventative care. There is a particular need for in-home care and social support ser-

vices. Because of the increased prevalence of chronic disease and functional disability among the elderly, such specialized supportive services are needed to minimize the risk of nursing home placement. The continued rapid increase in the older population with chronic diseases and functional dependence will contribute significantly to the

Figure 124–2
A, The absolute increase in the number of persons between the ages of 65 and 74 yr and older than 75 yr between 1910 and the current time. The projected increase to the year 2030 is also shown. *B*, The percentage of the population over age 65 yr has significantly increased from 6% of the total population in 1940 to 11% at the current time. By the year 2030, it is projected that 16% of the population will be over the age of 65 yr. Thus, the increase in older persons is not merely a reflection of an overall rise in the total population.

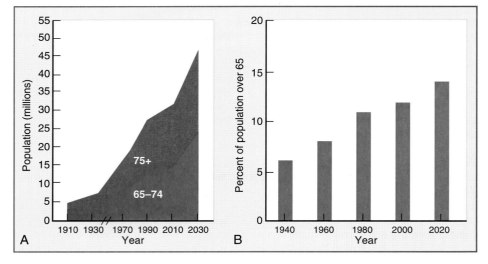

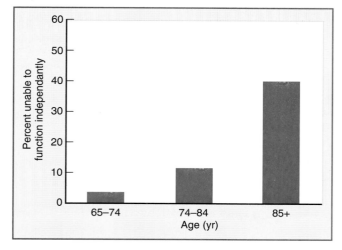

Figure 124-3
Percentage of the population with significant disabilities resulting in functional dependence and the need for assistance with activities of daily living.

current health care crisis and will certainly affect priorities and the way medicine is practiced in the near future.

ASSESSMENT OF THE OLDER PATIENT

Disease Presentation in the Elderly

The elderly patient presenting for a diagnostic evaluation must be assessed carefully. Clinical signs and symptoms of disease in the older patient are often blunted, absent, or atypical. A good example is thyrotoxicosis. Compared with the younger patient, who typically presents with a variety of classic signs and symptoms such as nervousness, weight loss, tremor, and tachycardia, elderly patients are more likely to present with cognitive dysfunction, anorexia, muscle weakness, atrial fibrillation, or congestive heart failure. Even a carefully obtained history may fail to elicit expected diagnostic clues. The older patient may not report chest pain with an acute myocardial infarction, dysuria with a urinary tract infection, or cough and shortness of breath with pneumonia. Often, only subtle and nonspecific signs and symptoms, such as a change in mental status, increased lethargy, a diminished appetite, or an increased frequency of falls, suggest that an underlying acute illness is present. Although psychiatric symptoms such as depressed mood, personality change, or inattentiveness may indicate the presence of infection, congestive heart failure, or a metabolic disorder, a true psychiatric problem such as depression may manifest with constitutional symptoms such as headache or weakness and dizziness.

Medications often add to the diagnostic confusion. The side effects of drugs can either mimic or blunt the symptoms of acute illness. Difficulties in identifying the cause of an elderly patient's clinical deterioration can even result when the symptoms of a chronic disease mask those of a new illness. There may be a delay in diagnosing an acute septic arthritis, when, for example, the patient has a history of chronic recurrent painful arthritis in the same joint. Potentially life-threatening diseases in the elderly can also present with initial manifestations that pose a diagnostic challenge for the clinician. For example, it is not uncommon for an older patient with pneumonia, urosepsis, or an intra-abdominal catastrophe to present with few identifying physical signs, a blunted or absent fever response, and a white blood cell count that is mildly elevated, in the normal range, or even low. A paradoxical fall in body temperature is usually a bad prognostic sign. The likelihood that disease will manifest atypically is increased in elderly patients who are cognitively impaired, malnourished, debilitated, or suffering from multiple chronic medical conditions. For this reason, these patients often present the greatest diagnostic challenge.

Assessment of Rehabilitation

The sequelae of disease may be particularly devastating in older individuals. Even a relatively minor illness can cause a significant deterioration in the elderly patient's cognitive or physical functioning. Furthermore, compared with that in younger patients, recovery in the elderly is likely to be slower, requiring longer and more intensive periods of recuperation and rehabilitation if return to the premorbid state is to be achieved. Loss of functional independence from either physical or cognitive disability places the elderly patient at high risk for institutionalization. For these reasons, an assessment that includes an evaluation of functional and cognitive status and the development of a treatment plan that attempts to restore independence must be included in any medical evaluation of the elderly patient. In addition, selected patients require an in-depth assessment of their social support structure (family, friends, relatives), economic status, and home environment in order to determine what resources would be required to allow the patient to return to or remain at home safely. Such comprehensive assessments of the patient represent the cornerstone of geriatric care. These assessments require a *comprehensive interdisciplinary evaluation* that includes input from physicians, nurses, social workers, physical and occupational therapists, pharmacists, and, depending on the patient's needs, many other health care professionals (Fig. 124–4). In collaboration with the various team members, a treatment plan must be developed that includes optimal medical management, minimal medication use, and, as needed, a long-term strategy for physical, cognitive, or nutritional rehabilitation (Table 124–2). For elderly patients who are assessed to have a reasonable potential for rehabilitation, numerous studies have shown that such a comprehensive strategy of evaluation and care is cost-effective, improves functional status, and allows a large fraction of patients to return to or remain in their own home.

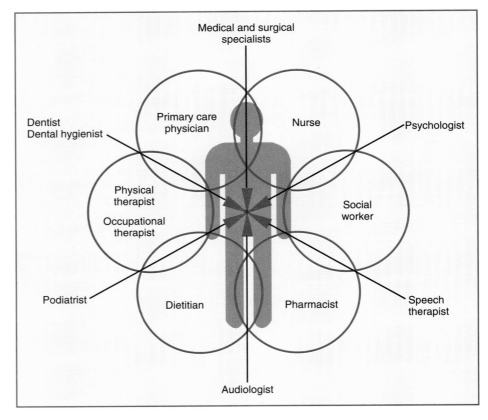

Figure 124-4
A diagrammatic illustration of health care professionals involved in the complex interdisciplinary assessment of frail elderly patients. The core health care team that should optimally evaluate every patient is shown in the circles. Consultative members of the team (shown outside the circles) contribute as needed. It must be emphasized that in many circumstances a consultant such as a dentist, psychologist, or medical subspecialist may be critically important in the development of a treatment and disposition plan.

COMMON AND OFTEN INADEQUATELY ASSESSED MEDICAL PROBLEMS OF THE ELDERLY

Polypharmacy

The elderly are at high risk of developing medication-related problems. One reason for this is the fact that the elderly tend to take multiple pharmaceuticals. The average patient over the age of 70 takes 4.5 prescription and 3.5 over-the-counter medications. The risk of both adverse drug reactions and poor compliance increases in relation to the number of medications taken. The probability of experiencing an adverse drug reaction, for example, increases from 2% for patients taking two or fewer medications to more than 13% for patients taking six or more. The often prohibitive cost of medications and the complexity of some treatment regimens contribute to poor compliance. The problem is compounded by the fact that elderly patients frequently see multiple physicians who are often unaware of medications prescribed by others. This leads to problems of overprescribing, duplicate prescriptions, and adverse drug-drug interactions.

In addition, medication-related problems often occur in the elderly owing to age-related alterations in both pharmacokinetics and pharmacodynamics. Compared with younger patients, the elderly take longer to clear many medications from their systems. They also are more likely to experience toxic manifestations of a drug even when the serum level is within a range considered normal for a younger patient. If prescribed dosages of certain medica-

tions are not reduced appropriately, an older patient can quickly develop a toxic reaction. The proper use of drugs, avoidance of unnecessary medications, and ensuring that medications do not aggravate existing disease are particularly important in the older patient.

TABLE 124-2	Principles of Comprehensive Geriatric Assessment

1. Identify treatable medical conditions
2. Screen for depression and memory loss
3. Minimize drug use
4. Avoid restraints if possible, both chemical and physical
   a. Discuss options with family or caregivers
   b. Consider nonrestraining alternatives
5. Assess functional status
   a. Activities of daily living (bathing, dressing)
   b. Instrumental activities of daily living (shopping)
6. Set rehabilitation goals
   a. Assess rehabilitation potential with consideration of the following:
     (1) Medical prognosis
     (2) Cause and duration of functional debilitation
     (3) The patient's and family's expectations or desires
   b. Develop rehabilitation program tailored to patient's needs
7. Develop a disposition plan
   a. Assess the patient's ability to return to work or remain at home. Include assessment of the following:
     (1) Family and informal community support networks
     (2) Financial resources and availability of private community services
     (3) Eligibility for sponsored programs or support services
   b. Evaluate need for short- or long-term placement in an institution
     (1) Geriatric rehabilitation center
     (2) Nursing home

Falls and Decreased Mobility

Difficulties with walking, gait, and balance occur frequently among older persons. As a consequence, approximately 30% of subjects over the age of 70 fall once or more annually. This results in a high incidence of hip fracture and other injuries that confine patients to their beds, increasing the risks of developing other medical complications, such as dehydration, pneumonia, urinary retention, and infections. Usually, the etiology of falls is multifactorial and includes visual impairment, neurologic or vestibular disease, postural hypotension, decreased muscle mass, joint disease, and various foot disorders. Falls often occur at night, are more common in dementia, and are increased in frequency by medication use. Recent reports have suggested that rehabilitation and strength training can improve muscle mass, balance, and gait and can decrease the risk of falls.

Delirium

Delirium is an acute confusional state that is commonly observed in hospitalized older persons. The diagnosis, which must be made clinically, should be suspected in any older person who has confusion that is of recent onset and is accompanied by a fluctuating level of consciousness. A decreased ability to maintain attention, daytime sleepiness, hallucinations, disorientation, and memory loss may all be part of the presenting clinical picture. Virtually any disorder can manifest with delirium in the elderly. Common causes include dehydration, congestive heart failure, myocardial infarction, pulmonary or urinary tract infections, and numerous drugs (Table 124–3). In addition to drugs that have known central nervous system effects, delirium has been reported with penicillin, digoxin, cimetidine, and nonsteroidal anti-inflammatory agents such as aspirin and ibuprofen. In older persons, delirium may occur at a dose that would not usually be considered toxic.

Elderly patients can develop delirium even as a result of a change in their living environment, such as occurs with hospitalization or placement in a nursing home. Postoperative delirium is also very common in the elderly, occurring, for example, in 50% of patients following hip surgery. In this setting, the etiology is multifactorial and often includes drugs and infection. Delirium is more common in patients who have baseline disorders of cognition. Because delirium is potentially reversible, it should not be ignored as "senile dementia" or "organic brain syndrome." Management involves accurate diagnosis and treatment of underlying diseases stopping or changing all drugs that could be contributory, and aggressively treating dehydration. When agitation is severe, sedatives or tranquilizers may be required. Although not ideal, haloperidol is the drug of choice. The usual initial dose is 0.5 mg administered intramuscularly or orally and repeated at 30-minute intervals as needed. Although this drug is usually well tolerated, a rare but potentially fatal side effect is the development of the neuroleptic malignant syndrome, which is characterized by fever and extra-pyramidal signs. In conjunction with haloperidol, benzodiazepines (e.g., lorazepam) have also been recommended as therapy for delirium. However, it is important to keep in mind that drugs themselves are often the cause of delirium. Sedatives should be avoided in the drowsy patient, and they should never be given for prolonged periods. Although pharmacologic and physical restraints are used commonly in patients with delirium, they are both associated with an increased risk of morbidity and should be avoided if at all possible.

For a discussion of dementia, see Chapter 112 (Fig. 122–5).

Benign Prostatic Hyperplasia (BPH)

BPH is a benign age-related enlargement of the prostate gland that may or may not lead to voiding problems in older persons. Until recently surgery was the only realistic therapeutic modality. However, newer medical approaches capable of reversing the prostatic enlargement and relieving symptoms now make it essential that the primary care physician assume an important role in assessment and treatment. Defined on the basis of a prostate >20 g, urinary symptoms, and/or a peak flow of <15 ml/sec, the prevalence of BPH is 430 out of 1000 men between the ages of 60 and 70. Irritative symptoms in-

TABLE 124–3	**Causes of Delirium in the Elderly**

Organ Failure
  Respiratory failure
  Congestive heart failure
  Hepatocellular failure

Infections
  Acute bronchitis
  Bronchopneumonia
  Bladder infections
  Septicemia

Metabolic
  Dehydration
  Hyponatremia
  Hypernatremia

Drugs
  Anticholinergics
  Antibiotics
  Anticonvulsants
  Digitalis
  Alcohol
  Alcohol withdrawal

Neurologic Causes
  Subdural hematoma
  Cerebrovascular accident
  Raised intracranial pressure
  Cerebral infections

Miscellaneous
  Postoperative delirium
  Sensory deprivation
  Recent institutionalization
  Change of living arrangement

Figure 124-5

A, Normal aging is not associated with a significant decline in cognitive function; the progressive and steady decline in memory seen in patients with Alzheimer's disease is contrasted with the stepwise decreases seen in patients with multi-infarct dementia. *B,* Modest, temporary declines in cognitive function can occur in normal elderly subjects during periods of acute illness. In patients with Alzheimer's disease or other disorders associated with memory loss, an acute medical illness can result in a much greater loss of cognitive function, which may or may not return to the pre-illness level.

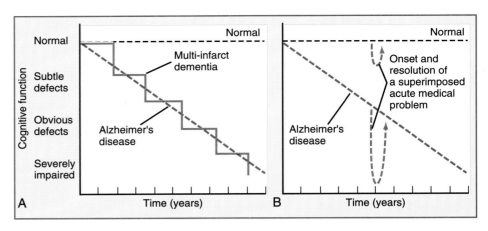

clude nocturia, frequency, urgency, dysuria, and incontinence. Obstructive symptoms include decreased force, hesitancy, terminal dribbling, double voiding, and straining to urinate. Decisions regarding workup and therapy depend on an evaluation of the severity of the disease. Symptom assessment by questionnaires that can be completed by the patient make it possible to identify mild, moderate, and severe disease. A rectal examination should be performed to evaluate prostate size and to exclude the presence of nodules. Further work-up should include a urinalysis to exclude an infection and a serum creatinine to exclude renal impairment. Prostatic specific antigen (PSA) should be obtained if a nodule is found on rectal exam. If significant obstructive symptoms are present, post-void residual urine volume should be determined either by ultrasound or catheterization.

Treatment options include watchful waiting, medical therapies, or surgery. For patients with mild to moderate disease, a period of observation is often warranted. Frequently, symptoms improve without any interventions. Medical therapy is an option for the patient with moderate to severe disease who has no evidence of urinary obstruction or renal impairment. Alpha-adrenergic receptor blockers relieve symptoms by reducing smooth muscle tone. Recent studies have shown significant symptomatic benefit. Adverse effects include dizziness, postural hypotension, and fatigue. Finasteride, a $5\alpha1$-reductase inhibitor, blocks the conversion of testosterone to dihydrotestosterone and causes a 30% reduction in prostate size within 6 months of commencing therapy. The drug has been shown to cause symptomatic relief of both irritative and obstructive symptoms. Side effects are rare and include impotence and problems with ejaculation. Patients with refractory urinary retention, an increased post-void residual volume, recurrent or persistent gross hematuria, bladder stones, or renal insufficiency should be referred for surgery.

Urinary Incontinence

Incontinence is defined as loss of urine of sufficient severity to be a social or health problem. The incidence is 5 to 10% of ambulatory older persons, 30% of hospitalized geriatric patients, and 60% of nursing home residents. *Stress incontinence* is the commonest cause in women

TABLE 124-4	**Causes, Etiology, and Treatment of Urinary Incontinence**		
Type	**Definition**	**Etiology**	**Treatment**
Stress	Leakage associated with increased intra-abdominal pressure (coughing, sneezing)	Hypermobility of the bladder base frequently caused by lax perineal muscles	Pelvic muscle exercise; timed voiding; alpha-adrenergic drugs; estrogens; surgery
Urge	Leakage associated with a precipitous urge to void	Detrusor hyperactivity (outflow obstruction, bladder tumor, detrusor instability); idiopathic (poor bladder); compliance (radiation cystitis); hypersensitive bladder	Bladder training; pelvic muscle exercise; bladder relaxant drugs (anticholinergics, oxybutynin, imipramine)
Overflow	Leakage due to a mechanically distended bladder	Outflow obstruction; enlarged prostate; stricture; prolapsed cystocele; acontractile bladder (Idiopathic, neurologic [spinal cord injury, stroke, diabetes])	Surgical correction of obstruction; intermittent catheter draining
Functional	Inability or unwillingness to void	Cognitive impairment; physical impairment; environmental barriers (physical restraints, inaccessible toilets); psychologic problems (depression, anger, hostility)	Prompted voiding; garment and padding; external collection devices

under age 75, whereas *urge incontinence* is the commonest cause in patients over age 75. *Overflow incontinence* is less common but must be diagnosed because of an increased incidence of urinary tract infections and impaired renal function. *Functional incontinence* is common in the nursing home and is diagnosed by exclusion. (Table 124–4) lists the mechanisms, causes, and approaches to treatment of this common clinical problem. A history is important in obtaining an accurate diagnosis. Leakage with coughing or sneezing is suggestive of stress incontinence. In urge incontinence the patient is aware of the need to void but cannot make it to the toilet in time. Overflow should be considered in those patients with neurologic deficits, including the autonomic dysfunction that accompanies medication use and diabetes. Physical examination should focus on the detection of neurologic or metabolic diseases that could result in incontinence and rectal examination as a measure of perineal floor tone and, in men, to evaluate the prostate. Pelvic examination should be performed in women to exclude pelvic prolapse. A urinalysis is needed to screen for diabetes, hematuria, and infection. In patients with features suggestive of obstruction, a post-void residual urine volume should be measured, either by catheterization or ultrasound. Referral for further work-up should be considered in patients with recurrent urinary tract infections, a prostatic mass (in males), pelvic prolapse (in females), a neurologic disorder that could make an accurate diagnosis difficult, hematuria, or an increased post-void residual volume.

Initial treatment should be directed at correcting treatable conditions that can aggravate incontinence. Examples include medication use (diuretics and alcohol), fecal impaction, delirium, infections, and restricted mobility. Specific treatment for stress incontinence includes exercises to increase pelvic muscle strength (see Table 124–4). The use of biofeedback has been shown to be effective in helping women perform the exercises appropriately. Timed voiding assists in preventing a full bladder. Estrogen replacement should be considered to strengthen periurethral tissues. In some patients the use of an alpha-adrenergic agonist should be considered to stimulate urethral smooth muscle contraction. Exercises, biofeedback, and timed voiding should also be used in patients with urge incontinence. A bladder relaxant such as oxybutynin may also be considered. Patients with overflow incontinence are at great risk for developing infections. Mechanical obstruction should be treated surgically. Patients with neurogenic bladder require intermittent or chronic indwelling catheterization. Functional incontinence, common in the nursing home, is best treated by attempting to correct the underlying cause and by prompted voiding. Pads and external catheters should be used with caution as they may increase the risk of functional dependency. Chronic indwelling catheters should be used only in patients with skin disorders.

REFERENCES

Appelgate WB, Blass, JP, Williams TF: Instruments for the functional assessment of older patients. N Engl J Med 1990; 322:1207–1214.

Francis J, Martin D, Kapoor WN: A prospective study of delirium in hospitalized elderly. JAMA 1990; 263:1097–1101.

Grisso JA, Kelsley JL, Strom BL, Chiu GY, Maislin G, O'Brien LA, Hoffman S, Kaplan F: Risk factors for falls as a cause of hip fractures in women. N Engl J Med: 1991; 324:1326–1331.

Hazzard WR, Bierman EL, Blass JP, Ettinger WH, Halter JB: Principles of Geriatric Medicine and Gerontology. 3rd ed. New York, McGraw-Hill Book Co., 1994.

Katzman R, Jackson JE: Alzheimer's disease: Basic and clinical advances. J Am Geriatr Soc. 1991; 39:516–525.

Katzman R: Apolipoprotein E and Alzheimer's disease. Curr Opin Neurobiol 1994; 4:703–707.

McConnel JD: Benign prostatic hyperplasia: Treatment guidelines and patient classification. Br J Urol 1995; 76 Suppl 1:29–46.

Oesterling JE: Benign prostatic hyperplasia. Medical and minimally invasive treatment options. N Engl J Med 1995; 332:99–109.

Ouslander JG: Geriatric urinary incontinence. Disease-A-Month 1992; 38:65–149.

Schneider LS, Tariot PN: Emerging drugs for Alzheimer's Disease. Med Clin North Am 1994; 78:911–934.

Schor JD, Levkoff SE, Lipsitz LA, Reilly CH, Cleary PD, Rowe JW, et al.: Risk factors for delirium in hospitalized elderly. JAMA 1992; 267:827–831.

Tinetti ME, Baker DI, McAvay G, Claus EB, Garret P, Gottschalk M, Koch ML, Trainor K, Horwitz RI: A multifactorial intervention to reduce risk of falling among elderly people living in the community. N Engl J Med 1994; 331:821–827.

Urinary Incontinence Guidelines Panel: Urinary incontinence in adults. Clinical practice guideline. AHCPR Pub No 92-0038. Rockville MD, Agency for Health Care Policy and Research, US Department of Health and Human Services, March 1992.

Whitehouse PJ, Geldmacher DS: Pharmacotherapy for Alzheimer's Disease. Clin Geriatr Med 1994; 10:339–350.

Substance Abuse

Section XVI

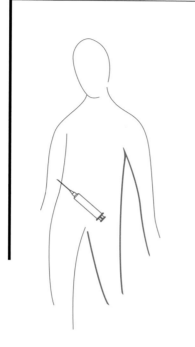

125   ALCOHOL AND SUBSTANCE ABUSE

125

Alcohol and Substance Abuse

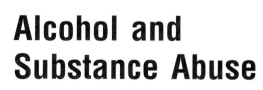

Alcohol and substance abuse are enormous economic and medical problems worldwide. It is estimated that 15 to 20 million Americans are either problem drinkers or alcoholics. Around 10 million use marijuana regularly and about 2 million use cocaine. Many deaths from overdose, suicide, homicide, motor vehicle accidents, or infectious diseases occur annually due to illicit drug use.

Drug abuse is best understood in behavioral terms; it is a maladaptive pattern in the use of any substance that persists despite adverse social, psychological, or medical consequences. *Tolerance* is the body's ability to adapt to repeated uses of the drug and thus mitigate the drug's pharmacologic action. As tolerance increases, higher doses and more frequent administration are required to achieve the desired effect. *Physical dependence* can occur and results in a physiologic withdrawal syndrome after cessation of drug use. *Psychological dependence* also occurs and can result in alcohol or drug craving and associated behaviors to obtain the drug.

SCREENING

Physicians have a unique opportunity to identify patients with alcohol and substance abuse and initiate treatment before serious social, medical, or psychiatric problems develop. Historical clues to possible drug abuse include infections such as endocarditis, hepatitis B or C, tuberculosis, frequent sexually transmitted diseases, recurrent pneumonias, skin abcesses, and human immunodeficiency virus (HIV) infection. Other clues include frequent emergency department visits for chest pain for young persons, insomnia, mood swings, chronic pain, repetitive trauma, and behavioral or social problems. Physical findings are usually nonspecific but may include needle marks (often obscured by tatoos), upper extremity edema, chronic sinusitis or a scarred or perforated nasal septum from cocaine use, and the presence of withdrawal symptoms.

Objective screening tools for alcohol use include the Michigan Alcoholism Screening Test and the CAGE questionnaire (need to "cut" down on drinking; "annoyed" by criticism of drinking; "guilty" feelings about drinking; and need for early morning "eye-opener" drink). For the CAGE questionnaire, two positive answers identify 75% of alcoholics with 95% specificity. Similar questionnaires can screen for other types of substance abuse.

Screening through blood and urine tests is helpful but usually cannot be obtained without consent of the patient. Urine tests can screen for marijuana, cocaine, opioids, phencyclidine, barbiturates, benzodiazepines, and amphetamines; positive screening results must be confirmed by gas chromatography–mass spectrometry. These tests can indicate use in a specific time period but cannot disclose the pattern of use or the existence of dependence.

TOBACCO AND ALCOHOL ABUSE

Nicotine

Tobacco smoking is society's greatest health burden and the most preventable cause of death in the United States. It is estimated by the Centers for Disease Control and Prevention to be responsible for over 420,000 deaths each year. It has been causally linked to lung cancer and other malignancies, cardiovascular disease, chronic obstructive pulmonary disease, pregnancy complications, gastrointestinal disorders, and other diseases. Passive smoking is implicated in lung cancer, cardiovascular disease, and other pulmonary disorders.

Nicotine is a highly addictive stimulant that can lead to dependence, tolerance, and withdrawal. The withdrawal syndrome is highly variable but usually involves irritability, impatience, anxiety, difficulty concentrating, sleep disturbance, increased appetite, and craving. Early addiction is the key factor for the continuing use of cigarettes.

Since 1965, the prevalence of smoking among adults has decreased from 42.2% to 25.5% in 1994. Despite this promising result, the actual number of smokers has declined only slightly due to the increase in the United States population since 1965. The prevalence rates have plateaued sinced 1993. Among adolescents, the smoking initiation rate increased from 1984 through 1989, adding around 600,000 adolescents to the ranks of smokers. This is crucial, since over 80% of adult smokers begin smoking as adolescents. A major reason for the increase in adolescent smoking has been the effective marketing campaigns of the tobacco industry. From 1980 to 1991, the total annual advertising and promotional expenditures increased from $2.1 billion to $4.6 billion. The Food and Drug Administration is now considering further restrictions on advertising and adolescent cigarette consumption.

Alcoholism

Alcohol's toll on society is great; it causes about 100,000 deaths per year in the United States; half from trauma. Alcohol use is implicated in about half of all traffic-related deaths and it plays a major role in homicides, suicides, domestic violence, and homelessness. Complications of alcohol use cost society in excess of $130 billion each year in the United States. Recognition of the problem is critical, since early diagnosis and treatment improve the prognosis for recovery.

Pharmacology

Alcohol is absorbed rapidly and may be detected in the blood within minutes. Ethanol is a small molecule soluble in water and lipids; it readily crosses biologic membranes

and permeates all tissues of the body. Ninety percent is metabolized by the liver and the remainder is excreted by the kidneys, lungs, and skin. Its elimination is independent of concentration; a 70 kg man can metabolize 5 to 10 gm/hr. Once drinking ceases, blood levels fall about 10 to 25 mg/dl/hr.

Metabolism

Many of the effects of chronic alcohol use result from its metabolism by the alcohol dehydrogenase pathway and the microsomal ethanol oxidizing system (Fig. 125–1). The alcohol dehydrogenase pathway metabolizes alcohol to acetaldehyde, which is then converted to acetate. In both these reactions, nicotinamide-adenine dinucleotide (NAD) is reduced to NADH. Excess NADH produces a number of metabolic problems, including elevated lactic

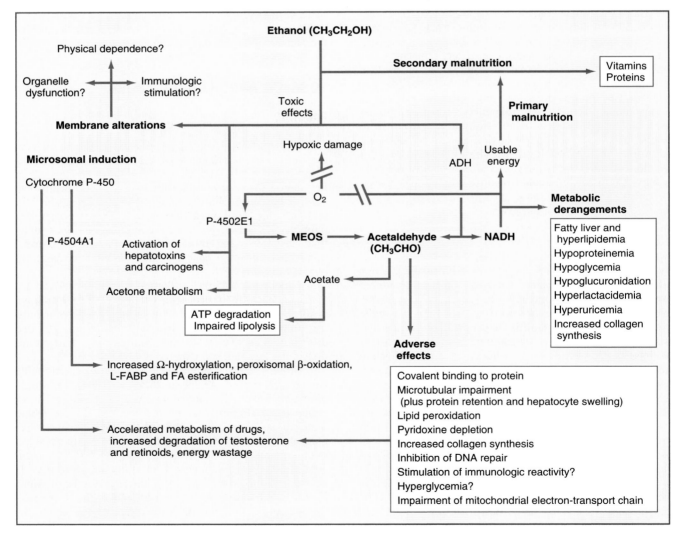

Figure 125–1

Toxic and metabolic effects of alcohol abuse. ADH = alcohol dehydrogenase; FA = fatty acids; L-FABP = liver fatty acid–binding protein. NADH = reduced nicotinamide-adenine dinucleotide. (From Lieber, CS: Medical disorders of alcoholism. N Engl J Med 1995; 333(16): 1060. Reprinted with permission.)

acid and uric acid levels, hyperlipidemia, hypoglycemia (through a block in gluconeogenesis), hypoproteinemia, and increased collagen synthesis. Acetaldehyde itself has toxic effects and can promote cellular death. It can block secretion of proteins from hepatocytes; the resulting increases in proteins, lipids, and water can cause hepatocytes to "balloon," a finding in alcoholic liver disease. Finally, acetaldehyde can cross the placenta and impair fetal DNA methylation, contributing to the fetal alcohol syndrome.

Long-term use of alcohol induces the microsomal ethanol oxidizing system and cytochrome P-4502E1, a key enzyme in the oxidation of ethanol. This contributes to the development of tolerance and increases the metabolism of many drugs, including pentobarbital, propanolol, tolbutamide, warfarin, and diazepam. Cytochrome P-4502E1 converts many foreign substances (solvents, anesthetic agents, cocaine, isoniazid, acetaminophen) into highly toxic metabolites. It activates carcinogens and, coupled with vitamin A deficiency and the increased mutagenicity of tobacco caused by alcohol, may lead to increased incidence of cancers of the gastrointestinal tract, lung, and breast. Finally, in contrast to chronic use, short-term consumption can inhibit the metabolism of many drugs due to direct competition for the cytochrome P-4502E1 system.

Medical Effects

The medical consequences of long-term alcohol use are listed in Table 125–1. Many of these problems result from nutritional depletion. Alcohol's energy content is 7.1 kcal/gm and may account for half of an alcoholic's caloric intake. Malnutrition results when alcohol displaces normal nutrients and when malabsorption occurs from gastrointestinal problems such as pancreatic insufficiency. Levels of folate, thiamine, and other vitamins are reduced. The most common nutritional related disorders include peripheral neuropathy, myopathy, and the Wernicke-Korsakoff syndrome.

Many of these medical problems are more severe in women and in the elderly. Blood levels tend to be higher in women due to their smaller size, higher proportion of body fat, and less gastric alcohol dehydrogenase activity in younger women. Liver injury, cirrhosis, and cerebral atrophy progress faster among women than men with similar histories of alcohol use.

Genetics

Genetic factors play a large role in the development of alcoholism in certain individuals. Studies of siblings and adoptees suggest a genetically transmitted susceptibility for alcoholism. Earlier work implicated the gene for the dopamine D2 receptor but this was not confirmed in other work. The exact nature is still unknown. Differences in the rate of ethanol metabolism and the severity of alcohol-related liver disease are also, in part, genetically determined. Levels of gastric alcohol dehydrogenase differ among ethnic groups; for example, a majority of Japanese

TABLE 125–1	Alcohol-Related Medical Disorders
Affected Organ or System	**Disorder**
Nutrition	Deficiencies of:
	Folate, thiamine, pyridoxine, niacin, and riboflavin
	Magnesium, zinc, calcium
	Protein
Brain	Hepatic encephalopathy
	Wernicke-Korsakoff syndrome
	Cerebral atrophy
	Amblyopia
	Central pontine myelinolysis
	Marchiafava-Bignami disease
Nerve	Neuropathy
Muscle	Myopathy
Liver	Fatty liver
	Hepatitis
	Cirrhosis
	Hepatoma
Heart	Hypertension
	Cardiomyopathy
	Arrhythmia
Blood	Anemia
	Leukopenia
	Thrombocytopenia
	Macrocytosis
Gut	Esophagitis and gastritis
	Pancreatitis
Metabolite and electrolytes	Hypoglycemia
	Hyperlipidemia
	Hyperuricemia
	Ketoacidosis
	Hypomagnesemia
	Hypophosphatemia
Endocrine	Pseudo-Cushing's syndrome
	Testicular atrophy
	Amenorrhea
Bone	Osteopenia

From Diamond I: Alcoholism and alcohol abuse. *In* Wyngaarden JB, Smith LH, Jr [eds.]: Cecil's Textbook of Medicine. 18th ed. Philadelphia, WB Saunders, 1992, p 45; with permission.

lack an isoenzyme of alcohol dehydrogenase and thus can have increased blood acetaldehyde levels and an alcohol flush reaction if they drink.

Acute Alcohol Intoxication

Since there is virtually no blood-brain barrier to alcohol, uptake into the brain is rapid and is limited primarily by cerebral blood flow and capillary perfusion. Within a short time after drinking, the concentration of ethanol in the brain is nearly that in the blood. Signs and symptoms are listed in Table 125–2. These vary with the rate of consumption and are more severe when the alcohol level is rising than falling. As blood levels rise, patients may develop slurred speech, ataxia, incoordination, and slow or irregular eye movements. At higher blood levels, central nervous system (CNS) depression and deterioration of cerebellar and vestibular function produce dysarthria, ataxia, nystagmus, diplopia, decreased respirations, vomiting, and pulmonary aspiration. For nondrinkers, stupor and coma may develop at 400 mg/dl and fatalities can occur at 500 mg/dl from respiratory depression, hypoten-

TABLE 125-2	Blood-Alcohol Levels and Symptoms	
Level (mg/dl)	Sporadic Drinkers	Chronic Drinkers
50 (party level)	Congenial euphoria	No observable effect
75	Gregarious or garrulous	Often no effect
100	Incoordinated; legally intoxicated	Minimal signs
125–150	Unrestrained behavior; episodic dyscontrol	Pleasurable euphoria or beginning incoordination
200–250	Alertness lost → lethargic	Effort required to maintain emotional and motor control
300–350	Stupor or coma	Drowsy and slow
>500	Some die	Coma

sion, and acidosis. Alcoholic blackouts (amnesia) can occur after consuming large amounts of alcohol and are a sign of serious intoxication and probable dependence.

Mild drunkenness requires no treatment other than observation. Those with marked drowsiness or stupor require close evaluation, especially if other drug use may have occurred. Other diagnostic possibilities such as hypoglycemia, acidosis, meningitis, and subdural hematomas must be considered. Evidence of head trauma or focal neurologic signs require computed tomography (CT) scanning to exclude intracranial pathology. Intubation may be necessary for severe hypoventilation or comatose patients. Hemodialysis may be needed if the blood alcohol level exceeds 600 mg/dl.

Withdrawal Syndrome

Alcohol withdrawal syndrome can be divided into several stages depending on the severity of physical dependence. Minor withdrawal symptoms may begin in 8 to 12 hours and may last 3 to 5 days. Patients may experience tremors, sweating, anxiety, tachycardia, nausea, diarrhea, and insomnia. These symptoms reflect a state of central adrenergic hyperexcitation that begins as the inhibitory influence of alcohol dissipates. Generally, observation suffices. Those patients with marked alcohol dependence may develop more profound symptoms 12 to 24 hours after the last drink. These include marked tremulousness, hyperactivity, tachycardia, increased startle response, insomnia, nightmares, visual hallucinations, and alcohol craving. Withdrawal seizures (rum fits) may occur 12 to 48 hours after abstinence and can be single or multiple episodes of tonic-clonic seizures. Status epilepticus is seen in less than 3% of patients. If the seizures are focal, or accompanied by a fever or status, then further evaluation is necessary.

The most severe stage is delirium tremens, which typically occurs 72 to 120 hours after cessation in about 5% of patients after a decade or more of fairly heavy drinking. These patients have acute delirium, confusion, fear, agitation, gross tremor, insomnia, incontinence, hy-

pertension, tachycardia, profuse sweating, and fever (often 40°C or higher). Patients may be combative, destructive, and dangerous. Many patients are malnourished and may have signs of hepatic insufficiency, gastritis, dehydration, infection, polyneuropathy, or Wernicke's syndrome. Delirium tremens may last several days and is a medical emergency.

Management

Patients with mild withdrawal symptoms can be managed as outpatients. However, those patients with hyperactivity, concurrent medical problems, and previous history of withdrawal problems should be hospitalized. Management principles are aimed at controlling suffering and preventing severe complications (Table 125–3). Vital signs should be normalized and moderate sedation begun with another sedative hypnotic. Chlordiazepoxide and diazepam are long acting benzodiazepines and are very effective in this setting. In patients with significant liver disease, lorazepam or oxazepam can be used, since these agents are not extensively metabolized by the liver. Benzodiazepines can be given intravenously but intramuscular use is to be avoided (except for lorazepam) due to erratic absorption. The adequacy of management can be judged by heart rate, blood pressure, and the degree of tremor, agitation, or insomnia. Barbiturates (phenobarbital) can substitute for benzodiazepines.

For hallucinations or extreme agitation, haloperiodol can be used cautiously but must be given with benzodiazepines since it lowers the seizure threshold. It is best used after 48 hours when the risk for seizures has lessened. Thiamine must be given before administering a glucose load in intravenous fluids to prevent precipitation of the Wernicke-Korsakoff syndrome. Beta-blockers and clonidine can be used to reduce adrenergic signs and may reduce the hospital stay and the total dose of benzodiazepines.

Treatment of withdrawal seizures remains controversial. While long-term use of phenytoin is not thought to be helpful, it is reasonable to consider the short-term use of phenytoin for withdrawing patients with a documented history of either nonalcohol-related seizures or withdrawal seizures.

TABLE 125-3	Management of Alcohol Withdrawal

Observe and normalize vital signs
Replace fluid and electrolytes
Begin sedation with benzodiazepines or barbiturates (chlordiazepoxide 25–100 mg orally q4h as needed or diazepam)
Use haloperidol (1–2 mg orally q4h as needed) cautiously for hallucinations or agitation
Replace folic acid (1 mg orally daily) and thiamine (100 mg intramuscularly and then 100 mg orally q day × 3–5 days. Give before glucose load.)
Measure and replace calcium and phosphate
Give multivitamin with zinc daily
Begin beta-blocker (atenolol 50 mg) or clonidine (0.2 mg orally twice daily) to reduce adrenergic signs

Delirium tremens carries a mortality rate of 20 to 40% for those not receiving treatment. These patients should be admitted to the intensive care unit with close attention to the general principles for withdrawal management. Physical restraint should be avoided, if possible, but sufficient sedation must be used to prevent self-inflicted injury. Five to ten milligrams of diazepam can be given every 5 to 15 minutes until the patient is calm, and maintenance therapy is continued every 1 to 4 hours as needed. Some patients may require up to 1200 mg of diazepam in the first 3 to 4 days of therapy.

The recidivism rate for alcoholism is high. After detoxification, patients should be referred to a multidisciplinary rehabilitation program. Family members, friends, and peers must be involved and support groups such as Alcoholics Anonymous and Al-Anon can be helpful. Those patients with alcohol problems identified through outpatient screening tests will need further assessment to establish alcohol dependence. Those with moderate dependence problems should be referred to outpatient treatment facilities, whereas those with more severe dependence may need inpatient management.

Pharmacotherapies that may help include the newer serotonin reuptake inhibitors (e.g., fluoxetine), which have been shown to reduce alcohol intake, probably from alleviation of depression. Other agents include the narcotic antagonist naltrexone, which helps reduce craving. It can be given once daily for 12 weeks but may precipitate opioid withdrawal if patients are dependent on opioids. Disulfiram is used to prevent relapse by blocking aldehyde dehydrogenase, leading to increased concentrations of acetaldehyde. Those taking disulfiram who drink will experience flushing, tachycardia, palpitations, headache, and dyspnea. These symptoms, though uncomfortable, are self-limited and usually without risk to the patient. Alcoholics who are daily drinkers and committed to treatment are good candidates for supervised disulfiram treatment, but it should be avoided in those with heart disease, seizures, cirrhosis, diabetes, pregnancy, and elevated transaminase levels.

PRESCRIPTION DRUG ABUSE

Benzodiazepines

Benzodiazepines are commonly prescribed and can produce both physical and psychological dependence and a potentially dangerous withdrawal syndrome. The effects of these drugs are additive with other CNS depressants such as alcohol and barbiturates.

Benzodiazepines are available as *short-acting agents* such as temazepam and triazolam; *intermediate-acting agents* such as alprazolam, lorazepam, and oxazepam; and *long-acting agents* such as chlordiazepoxide, diazepam, flurazepam, and clonazepam. Flunitrazepam ("roach" or "roofies") is becoming a popular benzodiazepine of abuse in the southern United States. It is not available in the United States but enters the country through Mexico, Central and South America, and other countries. In general, those agents with shorter half-lives have a more intense withdrawal syndrome. Older age, certain medica-

tions (cimetidine), and liver dysfunction can impede metabolism.

Withdrawal symptoms depend on the half-life of the agent, duration of use, and dosage. The onset of withdrawal symptoms usually peaks in 2 to 4 days for the short-acting drugs and in 5 to 6 days for the longer-acting drugs. Withdrawal is characterized by intense anxiety, insomnia, irritability, weight loss, muscle spasms, palpitations, diarrhea, sensitivity to light and sound, perceptual changes, tremors, and seizures. Panic attacks and disturbing nightmares may occur after long-term use and may wax and wane for months.

Treatment is difficult due to the intense symptoms and protracted course of withdrawal. Detoxification requires a change to a longer-acting benzodiazepine such as clonazepam or diazepam and a tapering regimen of 7 to 10 days for short-acting drugs and 10 to 14 days for longer-acting drugs. Propranolol can be used to decrease tachycardia, hypertension, and anxiety. In acute overdose, flumazenil, a competitive antagonist of benzodiazepines, can be given intravenously but may precipitate seizures if tricyclic antidepressants or cocaine has been used.

Barbiturates

Barbiturates include a large group of sedative drugs with varied half-lives. The ones most abused include the short-acting drugs pentobarbital and secobarbital and the intermediate-acting drugs amobarbital, aprobarbital, butabarbital, and butalbital. Patients acutely intoxicated show sluggishness, difficulty thinking, slurred speech, poor memory and judgment, nystagmus, diploplia, and vertigo.

Withdrawal syndromes resemble those with alcohol. Those drugs with short half-lives (8 to 24 hours) will produce a rapidly evolving withdrawal syndrome whereas those with longer half-lives will have less severe symptoms. Symptoms include restlessness, tremors, tachycardia, anxiety, insomnia, hyperpyrexia, vomiting, abdominal cramps, and hyperactive reflexes. Psychoses and generalized seizures are rare. Treatment requires estimating the daily dose of the abused drug and using an equivalent phenobarbital dose to stabilize the patient. The dose is then tapered over 4 to 14 days, depending on the half-life of the abused drug. Benzodiazepines can also be used for detoxification and propanolol and clonidine can help reduce symptoms. For acute overdose, oral charcoal and alkalinization of the urine (pH > 7.5) with forced diuresis can be effective.

Opioids

Opioids include the natural and semisynthetic alkaloid derivatives from opium and the purely synthetic drugs that mimic heroin. Commonly abused drugs in this class include heroin, morphine, codeine, oxycodone, meperidine, and fentanyl (Table 125–4). Abuse develops as patients seek treatment for legitimate reasons and then progressively require stronger opioids for worsening pain or for addiction purposes and relief of anxiety and depression. Others intentionally misuse opioids for their eu-

TABLE 125–4	Commonly Prescribed Opioids

Agonists

Morphine
Methadone
Meperidine (Demerol)
Oxycodone (Percodan)
Propoxyphene (Darvon)
Heroin
Hydromorphone (Dilaudid)
Fentanyl (Sublimaze)
Codeine

Mixed Agonist-Antagonists

Pentazocine (Talwin)
Nalbuphine (Nubain)
Buprenorphine (Buprenex)
Butorphanol (Stadol)

Antagonists

Naloxone (Narcan)
Naltrexone (Trexan)

From O'Brien C: Drug abuse and dependence. *In* Wyngaarden JB, Smith LH, Jr [eds.]: Cecil's Textbook of Medicine. 18th ed. Philadelphia, WB Saunders, 1992, p 45; with permission.

phoria-producing abilities. The incidence of opioid addiction among physicians and nurses is higher than in other groups with similar educational backgrounds. Intravenous heroin use, particularly when combined with cocaine ("speedball"), is increasing and represents a high-risk behavior for HIV infection.

Opioids can be classified as *agonists, mixed agonist-antagonists,* and *antagonists.* They act at specific receptors that are widely distributed. Opioids are thought to act by inhibiting neurons that tonically inhibit dopaminergic neurons, resulting in the increased release of dopamine. Potency depends on receptor affinity and metabolism; for example, heroin has high lipid solubility and enters the brain rapidly. Those drugs with mixed action will act as agonists at certain opiate receptors and relieve pain but can displace morphine from other receptors and precipitate withdrawal. The pure antagonists have no opiate effect but can reverse overdose and precipitate withdrawal.

Acute opioid overdose occurs when a user takes a higher dose than expected or a former user loses tolerance and begins usage at previous dosages. The acute syndrome (usually from injected heroin) is marked by cyanosis, pulmonary edema, respiratory distress, and mental status changes progressing to coma. Other findings include increased intracranial pressure, seizures, fever, and pinpoint pupils. The acute syndrome is thought to result mainly from adulterants in the mixture rather than to the opiate itself. Unsterile intravenous practices can lead to skin abcesses, cellulitis, meningitis, thrombophlebitis, endocarditis, hepatitis, and human immunodeficiency virus infection. Neurologic complications from intravenous heroin include transverse myelitis, inflammatory polyneuropathy, and peripheral nerve lesions.

For acute overdose, naloxone should be administered intravenously and repeated at 2- to 3-minute intervals. Patients should respond within minutes with increases in pupil size, respiratory rate, and level of alertness. If no response occurs, opioid overdose is excluded and other causes must be sought. Naloxone should be titrated carefully, since it can precipitate acute withdrawal symptoms in dependent patients.

Withdrawal symptoms develop 6 to 10 hours after the last injection of heroin. Feelings of drug craving, anxiety, restlessness, irritability, rhinorrhea, lacrimation, sweating, and yawning develop early and are followed by dilated pupils, piloerection, anorexia, nausea, vomiting, diarrhea, muscle spasms, abdominal cramps, bone pain, myalgias, tremors, sleep disturbance, and, rarely, convulsions. These symptoms peak at about 36 to 48 hours and then subside over 5 to 10 days, if untreated. There can be a protracted abstinence syndrome up to 6 months, characterized by mild anxiety, sleep disturbance, bradycardia, hypotension, and decreased responsiveness. Withdrawal can be managed with methadone, a long-acting synthetic agonist drug that prevents the sudden onset of CNS effects. After test doses, methadone can be given twice daily and tapered over 7 to 10 days. Levomethadyl acetate, a long-acting agonist, and buprenorphine, a partial agonist, can each be given 3 times a week. Clonidine can reduce autonomic hyperactivity and is especially effective if combined with a benzodiazepine.

Patients with repeated relapses can be maintained on methadone, usually in doses of 60 mg or more daily. Methadone has been shown to reduce opioid use and criminal behavior and improve health and employment status. It may be used for years with appropriate supervision. Naltrexone is a long-acting opioid antagonist that blocks impulsive opioid use. It can be given daily or 2 to 3 times weekly but only after the patient is thoroughly detoxified, since it can precipitate withdrawal. Pharmacotherapies must be combined with psychotherapy and rehabilitation programs for optimal outcomes.

Amphetamines

The most frequently abused amphetamines are dextroamphetamine, methamphetamine, methylphenidate, ephedrine, propylhexadrine, and phenmetrazine. They have been used for weight reduction, attention deficit disorder, and narcolepsy, although use is now strictly limited. They inhibit dopamine reuptake and release dopamine from intracellular stores.

Tolerance develops rapidly to the stimulant effects, and toxic effects can occur with higher doses. Toxic effects resemble acute paranoid schizophrenia with delusions and hallucinations. Withdrawal symptoms are similar to those seen with cocaine. There is a reduction in appetite but patients usually gain weight when amphetamines are discontinued. In the early 1990s, crystalline methamphetamine ("ice") was developed which, when heated and inhaled, produces a lasting and more dangerous state of intoxication.

Acute amphetamine toxicity is characterized by excessive sympathomimetic effects with tachycardia, tremors, hypertension, hyperthermia, and possible arrhythmias. There may be stereotyped compulsive behavior and tactile, visual, or auditory hallucinations. Chronic users may have an increased incidence of schizophrenia. There is evidence of neuronal degeneration in dopamine-rich areas of the brain, probably from formation of the neurotoxin 6-hydroxydopamine, which may increase the risk for the later development of Parkinson's disease. Treatment principles include a quiet environment and benzodiazepines for anxiety. Urine acidification with ammonium chloride may accelerate amphetamine excretion.

ILLICIT DRUG ABUSE

Cocaine

Cocaine is a naturally occuring alkaloid derived from the coca plant. It was introduced into the United States in the late 19th century as a local anesthetic and as an ingredient in teas, beverages, and patented medicines. Its abuse led to its ban in 1914 from proprietary use and strict limitations were placed on its medical use.

Cocaine use has increased most dramatically among adolescents and young adults and is a frequent cause of drug-related visits to emergency rooms. Over the past decade the use has shifted from the powder form to the freebase form and "crack" form—so-called from the cracking or popping sound it makes when heated. It is highly addictive.

Cocaine can be ingested orally or by snorting, injecting intravenously, or smoking crack. The blood half-life is about 1 hour. Its major metabolite is benzoylecogonine, which can be detected in the urine for 2 to 3 days after a single dose. Through smoking, high brain levels are obtained within seconds, due to the vast pulmonary vascular bed. An intense, pleasurable reaction lasting about 20 to 30 minutes is followed by rebound depression, agitation, insomnia, and anorexia and later by fatigue, hypersomnolence, and hyperphagia (the "crash"). This typically lasts 9 to 12 hours but may last up to 4 days. Users repeat the sequence at short intervals to recapture the euphoric state and avoid the crash. Medical complications increase as the pattern of abuse is intensified. Alcohol and other sedatives are often used concurrently to lessen anxiety and irritability. The combination of cocaine and heroin, injected intravenously, has resulted in some deaths.

Cocaine has a powerful effect on the central and sympathetic nervous systems. It blocks the reuptake of dopamine by binding strongly to the dopamine reuptake transporter at presynaptic nerve endings, leaving excess dopamine in the synapse to affect adjacent neurons. Physiologic responses are related to catecholamine excess: tachycardia, hypertension, hyperthermia, agitation, peripheral vasoconstriction, seizures, tachypnea, pupillary dilatation, and anorexia. Medical complications are listed in Table 125–5.

The most devastating medical complications relate to the cerebrovascular and cardiovascular effects of cocaine. Cocaine causes potent vasoconstriction of cerebral arteries and may result in acute strokes. It is associated with myocardial ischemia and arrhythmias, and rarely, with acute myocardial infarction (MI) in young people with normal or near normal coronary arteries. The principal mechanisms are coronary artery vasoconstriction, thrombosis, platelet aggregation, plasminogen-activator inhibi-

TABLE 125–5	Complications Associated with Cocaine Use

Cardiac	**Pulmonary**
Chest pain	Pneumothorax
Myocardial infarction	Pneumomediastinum
Arrhythmias	Pneumopericardium
Cardiomyopathy	Pulmonary edema
Myocarditis	Exacerbation of asthma
Endocrine	Pulmonary hemorrhage
Hyperprolactinemia	Bronchiolitis obliterans
	"Crack lung"
Gastrointestinal	**Psychiatric**
Intestinal ischemia	Anxiety
Gastroduodenal perforations	Depression
Colitis	Paranoia
Head and Neck	Delirium
Erosion of dental enamel	Psychosis
Gingival ulceration	Suicide
Keratitis	**Renal**
Corneal epithelial defects	Rhabdomyolysis
Chronic rhinitis	**Obstetric**
Perforated nasal septum	Placental abruption
Aspiration of nasal septum	Lower infant weight
Midline granuloma	Prematurity
Altered olfaction	Microcephaly
Optic neuropathy	**Others**
Osteolytic sinusitis	Sudden death
Neurologic	Sexual dysfunction
Headaches	Hyperpyrexia
Seizures	
Cerebral hemorrhage	
Cerebral infarctions	
Cerebral atrophy	
Cerebral vasculitis	

From Warner E: Cocaine abuse. Ann Intern Med. 1993; 19, 3:229. Reprinted with permission.

tion, increased oxygen demand, and accelerated atherosclerosis. Those presenting with acute MI need aggressive treatment with heparin, nitrates, thrombolytics, or invasive procedures. Use of beta-blockers is controversial since the ischemia may be worsened by unopposed, alpha-mediated vasoconstriction. Benzodiazepines, nitrates, and the alpha-antagonist phentolamine have been used successfully to treat myocardial ischemia. Those patients with a normal electrocardiogram or nonspecific changes can be safely managed without intensive care and some require only about 12 hours of observation. For those with cocaine-induced hypertension or tachycardia, metoprolol or labetolol is effective.

Immediate treatment measures for acute intoxication include obtaining vascular and airway access, if needed, and electrocardiogram monitoring. Benzodiazepines can be given intravenously and repeated at 5-minute intervals to control CNS agitation. Withdrawal requires a supportive environment but detoxification is not required since there are few physical signs of true dependence. Most patients suffer psychological dependence with intense craving for cocaine, along with fatigue and depression. Relapse is common and very difficult to treat. Recent work has centered on the short-term use of dopamine agonists (bromocriptine) or tricyclic antidepressants (primarily desipramine) to decrease the severe craving for cocaine and the fatigue and depression that follow. Other early research is looking at "vaccine" strategies—injecting protein-conjugated analogues of cocaine to produce anti-cocaine antibodies to bind cocaine and prevent its passage across the blood-brain barrier.

Cannabis

The cannabinoid drugs include *marijuana* (the dried flowering tops and stems of the resin-producing hemp plant) and *hashish* (a resinous extract of the hemp plant). Most of their pharmacological effects come from metabolites of delta-9-tetrahydrocannabinol. This drug is intensely lipophilic and is trapped on the surfactant lining of the lung and absorbed. Metabolites can be detected in the urine for 2 to 3 days following casual drug use and up to 4 weeks for chronic users. Other drugs or chemicals, such as opium or cocaine paste, may be mixed with marijuana to increase its effect.

The primary mode of ingestion is smoking; mood altering and intoxicating effects can be felt within 3 minutes with peak effects in about 1 hour. The acute physiologic effects are dose-related and may include an increase in heart rate, conjunctival congestion, decreased intraocular pressure, bronchodilation, peripheral vasodilation, dry mouth, fine tremor, muscle weakness, and ataxia. Psychoactive effects include euphoria, enhanced perception of colors and sounds, drowsiness, inattentiveness, and inability to learn new facts. Motor vehicle driving is impaired. Tolerance and physical dependence do occur, and chronic users may experience mild withdrawal with irritability, restlessness, anorexia, insomnia, or mild hyperthermia. Rarely, acute psychosis with panic reactions can occur. Treatment is supportive and reassuring; benzodiazepines can be used in more severely agitated patients. Some chronic users may experience poor academic performance, lethargy, poor concentration, and poor motivation (amotivational syndrome).

Medical uses of cannabinoids include antiemetic agents for cancer chemotherapy patients (dronabinol), weight stimulation (particularly effective in cancer and HIV disease patients), and in treating glaucoma and muscle spasticity.

Psychedelics

The major psychedelic-hallucinogenic drugs include lysergic acid diethylamide, (LSD), phencyclidine (PCP), mescaline, psilocybin, 5-methoxy-3,4-methylene dioxyamphetamine (MMDA), and dimethyltryptamine. These drugs reliably produce distortions in perception or thinking, even at low doses.

Lysergic acid diethylamide is the most potent psychedelic drug known. It interacts with several serotonin receptors in the brain but the actual psychoactive mechanism is unknown. Within 20 minutes of oral ingestion, sympathomimetic effects of mydriasis, hyperthermia, tachycardia, elevated blood pressure, increased alertness,

tremors, and occasional nausea and vomiting occur. Within 2 hours, psychoactive effects occur with heightened perceptions, body distortions, variable mood, and possible visual hallucinations. After 12 hours the syndrome starts to clear but fatigue and tension may persist for another day. Tolerance develops in a few days, but recovery is rapid. An acute panic or psychotic reaction may occur and occasionally has led to self-injury or suicide. Flashbacks, or brief reappearances of the hallucinations, may occur days or weeks after the last dose, but tend to disappear without treatment. Acute panic reactions are best treated in a supportive environment; benzodiazepines can be used for severely agitated patients.

Phencyclidine is another potent hallucinogen and is now the most widely abused of this group. It was developed as an anesthetic but its use was discontinued in 1965 due to bizarre effects. It produces a prompt stimulant effect similar to that of amphetamines with feelings of euphoria, power, and invincibility. Patients may present with hypertension, tachycardia, bidirectional nystagmus, hyperthermia, hallucinations, extreme agitation, ataxia, and slurred speech. With more severe reactions, patients may present in a comalike state with open eyes that are partially dilated, decreased pain response, brief periods of excitation, and muscle rigidity. Patients can have hypertensive crises, seizures, and bizarre, often violent behavior. Overdosing can result in death. Tolerance and mild withdrawal symptoms have been seen in daily users, but the major problem is drug craving.

Treatment entails a quiet environment, sedation with benzodiazepines, hydration, and haloperidol for terrifying hallucinations. Continuous gastric suction and acidification of the urine with intravenous ammonium chloride or ascorbic acid may aid excretion, but acidification may increase risk of renal failure if significant rhabdomyolysis or myoglobinuria exist.

Inhalants

The major groups of inhalants are *organic solvents, organic nitrites* such as amyl nitrite or amyl butyl, and *nitrous oxide*. Organic solvents include toluene (airplane glue), kerosene, gasoline, carbon tetrachloride, acrylic paint sprays, shoe polish, and degreasors. These solvents, particularly toluene, are most often inhaled by children or young adolescents and can produce dizziness and intoxication within minutes. Prolonged exposure or daily use can cause bone marrow depression, cardiac arrhythmias, cerebral degeneration, and damage to the liver, kidney, and the peripheral nervous system. Rarely, death may occur, most likely from cardiac arrhythmias.

Amyl nitrite is a yellowish, volatile liquid that dilates smooth muscle and is used as a sexual enhancer. It is usually sprayed into the nose and can produce flushing, dizziness, and a feeling of a rush. Adverse effects include palpitations, postural hypotension, and headache, but no chronic toxicity has been reported. Detoxification is rarely required for the solvents but specific psychiatric treatment may be needed to prevent relapse.

Designer Drugs

Designer drugs refers to illicit synthetic drugs that are manufactured in "underground" laboratories. These drugs are created by slight alterations in the molecular structure of existing drugs and often have markedly increased potency over the parent compound. The most common designer drugs include analogues of fentanyl, meperidine, methamphetamines, and phencyclidine.

The major *meperidine derivatives* are 1-methyl-4-phenyl-4-propionoxypiperidene (MPPP) and 1-methyl-4-phenyl-1,2,3,6-tetrahydropyridine (MPTP). These drugs are capable of producing a euphoria similar to heroin. MPTP was found to produce an irreversible form of Parkinson's disease in some users, probably related to neuronal enzyme inactivation in the substantia nigra. The best known fentanyl derivatives are alpha-methyl fentanyl (China white) and 3-methyl fentanyl. These drugs are about 1000 times more potent than heroin and fatal overdoses from respiratory depression have occurred.

The *mescaline-methamphetamine analogues* include 3,4-methylenedioxymethamphetamine (MDMA or "ecstacy"), 3,4-methylenedioxyamphetamine (MDA or "love drug") and 3,4-methylenedioxyethamphetamine (MDEA or "Eve"). MDMA is a CNS stimulant and produces a positive state of mind, with elevated mood and increased self-esteem. However, it may cause acute panic, anxiety, paranoia, hallucinations, tachycardia, nystagmus, ataxia, and tremor. Deaths in some users have been attributed to cardiac arrhythmias, hyperthermia with seizures, or intracranial hemorrhage.

Patients often present with signs and symptoms of narcotic overdose. Management principles are identical to those for narcotic abuse except the doses of naloxone will be much higher; some patients may require a continuous naloxone infusion. The parkinsonian symptoms can be managed with levodopa or carbidopa, but the syndrome is irreversible. The acute psychosis can be managed by a low-stimulus environment and haloperidol or benzodiazepines, if needed. Cooling blankets and ice baths can be used for hyperpyrexia, and alpha-blockers or alpha/beta-blockers (labetolol) can be used for hypertension.

REFERENCES

Diamond I: Alcoholism and alcohol abuse. *In* Bennett JC, Plum F (eds.): Cecil Textbook of Medicine. 20th ed. Philadelphia, WB Saunders, 1996, pp 44–47.

Hollander JE: The management of cocaine associated myocardial ischemia. N Engl J Med 1995; 333:1267–1272.

Jaffe JH: Drug addiction and drug abuse. *In* Goodman & Gilman's The Pharmacological Basis of Therapeutics. Elmsford, NY, Pergamon Press, 1990, pp 522–573.

Lieber CS: Medical disorders of alcoholism. N Engl J Med 1995; 333: 1058–1065.

Mendelson JH, Mello NK: Management of cocaine abuse and dependence. N Engl J Med 1995; 334:965–972.

Morbidity and Mortality Weekly Report. Centers for Disease Control and Prevention. Vol 43, No 55–3. November 18, 1994.

O'Brien CP: Drug abuse and dependence. *In* Bennett JC, Plum F (eds.): Cecil Textbook of Medicine. 20th ed. Philadelphia, WB Saunders, 1996, pp 47–55.

Warner E: Cocaine abuse. Ann Intern Med 1993; 119:226–235.

APPENDIX
Commonly Measured Laboratory Values

This appendix lists basic serum and urinary laboratory values measured commonly in clinical medicine. The values are presented in conventional units (CUs) and standard international (SI) units. The table also includes conversion factors (CFs) for interchanging conventional and standard international units using the following formula:

$$\text{SI units} = \text{CU} \times \text{CF}$$

This collection of laboratory values is not intended to be exhaustive. Most of the laboratory values are from the following sources: Wyngaarden JB, Smith LH, Bennett JC (eds): *Cecil Textbook of Medicine*, 19th ed, Philadelphia, WB Saunders Co, 1992, pp 2370–2377; and Henry JB (ed): *Clinical Diagnosis and Management by Laboratory Methods*, 18th ed, Philadelphia, WB Saunders Co, 1991, pp 1366–1382. These two sources also provide more comprehensive listings of laboratory measures. Laboratory values found in this appendix but not in either of the above references are from the clinical laboratories of University Hospital, University of Arkansas for Medical Sciences, Little Rock, Arkansas.

Commonly Measured Laboratory Values

Test	Conventional Units	Conversion Factor	SI Units
Arterial Blood Gases			
pH (37°C)	—	—	7.35–7.45
Oxygen (Po_2)	83–100 mm Hg	0.133	11–14.4 kPa
Oxygen saturation	95–98%	—	Fraction: 0.95–0.98
Carbon dioxide (Pco_2)	23–29 mEq/L	1	23–29 mmol/L
Serum Electrolytes			
Sodium	136–146 mEq/L	1	136–146 mmol/L
Potassium	3.5–5.1 mEq/L	1	3.5–5.1 mmol/L
Chloride	98–106 mEq/L	1	98–106 mmol/L
Bicarbonate	18–23 mEq/L	1	18–23 mmol/L
Anion gap [$Na - (Cl + HCO_3)$]	7–14 mEq/L	1	7–14 mmol/L
Calcium			
Total	8.4–10.2 mg/dL	0.25	2.1–2.55 mmol/L
Ionized	4.65–5.28 mg/dL	0.25	1.16–1.32 mmol/L
Magnesium	1.3–2.1 mEq/L	0.50	0.65–1.05 mmol/L
Phosphorus	2.7–4.5 mg/dL	0.323	0.87–1.45 mmol/L
Commonly Measured Serum Nonelectrolytes			
Urea nitrogen	7–18 mg/dL	0.357	2.5–6.4 mmol/L
Creatinine	M: 0.7–1.3 mg/dL	88.4	62–115 μmol/L
	F: 0.6–1.1 mg/dL	88.4	53–97 μmol/L
Uric acid	M: 3.5–7.2 mg/dL	0.059	0.21–0.42 mmol/L
	F: 2.6–6.0 ng/dL	0.059	0.15–0.35 mmol/L
Glucose	70–105 mg/dL	0.055	3.9–5.8 mmol/L
Osmolality	—	—	275–295 mOsm/kg
Serum Endocrine Tests			
ACTH	0800 h: 8–79 pg/mL	1	8–79 ng/L
	1600 h: 7–30 pg/mL	1	7–30 ng/L
Aldosterone	Supine: 3–10 ng/dL	0.0277	0.08–0.28 nmol/L
	Upright: 5–30 ng/dL	0.0277	0.14–0.83 nmol/L
Chronic (β-hCG) gonadotropin	<5.0 mU/mL	1	<5.0 IU/L
Cortisol	0800 h: 5–23 μg/dL	27.6	138–635 nmol/L
	1600 h: 3–15 μg/dL	27.6	82–413 nmol/L
C-peptide	0.78–1.89 ng/mL	0.328	0.26–0.62 nmol/L
Estrogen	M: 20–80 pg/mL	1	20–80 ng/L
	F: Follicular phase, 60–200 pg/mL	1	60–200 ng/mL
	Luteal phase, 160–400 pg/mL	1	160–400 ng/L
	Postmenopausal, ≤130 pg/mL	1	≤130 ng/L
Follitropin (FSH)	M: 4–25 mIU/mL	1	4–25 IU/L
	F: Follicular phase, 1–9 mU/mL	1	1–9 U/L
	Ovulatory peak, 6–26 mU/mL	1	6–26 U/L
	Luteal phase, 1–9 mU/mL	1	1–9 U/L
	Postmenopausal, 30–118 mU/mL	1	30–118 U/L
Gastrin	<100 pg/mL	1	<100 ng/L
Growth hormone	M: <2 ng/mL	1	<2 μg/L
	F: <10 ng/mL	1	<10 μg/L
Hemoglobin A_{1c}	5.6–7.5% of total Hg (whole blood)	0.001	Fraction: 0.056–0.075
Insulin (12-h fasting)	6–24 μIU/mL	7.0	42–167 pmol/L
Lutropin (LH)	M: 1–8 mU/mL	1	1–8 U/L
	F: Follicular phase, 1–12 mU/mL	1	1–12 U/L
	Midcycle, 16–104 mU/mL	1	16–104 U/L
	Luteal, 1–12 mU/mL	1	1–12 U/L
	Postmenopausal, 16–66 mU/mL	1	16–66 U/L
Progesterone	M: 0.13–0.97 ng/mL	3.2	0.4–3.1 nmol/L
	F: Follicular phase, 0.14–1.61 ng/mL	3.2	0.5–2.2 nmol/L
	Luteal phase, 2–25 ng/mL	3.2	6.4–79.5 nmol/L
Prolactin	Postmenopausal, 0–20 ng/mL	1	0–20 μg/L
Renin	Supine: 1.6 ± 1.5 ng/mL/h	1	1.6 ± 1.5 μg/L/h
	Standing: 4.5 ± 2.9 ng/mL/h	1	4.5 ± 2.9 μg/L/h
Testosterone			
Free	M: 52–280 pg/mL	3.5	180.4–971.6 pmol/L
	F: 1.6–6.3 pg/mL	3.5	5.6–21.9 pmol/L
Total	M: 300–1000 ng/dL	0.035	10.4–34.7 nmol/L
	F: 20–75 ng/dL	0.035	0.69–2.6 nmol/L
Thyrotropin (TSH)	2–10 μU/mL	1	2–10 μU/L
Thyrotropin-releasing hormone (TRH)	5–60 pg/mL	1	5–60 ng/L

Commonly Measured Laboratory Values *Continued*

Test	Conventional Units	Conversion Factor	SI Units
Serum Endocrine Tests *(Continued)*			
Thyroxine			
Free (FT$_4$)	0.8–2.4 ng/dL	13	10–31 pmol/L
Total (T$_4$)	5–12 μg/dL	13	65–155 nmol/L
Tri-iodothyronine resin uptake (T$_3$RU)	24–34%	1	24–34 AU (arbitrary units)
Urine Endocrine Tests			
Catecholamines	24 h: <100 μg/d	0.059	<5.91 nmol/d
5-Hydroxyindole-acetic acid	24 h: 2–6 mg/d	5.2	10.4–31.2 μmol/d
Metanephrines	24 h: 0.5–1.2 μg/mg creatinine	0.58	0.03–0.69 mmol/mol creatinine
Vanillylmandelic acid (VMA)	24 h: 2–7 mg/d	5.05	10.1–35.4 μmol/d
17-Hydroxycorticosteroids	24 h: M: 3–10 mg/d	2.76	8.3–27.6 μmol/d
	F: 2–8 mg/d	2.76	5.5–22.1 μmol/d
17-Ketosteroids	24 h: M: 9–22 mg/d	3.44	31–76 μmol/d
	F: 6–15 mg/d	3.44	21–52 μmol/d
Serum Markers of Gastrointestinal Absorption			
β-Carotene	10–85 μg/dL	0.0186	0.19–1.58 μmol/L
Vitamin B$_{12}$	100–700 pg/mL	0.74	74–516 pmol/L
Folate			
Serum	3–16 ng/mL	2.27	7–36 nmol/L
Red blood cells (RBCs)	130–628 ng/mL packed cells	2.27	294–1422 nmol/L
Serum Lipids			
Cholesterol	Recommended: <200 mg/dL	0.026	<5.18 mmol/L
	Moderate risk: 200–239 mg/dL	0.026	5.18–6.19 mmol/L
	High risk: ≤240 mg/dL	0.026	≥6.22 mmol/L
Fatty acids, free	8–25 mg/dL	0.0356	0.28–0.89 mmol/L
HDL-Cholesterol	M: >29 mg/dL	0.026	>0.75 mmol/L
	F: >35 mg/dL	0.026	>0.91 mmol/L
LDL-Cholesterol	Recommended: <130 mg/dL	0.026	<3.37 mmol/L
	Moderate risk: 130–159 mg/dL	0.026	3.37–4.12 mmol/L
	High risk: ≥160 mg/dL	0.026	≥4.14 mmol/L
Triglycerides	M: 40–160 mg/dL	0.011	0.45–1.81 mmol/L
	F: 35–135 mg/dL	0.011	0.4–1.52 mmol/L
Serum Liver/Pancreatic Tests			
Alanine aminotransferase (ALT, SGPT)	—	—	8–20 U/L
Aspartate aminotransferase (AST, SGOT)	—	—	10–30 U/L
γ-Glutamyltransferase (GGT)	—	—	M: 9–50 U/L
			F: 8–40 U/L
Alkaline phosphatase	—	—	M: 53–128 U/L
			F: 42–98 U/L
Bilirubin			
Total	0.2–1.0 mg/dL	17.1	3.4–17.1 μmol/L
Conjugated	0–0.2 mg/dL	17.1	0–3.4 μmol/L
Amylase	—	—	25–125 U/L
Lipase	—	—	10–140 U/L
Serum Markers for Cardiac or Skeletal Muscle Injury			
Aldolase	—	—	1.0–7.5 U/L
Lactate dehydrogenase (LDH)	—	—	208—378 U/L
Isoenzymes (%)	Fraction 1: 18–33	—	0.18–0.33
	Fraction 2: 28–40	—	0.28–0.40
	Fraction 3: 18–30	—	0.18–0.30
	Fraction 4: 6–16	—	0.06–0.16
	Fraction 5: 2–13	—	0.02–0.13
Creatine kinease (CK)	—	—	M: 38–174 U/L
			F: 26–140 U/L
Isoenzymes (%)	Fraction 2 (MB): <4–6% of total	—	<0.04–0.06
Myoglobin	—	—	M: 19–92 μg/L
			F: 12–76 μg/L
Serum Markers for Neoplasia			
Acid phosphatase	—	—	M: 2.5–11.7 U/L
Carcinoembryonic antigen (CEA)	Nonsmokers: <2.5 ng/mL	1	<2.5 μg/L
α-Fetoprotein	<10 ng/mL	1	<10 μg/L
Prostate-specific antigen (PSA)	0–4 ng/mL	0.001	0–4 μg/L

Continued on following page

Commonly Measured Laboratory Values *Continued*

Test	Conventional Units		Conversion Factor	SI Units	
Serum Proteins					
Albumin	3.5–5.0 g/dL		10	35–50 g/L	
Immunoglobulins	IgA: 40–350 mg/dL		10	400–3500 mg/L	
	IgD: 0–8 mg/dL		10	0–80 mg/L	
	IgE: 0–380 IU/mL		1	0–380 KIU/L	
	IgG: 650–1600 mg/dL		0.01	6.5–16 g/L	
	IgM: 55–300 mg/dL		10	550–3000 mg/L	
Protein					
Total	6.4–8.3 g/dL		10	64–83 g/L	
Electrophoresis	α_1-globulin: 0.1–0.3 g/dL		10	1–3 g/L	
	α_2-globulin: 0.6–1.0 g/dL		10	6–10 g/L	
	β-globulin: 0.7–1.1 g/dL		10	7–11 g/L	
	γ-globulin: 0.8–1.6 g/dL		10	8–16 g/L	
Complete Blood Count					
Hemoglobin (Hb)	M: 13.5–17.5 g/dL		0.155	2.09–2.71 mmol/L	
	F: 12–16 g/dL		0.155	1.86–2.48 mmol/L	
Hematocrit (Hct)	M: 39–49%		—	0.39–0.49	
	F: 35–45%		—	0.35–0.45	
Mean corpuscular Hb concentration (MCHC)	31–37% Hb/cell, or g Hb/dL RBC		0.155	481–5.74 mmol Hb/L	
Mean corpuscular volume (MCV)	—		—	80–100 fL	
Leukocyte count	$4.5–11 \times 10^3$ cells/μL		—	$4.5–11 \times 10^9$ cells/L	
Differential count	%	Cells/μl	—	Fraction	Cells $\times 10^6$/L
Myelocytes	0	0	—	0	0
Neutrophils—bands	3–5	150–400	—	0.03–0.05	150–400
Neutrophils—segmented	54–62	3000–5800	—	0.54–0.62	3000–5800
Lymphocytes	23–33	1500–3000	—	0.25–0.33	1500–3000
Monocytes	3–7	285–500	—	0.03–0.07	285–500
Eosinophils	1–3	50–250	—	0.01–0.03	50–250
Basophils	0–0.75	15–50	—	0–0.0075	15–50
CD$_4$ (T$_H$) count	36–54	660–1500	—	0.36–0.54	660–1500
CD$_8$ (T$_S$) count	19–33	360–850	—	0.19–0.54	360–850
T$_H$/T$_S$ ratio	1.1–2.9		—	1.1–2.9	
Platelet count	$150–450 \times 10^3$/μL (mm^3)		—	$150–450 \times 10^9$/L	
Anemia Tests					
Reticulocyte count	0.5–1.5% of erythrocytes		—	0.005–0.015	
Iron	M: 65–175 μg/dL		0.179	11.6–31.3 μmol/L	
	F: 50–170 μg/dL		0.179	9.0–30.4 μmol/L	
Ferritin	M: 20–250 ng/mL		1	20–250 μg/L	
	F: 10–120 ng/mL		1	10–120 μg/L	
Total iron-binding capacity	250–450 μg/dL		0.179	44.8–80.6 μmol/L	
Hemoglobin electrophoresis	HbA: >95%		—	>0.95	
	HbA$_2$: 1.5–3.5%		—	0.015–0.035	
	HbF: <2%		—	<0.02	
	HbS: 0%				
Coagulation Tests					
Prothrombin time (PT)	9–13 sec		+9 sec	18–22 sec	
Partial thromboplastin time (PTT)	—		—	60–85 sec	
Activated PTT	—		—	25–35 sec	
Bleeding time					
Ivy	—		—	Normal: 2–7 min	
				Borderline: 7–11 min	
Simplate				2.75–8 min	
Clotting time (Lee-White)	—		—	5–8 min	
Thrombin time	—		—	Time of control ±2 sec when control is 9–13 sec	
Disseminated Intravascular Coagulation Tests					
Fibrinogen	200–400 mg/dL		0.01	2.0–4.0 g/L	
Fibrin degradation products	<10 μg/mL		1	<10 mg/L	
Hemolysis Tests					
Haptoglobin	26–185 mg/dL		10	260–1850 mg/L	

ACTH = Corticotropin; F = female; FSH = follicle-stimulating hormone; β-hCG = β-human chorionic gonadotropin; HDL = high-density lipoprotein; LDL = low-density lipoprotein; LH = luteinizing hormone; M = male; SGOT = serum glutamic-oxaloacetic transaminase; SGPT = serum glutamate pyruvate transaminase.

Index

Note: Page numbers in *italics* refer to illustrations;
page numbers followed by t refer to tables.

I